The Non-Hodgkin's Lymphomas

The Non-Hodgkin's Lymphomas

Second Edition

Edited by

IAN T. MAGRATH

MB BS FRCP FRCPath

Chief, Lymphoma Biology Section,
Pediatric Branch, National Cancer Institute;
Professor of Pediatrics,
Uniformed Services University of the Health Sciences,
Bethesda, Maryland, USA

A member of the Hodder Headline Group
LONDON • SYDNEY • AUCKLAND
Copublished in the USA by Oxford University Press, Inc., New York

First published in Great Britain in 1997 by Arnold,
a member of the Hodder Headline Group,
338 Euston Road, London NW1 3BH

Co-published in the United States of America by
Oxford University Press, Inc.,
198 Madison Avenue, New York, NY10016
Oxford is a registered trademark of Oxford University Press

British Library Cataloguing in Publication Data
A catalogue record for this book is available from the British Library

Library of Congress Cataloging-in-Publication Data
A catalog record for this book is available from the Library of Congress

ISBN 0 340 55793 1

Typeset by Keyboard Services, Luton, Bedfordshire
Printed and bound in Great Britain
by The Bath Press

Contents

Colour plate sections fall between pages 80 and 81
and between pages 144 and 145

Contributors

Manzoor Ahmad HI(M) MB BS FRCPS(Pak) FRCP(Edin)
Surgeon General and Deputy General of Medical Sciences, Armed Forces Institute of Pathology, Rawalpindi, Pakistan

Richard Ambinder MD PhD
Associate Professor of Oncology, Hematological Malignancies, Johns Hopkins Oncology Center, Baltimore, Maryland, USA

Peter D. Aplan MD
Cancer Research Pediatrician, Departments of Pediatrics and Molecular Medicine, Roswell Park Cancer Institute, Buffalo, New York, USA

James O. Armitage MD
Professor and Chairman, Internal Medicine, University of Nebraska Medical Center, Omaha, Nebraska, USA

Yves Bastion MD
Attending Physician, Department of Hematology, Centre Hospitalier Lyon-Sud, Lyons, France

Kishor Bhatia PhD
Senior Investigator, Pediatric Branch, National Cancer Institute, Bethesda, Maryland, USA

Jacob D. Bitran MD
Chief, Division of Hematology/Oncology, Lutheran General Hospital, Park Ridge, Illinois, USA

William A. Blattner MD
Chief, Viral Epidemiology Branch, National Cancer Institute, Bethesda, Maryland, USA

Gianni Bonadonna MD
Director, Division of Medical Oncology, Instituto Nazionale Tumori, Milan, Italy

Murray F. Brennan MD
Chairman, Department of Surgery, Memorial Sloan–Kettering Cancer Center, New York, USA

David Brodeur MD PhD
Fellow, Department of Medicine, Division of Hematologic Oncology and Molecular Biology Program, Memorial Sloan–Kettering Cancer Center, New York, USA

Wolfram Brugger MD
Assistant Professor, Department of Hematology/Oncology, University of Tübingen, Tübingen, Germany

Jean-Noël Bruneton MD
Professor and Chief, Department of Radiology, Hôpital Pasteur, Nice, France

Fernando Cabanillas MD
Chief, Department of Hematology, The University of Texas MD Anderson Cancer Center, Houston, Texas, USA

Jorge A. Carrasquillo MD
Deputy Chief, Nuclear Medicine Department, Warren G. Magnusen Clinical Center, National Institutes of Health, Bethesda, Maryland, USA

Giorgio Cattoretti MD
Pathology Fellow, Division of Oncology, Columbia University, New York, USA

Franco Cavalli MD
Director, Division of Oncology, Ospedale San Giovanni, Bellinzona, Switzerland

Clara C. Chen MD
Senior Staff Fellow, Nuclear Medicine Department, Warren G. Magnusen Clinical Center, National Institutes of Health, Bethesda, Maryland, USA

Bertrand Coiffier MD PhD
Professor of Medicine, Université Claude Bernard, and Head, Department of Hematology, Centre Hospitalier Lyon-Sud, Lyons, France

Carlo M. Croce MD
Director, Jefferson Cancer Institute, Jefferson Cancer Center, Philadelphia, Pennsylvania, USA

Riccardo Dalla-Favera MD
Professor of Pathology and Genetics and Development, Division of Oncology, Columbia University, New York, USA

Alain Delmer MD
Assistant, Department of Hematology, Hôtel-Dieu de Paris, Paris, France

Steven W. Falen MD PhD
Professor, Department of Radiology, Bowman Gray School of Medicine, Winston-Salem, North Carolina, USA

Alexandra H. Filipovich MD
Director, Immunodeficiency Program, Division of Hematology/Oncology, Children's Hospital Medical Center, Cincinnati, Ohio, USA.

Richard I. Fisher MD
Professor of Oncology, and Director, Division of Hematology/Oncology, Loyola University Medical Center, Maywood, Illinois, USA

Nicola S. Fracchiolla MD
Laboratory of Experimental Hematology and Molecular Genetics, Institute of Medical Science, University of Milan, Milan, Italy

Glauco Frizzera MD
Professor of Pathology, and Director, Hematopathology, New York University Medical Center, New York, USA

Ellen R. Gaynor MD
Associate Professor of Medicine, Division of Hematology/Oncology, Loyola University Medical Center, Maywood, Illinois, USA

Antoine Gessain MD PhD
Professor, Epidemiology of Oncogenic Viruses Unit, Institut Pasteur, Paris, France

A. Massimo Gianni MD
Director, Division of Bone Marrow Transplantation, Istituto Nazionale Tumori, Milan, Italy

Eli Glatstein MD
Professor, Department of Radiation Oncology, Hospital of the University of Philadelphia, Philadelphia, Pennsylvania, USA

James R. Gray MD
Assistant Professor, Division of Radiation Oncology, Uniformed Services University of the Health Sciences, National Naval Medical Center, Bethesda, Maryland, USA

Henrik Griesser MD
Chief, Division of Applied Cytology; Professor, Department of Pathology, Julius-Maximilian-University, Würzburg, Germany

Reinhard Henschler MD
Assistant Professor, Department of Hematology/Oncology, Freiburg University Medical Center, Freiburg, Germany

Richard T. Hoppe MD
Professor and Acting Chair, Department of Radiation Oncology, Stanford University Medical Center, Stanford, California, USA

Sandra J. Horning MD
Associate Professor, Department of Medicine, Stanford University Medical Center, Palo Alto, California, USA

Elaine S. Jaffe MD
Chief, Hematopathology Section, Laboratory of Pathology, National Cancer Institute, Bethesda, Maryland, USA

Dennie V. Jones Jr MD
Genentech Inc., Mailstop 59, 460 Point San Bruno Boulevard, South San Francisco, California, USA

Marshall E. Kadin MD
Associate Professor of Pathology, Harvard Medical School, Director of Pathology, Beth Israel Hospital, Boston, Massachusetts, USA

Lothar Kanz MD PhD
Professor and Head, Department of Hematology/Oncology, University of Tübingen, Tübingen, Germany

John D. Kemp MD
Professor, Departments of Pathology and Microbiology, College of Medicine and Veterans' Affairs Medicine Center, University of Iowa, Iowa City, Iowa, USA

Youn H. Kim MD
Assistant Professor, Departments of Dermatology and Radiation Oncology, Stanford University School of Medicine, Palo Alto, California, USA

Marsha C. Kinney MD
Assistant Professor, Department of Pathology, Vanderbilt University Medical Center, Nashville, Tennessee, USA

Ilan R. Kirsch MD
Section Chief, National Cancer Institute, Navy Medical Oncology Branch, Bethesda, Maryland, USA

Tadamitsu Kishimoto MD
Professor, Department of Medicine III, Osaka University Medical School, Osaka, Japan

Daniel M. Knowles MD
Professor and Chairman of Pathology, New York Hospital – Cornell Medical Center, New York, USA

Turid Knutsen MT(ASCP) CLSp(CG)
Cytogenetic Technologist, Medicine Branch, National Cancer Institute, Bethesda, Maryland, USA

Gerrit Koopman PhD
Immunologist, Department of Pathology, Academic Medical Center, University of Amsterdam, Amsterdam, The Netherlands

Larry W. Kwak MD PhD
Senior Investigator, Biological Response Modifiers Program, Division of Cancer Treatment, National Cancer Institute – Frederick Cancer Research and Development Center, Frederick, Maryland, USA

Karl Lennert MD
Professor Emeritus, Zentrum Pathologie und Angewandte Krebsforschung, Kiel, Germany

Alexandra M. Levine MD
Professor of Medicine, Chief, Division of Hematology, University of Southern California School of Medicine, Norris Cancer Hospital, Los Angeles, California, USA

Jonathan J. Lewis MD
Attending Surgeon, Department of Surgery, Memorial Sloan–Kettering Cancer Center, New York; Assistant Professor, Cornell University Medical College, New York, USA

T. Andrew Lister MD FRCP FRCPath
Professor of Medical Oncology, Department of Medical Oncology, St Bartholomew's Hospital, London, UK

Dan L. Longo MD
Scientific Director on Aging, Gerontology Research Center, Baltimore, Maryland, USA

Ian T. Magrath MB FRCP FRCPath
Chief, Lymphoma Biology Section, Pediatric Branch, National Cancer Institute, Professor of Pediatrics, Uniformed Services University of the Health Sciences, Bethesda, Maryland, USA

Tak W. Mak PhD
Director, Amgen Institute, Ontario Cancer Institute; Professor, Departments of Medical Biophysics and Immunology, University of Toronto, Toronto, Canada

Imtiaz A. Malik MD
Director, National Cancer Institute; Senior Lecturer, Aga Khan University, Karachi, Pakistan

Angela Manns MD MPH
Senior Clinical Investigator, Viral Epidemiology Branch, National Cancer Institute, Bethesda, Maryland, USA

Pierre-Yves Marcy MD
Professor, Department of Radiology, Hôpital Pasteur, Nice, France

Roland Mertelsmann MD PhD
Professor and Head, Department of Hematology/ Oncology, Freiburg University Medical Center, Freiburg, Germany

Ann Mertens PhD
Assistant Professor, Department of Pediatrics, Division of Epidemiology and Clinical Research, University of Minnesota Hospital and Clinics, Minneapolis, Minnesota, USA

Michel-Yves Mourou MD
Chief, Department of Radiology, Hôpital Princesse Grâce, Monaco

Antonino Neri MD
Investigator, Laboratory of Experimental Hematology and Molecular Genetics, Institute of Medical Science, University of Milan, Milan, Italy

Ronald D. Neumann MD
Chief, Nuclear Medicine Department, Warren G. Magnusen Clinical Center, National Institutes of Health, Bethesda, Maryland, USA

Gerald Niedobitek MD MRCPath
Lecturer in Pathology, University of Birmingham, Birmingham, UK

Bernard Padovani MD
Professor, Department of Radiology, Hôpital Pasteur, Nice, France

Steven T. Pals MD PhD
Professor of Immunology and Hematopathology, Academic Medical Center, University of Amsterdam, Amsterdam, The Netherlands

Alejandro Preti MD
Assistant Professor of Medicine, Lymphoma Section, Departments of Medical Oncology and Hematology, The University of Texas MD Anderson Cancer Center, Houston, Texas, USA

Charles S. Rabkin MD Sci
HIV Cancer Coordinator, Viral Epidemiology Branch, National Cancer Institute, Bethesda, Maryland, USA

Mark Raffeld MD
Senior Investigator, Hematopathology Section, Laboratory of Pathology, National Cancer Institute, Bethesda, Maryland, USA

Bracha Ramot MD
Professor of Medicine, The Gregorio and Dora Shapiro Chair for Hematologic Malignancies, Sackler School of Medicine, Chaim Sheba Medical Center, Affiliated to the Tel-Aviv University, Tel-Hashomer, Israel

Gideon Rechavi MD PhD
Head, Pediatric Hemato-Oncology Department, Sackler School of Medicine, Chaim Sheba Medical Center, Affiliated to the Tel-Aviv University, Tel-Hashomer, Israel

Alfred Reiter MD
Professor, Medizinische Hochschule Hannover, Department of Pediatric Hematology/Oncology, Hannover, Germany

Hansjörg Riehm, MD
Professor of Pediatrics, Medizinische Hochschule Hannover, Department of Pediatric Hematology/Oncology, Hannover, Germany

Leslie Robison PhD
Professor, Departments of Pediatrics and Epidemiology, Division of Epidemiology and Clinical Research, University of Minnesota Hospital and Clinics, Minneapolis, Minnesota, USA

Ama Rohatiner MD FRCP
Reader in Medical Oncology and Consultant Physician, Department of Medical Oncology, St Bartholomew's Hospital, London, UK

Philip A. Salem MD
Director, Cancer Research Program, Medical Oncology, Salem Oncology Centre, Houston, Texas, USA

Gilles Salles MD PhD
Assistant Professor of Medicine, Department of Hematology, Centre Hospitalier Lyon-Sud, Lyons, France

John T. Sandlund MD
Associate Member, Department of Hematology/Oncology, St Jude Children's Research Hospital, Memphis, Tennessee, USA

Steven A. Schichman MD PhD
Research Instructor, Jefferson Cancer Institute, Thomas Jefferson University, Philadelphia, Pennsylvania, USA

Aziza T. Shad MD
Assistant Professor, Department of Pediatrics, Division of Hematology/Oncology, Vincent T. Lombardi Cancer Center, Washington, DC, USA

Ralph S. Shapiro MD
Immunologist, Midwest Immunology Clinic, Wayzata, Minnesota, USA

Lena Specht MD PhD
Senior Consultant and Chief Oncologist, Herlev Hospital, University of Copenhagen, Herlev, Denmark

Michael Stevens MD FRCP
Consultant Paediatric Oncologist and Senior Clinical Lecturer, The Children's Hospital, Birmingham, UK

Haruo Sugiyama MD
Professor, Department of Medicine III, Osaka University Medical School, Osaka, Japan

Guy de Thé MD PhD
CNRS Research Director, Professor, Pasteur Institute, Head, Epidemiology of Oncogenic Viruses Unit, Institut Pasteur, Paris, France

John E. Ultmann MD
Professor of Medicine, University of Chicago, Division of Biological Sciences, Pritzker School of Medicine, Chicago, Illinois, USA

Laura Virgilio MD
Postdoctoral Fellow, Department of Microbiology and Immunology, Jefferson Cancer Institute, Thomas Jefferson University, Philadelphia, Pennsylvania, USA

Julie M. Vose MD
Assistant Professor, Department of Oncology/Hematology, University of Nebraska Medical Center, Omaha, Nebraska, USA

Mary H. Ward PhD
Epidemiologist, Environmental Epidemiology Branch, National Cancer Institute, Bethesda, Maryland, USA

Ronald E. Weiner PhD
Associate Professor, Nuclear Medicine Department, University of Connecticut Health Center, Farmington, Connecticut, USA

Jacqueline Whang-Peng MD
Director, Cancer Clinical Research Center, Institute of Biomedical Sciences, Academia Sinica, Tai Pei, Taiwan

Wyndham H. Wilson MD PhD
Senior Investigator, Medicine Branch, National Cancer Institute, Bethesda, Maryland, USA

Dennis H. Wright BSc MD FRCPath
Professor, University Department of Pathology, Southampton General Hospital, Southampton, UK

Lawrence S. Young BSc PhD
Professor of Cancer Biology, Departments of Pathology and Cancer Studies, University of Birmingham, Birmingham, UK

Andrew D. Zelenetz MD PhD
Chief, Lymphoma Service, Division of Hematologic Oncology and Molecular Biology Program, Memorial Sloan-Kettering Cancer Center, New York, USA

Robert A. Zittoun, MD
Chief, Department of Hematology, Hôtel Dieu de Paris, Paris, France

Preface to the second edition

In the several years since the publication of the first edition of this book, there has been considerable progress in attempts to understand the pathobiology of the non-Hodgkin's lymphomas, but rather less tangible success with respect to the therapy of these diseases. Indeed, while the gains in survival rates in the childhood lymphomas of the last decade have been consolidated, little progress has been made in the treatment of adult lymphomas. The apparent advances achieved with so-called 'third-generation regimens' in the diffuse aggressive lymphomas, for example, have been refuted by the results of a randomized clinical trial conducted by the South West Oncology Group in the USA. Whether this difference in results of treatment between children and adults relates primarily to differences in the treatment regimens employed, or to differences in the biology of the diseases, is a question worthy of study. Similarly, the goal of demonstrating cure in the histological categories listed as *low-grade* in the now beleaguered *Working Formulation for Clinical Usage* remains elusive, even with the use of very high dose therapy supported by autologous bone marrow transplantation (ABMT). Perhaps expectations with respect to the value of very high dose therapy have also been too high in the diffuse aggressive lymphomas. While the long-awaited results of the PARMA study have demonstrated, to the satisfaction of most, that this approach is superior to continuation of the dexamethasone, high-dose ara-C, cis-platinum (DHAP) salvage regimen in patients with chemosensitive recurrent disease, the apparent failure of ABMT to date to influence survival rates when moved from second to first remission in patients in poor prognostic categories does not augur well for its overall contribution to the therapy of this subset of lymphomas.

The role of bone marrow transplantation is, in any event, beginning to undergo, if not a revolution, at least a conceptual reformation. The use of repeated infusions of hematopoietic stem cells obtained from peripheral blood for hematopoietic support after high-dose therapy is likely to lead to changes in the chemotherapy regimens traditionally associated with stem cell support. As a result they will probably more closely resemble existing combination regimens, but be much more intensive – a strategy that is strikingly similar to that which has already been used to advantage, without stem cell support, in the pediatric lymphomas. In addition, much more emphasis is being given to the immunotherapeutic elements inherent in allogeneic transplantation, and the use of donor T-cell infusions posttransplant is becoming increasingly common – both as a form of immunotherapy against tumor cells and as a means of preventing some of the complications of immuno-suppression, including cytomegalovirus infection and Epstein–Barr virus-associated lymphoprolifera-tive disease. The degree to which these newer approaches will influence treatment results in the non-Hodgkin's lymphomas is a question that may be answered within the next few years.

Advances in treatment are often saltatory – previous success slows further progress, for not only is it necessary to ensure that patients receive the best available treatment (however limited such success may be), but the comfort of traditional approaches contrasts starkly with the censure that awaits unsuc-cessful innovation. Treatment advances will also be slowed if the trend of recent years to emphasize the economic (even business) aspects of health care is continued, with the consequent detrimental influence on clinical research that this will entail. Medicine without research dooms populations to the inade-quacies of present knowledge and technology, while the absence of the spirit of enquiry in those who provide health care is likely to lead rapidly to medical mediocrity. This mistake is not a new one. It was made, perhaps for the first time in recorded human history, by the ancient Egyptians, although for a different reason. They considered their once supreme medical knowledge to be of divine origin and therefore already perfect! The present volume represents the antithesis of this philosophy – as evidenced by the marked increase in its size over the first edition. In addition, considerable space has been devoted to pathobiology for, without an understanding of the nature and origins of the non-Hodgkin's lymphomas, we shall remain confronted by the Faustian dilemma that continues to sour our present empirical treatment approaches (the cure is poisonous*), however successful some of them have been.

Recent advances in our understanding of the non-Hodgkin's lymphomas are reflected in the publication of the new Revised European–American Lymphoma (REAL) classification of lymphoid neoplasms, an event that was received with mixed emotions by pathologists, and which has provided new grounds to bewail the purported obfuscation that pervades lymphoma classification (a bewailing that has continued for more than a century), much of which has been occasioned simply by the multiplicity of classification schemes. Yet as progress is made, new schemes must replace the old. The REAL classification is an attempt on the part of an *ad hoc* assembly of European and American pathologists to identify and characterize as objectively as possible, using immunophenotyping as well as molecular genetics, the individual disease entities that comprise the malignant lymphomas – an endeavor that would appear to be an essential prerequisite to the development of optimal treatment approaches, and further, to move beyond present empiricism into the realm of tumor-targeted therapy. In this respect it is clearly superior to the Working Formulation and is seriously rivaled only by the widely used European scheme, the Kiel classification, which has been modified at intervals throughout the more than 20 years of its existence. Further, as a genuine attempt by pathologists from many countries to reach agreement, the REAL classification could help to eliminate much of the cause for confusion over lymphoma taxonomy.

However, an understanding of lymphoid neoplasia does not stop at diagnosis and treatment. The

challenge to relate environmental factors to the derangements of the immune system that precede lymphoma development – either in terms of epidemiological relationships, or better still, in terms of defined molecular genetic pathways – cannot be ignored, for such information could ultimately lead to methods to detect patients or populations at very high risk, and even to prevent lymphoma development. The inherited and acquired immunodeficiency syndromes, with their associated increased risk of lymphoma, provide one model system for understanding changes in the microenvironment that are relevant to lymphomagenesis, but another opportunity – one likely to be even more fruitful in the context of the lymphomas that develop *de novo* – is provided by the vast range of life styles and environments that exist throughout the world. This global laboratory is certainly underutilized, to the detriment of our comprehension of lymphoid neoplasia. It can only be hoped that the recent exponential improvement that has occurred in communications will lead to improved collaboration between industrial and developing nations, with consequent benefits to all.

The present volume, then, is a markedly expanded version of the first edition, and, like the first edition, represents an attempt to summarize our present understanding of the histopathology, immunopathology, molecular genetics, epidemiology, clinical features and treatment of the non-Hodgkin's lymphomas. The book has been extensively revised; most chapters have been completely rewritten and many new chapters have been added. While every effort has been made to make the book as up-to-date as possible, inevitably some new advances will have occurred since going to press. The book should, nevertheless, provide a firm foundation on which such new advances will fall more readily into place and it is to be hoped, for this reason, that it will serve a useful purpose for a number of years. Its contributors have been selected from the most expert and original in their fields and my thanks are due to all of them for their willingness to give so much of their precious time to this project. Any success that the book may enjoy will be entirely due to their efforts, while any imbalance, omissions or other deficiencies are due to my own shortcomings.

Finally, I am inestimably indebted to Laurene Kuhar, whose superlative administrative support has made a daunting task, superimposed on an already overwhelming schedule, manageable.

* Es ist so schwer den falschen Weg zu meiden,/ Es liegt in ihr so viel verborgnes Gift,/ Und von der Arzenei ist's kaum zu unterscheiden. (It is so difficult to avoid the wrong path,/ Concealed therein is so much poison,/ And it's scarcely possible to distinguish the poison from the cure.)

Ian T. Magrath
1996

Preface to the first edition

The exponential increase in scientific knowledge which has occurred throughout this century has dramatically changed the face of medicine. While the treatment of bacterial infections provides one of the most dramatic success stories, the broad compass of scientific progress can have had no greater impact than it has in the field of cancer.

Modern diagnostic methods include the use of computerized tomography, magnetic resonance imaging, radionuclide scanning, immunophenotyping, cytogenetics and, increasingly, molecular biology. Conventional treatment currently includes an array of the most sophisticated surgical, radiotherapeutic and pharmacological techniques, while experimental therapy is designed to explore the utility of a broad range of 'biological response modifiers' (BRMs), i.e. molecules which have an effect on cell differentiation or proliferation either by influencing host cellular regulatory mechanisms, or by acting directly on tumour cells via pathways which are utilized by normal cells. Such BRMs include monoclonal antibodies and various cytokines such as interleukin-2 and interferons, the latter frequently produced by means of recombinant DNA technology. In the laboratory, progress towards understanding the pathogenesis of cancer has been made with the help of a wide variety of advanced technologies encompassing the fields of biochemistry, immunology and molecular genetics.

One of the groups of tumours which has benefited the most, or, perhaps more accurately, which has provided the most fertile soil for progress, has been the non-Hodgkin's lymphomas. Yet paradoxically, the current therapeutic success which has been achieved with malignant non-Hodgkin's lymphomas is the result of empirical studies carried out over the last 25 years, and so far, little therapeutic benefit has been gained from recent progress in understanding the genetic and biochemical abnormalities of the tumour cell. Similarly, knowledge of the mechanisms of drug-induced cytotoxicity or drug resistance and of the regulation of cellular growth and differentiation has yet to provide tangible benefit to the patient. It seems highly probable, however, that in the near future this burgeoning growth of the science of oncology will have developed to the point where it will begin to have considerable impact upon the management of patients with malignant lymphomas. Moreover, it is likely that therapeutic advances of considerable magnitude will be seen, whereby more specific biochemical targets will be utilized with a resultant increase in therapeutic efficacy and decrease in toxicity. At the same time, we must accept that our present concepts of disease entities are likely to change considerably. New tools will enable us to perceive similarities and differences hitherto unrecognized. Yet the old, as always, will continue to exist beside the new, and the transition will be gradual.

Nomenclature is likely, for the foreseeable future, to continue to be confusing, since it will derive from an increasing number of perspectives and disciplines and, in the absence of international agreement, multiple terms will coexist with varying degrees of synonymity. This process has occurred throughout history, although at markedly different rates in different eras. We live in the most rapidly changing era that mankind has ever experienced, and as such must be more willing than our forebears to give up outmoded concepts, and replace, where necessary, the familiar with the unfamiliar. But this is a small price to pay for the rewards of witnessing, in the course of a professional lifetime, the transition from a purely descriptive morphological view of lymphomas to one which encompasses an understanding of the precise nature of the cell of origin and of the genetic and biochemical changes which lead to malignant behaviour.

This book attempts to convey something of the excitement of the era in which we live, and to deal with the malignant non-Hodgkin's lymphomas, wherever possible, from a biological perspective rather than from a purely clinical and therapeutic one. As a consequence, a large proportion of the book is devoted to the nature of the diseases themselves, and their pathogenesis, representing the foundation upon which future diagnostic and treatment approaches will be built. As such, the practicing oncologist, and even more, the clinical researcher responsible for the design and analysis of clinical trials, will need to become familiar with the broad range of techniques currently available for the characterization of the non-Hodgkin's lymphomas.

Ian T. Magrath
1989

PART 1

Introduction

CHAPTER 1

Introduction: concepts and controversies in lymphoid neoplasia

IAN T. MAGRATH

Our understanding of any natural phenomenon will never be complete, but it will grow and develop as we improve the tools that extend the reach of our four limbs and five senses.

John Rovert Rathgam (1994)

Nature and definition of lymphoid neoplasia

The lymphoid neoplasms are particularly fascinating, perhaps paradoxical neoplasms, since they arise from cells whose primary function is to maintain the integrity of the organism. Indeed, lymphomas and lymphoid leukemias can be simply defined as malignant neoplasms of the immune system, or more specifically, neoplasms of lymphocytes and their precursor cells, the principal cellular elements of the immune system. As such, our understanding of the cellular origins of lymphoid neoplasia has its foundations in the science of immunology, a discipline that evolved from attempts to understand biological defenses against microorganisms. However, because lymphoid neoplasms represent the outgrowth of single cell clones (in a sense, ready-made biological reductionism), the study of the non-Hodgkin's lymphomas has also contributed greatly to our knowledge of the tissues, cells and molecules that mediate immune responses.

Lymphomas, for most of this century, have been subdivided (classified) on the basis of their cytology and histology, an approach which gradually superceded clinical classification in importance, and which inescapably led to the assumption that the various subtypes of lymphoma arise from different normal cell types even before the function of the normal counterpart cells was known. This assumption has been amply confirmed by the more recent immunological and genetic characterization of lymphoma cells but, at the same time, these new tools have demonstrated the shortcomings of a purely morphological approach to classification. Gradually, although not without protest, classifications based ultimately on the appearances of cells – the most basic being cell size (small or large, lymphocytic or lymphoblastic, lymphosarcoma or reticulum cell sarcoma) – and architecture (nodular or diffuse), have been replaced, or at least greatly enhanced, by those that emphasize cell lineage (B-cell or T-cell) and state of differentiation, or functional role, as the framework on which to build (cell size being now understood, in the context of lymphoid cells at least, to be largely a correlate of cell proliferation). A great deal can be inferred about lineage, differentiation state and function by immunophenotypic characterization with monoclonal antibodies, so that pathologists increasingly utilize these reagents in making a diagnosis. Thus, in contrast to former times (e.g., when large-cell lymphomas were collectively referred to as reticulum cell sarcoma or histiocytic lymphoma), we recognize that there are large pathobiological differences among lymphomas that superficially resemble each other because of their similar cell size.

The recognition that many lymphomas are associated with the presence of nonrandom (i.e., reproducibly demonstrable) cytogenetic abnormalities has been instrumental in identifying the causes of the altered growth and differentiation that characterize the behavior of neoplastic cells. The identification of the genes situated at the sites of gross chromosomal abnormalities, such as translocations or deletions (by means of various molecular cloning strategies), has led to the recognition that the inappropriate expression or loss of function (a consequence of genetic deletion or mutation) of genes that participate in the biochemical pathways that regulate cell proliferation, differentiation and life span is the immediate cause of the abnormal accumulation and behavior of the neoplastic cell clone. These genetic changes simulate, or have similar molecular consequences to, the normal signals from growth or differentiation factors (i.e., antigen and cytokines), but in addition (hence the need for multiple genetic abnormalities) provide the cell with a means to pass through 'check points' that normally prevent the continued existence of cells that are defective in some way. For example, check points in the G_1 phase of the cell cycle prevent entry into S phase if there is damaged DNA, and check points in G_2 prevent entry into M phase if the mitotic apparatus is in any way defective. Thus, identification of the genetic abnormalities associated with a lymphoma, unlike immunological characterization, can provide insights into the molecular basis of the neoplastic state and, thereby, an even more precise means of characterizing individual diseases than current immunophenotyping. Because of this, molecular characterization will become increasingly important both to lymphoma classification and eventually, doubtless, to therapy, since it should permit the development of targeted, i.e., lymphoma-subtype-specific, treatment approaches.

Inappropriate accumulation of a specific cell type can result either from increased production of cells (i.e., proliferation) or decreased cell losses (i.e., increased cell life span) compared to the normal situation. Increased proliferation is caused primarily by inappropriate expression of oncogenes (e.g., c-*myc*) and, although loss of growth regulation by tumor suppressor genes is doubtless also important, in the context of lymphomas this has been less often recognized, to date, than in many other types of cancer. Lymphomas in which increased proliferation is the primary cellular defect are generally associated with medium to large-sized cells and 'aggressive' behavior, i.e., relatively rapid growth and a correspondingly short natural history (although patients with such tumors can be cured by chemotherapy). In contrast, increased expression of genes that inhibit apoptosis or programmed cell death (e.g., *bcl*-2), which is a crucially important aspect of the regulation of both ontogeny and immune responses, prolongs cellular life span such that there is relatively slow accumulation of neoplastic cells (small to medium in size) and indolent clinical behavior, i.e., a long natural history (although patients with such tumors appear to be, for the most part, incurable).

These broad characterizations must be qualified by the recognition that within individual pathological entities the degree of clinical aggressiveness varies (one has only to think of localized versus disseminated disease), and that there is no sharp dividing line between 'aggressive' and 'indolent' lymphomas. Indeed, indolent lymphomas often undergo clonal evolution (by developing additional genetic changes) and may either present as a more aggressive tumor, the indolent phase having been subclinical or very short in duration (e.g., the blastic variant of mantle cell lymphoma and an unknown fraction of large-cell lymphomas of both T- and B-lineages), or undergo transformation after a variable interval into a more rapidly progressive and cytologically different neoplasm.

The interaction of inherited and environmental factors that give rise to the set of functional changes necessary to the emergence of a lymphoma is only dimly perceived at present. While, doubtless, more or less drastic revisions of our pathogenetic paradigms will occur as new tools emerge, we can identify three elements to our present conceptual framework of lymphomagenesis. These include the factors, inherited and environmental, that predispose to the development of pathogenetically relevant genetic changes, the cell type in which the genetic changes occur and the molecular consequences of the genetic changes themselves. We can surmise that it is highly likely that inherited genetic variations involving multiple genes influence the exposure of the DNA of lymphoid cells to environmental agents and therefore also influence the likelihood of any individual in a population developing a lymphoid neoplasm. Such polygenetic factors include those relevant to the handling of infectious agents (e.g., phagocytosis and immune responsiveness) and potential carcinogens (e.g., intestinal absorption, hepatic detoxification, and membrane pumps). Other polygenetic factors influence the degree of DNA damage caused by chemical agents (e.g., free radical scavenging systems, DNA repair processes) and the likelihood of errors occurring during physiological recombination of antigen receptor genes. Environmental factors themselves may influence the ability to deal with other environmental agents. For example, resistance to microorganisms may be lessened by nutritional status or by immunosuppression caused by another infectious process. Moreover, because of the huge differences in life style and environment among countries, we ought to expect to find geographical differences in the distribution of lymphoma subtypes – and this is, indeed, the case. Such geographical variation should provide clues to pathogenesis (as has been demonstrated in the case of human T-cell lymphotrophic virus-1 (HTLV-1), and adult T-cell leukemia-lymphoma in Japan and the Caribbean) which could lead to the development of preventive measures in high-risk populations.

CELLULAR ORIGINS OF NON-HODGKIN'S LYMPHOMAS

With the exception of lymphoid neoplasms arising from stem cells, which retain the capacity to differentiate along more than one pathway, lymphomas can be readily divided into those of the B- and T-cell lineages (rarely of natural killer (NK) or even histiocyte lineage). Using a combination of cytological features and immunophenotype, most lymphoid neoplasms can also often be identified as belonging to one of the two lymphocyte differentiation sequences, the primary, antigen-independent sequence that encompasses differentiation from lymphoid stem cells into functionally mature cells (e.g., lymphoblastic lymphoma), or the secondary sequence in which mature lymphoid cells are activated by a specific immunological challenge, i.e., by antigen, or via nonspecific pathways, i.e., by cytokines (e.g., lymphomas of follicle center cell origin) (Figure 1.1). Identification of the cell of origin of a neoplasm, i.e., the cell type in which the pathogenetic changes occurred, can often be difficult, since differentiation may occur either after malignant transformation, or during the process of malignant transformation such that the predominant cell in the clinically apparent lymphoma is not that in which the neoplastic

transformation took place. This perhaps particularly applies to lymphomas in which the antigen receptor genes are involved in chromosomal translocations, since this implies that the translocation occurred in a precursor cell, although many such lymphomas have the phenotype of mature (i.e., immunocompetent or activated) lymphoid cells. In addition, since full neoplastic transformation requires multiple genetic events, it is not unlikely, in some cases, that genetic changes are accumulated over several differentiation stages. Follicular lymphomas, in which 14;18 translocations cause persistent and inappropriate expression of *bcl*-2, and consequently are protected against apoptosis, provide an excellent paradigm for the understanding of neoplasia in the context of normal lymphocyte differentiation.

The paradigm of follicular lymphoma

There are molecular grounds for believing that the 14;18 translocation occurs in a presursor B-cell (one in which immunoglobulin gene rearrangement is occurring), yet follicular lymphomas cytologically resemble cells present in normal germinal centers, including both the smaller (centrocytes) and larger (centroblasts) follicular center cells. It is possible, indeed probable, based on the detection by PCR of 14;18 translocations in normal individuals (even children), that the 14;18 translocation does not cause neoplastic transformation of immature cells. Instead, 14;18-bearing precursor cells become resting 'virgin' lymphocytes. Such clones, relatively few in number, persist but do not necessarily expand. This differs little from the normal long-term persistence of clones of memory cells, although the translocated cells have, presumably, never encountered antigen. Only if the cell encounters antigen (or perhaps is nonspecifically activated) and begins to proliferate does the translocation become important. A role for antigen could explain why all follicular lymphomas express immunoglobulin and perhaps why the majority of normal individuals with detectable 14;18 translocations do not develop follicular lymphoma. The presence of a 14;18 translocation should confer immortality on a cell, even though it does not succeed in generating a functional immunoglobulin gene (a situation that normally leads to apoptosis), but such cells would never become follicular lymphomas since they cannot be activated by antigen. The progeny of normal activated B-cells undergo somatic mutation of their immunoglobulin genes in the germinal follicle and switch off *bcl*-2 expression in order that clones with lower affinity to the antigen (present on the processes of follicular dendritic cells as antigen–antibody complexes) are deleted by apoptosis. The presence of the translocation, however, would prevent this and all progeny cells of the

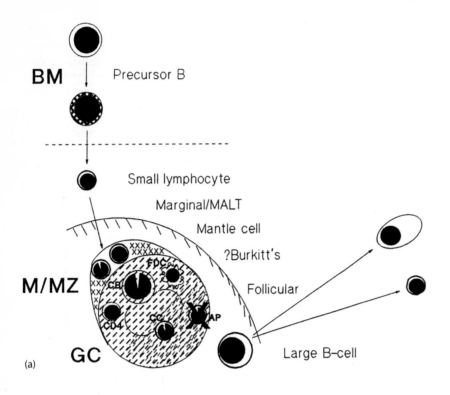

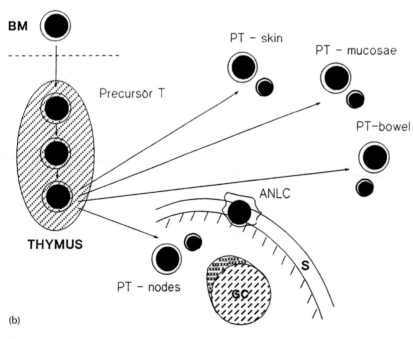

Figure 1.1 Cellular origins of non-Hodgkin's lymphomas. (a) Relationship of various B-lineage lymphomas to the normal ontogenetic and activation pathways of B-cells. BM, bone marrow; GC, germinal follicle; M/MZ, marginal/mantle zone – the marginal zone surrounds the follicle in Peyer's patches and spleen, but is mingled with the mantle zone in lymph nodes; FDC, follicular dendritic cell; CB, centroblast; CC, centrocyte; CD4, helper T-cell; AP, cell undergoing apoptosis, PC, plasma cell. (b) Relationship of various T-lineage lymphomas to the T-lymphocyte differentiation pathway. BM, bone marrow; GC, germinal center; PT, peripheral T-cell lymphoma; ANLC, anaplastic large-cell lymphoma.

clone would accumulate. It is easy to see why the immunohistochemical detection of *bcl*-2 expression clearly distinguishes follicular lymphoma from non-neoplastic hyperplastic follicles. Protected from apoptosis, follicular lymphoma cells are able to continue to accumulate somatic mutations in their immunoglobulin genes, as normal follicular center cells would. At the same time, of course, the persistent clones could undergo additional genetic changes with the effect of further increasing the proliferation of the abnormal cell clone. This would be manifest as an alteration in the fraction of large cells in the lymphoma (see discussion of grade below).

The role of follicular dendritic cells

The role of follicular dendritic cells as antigen presenting and storing cells may be crucial to an understanding of the pathogenesis of neoplasms of follicular cell origin. In addition to their role in lymphocyte activation, follicular dendritic cells appear to have an important role in the maintenance of immunological memory. It has been suggested, for example, that, in the absence of re-exposure to antigen stored on the dendritic processes of follicular dendritic cells as antigen–antibody complexes, even memory cells may have a life span of only 3 weeks. The presence of a tight web of dendritic reticulum cells is closely associated with a follicular architecture and follicular dendritic cells are absent in small cell lymphocytic lymphoma (chronic lymphocytic leukemia), which is believed to be of pregerminal center cell origin. Similarly, large B-cell lymphomas (centroblastic), even if they are of germinal center cell origin, are already the equivalent of activated cells and thus no longer dependent upon follicular dendritic cells, which are also absent from these tumors. Mantle cell lymphomas contain a disorganized meshwork of follicular dendritic cells. Whether follicular dendritic cells are relevant only to the architecture of follicular lymphomas or also have a role in the maintenance of the neoplastic state is not known.

Histological transformation

The concept of neoplastic clones retaining some capacity to differentiate is also relevant to the phenomenon of histological transformation, whereby a small cell lymphoma is transformed to a lymphoma consisting predominantly of large cells. In the case of transformation in follicular lymphomas, transformed lymphomas also lose their follicular architecture. Transformation is usually associated with the accumulation of additional genetic changes (probably always so, even if not detected) and the transformed lymphoma also exhibits more aggressive clinical behavior, probably because the cell is forced to progress further along lymphocyte activation pathways. Transformation can only occur in a 'small-cell' or less highly proliferative lymphoma, i.e., it can be thought of, at least in many cases, as the neoplastic counterpart of the normal activation process. In other words, only cells that retain a significant capacity to differentiate and that are not already rapidly proliferating can undergo transformation.

Lymphomas of uncertain provenance

Sometimes a corresponding normal counterpart cell to a particular, well-defined lymphoma cannot be definitely identified. This could either be because the normal cell counterpart has yet to be identified or because the neoplastic variant has diverged greatly from the cell type to which it is most closely related. This may be the case in Burkitt's lymphoma. It has been suggested that the normal counterpart of this highly proliferative tumor, which cytologically resembles either an immature lymphocyte precursor or activated lymphocyte is actually a *resting* lymphocyte. The deregulated expression of c-*myc* forces the cell to proliferate and, as a corollary of its proliferative state, to take on the cytological appearance of such a cell. However, some investigators believe that Burkitt's lymphoma is the malignant counterpart of a centroblast, differing from other neoplasms of centroblast origin because of the nature of the genetic changes it possesses.

Pleomorphism and normal cell admixtures

Another difficulty that often arises in attempting to identify a single normal counterpart cell is the presence of marked pleomorphism among the tumor cells (predominantly reflected in differences in cell size). It is probable that this is the result of the component lymphoma cells being at different stages of differentiation. If so, lymphomas might be better thought of as the neoplastic counterparts of a particular 'window' of differentiation, which includes several stages in the sequence and not of a single cell type. This is also well demonstrated in the follicular lymphomas and peripheral T-cell lymphomas, which both contain variable mixtures of cell types. The relative proportions of different sized cells may vary from one anatomical location to another, presumably resulting from differences in the local environment that favor growth of one or other of the constituent cell types.

The concept that some lymphomas are the neoplastic equivalent of an immune reaction helps to explain another phenomenon – the presence of numerous normal cells in some lymphomas – not simply residual cells belonging to the tissue being invaded, but cell types that are present in the lymphoma regardless of the tissue in which it occurs. Since immune responses require the participation of numerous cell types, which are attracted or activated by the release of cytokines, we might intuitively surmise that the cellular composition of lymphomas is likely to be much more varied in tumors that originate from activation pathways than those that derive from lymphocyte precursor cells. By the same token, T-cell lymphomas, being derived from cells involved in the regulation of other cell behavior, are more likely to include infiltrations of many normal cell types – of B-cells, of macrophages, granulocytes, epithelial cells, endothelial cells organized into blood vessels, or various mixtures of such cells. One B-cell lymphoma in which there is infiltration by normal lymphocytes, however, is the large B-cell lymphoma variant known as T-cell-rich B-cell lymphoma. T-cell neoplasms are also more likely than B-cell neoplasms to produce sufficiently large quantities of cytokines to induce systemic effects such as fever, weight loss, malaise, hypercalcemia, effects on erythroid and myeloid differentiation, or activation of macrophages with resultant hemophagocytosis. Molecular genetic changes may, of course, result in the production of cytokines not made by the normal counterpart cells.

LYMPHOMA CELL TROPISM – NODAL AND EXTRANODAL LYMPHOMAS

Because lymphoma cells retain many of the characteristics of their normal counterpart cells, they tend to reside in or recirculate through (prior to complete effacement) specific compartments of lymphoid tissue – whether nodal or extranodal. Thus, T-cell lymphomas, particularly if expressing a cytotoxic/ suppressor phenotype (CD8), will tend to involve the paracortical regions of lymph nodes and the periarteriolar sheaths of white pulp in the spleen, while B-cell lymphomas frequently involve or reiterate the follicles of lymphoid tissue, in some cases expanding certain components of these structures (e.g., the mantle or marginal zones, or the germinal centers), in others selectively invading the germinal follicles. Germinal follicles are the the normal site of B-cell activation, where B-cells come into contact with antigen presented by follicular dendritic cells and, as discussed, it appears that the follicular architecture of follicular lymphomas is dependent upon the presence of the dendritic reticulum cells. Tumors that are the counterpart of postfollicular center cells do not form follicles and tend to efface the normal architecture of lymphoid tissue.

Many lymphomas also retain the tropism of their normal cell counterparts, and selectively involve certain tissues such as skin, e.g., the cutaneous T-cell lymphomas, or mucosae of gut, respiratory tract, etc., e.g., lymphomas of mucosa-associated lymphoid tissue (MALT). It is highly likely that the cells of these neoplasms retain their homing mechanisms as a consequence of the expression of particular surface molecules (as has been shown, for example, in the case of intestinal T-cell lymphoma, which is usually associated with enteropathy). Lymphomas that present in lymph nodes are referred to as nodal lymphomas and those that involve organs or tissues rather than lymph nodes as extranodal. With the treatment regimens presently employed, extranodal lymphomas tend to have a worse prognosis than nodal lymphomas (at least in adults) and it is likely that this indicates a difference in biology. However, there is no sharp distinction between nodal and extranodal lymphomas, and both nodal and extranodal sites may be involved in the same patient. This is not surprising, since normal lymphocytes migrate between nodal and extranodal tissue, although there is a strong association between the gut and lymphocytes which express immunoglobulin (Ig) A. The current debate over the relationship between monocytoid B-cell lymphomas, which tend to involve organized lymphoid tissue, and MALT lymphomas, which involve epithelia, exemplifies this point. Many pathologists believe that these lymphomas are not truly separate entities and classify both as marginal zone lymphomas.

Selectivity of nodal regions, and organ and tissue involvement are more pronounced with more indolent lymphomas; in aggressive lymphomas, not only are normal homing mechanisms and dependence upon external growth or viability factors often lost but these highly proliferative tumors outgrow the physical confines of the compartments in which they would otherwise reside. The factors that govern the anatomical distribution of lymphomas are further discussed below.

CLONALITY OF LYMPHOID NEOPLASMS

The fact that multiple genetic changes are required in a single cell to give rise to neoplasia and that such changes, for the most part, occur sequentially (although not necessarily always in the same order) is entirely consistent with the observation that neoplasia is monoclonal – the chance that the same set of genetic changes will occur in more than one cell clone is highly unlikely unless the individual is at very high risk for malignancy. In the lymphoid neoplasms, clonality is usually easily assessed with reference to the antigen receptor genes. Since these genes are assembled by combining, during the early phases of lymphocyte differentiation, particular segments from the multiple elements present in germline DNA in order to generate specificity (in the case of B-cells, the antigen receptor is also secreted as antibody) each molecule is unique and can be used as a clonal marker. In many cases, structural rearrangements of specific genes, which arise as a result of the pathogenetically important chromosomal translocations or deteletions, or the presence of a particular pattern of mutations can also be used as highly specific markers of the malignant clone. However, not all potentially lethal diseases are monoclonal. Polyclonal or oligoclonal lymphoproliferative syndromes arising in individuals with inherited or acquired immunodeficiency syndromes, in which genetic changes are frequently not apparent, pose a semantic problem. Such syndromes are frequently (but not always) associated with the presence of Epstein–Barr virus (EBV) genomes in the proliferating cells. There also seems little doubt (see Chapter 45) that they arise as a consequence of failure of the immunodeficient individual to mount a normal – and usually effective – immune response against EBV-infected (or otherwise pathologically driven) lymphocytes, or to regulate the size of specific lymphocyte subpopulations. These immunodeficiency-associated lymphoproliferative syndromes thus appear to arise as a consequence of the immunological defects rather than from genetic changes occurring in a cell clone, although hyperplasia of lymphocyte subpopulations almost certainly predisposes to the development of genetic changes and, thus, to what we might call 'true neoplasia'. Interestingly, it is not infrequent in some immunodeficiency syndromes, e.g., Wiskott–Aldrich syndrome, for single clones of cells to intermittently become clinically manifest – sometimes associated with a measurable monoclonal Ig paraprotein in the peripheral blood. Such clones are usually self-limited and are not truly neoplastic (compare benign monoclonal gammopathy occurring in nonimmunosuppressed individuals). Thus, monoclonality is not always a sign of neoplasia, nor is polyclonality or oligoclonality evidence that the lymphoproliferative process is necessarily benign – death can result as readily from uncontrolled polyclonal lymphoproliferation as it can from monoclonal proliferation.

One potential pitfall for the unwary is inherent in the definition of clonality. A single rearranged band on a Southern blot probed with an antigen receptor gene does not necessarily indicate that the tumor is composed entirely of a single clone – only that the clone bearing the rearranged gene comprises a sufficiently high proportion of the cell population being examined to be detected – a proportion that need be no higher than 5–10%.

THE BORDERLANDS OF MALIGNANT LYMPHOMA

We have seen that, in essence, malignant lymphomas represent distortions of the normal processes of proliferation, differentiation and activation brought about by the occurrence of specific genetic changes in the biochemical pathways that regulate these processes. Malignant lymphomas are generally easy to recognize from their cytological and histological appearances. However, there are several borderlands

that provide both conceptual and practical difficulties. These include the boundaries between neoplastic and chronic inflammatory or benign lymphoproliferative processes, between lymphoid and nonlymphoid neoplasia, between leukemia and lymphoma, and between Hodgkin's disease and the non-Hodgkin's lymphomas.

Neoplastic versus nonneoplastic lymphoproliferation

The borderland between chronic inflammation and lymphoid neoplasia is an area of imprecision that is confined almost exclusively to lymphomas developing in activated lymphocytes, which are, in effect, neoplastic immune reactions. Such lymphomas frequently contain mixtures of lymphoid and nonlymphoid cells as do normal immune reactions. Morever, it appears highly probable that chronic inflammatory processes predispose to the development of true lymphomas, although, since malignant transformation and progression in lymphoid cells is, like that in all cell types, a step-wise process, defining the point at which a nonneoplastic lesion has become neoplastic can sometimes be very difficult. These diseases further underline the probable truth that all lymphoid neoplasms arise from a pre-existing hyperplastic stage, generally environmentally induced, that may or may not be apparent, depending upon its anatomical location. It is entirely possible that some genetic lesions may cause a clonal abnormality that remains sufficiently responsive to normal regulators of growth and differentiation (or simply prolongs the life span of the cell) that accumulation of the clone is subclinical, or of minimal clinical significance – at least until additional genetic changes occur and the process becomes more aggressive. The transition from 'benign' to 'malignant' neoplasia is perhaps more an issue of definition and semantics than biology, and does not necessarily have a bearing on treatment approaches.

This problem area is well illustrated by a number of mucosa-associated processes including the necrotizing lesions of the respiratory tract (sometimes referred to collectively as the lethal midline granuloma syndrome), which merge with, for the most part, peripheral T-cell lymphomas. A characteristically nodal process (i.e., arising in lymph nodes) that has also been considered to be a nonneoplastic process that frequently evolves into an overt T-cell lymphoma is angioblastic lymphadenopathy (AILD), although current opinion is that this disease is neoplastic from the outset. Relatively indolent B-lineage tumors of MALT of the respiratory or gastrointestinal tracts and immunoproliferative small intestinal disease can, in their early stages, be treated with antibiotics, but may also evolve into more malignant processes. The lymphoproliferative syndromes occurring in immunodeficient states (predominantly of B-cell origin), provide an excellent example of evolution from lymphoid hyperplasia to overt neoplasia, and other nonimmunodeficiency-related lymphoid hyperplasias may also evolve into neoplasia.

Midline granuloma syndrome

This rare disease, or collection of diseases, suffers from the familiar problems of classification – the existence of a plethora of designations and descriptions that sometimes artificially divide a single entity into several different diseases, but which may also include different pathological processes in the same disease category. The lack of pathogenetic information and the uncertainty as to the relevance of clinical features to diagnosis add to the difficulties, as they have to lymphoma classification in general.

Midline granulomas, i.e., necrotizing processes of the upper respiratory tract, sometimes contain 'atypical cells' and sometimes do not. Those that do not are generally diagnosed as a localized form of Wegener's granulomatosis, while those that do have been referred to either as Stewart's granuloma or polymorphic reticulosis (in homage to the possibility that the atypia was indicative of neoplasia) [1]. Both of the latter diseases appear to be identical histologically to lymphomatoid granulomatosis, an entity originally described as predominantly involving the lung. While the pleomorphic cellular infiltrate, granulomatous appearance and necrosis of lymphomatoid granulomatosis/polymorphic reticulosis invite classification as an inflammatory rather than a neoplastic disease, the presence of 'atypical cells', the tendency of some cases to evolve into overt lymphoma and the recent demonstration that single clones can predominate in the lesion, have suggested that lymphomatoid granulomatosis is actually a relatively indolent lymphoma, which sometimes evolves – like other lymphomas of a low degree of aggressivity – into a more aggressive process. Hence the proposal to use the term 'angiocentric lymphoma' for all of these processes [2]. If truly neoplastic from the outset, then it is probable that cytokine production by malignant cells causes infiltration of the lesion by normal cells. This is supported by the observation that some cases, at least, of lymphomatoid granulomatosis appear to consist of EBV-containing neoplastic cells of B-cell origin, with a marked infiltration of T-cells [3]. The necrotic element appears to be related to the angiocentricity, which leads to vascular obliteration.

There is, however, a spectrum of overlapping morphological appearances among this broadly defined group of angiocentric lymphomas, and some continue to differentiate between lymphomatoid granulomatosis and angiocentric lymphomas, while others refer to grades of angiocentric lymphoma.

Angioimmunoblastic lymphadenopathy

Angioimmunoblastic lymphadenopathy (AILD) is a systemic disease associated with lymph node enlargement and splenomegaly rather than involvement of mucosal tissue. Here, the recent application of interphase cytogenetics, using fluorescence *in situ* hybridization (FISH), to cases diagnosed as 'AILD type of T-cell lymphoma' has shed some light on the problem [4]. Multiple aberrant clones are present in this disease even though classical metaphase cytogenetics often fails to reveal them. Many of these clones appear to be unrelated – a finding which may be relevant to the frequent occurrence of both T- and B-cell receptor rearrangements in this disease. While it is important not to fall into the trap of presuming that aberrant cytogenetics always signify neoplasia (the functional consequence of the cytogenetic changes is what matters in this context), the inferred genetic instability is one of the hallmarks of malignancy. Depending upon the genetic changes that arise and may continue to arise, the behavior of the disease may be more or less aggressive.

Lymphomas of MALT

MALT lymphomas, formerly frequently referred to as 'pseudolymphomas', also appear to encompass reactive and neoplastic processes. The response of α-heavy chain disease and MALT lymphoma of the stomach to antibiotic therapy would seem to indicate that, in the early stages of evolution, such neoplasms remain dependent upon an external drive – presumably an environmental antigen, which, if removed, will lead to regression of the proliferative process. Indeed, there is now very good evidence that, in the case of MALT lymphomas, the antigen(s) in question is derived from the bacterium, *Helicobacter pylori* [5].

Lymphoproliferation in the context of immunodeficiency

A separate situation arises in the context of the variety of lymphoid hyperplasias that arise in the setting of immunodeficiency (whether inherited or acquired). Here, virus-infected cells or otherwise deregulated cells (many, but not all of these processes are associated with EBV) may proliferate in the absence of normal immunological regulation. Interestingly, it is possible that the proliferation of these cells may sometimes actually require signals from regulatory T-cells and the broad spectrum of syndromes observed (ranging from localized processes to rapidly progressive, widespread diseases) is probably a consequence, at least initially, of qualitative and quantitative differences in the immunosuppression. Genetic changes may, of course, occur in these hyperplastic cells, leading to independence from regulatory processes and true neoplasia.

Lymphadenopathies of uncertain origin

Finally, there are a large number of lymphadenopathic processes (i.e., characterized by lymph node enlargement) of uncertain origin. These include such histologically defined entities as massive lymphadenopathy with sinus histiocytosis (Rosai–Dorfman disease), Castleman's disease, the hemophagocytic syndromes and other diseases, which are sufficiently uncommon or have sufficiently varied characteristics that they defy all attempts at classification. The definition of these entities is not always precise. In this context, Castleman's disease may be used as an example. The localized form of this disease, usually diagnosed histologically as the 'hyaline variant' (derived from the appearance of germinal follicles from which there is progressive loss of cellularity) appears to be a hamartoma and is readily cured by surgical excision. In contrast, the systemic subtypes, often characterized by pronounced plasma cell infiltration (which has been related to interleukin-6 production within the lesions), sometimes evolve into more aggressive diseases. As with so many other diseases on the borderland of inflammation and neoplasia, predicting which lesions will progress in this way is hazardous at best. It seems likely that the systemic 'disease' is not a single entity in spite of the apparent histological uniformity but a convergent picture caused by a similarity in the pattern of cytokine production by cells within the lesions.

Viruses and the borderland of lymphoid neoplasia

Interestingly, some of the diseases at the interface between neoplasia and inflammatory or hyperplastic conditions are not infrequently associated with EBV, although the virus is usually present in only a fraction of the cells. This applies to both the T-cell processes, angiocentric lymphomas and angioimmunoblastic lymphadenopathy, and the B-cell lymphoproliferative syndromes associated with immunodeficiency. Unlike the B-cell lymphoproliferations, however, the T-cell diseases often contain

EBV in only a fraction of the tumor cells [6]. This means that it is difficult to invoke a pathogenetic role for EBV unless one postulates that the virus-infected cell population is the only truly neoplastic population in the lesion – and presumably induces the migration of other cell types into the lesion by cytokine production. The most extreme example of this paradigm is Hodgkin's disease. The alternative possibility – that EBV infects an already neoplastic cell – cannot be excluded, and it remains possible that EBV infection is the equivalent of a genetic change associated with progression from a less to a more aggressive process.

HTLV-1, a retrovirus associated with adult T-cell leukemia/lymphoma, is also associated with a range of diseases, varying in aggressivity. At its most benign, the virus simply causes subclinical hyperplasia of multiple T-cell clones. Only if additional genetic changes are superimposed on this clone does malignancy develop.

Lymphoid versus nonlymphoid neoplasia

Even the definition of the lymphocyte lineage must, at the borders, entail arbitrary decisions. There can be little doubt that cells that have functionally rearranged their antigen receptor genes are lymphocytes, for the hallmark of most cells that are considered to be lymphocytes (natural killer cells may be an exception) is an ability to mount a specific response to an antigen, made possible by the presence of antigen–receptor complexes at the cell surface. However, plasma cells – the terminal differentiation step of the B or humoral lymphocyte lineage, which secrete large amounts of immunoglobulin – are not usually considered as lymphocytes, nor myelomas as lymphomas. This apparently capricious quirk of classification is of historical origin (plasma cells were not initially recognized for what they are) and need concern us only with respect to the generally (but not invariably) accepted exclusion of myeloma from consideration with the lymphoid neoplasms (although neoplastic cells with a 'lymphoplasmacytoid' appearance are considered to be lymphomas). Similarly, at the other extreme of the lymphocyte differentiation pathway, the ability to distinguish lymphocyte precursors from cells with multiple differentiating potential, including that of developing into cells of other lineages, has not yet been accomplished. In fact, some lymphoid neoplasms appear to result from genetic abnormalities occurring in such multipotential cells, since cells that are present in the blast crisis of chronic myeloid leukemia are frequently of lymphoid origin, while mixed lineage leukemias (in which either two lineages, or cells of mixed myeloid and lymphoid phenotype, are present) are well recognized.

Histiocytic neoplasms

One of the histological categories in Rappaport's classification was 'histiocytic lymphoma'. Lymphomas that would have fallen into this category are now referred to as large-cell lymphomas, since immunophenotyping and molecular studies have shown them to be almost exclusively of lymphoid rather than histiocyte origin. While most such lymphomas have been shown to be of the B-cell lineage, it is now clear that several subtypes of T-cell lymphoma had, until the demonstration of immunophenotypic and molecular characteristics (i.e., T-cell receptor gene rearrangements) indicating a T-cell origin, been considered on morphological grounds to be of histiocytic origin. These include anaplastic large-cell lymphomas (which have been confused with a wide range of both neoplastic and nonneoplastic entities), and intestinal T-cell lymphoma, which is usually associated with gluten-sensitive enteropathy. Some neoplasms have been wrongly diagnosed as of histiocytic origin because of a marked histiocytic reaction to an underlying lymphoma, usually of T-cell origin. This doubtless results from the profile of cytokines produced by the lymphoma cells. Such patients may present with a hemophagocytic syndrome manifested by pancytopenia including microangiopathic anemia, disseminated intravascular coagulation, jaundice, fever, hepatosplenomegaly and lymphadenopathy. Occasionally such patients are misdiagnosed as histiocytic medullary reticulosis, now more often referred to as malignant histiocytosis, a rare and indistinct disease, in which hemophagocytosis occurs in apparently malignant histocytes.

It is clear that the majority of what were formerly considered to be histiocytic neoplasms are, in fact, of lymphoid origin. However, not all such neoplasms fall into this category. A small number of 'large-cell' lymphomas (less than 1%) do appear to have phenotypic characteristics consistent with an origin from histiocytes and lack the molecular hallmarks of the T-cell lineage. Whether or not such tumors should be considered lymphomas is a semantic point that depends upon whether or not the latter term is to be used only for the neoplasms of lymphocytes and their precursor cells, or, as originally conceived, for all tumors that arise in lymphoid tissue. While not of lymphoid origin, these cells have a crucial role in the immune response (a subset of such cells, the Langerhans cells and dendritic cells, have an important role in antigen presentation, while monocytes and macrophages are phagocytes, and are an integral component of lymphoid tissue). Some histiocytic lymphomas could be rare manifestations of monocytic leukemias in which a bone marrow component is not evident at a microscopic level, comparable to a pre-B-cell lymphoblastic lymphoma. Alternatively, they could be true neoplasms of tissue histiocytes or dendritic cells.

Leukemia versus lymphoma

Other taxonomic difficulties relevant to the definition of non-Hodgkin's lymphoma exist. For example, the dividing line between leukemia and lymphoma is not generally agreed upon – largely because the terms themselves do not have precise definitions. Leukemia was a term originally devised by Virchow (in German, Weisses Blut) to reflect a gross pathological appearance, namely 'white blood' caused by a very high white blood cell count (originally believed to be the result of 'suppuration'). The term is now generally used to indicate neoplasms arising from the lymphohematopoietic cells of the bone marrow, regardless of the circulating white cell count. Confusion arises with the lymphoid neoplasms since both T- and B-lymphocyte precursors originate in the bone marrow, which is, therefore, a primary lymphoid organ, while differentiated lymphocytes and plasma cells recirculate through the bone marrow (albeit in separate microanatomic locations) such that it is also a secondary lymphoid organ. Thus, while neoplastic diseases in which the cell has an immature phenotype usually involve the bone marrow, and not infrequently the peripheral blood, a variety of mature lymphoid neoplasms may also involve the bone marrow – in the case of Sézary syndrome, first entering the peripheral blood from the skin.

Not all neoplasms of lymphocyte precursors arise from, or at least overtly involve, the bone marrow. T-cell precursors, for example, undergo much of their differentiation in the thymus, so that a fraction of precursor T-cell neoplasms present as an anterior superior mediastinal mass and may not involve the bone marrow. If extensive disease is present in the bone marrow at presentation, such tumors are normally referred to as acute lymphoblastic leukemia. Relapse may or may not involve the bone marrow, regardless of whether it was involved at presentation. Even precursor B-cell malignancies may occasionally present as localized lymph node or bone involvement without overt marrow disease (although techniques more sensitive than microscopy may permit detection of marrow involvement), while small noncleaved cell lymphoma with extensive bone marrow involvement is usually referred to as 'acute B-cell leukemia' or L3 type of acute lymphoblastic leukemia. Marrow involvement is usually present in a number of lymphomas, for example, follicular lymphomas, but such tumors have not generally been referred to as leukemia unless there is a significant fraction of circulating tumor cells.

Thus, neither the simple criterion of bone marrow involvement, nor the demonstration that a lymphoid neoplasm is the malignant counterpart of lymphocyte precursors, provides a clear dividing line between leukemias and lymphomas. Indeed, from the pathobiological perspective, there is no clear dividing line – the terms are hangovers from an earlier period of clinical and gross pathological classification performed without the benefit of bone marrow examination, or even, initially, peripheral blood examination, during life (the terms were originally coined on the basis of post-mortem examinations). To avoid confusing the uninitiated, they ought either to be discarded (unlikely, in the near future, since they appear to be deeply entrenched) or redefined in the context of lymphoid neoplasia. A more rational use of the term leukemia might be to limit it to diseases of myeloid (including monocytes) and erythroid cells, and to classify all diseases of lymphoid origin, including acute lymphoblastic leukemia and chronic lymphocytic leukemia, as lymphoma, or simply lymphoid neoplasia. An alternative designation chosen from the plethora of previously used terms such as lymphosarcoma, leukosarcoma, lymphomatosis, or even a combination of terms such as lymphoblastosis and lymphocytosis (or lymphoblastoma and lymphocytoma), would be unlikely to be widely accepted, but could be put to the test at an international conference of high standing.

Pediatric oncologists generally use an arbitrary definition of leukemia, in the context of lymphoid neoplasia, of 25% or more neoplastic cells in the bone marrow, and adult oncologists sometimes use a cutoff of 30%, but it is not clear that either of these limits has prognostic importance and even less so that they have pathobiological significance beyond the surface characteristics relevant to proliferation or lodging in the bone marrow. Nor can the distinction between leukemia and lymphoma, based on such a criterion, be used in making treatment decisions – bone marrow involvement should be considered of importance only insofar as it has been shown to be a prognostic factor within each separate pathologic entity rather than assuming that bone marrow involvement signifies a completely different disease requiring different principles of treatment. Perhaps this nomenclature issue will be resolved as classification schemes are more drastically overhauled at such time as molecular and/or etiological criteria are used as a taxonomic framework.

Hodgkin's disease versus non-Hodgkin's lymphoma

Even the often presumed clear-cut distinction between Hodgkin's disease and the non-Hodgkin's lymphomas is not nearly as sharp as is generally believed and, as a consequence, is also rather arbitrary [7]. It has been estimated, for example, that 10–15% of patients who would have been diagnosed as having Hodgkin's disease 30–40 years ago are today diagnosed as having non-Hodgkin's lymphomas. The occurrence of both diseases in the same patient, either simultaneously or sequentially (in either order), occurs more frequently than can be accounted for by chance alone. Sequential occurrence could result from predisposition occasioned by immunosuppression or previous treatment, but this explanation does not hold for composite non-Hodgkin's lymphoma/Hodgkin's disease in which both diseases are present simultaneously in the same tumor or organ. Moreover, anaplastic large-cell lymphoma (ALCL) merges imperceptibly, both morphologically and immunophenotypically, with Hodgkin's disease. Some authors refer to a Hodgkin's-like variety of ALCL and ALCL may arise in patients diagnosed as having Hodgkin's disease. It can also be superimposed upon mycosis fungoides/Sézary syndrome, as can Hodgkin's disease, or develop in patients with 'low-grade' (more indolent) peripheral T-cell lymphomas. ALCL thus appears to represent a kind of blastic transformation common to many T-cell neoplasms, a parallel to the large B-cell lymphoma that may evolve from relatively indolent B-cell lymphomas. These findings suggest that a fraction of cases of Hodgkin's disease may be of T-cell origin.

There is more evidence that some cases of Hodgkin's disease are of B-cell origin, for the nodular lymphocyte predominant subtype of Hodgkin's disease (sometimes now referred to as nodular paragranuloma), occasionally evolves into a B-cell type of non-Hodgkin's lymphoma and differs histologically, immunophenotypically and with respect to its behavior from other types of Hodgkin's disease. In nodular paragranuloma, the 'Reed–Sternberg' cells have a different appearance from those of other histological subtypes of Hodgkin's disease, and are referred to as L and H, or 'popcorn' cells, while the Hodgkin's cells and infiltrating lymphocytes express B-cell characteristics. Some diffuse non-Hodgkin's lymphomas – T-cell or histiocyte-rich B-cell lymphomas – closely resemble nodular paragranuloma with respect to the morphology and immunophenotype of the malignant cells, and could represent more aggressive varients of nodular paragranuloma.

Hodgkin's disease may also arise in patients with other lymphoid neoplasms, e.g., chronic lymphocytic leukemia. This applies particularly to the variant in which morphologically and immunologically typical Reed–Sternberg cells are observed amidst otherwise typical (morphologically and immunologically) B-cell chronic lymphocytic leukemia cells, and, interestingly, EBV is usually present in the Reed–Sternberg cells in this situation.

Evidence that the Reed–Sternberg cells of Hodgkin's disease are of lymphoid origin – even excepting the L and H cells of nodular paragranuloma – is mounting [7a], and it would appear that the cellular infiltrates that produce the characteristic histological appearance of some types of Hodgkin's disease result from the production of lymphokines by Reed–Sternberg cells. Lymphokine production has also been well documented in ALCL, and there is little doubt that such molecules are responsible for the systemic effects that are frequently observed in both ALCL and Hodgkin's disease. Clearly, ALCL lymphoma might well have been classified as a form of Hodgkin's disease in which large cells (occasional varients of which may be essentially indistinguishable from Reed–Sternberg cells) predominate (the former Hodgkin's sarcoma?), rather than a variety of non-Hodgkin's lymphoma. Similarly, nodular paragranuloma could easily be conceptualized as a relatively indolent B-cell lymphoproliferative syndrome that can evolve into a more malignant B-cell lymphoma. As with so many other dividing lines made before objective criteria based on pathogenesis were available, that between Hodgkin's disease and the non-Hodgkin's lymphomas is arbitrary.

Classification of lymphoid neoplasia

As with all branches of knowledge, a thorough understanding of the pathology of lymphoid neoplasms involves the reductive process of classification, an endeavor that requires a framework, tools with which to discern the place of individual diseases within the framework and a system of nomenclature. As with many taxonomic systems, that of lymphoid neoplasia suffers from the persistence of framework concepts and nomenclatures used at earlier times in its evolution (see Chapter 2). Nomenclature is strongly influenced by extant prejudices regarding the dividing lines between different entities, the level of pathogenetic understanding, and the biases of those who propose new or modified terminology. This has led to the existence of numerous classifications at any given point in history with varying degrees of congruence, and hence varying degrees of equivalence between the terms from one scheme and those of another. The names applied to individual diseases may be descriptive of tissue of origin (e.g., MALT lymphoma), of tissue architec-

ture (e.g., mantle zone lymphoma, follicular lymphoma), of cytomorphology (e.g., small noncleaved cell lymphoma, anaplastic large-cell lymphoma), of lineage or immunophenotype (e.g., T- or B-cell lymphoma), of stage of differentiation (e.g., pre-B-cell leukemia, immunoblastic lymphoma), of geographic origin (e.g., Mediterranean lymphoma), of clinical course (e.g., chronic lymphocytic leukemia) or eponymic (e.g., Hodgkin's disease, Burkitt's lymphoma, Lennert's lymphoma). Many descriptive terms, derived from gross pathological appearances or presumed cellular origins (e.g., lymphosarcoma, reticulum cell sarcoma, stem cell lymphoma) have largely become obsolete. Numerous other descriptive terms that encompass groups of diseases or that are supplementary to classification systems (e.g., low-grade lymphoma, extranodal lymphoma, peripheral T-cell lymphoma, gastric lymphoma) are widely used.

Needless to say, the existence of multiple classification schemes, each using different frameworks and nomenclatures, sometimes overlapping, and the evolution of more precise tools with which to identify pathological entities (immunophenotyping and the detection of cytogenetic and/or molecular genetic abnormalities) has led to considerable confusion and a great deal of difficulty in communication. Indeed, the National Cancer Institute Working Formulation for Clinical Usage (which is an exclusively histological classification system) was proposed (tongue in cheek?) as a system that would permit translation among the major extant classification systems [8]. Not surprisingly, the Working Formulation has been primarily used as a classification system in its own right, but today clearly suffers from the disadvantage that many of its categories include several discrete pathological entities that have been recently recognized, or at least accepted, because of more detailed immunophenotypic and/or genetic studies (Figure 1.2). Other well-known classification systems, which have persisted alongside the Working Formulation, such as the Lukes and Collins [9] and Kiel schemes [10], while having the advantage over the Working Formulation that they are based on immunological concepts, remain essentially histological schemes. No classification system has yet been proposed that is based on the nature of the molecular genetic lesions present in the tumor cells (presumably because there is still insufficient information to be able to do this), although genetic information, along with immunophenotypic data, has been incorporated into the recently published Revised European–American Lymphoma (REAL) classification [11].

In view of the lack of a standard taxonomic framework, recently recognized entities have been named according to any of the previously used

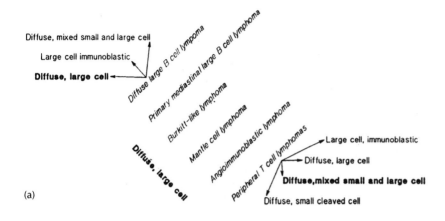

(a)

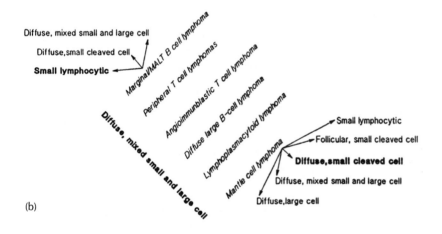

(b)

Figure 1.2 Heterogeneity of selected Working Formulation (WF) categories (Roman script) with respect to more recent entities recognized in the REAL classification (italic script). (a) Diffuse large-cell lymphoma. (b) Diffuse, mixed small and large cell lymphoma. Four of the entitites listed in the REAL classification are exploded (arrows) to show WF categories into which they would fall – the most likely in bold face print.

frameworks (e.g., monocytoid cell B-cell lymphoma, splenic marginal zone lymphoma, MALT lymphoma, anaplastic large-cell lymphoma). The REAL classification does not attempt to introduce a radically new system but provides, in effect, a list of all presumptive pathological entities. It does have, as an underlying theme, the separation of T- and B-cell lineages on the one hand, and precursor versus mature cell types on the other. It also provides information, for each entity, on immunophenotype and genetics as well as morphology. Finally, unlike other schemes, it gives an indication as to whether the entity is generally accepted to be a single disease or not.

The inclusion of a variety of different characteristics in the definition of individual lymphomas provides tacit recognition of the fact that no single descriptor (histology, immunophenotype, genotype, anatomical location or clinical behavior) is sufficient, at present, to define an entity precisely, although, for the most part, histology, frequently supplemented by immunophenotyping, remains the pre-eminent diagnostic technique. The same cytogenetic and molecular changes can be found in lymphomas in which the histology clearly differs, while apparently quite different molecular genetic findings may be observed within a single histological category (e.g., 14;18 and 8;14 translocations in both small noncleaved cell and large-cell lymphomas). This could be interpreted as indicating that morphological distinctions are often incorrect but more study will be needed to determine whether this is, in fact, the case – the same genetic abnormality, for example, in a different cell could produce a different 'phenotype'. Similarly, apparently identical diseases may or may not be associated with a virus (e.g., EBV, HTLV-1), while the same virus may be associated with quite different diseases (e.g., EBV in small noncleaved cell and anaplastic large-cell lymphoma, and Hodgkin's disease). Thus, an etiological diagnosis in the sense that it is used in infectious diseases (tuberculosis, anthrax) may not be feasible.

LYMPHOMAS IN THE CONTEXT OF LYMPHOCYTE ONTOGENY AND ACTIVATION

The most logical conceptual framework for the understanding of lymphomas is to classify them according to the normal cells that they most closely resemble. Most lymphomas fall naturally into one of four main divisions according to whether their normal counterpart cells are within the B- or T-cell lineages, and whether they are immature cells, i.e., in the process of differentiating from stem cells (the primary differentiation pathway), or immunocompetent cells (Figure 1.1). The latter often resemble antigen/mitogen-activated lymphocytes (the secondary differentiation pathway). Thus, knowledge of the events that occur during ontogeny and their anatomical locations, as well as an understanding of lymphocyte activation pathways – both in terms of the molecular events and the compartments within lymphoid tissue in which they take place – is crucial to a comprehension of both the principles that govern lymphomagenesis and the expression of any given tumor as a particular cell type.

Most of the more indolent (low-grade) lymphomas, in particular, are remarkably similar, with respect to their morphology and immunophenotype, to cells that are present in specific regions of lymphoid tissue (witness marginal zone lymphomas, MALT lymphomas, mantle cell lymphomas, follicular lymphomas) [12]. It is important to recognize that the majority of these pathological entities are derived from the B-cell lineage, and that B-cell lymphomas comprise perhaps 80% of the non-Hodgkin's lymphomas in North America, Europe and Australasia. It appears that, in these countries, the predominant lymphoma subtypes are the neoplastic counterparts of cells of the lymphoid follicles (including mantle zones, marginal zones and germinal centers) through which B-cells pass when activated by antigen. Perhaps not surprisingly, the majority (at least two-thirds, and probably more) of diffuse large B-cell lymphomas in adults also appear to be of follicular center cell origin. This has relevance to both the etiology and pathogenesis of these tumors. Knowledge of the check points and signals involved in the process of lymphocyte activation is likely to lead to a much more comprehensive understanding of the significance of the genetic lesions that permit the neoplastic cell to survive, and cause it to resemble one or other of the various cell types involved in the B-cell immune response (i.e., the mechanisms of neoplasia). In the germinal follicle, for example, competition by centrocytes for antigen expressed on a follicular dendritic cell results in apoptosis of cells with lower affinity antibodies. The cells that survive, because mutation of the hypervariable region of the immunoglobulin molecule has produced a higher affinity (more competitive) antibody, are reactivated, express Bcl-2, and respond to signals that determine whether they will become plasma cells or memory cells. These signals probably include interleukin-4 (IL-4) and the CD40 ligand (expressed on T4 cells, which may interact only with B-cells that present the cognate antigen), in the context of memory cells, and interleukin-1α (IL-1α) and soluble CD23 in the context of plasma cells. At present, the relationship of T-cell lymphomas that resemble immunocompetent or activated T-cells to the normal events involved in T-cell activation is much less well understood. Their role as regulatory cells of innumerable processes within the immune and hematopoietic systems increases the complexity of the resultant networks enormously. The production of cytokines by T-cell neoplasms, however, and their influence on systemic symptoms, and the histology of T-cell neoplasms, is entirely consistent with the regulatory role of T-cells. In addition, the frequency with which subtypes of T-cell lymphomas occur at extranodal sites, particularly skin and bowel (both surfaces in contact with the exterior), is consistent with their importance as 'guardians of the tissues' in contrast to the humoral role of antibody-producing B-cells. While division into cytotoxic and helper neoplasms has not been of great value, the differences in the role of α/β versus γ/δ T-cells may lead to useful separations (e.g., the latter cells appear to be more involved with chronic inflammatory processes).

In the ontogenic pathways, similar check points exist. Precursor B-cells, for example undergo apoptosis if they do not develop a set of functional antigen receptor genes (and possibly coreceptor molecules). In the thymus, similarly, successful rearrangement of T-cell receptor β (TCRβ) permits differentiation to an IL-2 receptor-negative CD4+/CD8+ cell, which, after successful expression of a TCRα chain and binding to the relevant major histocompatibility complex (MHC) antigen class, then develops into a mature IL-2 receptor expressing CD4+ (MHC class II) or CD8+ cell (MHC class I). Cells that fail to pass relevant check points are eliminated by apoptosis. Thus, precursor lymphoid neoplasms must either not progress to the point that a check point must be encountered, comply with the check point requirements, or avoid the consequences of not complying through the presence of relevant genetic lesions that prevent apoptosis in this context.

Thus, study of the signals and responses (largely encompassed by immunology) and of the molecules that mediate those signals (the domain of molecular biology) is likely to lead to considerable increments in the understanding of the mechanims of neoplasia, while, in turn, the identification of the functional consequences of the genetic aberrations of neoplastic cells will lead to a better understanding of the signalling processes.

HISTOLOGICAL CLASSIFICATION

Shortcomings of purely histological classification

Histological diagnosis is an essentially subjective skill, which consequently suffers from the lack of precise disease definitions and, consequently, from a lack of reproducibility – particularly among different histopathologists. Moreover, the histopathologist is faced with a number of difficulties, including technical artefacts, usually arising from differences in fixation techniques, which may alter the appearance of the tissue section, as well as the possibility that sampling is unrepresentative. Early histological classification schemes were hindered by the lack of parallel tools to justify separation of morphologic subtypes, but with the advent of immunophenotyping and, more recently, molecular characterization, it has been possible to confirm the existence of histological subtypes within larger histological categories (e.g., lymphoblastic lymphoma within the former diffuse poorly differentiated lymphocytic lymphoma of Rappaport). Indeed, there can no longer be any doubt that the majority of the categories in the Working Formulation are heterogeneous. However, while some of the heterogeneity is readily discerned by simple determination of lineage (T versus B), sometimes even immunophenotype is insufficient, in the absence of additional corroboration, to distinguish among several entities that belong to the same lineage and have the same histological appearances. For example, while the majority of large B-cell lymphomas may be closely related, i.e., predominantly of follicular center cell origin, there are at least three (and probably more) variants based on the presence of molecular abnormalities that involve different genes (namely *bcl*-2, *bcl*-6 and *myc*).

Another problem is the merging of one histological appearance with another such that the distinction between entities becomes arbitrary and difficult to reproduce. Imprecise boundaries of this kind include those between the three subtypes of follicular lymphoma included in the Working Formulation, those between the Working Formulation subtypes of small noncleaved cell lymphoma, and those between small noncleaved lymphoma and large B-cell lymphomas (Figure 1.3). The distinction between large B-cell (centroblastic) and B-cell immunoblastic lymphoma has also been shown not to be reproducible, and is not made in the REAL classification [11].

While separation of one lymphoma from another can sometimes be difficult, close relationships between histologically distinct lymphomas may also be obscured, either because of significant cytological variability within the entity or because of the variable infiltration (caused by cytokine production?) of normal cells, thus altering the histological appearance. Similarly, slightly different biological charac-

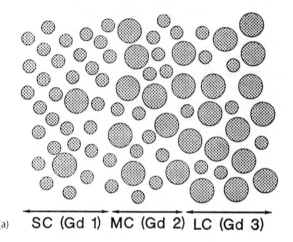

(a) SC (Gd 1) MC (Gd 2) LC (Gd 3)

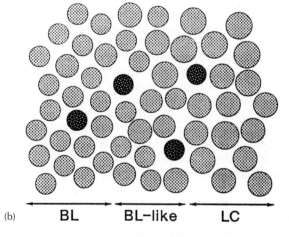

(b) BL BL-like LC

Figure 1.3 Illustration of the subjective determination of borderlines between selected histological categories. (a) Small, mixed small- and large-cell and large-cell variants of follicular lymphoma. (b) Burkitt's lymphoma, Burkitt-like lymphoma and large B-cell lymphoma. Macrophage nuclei are shown for size comparison – large-cell lymphoma nuclei are larger than macrophage nuclei.

teristics may alter the anatomical distribution of the lymphoma, e.g., cause a lymphoma to be extranodal rather than nodal or to proliferate in one tissue rather than another. Location of morphologically similar lymphomas at different sites – particularly nodal versus extranodal – may cause pathologists to consider them to be separate entities (e.g., monocytoid B-cell lymphoma and MALT lymphoma), while the same lymphoma may sometimes take on a different histological appearance in different tissues. Sometimes histological diagnosis may be confounded by differences in the degree to which otherwise identical tumors undergo 'differentiation' (or perhaps the neoplastic equivalent of 'activation'), leading some to separate the 'entity' into two or more categories, and others to recognize only a single category. Mantle cell lymphomas, for example, contain cells that resemble small lymphocytes, others that have the appearance of the small cleaved cells (centrocytes) of the follicle center, and others that have a plasmacytoid appearance. Such tumors, prior to their recognition as an entity, were therefore variably diagnosed as small lymphocytic, centrocytic (small cleaved cell) or lymphoplasmacytoid lymphomas, while the blastic variant of mantle cell lymphoma was considered either to be a diffuse, mixed large- and small-cell lymphoma, or a diffuse large-cell lymphoma (Figure 1.2). The possibility of placing what is now considered a single entity into any of five different histological categories emphasizes the failings of purely histological diagnosis, although now that mantle cell lymphoma has been recognized and well characterized, a diagnosis based solely on histology can frequently be made.

Prominent histological features

Histological classification is based on the cytological appearance and size of the predominant cell type, the cytoarchitecture and the way in which the tumor cells invade surrounding tissue. While histology alone has major shortcomings as a means of understanding the cellular origins and classification of lymphoid neoplasms, cell size and appearance do have important implications with respect to clinical behavior and it is possible to divide non-Hodgkin's lymphomas into three main categories according to whether the tumor is composed of small cells (i.e., similar to, or only slightly larger in size than, a normal lymphocyte), large cells (equal to or greater than the size of lymphoblasts), or a mixture of large and small cells (Table 1.1). However, some entities do cross over between these categories, reflecting the size transitions that are made by their normal counterpart cells during lymphocyte activation.

Table 1.1 Major subtypes of non-Hodgkin's lymphomas based on cell size*

I. Small-cell lymphomas (i.e., approximately the size of a mature lymphocyte)
(a) B-Cell subtypes
Small lymphocytic lymphoma/leukemia
    B-Cell variant
Lymphoplasmacytoid lymphoma
Mantle cell lymphoma (centrocytic lymphoma)
    Nodular (mantle zone) variant
Marginal zone lymphomas
    MALT lymphoma
    Monocytoid B-cell lymphoma
    Splenic marginal zone lymphoma (splenic lymphoma with villous lymphocytes)
(b) T-Cell subtypes
Small lymphocytic lymphoma/leukemia
    T-Cell variant

II. Mixed small-T and large-cell lymphomas
(a) B-Cell subtypes
Variants of small-cell lymphomas
    Paraimmunoblastic/prolymphocytic variant of small lymphocytic lymphoma
    Blastic or lymphoblastoid variant of mantle cell lymphoma
Follicular lymphoma (centroblastic/centrocytic lymphoma)
    Small cleaved, mixed, large-cell 'variants'
(b) T-Cell subtypes
Peripheral T-cell lymphomas
    Unspecified
    Angiocentric lymphomas
    Angioimmunoblastic lymphomas
    Lymphoepitheloid lymphoma (?)†
    Adult T-cell leukemia/lymphoma (HTLV-1 associated)
    Intestinal T-cell lymphoma
    Mycosis fungoides/Sézary syndrome

III. Large-cell lymphomas (nucleus at least as large as that of a lymphoblast)
(a) B-Cell subtypes
Burkitt's lymphoma
    Burkitt-like variant?
Large B-cell lymphoma (centroblastic, immunoblastic lymphomas)
    Burkitt-like variant?
    Large cleaved and noncleaved variants
    Large B-cell lymphoma rich in T-cells‡
    Primary mediastinal large B-cell lymphoma
(b) T-Cell subtypes
Lymphoblastic lymphoma
Large (peripheral) T-cell lymphomas
    Unspecified
    Anaplastic large-cell lymphoma

*Based primarily size of the neoplastic cells, secondarily on cell lineage – B- or T-cell.
†While other peripheral T-cell lymphomas may contain admixed epitheloid cells, this probable entity contains large numbers of such cells.
‡Classified as large cell rather than mixed because the small infiltrating cells are not believed to be neoplastic.

Significance of cell size

Cell size gives a rough index of the growth fraction of lymphomas, since proliferating lymphoid cells (whether in the primary or secondary differentiation pathways) are larger than resting cells. Lymphomas consisting predominantly of large cells (i.e., significantly larger than a mature lymphocyte and usually with nuclei larger than those of a macrophage) are, correspondingly, generally associated with a more rapidly progressive clinical course than those that consist primarily of small cells (i.e., similar in size to, or only slightly larger than, a mature lymphocyte). The latter tend to contain fewer mitoses, to have a smaller fraction of cells in S phase, measured by a variety of techniques, and to be clinically relatively indolent. These neoplasms might be thought of as the normal counterparts of immunocompetent cells, which have not been immunologically activated or have been only partially activated, an assumption that is borne out by the phenomenon of transformation from a small-cell to a large-cell lymphoma.

Lymphomas that consist exclusively or predominantly of large cells, including neoplasms of lymphoid precursor cells (e.g., lymphoblastic lymphoma) and activated lymphoid cells (large-cell lymphomas), have in the past tended to have a poor prognosis with rapid demise (as opposed to most patients with small-cell lymphomas, who usually live for several years). Although of very different cellular origins, and including both B- and T-cell lymphomas, the large-cell lymphomas are, therefore, often lumped into a category frequently used by clinicians for purposes of deciding therapy, namely, 'diffuse aggressive lymphomas'. In more recent years, with the development of effective chemotherapy regimens, it has become clear that at least a fraction of the lymphomas that fall into this group are curable (generally not the case with small-cell lymphomas) when treated with appropriate combination chemotherapy regimens. The frequent inclusion of *small* noncleaved cell lymphomas with the diffuse aggressive lymphomas is explained by the perhaps inappropriate characterization of this lymphoma type as a 'small'-cell tumor, since the nuclei of these cells are significantly larger than those of mature lymphocytes. This tumor is the most rapidly progressive of all lymphomas. However, because of their rather poor responsiveness to the regimens used for the diffuse aggressive lymphomas, many investigators now exclude both small noncleaved cell lymphomas and lymphoblastic lymphomas from this clinical catogory for treatment purposes.

Morphological correlates of lineage

Large- and small-cell lymphomas encompass neoplasms of both T- and B-lineages, and some morphological features appear to be 'lineage specific', although there are numerous exceptions to this and determining lineage on the basis of morphology alone is hazardous. T-cell lymphomas, for example, may have convoluted – even cerebriform (as in the cutaneous T-cell lymphomas) – nuclear morphology, which is not observed in B-cell lymphomas. B-cell lymphomas may take on a 'plasmacytoid' appearance, with an eccentric nucleus and a lower nucleus to cytoplasm ratio, when significant quantities of immunoglobulin are synthesized, although this may apply to both large- and small-cell lymphomas. Follicular lymphomas, in which the neoplastic cells form aggregates that resemble normal germinal follicles, are always of B-cell origin, since they are the neoplastic counterpart of germinal center cells. Similarly, other B-cell lymphomas, such as mantle cell and marginal zone lymphomas, are characterized morphologically by expansions of the corresponding regions of lymph nodes or spleen.

Cleaved and noncleaved cells

Lennert and colleagues, and Lukes and Collins, in particular, carefully studied the cells of normal germinal centers and attempted to equate their morphological appearances with those of lymphoma cells. Lukes and Collins observed that some stages of activated B-cells have cleft nuclei (hence the terms cleaved and noncleaved), and categorized lymphomas of germinal center origin according to the predominant cell size, whether they had cleaved nuclei or not, and whether the architecture was follicular or diffuse. It is not clear that clefts in the nuclei of large-cell lymphomas have clinical or biological significance. Small noncleaved cell lymphoma and small cleaved cell lymphoma, however, are very different entities. Small noncleaved cell lymphomas, for example, are never follicular and, if untreated, have uniformly aggressive clinical behavior. In contrast, the histological category of small cleaved cell lymphomas includes several different entities, including mantle cell lymphomas (centrocytic lymphomas in the Kiel classification) and follicular lymphomas (centroblastic–centrocytic in the Kiel classification). The latter may be quite indolent, although mantle zone lymphomas, particularly the blastic variant, tend to have a significantly worse prognosis.

Histological classification systems

The major histological classification schemes and their evolution are provided elsewhere in this book.

THE CONCEPT OF 'GRADE'

For more than a century, it has been observed that some patients with lymphoma have a short survival while others have a longer survival. Follicular lymphomas, first recognized in the late 1920s (perhaps partly related to an increasing incidence of these neoplasms), were initially considered to be examples of 'hyperplasia' rather than true neoplasms because of their relatively indolent course – even with the limited therapies then available (surgery and kilovolt radiation) such patients generally survived for several years. Thus, the concept of indolent and malignant lymphomas developed – recognized, for example, by Robb Smith in his division of lymphoid neoplasia (diseases of the reticuloendothelial system) into the *reticuloses* and *reticulum cell sarcoma*, and by the nodular and diffuse categories of Rappaport's classification system. This notion has, more recently, been expressed as lymphoma grade, i.e., low and high grade, whereby histologically defined lymphomas of greater or lesser degrees of clinical aggressiveness have been grouped together. Thus a 'grade' has become equivalent to a prognostic group and as such, has governed, to a considerable extent, the type of treatment that will be administered.

In the Kiel classification, two grades are specified, while in the Working Formulation there are three grades – low, intermediate and high. In essence, the Working Formulation intermediate- and high-grade categories together make up the high-grade category of the Kiel classification. While these terms are useful in that they provide an indication of the anticipated clinical behavior, it may not be appropriate to use them as treatment groupings, i.e., to use the same treatment approach for all lymphomas in a given grade. During periods in which treatment approaches have been limited and long-term survivors few, this tendency has had little consequence. Today, as more refined diagnostic methods are demonstrating the heterogeneity of many histological categories and when dramatic improvements in survival have been demonstrated in at least some subgroups by gradual improvement of combination chemotherapy regimens (particularly childhood lymphomas), the tendency of clinicians to rely, to a large extent, upon the composite groupings that make up different grades as a guide to treatment may prove to be deleterious, since it is entirely possible that different treatment protocols may be required for different pathological entities. This is exemplified by the Working Formulation high-grade lymphomas. Perhaps not surprisingly, the 5-year survival rate of immunoblastic lymphoma (a high-grade lymphoma) in the National Cancer Institute (NCI) study (32%) was similar to that of large-cell intermediate-grade lymphomas (35%), from which (it was recently decided), it cannot be reproducibly distinguished [11]. Survival rates for small noncleaved cell lymphomas and lymphoblastic lymphomas (the other high-grade lymphomas) were 26% and 23%, respectively. These 1982 survival rates in patients with 'high-grade' lymphomas who did not receive uniform treatment are much worse than those obtained today, particularly in children, in whom the prognosis is now excellent – 70–90% cure rates have been reported by several groups of investigators, although lymphoblastic and small noncleaved cell lymphomas are usually treated differently. In contrast, there has been no definite improvement in the treatment of intermediate-grade lymphomas, which now, therefore, have a worse prognosis than high-grade lymphomas. Low-grade lymphomas remain essentially incurable.

The grading of T-cell lymphomas poses particular problems since some 80% of non-Hodgkin's lymphomas in the USA and Europe are of B-cell origin, and classification schemes have been directed primarily towards the B-cell lymphomas. The T-cell lymphomas, with their markedly varied cytology (adult T-cell leukemia/lymphoma, for example, encompasses the morphological appearances of four of the categories in the Working Formulation, in both intermediate and high grades) defy simple correlation of cyotomorphology with clinical behavior. Probably because of the nature of the T-cell arm of the immune system, the pattern of organ or tissue involvement in T-cell lymphomas often provides a better means of predicting clinical behavior than the cytomorphology of the cells (e.g., nasal lymphomas, cutaneous lymphomas, intestinal T-cell lymphomas, etc.).

Because of the uncertain and temporally variable correlation of histology with treatment outcome (in part, because of the crucial importance of the treatment itself), the REAL classification does not assign subsets of lymphomas to a different grade, but instead uses the term 'grade' in the context of the follicular lymphomas to indicate variations in histology (i.e., increasing grade, from 1 to 3, indicates increasing proportions of large cells). However, it cannot be denied that there are more and less clinically aggressive lymphomas, and the concept of broad divisions of lymphomas should not, perhaps, be perfunctorily discarded. An alternative would be to group lymphomas into categories on the basis of the functional consequence of the causal genetic abnormalities (e.g., protection against apoptosis versus inappropriate expression of genes involved in cell proliferation), subdivided according to the presence or absence of secondary genetic lesions, e.g., p53 mutations. This would have the advantage of directing more attention to the genetic lesions, which may, after all, be relevant to the treatment approach which is adopted and are likely to become increasingly so. This is discussed further below. In the meantime, for convenience, the terms low, intermediate and high grade will be used in the Working Formulation sense throughout the remainder of this chapter.

IMMUNOPHENOTYPE IN LYMPHOMA CLASSIFICATION

The recognition of the two major lineages of the immune system, B- and T-lymphocytes, provided the first possibility of moving beyond histopathology as a means of classifying lymphomas, and, of course, the development of ever-increasing numbers of monoclonal antibodies provided a powerful tool for further subdividing lymphocyte lineages and, hence, lymphoma categories. This is exemplified by the heterogeneity of several of the Working Formulation categories, even when simply characterized as B- or T-cell lymphomas (Table 1.2). While immunophenotyping is unlikely to replace histology as a diagnostic tool, because there is considerable immunophenotypic overlap among different lymphoma subtypes, it can often provide assistance in differentiating between subtypes of lymphoma. Not only are B- and T-cell lineage lymphomas usually clearly differentiated but within these categories subtypes can often be readily distinguished, while neoplasms of precursor cells are readily separable from lymphomas of more mature lymphoid cells. Immature lymphoid cells and their neoplastic counterparts, for example, express terminal deoxynucleotidyl transferase (TdT) in both B- and T-cell lineages, but this enzyme, an important element of the generation of antigen receptor diversity, is never associated with mature neoplasms. CD10, also known as the common acute lymphoblastic leukemia antigen, however, is expressed not only by immature lymphoid neoplasms (e.g., a majority of precursor B-cell acute lymphoblastic leukemias and a minority of precursor T-cell acute lymphoblastic leukemias), but also by Burkitt's lymphoma, by follicular lymphomas and by some large-cell lymphomas. This is because this antigen is expressed both on lymphocyte precursors and on germinal center cells. Among the small-cell B-cell lymphomas, immunophenotyping can be particularly useful (Table 1.3), a 'pivotal' antigen being CD5, which probably identifies a subset of virgin B-cells that express antibodies capable of reacting at low affinity with multiple epitopes – in some senses, a precursor antibody that can be mutated to react to a single epitope with high affinity. CD5 is expressed by small lymphocytic lymphoma cell (chronic lymphocytic leukemia) and mantle cell lymphomas, but not by marginal zone lymphomas or follicular lymphomas. Among CD5-positive lymphomas, mantle cell lymphomas do not express CD23, whereas small-cell lymphocytic lymphoma does. Among the T-cell lymphomas, CD30 expression is expressed by most anaplastic large-cell lymphomas, although this category does not appear to be completely homogeneous.

Immunophenotyping has, historically, been associated with the detection of 'marker' antigens, i.e., proteins of unknown function (usually), that have been empirically associated with lymphocyte subsets. The function of many of these antigens has now been identified (e.g., CD3, CD30), leading to a much improved understanding of their cell type specificity (or lack of it). Some important proteins, however, have been identified because of the analysis of the molecular lesions associated with lymphoid neoplasms and the cellular patterns of expression identified in

Table 1.2 Classification of Working Formulation categories into B- and T-lineage lymphomas*

	B-Lineage (%)	T-Lineage (%)
Low-grade and follicular large-cell (categories A–D)	100	0
Diffuse, small cleaved cell (E)	92	8
Diffuse, mixed small and large cell (F)	36	64
Diffuse, large cell (G	94	6
Large cell, immunoblastic (H)	73	27
Lymphoblastic (I)	17	83
Small noncleaved cell (J)	100	0
Total	88	12

*Data from 1160 cases in the Nebraska Lymphoma Study Group Registry [12a].

Table 1.3   Immunophenotypes of low-grade B-cell lymphomas*

Lymphoma	Immunophenotype				
Small lymphocytic	SIgM/IgD	CD5+	CD10–	CD23+	CD43+
Mantle cell	SIgM/IgD	CD5+	CD10±	CD23–	CD43+
Marginal zone (MALT, monocytoid)	SIgM	CD5–	CD10–	CD23±	CD43±
Follicular	SIgM/G	CD5–	CD10+	CD23±	CD43–

*All four subtypes express B-cell antigens such as CD19, CD20, CD79a.

the process of attempting to understand the function of the protein. Examples of this kind include Bcl-2 and Bcl-6. Thus, antibodies to such proteins have entered the immunophenotyping repertoire and recognition of their expression may be of particular importance because of their relevance to pathogenesis. Bcl-2, for example, is expressed by follicular lymphomas and mantle cell lymphomas as well as the large-cell lymphoma variants which arise from them, but not by MALT lymphomas, marginal zone lymphomas or the vast majority of small noncleaved cell lymphomas. Approximately 30% of large B-cell lymphomas have 14;18 translocations and express Bcl-2, and an even higher percentage have *bcl*-6 rearrangements and express Bcl-6.

CYTOGENETICS AND MOLECULAR GENETICS IN LYMPHOMA CLASSIFICATION

In recent years, the identification of cytogenetic and subsequently molecular abnormalities that are characteristic of specific cytomorphological entities (Table 1.4) has led to a quantum leap in the understanding of the pathogenesis of these diseases, but also to a dilemma – cytomorphology and cytogenetics (or molecular genetic changes) are not always congruent. Perhaps this indicates that the histological limits of some pathological entities are artificially drawn, a point that may be crucial if progress is to

be made in the development of optimal treatment approaches for these diseases. For example, most follicular lymphomas contain a 14;18 translocation, regardless of whether they have small cleaved cell, mixed small- and large-cell, or large-cell morphology. These histological categories, which also have very similar clinical behavior patterns, probably do not, therefore, reflect different diseases (although they may reflect different degrees of aggressiveness of the same disease). In addition, some diffuse large B-cell lymphomas contain 14;18 translocations, strongly suggesting that they are closely related to follicular lymphomas. It seems highly probable that some large-cell lymphomas that present *de novo*, are in fact transformed follicular lymphomas (which, in general, have a very poor prognosis with current combination chemotherapy regimens). Other diffuse large B-cell lymphomas, however, may contain 8;14 translocations or translocations involving 3q27. The former are probably closely related to small non-cleaved cell lymphomas, the latter more to follicular lymphomas, since the protein encoded by the gene on band 3q27, which is deregulated by fusion with a variety of heterologous promoters from other chromosomes, is expressed in germinal follicle cells. Thus, the grouping of all diffuse large-cell lymphomas together for treatment purposes may not be appropriate, as is suggested by several recent series that indicate differences in prognosis among these molecular subtypes [13,14]. Treatment approaches could undergo a minor revolution if, instead of

Table 1.4   Association of various non-Hodgkin's lymphomas with specific cytogenetic abnormalities

Lymphoma	Chromosomal abnormality	Relevant gene(s)
Small lymphocytic (B-cell)	Trisomy 12	Unknown
Small lymphocytic (T-cell)	Inversion 14	TCRα, IgH
Mantle cell	t(11;14)	Cyclin D1
Follicular	t(14;18)	*bcl*-2
Small noncleaved cell	t(8;14), t(8;22), t(2;8)	c-*myc*
Large B-cell	t(14;18), t(8;14), t(3;14)*	*bcl*-2, c-*myc*, *bcl*-6
Anaplastic large cell	t(2;5)	*alk*

*Many partner chromosomes have been associated with translocations involving q27 of chromosome 3.

lumping together a group of mixed small- and large-cell, and large B-cell lymphomas into the category of 'diffuse aggressive lymphomas' (Table 1.5), separate treatment approaches were developed for histologically immunophenotypically different diseases, or for histologically immunophenotypically similar diseases with different genetic lesions. Already, the recognition of the heterogeneity of the Working Formulation entities ought to have led to a refinement of the composition of this category. This could, of course, result in an apparent improvement in results with the same (or equivalent) therapy, such that the spectrum of diseases in clinical trials will need to be much more carefully scrutinized in future.

While genetic studies may permit the recognition of the heterogeneity of histological categories, they may also lead to the identification or confirmation of the existence of an entity that is morphologically heterogeneous, and thus difficult to define by histology alone. A good example of this kind is mantle cell lymphoma. Here, the identification of the 11;14 translocation has been instrumental in leading to general acceptance of an entity imperfectly defined on histological grounds (as centrocytic lymphoma or lymphocytic lymphoma of intermediate differentiation). In addition, the presence of this translocation in tumors that would not be classified by most pathologists as mantle cell lymphoma (e.g., in some small lymphocytic lymphomas) strongly suggests that such tumors are in fact mantle cell lymphomas. Routine detection of the 11;14 translocation (by

cyclin D_1 histochemistry) could, therefore, lead to much more precise definition of this entity, thus aiding the interpretation of treatment results.

As understanding of the molecular consequences of the nonrandom cytogenetic abnormalities present in lymphomas cells increases, we shall be confronted more and more with an issue that has been present throughout the history of lymphoma classification – what are the defining characteristics of individual diseases? While in an earlier era the debate centered on the relative importance of clinical versus histological or cytological features, today immunophenotype and genetic lesions have been added to this list. Perhaps no one of these perspectives will prove to be sufficient, although it must surely be true that a catalogue of all relevant molecular lesions and their functional consequences in a given tumor would provide the most complete description possible. Since the major molecular abnormalities have yet to be identified or understood in a number of presumptive pathobiological entities, and detailed molecular analysis has not yet become an element of routine diagnosis in most pathology departments, we are far from a complete description of this kind for any tumor, although in many cases a great deal of detailed information exists. Nonetheless, there can be no question that the identification of molecular abnormalities will play an integral role in the refinement of our ideas as to the definition of disease entities, or perhaps the spectrum of manifestations of a given disease, and that information of this kind

Table 1.5 Pathobiological heterogeneity of diffuse aggressive lymphomas

Working Formulation category	Presently recognized entities that may fall within the WF category*
Diffuse, mixed small and large cell	Lymphoplasmacytoid lymphoma Mantle cell lymphoma MALT lymphoma Marginal zone B-cell lymphoma Peripheral T-cell lymphomas
Diffuse large-cell lymphoma	Diffuse, large B-cell lymphoma Primary mediastinal B-cell lymphoma Burkitt-like lymphoma
Immunoblastic lymphoma	Diffuse, large B-cell lymphoma Primary mediastinal B-cell lymphoma Burkitt-like lymphoma
Small noncleaved cell lymphoma	Burkitt's lymphoma Burkitt-like lymphoma
Lymphoblastic lymphoma	Lymphoblastic lymphoma

*Not all lymphomas in each of these categories would have been included – only the subfraction that would have met the histological criteria for the Working Formulation catogories, e.g., blastic and paraimmunoblastic (prolymphocytic) variants of mantle cell and lymphoplasmacytoid lymphomas, respectively.

should be continually sought, and utilized in the design and analysis of clinical trials.

Epidemiology and pathogenesis of lymphoid neoplasia

THE INCREASING INCIDENCE OF LYMPHOMA

In almost all countries in the world for which good registry information is available, the average annual incidence rate of the non-Hodgkin's lymphomas has been increasing [15,16]. In the USA, for example, the rate of increase has averaged 3–4% per year since the early 1970s. In 1950, the average annual incidence of non-Hodgkin's lymphoma in the USA was 5.9 per 100 000, whereas in 1989 it was 13.7. This increase has included both sexes, all ages and all ethnic groups, although the largest increase in incidence has been in the elderly, i.e., in individuals aged 75 years or above. In absolute terms, because non-Hodgkin's lymphomas more often present in lymph nodes (30–40%) than in extranodal sites, the increase in incidence has been greatest in nodal disease. However, the greatest relative increase in incidence has been in extranodal lymphomas, and the most rapidly increasing anatomical locations of lymphoma have been the stomach, intestines, skin (50–67% increase since 1973), eye (140%) and primary brain lymphoma (240–250%). Increases have been observed in all histological types of non-Hodgkin's lymphomas, but the largest increases have occurred in diffuse large-cell lymphomas.

While this increased incidence rate is at least partly the result of the increased longevity of the population and improved diagnosis, as well as the acquired immunodeficiency syndrome (AIDS) epidemic with its associated lymphomas, these factors do not appear to be sufficient to account for all of the increased incidence. It seems likely that multiple factors are involved, one of which may well be the increasing exposure of the world's population to a wide variety of chemical compounds (see below). Altered exposure to infectious agents such as human immunodeficiency virus (HIV) and *Helicobacter pylori*, dietary habits and smoking are likely to have made smaller contributions.

ENVIRONMENTAL FACTORS RELEVANT TO PATHOGENESIS

It appears likely that genetic changes, including chromosomal translocations, accumulate in all individuals throughout life. This has clearly been shown in the case of 14;18 translocations, which can even be detected in hyperplastic lymphoid tissue obtained from children, and which are increasingly easily detected, using polymerase chain reaction (PCR) techniques, with advancing age [17]. This is consistent with the observation that chromosomal aberrations detectable in normal lymphocytes increase with age and with exposure to environmental toxins [18], providing an important clue to the observed increase with age in the frequency of 14;18-associated germinal center cell lymphomas. Moreover, since follicular lymphoma has a very low incidence in some world regions (the developing countries and Japan), the examination of the frequency of 14;18 translocations in normal lymphocytes in different populations and geographic regions could provide further important insights into the pathogenesis of lymphoma subtypes associated with it. In Japan, the frequency of 14;18 translocations in normal individuals is similar to that in the USA, suggesting that factors other than the occurrence of the translocation account for the difference in the incidence of follicular lymphomas in these two countries.

The molecular genetic abnormalities present in lymphoid neoplasms arise as a consequence of errors in DNA replication, which, at their naturally low basal rate, may occur stochastically, but which are likely to be increased by specific environmental factors that vary with geography and life style. The latter include infectious diseases – bacterial, viral, protozoal and perhaps parasitic infestations, and chemicals. Perhaps the best documented example of the induction of non-Hodgkin's lymphoma by chemical agents is their occurrence in cancer patients treated with chemotherapy, particularly alkylating agents, a finding that is consistent with the possibility that exposure to chemicals may be relevant to lymphomagenesis in the general population. However, a number of occupations have been associated with an increased risk of developing non-Hodgkin's lymphomas, including farmers, forestry and lumbar workers, applicators of pesticides and fungicides, chemists, printers, and workers in the petrochemical, rubber and plastics industries. There is little doubt that the increased risk associated with these occupations results from repeated exposure to particulate material, such as wood and cotton dusts, and to various chemicals and solvents, including benzene, formaldehyde, creosote, herbicides such as 2,4-D, fungicides, hair dyes, various paint thinners and oils. There is some evidence that a high dietary intake of citrus fruits, and green and yellow vegetables has a protective effect.

Pathogenetic pathways

Environmental factors may be considered in two broad categories, which are not, however, mutually exclusive – (a) 'lymphomagens', which act on the cell genome directly and cause changes that influence cell behavior, e.g., chemicals and viruses, and (b) predisposing factors which increase the risk of the development of a genetic change by altering the numerical proportions of particular cell populations (i.e., causing hyperplasia), either specifically or nonspecifically, and either directly or indirectly, e.g., bacterial and parasitic infections. Hyperplastic cell populations are more likely to develop additional genetic changes that may convert the hyperplasia to malignant neoplasia. In each of these circumstances, increased cell numbers (generated by increased proliferation), increase the chance that a mutation or cytogenetic change (generated during DNA replication) will arise in an individual. Exposure to chemical lymphomagens at the same time is likely to considerably increase this risk.

Chemical agents may act either as antigens, mitogens or as mutagens, and perhaps as all three. There is accumulating evidence, however, that genetic changes do arise from exposure to certain chemicals. For example, there is a temporal association between an increased frequency of inversions of chromosome 7 (occurring between the TCRβ and TCRγ receptors) in peripheral blood lymphocytes and exposure to herbicide in agricultural workers [19]. Other chromosomal abnormalities, some of which are known to be associated with non-Hodgkin's lymphoma, have also been described in workers who apply pesticides and it seems probable that the detected abnormalities simply point to the presence of certain types of genetic instability that may be relevant to lymphomagenesis.

Infectious diseases or parasitic infestations may chronically expose the patient's immune system to antigens (e.g., via the intestinal mucosa) such that there is chronic hyperplasia of one or more lymphocyte subpopulations. In some cases, microorganisms may provide superantigens, which, by binding to parts of antigen receptors other than or in addition to the variable regions, are able to activate greater numbers of lymphocytes than normal antigens. Bacterial infections appear to be involved in the pathogenesis of some mucosa-associated lymphoid neoplasms, e.g., *Helicobacter pylori* in the context of gastric lymphoma. Bacteria also appear to be relevant to the genesis of immunoproliferative small

intestinal disease (IPSID), since antibiotics can cause regression in the early stages. Malaria, and perhaps other infections or infestations, may well increase the likelihood that Burkitt's lymphoma will develop, probably by inducing hyperplasia of B-cell precursors. Molecular evidence (the presence of somatic mutations in their immunoglobulin genes) suggests that follicular lymphomas may arise because of chronic antigenic stimulation, although the nature of the antigens involved is unknown. In the context of T-cell receptors, somatic mutations do not occur, so that this potential indicator of a role for antigen cannot be used in T-lineage lymphomas.

Interaction of environmental agents with the cell genome

A pointer to the molecular mechanisms involved in the generation of genetic changes is provided by examination of the DNA sequences adjacent to chromosomal translocations. These may include sequences that resemble, to a greater or lesser extent, the signal sequences (heptamer–nonamers) at which recombination of antigen receptor genes occur, repetitive DNA sequences that are widely dispersed throughout the genome (e.g., *alu* and *line* sequences), chi-like sequences, that have also been associated with DNA recombination, matrix attachment elements (that may be necessary to genetic recombination) and topoisomerase II sites. The latter enzyme is responsible for permitting DNA loops to pass through each other, a process that entails staggered DNA strand cleavage and religation. Topoisomerase II inhibitors such as the epipodophyllotoxin drugs (which are natural products) appear to increase the likelihood of chromosomal translocation, providing a paradigm for the mechanisms whereby some types of environmental agents may increase the likelihood of translocation [20]. Agents that influence the concentration or activity of recombinases could also increase the risk of translocations or other erroneous recombinational events.

MOLECULAR GENETICS

While the proximate causes of genetic abnormalities are ultimately stochastic, cells of different lineages and levels of differentiation are susceptible, by virtue of the sets of genes that are expressed, to a limited number of genetic changes. This applies both to the likelihood that any given genetic change will occur and also to the likelihood that a genetic change will have a functional consequence. Genetic changes in genes that are not expressed can have no effect unless they lead to aberrant expression. It is because the range of functionally relevant genetic changes is limited by the cell type, and because the genetic changes are also the direct cause of the characteristic clinical behavior of the resultant tumor, that the genetic lesions present in lymphoma cells provide an important aid to classification and diagnosis.

Frequent involvement of antigen receptor genes

A theme of the chromosomal translocations that occur in lymphoid neoplasms is the frequent involvement of antigen receptor genes – the heavy chain immunoglobulin locus on chromosome 14q32, the light chain immunoglobulin loci on chromosomes 2p12 and 22q11, or the T-cell receptor loci on chromosomes 14q11, 7q13 and 7p35 [21]. This suggests that such regions are highly susceptible to the required breakage and inappropriate religation that constitutes a chromosomal translocation, and, further, that enhancer or promoter elements in these loci can influence the expression of oncogenetically relevant genes that are juxtaposed by virtue of the rearrangement. Enhancers are regulatory elements that increase transcription from an adjacent promoter. They are often tissue or even differentiation-stage specific, so that in any given type of malignancy, the genes involved in a translocation are likely to be drawn from a limited pool. It should, perhaps, not be a surprise, therefore, that, in the case of lymphoid cells, the regulatory elements of B- and T-cell antigen receptor genes, which are expressed through most of the life span of the cell, are frequently involved. However, if this is so, there is an additional implication – that the translocation is more likely to have occurred in an immature cell at, or close to, the time when antigen receptor gene rearrangment is occurring. The predominant cell type in the neoplasm, however, is not necessarily the same cell type in which the translocation occurred – further differentiation may occur before the cell reaches a stage at which the accumulated genetic changes are sufficient to render the cell neoplastic.

Deregulation of transcription factors – a characteristic of clinically aggressive lymphomas

Alterations in the expression of transcription factors are among the most frequently observed genetic changes in lymphoid neoplasms. This is, perhaps, not surprising, since transcription factors often influence the expression of multiple target genes relevant to the complex processes of differentiation and proliferation. Hence, the deregulation or inactivation of a single gene could result in altered expression of a range of genes relevant to a particular functional pathway (e.g., cell proliferation). Aberrant expression of transcription factors is usually a consequence of major structural alterations in the genome (generally, chromosomal translocations), whereby a transcription factor is separated from its regulatory elements and brought under the control of other regulatory elements – either enhancers or promoters (Figure 1.4). Sometimes, a translocation may result in the formation of fusion genes, i.e., the promoter region of one gene that is normally expressed in the cell type is fused to the dimerization, DNA binding and transactivating regions of a transcription factor that is not normally expressed in the cell such that the set of genes regulated by the transcription factor are transcribed inappropriately. Alternatively, the transactivating region of one transcription factor is fused to the DNA binding region of another such that the chimeric protein, in effect, transactivates the wrong set of genes (or sometimes inhibits activation of a set of genes). One requirement for a pathogenetic effect is that there must be chromosomal access (a consequence of chromatin structure) to the target genes of the aberrantly expressed transcription factor and the presence of other proteins (e.g., dimerization partners or co-transcription factors) that are required for the function of the aberrantly expressed gene (Figure 1.4). Genetic changes resulting in the aberrant expression of a transcription factor (e.g., c-*myc*, *bcl*-6) are usually associated with rapidly growing lymphomas, since they result in profound alterations of cell proliferation and differentiation. Sometimes, fusion genes cause the aberrant expression of a protein kinase (e.g., *alk* in the 2;5 translocation).

Promiscuous and continent translocation

One conspicuous difference among translocation partners is that some genes (e.g., c-*myc* and *bcl*-2) appear to be involved in translocations with a limited set of genes – in the case of c-*myc*, to antigen receptor genes (of both T- and B-cell lineages). In contrast, some genes, such as *bcl*-6 and *all*-1, participate in a variety of translocations – i.e., involving as many as 20 or 30 different partner chromosomes. The reasons for this are largely speculative but may relate to the timing of the translocation in the context of lymphocyte differentiation, or to the required functional result of the translocation. Some translocations, for unknown reasons but possibly related to chromatin patterns (i.e., the availability of a gene for translocation), may be much more likely to occur at a specific cell stage. If this is the case, the number of possible translocational events that can give rise to the

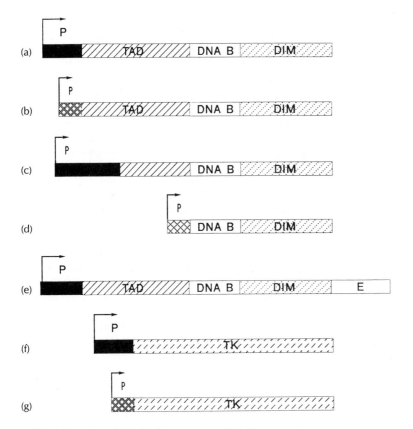

Figure 1.4 Diagrammatic depiction of some of the possible consequences of chromosomal translocations. (a) Normal transcription factor.
(b) Translocation-mediated fusion of a heterologous promoter with the transcription factor, resulting in inappropriate expression and transactivation of target genes.
(c) Translocation-mediated fusion of a heterologous promoter with the transcription factor, resulting in inactivation of the transactivation region and inhibition of expression of target genes (dominant negative effect). (d) Translocation-mediated fusion of a heterologous promoter to a protein which can form a heterodimer with a transcription factor – with a resultant positive or negative effect on transcription.
(e) Translocation-mediated juxtaposition of an enhancer element to a transcription factor resulting in deregulation of its expression. (f) Normal kinase gene.
(g) Translocation-mediated fusion of a heterologous promoter to kinase gene, resulting in inappropriate kinase activity. TAD, transactivation domain; DNA B, DNA binding domain; DIM, dimerization domain; E, enhancer element; TK, tyrosine kinase.

required functional abnormality may be limited, or alternatively, the chance of a particular chromosomal translocation occurring may be greatly increased, e.g., translocations occurring early in ontogeny may be extremely likely to involve antigen receptor genes. As long as the translocation brings about a lymphogenetic functional change, it may simply be the relative likelihood of occurrence that leads to the observation of restricted translocation partners. Thus, it could be argued that translocations that occur in immature lymphoid cells are much more likely to involve the loci of antigen receptor genes than loci on other chromosomes. Perhaps their occurrence in an immature cell is necessary to lymphomagenesis, or, alternatively, the expression of the translocated gene in immature cells is a requirement for the translocation. The translocations involving c-*myc* fall into this category.

In contrast, translocations that occur in more mature cells may be very unlikely to involve antigen receptor genes – perhaps because of suppression of recombinational events at these loci. Perhaps too, the translocation is unlikely to occur in an immature cell because of lack of expression of the relevant gene in

such cells. In such a case, there may be a number of possible partner genes that can bring about the same functional end result. For example, deregulation of expression may simply require fusion of the coding region of the gene to any of a wide range of promoters belonging to other genes – the only provision being that the promoter must belong to a gene that is expressed at the differentiation stage in question. Translocations involving *bcl*-6 – there are as many as 25 – may fall into this category. Sometimes a gene that is involved in translocations associated with diseases of different cell lineages may have different sets of partners in each disease, e.g., the *all*-1 gene on chromosome 11q23 and lymphoid versus myeloid leukemias. This also suggests that the differentiation status may limit the availability of partner genes, but it could also be a consequence of the alternative explanation for the degree of promiscuity observed – that different translocations are associated with subtle distinctions at a functional level (pertaining either to regulatory elements or to the functional domains required in the chimeric protein created by the translocation).

Inhibition of apoptosis – a characteristic of clinically indolent lymphomas

Relatively slowly growing lymphomas, which sometimes give rise to few or no symptoms for many years, are clearly the consequence of a different set of genetic changes from those that result in rapidly proliferating neoplasms. The best studied of these is the 14;18 translocation, which is present in the majority of follicular lymphomas. This translocation results in the persistent expression of high levels of Bcl-2, a protein that inhibits programmed cell death or apoptosis. Cells containing such translocations accumulate inappropriately – perhaps only as a consequence of antigen stimulation. Interestingly, most low-grade lymphomas, perhaps most prominently mantle zone lymphomas, express significant levels of Bcl-2 even though they lack 14;18 translocations [22]. Either Bcl-2 is deregulated by another mechanism in these tumors, or the high level of Bcl-2 expression simply reflects the situation in their normal counterpart cells. In either case, the characteristic feature of the low-grade lymphomas appears to be prolongation of life span rather than rapid proliferation.

Avoiding check points – the need for multiple genetic abnormalities

It is generally believed that cells must accumulate multiple genetic abnormalities for transformation to the fully neoplastic phenotype. At one level, this can be considered from the perspective of the need for the simultaneous activation of growth-promoting genes, and inactivation of growth suppressor and apoptosis-inducing genes. At another, multiple genetic defects may be required for complete deregulation of even a single gene (transcription factors, for example, are usually regulated at transcriptional, translational, posttranslational and functional levels). Teleologically, the need for so many levels of regulation can be summed up in the word 'homeostasis'. In the context of the life of cells, this pertains to maintenance of the integrity of the genome during cell division, the orderly and appropriate entry and passage through the cell cycle, and orderly and appropriate differentiation. Further, cell populations, whether in the context of a clone of cells capable of responding to a specific antigen or cells which have a supporting (structural or functional) role, must be maintained within certain limits if the health of the organism is to be preserved. The pathways of cell proliferation and differentiation are thus punctuated by check points for DNA integrity and gene expression.

Such check points in the G_1 and G_2 phases of the cell cycle are predominantly concerned with the integrity of the genome and the appropriateness of cell proliferation, e.g., whether both primary and accessory signals are 'switched' to 'go'. In the presence of DNA damage, for example, p53 is expressed, which in turn induces the expression of the cyclin-dependent kinase (cdk) inhibitor p21 (also known as Waf-1 or Cip-1). p21 inhibits the phosphorylation of the retinoblastoma protein by the cyclin D–cdk4 complex, such that Rb continues to sequester the transcription factor E2F, required for further cell cycle progression. In effect, the DNA damage led to a block to cell cycle progression. This enables the cell to repair the damage or causes it to enter the pathway leading to programmed cell death. Similarly, cells that express high levels of c-*myc* in the absence of growth factors also undergo apoptosis.

Check points related to B-cell differentiation exist both in primary and secondary differentiation pathways – lack of a functional immunoglobulin gene will lead to attempts to create one by further recombinational events, or to apoptosis; cells responding to antigen will undergo apoptosis in the germinal follicle if they cannot compete effectively for antigen and thus be further activated via surface immunoglobulin (antigen receptor). Similar check points exist in the context of T-cells.

Neoplastic cells, which are neither responding normally to growth signals nor differentiating normally and which, by virtue of genomic instability or the effects of therapy, frequently contain damaged DNA, would presumably be recognized as abnormal at multiple check points and diverted to apoptotic pathways. Thus, the neoplastic state is only achieved by avoidance of check point controls while tumor progression is associated with additional mechanisms for the circumvention of check points, e.g., p53 mutation. Clearly, deregulation of a single growth-promoting gene would be quite insufficient to lead to neoplasia and it is likely, also, that expression of effective levels of anti-apoptotic genes such as *bcl-2* may be insufficient to permit survival of neoplastic cells. Certainly, Bcl-2 expression alone, without some form of proliferative drive, would not lead to cell accumulation. Whether Bcl-2 deregulation as a single genetic lesion, in conjunction with a normal antigen stimulus, might account for some indolent follicular lymphomas remains unknown at this time, although the progression of follicular lymphomas is associated with the accumulation of additional genetic defects.

Viruses and lymphomagenesis

Viruses may predispose to lymphoma development in a variety of ways. They may, theoretically, act as a chronic antigenic stimulus, although this mechanism has not been demonstrated. They may also have a suppressive effect on the immune system (e.g., EBV, HIV) such that there are alterations in the absolute numbers and proportions of various subpopulations of lymphoid cells (decreases in some, consequent increases in others). Either effect is likely to increase the risk that genetic changes will occur in the expanded cell population. Alternatively, viruses may more directly affect the proliferative capacity of lymphoid cells by effecting (through expression of their own genes) the expression or function of cellular genes. EBV, for example, can transform B-cells and render them immortal *in vitro*, and could result in expansion of B- (or T-cell) subpopulations, while HTLV-1 has a similar capability in the context of T-cells. This effect of viral genes is the equivalent of genetic damage but, like other genetic changes, is presumably insufficient, in the absence of other genetic changes, to cause malignant transformation. The ability of viruses to assist cells avoid check point controls is also evident – some DNA viruses (none known to be associated with human lymphoid neoplasia) such as adenovirus, SV40 and papilloma viruses inhibit the ability of the retinoblastoma protein and p53 to cause G_1 arrest, while EBV can inhibit apoptosis – it contains both a homologue of *bcl*-2, BHRF-1 and can also, in some circumstances, via the mediating effect of one of its latent genes, *LMP*-1, increase Bcl-2 expression.

A feature that appears to influence the oncogenic potential of both EBV and HTLV-1 is the age of infection. In both cases, infection early in childhood appears to increase the risk of lymphoma development greatly.

FAMILIAL LYMPHOMAS

The risk of developing a hematopoietic malignancy is only slightly increased (odds ratio approximately two) among the siblings of patients with a leukemia or lymphoma [23]. Whether this increased risk is inherited or indicates exposure to similar environmental factors is unknown. However, there is evidence for an inherited predisposition to lymphoid neoplasia. In families with the Li Fraumeni syndrome (who have an inherited predisposition to certain cancers including adrenocortical cancer, breast cancer and sarcomas), there is an increased incidence of leukemias and, to some extent, lymphomas. Some of these families have inherited mutations in the p53 gene. There is also a markedly increased incidence of Hodgkin's disease (approximately 100 times greater than expected) among the monozygotic twins of young patients (less than 50 years) with Hodgkin's disease in the USA [24]. The lack of a similar increased incidence of Hodgkin's disease among the dizygotic twins of patients with Hodgkin's disease and the lack of an increased incidence of other cancers (two-fold greater at most)

clearly indicates that genetic factors, at least in part, are responsible for increased susceptibility to Hodgkin's disease in young people. However, the explanation for the observed susceptibility is unknown and may include a role for environmental factors.

AGE-RELATED DIFFERENCES IN THE PATTERN OF LYMPHOID NEOPLASIA

The non-Hodgkin's lymphomas increase in incidence throughout life. In children less than the age of 15, the average annual incidence rate in the period 1989–1990 was 0.8 per 100 000 in the USA. In individuals less than age 65, the average annual incidence rate was 8.5 per 100 000 in the period 1987–1991, while in persons over the age of 65 it was 68.8 per 100 000 – eight-fold higher [25]. The increasing incidence of the non-Hodgkin's lymphomas with age parallels the increasing incidence of cancer in general and is probably best explained by a combination of exposure to environmental agents – the longer the duration of exposure, the more likely the risk of developing a malignant disease – and age-related alterations in the immune system. It seems probable that the increase in chromosomal abnormalities that has been associated with increasing age is also a result of environmental factors and it is likely that the gradual accumulation of genetic defects in lymphoid cells or their precursors is the proximate cause for the increasing incidence of cancer with age, although only a tiny proportion of such defects is likely to be relevant to the development of lymphoid neoplasia.

Age is not only relevant to the incidence rate of the non-Hodgkin's lymphomas but also influences the pattern, i.e., the relative incidence of various subtypes of lymphoid neoplasia. This (and perhaps also, in part, the incidence of lymphomas at different ages) probably relates to age-related differences in the immune system. The lymphoid system may be thought of as undergoing three major stages of development: differentiation in the fetus; postnatal maturation to the level of the adult immunological repertoire; and, finally, gradual involution. These stages are characterized by differences in the size of various lymphocyte compartments, most obviously demonstrated by the size of the thymus in childhood compared to adults. At each of these stages, differentiated progeny are produced from precursor cells, although there are differences with respect to the cell population in which the major imunological reserve resides. For example, children recovering from acquired immunosuppression can often rapidly regenerate a T-cell repertoire from thymocytes, whereas in adults regeneration appears to take place predominantly from peripheral T-cells [26]. In addi-

Chronic inflammatory diseases

Sjögrens disease and Hashimoto's thyroiditis are associated with a markedly increased risk (40–60-fold) for the development of lymphomas, while lymphomas that arise in MALT are believed to result from chronic antigenic stimulation or lymphoid hyperplasia induced by bacterial infection. The problems in differentiating chronic inflammatory processes from lymphomas has already been discussed in the context of the midline granuloma syndrome, but in tissues or organs associated with specific inflammatory processes, there may be particular difficulty (for example, Hashimoto's thyroiditis and myoepithelial sialoadenitis may be difficult to distinguish from low-grade marginal zone lymphoma, which is not infrequently superimposed on these conditions).

Inherited and acquired immunodeficiency

A well-known underlying cause for an increased risk of lymphoma development is the presence of an inherited or acquired immunodeficiency syndrome. This is presumably a consequence of altered regulation of the size and proliferative pool of various lymphoid subpopulations, and there is no doubt that impaired immunological contol of EBV-infected B-lymphocytes is an important element in the development of lymphoproliferative processes in such patients. In some inherited diseases associated with a predisposition to the development of lymphomas, however, such as Bloom's syndrome, the underlying inherited abnormality is increased chromosome fragility or defective DNA repair. Such abnormalities may well predispose to the genetic changes associated with lymphomagenesis. In this context, the increased proportion of circulating lymphocytes with inappropriately rearranged T-cell receptor genes in ataxia telangiectasia is likely to be linked to the increased risk of lymphomagenesis in this disease.

There is some evidence that the nature of the immunodeficiency may be relevant to the pathogenesis of lymphomas arising in the immunocompromised host. Thus, in HIV-infected individuals, small noncleaved lymphomas are more likely to arise early in the disease, when the immune system is relatively intact, while large-cell lymphomas (more often associated with EBV in this context than are the small noncleaved cell lymphomas associated with HIV infection) are more likely to occur in the later stages of the disease when there is profound immunosuppression. Small noncleaved cell lymphomas also have their highest incidence in young patients with HIV infection – just as they do in the

normal population. Thus, HIV infection seems to predispose to small noncleaved cell lymphomas but may introduce a new pathogenetic process for large-cell lymphomas. In contrast, the incidence of central nervous system (CNS) lymphomas, which are invariably associated with EBV in HIV-infected individuals, is similar at all ages [30].

Interestingly, the types of progressive B-cell polyclonal lymphoproliferative syndromes common in allograft recipients appear to be less common in patients with HIV infection. In severe combined immunodeficiency (SCID) mice, the outgrowth of EBV-containing lymphoproliferations requires the presence of T-cells – presumably CD4-positive cells [31]. It is possible that the disturbances of CD4 populations in HIV-infected individuals accounts for the relative paucity of this particular type of lymphoproliferation – those that do arise may have already undergone genetic changes that obviate the need for T-cell help and present as EBV-associated immunoblastic lymphomas.

Secondary lymphomas

Secondary non-Hodgkin's lymphomas, i.e., lymphomas that arise following treatment for another neoplasm (e.g., Hodgkin's disease), sometimes arise as a consequence of the carcinogenic properties of the delivered therapy for the primary condition, but in other cases may represent pathological evolution – as is clearly the case for diffuse lymphoma superimposed on follicular lymphoma (which does not appear to be greatly influenced by therapy) and B-cell lymphoma arising in nodular paragranuloma. Even when the secondary lymphoma does not appear to be related to the first, it remains possible that the patient has an inherited predisposition to the development of lymphoma – one that may only become apparent on exposure to DNA damaging agents.

Clinical characteristics and management of lymphoid neoplasia

PRESENTATION

Patients with lymphoma may present with a wide variety of symptoms, the most common of which are swelling of peripheral lymph nodes or symptoms (pain and/or swelling) relating to a mass (nodal or extranodal) in the abdomen or chest. Since almost any organ or tissue in the body may be infiltrated by lymphoma cells, presentations can be equally protean. Serous effusions, pharyngeal or nasal sinus involvement, facial swellings, testicular swelling, malabsorption, skin nodules, plaques or ulcers, bleeding or infection consequent upon marrow involvement (or, more rarely, bleeding diatheses or immunodeficiency), jaundice and systemic symptoms (owing to cytokine production) including fever, malaise, weight loss, as well as peripheral or cranial neuropathy from direct involvement or compression of nerves, paraplegia or CNS symptomatology may all be manifestations of non-Hodgkin's lymphoma. Occasionally, autoimmune hemolytic anemia or hemophagocytic syndromes (which may include severe systemic symptoms, jaundice, hemolytic anemia and disseminated intravascular coagulopathy), may precede the development of overt lymphoma.

Factors governing anatomical location

Some 60–70% of non-Hodgkin's lymphomas in adults present with disease in lymph nodes, whereas in children, the majority of patients present with extranodal disease. There seems little doubt that the site(s) at which lymphoma cells flourish are a consequence of the expression of surface molecules on the tumor cells (adhesion molecules, homing molecules, growth factor receptors, etc.), and the presence of corresponding ligands or growth factors in the infiltrated tissue. Some evidence in support of a role for homing molecules has been obtained. In B-cell lymphomas, for example, the lack of ICAM-1 (CD54) expression has been associated with bone marrow or peripheral blood involvement [32], while extranodal but not nodal T-cell lymphomas often express N-CAM [33]. CD54 and VCAM-1 are both expressed by follicular dendritic cells in germinal follicles and appear to be necessary for the interaction of centrocytes (through CD11a/CD18 and VLA-4, respectively) with these cells, and may be important to the interaction between centrocytes and follicular dendritic cells in follicular lymphomas. It is possible, however, that the presence of growth factors is equally or even more important – at least in the context of more proliferative tumors – since in some circumstances, their absence may lead to apoptosis as the cell passes through growth or differentiation check points. Thus, the tissue or location at which a lymphoma presents is not necessarily that in which neoplastic transformation occurred but this does sometimes appear to be the case. There seems little doubt, for example, that acute lymphoblastic leukemia arises from bone marrow precursor cells, while lymphoblastic lym-

phoma, which is predominantly of T-cell lineage, frequently arises in the thymus. These locations are conducive to the growth of lymphoid neoplasms that arise there and retain the characteristics of precursor cells. In the case of Burkitt's lymphoma, however, there is evidence that the pathogenetically relevant translocations occur in immature cells – presumably in the bone marrow – but that differentiation into mature B-cells is necessary for full neoplastic transformation. In this case, the site of tumor growth will depend upon the external milieu, which may not include the bone marrow after the cell has undergone further differentiation. Histopathological examination of the jaw, a frequent location in young African children, has clearly demonstrated the association of the lymphoma with the developing molar teeth, and, presumably, with growth factors relevant to tooth eruption. Jaw involvement is much less frequent in older children and adults in whom molar tooth eruption is complete. Similarly, if Burkitt's lymphoma involves the breasts, it does so in pubertal or lactating females, again suggesting that growth factors in the immediate environment favor the proliferation of the lymphoma cells.

To some extent, the surface characteristics of lymphoma cells that are responsible for determining organ and tissue distribution are a function of lymphoma subtype, such that different lymphomas have different characteristic distributions. For example, small noncleaved cell lymphomas and lymphomas associated with small intestinal lymphoproliferative disease (IPSID) both frequently involve small bowel (interestingly, both mantle cell and small noncleaved cell lymphomas in particular frequently involve the ileocecal region and adjacent colon), some T-cell lymphomas occur predominantly in skin, while MALT lymphomas are frequently observed in the stomach (almost all low-grade lymphomas of the stomach are of MALT origin). However, the majority of lymphomas, and quite probably all, may be observed in both nodal and extranodal sites, while within a single lymphoma subtype there is a broad range of tissue and organ locations. It seems likely that the genetic lesions associated with progression permit survival in a wider range of tissue locations.

There is some debate whether lymphomas, which are morphologically similar or identical but which present differently (i.e., nodally versus extranodally), are the same pathogenetic entity. Monocytoid B-cell lymphoma and MALT lymphoma, for example, are very similar morphologically, and both appear to be derived from marginal zone lymphocytes, but the former is nodal and the latter extranodal. The marginal zone is a B-cell region external to the mantle zone of germinal follicles, and occurs in spleen and Peyer's patches. Marginal zone cells are also present in lymph nodes, but here are inter-mingled with mantle cells in the mantle zone. In the REAL classification, MALT lymphomas are classified as a variety of marginal zone lymphomas.

Prognostic significance of organ/tissue involvement

The anatomical location at presentation may have prognostic significance beyond its relationship to lymphoma subtype. For example, in diffuse aggressive lymphomas, the number of extranodal sites has been shown to be of prognostic significance. This may result from secondary genetic changes that lead to the development of a greater degree of autonomy, which is manifested as more widespread disease and associated with greater resistance to chemotherapy. While it is probable that this is generally true, diffuse aggressive lymphomas are generally heterogeneous, and an increased tendency to spread beyond lymph nodes may also indicate primary genetic differences that are not reflected in the morphological appearance. This is supported by the finding that 8;14 translocations (which are associated with a poorer prognosis when treated with many of the more frequently used drug combinations in adults) occur more commonly in extranodal (particularly gastrointestinal) than in nodal large B-cell lymphomas [34].

Widely disseminated disease and a high tumor burden often go together, and usually connote a poor prognosis. This probably reflects, as discussed, genetic aberrations that permit lymphoma cells to flourish in a wider range of tissues but in treated patients may result from poor accessibility of chemo-therapeutic agents (in the case of CNS disease and possibly testicular involvement). Factors that influence the kinetics of lymphoma cell proliferation, including the presence of various growth, or viability-promoting or suppressing factors in the invaded tissue (as long as cognate receptors are present on the lymphoma cells), could influence the response to chemotherapy. Elevated serum levels of IL-6, IL-10 and IL-2 receptor levels have been shown to correlate with a poor prognosis [35–37], but it seems likely that this is because these molecules are produced by the tumor cells, such that, like β_2-microglobulin and lactate dehydrogenase (LDH), they are surrogate markers of total tumor burden.

DIAGNOSIS AND MANAGEMENT

A diagnosis of non-Hogkin's lymphoma cannot be established, at the present time, without the examination of tissue obtained at biopsy. Most frequently an enlarged lymph node or group of lymph nodes, usually in the cervical region, will be the presenting symptom. Failure to determine the cause of pathological lymphadenopathy within 1–4 weeks, depending upon circumstances (rate of growth, site, presence of other symptoms or signs), should lead to biopsy. In the absence of lymphadenopathy, lymphoma may not be initially suspected (although certain presentations relating to a mass are characteristic), in which case hematological and biochemical tests, imaging studies or even exploratory laparotomy may precede biopsy. In the presence of an underlying condition known to predispose to lymphoma, however, such as an immunodeficiency syndrome, or a chronic inflammatory process, the index of suspicion should be high.

In some circumstances, a diagnosis may have to be based solely on the examination of cytological preparations made from aspirated cells from a serous effusion or bone marrow, rarely from examination of a peripheral blood smear. Cytology alone cannot provide information on cytoarchitecture – information that may be crucial to the determination of whether a disease is follicular or diffuse, or that often provides ancillary strongly supportive evidence for a diagnosis, e.g., involvement of the lymph node sinus in anaplastic large-cell lymphoma. Support from immunophenotyping and cytogenetics or molecular studies (clonality, presence of recognized molecular genetic abnormalities), whether or not histological material is also available, may substantially improve the degree of confidence in the diagnosis, or may be crucial to research – e.g., in determining whether the molecular subtype of large-cell lymphomas is of prognostic importance. For this reason, wherever facilities permit, part of the tissue obtained should be studied by those techniques immediately or frozen for future studies.

Medical emergencies

Patients with lymphoid malignancies may present with a wide spectrum of medical emergencies that result from compression or infiltration of an equally wide range of tissues or organs. Among the more common are gastrointestinal obstruction, perforation or bleeding, respiratory impairment from tracheal compression or massive pleural effusions, renal failure from rapid tumor cell turnover with oxy-purine production and/or renal outflow obstruction, paraplegia from epidural cord compression, cranial nerve palsies, hemorrhage and/or infection from bone marrow failure or disseminated intravascular coagulation, or metabolic abnormalities including hypercalcemia and, very rarely, hypoglycemia. While each of these problems may require emergency management, this will usually be combined with or rapidly followed by specific therapy for the non-Hodgkin's lymphoma, since the underlying cause of the emergency must be removed as soon as possible.

Staging and prognostic factors

Staging studies, i.e., studies primarily designed to determine the extent of disease, are important for several related reasons. Firstly, the extent of disease is of prognostic significance and estimates of survival rates can be made when this information is coupled to knowledge of the subtype of lymphoma. Secondly, optimal therapy usually varies with the extent of disease. In a research setting, patients with a poor prognosis with standard treatment approaches can be selected for more experimental therapies. In addition, realistic comparison of the outcome of different treatment approaches requires that patient series can be compared for stage and other prognostic factors.

Perhaps the most important determinant of outcome is the treatment itself. Close behind is the total tumor burden. Clinical staging studies ought, therefore, to provide a shorthand notation of tumor burden. In practice this is only partially the case, since the most commonly used staging system is the Ann Arbor system, originally designed for Hodgkin's disease and not very suitable for the non-Hodgkin's lymphomas. Even newer staging systems tend to be based on the Ann Arbor scheme since this has been in use for a sufficient period of time and is sufficiently widely used to make it 'traditional'. Staging systems devised for childhood non-Hodgkin's lymphomas probably more accurately represent tumor volume but they still have inadequacies – as will any shorthand notation. One difficulty is that staging systems are usually applied to a wide variety of lymphoma subtypes with different patterns of disease presentation, although separate staging systems have been devised for lymphoma involvement of certain organs, for example, for the cutaneous T-cell lymphomas and stomach lymphomas. While disease-specific staging schemes would be more logical – at least for disease entities that can be precisely defined – the introduction of a plethora of staging schemes would be likely to create confusion unless agreed upon at international meetings.

Disadvantages of the Ann Arbor staging system

In Hodgkin's disease, a lymphoma of primarily nodal origin, spread is predominantly via lymphatic vessels, such that nodal groups contiguous with or adjacent to known sites of disease have a high probability of being involved, even if at a sub-microscopic level. Thus, the distance between involved nodes is a crude measure of the tumor burden, and is hence the fulcrum of this staging scheme; stages I and II are divided from stage III according to whether (III) or not (I or II) nodes both above and below the diaphragm are involved. Stage IV indicates patients with a spread of Hodgkin's lymphoma outside the lymph nodes, i.e., diffuse extranodal disease, and, in Hodgkin's disease, usually does correlate with both widespread and bulky disease. However, in the case of non-Hodgkin's lymphomas, which do not primarily spread by lymphatics, patients with a small tumor volume may sometimes have extranodal tumor or widely separated disease sites, while tumor confined to the abdomen or to the chest may be very extensive indeed. Thus, the unmodified Ann Arbor staging scheme cannot be applied to patients with primary extranodal lymphoma (common in particular lymphoma subtypes) and, although it crudely separates patients with limited versus extensive disease, its theoretical disadvantages coupled to its frequent lack of prognostic value suggest that there is a need for the development of a completely new approach to the measurement of tumor burden and other potential prognostic markers in the non-Hodgkin's lymphomas. This has recently been recognized and a broad range of potential prognostic indicators have been examined and combined in staging indexes, which can give a quite accurate assessment of prognosis. However, it should be recognized that many of these factors are simply alternative measures of tumor burden.

To determine the extent of disease, heavy reliance is presently placed, after the clinical examination, on computerized axial tomography. This is supplemented by ultrasound, magnetic resonance imaging and nuclear medicine scans. Examination of the bone marrow and cerebrospinal fluid (CSF) is usually indicated, and, in special circumstances, endoscopic procedures supplemented by biopsy or other radiological studies may be important. Staging laparotomy is not indicated but, when surgery is an element of treatment, an opportunity to examine the extent of local spread directly is presented, and can provide useful prognostic information.

Other clinical prognostic factors and prognostic indexes

Recently, perhaps stimulated by the lack of progress in the treatment of patients with diffuse aggressive lymphomas (prognostic indicators are difficult to identify and of limited value when therapy results in cure of nearly all patients), attempts to divide patients more effectively into different prognostic groups have focused on the identification of clinical parameters that correlate with survival [38]. Such factors, may, of course, vary from one disease to another, depending upon relative sensitivity to chemotherapy, so that all systems that are designed to be applied to all non-Hodgkin's lymphomas, or to broad subgroups such as low-grade or diffuse aggressive lymphomas, are likely to be less than ideal in some situations. It is likely, however, that the concept that total tumor burden is a major determinant of prognosis will hold for all diseases except the most sensitive or most resistant to therapy, such that improved means of determining tumor volume (ranging from improved imaging to the measurement of serum levels of molecules synthesized by tumor cells), if not too complex or expensive, could prove to be of general application.

Prognostic indexes that have been described recently include that of the Groupe d'Études des Lymphomes Agressifs [38] and the International Prognostic Index [39]. Such indexes are based on measurements of a broader range of possible prognostic factors than stage alone, including histology, stage, tumor size, serum LDH and β-microglobulin levels, site, number of extranodal sites, age, performance status, presence of systemic symptoms, etc. followed by statistical analysis to determine their relative influence on outcome when a single treatment approach is used. The most important factors are combined to create a numerical index that is predictive of prognosis with the same or similar treatment. These indexes, in essence, provide improved measures of the total tumor volume and a prediction of the amount of treatment that is likely to be deliverable. The former is based on the extent of the tumor (localized versus advanced), tumor size, the number of extranodal sites involved and the serum LDH level. The latter is an estimate of the ability of the host to tolerate chemotherapy – largely age and performance status. Performance status is often a more subjective measurement than tumor burden, while 'tolerance' to chemotherapy is, to a degree, subjective and a question of what toxicity the oncologist (or the patient!) is willing to accept.

One of the most useful purposes of prognostic indexes is to permit risk-adapted therapeutic approaches (i.e., lower treatment intensity for patients with a good prognosis than for patients with a poor prognosis) and the investigation of newer approaches in patients with a poor prognosis. To date, however, prognostic indexes have not led to significant advances in treatment. As therapeutic results improve, all prognostic factors will cease to be important, but risk assessment may still be valuable (where there is significant toxicity) to stratify patients for more and less intensive therapy. One issue that must be considered is what is an 'accept-

able' cure rate, since this will determine whether more or different therapy should be given to each prognostic group. Of course, even if a treatment approach is highly successful, efforts to lessen its toxicities (immediate or late) are almost always appropriate. At present, the trend in diffuse aggressive lymphomas is to continue to treat patients with a better prognosis with current therapies (e.g., CHOP – cyclophosphamide, Adriamycin, vincristine and prednisone), on which the prognostic indexes were based, and to use novel approaches in patients with a poor prognosis.

Age

A special word is necessary in the context of age. While age has been shown to be an important determinant of outcome in patients with diffuse aggressive lymphomas treated with a standard chemotherapy regimen, it is also widely believed that older patients tolerate therapy less well. Oncologists, therefore, frequently lower drug doses arbitrarily in older patients – a practice that certainly prejudices outcome. There are, of course, other reasons why elderly patients (above 60 years) could have a worse prognosis, including the possibility that the spectrum of lymphoma subtypes (particularly when assessed at a molecular level) may differ. Although comorbidity (e.g., renal, cardiac or hepatic impairment), which increases with age, may alter the handling or increase the impact of toxicities of specific drugs, and while psychological factors may sometimes decrease the willingness of patients to undergo intensive chemotherapy (or their doctors to adminster it), age itself does not necessarily lead to impaired ability to tolerate standard chemotherapy; many elderly patients are able to tolerate the rigors of remission induction in acute myeloid leukemia!

It is entirely possible that additional supportive care, possibly including the use of colony-stimulating factors, the development of an improved antibiotic policy, the development of approaches to minimize toxicity (e.g., cardioprotective agents) or avert fatalities when severe toxicities unexpectedly supervene (e.g., the use of carboxypeptidase in patients who develop renal failure during or immediately after the administration of high-dose methotrexate [40]), coupled to improved psychological support, could lead to a higher fraction of older patients receiving full-dose therapy with a resultant improvement in outcome. At the very least, this issue is worthy of further study.

In contrast to the diffuse aggressive lymphomas, in elderly patients with low-grade lymphomas, in which there appears to be no reasonable chance of cure with present approaches, it may be entirely reasonable to avoid therapy if possible (i.e., to employ a 'watch and wait' approach), or to favor simple chemotherapy regimens or even biological response modifiers.

Risk-adapted therapy

While the concept of risk-adapted therapy based on clinically defined prognostic groups appears logical, it is relatively easy to define a poor-risk group with any given therapy but not an easy task to develop more effective therapy, since poor prognosis *per se* does not provide any information relevant to the improvement of the unsuccessful treatment regimen or to the development of a new approach. The requirement that only poor-risk patients (based on present prognostic indexes) be subjected to more experimental therapy is not unwise, but the value of this approach depends on how experimental or how toxic the therapy is likely to be, and it must be borne in mind that risk factors may differ with newer therapies. It should also be pointed out that the International Non-Hodgkin's Lymphoma Prognostic Factor Index divides patient into four groups, which have predicted 5-year survival rates of 73%, 51%, 43% and 26% (these figures are higher in patients less than 60 years old) [39]. Thus, one could argue that *all* patients currently receive inadequate therapy and that unless the 'experimental' therapy involves a considerable departure from accepted approaches, or a particularly high risk (e.g., the use of bone marrow support following very high dose therapy), clinical trials ought to be inclusive of as many patients as possible. There would then be no need to utilize relatively imprecise prognostic factors in determining patient entry, although these could be used to compare the results of different clinical trials.

It is important to recognize that, since present prognostic categories include multiple pathobiological entities, it is entirely possible that outcome from a new treatment approach would not correlate with the risk categories identified from present clinical trials. Therefore, considerable effort ought to be put into attempting to define individual diseases as accurately as possible (including the use of genetic markers) and it is at least as important to analyze the results of clinical trials by individual pathological entities as it is by clinically defined prognostic groups. Crude immunophenotype (B- versus T-cell lineage) is unlikely to be sufficient to subdivide clinically defined prognostic groups. While there is some evidence that patients with T-cell lymphomas have a worse prognosis with at least some current treatment approaches, the large number of distinct entities that can arise from each lineage indicates that immunophenotype is likely to be of greatest value when used

as one element in the definition of individual disease entities.

Prognostic relevance of biological 'progression' factors

Not all genetic lesions are related to pathogenesis. Some arise late, i.e., they are associated with tumor progression, and often, therefore, with a worse prognosis. This is probably because greater autonomy also implies the ability of tumor cells to bypass check points, perhaps the most important in this context being those in G_1 and G_2 of the cell cycle. In effect, cells with damaged DNA are able to survive instead of being directed into the apoptosis pathway. It has become clear that one reason for the death of cells exposed to radiation or chemotherapy is that the damage conferred upon their DNA induces programmed cell death at these cell cycle check points. If the cell is able to bypass the check points, it will therefore be more resistant to therapy (at least, therapy that damages DNA). In addition, the increased genetic instability of the clone is likely to increase the likelihood that cells bearing genetic changes relevant to other mechanisms of therapy resistance will survive.

One lesion that permits cells to circumvent the G_1 check point is a mutation in p53. *In vitro*, Burkitt's lymphoma cells carrying p53 mutations do not arrest in G_1 or undergo apoptosis following DNA damage, and are, as anticipated, associated with resistance to radiation and many chemotherapeutic drugs (but not spindle active agents) [41,42]. p53 appears to be an important determinant of prognosis in at least some diffuse aggressive lymphomas, including Burkitt's lymphoma, and the measurement of p53 expression by immunohistochemistry, which in this context at least correlates well with the presence of p53 mutations (which elevate p53 levels by stabilizing the protein), could prove to be a valuable means of stratifying patients, in at least some histological categories, for different treatment approaches. The frequent association of p53 mutations with transformed follicular lymphomas may also be relevant to the generally poor prognosis of these tumors.

An alternative mechanism that can be utilized by tumor cells to avoid apoptosis is the expression of Bcl-2. Indeed, the expression of Bcl-2 could well be relevant to the apparent inability of standard chemotherapy to cure follicular and mantle cell lymphomas, and may be an important prognostic determinant in large B-cell lymphomas [43], some of which may arise from clinically apparent low-grade lymphomas, as evidenced by the occasional finding of what appears to be follicular lymphoma in the bone marrow of patients presenting with primary large-cell lymphoma [44]. Such patients appear to be at continuous risk of relapse, like patients with follicular lymphoma *per primam. In vitro*, Bcl-2 has been shown to protect against cell death induced by reactive oxygen ions and to increase toxicity from Ara-C.

Undoubtedly, there are other biochemical attributes or changes relevant to therapeutic effect (e.g., Mdr-1 amplification), which may need to be taken into account when devising appropriate risk-adapted treatment strategies. These attributes, if a high degree of resistance to specific drugs results, may be independent of tumor burden to the extent that the drugs in question represent important elements of the overall treatment regimen. However, in contrast to therapy adapted to clinically identified risk factors, a knowledge of the genetic lesions that may be associated with drug resistance should permit more rational design of therapy. For example, in lymphomas that contain p53 mutations or high levels of Bcl-2, more emphasis may be put on drugs (e.g. mitotic spindle inhibitors) that do not kill cells by inducing DNA damage. Attempts to block the membrane pump, Mdr-1, with various drugs are presently under study. Secondary genetic lesions also provide potential targets for novel therapeutic approaches.

Detection of minimal residual disease

One promising approach, still being evaluated, to predicting relapse is to assay for the presence of small numbers of tumor cells by PCR detection of a clonal marker (i.e., antigen receptor gene rearrangement) or a molecular genetic abnormality (e.g., a chromosomal translocation) in peripheral blood or bone marrow after the induction of remission and subsequently. The ability of PCR to detect 'minimal residual disease' and the value of this may vary from one disease to another even though, in a given sample, the assay can permit the detection of one tumor cell per 10^5 or 10^6 normal cells. For example, it requires involvement of the bone marrow or peripheral blood for practical (sampling) reasons and, in low-grade lymphomas, where cure is not possible, the persistence of disease after clinical remission is assumed. However, increasing ease of detection during remission (quantitative or semi-quantitative PCR is valuable in this context) may indicate disease progression and impending relapse. The persistence of a given genetic abnormality cannot always be assumed to predict for relapse. Translocations involving *bcl*-2, for example, are more easily detected in normal individuals with advancing age and a specific translocation has been detected in patients after 17 years of disease-free survival [45,46]. Similarly, the AML-1/ETO fusion gene that results from 8;21 translocations in acute myeloid leukemia can be detected by PCR after years of complete clinical remission.

PRIMARY TREATMENT MODALITIES

Because of the physiological role of the cells from which they arise, most non-Hodgkin's lymphomas can be considered as disseminated diseases even when they appear to be localized – only a fraction of patients with localized disease can be cured with radiation therapy or surgery, depending upon the site. Thus, the primary approach to therapy should be systemic. However, radiation and, in special circumstances, surgery (e.g., localized gastro-intestinal lymphoma) were once the only treatment modalities that could cure any patients, albeit few in number, such that a tradition of radiation therapy evolved upon which systemic approaches were initially grafted. Surgery may still have a role in the treatment of localized gastrointestinal lymphoma, but this is a controversial area and there is increasing advocacy for a primary chemotherapeutic approach.

Radiation is an important treatment modality in patients with low-grade lymphomas and cutaneous lymphomas, but its value in the intermediate lymphomas is controversial, while in high-grade lymphomas radiation is no longer a component of therapy for most patients. Even in patients with primary CNS lymphoma, very good results have been achieved without the use of radiation therapy, suggesting that the presence of parenchymal brain lymphoma may no longer be an absolute indication, in the intermediate- and high-grade lymphomas, for radiation therapy. Radiation should also be reconsidered as the standard approach in emergency situations such as paraplegia or superior vena caval obstruction. This must be judged with respect to the relative degree of radiosensitivity versus chemosensitivity and the role of radiation therapy in the overall treatment of the disease. In the small noncleaved cell lymphomas, for example, in which radiation therapy is relatively ineffective and chemotherapy highly effective, the balance favors chemotherapy.

The range of subtypes, presentations and responses to various therapeutic modalities is sufficiently variable that the non-Hodgkin's lymphomas cannot be considered as a single entity for therapeutic purposes. While the development of separate treatment approaches for each histological subtype, let alone cytogenetic or molecular subtype, would pose logistic problems in the conduct of clinical trials, it is quite possible that much better results would be obtained if present 'therapeutic groupings' were subdivided and therapeutic approaches separately evolved. At present, although low-grade lymphomas are managed quite differently from intermediate- and high-grade lymphomas, there is a tendency to develop separate treatment approaches for different anatomical sites of disease. This is eminently justifiable for the cutaneous lymphomas and brain lymphomas, but less so for other extranodal lymphomas such as those of gastrointestinal origin.

Present treatment approaches

The most important innovation since the introduction of drug therapy for lymphoid neoplasia has been the use of combination regimens. The identification of successful regimens has, however, of necessity been based on empirical observations. There is still controversy over the importance of dose intensity (dose of drug administered per unit time, e.g., per week), the number of drugs that should be included and the duration of therapy. More drugs are not necessarily better. If relatively inactive agents are included in a regimen, their toxicity may preclude the administration of higher doses of the more effective agents. An additional issue is the degree of toxicity (and risk of dying as a consequence of treatment) that is considered 'acceptable'. This may appropriately vary with the prognosis of the patient, but this also begs the question as to what is meant by a 'good' or 'poor' prognosis. Clearly, multiple factors other than simply the disease the patient has, including age, comorbidity, financial cost, available facilities and expertise, etc., must be taken into consideration when deciding appropriate therapy, particularly in the context of a research protocol.

Today treatment differs according to the lymphoma grade (Working Formulation) and a brief outline of the main approaches for each grade is provided.

Low-grade non-Hodgkin's lymphomas

The current treatment of low-grade lymphomas ranges from nothing at all – so-called watchful waiting – in patients without rapidly progressive or symptomatic tumors, to bone marrow transplantation, following induction of remission by chemotherapy, either for a first or a second time. There is no evidence that waiting until the patient needs symptomatic relief is disadvantageous or that combination therapy has any advantage over single agent chemotherapy (e.g., chlorambucil) in terms of survival, although anthracycline-containing regimens, e.g., CHOP, are associated with a higher response rate. In addition, younger patients may sometimes achieve long remissions, whereas in older patients comorbidity may lead to increased toxicity, so that age must be taken into consideration when deciding

the optimal treatment approach. In addition, total body irradiation or biological therapies, such as α-interferon, used as single agents can induce responses in a significant number of patients. Several recent randomized studies have demonstrated an advantage (in time to progression, and in one trial, in overall survival) to the addition of α-interferon to combination chemotherapy – whether used as part of the remission induction regimen or maintenance [47–49]. More recently, the newer purine analogues, including fludarabine monophosphate, chlorodeoxyadenoside and deoxycorfomycin (pentostatin), have been shown to be useful in the treatment of a variety of low-grade lymphomas.

Transformed low-grade lymphomas occur in 20–60% of patients by 8 years, as a result of the acquisition of new genetic changes, including, in the case of follicular lymphomas, the development of an 8;14 translocation or of a p53 mutation. The additional genetic changes may be responsible for the generally poor prognosis that such patients have when treated with standard regimens used in intermediate-grade lymphomas. Some patients (less than 20%) do, however, achieve long-term survival [50] and it will be important to determine whether prognostic groups can be identified on the basis of the genetic abnormalities present.

Cutaneous T-cell lymphomas

In cutaneous T-cell lymphomas (mycosis fungoides and Sézary syndrome), systemic chemotherapy, at least as adminstered to date, is of limited value. Because the skin may be the only site of disease for long periods of time, local therapy has an important role. Even patients with extensive skin disease can benefit from radiation therapy, e.g., total skin irradiation with electrons. Ultraviolet radiation, usually with photosensitizing agents such as psoralens, can also produce responses, including complete responses, and the local application of nitrogen mustard may provide considerable relief. Combined modality approaches are frequently used when disease is extensive.

Intermediate-grade non-Hodgkin's lymphomas

The development of effective chemotherapy regimens for intermediate-grade lymphomas through empirical clinical trials has been a slow process. In the late 1970s, several combination regimens, including C-MOPP, BACOP and CHOP, were shown to result in the cure of perhaps 30–40% of patients. Today, CHOP has been shown to be as effective as more recently developed regimens (e.g., ProMACE-

CytaBOM, m-BACOD, MACOP-B) (Chapter 42), which were initially thought to be superior to CHOP [51].

There are several possible reasons for the failure of the SWOG/EOG (Southwest Oncology/Eastern Oncology Group) trial to demonstrate the superiority of the third-generation regimens. Firstly, as can be seen from Table 1.6, the incremental increase in intensity of the newer regimens, whether measured as planned dose intensity (i.e., mg/M^2/week) of the presumed major drugs (cyclophosphamide and Adriamycin) or taking into account the addition of other drugs, such as etoposide and bleomycin, is actually quite small. This table also demonstrates that the doses used in any of the regimens designed for adults (first four) are considerably less than those used in protocols designed for childhood B-cell lymphomas (last three). Secondly, a number of histologically and, perhaps more importantly, biologically different adult lymphomas are often lumped together for treatment purposes (Table 1.5) – it is possible that some respond to one treatment regimen and others to another. This does not seem to be the case when histological categories alone are considered but there

is evidence that molecular abnormalities, i.e., rearrangements of the *bcl*-6, *bcl*-2 or c-*myc* genes, correlate with outcome [13,14]. The possible prognostic significance of p53 mutations has already been discussed. It will be important to explore further the relevance of these genetic abnormalities to prognosis, since it may be necessary to develop a different therapeutic regimen for each of these subgroups.

In adults with localized intermediate-grade lymphoma, chemotherapy clearly increases the disease-free survival rate compared to radiation alone but whether radiation adds therapeutic benefit to chemotherapy in these patients has yet to be studied.

High-grade non-Hodgkin's lymphomas

In the high-grade B-cell lymphomas (small non-cleaved cell lymphomas and, in children at least, large B-cell lymphomas) survival rates in the range of 80–90% prolonged disease-free survival have been reported in children with several recent protocols [52–54]. These results have been obtained by increasing both dose intensity and the number of

Table 1.6 Comparison of doses/dose intensity per cycle in various treatment regimens used in lymphomas that are included among the diffuse aggressive lymphomas (intermediate and high grade, predominantly B-cell)

Drug regimen	Dose/dose intensity of CTX	Dose/dose intensity of ADR	Dose/dose intensity of VCR	Dose/dose intensity of MTX	Dose/dose intensity of VP16	Dose/dose intensity of Ara-C	Other drugs
CHOP	750 mg/M^2/ 250 mg/M^2	50 mg/M^2/ 18 mg/M^2	1.4 mg/M^2/ 0.46 mg/M^2	None	None	None	Prednisone
m-BACOD	600 mg/M^2/ 200 mg/M^2	45 mg/M^2/ 15 mg/M^2	1.4 mg/M^2/ 0.46 mg/M^2	200 mg/M^2/ 100 mg/M^2	120 mg/M^2/ 40 mg/M^2	300 mg/M^2/ 100 mg/M^2	Dexamethasone, bleomycin
ProMACE-CytaBOM	650 mg/M^2/ 217 mg/M^2	25 mg/M^2/ 8.3 mg/M^2	1.4 mg/M^2/ 0.46 mg/M^2	120 mg/M^2/ 40 mg/M^2	None	None	Prednisone, bleomycin
MACOP-B	350 mg/M^2/ 125 mg/M^2	50 mg/M^2/ 25 mg/M^2	1.4 mg/M^2/ 0.7 mg/M^2	400 mg/M^2/ 100 mg/M^2	None	None	Prednisone, bleomycin
BFM 86	1000 mg/M^2/ 500 mg/M^2	50 mg/M^2/ 25 mg/M^2	1.5 mg/M^2/ 0.75 mg/M^2	5000 mg/M^2/ 2500 mg/M^2	200 mg/M^2/ 100 mg/M^2	600 mg/M^2/ 200 mg/M^2	Ifosfamide, dexamethasone
SFOP LMB89	1500 mg/M^2/ 500 mg/M^2	60 mg/M^2/ 20 mg/M^2	2 mg/M^2/ 0.63 mg/M^2	8000 mg/M^2/ 2666 mg/M^2	800 mg/M^2/ 266 mg/M^2	9000 mg/M^2/ 3000 mg/M^2	Prednisone
CODOX-M/ IVAC	1600 mg/M^2/ 533 mg/M^2	40 mg/M^2/ 13 mg/M^2	1.4 mg/M^2/ 0.93 mg/M^2	6720 mg/M^2/ 2240 mg/M^2	300 mg/M^2/ 100 mg/M^2	8000 mg/M^2/ 2666 mg/M^2	Ifosfamide

MTX in MACOP-B is given on days 8, 36 and 64.
Dose intensity is expressed as *planned* dose intensity.
Dose intensities in BFM, SFOP and CODOX-M/IVAC are calculated as mg/M^2 per week for cycles in which the drug is included.
Doses for SFOP LMB89 and BFM 86 are given for the highest risk groups.
When a drug is given daily for 2 or more days, the total dose is given.
In some protocols (MACOP-B, LMB89) the maximum dose of vincristine allowed is 2 mg per dose.
BFM 86 uses VM26 (teniposide) rather than VP16 (etoposide). The dose of teniposide is given.
BFM 86, SFOP LMB89 and CODOX-M/IVAC are regimens used for B-cell lymphomas in children. SFOP LMB89 and CODOX-M/IVAC have also been used successfully in adults.

drugs, but the duration of therapy can be as short as 3–4 months in patients with extensive disease and even less in patients with limited disease. It appears that more than four or five drugs (the standard agents being cyclophosphamide, Adriamycin, vincristine and methotrexate, usually with corticosteroid) are necessary to cure the majority of patients with extensive disease (etoposide and ifosfamide are usually added today, at least for patients with extensive disease), and that high-dose S phase agent therapy (methotrexate and Ara-C) also has an important role – both for the control of systemic disease and for the prevention or treatment of CNS disease.

There is evidence that adult patients with small noncleaved cell lymphomas have a similar prognosis to children when treated with the same protocols and it is possible that these drug combinations might prove superior to CHOP in adult patients with other diffuse aggressive lymphomas. In children with localized non-Hodgkin's lymphoma, a randomized clinical trial has demonstrated that radiation adds toxicity to chemotherapy but no measurable therapeutic advantage.

Lymphoblastic lymphomas are still generally treated with long-duration therapy based on or identical to acute lymphoblastic leukemia protocols, but similar results, at least in patients without marrow involvement, have been obtained with regimens based on repeated cycles of cyclophosphamide, Adriamycin, vincristine and prednisone with or without high-dose methotrexate.

Anaplastic large-cell lymphomas may be treated with either of the approaches discussed for other high-grade lymphomas. There would appear, however, to be a practical advantage to the use of short-duration intensive therapy as currently employed for high-grade B-cell lymphomas.

BONE MARROW TRANSPLANTATION AND STEM CELL INFUSIONS

The role of bone marrow transplantation in the treatment of the non-Hodgkin's lymphomas is a subject of much topical interest – perhaps particularly in view of the lack of progress that has been made in the treatment of the adult diffuse aggressive lymphomas in recent years. In general, autologous bone marrow transplantation (ABMT), which in essence permits much higher doses of drugs (and, often, total body irradiation) to be given because potentially fatal myelotoxicity is averted by 'hematopoietic rescue', has been used in two situations – after relapse, or in patients considered to be at particularly high risk for failure of primary therapy. The rationale

for this approach is the steep dose–response curve of lymphomas to chemotherapy and radiation, but the number of drugs in which dose-limiting toxicity is myelopoietic (the only agents for which hematopoietic rescue from toxicity makes sense) is limited. Total body irradiation (TBI) has, in the past, generally been a part of bone marrow transplantation regimens. However, evidence that it adds no therapeutic advantage to some regimens and in others can be replaced by higher doses of alkylating agent, coupled to its late effects (particularly in children), have led to a swing away from its incorporation in current preparative regimens. Although in the non-Hodgkin's lymphomas autologous transplantation has been used much more than allogeneic transplantation, there is evidence that allografting is associated with fewer relapses, presumably because of the ability of donor-derived immunocompetent cells to eliminate tumor cells.

The application of bone marrow transplantation is limited by age – patients over 55 or 60 years are rarely transplanted because of increased toxicity, while allogeneic transplantation is also limited by donor availability – only approximately one in three siblings will be histocompatible, but the possibility of finding a matched or partially matched unrelated donor now exists through national and international donor registries. A theoretical problem with ABMT is that of reinfusing tumor cells present in the autologous marrow. Purging, for example with monoclonal antibodies, should theoretically lessen this risk but there are no clinical data to support an advantage to purging. In general, only patients who have a good response to salvage therapy after relapse (or to primary therapy if transplantation is to be performed in first remission) are considered candidates for transplantation since results in patients with resistant disease are particularly poor. Patients in whom the bone marrow was involved are not usually considered candidates for autologous transplantation.

A relatively recent approach to hematopoietic support is the use of peripheral stem cells, harvested after chemotherapy and administration of a colony-stimulating factor, to permit hematopoietic rescue after a single or repeated cycles of high-dose therapy [55,56]. Peripheral stem cells appear to be at least as effective as and possibly more effective than bone marrow stem cells at replenishing the hematopoietic system after high-dose therapy, and can even be expanded *in vivo* [57]. An approach in which repeated cycles of therapy are given with peripheral stem cell support includes the psychological advantage that it appears to be an extension of conventional therapy rather than a completely different approach. Oncologists may be readier to use the prop of stem cell support while exploring more vigorously the principles of combination therapy, which has led to significant advances in the intermediate, and particularly in the high-grade non-Hodgkin's lymphomas.

Bone marrow transplantation for diffuse aggressive lymphomas

Bone marrow transplantation, whether autologous or allogeneic, has resulted in the cure of a proportion of patients with intermediate-grade lymphomas who have progression of their disease after treatment with conventional chemotherapy. Recently, the long-awaited results of the PARMA randomized study have been reported. The event-free survival rate of patients who do not have CNS or bone marrow involvement at the time of relapse, are less than 55 years old and who have a good response to salvage therapy with the DHAP regimen (dexamethazone, high-dose cytosine arabinoside and cisplatin) was 46% at 5 years (overall survival 53%) after random assignment to ABMT, while the corresponding figure for patients randomized to continue with DHAP was 12% at 5 years (overall survival 32%) [58]. In interpreting these results, it should be borne in mind that they apply only to the patient group selected and to the treatment comparisons made. In addition, the benefit of ABMT in this setting has not translated into a benefit to high-risk patients transplanted in first remission [59]. The reason for this is unclear but may relate to differences in the efficacy of the primary regimens used in these studies, or perhaps DHAP selects only a small subset of patients who still have particularly sensitive tumors.

There is also evidence that ABMT in first remission provides no advantage, compared to CHOP, to slowly responding patients with aggressive non-Hodgkin's lymphomas [60], and may give a worse result than conventional chemotherapy in the small noncleaved cell lymphomas – perhaps because of the limitations of the preparative regimens [61]. These data, overall, suggest that ABMT is not likely to provide a means of markedly improving overall survival in the non-Hodgkin's lymphomas.

Bone marrow transplantation for low-grade lymphomas

Because of the much longer life expectancy of patients with low-grade lymphomas – even though few achieve a true complete response – there has been an appropriate reluctance to subject them to unproven and highly toxic therapy. In addition, ABMT has been inhibited by the high frequency of bone marrow involvement. The latter obstacle has been addressed by the use of purging techniques. Results in patients with relapsed low-grade non-Hodgkin's lymphoma (predominantly follicular lymphoma) are somewhat controversial, largely because the studies were not randomized comparisons. In addition, the median age of these patients is lower than that in unselected series of conventionally treated patients. Some 9 years after the start of the two major studies that have been performed (at the Dana Farber Cancer Institute, Boston, and St Bartholomew's Hospital, London), it can be stated that treatment-related mortality is less than 5%, that the disease-free survival rate is approximately 40% at 5 years and that patients continue to relapse even after this time, as do patients who receive only conventional therapy [62]. Perhaps not surprisingly, the detection of 14;18 translocations by PCR in bone marrow or peripheral blood (positivity in bone marrow was more predictive) after transplant correlated with a worse prognosis in patients in second or greater remission [63,64]. The ability to detect the 14;18 translocation in the purged marrow that was infused (99% of marrows were positive before purging, 55% after) was also of prognostic significance, and these cells (presumptively) could be detected in the peripheral blood within 2 hours of the infusion of bone marrow and, in many patients, for extended periods thereafter [64,65]. Similar contamination of peripheral blood stem cells used to reconstitute patients after intensive therapy has been observed [66]. These findings suggest that reinfusion of lymphoma cells may contribute to recurrence but the possibility that the presence of residual cells in the purged bone marrow simply reflects the residual tumor burden, and that this is the primary determinant of the duration of disease-free survival, cannot be excluded.

ABMT has also been employed as a component of primary therapy in patients in first remission or good partial remission after combination chemotherapy [67,68]. Once again, there is no evidence, to date, that this approach can result in cure, and disease-free survival does not appear to be significantly different from unselected conventionally treated patients – and could prove to be worse than that of patients treated with similar conventional chemotherapy and additional α-interferon [47–49].

FUTURE PROSPECTS FOR LYMPHOMA CONTROL

While there can be little doubt that a more thorough understanding of the nature of the non-Hodgkin's lymphomas, i.e., the genetic changes that result in their disordered growth and differentiation, and that permit abnormal cells to pass the check points on these pathways, will ultimately lead to more effective intervention. This will take many years and the degree of success that will be achieved is uncertain. In the meantime, empirical approaches have resulted in considerable improvement in the outcome of therapy for virtually all the non-Hodgkin's lymphomas, and particularly the childhood lymphomas, where almost all patients (80–90%) can now be cured, even those with very extensive disease involving the bone marrow and CNS. Further refinement and broader application of these results represents an appropriate research direction. The most immediate use to which our ever-increasing knowledge of the genetic abnormalities that lead to lymphoid neoplasia can be put is to improve our ability to separate disease entities, and to examine the relevance of specific genetic abnormalities to prognosis with current therapeutic approaches. Improvements in the results with available chemotherapeutic agents (or new drugs) may be achieved by better adaptation of treatment approaches to risk, and possibly, using genetic information, such as the presence of p53 mutations or *bcl*-2 expression, in the choice of regimens. Improvements may also be achieved by strategies designed to lessen toxicity, e.g., the use of growth factors of various kinds that may lessen the degree or duration of injury to a variety of tissues including the bone marrow, epithelia and nerves.

At the same time as conventional treatment is refined, it will be important to continue to attempt to understand the consequences of the genetic lesions that cause lymphoid neoplasia, and to begin to develop novel treatment approaches targeted to lymphoma cells (and therefore, by definition, less toxic). Two themes are worthy of special mention. The first is the use of molecules such as cytokines known to be relevant to the regulation of the growth and differentiation of normal lymphoid cells. These may be much more likely to be successful in the low-grade lymphomas, which appear to remain subject to some form of regulation by physiological mechanisms. The now clearly demonstrated advantage, at least with respect to freedom from progression, of α-interferon in combination with chemotherapy in the follicular lymphomas is an important step towards the development of even more effective therapies of this type. The second is to attempt to use the pathogenetically relevant molecular abnormalities of lymphoma cells (or resident viral genomes) as targets for therapy – either by using them as 'hooks' and 'switches' for antibody or virus-directed prodrug, toxin or radionuclide treatment, or by developing therapies that will reverse or bypass the biochemical abnormalities that they create. These genetic changes, which are unique to tumor cells or their precursors,

provide, in effect, the tumor-specific markers that have for so long been sought. A variety of approaches can be envisaged, as described in Chapter 51. If these approaches, or their successors, prove to be highly effective, the most important element of lymphoma classification in the future could prove to be the identification of the causal genetic lesions.

Finally, a knowledge of the epidemiology and pathogenesis of lymphomas should permit attempts to prevent lymphomagenesis. This could be important in subpopulations at a very high risk of developing lymphoma, including people living in certain world regions (males in northern Pakistan, children in equatorial Africa), elderly persons, individuals exposed to known lymphomagens such as solvents and agricultural chemicals, individuals with inherited immunological deficiencies or other lymphoma-predisposing syndromes or diseases, and patients undergoing organ or tissue allografting. An important step forward has been recently made in the use of donor leukocytes to prevent or treat EBV-related lymphoproliferative processes in bone marrow allograft recipients [69]. This same technique, or variations on this theme, also has promise as a form of immunotherapy against the underlying malignancy in patients with relapsed tumors. In the context of virus-related lymphomas (EBV or HTLV-1) the possibility of vaccination holds promise as a means of prevention. Viral vaccines of this kind would, of course, provide additional benefits in that they should also prevent all of the diseases related to infection with the virus in question, in the case of EBV, a gradually lengthening list of lymphomas and epithelial tumors (nasopharyngeal carcinoma, stomach cancer and breast cancer), as well as infectious mononucleosis and its rare, but sometimes serious, sequelae.

References

1. Costa J, Delacretaz F. The midline granuloma syndrome. *Pathol. Annu.* 1986, **21**: 159–171.
2. Lipford E, Margolich JB, Longo DL, et al. Angiocentric immunoproliferative lesions: A clinicopathological spectrum of post-thymic T-cell proliferations. *Blood* 1988, **72**: 1674–1681.
3. Guinee D, Kingma D, Fishback N, et al. Pulmonary lesions with features of lymphomatoid granulomatosis/angiocentric immunoproliferative lesion (LYG/AIL); evidence for Epstein–Barr virus within B lympocytes (abstract). *Mod. Pathol.* 1994, **7**: 151.
4. Schlegelberger B, Zhang Y, Weber-Matthiesen K, et al. Detection of aberrant clones in nearly all cases of angioimmunoblastic lymphoadenopathy with dysproteinemia-type of T-cell lymphoma by combined inter-

phase and metaphase cytogenetics. *Blood* 1994, **84**: 2640–2648.

5. Parsonnet J, Hansen S, Rodriguez L, et al. *Helicobacter pylori* infection and gastric lymphoma. *N. Engl. J. Med.* 1994, **330**: 1267–1271.

6. Palleson G, Hamilton-Dutoit SJ, Zhou X. The association of Epstein–Barr virus (EBV) with T-cell lymphoproliferations and Hodgkin's disease: Two new developments in the EBV field. *Adv. Cancer Res.* 1993, **62**: 179–239.

7. Jaffe ES, Zarate-Osorno A, Kingma DW, et al. The interrelationship between Hodgkin's disease and non-Hodgkin's lymphoma. *Ann. Oncol.* 1994, **5** (Suppl. 1): S7–S11.

7a. Kuppers, R, Rajewsky K, Zhao M, et al. Hodgkin disease: Hodgkin and Reed–Sternberg cells picked from histological sections show clonal immunoglobulin gene rearrangements and appear to be derived from B cells at various stages of development. *Proc. Nat. Acad. Sci. USA* 1994, **91**: 10962–10966.

8. National Institute sponsored study of classifiations of non-Hodgkin's lymphomas. Summary and description of a working formulation for clinical usage. *Cancer* 1982, **49**: 2112–2135.

9. Lukes RJ, Collins RD. Immunological characterization of human malignant lymphomas. *Cancer* 1974, **34**: 1488–1503.

10. Stansfeld AG, Diebold J, Noel H, et al. Updated Kiel classification for lymphomas. *Lancet* 1988, **1**: 292–293.

11. Harris NL, Jaffe ES, Stein H, et al. A proposal for an international consensus on the classification of lymphoid neoplasms. *Blood* 1994, **84**: 1361–1392.

12. Zukerberg LR, Medeiros JL, Ferry JA, et al. Diffuse low grade B-cell lymphomas. *Am. J. Clin. Path.* 1993, **1001**: 373–385.

12a. Weisenberger DD. Epidemiology of non-Hodgkin's lymphoma: Recent findings regarding an emerging epidemic. *Ann. Oncol.* 1994, **5**: 519–524.

13. Offit K, Lo Coco F, Louie DC, et al. Rearrangement of the *bcl-6* gene as a prognostic marker in diffuse large-cell lymphoma. *N. Engl. J. Med.* 1994, **331**: 74–78.

14. Bastard C, Deweindt C, Kerckaert JP, et al. LAZ3 rearrangements in non-Hodgkin's lymphoma: Correlation with histology, immunophenotype, karyotype and clinical outcome in 217 patients. *Blood* 1994, **83**: 2423–2427.

15. Weisenburger DD. Epidemiology of non-Hodgkin's lymphoma: Recent findings regarding an emerging epidemic. *Ann. Oncol.* 1994, **5** (Suppl. 1): S19–S24.

16. Devesa SS, Fears T. Non-Hodgkin's lymphoma time trends: United States and international data. *Cancer Res.* 1992, **52**: 5432s–5440s.

17. Liu Y, Hernandez AM, Shibata D, Cortopassi GA. BCL2 translocation frequency rises with age in humans. *Proc. Nat. Acad. Sci. USA* 1994, **91**: 8910–8914.

18. Au WW, Walker DM, Ward JB Jr, et al. Factors contributing to chromosome damage in lymphocytes of cigarette smokers. *Mutat. Res.* 1991, **260**: 137–144.

19. Kirsh IR, Lipkowitz S. A measure of genomic instability and its relevance to lymphomagenesis. *Cancer Res.* 1992, **52**: 5545s–5546s.

20. Felix CA, Hosler MR, Winick NH, et al. ALL-1 gene rearrangements in DNA topoisomerase II inhibitor-related leukemia in children. *Blood* 1995, **85**: 3250–3256.

21. Magrath IT. Molecular basis of lymphomagenesis. *Cancer Res.* 1992, **52**: 5529s–5540s.

22. Pezzella F, Tse A, Cordell J, et al. Expresion of the Bcl-2 oncogene is not specific for the 14;18 chromosomal translocation. *Am. J. Pathol.* 1990, **137**: 225–232.

23. Pottern LM, Linet M, Blair A, et al. Familial cancers associated with sutypes of leukemia and non-Hodgkin's lymphoma. *Leuk. Res.* 1991, **15**: 305–314.

24. Mack TM, Cozen W, Shibata D, et al. Concordance for Hodgkin's disease in identical twins suggesting genetic susceptibility to the young-adult form of the disease. *N. Engl. J. Med.* 1995, **332**: 413–418.

25. National Cancer Institute. *Cancer Statistics Review, 1973–1991.* NIH publication, Bethesda, MD, National Cancer Institute, 1994.

26. Mackall CL, Fleisher TA, Brown M, et al. Age, thymopoiesis and CD4+ lymphocyte regeneration. *N. Engl. J. Med.* 1995, **332**: 143–149.

27. Shih LY, Liang DC. Non Hodgkin's lymphomas in Asia. *Hematol. Oncol. Clins. N. America* 1991, **5**: 983–1001.

28. Ramot B, Magrath IT. Hypothesis: The environment is a major determinant of the immunological sub-type of lymphoma and acute lymphoblastic leukemia in children. *Br. J. Haematol.* 1982, **50**: 183–189.

29. Kamel AM, Ghaleb FM, Assem NM, et al. Phenotypic analysis of T-cell acute lymphoblastic leukemia in Egypt. *Leuk. Res.* 1990, **14**: 601–609.

30. Beral V, Peterman T, Berkelman R, Jaffe H. AIDS associated non-Hodgkin's lymphoma. *Lancet* 1991, **337**: 805–809.

31. Veronese ML, Veronesi A, Bruni L, et al. Properties of tumors arising in SCID mice injected with PMC from EBV positive donors. *Leukemia* 1994. **8**: S214–217.

32. Nozawa Y, Yamaguchi Y, Tominaga K, et al. Expression of leukocyte adhesion molecules (ICAM-1/LFA-1) related to clinical behavior in B-cell lymphomas. *Hematol. Oncol.* 1992, **10**: 189–194.

33. Kern WF, Spier CM, Hanneman EH, et al. Neural cell adhesion molecule positive peripheral T-cell lymphoma: A rare variant with a propensity for unusual sites of involvement. *Blood* 1992, **79**: 2432–2437.

34. Van Krieken JHJM, Raffeld M, Raghoebier S, et al. Molecular genetics and gastrointestinal non-Hodgkin's lymphomas: Unusual prevalence and pattern of c-*myc* rearrangements in aggressive lymphomas. *Blood* 1990, **76**: 797–800.

35. Wagner D, Kiwanuka J, Edwards B, et al. Soluble interleukin-2 receptor levels in patients with undifferentiated and lymphoblastic lymphomas. Correlation with survival. *J. Clin. Oncol.* 1987, **5**: 1262–1274.

36. Blay JY, Burdin N, Rousset F, et al. Serum interleukin-10 in non-Hodgkin's lymphoma: A prognostic factor. *Blood* 1993, **82**: 2169–2174.

37. Kurzrock R, Redman J, Cabanillas F, et al. Serum interleukin-6 levels are elevated in lymphoma patients and correlated with survival in advanced Hodgkin's disease and with B-symptoms. *Cancer Res.* 1993, **53**: 2118–2122.

38. Coiffier B, Gisselbrecht, Vose J, et al. Prognostic factors in aggressive malignant lymphomas: Description and validation of a prognostic index that could identify patients requiring a more intensive therapy. *J. Clin. Oncol.* 1991, **9**: 211–219.

39. The International Non-Hodgkin's Lymphoma Prognostic Factors Index Project. A predictive model for aggressive non-Hodgkin's lympoma. *N. Engl. J. Med.* 1993, **329**: 987–994.

40. Widemann BC, Hetherington ML, Murphy R, et al. Carboxypeptidase-G-2 rescue in a patient with high dose methotrexate-induced nephropathy. *Cancer* 1995, **76**: 521–526.

41. O'Connor PM, Jackman J, Jondle D, et al. Role of the p53 tumor suppressor gene in cell cycle arrest and radiosensitivity of Burkitt's lymphoma cell lines. *Cancer Res.* 1993, **53**: 4776–4780.

42. Fan S, El-Deiry WS, Bae I, et al. p53 gene mutations are associated with decreased sensitivity of human lymphoma cells to DNA damaging agents. *Cancer Res.* 1994, **54**: 5824–5830.

43. Jacobson JO, Wilkes BM, Kwiatkowski DJ, et al. *bcl*-2 rearrangements in de novo diffuse large cell lymphoma: Association with distinctive clinical features. *Cancer* 1993, **72**: 231–236.

44. Robertson LE, Redman JR, Butler JJ, et al. Discordant bone marrow involvement in diffuse large-cell lymphoma: A distinct clinical–pathologic entity associated with a continuous risk of relapse. *J. Clin. Oncol.* 1991, **9**: 236–242.

45. Price CCA, Meerabuz J, Murtagh S, et al. The significance of circulating cells carrying t(14;18) in long remission from follicular lymphoma. *J. Clin. Oncol.* 1991, **9**: 1527–1532.

46. Finke J, Slanina J, Lange W, et al. Persistence of circulating t(14;18) cells in long term remission after radiation therapy for localized-stage follicular lymphoma. *J. Clin. Oncol.* 1993, **11**: 1668–1673.

47. Smalley RV, Andersen JW, Hawkins MJ, et al. Interferon-α combined with cytotoxic chemotherapy for patients with non-Hodgkin's lymphoma. *N. Eng. J. Med.* 1992, **327**: 1336–1341.

48. Solal-Celigny P, Lepage E, Brousse N, et al. Recombinant interferon α-2b combined with a regimen containing doxorubicin in patients with advanced follicular lymphoma. Groupe d'Étude des Lymphomes de l'Adulte. *N. Engl. J. Med.* 1993, **329**: 1608–1614.

49. McLaughlin P. The role of interferon in the therapy of low grade lymphoma. *Leuk. Lymph.* 1993, **10** (Suppl.): 17–20.

50. Yuen AR, Kamel OW, Halpern J, et al. Long term survival after histologic transformation of low-grade follicular lymphoma. *J. Clin. Oncol.* 1995 **13**: 1726–1733.

51. Fisher RI, Gaynor ER, Dahlberg S, et al. Comparison of a standard regimen (CHOP) with three intensive chemotherapy regimens for advanced non-Hodgkin's lymphoma. *N. Engl. J. Med.* 1993, **328**: 1002–1006.

52. Patte C, Philip T, Rodary C, et al. High survival rate in advanced-stage B-cell lymphomas and leukemias without CNS involvement with a short intensive polychemotherapy: Results from the French Pediatric Oncology Society of a randomized trial of 216 children. *J. Clin.*

Oncol. 1991, **9**: 123–132.

53. Reiter A, Schrappe M, Parwaresch R, et al. Non-Hodgkin's lymphomas of childhood and adolescence: Results of a treatment stratified for biologic subtypes and stage – a report of the Berlin–Frankfurt–Münster Group. *J. Clin. Oncol.* 1995, **13**: 359–372.

54. Magrath I, Adde M, Shad A, et al. Adults and children with small noncleaved cell lymphoma have a similar excellent outcome when treated with the same chemotherapy regimen. *J. Clin Oncol.* 1996, **14**: 925–934.

55. Pettengell R, Morgenstern PJ, Woll J, et al. Peripheral blood progenitor cell transplantation in lymphoma and leukemia using a single apheresis. *Blood* 1993, **82**: 3770–3777.

56. Weaver CH, Peterson FB, Appelbaum FR, et al. High dose fractionated total body irradiation, etoposide, and cyclophosphamide followed by autologous stem-cell support in patients with malignant lymphoma. *J. Clin. Oncol.* 1994, **12**: 2559–2566.

57. Brugger W, Mocklin W, Heimfeld S, et al. *Ex vivo* expansion of enriched peripheral blood CD34+ progenitor cells by stem cell factor, interleukin-1β (Il-1β), Il-6, Il-3, interferon-gamma and erythropoietin. *Blood* 1993, **81**: 2579–2584.

58. Philip T, Guglielmi C, Chauvin F, et al. Autologous bone marrow transplantation (ABMT) versus (VS) conventional chemotherapy (DHAP) in relapsed non-Hodgkin lymphoma (NHL): Final analysis of the Parma randomized study (216 patients) [abstract]. *Proc. Am. Soc. Clin. Oncol.* 1995, **14**: 390.

59. Haioun C, Lepage E, Gisselbrecht C, et al. Comparison of autologous bone marrow transplantation with sequential chemotherapy for intermediate-grade and high-grade non-Hodgkin's lymphoma in first complete remission. A study of 464 patients. *J. Clin. Oncol.* 1994, **12**: 2543–2551.

60. Verdonck LF, Van Putten WLJ, Hagenbeek A, et al. Comparison of CHOP chemotherapy with autologous bone marrow transplantation for slowly responding patients with aggressive non-Hodgkin's lymphoma. *N. Engl. J. Med.* 1995, **332**: 1045–1051.

61. Soussain C, Patte C, Ostronoff M, et al. Small noncleaved cell lymphoma and leukemia in adults. A retrospective study of 65 adults treated with the LMB pediatric protocols. *Blood* 1995, **85**: 664–674.

62. Rohatiner AZ, Freedman A, Nadler L, et al. Myeloablative therapy with autologous bone marrow transplantation as consolidation therapy for follicular lymphoma. *Ann. Oncol.* 1994, **5** (Suppl. 2): 143–146.

63. Gribben JG, Neuberg D, Freedman AS, et al. Detection by polymerase chain reaction of residual cells with the bcl-2 translocation is associated with increased risk of relapse after autologous bone marrow transplantation for B-cell lymphoma. *Blood* 1993, **81**: 3449–3457.

64. Gribben JG, Neuberg D, Barber M, et al. Detection of residual lymphoma cells by polymerase chain reaction in peripheral blood is significantly less predictive for relapse than detection in bone marrow. *Blood* 1994, **83**: 3800–3807.

65. Gribben JG, Freedman AS, Neuberg D, et al. Immunologic purging of marrow asessed by PCR before autologous bone marrow transplantation for B-cell lymphoma. *N. Eng. J. Med.* 1991, **325**: 1525–1533.

66. Hardingham JE, Kotasek D, Sage RE, et al. Molecular detection of residual lymphoma cells in peripheral blood stem cell harvests and following autologous transplantation. *Bone Marrow Transplant* 1993, **11**: 15–20.

67. Morel P, Laporte JP, Noel MP, et al. Autologous bone marrow transplantation as consolidation therapy may prolong remission in newly diagnosed high-risk follicular lymphoma: a pilot study of 34 cases. *Leukemia* 1995, **9**: 576–582.

68. Gribben JG, Neuberg D, Barber M, et al. Detection of residual lymphoma cells by polymerase chain reaction in peripheral blood is significantly less predictive for relapse than detection in bone marrow. *Blood* 1994, **83**: 3800–3807.

69. Rooney CM, Smith CA, Ng CYC, et al. Use of gene modified virus-specific T-lymphocytes to control Epstein–Barr-virus related lymphoproliferation. *Lancet* 1995, **345**: 9–13.

CHAPTER 2

Historical perspective: the evolution of modern concepts of biology and management

IAN T. MAGRATH

Origins of modern concepts of malignant lymphomas

The foundations of modern pathology rest firmly upon the shoulders of Giovanni Battista Morgagni (1682–1771), Marie-Francois-Xavier Bichat (1771–1802), Johannes Müller (1801–1858) and Rudolph Virchow (1821–1905). Morgagni initiated the science of the study of gross morbid anatomy. His revolutionary notion that disease is caused by malfunction of one or more organs, based on 500 case histories and autopsies conducted at the University of Padua, and published in 1761 as *De sedibus et causis morborum per anatomen indagatis*, finally provided a sound replacement for the ancient humoral theory. Bichat, also a prodigious morbid anatomist (he is reputed to have performed 600 necropsies in a single winter, during which he lived in the autopsy room), established the importance of tissues as the matrix for disease processes, while Müller, utilizing the microscope extensively (which Bichat never did), began to

base the classification of tumors on their histological appearances and made a number of seminal observations on the nature of cancer. However, it is in the work of Virchow, a student of Müller, that our present concepts of neoplastic disease originated. As a young man, Virchow lived in an era when disease was generally considered to have a separate existence from the body, into which it could enter and live as a parasite. This idea was to change radically during the intellectual and political foment of the mid-19th century.

Virchow himself espoused careful observation and experiment as the fundamental tools of pathology rather than the then prevalent tendency, particularly in Germany, to formulate unsupportable (and therefore frequently replaced) hypotheses. His emphasis on the value of the experimental approach followed the earlier examples of John Hunter (1728–1793) and Claude Bernard (1813–1878). Virchow went beyond the organ and tissue theories of the origin of disease and, in establishing the science of cellular pathology, can be considered as the originator of our modern concepts of neoplasia. This momentous advance was made possible by the observations of Schleiden and Schwann (the latter also a student of Müller), who respectively demonstrated that the fundamental structural unit of plants and animals is the nucleated cell. Virchow's central idea, that diseases are disorders in the functioning of cells (and that cells arise from other cells), was expounded in a series of lectures in Berlin in the spring of 1858, which were subsequently assembled into a single volume entitled *Cellularpathologie*. Virchow also made important observations on the anatomy and function of the spleen and lymphoid tissues, and originated the terms leukemia and lymphoma. His Berlin lecture series on malignant tumors, given during the winter of 1862, was published as *Die krankhaften Geschwülste*, a work that launched the present era of neoplastic pathology [1]. Virchow's most distinguished pupil, Julius Cohnheim (1839–1884), was responsible for the first modern book on pathology, which emphasized the pathophysiology and experimental study of disease.

HODGKIN'S DISEASE AND PSEUDOLEUKEMIA

In the middle of the last century, international communication was remarkably slow by modern standards and it is, therefore, not surprising that the first glimmerings of a concept of lymphoid neoplasia appeared and evolved separately in the medical centers of Europe. Sporadic descriptions of generalised lymph node swelling of unknown cause, often associated with splenic enlargement, occur in the literature in the late 18th and 19th centuries, including those of Cruickshank, Craigie, Hodgkin, Wunderlich, Wilkes and Trousseau [2–7]. Various descriptive terms were used for this entity, slowly emerging from both clinical and gross pathological observationst – in England, Hodgkin's disease (an eponym first used by Wilkes [8], who independently described primary lymphadenopathy [5]), in France, l'adenie [7], and in Germany, Pseudoleukämie [9]. Craigie commented on a malignant lymphadenopathy referred to by other authors as 'scirrhus' and 'cancer' that he believed to originate as an inflammatory process. Hodgkin, in his classical paper of 1832, surmised that the lymph node enlargement he described was a primary process and not secondary to inflammation in adjacent tissue. We should bear in mind that the concept of malignant disease in the 19th century was very different from ours, and also, that we now believe that many malignant processes have their origins in persistent inflammation or hyperplasia. Consequently, it would be inappropriate to judge, as is sometimes done, which of these observers

most correctly perceived the nature of the 'disease' he was describing. The term 'Pseudoleukämie', first used by Cohnheim in 1862 [9], emphasized the lack of a high white blood cell count in a disease otherwise similar to the entity described by Virchow in 1845 as 'Weisses Blut' [10], subsequently to be renamed 'Leukämie'. Craigie and Bennett, had also independently observed pathological states characterized by a very high white cell count but had misinterpreted them as forms of suppuration of the blood [11,12].

Each of these designations – Hodgkin's disease, l'adenie and Pseudoleukämie – encompassed the whole range of malignant lymphomas (i.e., both Hodgkin's and non-Hodgkin's lymphomas) as we know them today, as well, quite probably, as acute leukemias with low white blood cell counts, and non-neoplastic lymphadenopathies without recognizable cause. Wunderlich, for example, in his work on Pseudoleukämie, describes a 21-year-old with an acute febrile illness associated with marked malaise, generalized lymphadenopathy, hepatosplenomegaly and tonsillitis who recovered after some 4–5 weeks – perhaps a case of infectious mononucleosis [13]. In Osler's textbook of medicine [14], published in 1892, all lymphomas are included under the general term 'Hodgkin's disease', which was stated to be synonymous with 'pseudoleukemia, general lymphadenoma and adénie'. Osler pointed out that a large majority of the cases arise without any recognizable cause and that recovery is very rare. Both he and Dreschfeld [15] drew attention to the extremely variable clinical course, and referred to acute and chronic cases of Hodgkin's disease, resorting to clinical subdivisions in the absence of other distinguishing features.

LYMPHOSARCOMA

Localized lymph-node swellings unrelated to a recognized disease entity such as tuberculosis, or to obvious pathology in the drainage area of a nodal group had also been recognized for some time. In Germany, diseases of this kind usually fell under the rubric of 'Lymphosarkoma', a term with its origins in antiquity, for the word 'sarcoma' was used in the second century by Galen to refer to any fleshy, superficial tumor. Virchow, in his *Die krankhaften Geschwülste* appears to have used the term for patients with generalized lymph node swelling who did not have leukemia. Thus, his lymphosarcoma subsequently became known as pseudoleukemia or Hodgkin's disease, and included all non-Hodgkin's lymphomas. Kundrat, in attempting to subdivide these diseases, classified Lymphosarkom with the other sarcomata, i.e., cellular growths arising in connective tissue, and separated it from 'lymphatic growths', a term he presumably applied to lymphatic swelling that was generalized from the outset, i.e., pseudoleukemia [16]. In Kundrat's experience, lymphosarcoma was confined to lymph nodes or lymphatic tissue in mucous membranes, although it tended to invade neighboring tissues and could spread directly from its local origin to other lymph node groups (in contrast to the bloodstream spread of pseudoleukemia). Involvement of the liver and spleen, if present, was nodular and involvement of the medulla of bone was rare. He referred to this progressive form as 'Lymphosarkomatosis', which he still considered, on clinical grounds (i.e., the evolution of the disease from a single site, and the lack of diffuse involvement of liver, spleen and bone marrow), to be distinct from Pseudoleukämia. Kundrat's categories do not correspond to any modern subdivisions, although his distinction between localized and generalized forms of the disease heralded our present separation of individual diseases into clinical stages. Clearly, Lymphosarkomatosis, as defined by Kundrat, like Cohnheim's Pseudoleukämia, included patients who would today be diagnosed as having Hodgkin's disease. In fact, his description of progressive anatomical involvement of other lymph node areas is more reminiscent of Hodgkin's disease than non-Hodgkin's lymphomas, which, ironically, later became known collectively as lymphosarcoma.

Kundrat's concept of lymphosarcoma and lymphosarcomatosis, a disease that began in one location and subsequently spread by way of direct tissue invasion and lymphatics, and which was intrinsically different from one that was generalized from the outset, persisted for over 50 years. Kundrat had paid only cursory attention to histology, and indeed, it was many years before the notion that histology provided grounds for distinguishing one disease from another was generally accepted. However, not everybody agreed with Kundrat's views, and considerable confusion appears to have reigned over the distinction, if any, between Lymphosarkomatosis and Hodgkin's disease/Pseudoleukämia. Dreschfeld's brave attempt to classify Hodgkin's disease, also on clinical grounds, provides some insight into this. He viewed malignant lymphoma, lymphosarcoma, lymphosarcomatosis, adénie, lymphadénie, lymphadenoma, lymphadenosis and pseudoleukemia as synonyms for Hodgkin's disease, but recognized differences in disease pattern and the rapidity of progression. Hodgkin's disease, he thought, was 'a specific inflammatory growth (a specific granuloma)' caused by an as yet unidentified infectious agent, which could present with local involvement that became generalized (similar to Kundrat's Lymphosarkoma-

tosis) or which could be generalized from the outset (Pseudoleukämia). He alluded to differences in the predominant location of the disease (superficial, thoracic or abdominal lymph nodes), but did not believe that there were fundamental 'structural differences' between benign and malignant lymphomas (referred to as lymphadenoma and lymphosarcoma, respectively) as had been proposed by others.

Acute Hodgkin's disease, he suggested, might better be called acute lymphosarcomatosis, which resembled one of the forms of chronic Hodgkin's disease (both presumably based on Kundrat's concept of a disease beginning in one region and spreading to others). In agreement with Stevens [17], he believed that a second form of chronic Hodgkin's disease (generalized *ab initio*) was closely related to leukemia in that it resulted from hyperplasia of the blood-forming organs (then thought to be the medulla of the bone, the spleen and the lymphatic glands). He suggested that such cases might 'more aptly be termed chronic pseudo-leukemia'. Like leukemia, the latter entity could be divided into lymphatic, splenic and myelogenic types, although the separate nature of the latter two, referring to primary involvement of the spleen and medulla (marrow) of the bones, respectively, remained in question. It is clear to the modern reader that these dimly perceived, and largely clinical, subtypes of 'Hodgkin's disease' must have overlapped considerably, and that then, as now, terms were used differently by different authors. Certainly, 'Hodgkin's disease' and 'lymphosarcoma' did not have the connotations that they subsequently took on.

While the terminology of malignant lymphomas at the turn of the century was confusing, the presence of slowly and rapidly progressive (compare our low-grade and intermediate-/high-grade categories), and localized and generalized subtypes were recognized, as were forms presenting with primary lymph node, primary intrathoracic (usually recognized to involve the mediastinum solely on the basis of dullness to percussion over the sternum) or primary intraabdominal involvement – often arising in the bowel. The difficulty of separating disease entities on largely clinical grounds was soon echoed by the struggle that ensued as histological examination slowly emerged as a taxonomic tool during the first half of the present century. For this was a period in which there were few insights into the physiology of lymphoid tissue and morphology was therefore paramount. Even now, in an era when the functional attributes of cell populations and the derangements caused by genetic anomalies are gradually being absorbed into lymphoma classification, it is likely that many of our 'pathological entities' do not represent individual diseases, and our concepts may prove, in some circumstances, to be as perplexing to our descendents as those of late 19th century authors are to us.

Evolution of histological classification

Although Bichat is often considered to be the father of histology, his work was at a macroscopic level, and he made little or no use of the microscope in spite of the clear indication of its value provided by the host of discoveries already made by its use. Marcello Malpighi (1628–1694), for example, who founded the science of microscopic anatomy, had discovered kidney glomeruli and the splenic corpuscles that bear his name a century before. Malpighi's work had been made possible by Anton Van Leeuwenhoek (1632–1723), who, in addition to his own discoveries, made more than 400 microscopes and donated many to scientific societies. Perhaps the curious failure of pathologists, prior to the 19th century, to exploit the extraordinary potential of the microscope resulted from the prevailing 'nonspecific' concepts of disease, which were based on theories dating from the preclassical era rather than on methodical observation and experiment. While Galen's ideas continued to exert sway until well into the 18th century, they were finally superceded by the new science of pathological anatomy, yet still there was little attempt to move beyond gross description. As late as 1842, Rokitansky's great *Handbuch der pathologischen Anatomie* made no use of histology, although the microscopic study of tissues, aided by the discovery of the achromatic lens in the 19th century was, by now, well advanced. This doubtless stemmed from Rokitansky's view that the formed elements of the body arose from lymph or 'body juices'. He even attempted to reinstate the classical humoral theory of disease. Histopathology owes much to Jacob Henle (1809–1885), another of Müller's protégés, who wrote the first text on microscopic histology, *Allgemeine Anatomie*, published in 1841. By this time, greatly improved techniques in the hardening, sectioning and staining of tissues had been developed. Eventually, the concept of cells as the ultimate pathological unit set the stage for rapid progress. Virchow devoted a third of his book, *Cellularpathologie*, to normal histology, while his student Cohnheim was one of the pioneers of modern experimental pathology. Conheim's book, *Vorlesungen über Allgemeine Pathologie*, written between 1877 and 1880, ultimately supplanted Virchow's earlier text.

HISTOLOGICAL PERSPECTIVE ON HODGKIN'S DISEASE AND LYMPHOSARCOMA

The value of histology as a means of classifying lymphomas was not widely recognized until the 20th century – perhaps a consequence of reluctance to abandon the traditional clinical classification and the novelty of the concept of cellular pathology. In future years, the reasons for the slow permeation of molecular genetics into lymphoma taxonomy may be similarly pondered. In spite of the emphasis on clinical classification, there was, in the late 19th century, no shortage of histological descriptions, even though these were subordinated to lengthy discussions of the gross pathology – just as today there is a great deal of information regarding molecular genetic abnormalities, but diagnostic pathology is still predominantly based on histology, with an increasing contribution from immunophenotyping. Wunderlich, for example, described the histological appearance of enlarged lymph nodes in a case of Pseudoleukämia, and mentioned the presence of binucleate and large multinucleate cells as early as 1858 [6]. It was Sternberg, however, who, having described the histology (including giant cells) of what he considered to be 'a peculiar type of tuberculosis masquerading as Pseudoleukämie' [18], suggested that a diagnosis of Pseudoleukämie should only be entertained after histological examination or even only after inoculation of involved tissue into animals failed to induce tuberculosis. Sternberg questioned, on both histological grounds and the ultimate development of tuberculosis in a high fraction of patients, whether, after separating clearcut cases of Lymphosarkom, most cases of Pseudoleukämia were not actually a manifestation of tuberculosis (the relationship between Pseudoleukämia and tuberculosis was not a new issue). This seemed consistent with Pel and Ebstein's delineation of what, on the basis of the presence of a characteristic chronic relapsing fever, they believed to be a separate disease entity [19,20].

Dorothy Reed [21] refuted Sternberg's contention that the tubercle bacillus was causally involved in Hodgkin's disease (although she favored an infectious origin), but also emphasized the association of particular clinical features with a specific histological appearance. She, like Sternberg, described giant cells with one or multiple nuclei and prominent nucleoli in the setting of a granuloma. Clinically, the cases she described nearly always began with cervical lymphadenopathy that rapidly spread to other nodal regions, the nodes being more mobile and discrete than is the case with sarcoma or tuberculosis. Of course, as pointed out by Coley [22], this clinical description was also sometimes seen in cases that had a histological appearance of 'round cell sarcoma', and Coley was of the opinion that Hodgkin's disease was a type of sarcoma (i.e., malignant) and might better be called lymphosarcoma. Thus, while confusion still reigned as to the use of these terms (the concept of histological definitions of disease entities had yet to be accepted), the precedent of histological examination as a component of diagnosis, and the existence of different histological appearances in different diseases, albeit with overlapping clinical features, had been set.

We might wonder why the term 'Hodgkin's disease', initially a general term that encompassed a wide range of lymphoid neoplasms, eventually became associated with the histological appearance that was well described by Paltauf and his student, Sternberg, as lymphogranulomatosis [23,24] – particularly since Reed's cases fitted more clearly with Kundrat's clinical description of lymphosarcomatosis. While there is no clear explanation, it is perhaps more by default than by design, for the term 'lymphosarcoma' had already gradually become associated with lymphomas in which the cells more or less resembled those present in normal lymph nodes. Virchow himself had described the appearance of the cells present in 'Lymphosarkom' as small round cells, although he had also recognized the existence of lymphosacomas in which the cells were of much larger size than a normal lymphocyte – a finding which others confirmed. Ghon and Roman, for example, had already, in 1916, begun to relate the cytology of lymphosarcomas to that of the cells of normal lymph nodes, and referred to lymphocytic and lymphoblastic forms [25]. They were aware, however, of significant differences in the appearance of the nuclei of lymphosarcoma cells compared to normal lymphoid cells, and also recognized that many tumors consisted of mixtures of cell types – not only large and small lymphoid cells, but also macrophage-like cells and plasma cells. Interestingly, not only did Ghon and Roman report that the number of cells in mitosis varied greatly from one tumor to another, but they also recognized 'dwarf cells' with a very dense, round nucleus – cells that would today be recognized as undergoing apoptosis. Presciently, Ghon and Roman wondered whether this appearance was a consequence of cell damage!

The term 'pseudoleukemia' gradually fell into disuse as histology took precedence over clinical characteristics, since most cases could, by the second decade of this century, be classified on the basis of histology either as lymphosarcoma or lymphogranuloma (the histological appearance associated with the term Hodgkin's disease by Reed). Pseudoleukemia simply implied lymphadenopathy and splenomegaly (and even involvement of the bone marrow) without an elevated white blood count. In addition, pseudoleukemia had often been observed to evolve into leukemia. Debate over the relationships and cellular origins of these various entities persisted, as did the question of whether Hodgkin's disease is an infectious process or a malignant disease. Similar debates continue in a more modern context.

RETICULUM CELL SARCOMA

In the early part of the 20th century, the increasing emphasis on histology led to the recognition of new entities, which fell under the general rubric of lymphosarcoma, although debate (mired in a semantic morass) continued on whether this entity was truly distinct from Hodgkin's disease [26]. Although no formal histological classification had been proposed, many pathologists recognized that lymphosarcoma, i.e., what was left after the exclusion of lymphogranuloma (Hodgkin's disease), because of its varied cytology, was probably a group of diseases rather than a single entity. As expressed by Ewing in 1939, amidst the confusion, there was at least recognition of small-cell and large-cell 'lymphosarcomas' [27]. This, of course, had already been recognized by Virchow in the previous century. However, histological examination of normal lymph nodes had also aroused curiosity regarding the cellular origins of lymph node tumors. The accepted canon was that lymphosarcomas could arise from any of the cell types present in lymph nodes. Apart from the lymphoid cells themselves, believed by many to arise from the germinal follicles, there were endothelial cells lining the lymph node sinuses and reticulum cells interspersed among the lymphoid cells. The term 'reticulum cell' was applied to the larger, 'stationary' cells scattered throughout the lymph node, and probably encompassed what would today be recognized as several cell types, including macrophages and dendritic reticulum cells. Both reticulum cells and endothelial cells were believed, by many pathologists, to be derived from a single precursor cell of mesenchymal origin (that also gave rise to lymphocytes) and to have phagocytic properties. Some believed they could recognize this precursor cell in lymph nodes; others thought the reticulum cell itself to be the 'mother cell'.

Considerable controversy has surrounded the tumors that were presumed to originate from these various cells and it is clear now that virtually all primary tumors of lymph nodes actually originate in lymphoid cells. Endothelial sarcoma or endothelioma of lymph nodes was a term used by many pathologists to denote a tumor of larger cell type believed to arise from the endothelial lining cells of the lymph node sinuses [28]. Oberling, in France, used the terms 'reticulosarcoma' and 'reticuloendotheliosarcoma' in the context of a subset of bone tumors, described shortly before by Ewing, which, he believed, arose in the reticuloendothelial tissue of bone marrow and thus were to be differentiated from other 'myelomas', i.e., tumors arising in the bone marrow. Oberling suggested that these bone marrow tumors had the same histogenesis as similar tumors arising in lymph nodes [29], although it is probable that the tumors he studied were not lymphomas at all, but bone sarcomas. Roulet, in Germany, set out to characterize more precisely the 'third' type of lymphosarcoma of lymph nodes, which he distinguished from the lymphocytic and lymphoblastic types, and referred to as 'Retothelsarkom' (after Rössle) rather than 'Retikuloendotheliosarkom', on the grounds that it arose not from the endothelial cells of the lymph node sinus but from the cells associated with the fibrous scaffolding (or reticulothelium) of the node, the reticulum cells [30]. Unfortunately, Roulet's descriptions were sufficiently broad that they did not enable this 'entity' to be sharply differentiated from other forms of lymphosarcoma. Nonetheless, the categorization of reticulum cell sarcoma as being of large-cell type, and its presumed different histogenesis, led some pathologists to refer to large- and small-cell lymphoid neoplasms as reticulum cell sarcoma and lymphosarcoma, respectively. Others continued to refer to all lymphoid tumors as lymphosarcomas but to subcategorize some large-cell lymphomas as reticulum cell lymphosarcomas. There was even a school of thought that considered all tumors of lymph nodes to be varieties of reticulum cell sarcoma. Meanwhile, the debate continued as to whether Hodgkin's disease (or lymphogranuloma) was a variety of lymphosarcoma or not.

GIANT FOLLICULAR LYMPHOMA

The occurrence of lymphomas with a follicular or nodular architecture had been recognized at least as early as 1902 [31], according to Ghon and Roman [25], but received only sporadic mention in the literature until the independent descriptions by Brill et al. and Symmers of patients with lymphadenopathy and splenomegaly in which histological studies revealed enlarged lymphoid follicles [32,33]. This disease, because of its generally protracted clinical course, also generated considerable controversy as to whether it was simply a chronic hyperplastic state, as originally believed to be the case by Brill et al. and Symmers, or a truly neoplastic condition (a debate not unlike that pertaining to a number of T-cell lymphomas today). That it could evolve into a rapidly

progressive malignant lymphoma was, however, accepted by all. Varying descriptions of the histology and clinical course of follicular lymphomas appear to reflect the range of diseases that originally fell under this rubric. Its relative rarity was such that it was difficult for any one individual to acquire a large experience. In fact, reports of series collected in the first half of this century suggest that follicular lymphoma comprised a considerably lower proportion of lymphoma cases than today, namely 4% and 13% of patients with non-Hodgkin's lymphoma in two large series reported in the USA [34,35]. It is probable that this reflects a truly lower incidence in the early part of this century, which would be consistent with the low frequency of follicular lymphomas in developing countries today, although the possibility of underdiagnosis because of the slow progression of this disease, at least before conversion to a diffuse lymphoma, cannot be excluded. It is also possible that many cases were diagnosed as reactive hyperplasia and excluded from series of lymphoma patients. Gall et al. [36] described four main histological forms of the disease, which correspond to categories that are still recognized. Types one, two and three were composed of follicles containing small cells, mixed small and large cells, and large cells, respectively. Type four referred to a variety in which there was a degree of confluence or 'rupture of follicles' such that a diagnosis of follicular lymphoma was sometimes difficult. Such cases may have been in transition to diffuse lymphoma and are well recognized today. It is interesting that the average duration of survival was roughly similar in all subtypes, when the duration of symptoms prior to biopsy (ranging from 2 to 4 years) was added to survival after biopsy (approximately 2 years), suggesting to Gall and colleagues that the subtypes represented successive phases in the development of the disease. These patients were treated almost exclusively with local kilovoltage radiation to 600 roentgens; doses as high as 1800 roentgens were occasionally used.

HISTOLOGICAL CLASSIFICATION SCHEMES

The recognition of several histological subtypes of lymphoma paved the way for classification schemes based on morphology alone, although the long tradition of clinical diagnosis, supplemented by gross pathology, ensured the persistence of clinical characteristics in classification for many years and, even now, the final traces have not been completely expunged (consider the issue of the borderland between lymphoma and leukemia). This reluctance to relinquish clinical classification (e.g., acute and chronic diseases) was supported by the lack of evidence that histology, with the exception of the separation of follicular lymphomas from the remainder, was able to predict either the natural history of the disease, or the outcome of treatment – confined in the first half of this century to either surgery or radiation. However, as an essential step in attempting to comprehend the nature of the lymphoid neoplasms, pathologists began to arrange the various histological appearances they were able to discern into classification schemes. From the early days, the American and European schools had a tendency to evolve separately. In the United States, the first purely histological classification scheme was published by Gall and Mallory in 1942 [37]. The lineage of this classification scheme led, over the course of 40 years, to the Working Formulation for Clinical Usage. In Europe, Robb-Smith built on the ideas of Pullinger to develop a rather complex histological classification of 'reticuloses' and 'reticulum cell sarcoma', which he considered to be less and more malignant subsets of diseases of the reticuloendothelial system – in effect, low and high 'clinical' grades. This classification scheme included both neoplastic and nonneoplastic lymphadenopathies as well as malignant lymphomas (see Table 2.4) [38]. Robb-Smith's classification, which was revised in 1947 and 1964, was eventually replaced by the Kiel classification, which also has low and high grade categories.

Gall and Mallory's classification superseded that provided by Callender in his review of the American College of Pathologist's Registry of Lymphatic Tumors. Callender's classification [39] was based on a mixture of cytological, gross anatomical and clinical characteristics and, like that of Robb-Smith, included leukemias, lymphomas and nonneoplastic lymphadenopathies (Table 2.1). Gall and Mallory created a much simpler scheme, which included only the malignant lymphomas. They recognized seven major types of lymphoma (Table 2.2): Hodgkin's lymphoma, Hodgkin's sarcoma, follicular lymphoma, lymphocytic, lymphoblastic and two types of reticulum cell (large-cell) sarcoma-stem cell lymphoma, which was believed to arise from an undifferentiated mesodermal cell able to give rise to all types of blood cell, and clasmatocytic lymphoma, which was thought to arise from cells with marked phagocytic properties, simulating monocytes. Since that time, and until very recently, histology has been the primary basis for classification, although the clinical features, immunophenotype and, in some cases, geographic distribution, viral association or molecular characteristics of the more recently recognized pathologic entities such as Burkitt's lymphoma,

Table 2.1 Callender's classification of tumors and tumor-like conditions arising from lymphocyte stem cells, and monocyte or reticuloendothelial stem cells

Adult cell type	Lymphocyte	Reticulum cell	
		Reticulocyte monocyte	Hodgkin's disease
I. Reactions	'Lymphoma' Lymphocytosis	Gaucher's disease Niemann–Pick disease	Localized (sclerosing)
II. Neoplastic proliferations	Leukemic lymphocytoma 1. Chronic 2. Acute	Leukemic reticulocytoma (syn. monocytic) leukemia)	
III. Neoplastic proliferations	Aleukemic lymphocytoma 1. Diffuse 2. Nodular	Aleukemic reticulocytoma	Generalized (cellular)
IV. Malignant tumors	Lymphosarcoma 1. Aleukemic 2. Leukemic (syn. lymphatic leukosarcoma)	Reticulum cell sarcoma	Sarcomatous

and which persists in the histological grades (low and high, or in the Working Formulation, low, intermediate and high) of today. He was able to confirm that in his series of 119 patients, those with follicular lymphoma (referred to as giant follicle lymphoma) survived considerably longer than most other patients (36.8% of untreated, and 43.8% of treated patients survived for 5 years as compared to 23% of treated patients with either lymphocytic or reticulum cell tumors), although he could discern no clear difference in survival between patients with lymphocytic versus reticulum cell lymphosarcoma. Surprisingly, 20% and 15%, respectively, of untreated patients in the latter groups survived 5 years, although less than 10% lived 10 years. He, like others before him, noted that among patients with follicular lymphomas, patients with a mixed follicular and diffuse pattern had a worse prognosis – survival was half that of patients with 'fully differentiated' follicular lymphosarcoma. He also recognized that extranodal lymphomas tended to have a better prognosis, in that 26% of 35 such patients were alive 10 years after treatment versus 7% of his 83 treated patients with nodal lymphomas. Most of these long-surviving extranodal lymphomas had primaries in the oral cavity, tonsil, nasopharynx, salivary glands and gastrointestinal tract, and presumably included what subsequently became known as 'pseudo-lymphomas' and, more recently, MALT lymphomas. They also more often had localized disease. Stout did not observe a difference in survival between reticulum cell and lymphocytic cell tumors, but did remark that childhood lymphomas and lymphomas complicated by leukemia had an almost invariably fatal course.

The difficulty of moving forward in the absence of knowledge of the cellular origins of lymphomas is illustrated by the Rappaport classification, published in 1956 [47,48]. This scheme represented an evolution from the classification of Gall and Mallory and the subsequent modification by Gall and Rappaport [44] (Table 2.4), and was based, as it subsequently proved, on largely erroneous concepts. Nonetheless, Rappaport's classification was widely used, particularly in the United States, and was favored by clinicians for its simplicity. Rappaport and his colleagues had questioned whether the follicles seen in giant follicular lymphoma were truly the neoplastic counterparts of germinal follicles of lymphoid tissue [47], and proposed using the designation 'nodular' instead of follicular, a term that had been used by Callender in his classification of lymphohematopoietic neoplasms in 1934 [39]. The new element of Rappaport's scheme was the division of the non-Hodgkin's lymphomas into two broad classes, nodular and diffuse, each of which consisted of three main types of tumor: those consisting mainly of small cells; those consisting mainly of large cells; and those in which there was a roughly equal mixture of small and large cells. Small cells were referred to as well-differentiated, intermediate as 'poorly differentiated' and large as histiocytic, following the former 'clasmatocytic' category of Gall and Mallory, and the long-held notion that the reticulendothelial system is a phagocytic system in which reticulum cells might be equated with monocytes, a concept also mentioned by Callender [39]. This system was subsequently modified to take into account the new tumors described in children (see below) [49], but without a sound basis for classification beyond histological or cytological appearance, it was not possible to progress very far, in spite of repeated efforts that extended into the 1970s [50–52].

It was in the 1970s, however, that a major advance was made in the understanding of the immune system – the division of lymphocytes into B- and T-cell subtypes, concerned with antibody-mediated and cell-mediated immunity, respectively. Immediately, attempts were made to incorporate this new understanding into lymphoma classification schemes, notably by Lukes and Collins in the USA, and

Table 2.4 Evolution of histological classification systems of non-Hodgkin's lymphomas in the United States

Custer and Bernhard	Gall and Mallory	Gall and Rappaport*	Rappaport*
Lymphosarcoma	Lymphocytic Lymphoblastic	Lymphocytic, WD Lymphocytic, PD Histiocytic/ lymphocytic	Lymphocytic, WD Lymphocytic, PD Histiocytic/ lymphocytic, mixed
Reticulum cell sarcoma	Stem cell Clasmatocytic	Stem cell Histiocytic } RCS	Histiocytic
Follicular	Follicular	Nodular (divided into all of the above subtypes)	Nodular (divided into all of the above subtypes)

*In these classifcation schemes, each cytological type of lymphoma is divided into diffuse and nodular forms (see text).
RSC, Reticulum cell sarcoma; WD, well differentiated; PD, poorly differentiated.

Lennert in Germany [53,54]. Although these classification systems were still based on histological appearances, immunological characterization of histological entities had become possible, just as, in an earlier era, histology had supplemented classifications based primarily on clinical and gross pathological characteristics. These newer classification schemes, in spite of considerable resistance to the incorporation of immunological concepts, continued to coexist with earlier schemes, such as Rappaport's. Indeed, although Lennert's classification, or rather, its derivative, the Kiel classification, was favored in Europe, Rappaport's continued to hold sway in North America – in spite of numerous proposals for alternative schemes on both sides of the Atlantic [50–52]. Extensive clinical correlations had not been made with these various classification schemes and no clear advantages to any of them in terms of predicting the outcome of therapy – by now entering the era of combination chemotherapy – had been shown. However, the profusion of different terms for histological entities that at least overlapped (e.g., poorly differentiated lymphocytic, small cleaved cell and centrocytic–centroblastic) led a group of experienced hematopathologists and hemato-oncologists to attempt to clarify the situation. In 1982, under the auspices of the US National Cancer Institute (NCI), 12 pathologists tested the reproducibility and clinical relevance of the six major extant classification systems, and attempted to devise a 'translation' system or 'formulation' [55] to 'facilitate clinical comparisons of case reports and therapeutic trials'. In this study, the histological slides and clinical records of 1175 cases of non-Hodgkin's lymphoma were examined by the participating pathologists (six of whom were identified with a major classification scheme) and the diagnoses made correlated with clinical information, primarily the outcome of therapy (although a variety of different treatments had been used). The Working Formulation separated lymphomas into ten major categories on the basis of morphology alone, each with a different survival expectancy. Although terms from the Lukes and Collins scheme were introduced, the Formulation was quite similar to the modified Rappaport classification. Survival curves for each of the ten subtypes were rather evenly spread between 29% and 70% alive at 5 years, but it was felt that three major prognostic groups could be discerned such that the subtypes were divided into low, intermediate and high grade. Perhaps not surprisingly, the Working Formulation was quickly used as a classification in its own right and largely replaced the Rappaport scheme in North America, although the Kiel classification continued to predominate in Europe.

One could argue that the basic concept of correlating prognosis with histological entities is flawed, because many histological 'entities' are biologically heterogeneous and, for that matter, have often proven to be histologically heterogeneous. In addition, similarity of prognosis cannot be assumed to indicate similarity of biology, while the single most important determinant of prognosis is the efficacy of therapy. Thus, as treatment approaches have evolved since the 1970s, when the patients included in the National Cancer Institute (NCI) study were treated, a paradox has developed whereby patients with high-grade lymphomas, for whom treatment has improved considerably, now have better long-term survival than patients with low-grade lymphomas, who, for the most part, remain incurable. Prognosis based on histology, then, is most useful when treatment is ineffective, such that the outcome is similar to that in the untreated patient. It is least useful when treatment is highly successful. Truly separate pathological entities might be expected to be associated with characteristic clinical syndromes, albeit frequently overlapping ones, which differ with respect to the anatomical distribution of disease, rate of progression in the absence of treatment, and sometimes, response to treatment.

Recently, European and American pathologists have again attempted to define common ground, an effort that has resulted in a proposal for a new classification, this time simply a list of what appear, on the basis of a combination of histology, immunophenotyping, viral association, cytogenetics and molecular genetics, to be separate pathological entities [56]. The degree of certainty that the categories do indeed represent separate entities varies and will, no doubt, be improved in future classifications. Meanwhile, although some clinicians are concerned at the complexity of this scheme and have questioned its clinical utility [44], there can surely be no doubt that continuing attempts to define discrete pathological entities, using all available tools, is a prerequisite for further progress to be made in both the understanding and treatment of the non-Hodgkin's lymphomas.

MORE RECENTLY RECOGNIZED LYMPHOMA SUBTYPES

Childhood lymphomas

While the occurrence of lymphomas in childhood had been reported upon since the 19th century, it was only quite recently that clinical and histological differences from adult lymphomas were recognized. As early as 1925, Liu noted that a high fraction of patients with lymphoid tumors of the intestines were children – six of the 12 patients he reported were less than 20 years, and five less than 10 [57]. Eleven of these 12 cases were in the ileocecal region and six had presented with intussusception – characteristic features of small noncleaved cell lymphomas. Both the relative infrequency of non-Hodgkin's lymphomas, and the paucity of the follicular subtype was commented upon by several authors in the 1940s and 1950s [37,58,59], but apart from the occasionally made, and often disputed, statement that reticulum cell sarcoma was less common in children, no histological differences from these tumors in adults were discerned in this era. Of relevance to the development of treatment approaches is the frequently noted morphological similarity between leukemia and lymphoma in children, but, interestingly, in spite of the recognition that overt leukemia often developed in children with lymphosarcoma, patients with bone marrow involvement at onset or a high peripheral blood white cell count were generally excluded from series of childhood lymphosarcoma.

Burkitt's lymphoma

It was the description of an unusual form of lymphoma in African children (subsequently designated Burkitt's lymphoma) that eventually led to the recognition that the histopathological spectrum of the non-Hodgkin's lymphomas in children differs from that in adults. This was largely a consequence of the high frequency of jaw tumors in Burkitt's lymphoma. This striking presenting feature appears to have been first observed by Sir Albert Cook, who, with his brother, established a mission hospital in Uganda in 1897 [58,59]. Evidence that lymphoma and/or facial 'sarcomas' have a high incidence in African children first came from ex-patriot pathologists working in Africa: Smith and Elmes, as early as 1934, noted ten 'round-cell sarcomas of the orbit' among 500 tumors from Lagos [60]; Edington, in the Gold Coast, commented on the high frequency of maxillary lymphosarcoma in children [61]; Thjis, working in the Belgian Congo, reported that 74 out of 145 children with malignant tumors had lymphosarcoma [62]; and De Smet, also in the Belgian Congo, mentioned the frequent involvement of multiple organ sites, including the maxilla, orbit and abdomen, in children with lymphosarcoma [63]. However, it was Denis Burkitt, a surgeon working in Uganda, who first emphasized the high frequency of jaw 'sarcomas' in African children [64]. Burkitt also noted that such patients often had tumors in multiple organ sites, particularly in the abdomen. He subsequently demonstrated, by making safaris and writing to outlying hospitals, that the tumor occurred at high frequency in a broad belt across Africa extending approximately 15° north and south of the equator with a southern prolongation to the east [65,66].

Meanwhile, O'Conor and Davies, in a review of the malignant tumors of children in the Kampala Cancer Registry in Uganda realized that malignant lymphoma accounted for some 50% of all childhood malignant tumors in the registry [67,68]. They were able to confirm that the jaw and abdominal tumors were histologically identical and that Burkitt's patients had a form of lymphoma. O'Conor, using a version of the Gall and Rappaport classification then accepted by the American Society of Clinical Pathologists, diagnosed the majority of these lymphomas as belonging to the lymphocytic, poorly differentiated subtype, but also described several distinctive features, such as the interspersed macrophages, giving rise to a 'starry sky' or 'water pot' appearance, and the vacuolated, basophilic cytoplasm apparent on touch preparations and Giemsa-stained sections [68]. Soon after these observations in Africa, O'Conor, Wright (who had also worked in Uganda) and others reported histologically indistinguishable tumors in children in the USA and Europe [69–71], finally raising the possibility that the spectrum of diffuse non-Hodgkin's lymphomas in childhood may differ from that in adults. Epstein–Barr virus (EBV) was discovered in 1964 in a cell line derived from a Burkitt's lymphoma [72], a finding which led to the recognition of the association of African Burkitt's lymphoma with EBV.

Lymphoblastic lymphoma

The occurrence of mediastinal 'hyperplasia' in pseudoleukemia was mentioned in Virchow's seminal work, *Die krankhaften Geschwülste* [1], and Ortner, somewhat later, described the association of thymic tumors with leukemia [73]. Sternberg described several patients with thymic sarcoma in 1905, although he believed them to be of myeloid origin [74]. Gall and Mallory mentioned that 20% of their lymphoblastic lymphomas (a term that may overlap but is not congruent with present usage) occurred in patients less than 20 years old [37]. Our modern concept of lymphoblastic lymphoma stems from the observations of Barcos and Lukes [75] and Nathwani et al. [76]. They described a discrete histological entity with a high frequency of mediastinal involvement occurring predominantly in children and young adults. This entity would previously have been diagnosed as a poorly differentiated lymphocytic lymphoma according to the Rappaport classification. Initially the presence of nuclear convolutions, present in approximately half of the cases described by Nathwani et al., was believed to be a characteristic feature (hence Lukes and Collins term, convoluted T-cell lymphoma) but, although some lymphoblastic lymphomas have prominent convolutions, this is a variable feature, and neither essential to the diagnosis, nor of prognostic significance. Nathwani et al. pointed out that these tumors are cytologically indistinguishable from acute lymphoblastic leukemia.

Large-cell lymphoma

Lymphomas with large cells have been described in children at least since the identification of reticulum cell sarcoma, although it is not at all clear how many of these cases would today be diagnosed as large-cell lymphoma [77]. Oberling, in his classical work on reticulum cell sarcomas of 1928, mentions two girls, of 8 and 14 years with femoral and tibial tumors, respectively [29], although it seems likely now that these were examples of what we now understand as Ewing's sarcoma. Gall and Mallory report that 4% of their stem cell lymphomas, and 2% of their clasmatocytic lymphomas occurred in patients less than 20 years old. In a review of cases of childhood lymphosarcoma (i.e., non-Hodgkin's lymphoma) seen between 1928 and 1952 at the Memorial Center for Cancer and Allied Diseases in New York, Rosenberg et al. state that 36% of their 69 patients aged 15 or less had reticulum cell sarcoma. They mention that 24% of the latter patients had bone lesions, mostly solitary, but the very different clinical characteristics of these patients and particularly 'late metastasis' suggests that many of these patients, again, may have had Ewing's sarcoma. It is likely that this confusion between Ewing's sarcoma and lymphoma is the origin of the erroneous notion, still extant, that malignant lymphoma of bone should be considered an entity in its own right.

More recently, the use of immunophenotyping has led to the separation of childhood large-cell lymphomas into those of B-cell origin, which merge, histologically, with small noncleaved cell lymphomas, and lymphomas of peripheral T-cell origin, the majority of which fall into the recently recognized category of anaplastic large-cell lymphoma. The latter was identified approximately 10 years ago by Stein and colleagues, with the help of a monoclonal antibody (Ki-1) they had developed against Reed–Sternberg cells [78]. Most anaplastic large-cell lymphomas are strongly positive for the CD30 receptor, recognized by Ki-1 or other monoclonal antibodies, and have characteristic histological features such as a parafollicular and sinus distribution in the lymph node. These tumors involve nodal and extranodal sites, not infrequently the skin. Prior to the recognition of this entity, anaplastic large-cell lymphomas appear to have been frequently misdiagnosed as nonlymphoid neoplasms – often as malignant histiocytosis, or even carcinoma or melanoma.

Low-grade lymphomas

The continuing evolution of our ability to recognize individual pathologic entities is well illustrated by the identification and acceptance of a number of new entities in the last 30 years. Some of these entities have been recognized initially on the basis of careful histological examination or because of a striking clinical syndrome, but nearly always the acceptance of the new disease as a true pathological entity has resulted from immunophenotypic and sometimes cytogenetic or molecular studies, as illustrated by the examples provided. As has been the case throughout the history of attempts to understand the lymphoid neoplasms, the same disease has often been described by different investigators, each of whom provides a different name. Subsequently there is much discussion as to whether or not these various entities are identical. This is not always easy to resolve, but is certainly easier today than it was prior to the age of immunophenotyping, cytogenetics and molecular biology.

Mantle cell lymphoma

Lennert's careful cytological analysis of the germinal center led to the recognition of two main cell types, the germinoblast (centroblast) and germinocyte (centrocyte) [79]. Subsequently, lymphomas believed to be of germinal center origin were divided, according to the Kiel classification system, into centrocytic and centrocytic–centroblastic lymphomas [53]. Centrocytic lymphoma, composed almost exclusively of centrocytes, was initially not widely accepted as an entity in North America. However, Berard and Dorfman in the United States described a diffuse or vaguely nodular 'lymphocytic lymphoma of intermediate differentiation' (i.e., one that was neither poorly nor well differentiated according to the Rappaport classification) [80], and subsequently, Weisenberger et al. described a 'follicular variant' of this disease, in which a follicular pattern was particularly prominent, which they called mantle zone lymphoma [81]. They reported that the cells of this neoplasm were similar to those in the normal mantle zone of secondary lymphoid follicles. Over the years there has been much discussion as to the relationship between these several diseases, but the recent identification of a characteristic chromosomal translocation common to all (t11;14), coupled to the similarity of immunophenotype and clinical course has finally led to widespread acceptance that centrocytic lymphoma, diffuse lymphocytic lymphoma of intermediate differentiation and mantle zone lymphoma are one and the same disease, the latter entities now being referred to in North America as 'mantle cell lymphoma' [82,83].

MALT lymphomas, monocytoid B-cell and marginal zone lymphomas

In 1983, Isaacson and Wright described a subtype of B-cell lymphoma that was associated with MALT of the bowel [84], particularly the stomach. Similar (histologically, immunophenotypically and behaviorally) lymphomas were subsequently described in lung, salivary gland, thyroid, breast, kidney and skin, and the male and female urogenital tracts [85]. The cells of these lymphomas are somewhat heterogeneous and include small lymphocytes, cells that resemble the cells of the mantle zone of germinal follicles (centrocytes), lymphoplasmacytoid cells and cells that resemble the cells of the marginal zone of lymphoid follicles (external to the mantle zone) in the spleen.

In 1986, Sheibani et al. described a type of lymphoma they referred to as a monocytoid B-cell lymphoma [86], the cells of which resemble those seen in the lymph node sinus in certain infectious conditions including toxoplasmosis and human immunodeficiency virus (HIV)-associated follicular hyperplasia. Both cytological and immunophenotypic similarities between the cells of this lymphoma and those of the splenic marginal zone have been described, and although the disease has been predominantly described as a nodal lymphoma, involvement of extranodal sites including salivary gland (particularly in patients with Sjögren's syndrome), spleen, stomach, breast and thyroid has been well documented [87]. Recently, the identification of patients with nodal monocytoid lymphoma and extranodal disease indistinguishable from MALT lymphoma, as well as monocytoid lymphoma in lymph nodes draining gastric MALT lymphomas has led to the conclusion that these lymphomas are likely to be closely related [88,89]. Both have a relatively broad cytological spectrum, which overlaps the Kiel 'immunocytoma', a tendency to colonize adjacent epithelium and reactive germinal centers, and a rather benign clinical course. They probably account for the majority of lymphoproliferations previously diagnosed as pseudolymphoma. More detailed understanding of the immunology and the genetic lesions associated with these diseases is likely to lead to a better understanding of their relationships, but their similarity has led to their being combined in a single diagnostic category, 'marginal zone B-cell lymphoma' in the Revised European–American Lymphoma (REAL) classification. This appears to be a separate entity from the splenic marginal zone lymphoma.

Enteropathy-associated T-cell lymphoma

Recently, a unique T-cell lymphoma, the neoplastic counterpart of intestinal mucosa-associated T-cells was described. This lymphoma is usually associated with a gluten-sensitive enteropathy (celiac disease or sprue) and was formerly called malignant histiocytosis of the intestine [90]. It is characterized by reactivity with a monoclonal antibody, HML-1, which also reacts with all intraepithelial T-cells and some 40% of T-cells in the intestinal lamina propria, but only occasionally with T-cells in lymph nodes, tonsils blood or skin [91].

Understanding the cellular origins of lymphomas

EARLY CONCEPTS OF HISTOGENESIS

Even a cursory consideration of the history of the classification of lymphoid neoplasms will rapidly lead to the conclusion that the identification of individual disease entities was generally not possible prior to the development of an understanding of the functional attributes of the normal counterpart cells of each neoplasm. The only exceptions to this were diseases in which the clinical manifestations or epidemiology were sufficiently unique that the existence of a true pathogenetic entity could be discerned. An excellent, but relatively recent example of this was the discovery of Burkitt's lymphoma in Africa. However, as has been emphasized already, early descriptions that could only be based on clinical features and gross pathology often encompassed several – often numerous – diseases as we now conceive them. As such, the nature of the disease could be discerned only vaguely, through its natural history, which was, in any event, often clouded by the presence of several quite different entities that on clinical grounds initially appeared to be one. Mycosis fungoides, recognized at about the same time as Hodgkin was describing primary disease of the absorbent glands, provides a good example of these problems. Alibert (1760–1837), a physician for skin diseases in Paris, first used the term 'mycosis fungoides' for what was formerly referred to as 'framboesia', a fungating skin condition first recognized in West Africa (as pian) and the West Indies (as yaws) [92]. As recorded by Kaposi (1837–1902) [93], Alibert believed the fungating condition of the face that he described to be related to syphilis. Kaposi, however, was confused by the observations that the disease may remain confined to the skin for long periods, but could also involve underlying structures and even, uncommonly, the viscera. He suggested that it was one of the 'sarcoid tumors' in which he included sarcomatosis but thought the more invasive forms might well be related, following Paltauf's suggestion, to pseudo-leukemia or lymphosarcoma. Kaposi's discussion, at the turn of the last century, highlights the prevailing uncertainty as to whether mycosis fungoides was an inflammatory skin condition or belonged to the sarcomas. In this same era, impassioned discussions were taking place regarding the nature of Hodgkin's disease and its relationship to tuberculosis. Until quite recently similar debates have continued in the context of a number of 'diseases', notably the angiocentric lymphomas (midline granuloma, lymphomatoid granulomatosis), and angioimmunoblastic lymphadenopathy, while the recent suggestion that Hodgkin's disease may sometimes be polyclonal [94], challenges our hard-won concepts regarding the neoplastic nature of that 'disease'. In these various conditions, as was the case in mycosis fungoides, the pathophysiology is still not understood. The presence of multiple cell types in a lesion brings uncertainty as to which, if any, are neoplastic cells, and it is probable that in many cases (including Hodgkin's disease), separate entities still reside under a single rubric.

The advent of histological examination provided a much more sensitive tool than clinical examination and gross pathology for classifying disease, and, in addition, at least the theoretical possibility of understanding the origins of neoplasms and their relationships to each other. Although greatly hampered in their endeavors by a lack of knowledge of the functional attributes of the normal cells observed in lymph nodes, pathologists made brave attempts to understand the cellular origins and pathogenesis of what they perceived as separate entities. Because of their almost exclusive dependence upon morphology, these efforts were largely confined to the liberal interpretation of morphological resemblances to normal cells. Differentiation pathways were surmised on the basis of the perception that some tumors had cytomorphology intermediate between different normal cell types, laced with a good deal of guesswork.

It was, perhaps, the greater interest in histological diagnosis, following Sternberg's and Reed's description of the histology of Hodgkin's disease, coupled to the development of the concept of a reticuloendothelial system [95], that led to the considerable interest in the histogenesis of tumors of the lymph nodes, spleen and bone marrow that was apparent in the first half of this century. In part, perhaps, because of the presence of some of the constituents of lymph

nodes (lymphocytes and monocytes, or macrophages) in the bloodstream, and the swelling of lymph nodes that accompanied leukemia – even, sometimes, of the myeloid type, the idea that all the elements of the blood were formed in the lymph nodes as well as the bone marrow persisted. At the same time, the notion of a protective system, based on phagocytosis, had emerged, stimulated, doubtless, by the developing concepts of the pathophysiology of inflammation and immunity that had begun to emerge in the last decades of the 19th century. The germ theory of the cause of disease had been well established by the work of Louis Pasteur (1822–1895) and Jacob Henle's student, Robert Koch (1843–1910), who, in 1882, had discovered the tubercle bacillus. Meanwhile, Elie Metchnikoff's (1845–1916) extensive studies on phagocytosis from 1885 [96], coupled to the absence of any understanding of immune mechanisms, were instrumental in the development of Aschoff's notions of a phagocytic reticuloendothelial system and in bringing them to prominence. By the 1920s, a detailed histological analysis of normal lymph nodes had been accomplished (Figure 2.1) and several cell types were well recognized. These included reticulum cells, endothelial cells (of the lymph node sinuses) and various

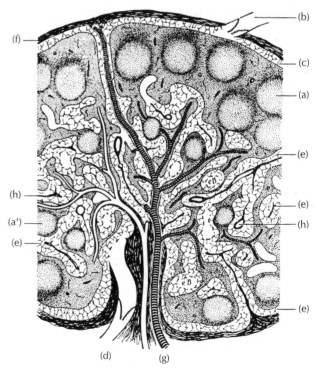

Figure 2.1 Normal lymph node (after Heudorfer [96a]. (a) Lymph follicle, (a') pseudofollicle, (b) afferent lymphatic, (c) cortical sinus, (d) efferent lymphatic, (e) medullary sinus, (f) capsule, (g) hilum vessels, (h) trabeculae. Taken from Robb-Smith [38].

and complexity of immune responses and the ontogeny of lymphocytes.

AN IMMUNOLOGICAL BASIS FOR UNDERSTANDING LYMPHOID NEOPLASMS

The field of immunology developed from attempts to
improve the diagnosis and therapy of bacterial
diseases, but it was not until the early 1960s that the
lymphocyte was recognized as the cell type involved
in the development of immunity. The discovery, in
1960, that the lymphocyte is not an end-stage cell,
but can undergo transformation to a large proliferating cell in response to mitogen, e.g., phytohemagglutinin, stimulation [105], led to dramatic advances
in the understanding of the physiological basis of
immunity and, simultaneously, to advances in the
understanding of the neoplasms of lymphocytes.
New tools with which to study lymphocytes and their
tumors were developed, initially reagents such as
polyclonal antibodies to detect surface immunoglobulin, sheep erythrocytes, either untreated or
coated with complement components [106], and
eventually, monoclonal antibodies [107], able to
react with exquisite specificity with various cellular
constituents and particularly valuable in the study of
surface markers. However, even before the full
impact of this biological revolution on the classification of lymphoid neoplasms had been felt, recognition that lymphocytes provide the cellular basis for
immunological reactions led to a conceptual change
in lymphoma taxonomy – at least, with respect to
the Rappaport classification system that had been
widely accepted in North America and, consequently, in many other countries in the world.

The reinstatement of follicular lymphoma

Follicular lymphomas have, since their recognition
in the late 1920s (albeit, initially considered to be
benign hyperplasias rather than neoplasms) occupied
an important – perhaps even a pivotal – role in
the classification of the non-Hodgkin's lymphomas.
This probably relates to the fact that the characteristic follicular pattern permitted reproducible separation from all other lymphomas – perhaps the only
reproducible and meaningful separation that could
be made in the first half of the present century – and
that these patients had a relatively good prognosis. It
is also true that the follicular lymphomas have made
up an increasing fraction of non-Hodgkin's lymphomas in North America and Europe as the century
has progressed, such that they have attracted increas-

ing attention. Today, these tumors account for less
than 10% of non-Hodgkin's lymphomas in developing countries, but as much as 40% in industrialized
nations. In Gall and Mallory's classic paper of 1942,
only 42 cases among the 389 (10.7%) non-Hodgkin's
lymphomas were observed, and it is quite likely that
the proportion was even lower in the 19th century –
Brill and his colleagues had been able to find at best a
single reported case in the earlier literature. It is
unlikely that pathologists able to recognize giant
cells in Hodgkin's disease would have failed to
observe the characteristic follicular pattern. This
alone might have suggested that the follicular
pattern indicated a disease, or group of similar
diseases, rather than being simply an alternative
manifestation of any of the non-Hodgkin's lymphomas. Indeed, this was the generally accepted
belief until Rappaport's reassessment in 1956 [47],
although Jackson had suggested that follicular lymphoma might represent an early form of lymphoma
that could become transformed into any other type
[108].

The term 'germinal centers' was proposed by
Flemming in 1885 [109], who believed them to be
the site of lymphocyte production – a view that
percolated into the pathology of lymphomas, since
many believed that lymphoid neoplasms, as opposed
to those derived from the reticuloendothelial elements of lymph nodes, might be considered to arise
from the germinal centers. Hellman, in contrast,
referred to germinal centers as 'Reaktionzentren',
i.e., the site of immunological reactions against
inflammatory or toxic insults [110]. Elements of
truth exist in both of these views but it was not until
the early 1970s that good evidence for the ability of
germinal center cells to synthesize antibodies was
provided [111]. Even before a functional understanding had been obtained, Lennert and his colleagues had performed a careful analysis of the cells
present in normal germinal centers and recognized
that these same cells were present in follicular
lymphomas [112–114]. Lennert referred to the smaller
lymphoid cells as 'germinocytes' (later, centrocytes) and the larger ones as 'germinoblasts' (later
centroblasts). He also recognized the presence of
immunoblasts and the desmosome-bearing dendritic
reticulum cell, a cell that had been described some
years earlier [115] and which appeared to be found
only in germinal centers. The dendritic reticulum cell
had already been associated, in some way, with
antigen [114]. Lennert concluded that germinocytes
and germinoblasts were transformed lymphocytes
and were, on the basis of morphological and cytochemical work conducted with several collaborators,
of lymphoid origin. These notions were supported by
the work of Lukes and Collins [116], and Kojima and
his collaborators [117]. In these studies, the exist-

ence of follicular lymphoma consisting of small lymphocytes was questioned.

These findings raised questions regarding the basis for Rappaport's classification scheme. Firstly, it appeared that follicular lymphomas probably did, after all, arise from germinal centers, and that the idea that all lymphomas are either nodular or diffuse was erroneous. Secondly, the notion that some lymphomas are mixtures of cells of histiocytic and lymphocytic origin, or indeed, that the large-cell types of lymphoma are of histiocytic origin was brought into question. Subsequent immunological evidence has confirmed that the large cells in the vast majority of large-cell lymphomas, or lymphomas consisting of mixed small and large cells, are of lymphoid origin, and that follicular lymphomas represent a single entity, or possibly a group of closely related entities that are of germinal center origin (or occasionally of mantle zone origin) [118–122]. This is entirely consistent with present immunological concepts whereby B-cells undergo an immune response in germinal follicles in relationship to antigen presenting cells (follicular dendritic cells, which appear to be important to the follicular architecture) and helper cells (T-cells). Some large-cell lymphomas in adults also appear to be comprised of large cells of germinal center origin as proposed by Lennert and Lukes. T-Cell lymphomas, like T-lymphocytes, never have a follicular pattern. Thus, the work of Lennert, Lukes, Kojima and colleagues did much to establish the concept, at a time of rapid advances in immunology, that lymphogenesis is closely related to the normal processes of lymphocyte activation and differentiation, providing a completely new way of understanding the lymphoid neoplasms (Table 2.6) [53,54]. Notwithstanding this new perspective, the Rappaport system, which had evolved prior to the era of rapid progress in immunological knowledge, was so well liked by clinicians – presumably largely because of its simplicity and familiarity – that it persisted until replaced by the Working Formulation. While it was frequently argued that the Rappaport scheme had clinical relevance, since patients with nodular lymphomas had a longer survival than those with diffuse lymphomas, in fact nodular variants of all lymphomas did not exist and the better survival of patients with follicular lymphoma was also observed in classifications that accepted this tumor as an entity originating from the germinal follicle.

Lymphocyte lineages and subpopulations

One of the most important immunological concepts from the perspective of lymphoma classification has been the division of the immune system, in the late 1960s, into cellular (T-cell-mediated) and humoral (B-cell-mediated) compartments, initially using surface immunoglobulin and sheep erythrocyte binding, and more recently, monoclonal antibodies. The latter have permitted finer and finer analysis of lymphocyte subpopulations in each of these arms of the immune system, and have been instrumental in the recognition of receptors and co-stimulatory molecules involved in lymphocyte activation, differentiation and homing. The application of immunological techniques to lymphoma classification has permitted not only improved separation of one entity from another, but the recognition that each lymphoma subtype can be equated with a subpopulation of lymphocytes or lymphocyte precursors, as postulated by Lennert and Lukes [53,54,123]. Even before monoclonal antibodies were used in classification, the B- or T-cell origin of a number of lymphomas and leukemias was established [106], while lymphoblastic lymphoma was demonstrated to be of precursor T-cell origin [124]. The old idea that large-cell lymphomas were derived from histiocytes was, in the vast majority of cases, quickly shown to be incorrect and it became possible to identify immunologically separate subtypes of lymphoma within what previously had been a single histological category. In some cases, monoclonal antibodies have permitted the recognition of lymphoma subtypes whose existence was not previously known, for example, anaplastic large-cell lymphoma, identified on the basis of strong reactivity with the Ki-1 antibody [78] that recognizes CD30, a receptor for a ligand belonging to the tumor necrosis factor family.

This process of identifying immunological subtypes of lymphoma has been continuously strengthened by the development of new monoclonal antibodies, and by the parallel evolution of the understanding of the immune system and its cellular compartments – major and minor. Considerable progress, for example, has been made recently in the understanding of the low-grade lymphomas (small-cell lymphomas in which survival is usually measured in years, even if patients are untreated). This should not, however, be solely attributed to the use of an ever-expanding arsenal of monoclonal antibodies but rather to the ability to bring several quite different disciplines to bear on the problem, including cytology, histology, immunological marker studies, and comparison with normal lymphocyte populations and their traffic patterns. With such evidence a substantial degree of certainty that a new entity has been defined can be provided and this will usually be accompanied by a characteristic clinical picture, although not necessarily a unique one.

In spite, however, of the power of modern analytical techniques for understanding the cellular origins of the non-Hodgkin's lymphomas, there remain many unresolved questions, perhaps par-

Table 2.6   The first classification systems based on immunological concepts (although histologically defined)

Lennert et al. (1974)	Lukes and Collins (1974)
Low-grade malignant lymphomas	
Lymphocytoma	
B-Cell types	B-Cell
CLL, hairy cell leukemia	Small lymphocytic (CLL)
T-Cell types	T-Cell
Sézary syndrome	Sézary's syndrome
(and mycosis fungoides?)	(and mycosis fungoides)
Others	
Immunocytoma (lymphoplasmacytoid)	
Lymphoplasmacytic	B-Cell
Lymphoplasmacytoid	Plasmacytoid lymphocyte
Polymorphic	
Germinocytoma (diffuse)	B-Cell
	Small cleaved FCC
	Large cleaved FCC
Germinoblastoma	
Follicular	Follicular
Follicular and diffuse	Follicular and diffuse
nonsclerotic	Diffuse
sclerotic (Bennett's type)	With or without sclerosis
High-grade malignant lymphomas	
Germinoblastic sarcoma	
	B-Cell
	Large noncleaved FCC
Lymphoblastic sarcoma (incuding ALL)	
B-Cell types	B-Cell
Burkitt's tumor	Small noncleaved FCC
Non-Burkitt's tumor	Burkitt type
T-Cell type	T-Cell
Convoluted type of Lukes	Convolute lymphocyte
Undefined	U-Cell (undefined)
Unclassifiable	Unclassifiable
Immunoblastic sarcoma	
	B-Cell
	Immunoblastic sarcoma
	T-Cell
	Immunoblastic sarcoma

ticularly within the area of T-cell lymphomas – lymphomas that are less common in Europe and the United States (although accounting for almost half of all lymphomas in some parts of Asia). This is because knowledge of the immune system remains incomplete with respect to the full complement of surface molecules that mediate the cellular interactions, activation and differentiation of lymphocytes, and the cellular traffic that mediates immunological responsiveness. There is little doubt that these gaps will be progressively filled in and, in the process, that some of our present concepts will need significant revision.

CYTOGENETICS AND MOLECULAR BIOLOGY

Improvements in cytogenetic techniques led to the recognition by Rowley in 1973 that the abnormally small G-group chromosome consistently present in chronic myeloid leukemia is caused by a translocation [125]. In 1982, Zech et al. [126] showed that the 14q+ abnormality discovered by Manolov and Manolova [127] in Burkitt's lymphoma is also caused by a chromosomal translocation and, in the same year, Yunis et al. recognized characteristic chromosomal abnormalities in follicular lymphomas and some large-cell lymphomas [128]. Thus it was demonstrated that specific genetic abnormalities are associated with particular neoplasms. The development of molecular cloning techniques led to the identification of the genes present at the breakpoints in each of these translocations, and, after identification of the functions of the genes concerned, to the elucidation, at least in essence, of the mechanisms whereby the genetic lesions in question lead to neoplastic behavior. Since these pioneering observations, many other genetic abnormalities have been detected in malignant lymphomas and our understanding of the molecular pathways involved in lymphomagenesis has continued to improve. These observations have refined our concepts of the nature of a pathological entity, but new questions have arisen because of the frequent lack of complete congruence of cytogenetic findings with histological or immunophenotypic findings. It is probable that former notions of clearly defined disease entities will, at least in some cases, need to give way to more flexible notions whereby lymphoid neoplasms undergo the same kind of cellular transformations as do their normal counterpart cells. In addition, the detection of several different types of chromosomal translocation in a single histological subtype (e.g., B-cell large-cell lymphoma [129]) should provide a tool beyond histology and even the present reach of immunophenotyping to separate individual pathological entities. This ought, eventually, to have a significant impact on therapy and to lead to the development of novel treatment approaches.

Molecular techniques have also proven valuable in other ways. Clonal rearrangements of antigen receptor genes can be used to determine lineage in cases where immunophenotyping is inconclusive (e.g., in the case of enteropathy-associated intestinal T-cell lymphoma [91], formerly believed to be of histiocytic origin) or to provide evidence of value in determining whether a pathological process is inflammatory or neoplastic (e.g., in angioimmunoblastic lymphadenopathy [130]). In all, there is little doubt that a combination of cytology, histology, immunophenotyping and molecular techniques has already led, and will continue to lead, to a more profound understanding of the nature of lymphoid neoplasia. While the number of recognized entities appears to be increasing rapidly, much to the dismay of clinicians who must not only become familiar with

each but be prepared to re-examine treatment approaches in attempting to define optimal therapy, there can be little doubt that the advances that have been made in understanding the pathogenesis of the non-Hodgkin's lymphomas – i.e., recognizing not only the genetic changes associated with malignant lymphomas, but their biochemical significance, will lead to further advances in classification and, perhaps of more pragmatic significance, eventually to tumor-specific approaches to therapy. Molecular analysis also shows promise of leading to an understanding of the mechanisms whereby environmental factors such as viruses and chemicals predispose to the development of malignant lymphomas [131,132].

Evolution of modern approaches to treatment

Active therapy for the malignant lymphomas has been available since the beginning of the 20th century, but it is only in the last 20 years that curative therapy for any patients except a fraction of those with localized disease could be contemplated. Prior to the development of therapeutic radiation facilities, arsenic, usually in the form of Fowler's solution, was frequently used, alongside various other medications, often given as 'tonics', but there is little or no evidence of any therapeutic efficacy of these measures [14]. Surgery can no longer be considered an appropriate modality of treatment when used in the absence of other therapy but, earlier in the century, the observation that a small number of patients with localized disease could be cured led to its advocacy by some [37,133]. In Gall and Mallory's series, only 10% of the 135 autopsied cases (which included Hodgkin's disease) had localized disease. Among 77 cases in whom surgery was attempted, resection was possible in only 33 and 12 of these patients lived an average of 7 years after the onset of their disease [37]. Gall subsequently reported on 39 patients with non-Hodgkin's lymphoma in whom surgery was considered possible [133]. Of these, complete removal of tumor was believed by the surgeon to have been accomplished in 17 patients. Some of these cases received subsequent adjuvant radiation. Gall concluded that surgical eradication improved survival for selected cases: 13 were alive beyond 5 years, and two for 10 years or more. Only four of these patients had primary lymph node disease, three of whom had follicular lymphoma, four had bone disease, and several had skin or eyelid disease. It is possible that some of these patients had MALT-type lymphomas, in which surgery remains the treatment of choice for localized disease. In Liu's series of ten patients with intestinal lymphoma who presented with intussusception, four were alive and free of disease 1.5–6 years after surgical resection [57], but in Cutler's series of children with intestinal lymphoma, only one out of five patients survived surgery and radiation [134]. These tiny series provide little more than anecdotes, but it is clear that patients with even potentially resectable lesions were few in number and the primary treatment modality for most of this century was therefore radiation, initially kilovoltage and subsequently megavoltage. Only recently has radiation largely been superseded by combination chemotherapy.

RADIATION THERAPY

The first report of the successful treatment of cancer by X-rays was published in 1899 by Sjögren [135], just 3 years after Roentgen (1845–1923) had discovered X-rays. In 1902, Pusey described the use of X-rays in a 24-year-old patient with a small round-cell sarcoma involving cervical lymph nodes, and in two cases of Hodgkin's disease [136]. All three patients had good responses, which must have been impressive in an era in which no therapy other than surgical excision had resulted in disease regression. The results in the early decades of radiation therapy, however, were usually temporary and recurrence in the radiation field or elsewhere was the rule. In addition, treatment was frequently associated with severe skin and soft tissue injury, and radiotherapy was further hindered by the unreliability of the early equipment. It was not until the invention of the Coolidge tube, in 1920, that 180 kV, and shortly thereafter, 200 and 250 kV machines became available for radiation therapy. The 250 kV machine became a standard that lasted until the era of megavoltage equipment (primarily ^{6}°-cobalt units and linear accelerators), which began in the 1950s.

Rather more success was obtained with radiotherapy in Hodgkin's disease in the 1930s and 1940s, largely by the irradiation of all known sites of disease followed by irradiation of adjacent healthy sites where recurrence, from experience, was likely. Then, in 1950, Peters reported an overall survival rate of 51% with rates of 88% for stage I and 72% for stage II Hodgkin's disease [137], but the results in the non-Hodgkin's lymphomas were much less promising, largely because of the less predictable pattern of spread. It was noted by Gall et al. in 1941 that follicular lymphomas appeared to be more sensitive to radiation than lymphosarcomas or reticulum cell sarcomas – 65% of 29 patients with follicular lymphoma had complete regression of lymphadeno-

pathy with long intervals between recurrences and an average survival duration after the commencement of therapy of 3.4 years [36]. Less than 10% of patients with the more aggressive lymphomas had such a response and about 35% had no response at all. In this series, patients received 600–1800 R with a 200 kV generator. Even in the megavoltage era, a high proportion of patients with localized diffuse aggressive lymphomas failed to achieve long-term disease-free survival, such that chemotherapy is indicated for such patients, while radiation alone can be considered only as palliative therapy in patients with more extensive disease [138]. In the small fraction of patients with low-grade lymphomas who have localized disease, radiation is generally considered to represent acceptable therapy, particularly in younger patients who have a high probability of remaining disease free at 10 years after radiation alone.

CHEMOTHERAPY

The modern era of chemotherapy could be said to have its beginnings in the Second World War, when, as part of a series of studies designed to examine the biological effects of chemical warfare agents, the lytic effect of the β-chloroethyl amines (nitrogen mustards) on lymphoid tissue and lymphosarcoma transplanted into mice was observed, and rapidly extended to the clinic [139,140]. In fact, the effect of mustard gas on the lymphoid organs and bone marrow had been known since the First World War [141], and was tragically confirmed in the Second World War when mustard gas was released from Allied ships bombarded in the harbour at Bari. In the 1940s, a number of trials of nitrogen mustards in the treatment of lymphosarcoma, Hodgkin's disease and leukemia were carried out in the United States [140,142,143]. Wintrobe, for example, reported a good effect (freedom from symptoms such that the patient could return to work for several months or more) of intravenous nitrogen mustard in 4 of 11 patients with lymphosarcoma and 17 of 28 patients with Hodgkin's disease [142]. In the 1950s, a series of alkylating agents, including chlorambucil and busulphan, were synthesized at the Chester Beatty Institute in London [144], and cyclophosphamide was developed in Germany [145].

Antimetabolites had also been developed in the 1940s and, in 1948, Farber reported disease regression (unfortunately, temporary) in acute leukemia for the first time, with the folate antagonist, aminopterine [146]. Aminopterine was soon replaced by methotrexate (amethopterine) and shortly after, the antimetabolites, 6-mercaptopurine and thioguanine (as well as allopurinol), were developed by Elion and coworkers [147]. When given in a continuous oral dosage of 75 mg/m^2, 6-mercaptopurine was shown to induce complete remissions in some 30–40% of children with acute lymphoblastic leukemia, a major advance [148]. Unfortunately, non-Hodgkin's lymphomas were not so successfully treated. In 1958, Rosenberg reported that 41.7% of 24 children with lymphosarcoma or reticulum cell sarcoma achieved an incomplete response (objective response lasting for more than a week) to antimetabolite drugs, but no complete responses were observed [35].

The vinca alkaloids were discovered in the late 1950s [149] and corticosteroids were also introduced into clinical trials in this decade, but with disappointing results, except in acute lymphoblastic leukemia, in which remission could be induced in 60–75% of patients [150,151]. During the 1960s, a number of additional newly synthesized drugs were tested, including the nitrosoureas [152], procarbazine [153] and the daunomycin [154], but by the end of the decade, the results of single agent therapy (with or without radiation) in the non-Hodgkin's lymphomas, even with the much larger armamentarium available, were still generally limited to temporary amelioration, although occasional dramatic results were obtained [155]. Somewhat more encouraging results were obtained in African Burkitt's lymphoma. Reports of long-term remissions in patients treated with only one or two doses of cyclophosphamide, or with orthomerphalan or melphalan [156,157] must have provided considerable encouragement to early chemotherapists, since it indicated that chemotherapy could, at least in some circumstances, eradicate disease completely.

In the 1960s, the exploration of simultaneous drug combinations was begun. This was a natural step following the observation that responses were often observed when a second drug was used after failure of a first, but was also based on theoretical considerations followed by experimental observations in the mouse models used by Goldin, Skipper, Bruce and others [158–161]. The principle of combination therapy is based upon synergy between agents whose toxicity is mediated via different pathways, and whose major side-effects are, at least to some extent, on different normal tissues. Initial combinations with three drugs, such as CVP (cyclophosphamide, vincristine and prednisone) produced good responses but poor long-term disease control. Meanwhile, investigators at the National Cancer Institute in Maryland explored a number of four-drug combinations in patients with various leukemias and lymphomas [162–166]. The initial combination, used in Hodgkin's disease – cyclophosphamide, methotrexate, vincristine and prednisone – resulted in prolonged survival in one out of five patients [162]. This was modified by replacing methotrexate with procarbazine and nitrogen mustard for cyclophosphamide, and alter-

ing the scheduling [163]. The resultant 'MOPP' regimen induced complete remission in 81% of 43 patients and at the time of the report, 17 patients remained in unmaintained remission for up to 52 months [166].

This dramatic result in Hodgkin's disease had a considerable influence on the drug combinations subsequently designed for the treatment of the non-Hodgkin's lymphomas in adults, particularly the diffuse large-cell (intermediate-grade) lymphomas. The substitution of cyclophosphamide for nitrogen mustard led to the combination called C-MOPP, which demonstrated, for the first time, that diffuse large-cell lymphomas (histiocytic lymphoma) were potentially curable [167]. The development of doxorubicin (Adriamycin) [168], bleomycin [169] and etoposide [170] in the 1970s permitted the successive introduction of the CHOP regimen (cyclophosphamide, doxorubicin, oncovin and prednisone) [171] and several variations, including BACOP [172], CHOP-Bleo [173] and COP-BLAM (see Chapter 28) [174]. Subsequently, the demonstration of the efficacy of (relatively) high-dose methotrexate with leucovorin rescue [175] led to its incorporation into additional drug combinations, e.g., M-BACOD [176], ProMACE-MOPP [177], ProMACE-CytaBOM [178] and MACOP-B (see Chapter 42) [179]. Initially, these newer regimens were believed to give increased survival rates compared to CHOP, but recent randomized studies have shown no advantage over CHOP; 40–50% of patients treated with any of these regimens survive without evidence of disease at 3 years [180–182]. Long-term survival (10 years or more) in diffuse large-cell lymphoma treated with CHOP (relapses may occur up to 7 years after the completion of therapy) appears to be approximately 30% [183]. These rather poor results have led to efforts to identify patients with a poor prognosis by detailed analysis of a variety of clinical factors at presentation, and to treat them with significantly more intensive therapy, e.g., by incorporating bone marrow transplantation into initial therapy (see below).

In the very aggressive childhood lymphomas, the greatest influences on the evolution of drug combinations came from the improving results in acute lymphoblastic leukemia and Burkitt's lymphoma rather than from Hodgkin's disease. The successful treatment – even apparent cures – achieved in African patients with Burkitt's lymphoma [156,157] led to similar strategies being employed at the National Cancer Institute in the USA, which had for some years collaborated with the University of Makerere in Kampala, Uganda, in the study of Burkitt's lymphoma. As in African children, some American patients with Burkitt's lymphoma, usually with limited disease, were cured with repeated doses of cyclophosphamide alone [184], and better results appeared to be achieved with three cycles of cyclophosphamide, methotrexate and vincristine [185]. At the same time, however, the high frequency of bone marrow recurrence in the childhood lymphomas (leukemic conversion), and the cytological similarities with acute lymphoblastic leukemias (particularly in the case of lymphoblastic lymphoma) seemed to indicate a close relationship between these diseases and suggested to many pediatric oncologists that similar types of therapy would be successful. Hence, in the 1970s, the use of the LSA_2L_2 and APO regimens (see Chapter 38) [186,187], both derived from treatment approaches used in acute lymphoblastic leukemia, were introduced and appeared to give good results – the former in all histological subtypes, the latter in lymphoblastic lymphomas. To determine which of these very different approaches was superior and whether histology was an important determinant of outcome, a randomized trial was initiated in 1977 by the Children's Cancer Study Group (CCG) of the USA. The 'lymphoma' treatment arm (COMP) (see Chapters 37 and 38) included cyclical drugs shown to be effective in Burkitt's lymphoma coupled to methotrexate with leucovorin rescue, after the demonstration by Djerassie of the efficacy of this approach in childhood lymphomas [188]. Unlike the treatments used in Burkitt's lymphoma, however, this regimen was continued for 18 months and radiation to sites of bulk disease was also given. The 'leukemia' treatment arm was LSA_2L_2, also continued for 18 months. The CCG trial demonstrated superiority for the LSA_2L_2 regimen in lymphoblastic lymphomas and better results with COMP in nonlymphoblastic lymphomas [189]. The results in nonlymphoblastic lymphomas, however, have since been greatly improved upon by the use of additional drugs and higher intensity therapy (with only a small number of treatment cycles and no radiation therapy) [190], and while very good results can be achieved with a leukemia type regimen in lymphoblastic lymphomas, it has also been shown that drugs in addition to COMP, particularly Adriamycin, considerably improve upon the results achieved with COMP.

In low-grade lymphomas, in contrast to intermediate- and high-grade lymphomas, combination regimens such as CVP and CHOP have shown only minor advantages (e.g., in complete remission rates), over single agent therapies and, overall, little progress has been made since the introduction of chlorambucil into therapy, at least for long-term survival. Thus, quite widely different approaches, ranging from no immediate treatment to bone marrow transplantation as a component of primary therapy, are currently being explored [191].

VERY HIGH-DOSE THERAPY

The principles of therapy determined in mouse models [158–160] suggested that, for most drugs, there is a linear relationship between drug dose and response rate of human tumors. In the high-grade lymphomas, combinations of drugs have been highly effective but, in the intermediate-grade lymphomas, a significant fraction of patients are not cured. Similarly, there is still no evidence that cure has been achieved in patients with low-grade lymphomas, excepting in those few that present with localized disease. In 1959, bone marrow grafting was shown to be capable of restoring normal hematopoiesis to patients accidentally irradiated to very high dosage [192]. A number of investigators subsequently explored the use of this approach in patients who had relapsed. It held promise of circumventing the potentially lethal marrow toxicity that would result from very high doses of myelotoxic agents and total body irradiation that might be necessary to cure such patients with disease demonstrably resistant to conventional doses of chemotherapy [193]. Reinfusions of bone marrow obtained from a matched (at histocompatibility loci) or partially matched allogeneic donor, or, as is more often the case in non-Hodgkin's lymphomas, from the patient (autograft) have been shown to be capable of curing a fraction of patients who relapse. It has become apparent that a poor response to salvage therapy predicts for a poor outcome to high-dose therapy with autologous bone marrow transplantation, while perhaps 40% of patients whose lymphoma is still responsive to salvage therapy are alive 2 years after an autologous bone marrow transplant [194]. These results have led to further exploration of the role of high-dose therapy and bone marrow transplantation as part of primary therapy (i.e., after remission induction) in patients unlikely to be cured by conventional approaches.

COLONY-STIMULATING FACTORS

Another possible means of permitting increased dose intensity of chemotherapeutic agents is to use naturally occurring factors that induce proliferation and differentiation in hematopoietic precursor cells. Attempts to understand hematopoiesis have been underway in the laboratory since the 1960s, but it was only after the developments in molecular biology that permitted the cloning and generation of large quantities of recombinant molecules that these factors became available for clinical use. The first clinical studies were conducted in 1986. While it is now clear that these factors can reduce the severity of myelosuppression and reduce the incidence of complications related to this in patients treated with intensive therapy, including bone marrow transplantation, it has yet to be shown that dose intensity can be sufficiently increased to result in higher rates of complete remission or lower rates of relapse. Colony-stimulating factors, however, have been shown to increase the level of circulating hematopoietic stem cells, particularly if given after chemotherapy, making possible the 'rescue' of patients treated with high-dose therapy by means of peripheral stem cells without the need for formal bone marrow transplant. Further, peripheral stem cell rescue after high-dose treatments can be used in individual patients on multiple occasions.

Whatever the value of high-dose therapy supported by stem cell infusions proves to be, perhaps more significant than the approach itself is the theoretical knowledge of hematopoiesis that has made it possible. Similarly, it is to be hoped that progress in understanding lymphopoiesis will not only lead to an improved understanding of lymphomagenesis, but also to improved classification of the lymphoid tumors, and to the development of novel therapies that are specific for lymphoma cells and have minimal toxicity. While this may seem, at first sight, to be the stuff of fantasy, what to the present generation of oncologists is routine – curative drug therapy, made possible, in part, by modern supportive care (antibiotic therapy, blood product support, which has not been discussed in this chapter but which is an essential element of modern therapy) – was surely the stuff of fantasy for our forebears, who labored with so little success to understand and treat the malignant lymphomas for much of the first half of the present century. Viewed, then, from an historical perspective, and based on the present rate of progress, it becomes clear that in the course of the next century, barring unanticipated human disasters, the development of highly effective, minimally toxic therapy, which will make our present attempts appear primitive, is not simply probable, it is inevitable.

References

1. Virchow R. *In Die krankhaften Geschwülste*. Dreissig Vorlesungen gehalten wahrend des Winter-semesters 1862–1863 an der Universitat zu Berlin. Hirschwald, Berlin 1864–1865, pp. 564–620.
2. Cruickshank W. *The Anatomy of the Absorbing Vessels of the Human Body*. London: G. Nicol, 1786.
3. Craigie D. *Elements of General Pathological Anatomy*. Edinburgh: Adam Black, 1828, p. 250.
4. Hodgkin T. On some morbid appearances of the absorbent glands and spleen. *Trans. Med. Chir. Soc. Lond.* 1832, **xvii**: 68–114.
5. Wilks S. Cases of lardaceous disease and some allied affections, with remarks. *Guy's Hosp. Rep.* 1856, **17** (Ser. II, vol. 2): 102–132.
6. Wunderlich CA. Zwei Fälle von progressiven muliplen Lymphdrüsenhypertrophien. *Arch. Physiol. Heilk.* 1858, **12**: 122–131.
7. Trousseau A. De l'adénie. *Clin. Méd. l'Hotel-Dieu Paris* 1865, **3**: 555–581.
8. Wilks S. Cases of enlargement of the lymphatic glands and spleen (or, Hodgkin's disease), with remarks. *Guy's Hosp. Gaz.* 1865, **23**: 528–532.
9. Cohnheim J. Ein Fall von Pseudoleukämia. *Virchows Arch.* 1862, **33**: 451–454.
10. Virchow R. *Weisses Blut*. Neue Notizen aus dem Gebiet der Natur und Heilkunde (Froriep's Neue Notizen) 1845, **36**: 151–156.
11. Craigie D. Case of disease of the spleen in which death took place in consequence of purulent matter in the blood. *Edinburgh Med. Surg. J.* 1845, **64**: 400–413.
12. Bennett JH. Case of hypertrophy of the spleen and liver, in which death took place from suppuration of the blood. *Edinburgh Med. Surg. J.* 1845, 64: 413–423.
13. Wunderlich CA. *Pesudoleukämie, Hodgin'sche Krankheit oder multiple Lymphadenome ohne Leukämie.* Arch. d. Heilkunde, 1866, 531–552.
14. Osler W. *The Principles and Practice of Medicine*. New York: Appleton and Company, 1892, pp. 704–708.
15. Dreschfeld J. Clinical lecture on acute Hodgkin's (or pseudoleucocythemia). *Br. Med. J.* 1882, **1**: 893–896.
16. Kundrat H. Über Lymphosarkomatosis. *Wiener kl. Wochenshr.* 1893, **6**: 211–213, 234–239.
17. Stevens. *Glasgow Med. J.* 1891.
18. Sternberg C. Über ein eigenartige unter dem Bilde der Pseudoleukämie verlaufende Tuberculose des Lymphatischen Apparates. *Z. Heilk.* 1898, **xix**: 21–90.
19. Pel PK. Pseudoleukämie oder chronisches Rückfallsfieber. *Berlin Klin. Wochenschr.* 1885, **24**: 644–646.
20. Ebstein W von. Das chronische Rückfallsfieber. *Berl. kl. Wochenschr.* 1887, **24**: 565–568.
21. Reed DM. The pathological change of Hodgkin's disease with special reference to its relation to tuberculosis. *Johns Hopkins Med. Rep.* 1902, **x**: 133–196.
22. Coley WB. Hodgkin's disease, a type of sarcoma. *N. York Med. J.* 1907, **lxxxv**: 577–583.
23. Paltauf R. Lymphosarkom (Lymphosarkomatose, Pseudoleukämia, Myelom, Chlorom). *Ergebn. allg. Path. path. Anat.* 1896, **3**: 652–691.
24. Sternberg C. Primärerkrankungen des lymphatischen und hämatopoetischen Apparates etc. *Erg. allgem. Path.* 1903, 9.
25. Ghon A, Roman. Über Lymphosarkom. *Frank Z. Path.* 1916, **xix**: 1.
26. Ginsburg S. Lymphosarcoma and Hodgkin's disease: Biologic characteristics. *Ann. Int. Med.* 1934, 14–36.
27. Ewing J. General pathology of lymphosarcoma. *Bull. N. York Acad. Med.* 1939, **15**: 92–103.
28. Oliver J. The relation of Hodgkin's disease to lymphosarcoma and endothelioma. *J. Med. Res.* 1913, **xxix**: 191–207.

29. Oberling C. Les réticulosarcomes et les réticuloendothéliosarcomes de la moelle osseuse (sarcomes d' Ewing). *Bull. Assoc. Franc étude Cancer* 1928, **17**: 250–256.

30. Roulet F. Das Primäre Retothelesarkom der Lymphknoten. *Virchows Arch. Path. Anat.* 1930, **277**: 15–47.

31. Borst M. *Die Lehre von den Geschwülsten.* Wiesbaden, 1902.

32. Brill NE, Baehr G, Rosenthal N. Generalized giant lymph follicle hyperplasia of the lymph nodes and spleen. *JAMA* 1925, **84**: 668–671.

33. Symmers D. Follicular lymphadenopathy with splenomegaly. A newly recognized disease of the lymphatic system. *Arch. Path. Lab. Med.* 1927, **3**: 816–820.

34. Evans TS, Doan CA. Giant follicle hyperplasia: A study of its incidence, histopathologic variability, and the frequency of sarcoma and secondary hypersplenic complications. *Ann. Intern. Med.* 1954, **40**: 851–880.

35. Rosenberg SA, Diamond HD, Dargeon HW, et al. Lymphosarcoma in childhood. *N. Engl. J. Med.* 1958, **259**: 505–512.

36. Gall EA, Morrison HR, Scott AT. The follicular type of malignant lymphoma: A survey of 63 cases. *Ann. Intern. Med.* 1941, **14**: 2073–2090.

37. Gall EA, Mallory TB. Malignant lymphoma. A clinico-pathological survey of 618 cases. *Am. J. Path.* 1942, **18**: 381–429.

38. Robb-Smith AHT. Reticulosis and reticulosarcoma: Histological classification. *J. Pathol. Bacteriol.* 1938, **47**: 457–480.

39. Callender GR. Tumors and tumor like conditions of the lymphocyte, the myelocyte, the erythrocyte and the reticulum cell. *Am. J. Path.* 1934, **10**: 443–465.

40. Stout AP. The results of treatment of lymphosarcoma. *N. York State J. Med.* 1947, **47**: 158–164.

41. Sugarbaker ED, Craver LF. Lymphosarcoma: A study of 196 cases with biopsy. *JAMA* 1940, **115**: 17–23, 112–117.

42. Warren S, Picena JP. Reticulum cell sarcoma of lymph nodes. *Am. J. Path.* 1941, **17**: 385–393.

43. Gall EA. Enigmas in lymphoma, reticulum cell sarcoma and mycosis fungoides. *Minnesota Med.* 1955, **38**: 674–681.

44. Gall EA, Rappaport H. Seminar on diseases of lymph nodes and spleen. In *Proceedings of the 23rd Annual Seminar of the American Society of Clinical Pathologists*, October, 1957. American Society of Clinical Pathologists, 1958.

45. Rosenberg SA. Classification of lymphoid neoplasms. *Blood* 1994, **84**: 1359–1360.

46. Carbone PP, Berard CW, Bennett JM, et al. NIH clinical staff conference: Burkitt's tumor. *Ann. Intern. Med.* 1969, **70**: 817–832.

47. Rappaport H, Winter WJ, Hicks EB. Follicular lymphoma. A re-evaluation of its position in the scheme of malignant lymphoma, based on a survey of 253 cases. *Cancer* 1956, **9**: 792–821.

48. Rappaport H. Tumors of the hematopoietic system. In *Atlas of Tumor Pathology*, Section III, Fascicle 8. Washington, DC: Armed Forces Institute of Pathology, 1966, pp. 97–161.

49. Rappaport H, Braylan RC. In Rebuck JW, Berard CW, Abell MR (eds) *The Reticuloendothelial System.* International Academy of Pathology Monograph, no. 16. Baltimore: Williams and Wilkins, 1975, pp. 1–19.

50. Bennett MH, Farrer-Brown G, Henry K, et al. Classification of non-Hodgkin's lymphomas. *Lancet* 1974, **2**: 405–406.

51. Dorfman RF. The non-Hodgkin's lymphomas. In Rebuck JW, Berard CW, Abell MR (eds) *The Reticuloendothelial System.* International Academy of Pathology Monograph, no. 16. Baltimore: Williams and Wilkins, 1975, pp. 262–281.

52. Mathé G, Rappaport H, O'Conor GT, et al. Histological and cytological typing of neoplastic diseases of hematopoietic and lymphoid tissues. *WHO International Classification of Diseases*, no. 14. Geneva: World Health Organisation, 1976.

53. Lennert K, Mohri N, Stein H, et al. The histopathology of malignant lymphoma. *Br. J. Haematol.* 1975, **31** (Suppl. II): 193–203.

54. Lukes RJ, Collins RD. Immunologic characterization of human malignant lymphomas. *Cancer* 1974, **34**: 1488–1503.

55. National Cancer Institute Sponsered Study of Classifications of Non-Hodgkin's Lymphomas. Summary and description of a working formulation for clinical usage. *Cancer* 1982, **49**: 2112–2135.

56. Harris N, Jaffe ES, Stein H, et al. A revised European–American classification of lymphoid neoplasms: A proposal from the international lymphoma study group. *Blood* 1994, **84**: 1361–1392.

57. Liu JH. Tumors of the small intestine, with especial reference to the lymphoid cell tumors. *Arch. Surg.* 1925, **xi**: 602–618.

58. Davies JNP, Elmes S, Hutt MSR, et al. Cancer in an African community, 1897–1956. An analysis of the records of Mengo Hospital, Kampala, Uganda, Part 1. *Br. Med. J.* 1964, **1**: 259–264.

59. Davies JNP, Elmes S, Hutt MSR, et al. Cancer in an African community, 1897–1956. An analysis of the records of Mengo Hospital, Kampala, Uganda, Part 2. *Br. Med. J.* 1964, **1**: 336–341.

60. Smith EC, Elmes BGT. Malignant disease in natives of Nigeria: An analysis of five hundred tumors. *Ann. Trop. Med. Parasit.* 1934, **28**: 461–512.

61. Edington GM. Malignant disease in the Gold Coast. *Br. J. Cancer* 1956, **10**: 595–608.

62. Thijs A. Considérations sur les tumeurs malignes des indigénes du Congo belge et du Ruanda-Urundi. A propos de 2536 cas. *Ann. Soc. Belge Med. Trop.* 1957, **37**: 483–514.

63. DeSmet MP. Observations cliniques de tumeurs malignes des tissus réticuloendothéliaux et des tissus hémolymphopoiétiques au Congo. *Ann. Soc. Belge Med. Trop.* 1956, **36**: 53–70.

64. Burkitt D. A sarcoma involving the jaws in African children. *Br. J. Surg.* 1958, **46**: 218–223.

65. Burkitt D, O'Conor GT. Malignant lymphoma in African children. I. A clinical syndrome. *Cancer* 1961, **14**: 258–269.

66. Burkitt D. Determining the climatic limitations of a children's cancer common in Africa. *Br. Med. J.* 1962, **2**: 1019–1026.

67. O'Conor GT, Davies JNP. Malignant tumors in African children with special reference to malignant lymphomas. *J. Pediat.* 1960, **56**: 526–535.
68. O'Conor G. Malignant lymphoma in African children. Cancer. II. A pathological entity. *Cancer* 1961, **14**: 270–283.
69. O'Conor G, Rappaport H, Smith EB. Childhood lymphoma resembling Burkitt's tumor in the United States. *Cancer* 1965, **18**: 411–417.
70. Dorfman RF. Childhood lymphosarcoma in St Louis, Missouri, clinically and histologically resembling Burkitt's tumor. *Cancer* 1965, **18**: 418–430.
71. Wright DH. Burkitt's tumor in England a comparison with childhood lymphosarcoma. *Int. J. Cancer* 1966, **1**: 503–514.
72. Epstein MA, Achong BG, Barr YM. Viral particles in cultured lymphoblasts from Burkitt's lymphoma. *Lancet* 1964, **i**: 702–703.
73. Ortner N. *Wien. Klin. Wochenschr.* 1890, **3**: 937–938.
74. Sternberg C. *Br. J Path.* 1905, **61**: 75–100.
75. Barcos MP, Lukes RJ. Malignant lymphoma of convoluted lymphocytes – a new entity of possible T-cell type. In Sinks JF, Godden JO (eds) *Conflicts in Childhood Cancer: An Evaluation of Current Management.* New York: Alan Liss, 1975, pp. 147–178.
76. Nathwani BN, Kim H, Rappaport H. Malignant lymphoma, lymphoblastic. *Cancer* 1976, **38**: 2121–2131.
77. Dargeon HW. Lymphosarcoma in childhood. *Adv. Pediat.* 1953: **6**: 13–32.
78. Stein H, Mason DY, Gerdes J, et al. The expression of Hodgkin's disease associated antigen Ki-1 reactive and neolastic lymphoid tissue: Evidence that Reed–Sternberg cells and histiocytic malignancies are derived from activated lymphoid cells. *Blood* 1985, **66**: 848–858.
79. Lennert K. *Pathologie der Halslymphknoten. Ein Abriss für Pathologen, Kliniker and praktizierende Ärtze.* Berlin: Springer, 1964.
80. Berard C, Dorfman R. Histopathology of malignant lymphomas. *Clin. Haematol.* 1974, **3**: 39–76.
81. Weisenberger DD, Kim H, Rappaport H. Mantle zone lymphoma: A follicular variant of intermediate lymphocytic lymphoma. *Cancer* 1982, **49**: 1429–1438.
82. Raffeld M, Jaffe E. bcl–1, t(1;14), and mantle cell-derived lymphomas. *Blood* 1991, **78**: 259–263.
83. Banks P, Chan J, Cleary ML, et al. Mantle cell lymphoma. A proposal for unification of mophologic, immunologic, and molecular data. *Am. J. Surg. Path.* 1992, **16**: 637–640.
84. Isaacson P, Wright DH. Malignant lymphoma of mucosa-associated lymphoid tissue. A distinctive type of B-cell lymphoma. *Cancer* 1984, **52**: 1410–1416.
85. Pelstring RJ, Essell JH, Kurtin PJ, et al. Diversity of organ site involvement among malignant lymphomas of mucosa-associated tissues. *Am. J. Clin. Pathol.* 1991, **96**: 738–745.
86. Sheibani K, Sohn C, Burke J, et al. Monocytoid B-cell lymphoma. A novel B-cell neoplasm. *Am. J. Pathol.* 1986, **124**: 310–318.
87. Shin SS, Sheibani K. Monocytoid B-cell lymphoma. *Am. J. Clin. Pathol.* 1993, **99**: 421–425.
88. Ortiz-Hidalgo, Wright DH. The morphological spectrum of monocytoid B-cell lymphoma and its relationship to lymphomas of mucosa-associated lymphoid tissue. *Histopathology* 1992, **21**: 555–561.
89. Nizze H, Cogliatti SB, Von Schilling C, et ai. Monocytoid B-cell lymphoma: Morphological variants and relationship to low-grade B-cell lymphoma of the mucosa associated lymphoid tissue. *Histopathology* 1991, **18**: 403–414.
90. Isaacson PG, Spencer J, Connolly CE, et al. Malignant histiocytosis of the intestine: A T-cell lymphoma. *Lancet* 1985, **ii**: 688–691.
91. Stein H, Dienemann D, Sperling M, et al. Identification of a T cell lymphoma category derived from intestinal-mucosa-associated T cells. *Lancet* 1988, **2**: 1053–1054.
92. Alibert JLM. *Description des maladies de la peau, observé á l'hôpital Saint-Louis, et expositions des meillieurs méthodes suivies pour le traitement.* Paris: Barrois L'Aine et Fils, 1806–1827.
93. Kaposi M. Mycosis fungoides (framboesia). In *Pathology and Treatment of Diseases of the Skin for Practitioners and Students.* New York: Willian Wood and Co., 1895, pp. 593–598.
94. Delabie J, Tierens A, Wu G. Lymphocyte predominance in Hodgkin's Disease: Lineage and clonality determination using a single-cell assay. *Blood* 1994, **84**: 3291–3298.
95. Aschoff L. *Das retikuloendotheliale System. Vorträge über Pathologie.* Jena, 1905.
96. Metchnikoff E. Untersuchungen über die intracelluläre Verdaung bei wirbellosen Thieren. *Arb. zool. Inst. Univ. Wien.* 1883, **5**: 141–168.
96.a Heudorfer. *Z. Anat. U. Entwickl.* 1921, **lxi**: 365.
97. Maximow AA. Relation of blood cells to connective tissues and endothelium. *Physiol. Rev.* 1924, **iv**: 431.
98. Klemperer P. Relationship of the reticulum to diseases of the hematopoietic system. In *Libman Anniversary Volumes*, Vol. 2. New York: The International Press, 1932, p. 665.
99. Ewing JJ . Endothelioma of lymph nodes. *J. Med. Res.* 1913, **28**: 1.
100. Ewing JJ. Diffuse endothelioma of bone. *Proc. N. York Pathol. Soc.* 1921, **21**: 17–24.
101. Willis RA. *The Spread of Tumors in the Human Body.* London: J and A Churchill Ltd, 1934.
102. Medlar EM. An interpretation of the nature of Hodgkin's disease. *Am. J. Path.* 1931, **7**: 499–513.
103. Rhoads CP. The reticulo-endothelial system. A general review. *N. Engl. J. Med.* 1928, **198**: 76–78.
104. Parker F Jr, Jackson H Jr. Primary reticulum cell sarcoma of bone. *Surg. Gynec. Obst.* 1939, **68**: 45–53.
105. Nowell PC. Phytohemagglutinin: An initiator of mitosis in cultures of normal human leukocytes. *Cancer Res.* 1960, **20**: 462–466.
106. Seligmann M, Grouet JC, Preud'Homme JL. The immunological diagnosis of human leukemias and lymphomas. An overview. In Thierfelder S, Rodt H, Thiel E (eds) *lmmunological Diagnosis of Leukemias and Lymphomas.* Berlin: Springer Verlag, 1977, pp. 1–16.

nating with standard agents (M-BACOD). *J. Clin. Oncol.* 1983, **1**: 91–98.

177. Longo DL, DeVita VT, Duffey PL, et al. Superiority of ProMACE-CytaBOM over ProMACE-MOPP in the treatment of advanced diffuse aggressive lymphoma: Results of a prospective randomized trial. *J. Clin. Oncol.* 1991, **9**: 25–38.

178. Fisher RI, DeVita VT, Hubbard SM, et al. Diffuse aggressive lymphomas: Increased survival after alternating flexible sequences of ProMACE and MOPP chemotherapy. *Ann. Intern. Med.* 1983, **98**: 304–309.

179. Klimo P, Connors JM. MACOP-B chemotherapy for the treatment of diffuse large cell lymphoma. *Ann. Intern. Med.* 1985, **102**: 596–602.

180. Gordon Ll, Harrington D, Andersen J, et al. Comparison of a second generation combination chemotherapeutic regimen (m-BACOD) with a standard regimen (CHOP) for advanced diffuse non-Hodgkin's lymphoma. *N. Engl. J. Med.* 1992, **327**: 1342–1349.

181. Cooper IA, Wolf MM, Robertson TI, et al. Randomized comparison of MACOP-B with CHOP in patients with intermediate-grade non-Hodgkin's lymphomas. The Australian and New Zealand Lymphoma Group. *J. Clin. Oncol.* 1994, **12**: 769–778.

182. Fisher RI, Gaynor ER, Dahlberg S, et al. Comparison of standard regimen (CHOP) with three intensive chemotherapy regimens for advanced non-Hodgkin's lymphoma. *N. Engl. J. Med.* 1993, **328**: 1002–1006.

183. Coltman CN Jr, et al. CHOP is curative in thirty percent of patients with large cell lymphoma: A twelve-year South West Oncology Group follow up. Advances in cancer chemotherapy. Update on treatment for diffuse large cell lymphoma. *Proceedings of the Symposia*, November 14–17, 1985, Marco Island, Florida, 1986, pp. 71–82.

184. Arseneau JC, Canellos GP, Banks PM, et al. American Burkitt's lymphoma – a clinicopathological study of 30 cases. I. Clinical factors relating to prolonged survival. *Am. J. Med.* 1975, **58**: 314–321.

185. Ziegler JL. Treatment results of 54 American patients with Burkitt's lymphoma are similar to the African experience. *N. Engl. J. Med.* 1977, **297**: 75–80.

186. Wollner N, Burchenal JH, Liebermann PH, et al. Non-Hodgkin's lymphoma in children. A comparative study of two modalities of therapy. *Cancer* 1976, **37**: 123–134.

187. Weinstein HJ, Cassady Jr, Levey R. Long-term results of the APO protocol (vincristine, doxorubicin [adriamycin] and prednisone) for treatment of mediastinal lymphoblastic lymphoma. *J. Clin. Oncol.* 1983, **1**: 537–541.

188. Djerassi I, Kim JS. Methotrexate and citrovorum factor rescue in the management of childhood lymphosarcoma and reticulum cell sarcoma (non-Hodgkin's lymphomas): Prolonged unmaintained remissions. *Cancer* 1976, **38**: 1043–1051.

189. Anderson JR. The results of a randomized therapeutic trial comparing a 4-drug regimen (COMP) with a 10-drug regimen (LSA₂L₂). *N. Engl. J. Med.* 1983, **308**: 559–565.

190. Reiter A, Schrappe M, Parwaresch R, et al. Non-Hodgkin's lymphomas of childhood and adolescence: Results of a treatment stratified for biologic subtypes and stage – a report of the Berlin-Frankfurt-Münster group. *J. Clin. Oncol.* 1995, **13**: 359–372.

191. Lister TA. The management of follicular lymphoma. *Ann. Oncol.* 1991, **2** (Suppl. 2): 131–135.

192. Jammet H, Pendic G, Schwarzenberg L, et al. Transfusions et greffes de moelle osseuse homologue chez des humains irradié á haute dose accidentellement. *Rev. Fr. Etude Clin. Biol.* 1959, **4**: 226–238.

193. Thomas D. The role of marrow transplantation in the eradication of malignant disease. *Cancer* 1982, **49**: 1963–1969.

194. Philip T, Armitage JO, Spitzer N, et al. High dose chemotherapy and ABMT in 100 adults with intermediate or high grade non-Hodgkin's lymphoma. *N. Engl. J. Med.* 1987, **316**: 1493–1497.

PART 2

Pathology

CHAPTER 3

Histopathology and immunopathology

ELAINE S. JAFFE

Introduction

The classification of the malignant lymphomas has undergone significant reappraisal over the past 40 years. These changes have resulted from insights gained through the application of immunological and molecular techniques, as well a better understanding of the clinical aspects of lymphoma through advances in diagnosis, staging and treatment. While at one point lymphomas were seen as no more than four or so generic types (lymphosarcoma, reticulum cell sarcoma, giant follicle lymphoma and Hodgkin's disease), currently many different distinct entities are recognized. Each variant can be distinguished by a combination of morphologic, immunophenotypic and genotypic analyses, and each is associated with a characteristic clinical behavior, pattern of spread and response to therapy.

Historically, the Rappaport classification, first introduced in 1956, divided lymphomas according to pattern, either nodular or diffuse, and then according to cell type, based on the degree to which the lymphoid cells morphologically resembled either normal lymphocytes or histiocytes [1]. The advances in immunology that occurred in the 1970s made it apparent that this approach was flawed and that the cells termed 'histiocytic' were for the most part transformed lymphocytes. In addition, the recognition of T-cells, B-cells and various other subsets made it reasonable to see lymphomas in functional terms, each deriving from a unique cell type. Both the Kiel classification, proposed by Karl Lennert and colleagues [2,3], and the Lukes–Collins scheme [4] were immunologically based, although at the time immunologic techniques were still in their infancy, and monoclonal antibodies as a diagnostic tool were not yet available.

By the 1970s, six different classifications had been proposed, and at least four were in use: the Rappaport (Table 3.1) and Lukes–Collins schemes in the United States; the Kiel classification (Table 3.2) in Europe; and the classification of the British National Lymphoma Investigation (BNLI) [5] in Great Britain. Although several meetings attended by both pathologists and clinicians were held in an attempt to reach consensus (in London, Florence, Italy and Airlie, Virginia), no agreement could be reached. The National Cancer Institute responded to this situation by sponsoring a study to test each of the classification schemes, using a data base containing clinical data from approximately 1200 cases of lymphoma treated on prospective clinical trials from four different institutions [6].

This study indicated that each of the schemes was capable of segregating the tumors into broad groups of low, intermediate and high clinical grade, as determined by survival, but no one scheme appeared superior to any other. Moreover, the study demonstrated both a relatively high lack of reproducibility by individual pathologists (0.53–0.93) when confronted by the same slides on a second review, as

Table 3.1   Modified Rappaport classification

Nodular
Lymphocytic, poorly differentiated
Mixed lymphocytic–histiocytic
Histiocytic

Diffuse
Lymphocytic, well differentiated
Lymphocytic, intermediate differentiation
Lymphocytic, poorly differentiated
Mixed lymphocytic–histiocytic
Undifferentiated, Burkitt's type
Undifferentiated, non-Burkitt's type
Histiocytic
Lymphoblastic

well as a low rate of concordance among the various pathologists (0.21–0.65) in trying to reproduce diagnoses within a given scheme. It should be noted that the pathologists were restricted to only routine hematoxylin and eosin-stained sections, and limited clinical information: age, sex and anatomic site. Nevertheless, the clinicians involved in this study reached the conclusion that 'clinical outcome' was a reasonable basis for a lymphoma classification scheme, since agreement could not be achieved regarding the individual pathologic entities.

The participants proposed the Working Formulation (WF) for the non-Hodgkin's lymphomas (NHLs) based on the clinical and pathological findings (Table 3.3). The original intent was to have the WF serve as a common language to translate among classifications and not to serve as a free-standing classification scheme. However, because it was a convenient guide to therapy, it quickly became popular among clinicians and was adopted for use in many centers in the USA for clinical trials. In reality the WF was in essence the Rappaport scheme. It

Table 3.2   Kiel (Lennert's) classification (1974)

Low-grade malignancy
Lymphocytic
Lymphoplasmacytoid
Centrocytic
Centroblastic–centrocytic
   Follicular
   Follicular and diffuse
   Diffuse

High-grade malignancy
Centroblastic
Lymphoblastic
   Burkitt's type
   Convoluted cell type
Immunoblastic

Table 3.3   Working Formulation for clinical usage

Working Formulation

Low-grade
A. Malignant lymphoma, small lymphocytic
   Consistent with CLL
   Plasmacytoid
B. Malignant lymphoma, follicular, predominantly small cleaved cell
   Diffuse areas
   Sclerosis
C. Malignant lymphoma, follicular, mixed, small cleaved and large cell
   Diffuse areas
   Sclerosis

Intermediate grade
D. Malignant lymphoma, follicular, predominantly large cell
   Diffuse areas
   Sclerosis
E. Malignant lymphoma, diffuse, small cleaved cell
   Sclerosis
F. Malignant lymphoma, diffuse, mixed, small and large cell
   Sclerosis
   Epithelioid cell component
G. Malignant lymphoma, diffuse, large cell
   Cleaved cell
   Noncleaved cell
   Sclerosis

High grade
H. Malignant lymphoma, large cell, immunoblastic
   Plasmacytoid
   Clear cell
   Polymorphous
   Epithelioid cell component
I. Malignant lymphoma, lymphoblastic
   Convoluted cell
   Nonconvoluted cell
J. Malignant lymphoma, small noncleaved cell
   Burkitt's
   Follicular areas

Miscellaneous
   Composite
   Mycosis fungoides
   Histiocytic
   Extramedullary plasmacytoma
   Unclassifiable
   Other

substituted the term 'large cell' for 'histiocytic' and divided the 'histiocytic' lymphomas of the Rappaport scheme into two subgroups: large cell and large cell immunoblastic. This separation split the 'histiocytic'

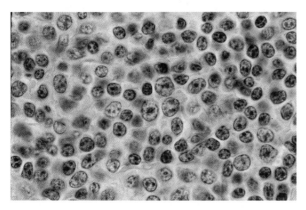

Plate 3.1 Chronic lymphocytic leukemia/small lymphocytic lymphoma. The cellular infiltrate in lymph nodes usually is comprised of small round lymphocytes, as well as prolymphocytes and paraimmunoblasts.

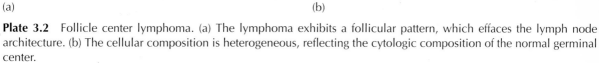

(a)   (b)

Plate 3.2 Follicle center lymphoma. (a) The lymphoma exhibits a follicular pattern, which effaces the lymph node architecture. (b) The cellular composition is heterogeneous, reflecting the cytologic composition of the normal germinal center.

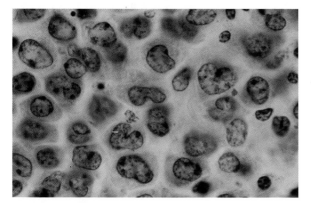

Plate 3.3 Large B-cell lymphoma. In most cases the cells resemble large noncleaved cells (centroblasts) and large cleaved cells.

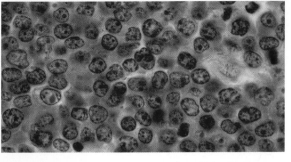

(a)

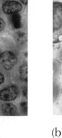

(b)

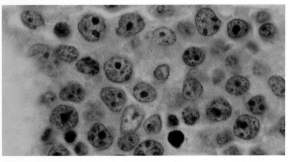

(c)

Plate 3.4 Burkitt and Burkitt-like lymphomas. (a) In classical Burkitt's lymphomas the cells are very uniform with small basophilic nucleoli. (b) In Wright–Giemsa-stained smears, intense basophilia of the cytoplasm is seen. Cytoplasmic vacuoles are prominent. (c) Burkitt-like lymphomas show greater variation in cell size and the nucleoli are usually more prominent.

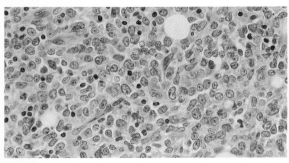

(a)

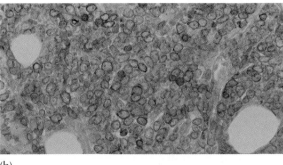

(b)

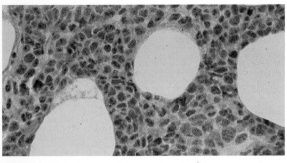

(c)

Plate 3.5 Lymphoblastic lymphoma, precursor T-cell phenotype. (a) The cells have sparse cytoplasm and finely distributed chromatin. (b) The cells contain cytoplasmic CD3, stained in paraffin sections by immunoperoxidase technique. (c) The cells also stain for TDT, with positive reactivity in nuclei.

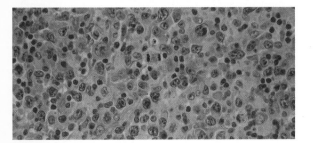

Plate 3.6 Peripheral T-cell lymphoma, unspecified. The infiltrate is polymorphous. Eosinophils are numerous. Some larger cells resemble Reed–Sternberg cells and variants.

Table 3.4 Updated Kiel classification of non-Hodgkin's lymphomas (1992)

B	T
Low-grade malignant lymphomas	
Lymphocytic	Lymphocytic
Chronic lymphocytic leukemia	Chronic lymphocytic leukemia
Prolymphocytic leukemia	Prolymphocytic leukemia
Hairy cell leukemia	Small cell, cerebriform
Lymphoplasmacytic/cytoid (immunocytoma)	Mycosis fungoides/Sézary's syndrome
Plasmacytic	Lymphoepithelioid (Lennert's lymphoma)
Centroblastic–centrocytic (follicular ± diffuse; diffuse)	Angioimmunoblastic (AILD)
Centrocytic (mantle cell)	T-zone lymphoma
Monocytoid, including marginal zone cell	Pleomorphic, small cell (HTLV-1 ±)
High-grade malignant lymphomas	
Centroblastic	Pleomorphic, medium-sized and large cell (HTLV-1 ±)
Immunoblastic	Immunoblastic (HTLV-1 ±)
Burkitt's lymphoma	Large-cell anaplastic (Ki-1+)
Large-cell anaplastic (Ki-1+)	
Lymphoblastic	Lymphoblastic

Other rare types of lymphoma may be separately identified for T- and B-cell lymphomas, respectively.

lymphomas among the intermediate- and high-grade categories, a division that has been controversial and not supported by subsequent analyses.

Another more basic flaw in the WF is that it is a classification based on treatment outcome, not the recognition of individual disease entities or cell of origin for a malignant neoplasm. This conceptual approach is a significant deviation from the way in which classification systems have been developed for other organ systems. It lumps diseases that share a similar cell size and survival into single categories, and splits diseases with variations in cytologic composition and clinical grade into separate categories.

Of the classifications originally tested in the National Cancer Institute study, only the Kiel classification has remained in widespread use, mainly in Europe and Asia. It is a functionally based classification, which divides tumors mainly according to their cell of origin, as well as other cytologic features. Several revisions have been published in recent years, with the addition of some of the more newly described entities, such as anaplastic large-cell lymphoma (ALCL) (Table 3.4).

However, several aspects of the Kiel scheme remain not universally accepted. For one, it is intended for nodal lymphomas only. It has become apparent that lymphomas arising in extranodal sites, whether they be of T- or B-cell origin, are often distinct and do not simply represent secondary spread of nodal disease. Moreover, its adherence to a relatively pure cytologic approach limits its utility in the delineation of certain diseases, such as nasal T-/natural killer (NK) cell lymphoma, and adult T-cell leukemia/lymphoma, both of which are delineated in part by their modes of presentation, epidemiology and respective viral associations, Epstein–Barr virus (EBV), and the human T-cell lymphotropic virus (HTLV)-1 [7,8]. Moreover, its failure to subclassify or grade follicular lymphomas has made it unpopular in the USA, where follicular lymphoma is the most common single disease, accounting for at least 40% of all NHLs. By contrast, it attempts to delineate several different subtypes of large B-cell lymphoma and several morphologic variants of node-based peripheral T-cell lymphoma. It remains to be shown that these distinctions are reproducible by others, and whether they are either biologically or clinically relevant.

In this chapter, the classification scheme proposed by the International Lymphoma Study Group (ILSG), which is a revision of former European and American schemes (Table 3.5) will be used. The authors of this scheme believe that the cell of origin, principally T-cell or B-cell, must be the starting point of any modern classification scheme. Stage of differentiation is also important, although in many instances the precise stage of differentiation is unknown. The classification delineates individual disease entities, based on morphologic features, immunophenotype and/or stage of differentiation, genotype, etiology, epidemiology and clinical behavior. In many instances several different entities that share some clinical characteristics, such as an indolent (low grade) or aggressive (intermediate or high grade) natural history are contained within a single WF category. Many of the entities are also

Table 3.5 Revised European–American lymphoma classification from the International Lymphoma Study group

B-Cell neoplasms

Precursor B-cell neoplasms
Precursor B-lymphoblastic leukemia/lymphoma

Peripheral B-cell neoplasms
1. B-Cell CLL/PLL/SLL
2. Lymphoplasmacytoid lymphoma/immunocytoma
3. Mantle cell lymphoma
4. Follicle center lymphoma, follicular
   Provisional cytologic grades: I (small), II (mixed), III (large)
   Provisional subtype: diffuse, predominantly small cell
5. Marginal zone B-cell lymphoma
   Extranodal (MALT ± monocytoid B-cells)
   Provisional category: nodal (± monocytoid B-cells)
6. Provisional entity: splenic marginal zone lymphoma
7. Hairy cell leukemia
8. Plasmacytoma/myeloma
9. Diffuse large B-cell lymphoma
10. Burkitt's lymphoma
11. Provisional entity: high-grade B-cell lymphoma, Burkitt-type

T-Cell and putative NK cell neoplasms

Precursor T-cell neoplasm
Precursor T-lymphoblastic lymphoma/leukemia

Peripheral T-cell and NK cell neoplasms
1. T-Cell CLL/PLL
2. Large granular lymphocyte leukemia
3. Mycosis fungoides/Sézary syndrome
4. Peripheral T-cell lymphomas, unspecified
   Provisional categories: medium, mixed, large, lymphoepithelioid
   Provisional subtypes
      Hepatosplenic γδ T-cell lymphoma
      Subcutaneous panniculitic T-cell lymphoma
5. Adult T-cell lymphoma/leukemia
6. Angioimmunoblastic T-cell lymphoma
7. Angiocentric lymphoma
8. Intestinal T-cell lymphoma (± enteropathy)
9. Anaplastic large cell lymphoma (T/null)
10. Provisional: ALCL Hodgkin's-like

Hodgkin's disease
1. Lymphocyte predominance (nodular ± diffuse)
2. Nodular sclerosis
3. Mixed cellularity
4. Lymphocyte depletion
5. Lymphocyte-rich classical HD (provisional subtype)

It should be noted that the ILSG classification also includes Hodgkin's disease (HD). It has become apparent that the cell of origin of HD is almost certainly a lymphoid cell. Moreover, a sharp distinction between HD and NHL is often not possible. Instances of composite HD/NHL and sequential HD/NHL further indicate a close relationship [9]. Therefore, while for clinical purposes we segregate HD and NHL, conceptually it is appropriate for them to be included in any classification scheme of lymphomas. The ILSG classification includes all lymphoid neoplasms. However, for the purposes of this chapter those entities other than the non-Hodgkin's lymphomas will be touched on only briefly, or in the case of HD, not discussed.

The authors of the ILSG classification recognize that many distinct lymphoma entities manifest a range of both histologic grades and degrees of clinical aggressiveness. This point is exemplified by the follicle center lymphomas (FCL) (follicular lymphoma in the WF). FCL is recognized as a single disease entity with a common molecular pathogenesis in the vast majority of cases. However, variations in cytologic grade are a valid basis for stratifying patients for therapy. The same applies to many of the entities in the ILSG scheme. To aid in deciding upon optimal therapy, the predominant clinical behavior for each of the subtypes is provided (Table 3.6). Patients could be stratified according to these clinical groupings for clinical trials, as is commonly done for the low-, intermediate-, and high-grade categories of the WF, and yet each disease entity could also be analyzed separately in order to observe differences in response to therapy, patterns of relapse or biologic parameters among different diseases.

B-Cell neoplasms

PRECURSOR B-LYMPHOBLASTIC LEUKEMIA/LYMPHOMA (BLBL/L)

(WF: malignant lymphoma, lymphoblastic; Kiel: lymphoblastic, B-cell type.)

While most BLBL/Ls present as leukemia, lymphomatous presentations occur in approximately 5–10% of cases [10–12] (Figure 3.1). Frequent sites of involvement include lymph nodes, skin and bone. Skin lesions in children frequently present in the head and neck region, including the scalp [10]. Progression to leukemia will occur in the vast majority of cases if a complete remission is not obtained. The disease is most common in children

recognized in the Kiel classification. Therefore, both the designation adopted by the ILSG as well as the most equivalent terms in the WF and Kiel classification will be provided.

Table 3.6 Suggested clinical groups of entities recognized by the ILSG classification

I. Indolent lymphomas
B-Cell
  B-CLL/SLL
  Lymphoplasmacytoid lymphoma
  Follicle center lymphoma, follicular (small and mixed)
  Marginal zone B-cell lymphoma
  Hairy cell leukemia
  Plasmacytoma/myeloma
T-Cell
  Large granular lymphocyte leukemia
  ATL/L (smoldering)
  Mycosis fungoides/Sézary syndrome

II. Moderately aggressive lymphomas
B-Cell
  B-PLL
  Mantle cell lymphoma
  Follicle center lymphoma (follicular large cell)
T-Cell
  T-CLL/PLL
  ATL/L (chronic)
  Angiocentric lymphoma
  Angioimmunoblastic lymphoma

III. Aggressive lymphomas
B-Cell
  Large B-cell lymphoma
T-Cell
  Peripheral T-cell lymphomas
  Intestinal T-cell lymphoma
  Anaplastic large-cell lymphoma

IV. Highly aggressive lymphomas
B-Cell
  Precursor BLBL/L
  Burkitt's lymphoma
  High-grade B-cell lymphoma, Burkitt-like
T-Cell
  Precursor TLBL/L
  ATLL (acute and lymphomatous)

and young adults. This disease is considered the solid tumor equivalent of common acute lymphoblastic leukemia and pre-B-cell acute lymphoblastic leukemia.

Cytologically, it is composed of lymphoblasts that are usually somewhat larger than a small lymphocyte but smaller than the cells of large B-cell lymphoma [13]. The cells have finely stippled chromatin with very sparse cytoplasm and inconspicuous nucleoli. The nuclei may be round or convoluted, but the presence or absence of nuclear convolutions is not useful in predicting immunophenotype in lymphoblastic malignancies. Mitotic figures are fre-

quent, in keeping with the high-grade nature of this neoplasm.

The differential diagnosis of BLBL/L includes the blastic variant of a mantle cell lymphoma (MCL) [14]. The cells of MCL usually have more abundant cytoplasm and some evidence of chromatin clumping. The clinical presentation is useful in that MCL is much more common in adults.

In some cases immunophenotypic studies will be required for the differential diagnosis. The blastic variant of MCL is terminal deoxynucleotide transferase (TdT)– and has a mature B-cell phenotype, in contrast to BLBL/L, which demonstrates an immature B-cell phenotype. The cells are TdT+ and usually express CD 10 and CD 19 [12,15]. CD 20 is present in fewer than 50% of cases. A very useful marker is CD 79a, which can be detected in paraffin sections [16].

B-CELL CHRONIC LYMPHOCYTIC LEUKEMIA (B-CLL), PROLYMPHOCYTIC LEUKEMIA (B-PLL) AND SMALL LYMPHOCYTIC LYMPHOMA (B-SLL)

(WF: small lymphocytic, consistent with CLL; Kiel: B-CLL, B-PLL, immunocytoma, lymphoplasmacytoid type.)

B-CLL/SLL usually presents in adults with generalized lymphadenopathy, frequent bone marrow and peripheral blood involvement, and often hepatosplenomegaly. Presentation as leukemia, i.e., B-CLL, is more common than as lymphoma, B-SLL. Even in patients with a lymphomatous presentation, careful examination of the peripheral blood may disclose a circulating monoclonal B-cell component. Nevertheless, there are some patients who will present with generalized lymphadenopathy and, while progression to leukemia is frequent, it does not necessarily occur in all cases [17].

Histologically, the lymph nodes involved by B-CLL/SLL show diffuse architectural effacement, although occasional residual naked germinal centers may be present. In this regard, the process may simulate a MCL but can usually be readily distinguished from MCL on cytologic grounds. While the predominant cell is a small lymphocyte with clumped nuclear chromatin, a spectrum of nuclear morphology is usually seen (Plate 3.1). Pseudofollicular growth centers or proliferation centers are present in the majority of cases [18]. These proliferation centers contain a spectrum of cells ranging from small lymphocytes to larger prolymphocytes and paraimmunoblasts. The prolymphocytes and paraimmunoblasts have somewhat more dispersed chromatin and usually centrally placed prominent nucleoli.

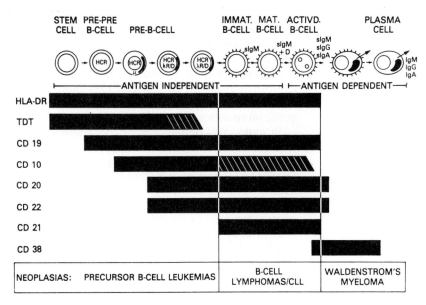

Figure 3.1 Schematic diagram of B-cell differentiation, as it relates to the malignant lymphomas and leukemias. Most NHL are at a mature B-cell stage and express monoclonal sIg. CD 79a, which is not pictured, is expressed at the stage of heavy-chain gene rearrangement (HCR), and is found in most plasma cells and approximately 50% of plasma cell malignancies. R, rearranged; D, deleted; IMMAT., immature; MAT., mature; ACTIVD., activated.

There is a moderate amount of amphophilic cytoplasm. Paraimmunoblasts are larger than prolymphocytes but in other respects are similar.

In some cases, the small lymphoid cells may show nuclear irregularity. This feature has caused confusion with MCL. However, the presence of pseudofollicles and paraimmunoblasts argues strongly in favor of a diagnosis of B-CLL/SLL over MCL. It has been shown that cases with cleaved nuclear morphology and pseudofollicles retain the indolent clinical behavior of B-CLL/SLL, and not the more aggressive clinical course of MCL [19,20]. If needed, immunophenotypic studies can be helpful in this differential diagnosis, since the cells of B-CLL/SLL are usually CD23+, whereas the cells of MCL are usually CD23− [21]. Surface immunoglobulin expression and expression of CD20 and CD22 are weaker in B-CLL/SLL than in MCL or FCL [22]. B-CLL/SLL is CD19+ and co-expresses CD5 [23, 24,25]. In paraffin sections, CD43 is co-expressed with CD20 and CD79a [26].

Mitotic rate has been shown to be prognostically important in B-CLL/SLL. While the presence of pseudofollicles does not necessarily indicate a more aggressive clinical course, a high mitotic rate (>30 mitoses per 20 high-powered fields) is associated with more aggressive disease and shortened survival [27]. As with B-CLL, prolymphocytic transformation may occur in lymph nodes and the end-point in this process is an aggressive large B-cell lymphoma, so-called Richter's syndrome [28]. However, some of the large B-cell malignancies occurring in B-CLL/SLL appear to be secondary, derived from a separate B-cell clone.

A Hodgkin's-like transformation has also been described in B-CLL/SLL. This transformation can take one of two forms. In some cases Reed–Sternberg cells and mononuclear variants are seen in a background of small, round B-lymphocytes, consistent with B-CLL [29]. The process lacks the rich inflammatory background characteristic of Hodgkin's disease, such as eosinophils, plasma cells and histiocytes. However, patients with this type of Hodgkin's transformation appear to progress to a process that is more typical of Hodgkin's disease, with loss of the B-cell small lymphocytic component. In other instances classical Hodgkin's disease of the mixed cellularity or nodular sclerosis subtype may be seen in patients with a history of B-CLL [30]. Studies have implicated EBV in the HD type of Richter's transformation [31]. The Reed–Sternberg cells and variants are EBV+ and the implication is that they are derived from the underlying B-cell clone.

In some cases of B-CLL/SLL, limited plasmacytoid differentiation may occur [32]. The overall cytology may resemble that of B-CLL/SLL, but the cells contain moderate amounts of cytoplasmic immunoglobulin. In such cases a small monoclonal immunoglobulin spike may be detected in the serum. These cases conform to the lymphoplasmacytoid subtype of immunocytoma in the Kiel classification [33]. However, because such cases retain the immunophenotype of classical B-CLL, they are regarded in the ILSG classification as a variant of B-CLL [34].

LYMPHOPLASMACYTOID LYMPHOMA/IMMUNOCYTOMA (LPL)

(WF: small lymphocytic, plasmacytoid; Kiel: immunocytoma, lymphoplasmacytic type.)

This tumor conforms in most cases to the clinical picture of Waldenström's macroglobulinemia. This is a disease of adult life that usually presents with generalized lymphadenopathy, vague constitutional symptoms, anemia and splenomegaly. Autoimmune hemolytic anemia is a common complication. IgM monoclonal gammopathy may be associated with increased serum viscosity leading to neurologic and vascular complications. Peripheral blood involvement with an absolute lymphocytosis is less common in LPL than in B-cell CLL/SLL.

The neoplastic cells in LPL show evidence of plasmacytic differentiation [35,36]. They have been referred to as 'lymphoplasmacytoid' because, while the cytoplasm assumes a distinctly plasmacytic appearance with amphophilic cytoplasm and a perinuclear *HOF*, the nucleus retains the condensed nuclear chromatin characteristic of a lymphocyte. Usually, a spectrum of plasmacytoid differentiation is seen, with the most plasmacytoid-appearing cells found in a perivascular and perisinusoidal location. Dutcher bodies are another characteristic cytologic feature of LPL. An interesting architectural feature of LPL is the tendency for lymphoid sinuses to be preserved, and even congested and distended. This apparent preservation of nodal architecture may cause problems in diagnosis. However, careful examination will usually reveal absence of follicles and paracortical regions, indicating architectural effacement by the lymphoid neoplasm.

Those cells showing plasmacytoid differentiation can usually be demonstrated to contain cytoplasmic immunoglobulin, even in paraffin section immunohistochemistry. Immunophenotypically, this tumor lacks CD5, in contrast to B-CLL/SLL and by analogy can be related to a late stage in B-cell differentiation, just prior to the plasma cell stage [21,37]. Conceptually, it can be related to a postfollicular medullary cord B-cell, in contrast to B-CLL/SLL, which appears to be prefollicular in its stage of differentiation [35]. CD20 expression is variable, as CD20 is lost at the mature plasma cell stage of development.

MANTLE CELL LYMPHOMA (MCL)

(WF: diffuse or follicular, small cleaved cell (rarely diffuse large cleaved cell); Kiel: centrocytic lymphoma.)

MCL is a distinct clinical pathologic entity that has been more precisely defined in recent years through the integration of immunophenotypic, molecular genetic and clinicopathologic studies [38,39]. This tumor had been recognized in the Kiel classification as centrocytic lymphoma and in the modified Rappaport scheme as lymphocytic lymphoma of intermediate differentiation. Early on it was noted that this tumor tended to surround residual naked germinal centers and a derivation from the follicular lymphoid cuff was postulated [40]. Tumors with a very conspicuous mantle zone pattern of growth were also termed 'mantle zone lymphoma' [41]. This tumor is not recognized in the WF, but most cases would fall within the category of diffuse small cleaved cell. However, a vaguely follicular pattern may lead to a diagnosis of follicular, small cleaved cell. The blastic variant, to be described below, would be considered as a large cleaved cell in the WF in some cases.

MCL occurs in adults, with a high male:female ratio. Most patients present with stage III or IV disease at diagnosis [42, 43]. Common sites of involvement include the lymph nodes, spleen, bone marrow and lymphoid tissue of Waldeyer's ring. Gastrointestinal tract involvement is frequent and is associated with the picture of lymphomatous polyposis [44]. Like the low-grade lymphomas in the WF, this tumor appears to be incurable with available treatment. Although initial complete remissions may be obtained, the relapse rate is high. However, the median survival is shorter than for most other low-grade lymphomas in the WF and is in the range of 3–5 years. The median survival of the blastic variant is less than 3 years [14]. The relatively short median survival places this tumor in the intermediate-grade category in the WF.

The hallmark of MCL is a very monotonous cytologic composition. Within a given case the cells are usually of comparable size and share similar cytologic features. In the typical case, the cells are slightly larger than a normal lymphocyte with finely clumped chromatin, scant cytoplasm and inconspicuous nucleoli (Figure 3.2). The nuclear contour is usually irregular or cleaved. However, in some cases nuclear irregularities may be minimal, leading to a diagnosis of small lymphocytic lymphoma in the WF. Transformed cells resembling centroblasts or immunoblasts are essentially absent, providing an important distinction from follicle center lymphomas. In addition, transformation to a large-cell lymphoma, a common event in many other low-grade lymphomas, is not seen.

Approximately 25% of cases of MCL have cells with large nuclei, more dispersed chromatin and a higher proliferation fraction. This cytologic variant has been termed the 'blastic' variant, because of the resemblance of the cells to lymphoblasts [14]. Indeed, immunophenotypic studies may be required

B-cell lymphoma (MALT lymphomas discussed but not included in classification scheme).)

Most lymphomas of marginal zone derivation present in extranodal sites and have the histopathologic and clinical features identified by Isaacson and Wright as part of the spectrum of MALT lymphomas [67,68]. MALT lymphomas are characterized by a heterogeneous cellular composition that includes marginal zone or centrocyte-like cells, monocytoid B-cells, small lymphocytes and plasma cells. In most cases, large transformed cells are infrequent. Reactive germinal centers are nearly always present. Therefore, it is not surprising that based on the heterogeneous cellular composition and presence of reactive follicles, most MALT lymphomas were diagnosed in the past as pseudolymphomas or atypical hyperplasias. However, recent studies have shown the majority to be composed of monoclonal B-cells. The follicles of involved lymph nodes usually contain reactive germinal centers, but the germinal centers may become colonized by neoplastic cells. When follicular colonization occurs, the process may simulate follicular lymphoma [69]. The plasma cells are usually found in the subepithelial zones and are monoclonal in up to 50% of cases.

MALT lymphomas have been described in nearly every anatomic site but are most frequent in the stomach, lung, thyroid, salivary gland and lacrimal gland [37,70]. Other less common sites of involvement include the orbit, breast, conjunctiva, bladder and kidney, and thymus gland [71]. Most patients present with localized disease, although regional lymph node involvement is common in gastric and salivary gland MALT lymphoma. The involved lymph nodes in those cases resemble monocytoid B-cell lymphoma, and it is thought that monocytoid B-cell lymphoma is the nodal equivalent of a MALT lymphoma [72–75]. Widespread nodal involvement is infrequent, as is bone marrow involvement. The clinical course is usually quite indolent and many patients are asymptomatic. MALT lymphomas tend to relapse in other MALT-associated sites. For example, a patient with a salivary gland lymphoma may relapse with lacrimal gland involvement or conjunctival disease [37].

MALT lymphomas of the salivary gland are usually associated with Sjögren's syndrome and a history of autoimmune disease. Similarly, MALT lymphomas of the thyroid are associated with Hashimoto's thyroiditis. *Helicobacter* gastritis is frequent in most patients with gastric MALT lymphomas, and it has been suggested that antigen stimulation is critical to both the development of a MALT lymphoma and the maintenance of the neoplastic state [76]. Indeed antibiotic therapy and eradication of *Helicobacter pylori* has led to the spontaneous

remission of gastric MALT lymphoma in some cases [77].

Isolated MALT lymphomas are usually treated with surgery or radiation, chemotherapy being reserved for more widespread disease. MALT lymphomas, when they disseminate, have a survival similar to other low-grade lymphomas [78]. As noted above, most MALT lymphomas are clinically low grade and contain a paucity of large transformed cells. However, histologic progression may occur, and the end-point in this progression is a diffuse large B-cell lymphoma.

Monocytoid B-cell lymphoma is seen most often in association with an extranodal MALT lymphoma [79]. However, the existence of the primary extranodal disease may not be immediately apparent. Relapses in nodal sites may occur many years after primary diagnosis. A morphologically similar but different phenomenon is monocytoid B-cell differentiation in a primary nodal lymphoma. Cells resembling monocytoid B-lymphocytes have been described in many low-grade lymphomas, most commonly FCL [80]. The monocytoid B-cell component appears to occupy the marginal zone. Nevertheless, the immunophenotype and genotype of the neoplastic cells is that of FCL. The monocytoid differentiation is an interesting morphologic variant but does not appear to have independent clinical or biological significance. The survival is that of FCL.

Immunophenotype is helpful in the differential diagnosis of MALT lymphomas from cytologically similar low-grade lymphomas such as B-CLL/SLL and MCL. MALT lymphomas are positive for B-cell-associated antigens CD19, CD20, and CD22, but are negative for CD5, in contrast to most systemic small lymphocytic malignancies [37]. MALT lymphomas also have a commonly recurring cytogenetic abnormality, and show trisomy 3 in 60% of cases, regardless of site of presentation [81]. Other cytogenetic changes including numerical abnormalities of chromsomes 7 and 12, and the t(11;18) have also been reported [82,83].

Many cutaneous B-cell lymphoma, particularly cutaneous immunocytomas, have features reminiscent of MALT lymphomas in other sites. These lymphomas tend to remain localized in the skin, with a low risk of systemic dissemination [66]. Cutaneous immunocytomas often present solitary or localized lesions affecting the extremities [84]. They often contain germinal centers and plasma cells and in the past had probably been considered 'pseudolymphomas' (Figure 3.3). However, immunophenotypic studies show evidence of monoclonality.

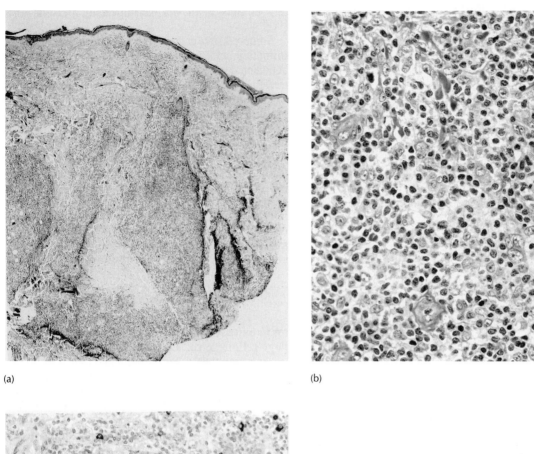

(a)

(b)

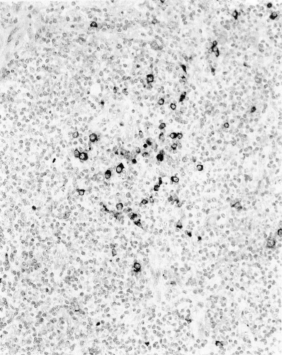

(c)

Figure 3.3 Cutaneous B-cell lymphoma (immunocytoma). (a) The infiltrate is extensive in the dermis, without epidermal involvement. (b) The cytologic composition resembles that of MALT lymphoma. (c) Plasmacytoid cells stain for kappa light chain by immunoperoxidase in paraffin sections.

SPLENIC MARGINAL ZONE LYMPHOMA (PROVISIONAL CATEGORY)

(WF: small lymphocytic, small lymphocytic plasmacytoid; Kiel: not listed.)

Recent studies have shown that small lymphocytic lymphomas presenting with predominant splenomegaly and minimal lymphadenopathy differ in their immunophenotype from those presenting primarily with lymph node and bone marrow involvement. Whereas typical B-CLL/SLL are CD5+, splenic small lymphocytic lymphomas are usually CD5– [85]. Careful attention to the cytologic features in these cases indicates that the cells have somewhat more abundant cytoplasm than those of typical B-CLL/SLL and resemble the lymphocytes of the normal splenic marginal zone. The nuclei are usually predominantly round but may be slightly irregular. They have a moderate amount of pale cytoplasm. Histologically, the spleen shows expansion of the white pulp, but usually some infiltration of the red pulp is present as well [86]. In early cases, preferential involvement of the marginal zone may be seen [87].

Splenic marginal zone lymphomas present in adults and are slightly more frequent in females than males. The clinical presentation is splenomegaly, usually without peripheral lymphadenopathy. The majority of patients have bone marrow involvement, but there is usually only a modest lymphocytosis, with elevations in the lymphocyte count usually less than seen in B-CLL. Some evidence of plasmacytoid differentiation may be seen and patients may have a small M component. The abundant pale cytoplasm evident in tissue sections may also be seen in peripheral blood smears. The cytologic features may be mistaken for hairy cell leukemia. The disorder described as splenic lymphoma with villous lymphocytes (SLVL) appears equivalent to splenic marginal zone lymphoma [88,89]. The course is reported to be indolent, and splenectomy may be followed by a prolonged remission.

PLASMACYTOMA/PLASMA CELL MYELOMA

(WF: extramedullary plasmacytoma; Kiel: plasmacytic lymphoma.)

Plasmacytomas are rare in lymph nodes but occur with some frequency in extranodal sites. Patients with localized plasmacytomas involving lymph nodes or other organs are at risk to develop systemic disease, i.e., plasma cell myeloma. The majority of localized plasmacytomas are well differentiated, clinically low grade and morphologically composed of normal-appearing plasma cells [90].

Some plasma cell malignancies are composed of immature cells with prominent central nucleoli and abundant deeply amphophilic cytoplasm [91]. Marked nuclear irregularity may be seen in rare cases [92]. This morphologic appearance has been termed 'anaplastic myeloma'. Patients with this high-grade histology are at greater risk to develop disease outside the bone marrow, e.g., lymph nodes, spleen, liver. In addition, anaplastic myeloma may be difficult to distinguish from large-cell immunoblastic lymphoma exhibiting plasmacytoid differentiation. The cells contain abundant monoclonal cytoplasmic immunoglobulin and may lack B-cell-associated antigens. The clinical behavior of these high-grade malignancies is more similar to aggressive lymphoma than typical multiple myeloma.

DIFFUSE LARGE B-CELL LYMPHOMA

(WF: diffuse mixed small and large cell, diffuse large cell, large cell immunoblastic; Kiel: centroblastic, immunoblastic, large-cell anaplastic (B-cell).)

Diffuse large B-cell lymphomas are composed of large, transformed lymphoid cells with nuclei at least twice the size of a small lymphocyte (Plate 3.3). The nuclei generally have vesicular chromatin, prominent nucleoli, basophilic cytoplasm and a moderate to high proliferation fraction. The cells have been likened by Lukes and Collins to either large cleaved or large noncleaved follicular center cells [4]. Marked variation in the nuclear contour may be seen. In the majority of cases, the cells are round to oval. However, in some cases the cells may be polylobated or cleaved [93]. Expression of B-cell-associated antigens, especially CD20, is a consistent feature. Therefore, staining for CD20 in paraffin sections is helpful for routine diagnosis. Because the neoplastic nature of the process is usually readily apparent, for practical purposes it is usually not necessary to show monoclonal Ig expression. Nevertheless, most cases can be shown to express a single light chain, if appropriately studied.

Diffuse large B-cell lymphomas may be associated with sclerosis, particularly in extranodal sites [6, 94]. Sclerosis is more common in those tumors with a large cleaved cell morphology and is also seen in mediastinal or thymic large B-cell lymphoma [95] (see below).

Some large B-cell lymphomas are rich in either small T-lymphocytes or histiocytes or both. Histologically, they may resemble peripheral T-cell lymphomas or Hodgkin's disease [96–98]. In the working formulation most such cases would be classified as diffuse mixed small- and large-cell lymphoma [64].

They are clinically aggressive with a prognosis comparable to that of diffuse large B-cell lymphoma [99]. The admixture of small lymphocytes and histiocytes is a variable phenomenon and the inflammatory background may be absent on second biopsies. These tumors have been referred to in the literature as 'pseudoperipheral T-cell lymphomas' [96] or T-cell-rich B-cell lymphoma [100]. T-Cell-rich B-cell lymphoma, as currently defined, does not appear to be a distinct clinical pathologic entity, but a variant that can be seen in association with several different subtypes of diffuse large B-cell lymphoma [101].

The WFs subdivided the 'histiocytic' lymphomas of Rappaport into two major subgroups: large cell and large cell immunoblastic [6]. Based on minor differences in median survival, the large-cell group was placed in the intermediate-grade category and the large-cell immunoblastic group placed in the high-grade category. Subsequent studies have not been able to justify the validity of this subclassification [102]. Moreover, it is exceedingly difficult for pathologists to make this distinction reliably and reproducibly [103,104]. Most aggressive lymphomas show a spectrum in cytologic appearance, and in any given field the predominant cell could be large cell or large cell immunoblastic. Similarly, the Kiel classification describes four different variants of centroblastic lymphoma: monomorphic, polymorphic, multilobated, and centrocytoid [105]. The designation of immunoblastic lymphoma of B-cell type is reserved for cases in which more than 90% of the cells have an immunoblastic appearance. If only 10% of the cells resemble centroblasts, the case is classified as a centroblastic lymphoma. Using these criteria only 4% of all NHLs are classified as B-immunoblastic [105].

Diffuse large B-cell lymphoma is one of the more common subtypes of NHL, representing up to 40% of cases. It has an aggressive natural history but responds well to chemotherapy. The complete remission rate with modern regimens is 75–80%, with long-term disease-free survival approaching 50% or more in most series [106]. This lymphoma may present in lymph nodes or in extranodal sites. Frequent extranodal sites of involvement include bone, skin, thyroid, gastrointestinal tract and lung. Some of these extranodal diffuse large-cell B-cell lymphomas may be MALT lymphomas with histologic progression, in which the low-grade component is not recognized. Nevertheless, once progression has occurred to a diffuse large B-cell lymphoma, the clinical approach is equivalent to that of node-based large B-cell lymphoma.

Because there is variation in the responsiveness to chemotherapy and because large B-cell lymphoma is one of the more common subtypes, there has been great interest over the years in identifying morphologic or immunophenotypic features that might be prognostically important. In most studies there is some suggestion that tumors composed of large cleaved or large noncleaved follicular center cells have a slightly better prognosis than those composed predominantly of immunoblasts [6,103]. However, the differences have been neither statistically significant nor consistently reproducible. Most data suggest that growth fraction is an important prognostic marker [107]. It is likely that in the future the use of immunophenotypic and/or genotypic markers may yield useful information in the subclassification of large B-cell lymphoma [107–110]. At present, while morphologic features are useful in identifying the spectrum of appearances that one may encounter diagnostically, morphologic features do not appear to be important prognostically.

PRIMARY MEDIASTINAL (THYMIC) LARGE B-CELL LYMPHOMA

(WF: large cell, large-cell immunoblastic; Kiel: discussed as 'rare and ambiguous subtype'.)

This lymphoma has emerged in recent years as a distinct clinicopathologic entity [95,111,112]. Cytologically, it resembles many other large B-cell lymphomas and is composed of large transformed cells that can resemble large noncleaved cells, large cleaved cells, multilobated cells and even immunoblasts. A constant feature is relatively abundant pale cytoplasm, often with distinct cytoplasmic membranes [112]. Many cases have fine compartmentalizing sclerosis, which may even lead to misdiagnosis as an epithelial tumor, such as thymoma. The tumor appears to be derived from medullary B-cells within the thymus gland [111,113,114]. These cells express CD20 and CD79a, but do not express surface Ig [114].

Clinically, mediastinal large B-cell lymphoma is much more common in females than males [115]. It is common in adolescents and young adults with a median age at presentation in the fourth decade. The clinical presentation is that of a rapidly growing anterior mediastinal mass with frequent superior venacaval syndrome and/or airway obstruction. Nodal involvement is uncommon at presentation and also at relapse. Frequent extranodal sites of involvement, particularly at relapse, include the liver, kidneys, adrenal glands, ovaries, gastrointestinal tract and central nervous system. Some studies suggested that the tumor was associated with an unusually aggressive clinical course with poor responses to conventional chemotherapy. More recent studies have reported cure rates similar to those seen for other large B-cell lymphomas.

BURKITT'S LYMPHOMA

(WF: small noncleaved cell, Burkitt's type; Kiel: Burkitt's lymphoma.)

Burkitt's lymphoma is most common in children and accounts for up to one-third of all pediatric lymphomas in the USA [116]. It is the most rapidly growing of all lymphomas with 100% of the cells in cell cycle at any time. It usually presents in extranodal sites. In nonendemic regions, such as the USA, frequent sites of presentation are the ileocecal region, ovaries, kidneys or breasts. Jaw presentations, as well as involvement of other facial bones, are common in African or endemic cases, and are seen occasionally in nonendemic regions. Rare cases present as acute leukemia with diffuse bone marrow infiltration and circulating Burkitt tumor cells (L3-ALL). Even in patients with typical extranodal disease, bone marrow involvement is a poor prognostic sign.

Burkitt's lymphoma is one of the more common tumors associated with the human immunodeficiency virus (HIV) [117]. It can present at any time during the clinical course. In some patients with HIV infection, Burkitt's lymphoma may be the initial acquired immunodeficiency syndrome (AIDS)-defining illness.

The pathogenesis of Burkitt's lymphoma is undoubtedly related to the translocations involving the c-*myc* oncogene which are seen in virtually 100% of cases [118,119]. Most cases involve the immunoglobulin heavy chain gene on chromosome 14. Less commonly the light chain genes on chromosomes 2 and 22 are involved in the translocation. African Burkitt's lymphoma occurs in regions endemic for malaria and it has been postulated that immunosuppression associated with malaria infection places patients at increased risk for Burkitt's lymphoma [55]. In this regard, the pathogenesis appears similar to that seen with HIV infection.

EBV is closely linked to Burkitt's lymphoma in endemic regions, but is less frequently seen (15–20%) in European and North American cases [116]. In other regions characterized by low socioeconomic status and EBV infection at an early age, Burkitt's lymphoma is often EBV-positive, in the range of 50–70% [120]. These data support the concept the EBV is a cofactor for the development of Burkitt's lymphoma. Differences in the proportion of cases associated with the two EBV strains (types 1 and 2) have also been shown in sporadic and endemic EBV-positive Burkitt's lymphomas [121].

Cytologically, Burkitt's lymphoma is exceedingly monomorphic. The cells are medium in size with round nuclei, moderately clumped chromatin, and multiple (2–5) basophilic nucleoli (Plate 3.4). The cytoplasm is deeply basophilic and moderately abundant. These cells contain cytoplasmic lipid vacuoles, which are probably a manifestation of the high rate of proliferation and high rate of spontaneous cell death. Lipid vacuoles are usually evident on imprints or smears, but not in tissue sections. The starry sky pattern characteristic of Burkitt's lymphoma is a manifestation of the numerous benign macrophages that have ingested karyorrhectic or apoptotic tumor cells.

Some cases of Burkitt's lymphoma are associated with a marked granulomatous reaction, which may even obscure the lymphoma in some cases. This reaction is often seen in patients with early stage but, even if the stage is more advanced at presentation, these patients usually have an excellent prognosis [122]. Thus, this granulomatous reaction may be a manifestation of host immune response to the disease. The reaction has also been described in Burkitt-like lymphomas [122].

Burkitt's lyphoma has a mature B-cell phenotype. The cells express CD19, CD20, CD22, CD79a and monoclonal surface Ig, nearly always IgM. CD10 is positive in nearly all cases, and CD5 and CD23 are consistently negative [123].

HIGH-GRADE B-CELL LYMPHOMA, BURKITT-LIKE (PROVISIONAL)

(WF: small noncleaved cell, non-Burkitt's; Kiel: not listed (centroblastic).)

The small noncleaved cell category of the WF includes tumors with cells similar in size and appearance to Burkitt's lymphoma, but with greater pleomorphism [6]. These lymphomas lack the monotonous cytology of Burkitt's lymphoma but are composed of cells that have nuclei roughly equivalent to the size of the nuclei of the starry sky macrophages. However, there is usually some variation in both cell size and shape. There may be multiple nucleoli or a single distinct prominent nucleolus.

In the WF small noncleaved cell, non-Burkitt's is a heterogeneous category and includes both B- and T-cell lymphomas. For example, some cases of adult T-cell leukemia lymphoma are composed of cells conforming to this description. However, in the ILSG classification high-grade B-cell lymphoma, Burkitt-like, is reserved for tumors with a B-cell phenotype. However, even in the ILSG scheme, this category is probably heterogeneous. A number of clinical studies have suggested that small noncleaved cell lymphomas, whether or not they conform to classic Burkitt's lymphoma, have a very high growth fraction and an aggressive clinical course [107,124]. It was felt that the separation of such tumors from diffuse large B-cell lymphoma may be warranted on clinical grounds. Using immunocytochemistry to detect the Ki-67 or MIB1 antigen, such tumors usually have a growth fraction in excess of 80%, which places them in a highly aggressive category. Nevertheless, with modern third-generation chemotherapeutic regimens, a complete continuous remission can be obtained in many cases [124].

On clinical grounds, Burkitt-like lymphomas share more similarities with large B-cell lymphomas than with true Burkitt's lymphomas. They usually present in adults, often with nodal as well as extranodal disease [125]. Review of data from the original WF project data base indicated a median survival of 1.5 years for large-cell lymphoma (LCL), 1.3 years for small noncleaved, non-Burkitt's (SNC-NB), but only 0.5 years for Burkitt's (unpublished data, CW Berard, personal communication). Similarly the 5-year survival rates for LCL and SNC-NB were 35% and 41%, in contrast to 20% for Burkitt's lymphoma, with complete remission rates of 59%, 57% and 42%, respectively. Therefore, based on these data, categorization of the Burkitt-like lymphomas with other large B-cell lymphomas would seem appropriate.

Biologically, these tumors appear to be more closely related to large noncleaved or centroblastic lymphomas than true Burkitt's lymphoma. A recent study showed that cases classified as small noncleaved non-Burkitt's lacked c-*myc* rearrangement but contained *bcl*-2 rearrangement with a frequency equivalent to that of large B-cell lymphoma [119]. Therefore, biologically these tumors also correspond to large-cell lymphoma. Given the improvement in prognosis with third-generation regimens, a distinction from large B-cell lymphoma may not be warranted in the future [124].

Burkitt's-like lymphomas occurring in the setting of HIV infection, by contrast, are biologically comparable to true Burkitt's lymphoma. They frequently contain c-*myc* rearrangements, despite their greater nuclear pleomorphism [117].

T-Cell and putative NK cell neoplasms

OVERVIEW OF THE CLASSIFICATION OF T-CELL NEOPLASMS

While the definition of precursor T-cell or lymphoblastic neoplasms is straightforward, the classification of peripheral T-cell lymphomas has been controversial. Most previously published classification schemes for the malignant lymphomas published in the United States or Europe have been based on B-cell malignancies, as these are far more common than their T-cell counterparts. The Rappaport classification and the original Kiel and Lukes–Collins classifications focus primarily on B-cell lymphomas. The WF, being based on the Rappaport scheme, also focuses almost exclusively on B-cell malignancies. Only mycosis fungoides is delineated as a specific entity and it is included in the miscellaneous category. The vast majority of peripheral T-cell lymphomas in the WF are classified as either diffuse, mixed, small, and large cell or large-cell immunoblastic. T-cell lymphomas composed predominantly of small atypical cells would be included in the diffuse small cleaved cell category or remain unclassified.

The revised Kiel classification does include T-cell lymphomas [105,126]. However, the ILSG Classification differs from the approach utilized in the Kiel scheme in several respects. For one, the ILSG classification recognizes adult T-cell leukemia/lymphoma (ATLL) as a distinct clinicopathologic entity [8]. The Kiel classification describes T-cell lymphomas in morphologic terms and notes independently the status as HTLV-1 positive or negative.

The ILSG classification also recognizes the distinctive nature of many extranodal T-cell lymphomas. These include the nasal and nasal-type angiocentric lymphomas, enteropathy-associated T-cell lymphoma and subcutaneous panniculitic T-cell lymphoma. Clinical features play an important role in the definition of many T-cell lymphoma entities, as it is felt that cytologic features alone are not sufficient to delineate many of these diseases.

Additionally, the Kiel classification divides T-cell lymphomas into low-grade and high-grade forms based on the cytologic features of the neoplastic cells. Low-grade lymphomas are composed of small- to medium-sized atypical cells, whereas large transformed cells predominate in the high-grade lymphomas. While these distinctions are valid cytologically, they do not necessarily relate to a more aggressive clinical course for the tumors composed of large cells [127]. For this reason, the ILSG classification does not divide T-cell lymphomas into low-grade and high-grade variants.

Finally, T-zone lymphoma and lymphoepithelioid cell lymphoma were not felt to be distinct clinico-pathologic entities, although they do represent morphologic variations that can be seen in peripheral T-cell lymphoma. In addition, previous studies have suggested that they are difficult to reliably distinguish from other nodal T-cell lymphomas [128]. Cytogenetic studies also have suggested overlap among these categories of low grade T-cell lymphoma in the Kiel classification [129]. Therefore, they were left within the category peripheral T-cell lymphomas, unspecified.

PRECURSOR T-LYMPHOBLASTIC LYMPHOMA/LEUKEMIA (TLBL/ALL)

(WF: lymphoblastic; Kiel: T-lymphoblastic.)

Most TLBL/ALL are cytologically indistinguishable from their B-cell counterparts. The cells usually are convoluted, but nonconvoluted forms also exist [13,130] (Plate 3.5). The cells have finely distributed chromatin, inconspicuous nucleoli and sparse, pale cytoplasm. Eighty-five per cent of patients with lymphoblastic lymphoma have a tumor of precursor T-cell phenotype. This is a disease of adolescents and young adults, with an increased male to female ratio. A total of 50–80% of patients present with an anterior mediastinal mass, usually with involvement of the thymus gland. This is a high-grade

lymphoma; the rapidly growing mass may be associated with airway obstruction. Bone marrow involvement is common and progression to a leukemic picture will occur in the absence of effective therapy. This tumor also has a high frequency of involvement of the central nervous system (CNS); CNS involvement is a poor prognostic sign.

TLBL is closely related to T-cell ALL, although the lymphomatous forms usually exhibit a more mature T-cell phenotype [131] (Figure 3.4). Both are TDT-postive in the vast majority of cases [132]. CD7 is the most consistently expressed T-cell-associated antigen, followed by CD5 and CD2 [133–135]. Cytoplasmic CD3 expression precedes surface CD3 positivity [136].

In lymph nodes TLBL has a diffuse leukemic pattern of infiltration. There is very little stromal reaction and the cells diffusely infiltrate the lymph node parenchyma. Streaming of cells in the medullary cords may be prominent, especially around vascular structures. Some residual follicles may be present but ultimately architectural effacement is the rule. A starry sky pattern is seen in approximately one-third of cases. Mitotic figures are readily observed.

Histologically, it is not possible to differentiate TLBL from BLBL. Immunophenotypic studies performed in paraffin or frozen sections can usually identify the cell of origin. In paraffin sections the two most useful markers are CD3 and CD79a, capable of distinguishing precursor T-cell and B-cell forms, respectively [16]. TDT can also be detected immunocytochemically in formalin-fixed but not B5-fixed tissue sections. TLBL may also simulate the blastic

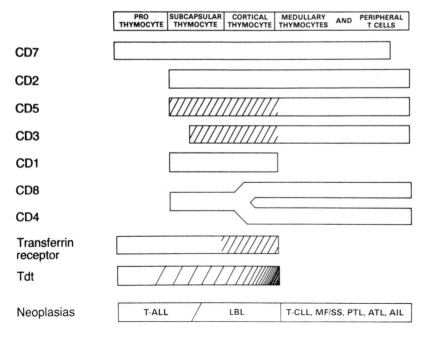

Figure 3.4 Schematic diagram of T-cell differentiation, as it relates to the malignant lymphomas and leukemias. T-ALL, T-cell acute lymphoblastic leukemia; LBL, lymphoblastic lymphoma; T-CLL, T-cell chronic lymphocytic leukemia; MF/SS, mycosis fungoides/Sézary syndrome; PTL, peripheral T-cell lymphoma; ATL, adult T-cell leukemia/lymphoma; AIL, angioimmunoblastic lymphadenopathy lymphoma.

variant of mantle cell lymphoma. The cells of mantle cell lymphoma usually show more chromatin clumping and have more abundant cytoplasm than either TLBL or BLBL.

T-CELL CHRONIC LYMPHOCYTIC LEUKEMIA/PROLYMPHOCYTIC LEUKEMIA (T-CLL/PLL)

(WF: small lymphocytic, consistent with CLL, diffuse small cleaved cell, unclassified; Kiel: T-cell CLL/PLL.)

T-CLL/PLL presents with leukemia, with or without lymphadenopathy, usually with markedly elevated white blood cell counts [137,138]. Instances of primary lymph node involvement are exceedingly rare. The lymph node involvement is diffuse, primarily paracortical, with sparing of the follicles. The cellular infiltrate is usually more monotonous than that of B-CLL and lacks pseudofollicular proliferation centers. Involvement of the spleen is associated with diffuse red pulp infiltration. Hepatomegaly is frequently present. Clinically, T-CLL/PLL is much more aggressive than B-CLL. In most cases, some cytologic atypia is present, so that the cells do not resemble small round normal-appearing lymphocytes. On this basis, they are more accurately classified as T-PLL.

LARGE GRANULAR LYMPHOCYTE (LGL) LEUKEMIA, T-CELL AND NK CELL TYPES

(WF: small lymphocytic, consistent with CLL; Kiel: T-CLL.)

These disorders are not generally considered with the malignant lymphomas, and will be discussed only briefly. The cells have more abundant pale cytoplasm than those of T-CLL. In smear preparations azurophil granules are readily identified. Most cases of T-LGL have been shown to be clonal, based on analysis of T-cell receptor gene rearrangement [139]. Clonality has not been convincingly shown in most cases of low-grade NK-LGL. In some cases, this may represent an atypical reactive, nonneoplastic lymphoproliferative disorder. Clonal disorders of T-LGL are more common. In addition to peripheral blood involvement, the cells infiltrate the marrow, splenic red pulp and liver. Lymphadenopathy is uncommon and the clinical course is indolent.

Two high-grade variants of NK cell leukemia have been described. One resembles acute myeloid leukemia [140]. The cells have a blastic or monomorphic appearance, and are usually negative for

EBV. The second variant is EBV-positive and may represent a leukemic form of angiocentric nasal T-/NK cell lymphoma (see below) [141]. It is much more common in Asia than in Western countries and pursues an aggressive clinical course. The cells are medium to large in size, contain hyperchromatic nuclei and demonstrate nuclear pleomorphism. Azurophil granules can be seen on smears, but the marked cytologic atypia readily permits distinction from the more indolent forms of T- and NK LGL.

MYCOSIS FUNGOIDES/SÉZARY SYNDROME (MF/SS)

(WF: mycosis fungoides; Kiel: small cell, cerebriform.)

MF/SS by definition present with cutaneous disease. Skin involvement may be manifested as multiple cutaneous plaques or nodules, or with generalized erythroderma. Lymphadenopathy is usually not present at presentation and, when identified, is associated with a poor prognosis [142]. In early stages enlarged lymph nodes may only show dermatopathic changes (LN1 or LN2) [143]. If malignant cells are present in significant numbers and are associated with architectural effacement (LN3 and LN4), the prognosis is significantly worse.

Cytologically, the small cells of MF/SS demonstrate cerebriform nuclei with clumped chromatin, inconspicuous nucleoli and sparse cytoplasm. The larger cells may be hyperchromatic or have more vesicular nuclei with prominent nucleoli. Nuclear pleomorphism is usually evident in the large cells. The cells have a mature T-cell phenotype, usually CD4+, with loss of CD7 in many cases [26,144]. Tumor stage MF is more frequently CD7− than earlier clinical forms.

PERIPHERAL T-CELL LYMPHOMAS (PTL), UNSPECIFIED PROVISIONAL CYTOLOGIC GRADES: MEDIUM-SIZED CELL, MIXED MEDIUM AND LARGE CELL, LARGE CELL

(WF: diffuse small cleaved, diffuse mixed small and large cell, large-cell immunoblastic; Kiel: T-zone lymphoma, lymphoepithelioid cell lymphoma, pleomorphic small, medium and large cell (HTLV-1 negative), immunoblastic (HTLV-1 negative).)

PTLs account for only 10–15% of all NHLs in the USA and Europe. Angioimmunoblastic T-cell lymphoma is the most common specific form. The majority of other PTLs arising in lymph nodes would fall in the unspecified category. PTL are characterized by a heterogeneous cellular composition. There is usually a mixture of small and large atypical lymphoid cells (Plate 3.6). An inflammatory background is frequent, consisting of eosinophils, plasma cells and histiocytes. If the epithelioid histiocytes are numerous and clustered, it fulfills criteria for lymphoepithelioid cell lymphoma or Lennert's lymphoma [145,146]. In the ILSG classification lymphoepithelioid cell lymphoma was considered a morphologic variant of PTL and not a distinctive clinicopathologic entity. It has not been associated with any immunophenotypic, cytogenetic or molecular features permitting distinction from other PTL [129].

PTL may show preferential involvement of the paracortical region of lymph nodes. In some cases this architectural pattern is striking, with sparing of follicles. Such cases have been referred to as T-zone lymphoma [126]. However, on cytologic grounds they resemble other peripheral T-cell lymphomas of medium or mixed cytologic types. The neoplastic cells usually have a moderate amount of pale cytoplasm. A conspicuous clear cell component is more characteristic of angioimmunoblastic T-cell lymphoma than PTL, unspecified.

Clinically, PTL present in adults. Most patients exhibit generalized lymphadenopathy, hepatosplenomegaly and frequent bone marrow involvement. Constitutional symptoms, including fever and night sweats, are common, as is pruritus. The clinical course is aggressive, although complete remissions may be obtained with combination chemotherapy [147–149]. However, the relapse rate is higher in PTL than in B-cell lymphomas of comparable histologic grade [149].

PTL, as defined in the ILSG classification, is heterogeneous. It is likely that individual clinicopathologic entities will be delineated in the future from this broad group of malignancies. Thus far, immunophenotypic criteria have not been helpful in delineating subtypes. Most cases have a mature T-cell phenotype, and express one of the major subset antigens: CD4>CD8. These are not clonal markers and antigen expression can change over time. Deletion of one of the pan-T-cell antigens (CD3, CD5, CD2 or CD7) is seen in 75% of cases, with CD7 most frequently being absent [26].

SUBCUTANEOUS PANNICULITIC T-CELL LYMPHOMA (PROVISIONAL)

(WF: diffuse mixed small and large cell, large-cell immunoblastic, small cleaved cell; Kiel: pleomorphic medium mixed and large cell (HTLV-1 negative).)

Subcutaneous panniculitic T-cell lymphoma is sufficiently distinct to warrant separation from other forms of peripheral T-cell lymphoma [150]. The disease usually presents with subcutaneous nodules, primarily affecting the extremities. The nodules range in size from 0.5 cm to several centimeters in diameter. Larger nodules may become necrotic. In its early stages the infiltrate may appear deceptively benign and lesions are often misdiagnosed as panniculitis [150, 151]. However, histologic progression usually occurs and subsequent biopsies show more pronounced cytologic atypia, permitting the diagnosis of malignant lymphoma.

As noted above, the cytologic composition of subcutaneous panniculitic T-cell lymphoma is extremely variable. The lesions may contain a predominance of small atypical lymphoid cells, large transformed cells with hyperchromatic nuclei or an admixture of several different cell types. Admixed reactive histiocytes are frequently present, particularly in areas of fat infiltration and destruction. The histiocytes are frequently vacuolated as a result of ingested lipid material. Vascular invasion may be seen in some cases, and necrosis and karyorrhexis are common.

A hemophagocytic syndrome is a frequent complication of subcutaneous panniculitic T-cell lymphoma [150]. Patients present with fever, pancytopenia and hepatosplenomegaly. It is most readily diagnosed in bone marrow aspirate smears where histiocytes containing phagocytosed erythrocytes and occasionally platelets may be observed. The hemophagocytic syndrome usually precipitates a fulminant downhill clinical course. However, if therapy for the underlying lymphoma is instituted and is successful, the hemophagocytic syndrome may remit. A hemophagocytic syndrome is the cause of death in the majority of patients with subcutaneous panniculitic T-cell lymphoma. Dissemination to lymph nodes and other organs is uncommon, and usually occurs late in the clinical course. The cause of the hemophagocytic syndrome appears related to cytokine production by the malignant cells. Both interferon gamma as well as granulocyte–monocyte colony-stimulating factor have been identified [151].

It is likely that subcutaneous panniculitic T-cell lymphoma is the process previously described as histiocytic cytophagic panniculitis. It had been thought that histiocytic cytophagic panniculitis was a malignant histiocytic proliferation. Although histiocytes may be numerous in these lesions, the malignant cells have a mature T-cell phenotype. Evidence for an association with EBV has been absent. The neoplastic cells are usually CD8+.

γδT-Cell lymphoma (provisional)

(WF: diffuse small cleaved cell, unclassified; Kiel: pleomorphic small cell, medium-size cell (HTLV-1 negative).)

The majority of peripheral T-lymphocytes belong to the αβ subset, whereas only a minority are γδT-cells. Similarly, most peripheral T-cell lymphomas are of αβT-cell derivation. However, there is a unique subtype of peripheral T-cell lymphoma that is derived from γδT-cells.

γδT-Cell lymphoma presents with marked hepatosplenomegaly [152]. This tumor has also been referred to in the literature as hepatosplenic T-cell lymphoma. The homing pattern manifested by the malignant cells is similar to that of normal γδT-cells, which preferentially involve the sinusoidal areas of the spleen and also the intestinal mucosa.

γδT-Cell lymphomas show a marked male predominance. Most patients are young adults [153]. The clinical presentation is that of marked hepatosplenomegaly in the absence of lymphadenopathy. Abnormal cells are usually present in the bone marrow but may be difficult to identify. They selectively infiltrate the bone marrow sinusoids and can be most easily recognized with immunohistochemical stains of bone marrow biopsy sections. A variant of γδT-cell lymphoma with cutaneous disease has also been reported [151].

The cells of γδT-cell lymphoma are usually moderate in size with a rim of pale cytoplasm. The nuclear chromatin is loosely condensed with small inconspicuous nucleoli. Usually some irregularity of the nuclear contour can be seen. The liver and spleen show marked sinusoidal infiltration, with sparing of both portal triads and white pulp, respectively. The neoplastic cells have a phenotype that resembles that of normal γδT-cells. The are negative for both CD4 and usually CD8. Although they are positive for CD3, they are negative for antigens such as βF1, expressed on αβ cells, but postive for TCRδ. CD56 is often positive, and the cells express cytotoxic molecules [152,153]. *In situ* hybridization for EBV has been negative [153].

Clinically, γδT-cell lymphoma is aggressive [153]. Although patients may respond initially to chemotherapy, relapse has been seen in the vast majority of cases and the median survival is less than 2 years.

ANGIOIMMUNOBLASTIC T-CELL LYMPHOMA (AILD)

(WF: diffuse mixed small and large cell, large-cell immunoblastic, AILD; Kiel: angioimmunoblastic.)

AILD was initially proposed as an abnormal immune reaction or form of atypical lymphoid hyperplasia with a high risk of progression to malignant lymphoma [154]. Because the majority of cases show clonal rearrangements of T-cell receptor genes, it is now regarded as a variant of T-cell lymphoma [155]. The median survival is generally less than 5 years, so that the designation as lymphoma is warranted on clinical grounds [156].

The nodal architecture is generally effaced, but peripheral sinuses are often open and even dilated. The abnormal infiltrate usually extends beyond the capsule into the surrounding adipose tissue. Hyperplastic germinal centers are absent. However, there may be regressed follicles containing a proliferation of dendritic cells and blood vessels. These regressed follicles are referred to as 'burned out'.

At low power there is usually a striking proliferation of postcapillary venules with prominent arborization. The cellularity of the lymph node usually appears reduced or depleted at low power. Clusters of lymphoid cells with clear cytoplasm may be seen. Their nuclei exhibit moderately condensed chromatin and a slightly irregular nuclear contour. These are admixed with a polymorphous cellular background containing small normal-appearing lymphocytes, basophilic immunoblasts, plasma cells and histiocytes, with or without eosinophils (Figure 3.5). The abnormal cells are usually CD4+ T-cells. In paraffin sections, a helpful diagnostic feature is the presence of numerous CD21+ dendritic reticulum cells, which are especially prominent around postcapillary venules [157]. Polyclonal plasma cells may be numerous.

AILD presents in adults. Most patients have generalized lymphadenopathy and prominent systemic symptoms with fever, weight loss and skin rash. There is usually a polyclonal hypergammaglobulinemia. Patients may respond initially to steroids or mild cytotoxic chemotherapy, but progression usually occurs. More aggressive combination chemotherapeutic regimens have led to a higher remission rate but patients are prone to secondary infectious complications [158]. Progression to a more monomorphic T-cell immunoblastic lymphoma occurs in some cases and the proportion of large immunoblastic cells appears to correlate with clinical course [159]. Rarely, B-cell immunoblastic lymphomas positive for EBV are seen [160]. These latter malignancies appear secondary to the underlying immunodeficiency.

ADULT T-CELL LEUKEMIA/LYMPHOMA (ATLL)

(WF: diffuse small cleaved, diffuse mixed small and large cell, large cell, large-cell immunoblastic, small

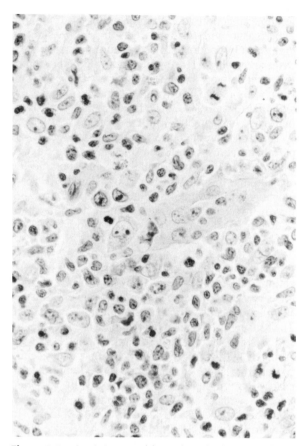

Figure 3.5 Angioimmunoblastic lymphadenopathy lymphoma. Postcapillary venules are prominent. The infiltrate is polymorphous, with frequent clear cells.

noncleaved non-Burkitt; Kiel: pleomorphic small cell, medium-sized and large cell, immunoblastic (HTLV-1 positive).)

ATLL is a distinct clinicopathologic entity originally described in southwestern Japan, which is associated with the retrovirus HTLV-1 [161,162]. HTLV-1 is found clonally integrated in the T-cells of this lymphoma. HTLV-1 is also endemic in the Caribbean, where clusters of ATLL have been described, predominantly among Blacks [163,164]. It is seen with lesser frequency in Blacks in the southeastern USA [165]. The median age of affected individuals is 45 years. Patients in the Caribbean tend to be slightly younger than those in Japan [166]. Patients may present with leukemia or with generalized lymphadenopathy. The leukemic form predominates in Japan, whereas lymphomatous presentations are more common in the Western hemisphere. Other clinical findings include lymphadenopathy, hepatosplenomegaly, lytic bone lesions and hypercalcemia [8]. The acute form of the disease is associated with a poor prognosis and a median survival of under 2 years [165]. Complete remissions

may be obtained but the relapse rate is nearly 100%.

Chronic and smouldering forms of the disease are seen less commonly [167]. These are associated with a much more indolent clinical course. There is usually minimal lymphadenopathy. The predominant clinical manifestation is skin rash, with only small numbers of atypical cells in the peripheral blood. In the chronic and smouldering forms HTLV-1 virus is also found integrated within the atypical lymphoid cells.

The cytologic spectrum of ATLL is extremely diverse. The cells may be small with condensed nuclear chromatin and markedly polylobated nuclear appearance [165,168] (Figure 3.6). Larger cells with dispersed chromatin and small nucleoli may be admixed and predominate in some cases. Reed–Sternberg-like cells can be seen, simulating Hodgkin's disease [169]. In the smouldering form of ATLL, the cells may show minimal cytologic atypia and may even be diagnosed as small lymphocytic lymphoma

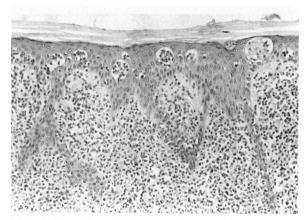

(a)

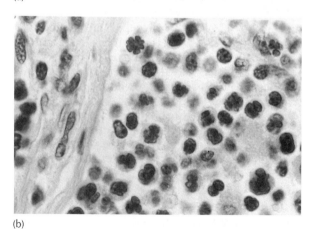

(b)

Figure 3.6 Adult T-cell leukemia/lymphoma. (a) The infiltrate in skin frequently involves the epidermis, producing Pautrier microabscesses. (b) Lymphoid cells are markedly polylobated, as seen in this lymph node sinus.

in the WF. The larger cells usually show abundant cytoplasmic basophilia.

The neoplastic cells, regardless of cytologic subtype, are usually CD4+ T-cells that strongly express the interleukin-2 receptor, CD25 [8]. High levels of soluble interleukin-2 receptors can also be found in the serum and can correlate with disease activity. CD7 is nearly always absent, but CD3 and other mature T-cell antigens are usually expressed.

ANGIOCENTRIC T-/NK CELL LYMPHOMA

(WF: diffuse small cleaved, mixed small and large cell, large-cell immunoblastic; Kiel: unclassified, pleomorphic small cell, medium and large cell (HTLV-1 negative).)

Angiocentric T-/NK cell lymphoma is a distinct clinicopathologic entity highly associated with EBV [170,171]. The most common clinical presentation is with a destructive nasal or midline facial tumor. Palatal destruction, orbital swelling and edema may be prominent [172]. Angiocentric lymphomas have been reported in other extranodal sites, including skin, soft tissue, testis, upper respiratory tract and gastrointestinal tract. A leukemic form of the disease also has been reported with similar morphologic, immunophenotypic and genotypic features [141].

Angiocentric T-/NK cell lymphoma is characterized by a broad cytologic spectrum (Figure 3.7). The atypical cells may be small or medium in size. Large atypical and hyperchromatic cells may be admixed, or may predominate. If the small cells are in the majority, the disease may be difficult to distinguish from an inflammatory or infectious process. In early stages there may also be a prominent admixture of inflammatory cells, further causing difficulty in diagnosis [173].

Because virtually all cases of nasal T-/NK cell

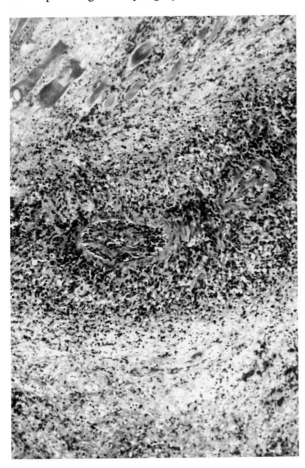

(a)

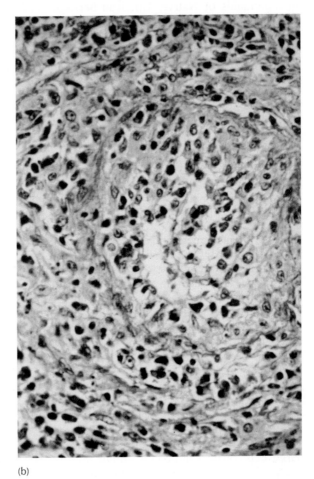

(b)

Figure 3.7 (a) Angiocentric lymphoma of T-/NK cell type involving buccal mucosa. Extensive tissue necrosis surrounds affected vessel. (b) Lymphomatoid granulomatosis. The pattern of vascular infiltration in the lung resembles that seen in angiocentric lymphomas.

lymphoma are positive for EBV, *in situ* hybridization studies with probes to EBV-encoded small nuclear RNA (EBER 1/2) may be very helpful in diagnosis and can detect even small numbers of neoplastic cells [174,175]. Although the cells express some T-cell associated antigens, most commonly CD2, other T-cell markers, such as surface CD3, are usually absent [174]. Cytoplasmic CD3 can be found in paraffin sections. However, cytoplasmic CD3 can be found in NK cells and is not specific for a T-cell lineage. In addition, molecular studies have not shown a clonal T-cell gene rearrangement, despite clonality being shown by other methods [174,176,177]. In favor of an NK-cell origin, the cells are nearly always CD56+; however, CD16 and CD57, other NK-cell associated antigens, are usually negative.

Angiocentric T-/NK cell lymphoma is much more common in Asians than in individuals of European background. Clusters of the disease have also been reported in Central and South America in individuals of Native American heritage [178], suggesting that genetic factors may play a role in the pathogenesis of angiocentric T-/NK cell lymphoma.

A hemophagocytic syndrome is a common clinical complication, which adversely affects survival in angiocentric T-/NK cell lymphoma [179]. It is likely that EBV plays a role in the pathogenesis of this complication.

Lymphomatoid granulomatosis (LYG) exhibits many similarities both clinically and pathologically to angiocentric T-/NK cell lymphoma [173]. Only recently it was considered to be part of the same disease spectrum, angiocentric immunoproliferative lesions (AIL). However, recent data indicate that LYG is an EBV-positive B-cell proliferation associated with an exuberant T-cell reaction [180]. LYG also presents in extranodal sites but the most common site of involvement is the lung [181]. The kidney and central nervous system are also frequently involved as are skin and subcutaneous tissue. The pattern of necrosis in both LYG and T-/NK cell lymphoma is very similar, emphasizing the likely importance of EBV in mediating the vascular damage.

INTESTINAL T-CELL LYMPHOMA (± ENTEROPATHY) (EATL)

(WF: diffuse small cleaved, diffuse mixed small and large cell, diffuse large-cell immunoblastic; Kiel: unclassfied, pleomorphic medium and large cell, immunoblastic (HTLV-I).)

EATL was originally termed malignant histiocytosis of the intestine [182]. However, the demonstration of clonal T-cell gene rearrangement indicated that it was a T-cell lymphoma. The small bowel usually shows ulceration, frequently with perforation. A mass may or may not be present. The infiltrate shows a varying cytologic composition with an admixture of small, medium and larger atypical lymphoid cells. The adjacent small bowel may show villous atrophy associated with celiac disease [183]. The neoplastic cells are CD3+, CD7+ T-cells, which also express the homing receptor CD103 (HML-1) [184]. The cells express cytotoxic molecules.

This disease occurs in adults, the majority of whom have a history of gluten-sensitive enteropathy. Patients usually present with abdominal symptoms such as pain, small bowel perforation and associated peritonitis. The clinical course is aggressive.

ANAPLASTIC LARGE-CELL LYMPHOMA (ALCL)

(WF: large cell, large-cell immunoblastic; Kiel: ALCL (Ki-1+ T-cell).)

Classical ALCL

ALCL is characterized by pleomorphic cells which have a propensity to invade lymphoid sinuses [185]. Because of the sinusoidal location of the tumor cells and their lobulated nuclear appearance, this disease was previously interpreted as a variant of malignant histiocytosis. Misdiagnosis as metastatic carcinoma or melanoma is also common.

A consistent feature is the expression of the CD30 antigen, which is a hallmark of this disease [186]. It has been referred to as Ki-1+ lymphoma [187]. However, antigen expression is not specific for ALCL and is also be seen in other forms of malignant lymphoma, including, of course, Hodgkin's disease [188].

ALCL can present in all age groups, but is relatively more common in children and young adults. A high incidence of cutaneous disease has been reported [189]. A primary cutaneous form of ALCL is associated with lymphomatoid papulosis and differs clinically, immunophenotypically, and at the molecular level [190–192]. Classical ALCL is associated with a characteristic chromosomal translocation, t(2;5) (p23;q35) [193,194]. Recently the genes involved in this translocation have been identified, and a polymerase chain reaction method has been developed to detect cells containing the fused *NPM/ALK* genes [195]. A monoclonal antibody to the protein product of the fused genes has also been made and it stains tumor cells containing the translocation [196].

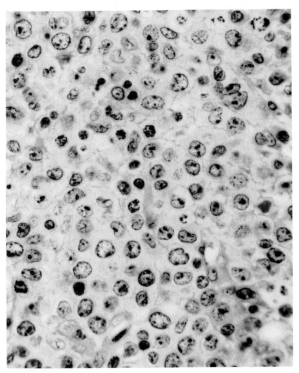

Figure 3.8 Anaplastic large-cell lymphoma. This case was positive for the NPM/ALK translocation by RT-PCR. The cells are large with abundant cytoplasm. Some nuclei are indented, but most are round in this relatively monomorphic case.

The cells of classic ALCL have large, often lobated nuclei (Figure 3.8). Nucleoli are present but tend not to be prominent, and are frequently basophilic. In some cases the nuclei may be round. The cytoplasm is usually abundant and amphophilic, and there are distinct cytoplasmic borders. A prominent Golgi region is usually apparent. Immunohistochemistry is very valuable in the correct diagnosis of ALCL. The prominent Golgi region usually shows intense staining for CD30 and epithelial membrane antigen (EMA) [197].

Recently, histologic variants of classic ALCL have been described. These may contain a prominent admixture of histiocytes, which may lead to misdiagnosis as an inflammatory condition [198]. In some cases the cells are small to medium in size with abundant cytoplasm [199]. In addition, there are more monomorphic variants, which may be difficult to distinguish from peripheral T-cell lymphomas that are unspecified and composed of large lymphoid cells [192,194,200]. Again, staining with antibodies to CD30 can serve to highlight the malignant cells. Although the cells of PTL may be

CD30+, staining is seldom as intense as in true ALCL.

Primary cutaneous ALCL

Primary cutaneous ALCL is a different disease and is closely related to lymphomatoid papulosis [201]. Indeed, lymphomatoid papulosis and cutaneous ALCL appear to represent a histologic and clinical continuum [191,202]. Small lesions are likely to regress. Patients with large tumor masses may develop disseminated disease with lymph node involvement. However, primary cutaneous ALCL is a more indolent disease than other T-cell lymphomas of the skin [203]. Most patients with primary cutaneous ALCL have multiple skin lesions. Because the skin nodules may show spontaneous regression, a period of observation is usually warranted before the institution of any chemotherapy. Cutaneous ALCL is CD30+ but usually EMA-negative. It also appears to lack the t(2;5) translocation [192].

ALCL HODGKIN'S-LIKE (PROVISIONAL)

(WF: Hodgkin's disease, large-cell immunoblastic; Kiel: ALCL, Hodgkin's disease.)

Hodgkin's-related ALCL has been described as a provisional form of lymphoma that is difficult to distinguish from Hodgkin's disease [204]. In many cases this process appears to be part of the spectrum of nodular sclerosing Hodgkin's disease (NSHD) [205]. It usually presents in young adults, often with a mediastinal mass. Skin lesions are not described. At low power, involved lymph nodes may show fibrous bands or capsular fibrosis resembling NSHD. An inflammatory background may be present focally but elsewhere there is sheeting out of the malignant cells in a monomorphic fashion. In these monomorphic areas, the cells may lack the prominent eosinophilic nucleoli of Reed–Sternberg cells. Intrasinusoidal growth of the malignant cells may also be present.

It is still uncertain whether Hodgkin's-like ALCL is part of the spectrum of Hodgkin's disease or a variant of non-Hodgkin's lymphoma [206]. It has been suggested that these patients respond poorly to conventional therapy for Hodgkin's disease but do respond to third-generation chemotherapy regimens used in the treatment of aggressive non-Hodgkin's lymphoma [204].

References

1. Rappaport H. Tumors of the hematopoietic system. In *Atlas of Tumor Pathology*. Washington, DC: Armed Forces Institute of Pathology, 1966.
2. Gerard-Marchant R, Hamlin I, Lennert K, et al. Classification of non-Hodgkin's lymphomas. *Lancet* 1974, **ii**: 406–408.
3. Lennert K, Mohri N, Stein H, et al. The histopathology of malignant lymphoma. *Br. J. Haematol.* 1975, **31** (Suppl.): 193–203.
4. Lukes R, Collins R. Immunologic characterization of human malignant lymphomas. *Cancer* 1974, **34**: 1488–1503.
5. Bennett MH, Farrer-Brown G, Henry, K, et al. Classification of non-Hodgkin's lymphomas. *Lancet* 1974, **2**: 405–406.
6. Non-Hodgkin's Lymphoma Pathologic Classification Project. National Cancer Institute sponsored study of classifications of non-Hodgkin's lymphomas: Summary and description of a Working Formulation for clinical usage. *Cancer* 1982, **49**: 2112–2135.
7. Chan JK, Yip TT, Tsang WY, et al. Detection of Epstein–Barr viral RNA in malignant lymphomas of the upper aerodigestive tract. *Am. J. Surg. Pathol.* 1994, **18**(9): 938–946.
8. Levine PH, Cleghorn F, Manns A, et al. Adult T-cell leukemia/lymphoma: A working point-score classification for epidemiological studies. *Int. J. Cancer* 1994, **59**(4): 491–493.
9. Jaffe ES, Zarate OA, Medeiros LJ. The interrelationship of Hodgkin's disease and non-Hodgkin's lymphomas – lessons learned from composite and sequential malignancies. *Semin. Diagn. Pathol.* 1992, **9**(4): 297–303.
10. Sander C, Medeiros L, Abruzzo L, et al. Lymphoblastic lymphoma presenting in cutaneous sites: A clinicopathologic analysis of six cases. *J. Am. Acad. Dermatol.* 1991, **25**: 1023–1031.
11. Haddy TB, Kennan AM, Jaffe ES, et al. Bone involvement in young patients with non-Hodgkin's lymphoma: Efficacy of chemotherapy without local radiotherapy. *Blood* 1988, **72**: 1141–1147.
12. Borowitz M, Croker B, Metzgar R. Lymphoblastic lymphoma with the phenotype of common acute lymphoblastic leukemia. *Am. J. Clin. Pathol.* 1983, **79**: 387–391.
13. Nathwani B, Diamond L, Winberg C, et al. Lymphoblastic lymphoma: A clinicopathologic study of 95 patients. *Cancer* 1981, **48**: 2347–2357.
14. Lardelli P, Bookman M, Sundeen J, et al. Lymphocytic lymphoma of intermediate differentiation. Morphologic and immunophenotypic spectrum and clinical correlations. *Am. J. Surg. Pathol.* 1990, **14**: 752–763.
15. Janossy G, Bollum F, Bradstock K, et al. Cellular phenotypes of normal and leukemic hematopoietic cells determined by selected antibody combinations. *Blood* 1980, **56**: 430–441.
16. Buccheri V, Mihaljevic B, Matutes E, et al. mb-1: A new marker for B-lineage lymphoblastic leukemia. *Blood* 1993, **82**(3): 853–857.
17. Pangalis G, Nathwani B, Rappaport H. Malignant lymphoma, well differentiated lymphocytic: Its relationship with chronic lymphocytic leukemia and macroglobulinemia of Waldenström. *Cancer* 1977, **39**: 999–1010.
18. Dick F, Maca R, The lymph node in chronic lymphocytic leukemia. *Cancer* 1978, **41**: 283–292.
19. Pombo de Oliveira MS, Jaffe ES, Catovsky D, Leukemic phase of mantle zone (intermediate) lymphoma: Its characterization in 11 cases. *J. Clin. Pathol.* 1989, **42**: 962–972.
20. Perry D, Bast M, Armitage J, et al. Diffuse intermediate lymphocytic lymphoma: A clinicopathologic study and comparison with small lymphocytic lymphoma and diffuse small cleaved cell lymphoma. *Cancer* 1990, **66**: 1995–2000.
21. Zukerberg L, Medeiros L, Ferry J, et al. Diffuse low-grade B-cell lymphomas: Four clinically distinct subtypes defined by a combination of morphologic and immunophenotypic features. *Am. J. Clin. Pathol.* 1993, **100**: 373–385.
22. Cossman J, Neckers LM, et al. Low-grade lymphomas: Expression of developmentally regulated B-cell antigens. *Am. J. Pathol.* 1984, **115**: 117–124.
23. Caligeris-Cappio F, Gobbi M, Bofill M, et al. Infrequent normal B lymphocytes express features of B chronic lymphocytic leukemia. *J. Exp. Med.* 1982, **155**: 623–628.
24. Spier CM, Grogan TM, Fielder K, et al. Immunophenotypes in 'well-differentiated' lymphoproliferative disorders with emphasis on small lymphocytic lymphoma. *Hum. Pathol.* 1986, **17**: 1126–1136.
25. Burns BF, Warnke RA, Doggett RS, et al. Expression of a T-cell antigen (Leu-1) by B-cell lymphomas. *Am. J. Pathol.* 1983, **113**: 165–171.
26. Picker L, Weiss L, Medeiros L, et al. Immunophenotypic criteria for the diagnosis of non-Hodgkin's lymphoma. *Am. J. Pathol.* 1987, **128**: 181–201.
27. Evans H, Butler J, Youness E, Malignant lymphoma, small lymphocytic type: A clinicopathologic study of 84 cases with suggested criteria for intermediate lymphocytic lymphoma. *Cancer* 1978, **41**: 1440–1455.
28. Richter M, Generalized reticular cell sarcoma of lymph nodes associated with lymphocytic leukemia. *Am. J. Pathol.* 1928, **4**: 285–292.
29. Williams J, Schned A, Cotelingam JD, et al. Chronic lymphocytic leukemia with coexistent Hodgkin's disease: Implications for the origin of the Reed–Sternberg cell. *Am. J. Surg. Pathol.* 1991, **15**: 33–42.
30. Brecher M, Banks P, Hodgkin's disease variant of Richter's syndrome: Report of eight cases. *Am. J. Clin. Pathol.* 1990, **93**: 333–339.
31. Momose H, Jaffe ES, Shin SS, et al. Chronic lymphocytic leukemia/small lymphocytic lymphoma with Reed–Sternberg-like cells and possible transformation to Hodgkin's disease. Mediation by Epstein–Barr virus. *Am. J. Surg. Pathol.* 1992, **16**(9): 859–867.
32. Ben-Ezra J, Burke J, Swartz W, et al. Small lymphocytic lymphoma: A clinicopathologic analysis of 268 cases. *Blood* 1989, **73**: 579–587.
33. Lennert K, Tamm I, Wacker H-H. Histopathology and immunocytochemistry of lymph node biopsies in

chronic lymphocytic leukemia and immunocytoma. *Leuk. Lymphoma* 1991, (Suppl.): 157–160.

34. Hall PA, D'Ardenne AJ, Richards MA, et al. Lymphoplasmacytoid lymphoma: An immunohistological study. *J. Pathol.* 1987, **153**(3): 213–223.

35. Jaffe ES, Raffeld M, Medeiros LJ. Histopathologic subtypes of indolent lymphomas: Caricatures of the mature B-cell system. *Semin. Oncol.* 1993, **20**: 3–30.

36. Harris N, Bhan A. B-Cell neoplasms of the lymphocytic, lymphoplasmacytoid, and plasma cell types: Immunohistologic analysis and clinical correlation. *Hum. Pathol.* 1985, **16**: 829–837.

37. Sundeen J, Longo D, Jaffe E. CD5 expression in B-cell small lymphocytic malignancies: Correlations with clinical presentation and sites of disease. *Am. J. Surg. Pathol.* 1992, **16**: 130–137.

38. Raffeld M, Jaffe ES. *bcl*-1, t(11;14), and mantle cell derived neoplasms. *Blood* 1991, **78**: 259–263.

39. Banks P, Chan J, Cleary M, et al. Mantle cell lymphoma: A proposal for unification of morphologic, immunologic, and molecular data. *Am. J. Surg. Pathol.* 1992, **16**: 637–640.

40. Jaffe E, Bookman M, Longo D. Lymphocytic lymphoma of intermediate differentiation – Mantle zone lymphoma. *Hum. Pathol.* 1987, **18**: 877–880.

41. Weisenburger DD, Kim H, Rappaport H. Mantle zone lymphoma: A follicular variant of intermediate lymphocytic lymphoma. *Cancer* 1982, **49**: 1429–1438.

42. Bookman MA, Lardelli P, Jaffe ES, et al. Lymphocytic lymphoma of intermediate differentiation: Morphologic, immunophenotypic, and prognostic factors. *J. Natl Cancer Inst.* 1990, **82**: 742–748.

43. Meusers P, Engelhard M, Bartels H, et al. Multicentre randomized therapeutic trial for advanced centrocytic lymphoma: Anthracycline does not improve the prognosis. *Hematol. Oncol.* 1989, **7**: 365–380.

44. O'Brian D, Kennedy M, Daly P, et al. Multiple lymphomatous polyposis of the gastrointestinal tract: A clinicopathologically distinctive form of non-Hodgkin's lymphoma of centrocytic type. *Am. J. Surg. Pathol.* 1989, **13**: 691–699.

45. Lennert K. *Histopathology of Non-Hodgkin's lymphomas: Based on the Kiel Classification.* New York: Springer-Verlag, 1981.

46. Weisenburger DD, Nathwani BN, Diamond LW, et al. Malignant lymphoma intermediate lymphocytic type: A clinicopathologic study of 42 cases. *Cancer* 1981, **48**: 1415–1425.

47. Swerdlow S, Habeshaw J, Murray L, et al. Centrocytic lymphoma: A distinct clinicopathologic and immunologic entity. *Am. J. Pathol.* 1983, **113**: 181–197.

48. Medeiros L, van Krieken J, Jaffe E, et al. Association of *bcl*-1 rearrangements with lymphocytic lymphoma of intermediate differentiation. *Blood* 1990, **76**: 2086–2090.

49. Raffeld M, Sander CA, Yano T, et al. Mantle cell lymphoma: An update. *Leuk. Lymphoma* 1992, **8**(3): 161–166.

50. Rosenberg C, Wong E, Petty E, et al. Overexpression of PRAD1, a candidate BCL1 breakpoint region oncogene in centrocytic lymphomas. *Proc. Natl Acad. Sci. USA* 1991, **88**: 9638–9642.

51. Bosch F, Jares P, Campo E, et al. PRAD-1/cyclin D1 gene overexpression in chronic lymphoproliferative disorders: A highly specific marker of mantle cell lymphoma. *Blood* 1994, **84**(8): 2726–2732.

52. Come ES, Jaffe ES, Andersen JC, et al. Non-Hodgkin's lymphomas in leukemic phase: Clinicopathologic correlations. *Am. J. Med.* 1980, **69**: 667–674.

53. Hu E, Trela M, Thompson J. Detection of B-cell lymphoma in peripheral blood by DNA hybridization. *Lancet* 1985, **2**: 1092–1095.

54. Mann R, Berard C. Criteria for the cytologic subclassification of follicular lymphomas: A proposed alternative method. *Hematol. Oncol.* 1982, **1**: 187–192.

55. Croce C, Nowell P. Molecular basis of human B-cell neoplasia. *Blood* 1985, **65**: 1–7.

56. Hockenbery D, Zutter M, Hickey W, et al. BCL2 protein is topographically restricted in tissues characterized by apoptotic cell death. *Proc. Natl Acad. Sci. USA* 1991, **88**: 6961–6965.

57. Pezzella F, Tse A, Cordell J, et al. Expression of the Bcl-2 oncogene protein is not specific for the 14–18 chromosomal translocation. *Am. J. Pathol.* 1990, **137**: 225–232.

58. Zutter M, Hockenbery D, Silverman G, et al. Immunolocalization of the Bcl-2 protein within hematopoietic neoplasms. *Blood* 1991, **78**: 1062–1068.

59. Gaulard P, d'Agay M, Peuchmaur M, et al. Expression of the *bcl*-2 gene product in follicular lymphoma. *Am. J. Pathol.* 1992, **140**: 1089–1095.

60. Jaffe E, Shevach E, Frank M, et al. Nodular lymphoma: Evidence for origin from follicular B lymphocytes. *N. Engl. J. Med.* 1974, **290**: 813–819.

61. Stein H, Gerdes J, Mason D. The normal and malignant germinal centre. *Clin. Haematol.* 1982, **11**(3): 531–559.

62. Harris N, Nadler L, Bhan A. Immunohistologic characterization of two malignant lymphomas of germinal center type (centroblastic/centrocytic and centrocytic) with monoclonal antibodies: Follicular and diffuse lymphomas of small cleaved cell types are related but distinct entities. *Am. J. Pathol.* 1984, **117**: 262–272.

63. Garvin AJ, Simon R, Young RC, et al. The Rappaport classification of non-Hodgkin's lymphomas: A closer look using other proposed classifications. *Semin. Oncol.* 1980, **7**: 234–243.

64. Medeiros L, Lardelli P, Stetler-Stevenson M, et al. Genotypic analysis of diffuse mixed cell lymphomas: Comparison with morphologic and immunophenotypic findings. *Am. J. Clin. Pathol.* 1991, **95**: 547.

65. Garcia CF, Weiss LM, Warnke RA, et al. Cutaneous follicular lymphoma. *Am. J. Surg. Pathol.* 1986, **10**: 454–463.

66. Santucci M, Pimpinelli N, Arganini L. Primary cutaneous B-cell lymphoma: A unique type of low-grade lymphoma. Clinicopathologic and immunologic study of 83 cases. *Cancer* 1991, **67**: 2311–2326.

67. Isaacson P, Wright D. Malignant lymphoma of mucosa associated lymphoid tissue. A distinctive B-cell lymphoma. *Cancer* 1983, **52**: 1410–1416.

68. Isaacson P, Spencer J. Malignant lymphoma of mucosa-associated lymphoid tissue. *Histopathology* 1987, **11**: 445–462.

69. Isaacson P, Wotherspoon A, Diss T, et al. Follicular colonization in B-cell lymphoma of mucosa associated lymphoid tissue. *Am. J. Surg. Pathol.* 1991, **15**: 819–828.

70. Pelstring R, Essell J, Kurtin P, et al. Diversity of organ site involvement among malignant lymphomas of mucosa-associated tissues. *Am. J. Clin. Pathol.* 1991, **96**: 738–745.

71. Parveen T, Navarro-Roman L, Medeiros L, et al. Low-grade B-cell lymphoma of mucosa-associated lymphoid tissue arising in the kidney. *Arch. Pathol. Lab. Med.* 1993, **117**: 780–783.

72. Shin S, Sheibani K, Fishleder A, et al. Monocytoid B-cell lymphoma in patients with Sjogren's syndrome: A clinicopathologic study of 13 patients. *Hum. Pathol.* 1991, **22**: 422–430.

73. Cogliatti S, Lennert K, Hansmann M, et al. Monocytoid B-cell lymphoma: clinical and prognostic features of 21 patients. *J. Clin. Pathol.* 1990, **43**: 619–625.

74. Ortiz-Hidalgo C, Wright DH. The morphological spectrum of monocytoid B-cell lymphoma and its relationship to lymphomas of mucosa-associate lymphoid tissue. Histopathology 1992, **21**: 555–561.

75. Nizze H, Cogliatti S, von Schilling C, et al. Monocytoid B-cell lymphoma: Morphological variants and relationship to low-grade B-cell lymphoma of the mucosa-associated lymphoid tissue. *Histopathology* 1991, **18**: 403–414.

76. Hussell T, Isaacson P, Crabtree J, et al. The response of cells from low-grade B-cell gastric lymphomas of mucosa-associated lymphoid tissue to *Helicobacter pylori*. *Lancet* 1993, **342**: 571–574.

77. Wotherspoon A, Doglioni C, Diss T, et al. Regression of primary low-grade B-cell gastric lymphoma of mucosa-associated lymphoid tissue type after eradication of *Helicobacter pylori*. *Lancet* 1993, **342**: 575–577.

78. Fisher RI, Dahlberg S, Nathwani BN, et al. A clinical analysis of two indolent lymphoma entities: Mantle cell lymphoma and marginal zone lymphoma (including the mucosa-associated lymphoid tissue and monocytoid B-cell subcategories): A Southwest Oncology Group study. *Blood* 1995, **85**(4): 1075–1082.

79. Sheibani K, Burke J, Swartz W, et al. Monocytoid B-cell lymphoma. Clinicopathologic study of 21 cases of a unique type of low grade lymphoma. *Cancer* 1988, **62**: 1531–1538.

80. Ngan B-Y, Warnke R, Wilson M, et al. Monocytoid B-cell lymphoma: A study of 36 cases. *Hum. Pathol.* 1991, **22**: 409–421.

81. Wotherspoon AC, Finn TM, Isaacson PG. Trisomy 3 in low grade B-cell lymphomas of mucosa-associated lymphoid tissue. *Blood* 1995, **85**(8): 2000–2004.

82. Horsman D, Gascoyne R, Klasa R, et al. t(11;18)(q21;q21.1): A recurring translocation in lymphomas of mucosa associated lymphoid tissue (MALT)? *Genes Chromosom. Cancer* 1992, **4**(2): 183–187.

83. Whang-Peng J, Knutsen T, Jaffe E, et al. Cytogenetic study of two cases with lymphoma of mucosa-associated lymphoid tissue. *Cancer Genet. Cytogenet.* 1994, **77**(1): 74–80.

84. Rijlaarsdam JU, van der Putte SC, Berti E, et al. Cutaneous immunocytomas: A clinicopathologic study of 26 cases. Histopathology 1993, **23**(2): 117–125.

85. Hollema H, Visser L, Poppema S. Small lymphocytic lymphomas with predominant splenomegaly: A comparison of immunophenotypes with cases of predominant lymphadenopathy. *Mod. Pathol.* 1991, **4**: 712–717.

86. Neiman R, Sullivan A, Jaffe R. Malignant lymphoma simulating leukaemic reticuloendotheliosis: A clinicopathologic study of ten cases. *Cancer* 1979, **43**: 329–342.

87. Schmid C, Kirkham N, Diss T, et al. Splenic marginal zone cell lymphoma. *Am. J. Surg. Pathol.* 1992, **16**: 455–466.

88. Melo J, Hegde U, Parreira A, et al. Splenic B cell lymphoma with circulating villous lymphocytes: differential diagnosis of B-cell leukaemias with large spleens. *J. Clin. Pathol.* 1987, **40**: 642–651.

89. Isaacson PG, Matutes E, Burke M, et al. The histopathology of splenic lymphoma with villous lymphocytes. *Blood* 1994, **84**(11): 3828–3834.

90. Callihan TT, Holbert JM, Berard CW. Neoplasms of terminal B-cell differentiation: The morphologic basis of functional diversity. In Sommers SC, Rosen PP (eds) *Malignant Lymphomas, Pathology Annual*. Norwalk, CT: Appleton-Century Crofts, 1983, pp. 169–268.

91. Falini B, De Solas I, Levine A, et al. Emergence of B-immunoblastic sarcoma in patient with multiple myeloma: A clinicopathologic study of 10 cases. *Blood* 1982, **59**: 923–933.

92. Zukerberg L, Ferry J, Conlon M, et al. Plasma cell myeloma with cleaved multilobated and monocytoid nuclei. *Am. J. Clin. Pathol.* 1990, **93**: 657–661.

93. O'Hara C, Said J, Pinkus G. Non-Hodgkin's lymphoma multilobated B-cell type. *Hum. Pathol.* 1986, **17**: 593–599.

94. Pettit C, Zukerberg L, Gray M, et al. Primary lymphoma of bone: A B cell tumor with a high frequency of multilobated cells. *Am. J. Surg. Pathol.* 1990, **14**: 329–334.

95. Lamarre L, Jacobson J, Aisenberg A, et al. Primary large cell lymphoma of the mediastinum. *Am. J. Surg. Pathol.* 1989, **13**: 730–739.

96. Jaffe E. Post-thymic lymphoid neoplasia. In Jaffe E (ed.) *Surgical Pathology of the Lymph Nodes and Related Organs*. W. B. Saunders: Philadelphia, 1985, pp. 218–248.

97. Chittal S, Brousset P, Voigt J, et al. Large B-cell lymphoma rich in T-cells and simulating Hodgkin's disease. *Histopathology* 1991, **19**: 211–220.

98. Delabie J, Vandenberghe E, Kennes C, et al. Histiocyte-rich B-cell lymphoma. A distinct clinicopathologic entity possibly related to lymphocyte predominant Hodgkin's disease paragranuloma subtype. *Am. J. Surg. Pathol.* 1992, **16**: 37–48.

99. Macon W, Williams M, Greer J, et al. T-cell-rich B-cell lymphomas. A clinicopathologic study of 19 cases. *Am. J. Surg. Pathol.* 1992, **16**(4): 351–363.

100. Ramsay A, Smith W, Isaacson P. T-cell-rich B-cell

lymphoma. *Am. J. Surg. Pathol.* 1988, **12**: 433–443.

101. Krishnan J, Wallberg K, Frizzera G. T-cell rich large B-cell lymphoma: A study of 30 cases supporting its histologic heterogeneity and lack of clinical distinctiveness. *Am. J. Surg. Pathol.* 1994, **18**: 455–465.

102. Nathwani B, Dixon D, Jones S, et al. The clinical significance of the morphological subdivision of diffuse 'histiocytic' lymphoma: A study of 162 patients treated by the Southwest Oncology Group. *Blood* 1982, **60**: 1068–1074.

103. Warnke RA, Strauchern JA, Burke JS, et al. Morphologic types of diffuse large cell lymphoma. *Cancer* 1982, **50**: 690–695.

104. Harris NL, Jaffe ES, Stein H, et al. A revised European–American classification of lymphoid neoplasms: A proposal from the International Lymphoma Study Group [see comments]. *Blood* 1994, **84**(5): 1361–1392.

105. Lennert K, Feller A. *Histopathology of Non-Hodgkin's Lymphomas*, 2nd edn. New York: Springer-Verlag, 1992.

106. Longo DL, Duffey PL, DeVita VJ, et al. Treatment of advanced-stage Hodgkin's disease: Alternating non-crossresistant MOPP/CABS is not superior to MOPP. *J. Clin. Oncol.* 1991, **9**(8): 1409–1420.

107. Miller TP, Grogan TM, Dahlberg S, et al. Prognostic significance of the Ki-67 associated proliferative antigen in aggressive non-Hodgkin's lymphomas: A prospective Southwest Onocology Group trial. *Blood* 1994, **83**: 1460–1466.

108. Hall PA, Richards MA, Gregory WM, et al. The prognostic value of Ki67 immunostaining in non-Hodgkin's lymphoma. *J. Pathol.* 1988, **154**(3): 223–235.

109. Gerdes J, Stein H, Pileri S, et al. Prognostic relevance of tumour-cell growth fraction in malignant non-Hodgkin's lymphomas [letter] [published erratum appears in *Lancet* 1987, Sep 26; **2**(8561): 756]. *Lancet* 1987, **2**(8556): 448–449.

110. Piris MA, Pezzella F, Martinez MI, et al. *p53* and *bcl-2* expression in high-grade B-cell lymphomas: Correlation with survival time [Published erratum appears in *Br. J. Cancer* 1994, **69**: 978]. *Br. J. Cancer* 1994, **69**: 337–341.

111. Addis B, Isaacson P, Large cell lymphoma of the mediastinum: A B-cell tumor of probable thymic origin. *Histopathology* 1986, **10**: 379–390.

112. Moller P, Moldenhauer G, Momburg F, et al. Mediastinal lymphoma of clear cell type is a tumor corresponding to terminal steps of B-cell differentiation. *Blood* 1987, **69**: 1087–1095.

113. Hofmann WJ, Momburg F, Moller P. Thymic medullary cells expressing B-lymphocyte antigens. *Hum. Pathol.* 1988, **19**: 1280–1287.

114. Kanavaros P, Gaulard P, Charlotte F, et al. Discordant expression of immunoglobulin and its associated molecule mb-1/CD79a is frequently found in mediastinal large B-cell lymphomas. *Am. J. Pathol.* 1995, **146**: 735–741.

115. Jacobson J, Aisenberg A, Lamarre L, et al. Mediastinal large cell lymphoma: An uncommon subset of adult lymphoma curable with combined modality therapy. *Cancer* 1988, **62**: 1893–1898.

116. Magrath I, Shiramizu B. Biology and treatment of small non-cleaved cell lymphoma. *Oncology* 1989, **3**: 41–53.

117. Ballerini P, Gaidano G, Gong JZ, et al. Multiple genetic lesions in acquired immunodeficiency syndrome-related non-Hodgkin's lymphoma. *Blood* 1993, **81**: 166–176.

118. Pelicci P, Knowles D, Magrath I, et al. Chromosomal breakpoints and structural alterations of the *c-myc* locus differ in endemic and sporadic forms of Burkitt lymphoma. *Proc. Natl Acad. Sci. USA* 1986, **83**: 2984–2988.

119. Yano T, Van KJ, Magrath IT, et al. Histogenetic correlations between subcategories of small non-cleaved cell lymphomas. *Blood* 1992, **79**: 1282–1290.

120. Cavdar AO, Gozdasoglu S, Yavuz G, et al. Burkitt's lymphoma between African and American types in Turkish children: Clinical viral (EBV) and molecular studies. *Med. Pediatr. Oncol.* 1993, **21**: 36–42.

121. Goldschmidts WL, Bhatia K, Johnson JF, et al. Epstein–Barr virus genotypes in AIDS-associated lymphomas are similar to those in endemic Burkitt's lymphomas. *Leukemia* 1992, **6**: 875–878.

122. Hollingsworth HC, Longo DL, Jaffe ES. Small noncleaved cell lymphoma associated with florid epithelioid granulomatous response. A clinicopathologic study of seven patients. *Am. J. Surg. Pathol.* 1993, **17**: 51–59.

123. Garcia C, Weiss L, Warnke R. Small noncleaved cell lymphoma: An immunophenotypic study of 18 cases and comparison with large cell lymphoma. *Hum. Pathol.* 1986, **17**: 454–461.

124. Longo DL, Duffey PL, Jaffe ES, et al. Diffuse small noncleaved-cell non-Burkitt's lymphoma in adults: A high-grade lymphoma responsive to ProMACE-based combination chemotherapy. *J. Clin. Oncol.* 1994, **12**: 2153–2159.

125. Miliauskas JR, Berard CW, Young RC, et al. Undifferentiated non-Burkitt's lymphomas (Burkitt's and non-Burkitt's types). The relevance of making this histologic distinction. *Cancer* 1982, **50**: 2115–2121.

126. Suchi T, Lennert K, Tu L-Y. Histopathology and immunohistochemistry of peripheral T-cell lymphomas: A proposal for their classification. *J. Clin. Pathol.* 1987, **40**: 995–1015.

127. Noorduyn LA, Van der Valk P, Van Heerde P, et al. Stage is a better prognostic indicator than morphologic subtype in primary non-cutaneous T-cell lymphoma. *Am. J. Clin. Pathol.* 1990, **93**: 49–57.

128. Hastrup N, Hamilton-Dutoit S, Ralfkiaer E, et al. Peripheral T-cell lymphomas: An evaluation of reproducibility of the updated Kiel classification. *Histopathology* 1991, **18**: 99–105.

129. Schlegelberger B, Himmler A, Godde E, et al. Cytogenetic findings in peripheral T-cell lymphomas as a basis for distinguishing low-grade and high-grade lymphomas. *Blood* 1994, **83**: 505–511.

130. Nathwani B, Kim H, Rappaport H. Malignant lymphoma lymphoblastic. *Cancer* 1976, **38**: 964–983.

131. Gouttefangeas C, Bensussan A, Boumsell L. Study of the CD3-associated T-cell receptors reveals further differences between T-cell acute lymphoblastic lymphoma and leukemia. *Blood* 1990, **74**: 931–934.

132. Braziel RM, Keneklis T, Donlon JA, et al. Terminal deoxynucleotidyl transferase in non-Hodgkin's lymphoma. *Am. J. Clin. Pathol.* 1983, **80**: 655–659.

133. Bernard A, Boumsell L, Reinherz L, et al. Cell surface characterization of malignant T-cells from lymphoblastic lymphoma using monoclonal antibodies: Evidence for phenotypic differences between malignant T-cells from patients with acute lymphoblastic leukemia and lymphoblastic lymphoma. *Blood* 1981, **57**: 1105–1110.

134. Weiss L, Bindl J, Picozzi V, et al. Lymphoblastic lymphoma: An immunophenotype study of 26 cases with comparison to T cell acute lymphoblastic leukemia. *Blood* 1986, **67**: 474–478.

135. Pittaluga S, Raffeld M, Lipford EH, et al. 3A1 (CD7) expression precedes T beta gene rearrangements in precursor T (lymphoblastic) neoplasms. *Blood* 1986, **68**: 134–139.

136. Pittaluga S, Uppenkamp M, Cossman J. Development of T3/T cell receptor gene expression in human pre-T neoplasms. *Blood* 1987, **69**: 1062–1067.

137. Matutes E, Brito-Babapulle V, Swansbury J, et al. Clinical and laboratory features of 78 cases of T-prolymphocytic leukemia. *Blood* 1991, **78**: 3269–3274.

138. Brouet J, Sasportes M, Flandrin G, et al. Chronic lymphocytic leukemia of T-cell origin. *Lancet* 1975, **ii**: 890–893.

139. Loughran T. Clonal diseases of large granular lymphocytes. *Blood* 1993, **82**: 1–14.

140. Scott AA, Head DR, Kopecky KJ, et al. HLA-DR– CD33+, CD56+, CD16– myeloid/natural killer cell acute leukemia: A previously unrecognized form of acute leukemia potentially misdiagnosed as French– American–British acute myeloid leukemia-M3 [see comments]. *Blood* 1994, **84**: 244–255.

141. Imamura N, Kusunoki Y, Kawa-Ha K, et al. Aggressive natural killer cell leukaemia/lymphoma: Report of four cases and review of the literature. Possible existence of a new clinical entity originating from the third lineage of lymphoid cells [see comments]. *Br. J. Haematol.* 1990, **75**: 49–59.

142. Colby T, Burke J, Hoppe R. Lymph node biopsy in mycosis fungoides. *Cancer* 1981, **47**: 351–359.

143. Burke J, Khalil S, Rappaport H. Dermatopathic lymphadenopathy. An immunophenotypic comparison of cases asssociated and unassociated with mycosis fungoides. *Am. J. Pathol.* 1986, **123**: 256–263.

144. Ralfkiaer E, Wantzin G, Mason D, et al. Phenotypic characterization of lymphocyte subsets in mycosis fungoides. *Am. J. Clin. Pathol.* 1985, **84**: 610–619.

145. Patsouris E, Noel H, Lennert K. Histological and immunohistological findings in lymphoepithelioid cell lymphoma (Lennert's lymphoma). *Am. J. Surg. Pathol.* 1988, **12**: 341–350.

146. Kim H, Jacobs C, Warnke R, et al. Malignant lymphoma with a high content of epithelioid histiocytes: A distinct clinicopathologic entity and a form of so-called 'Lennert's lymphoma'. *Cancer* 1978, **41**: 620–635.

147. Armitage J, Greer J, Levine A, et al. Peripheral T-cell lymphoma. *Cancer* 1989, **63**: 158–163.

148. Lippman S, Miller T, Spier C, et al. The prognostic significance of the immunotype in diffuse large-cell lymphoma: A comparative study of the T-cell and B-cell phenotype. *Blood* 1988, **72**: 436–441.

149. Coiffier B, Brousse N, Peuchmaur M, et al. Peripheral T-cell lymphomas have a worse prognosis than B-cell lymphomas: A prospective study of 361 immunophenotyped patients treated with the LNH-84 regimen. *Ann. Oncol.* 1990, **1**: 45–50.

150. Gonzalez C, Medeiros L, Braziel R, et al. T-cell lymphoma involving subcutaneous tissue: A clinicopathologic entity commonly associated with hemophagocytic syndrome. *Am. J. Surg. Pathol.* 1991, **15**: 17–21.

151. Burg G, Dummer R, Wilhelm M, et al. A subcutaneous delta-positive T-cell lymphoma that produces interferon gamma [see comments]. *N. Engl. J. Med.* 1991, **325**: 1078–1081.

152. Farcet J, Gaulard P, Marolleau J, et al. Hepatosplenic T-cell lymphoma: Sinusal/sinusoidal localization of malignant cells expressing the T-cell receptor $\gamma\delta$. *Blood* 1990, **75**: 2213–2219.

153. Cooke CB, Krenacs L, Stetler-Stevenson M, et al. Hepatosplenic T-cell lymphoma: A distinct clinicopathological entity of cytotoxic $\gamma\delta$T-cell origin. *Blood* (in press).

154. Frizzera G, Moran E, Rappaport H. Angio-immunoblastic lymphadenopathy with dysproteinemia. *Lancet* 1974, **i**: 1070–1073.

155. Weiss L, Strickler J, Dorfman R, et al. Clonal T-cell populations in angioimmunoblastic lymphadenopathy and angioimmunoblastic lymphadenopathy-like lymphoma. *Am. J. Pathol.* 1986, **122**: 392–397.

156. Feller A, Griesser H, Schilling C, et al. Clonal gene rearrangement patterns correlate with immunophenotype and clinical parameters in patients with angioimmunoblastic lymphadenopathy. *Am. J. Pathol.* 1988, **133**: 549–556.

157. Patsouris D, Noel H, Lennert K. AILD type of T-cell lymphoma with a high content of epithelioid cells. Histopathology and comparison with lymphoepithelioid cell lymphoma. *Am. J. Surg. Pathol.* 1989, **13**: 161–175.

158. Siegert W, Agthe A, Griesser H, et al. Treatment of angioimmunoblastic lymphadenopathy (AILD)-type T-cell lymphoma using prednisone with or without the COPBLAM/IMVP-16 regimen. A multicenter study. Kiel Lymphoma Study Group. *Ann. Intern. Med.* 1992, **117**: 364–370.

159. Nathwani BN, Rappaport H, Moran EM, et al. Malignant lymphoma arising in angioimmunoblastic lymphadenopathy. *Cancer* 1978, **41**: 578–606.

160. Abruzzo LV, Schmidt K, Weiss LM, et al. B-cell lymphoma after angioimmunoblastic lymphadenopathy: A case with oligoclonal gene rearrangements associated with Epstein–Barr virus. *Blood* 1993, **82**: 241–246.

161. Uchiyama T, Yodoi J, Sagawa K, et al. Adult T-cell leukemia: Clinical and hematologic features of 16 cases. *Blood* 1977, **50**: 481–492.

162. Poiesz B, Ruscetti F, Gazdar A. Detection and isolation of type C retrovirus particles from fresh and cultured lymphocytes of a patient with cutaneous T-cell lymphoma. *Proc. Natl Acad. Sci. USA* 1980, **77**: 7415–7419.

163. Swerdlow S, Habeshaw J, Rohatiner A, et al. Caribbean T-cell lymphoma/leukemia. *Cancer* 1984, **54**: 687–696.

164. Manns A, Cleghorn FR, Falk RT, et al. Role of HTLV-I in development of non-Hodgkin lymphoma in Jamaica and Trinidad and Tobago. The HTLV Lymphoma Study Group. *Lancet* 1993, **342**(8885): 1447–1450.

165. Jaffe E, Blattner W, Blayney D, et al. The pathologic spectrum of adult T-cell leukemia/lymphoma in the United States. *Am. J. Surg. Pathol.* 1984, **8**: 263–275.

166. Levine PH, Manns A, Jaffe ES, et al. The effect of ethnic differences on the pattern of HTLV-I-associated T-cell leukemia/lymphoma (HATL) in the United States. *Int. J. Cancer* 1994, **56**: 177–181.

167. Abrams M, Sidawy M, Novich M. Smoldering HTLV-associated T-cell leukemia. *Arch. Intern. Med.* 1985, **145**: 2257–2258.

168. Kikuchi M, Mitsui T, Takeshita M, et al. Virus associated adult T-cell leukemia (ATL) in Japan: Clinical histological and immunological studies. *Hematol. Oncol.* 1987, **4**: 67.

169. Duggan D, Ehrlich G, Davey F, et al. HTLV-I induced lymphoma mimicking Hodgkin's disease. Diagnosis by polymerase chain reaction amplification of specific HTLV-I sequences in tumor DNA. *Blood* 1988, **71**: 1027–1032.

170. Chan J, Ng C, Lau W, et al. Most nasal/nasopharyngeal lymphomas are peripheral T-cell neoplasms. *Am. J. Surg. Pathol.* 1987, **11**: 418–429.

171. Ho F, Choy D, Loke S, et al. Polymorphic reticulosis and conventional lymphomas of the nose and upper aerodigestive tract – a clinicopathologic study of 70 cases and immunophenotypic studies of 16 cases. *Hum. Pathol.* 1990, **21**: 1041–1050.

172. Ferry JA, Sklar J, Zukerberg LR, et al. Nasal lymphoma: A clinicopathologic study with immuno-phenotypic and genotypic analysis. *Am. J. Surg. Pathol.* 1991, **15**: 268–279.

173. Lipford E, Margolich J, Longo D, et al. Angiocentric immunoproliferative lesions: A clinicopathologic spectrum of post-thymic T cell proliferations. *Blood* 1988, **5**: 1674–1681.

174. Jaffe E, Chan J, Su I, et al. Report of the workshop on nasal and related extranodal angiocentric T/NK cell lymphomas: Definitions, differential diagnosis, and epidemiology. *Am. J. Surg. Pathol.* 1996, **20**: 103–111.

175. Tsang WY, Chan JK, Yip TT, et al. *In situ* localization of Epstein–Barr virus encoded RNA in non-nasal/nasopharyngeal CD56-positive and CD56-negative T-cell lymphomas. *Hum. Pathol.* 1994, **25**: 758–765.

176. Medeiros L, Peiper S, Elwood L, et al. Angiocentric immunoproliferative lesions: A molecular analysis of eight cases. *Hum. Pathol.* 1991, **22**: 1150–1157.

177. Ho F, Srivastava G, Loke S, et al. Presence of Epstein–Barr virus DNA in nasal lymphomas of B and T-cell type. *Hematol. Oncol.* 1990, **8**: 271–281.

178. Arber DA, Weiss LM, Albujar PF, et al. Nasal lymphomas in Peru. High incidence of T-cell immuno-phenotype and Epstein–Barr virus infection. *Am. J. Surg. Pathol.* 1993, **17**: 392–399.

179. Jaffe ES, Costa J, Fauci AS, et al. Malignant lymphoma and erythrophagocytosis simulating malignant histiocytosis. *Am. J. Med.* 1983, **75**: 741–749.

180. Guinee DI, Jaffe E, Kingma D, et al. Pulmonary lymphomatoid granulomatosis. Evidence for a proliferation of Epstein–Barr virus infected B-lymphocytes with a prominent T-cell component and vasculitis. *Am. J. Surg. Pathol.* 1994, **18**: 753–764.

181. Katzenstein A-L, Peiper S. Detection of Epstein–Barr genomes in lymphomatoid granulomatosis: Analysis of 29 cases by the polymerase chain reaction. *Mod. Pathol.* 1990, **3**: 435–441.

182. Isaacson P, Spencer J, Connolly C, et al. Malignant histiocytosis of the intestine: A T-cell lymphoma. *Lancet* 1985, **ii**: 688–691.

183. Chott A, Dragosics B, Radaszkiewicz T. Peripheral T-cell lymphomas of the intestine. *Am. J. Pathol.* 1992, **141**: 1361–1371.

184. Spencer J, Cerf-Bensussan N, Jarry A, et al. Entero-pathy-associated T-cell lymphoma is recognized by a monoclonal antibody (HML-1) that defines a membrane molecule on human mucosal lymphocytes. *Am. J. Pathol.* 1988, **132**: 1–5.

185. Stein H, Mason D, Gerdes J, et al. The expression of the Hodgkin's disease associated antigen Ki-1 in reactive and neoplastic lymphoid tissue: Evidence that Reed–Sternberg cells and histiocytic malignancies are derived from activated lymphoid cells. *Blood* 1985, **66**: 848–858.

186. Kadin ME, Sako D, Berliner N, et al. Childhood Ki-1 lymphoma presenting with skin lesions and peripheral lymphadenopathy. *Blood* 1986, **68**: 1042–1049.

187. Agnarsson B, Kadin M. Ki-1 positive large cell lymphoma: A morphologic and immunologic study of 19 cases. *Am. J. Surg. Pathol.* 1988, **12**: 264–274.

188. Piris M, Brown D, Gatter K, et al. CD30 Expression in non-Hodgkin's lymphoma. *Histopathology* 1990, **17**: 211–218.

189. Kaudewitz P, Stein H, Dallenbach F, et al. Primary and secondary cutaneous Ki-1+ (CD30+) anaplastic large cell lymphomas. Morphologic, immunohisto-logic, and clinical-characteristics. *Am. J. Pathol.* 1989, **135**: 359–367.

190. de Bruin P, Beljaards R, van Heerde P, et al. Differences in clinical behaviour and immunopheno-type between primary cutaneous and primary nodal anaplastic large cell lymphoma of T-cell or null cell phenotype. *Histopathology* 1993, **23**: 127–135.

191. Willemze R, Beljaards RC. Spectrum of primary cutaneous CD30 (Ki-1)-positive lymphoproliferative disorders. A proposal for classification and guidelines for management and treatment. *J. Am. Acad. Dermatol.* 1993, **28**: 973–980.

192. Wellman A, Otsuki T, Vogelbruch M, et al. Analysis of the t(2;5) (p23;q35) by RT-PCR in CD30-positive anaplastic large cell lymphomas, in other non-Hodgkin's lymphomas of T-cell phenotype, and in Hodgkin's disease. *Blood* 1995, **86**: 2321–2328.

193. Mason D, Bastard C, Rimokh R, et al. CD30-positive large cell lymphomas ('Ki-1 lymphoma') are associated with a chromosomal translocation involving 5q35. *Br. J. Haematol.* 1990, **74**: 161–168.

194. Bitter MA, Franklin WA, Larson RA, et al. Morphology

in Ki-1(CD30)-positive non-Hodgkin's lymphoma is correlated with clinical features and the presence of a unique chromosomal abnormality t(2;5)(p23;q35). *Am. J. Surg. Pathol.* 1990, **14**: 305–316.

195. Morris SW, Kirstein MN, Valentine MB, et al. Fusion of a kinase gene, ALK, to a nucleolar protein gene, NPM, in non-Hodgkin's lymphoma. *Science* 1994, **263**(5151): 1281–1284. [Published erratum appears in *Science* 1995, **267**(5196): 316–317.]

196. Shiota M, Fujimoto J, Takenaga M, et al. Diagnosis of t(2;5)(p23;q35)-associated Ki-1 lymphoma with immunohistochemistry. *Blood* 1994, **84**: 3648–3652.

197. Delsol G, Al Saati T, Gatter K, et al. Coexpression of epithelial membrane antigen (EMA) Ki-1 and interleukin-2 receptor by anaplastic large cell lymphomas: Diagnostic value in so-called malignant histiocytosis. *Am. J. Pathol.* 1988, **130**: 59–70.

198. Pileri S, Falini B, Delsol G, et al. Lymphohistiocytic T-cell lymphoma (anaplastic large cell lymphoma CD30+/Ki1+) with a high content of reactive histiocytes. *Histopathology* 1990, **16**: 383–391.

199. Kinney M, Collins R, Greer J, et al. A small-cell-predominant variant of primary Ki-1 (CD30)+ T-cell lymphoma. *Am. J. Surg. Pathol.* 1993, **17**: 859–868.

200. Chan JK, Ng CS, Hui PK, et al. Anaplastic large cell Ki-1 lymphoma. Delineation of two morphological types [see comments]. *Histopathology* 1989, **15**: 11–34.

201. McCarty MI, Vukelja SJ, Sausville EA, et al. Lymphomatoid papulosis associated with Ki-1-positive anaplastic large cell lymphoma. A report of two cases and a review of the literature. *Cancer* 1994, **74**: 3051–3058.

202. Kaudewitz P, Burg G, Stein H. Ki-1 (CD30) positive cutaneous anaplastic large cell lymphomas. *Curr. Probl. Dermatol.* 1990, **19**: 150–156.

203. Beljaards RC, Meijer CJLM, Scheffer E, et al. Prognostic significance of CD 30 (Ki-1/BerH2) expression in primary cutaneous large-cell lymphomas of T-cell origin: A clinicopathologic and immunohistochemical study in 20 patients. *Am. J. Pathol.* 1989, **135**: 1169–1178.

204. Pileri S, Bocchia M, Baroni C, et al. Anaplastic large cell lymphoma (CD30+/Ki-1+): Results of a prospective clinicopathologic study of 69 cases. *Br. J. Haematol.* 1994, **86**: 513–523.

205. Leoncini L, Del Vecchio M, Kraft R, et al. Hodgkin's disease and CD30-positive anaplastic large cell lymphomas – a continuous spectrum of malignant disorders. *Am. J. Pathol.* 1990, **137**: 1047–1057.

206. MacLennan K, Bennett M, Tu A, et al. Relationship of histopathologic features to survival and relapse in nodular sclerosing Hodgkin's disease. *Cancer* 1989, **64**: 1686–1693.

CHAPTER 4

The role of molecular analysis in lymphoma diagnostics

MARK RAFFELD

Introduction

The lymphomas comprise a diverse group of tumors with respect to their clinical behavior and pathogenesis. They form a spectrum of disease ranging from indolent small lymphocytic neoplasms to aggressive large-cell lymphomas and Burkitt's lymphoma. Histologic evaluation of these tumors is challenging and has driven the development of ancillary diagnostic techniques.

The application of immunohistologic techniques to study lymphoid proliferations was a major advance for lymphoma diagnosis. Once it was discovered that B-cell tumors produce only one type of immunoglobulin light chain, κ or λ, it became possible to use the new technique to assess clonality. By studying the surface expression of the immunoglobulin molecule, one could distinguish monoclonal lymphomas derived from B-cells from polyclonal reactive populations.

The explosion of information about normal B- and T-cell biology over the past 15 years led to the development of large panels of lymphoid markers that allow the accurate differentiation of B-cell lymphomas from T-cell lymphomas. Detailed immunophenotypic analysis has further assisted in discriminating among histologically similar subtypes of lymphomas. For example, classical small lymphocytic lymphoma can be distinguished from other lymphomas composed of small lymphocytes, such as mantle cell lymphoma and lymphomas arising in mucosa-associated lymphoid tissue (MALT), on the basis of its consistent CD5 and CD23 expression. While mantle cell lymphomas and some MALT lymphomas may express CD5, neither express CD23.

However, although immunologic marker studies have transformed diagnostic hematopathology, they have limited use in certain situations. First, the assessment of clonality requires the presence of surface or cytoplasmic immunoglobulin. Not all B-cell lymphomas express a complete immunoglobulin molecule. Secondly, there is no comparable immunologic marker for assessing clonality in T-cell neoplasms, which comprise 15–25% of all lymphomas. Although immunologic marker studies have been very useful in classifying different lymphoma subtypes, there are still situations in which the available markers are not sufficiently helpful and additional information is desirable.

Over the past decade molecular genetic analysis has become an important adjunct to classical histologic and immunohistologic approaches. Molecular analysis of both the immunoglobulin and T-cell receptor genes, using restriction fragment analysis or polymerase chain reaction (PCR), has supplanted immunohistochemistry as the technique of choice for clonal analysis. Molecular analysis does not require gene expression and has greatly expanded the information obtainable by immunohistologic approaches alone. In addition, molecular genetic analysis of the antigen receptor genes yields information regarding cell lineage.

Molecular genetic approaches have also been applied to study involvement of specific recurring chromosomal translocations in lymphomas. These translocations usually result in the activation of proto-oncogenes located near the translocation breakpoints, and are characteristic of particular subtypes of lymphomas. The molecular reconfiguration involved in a translocation can be analyzed with the same methods used to study gene rearrangements. The molecular analysis of cytogenetic abnormalities is often referred to as molecular cytogenetics. The information obtained from molecular cytogenetic techniques is a useful adjunct to classical cytogenetic analysis. 'Masked' translocations (i.e., not apparent on classical cytogenetic analysis) can be detected, it is less time consuming to perform and it is applicable to a wider range of specimens.

The molecular profile of a tumor includes more than the analysis of translocation breakpoint regions. Chromosomal amplifications involving oncogenes, and deletions and mutations involving tumor suppressor genes, can also be studied. Although these lesions are less commonly associated with specific subtypes of lymphomas, they form a part of the overall molecular profile of a tumor, and may contain information related to the biologic properties of the lymphoma, such as its proliferative potential or resistance to chemotherapy, which may have prognostic implications for the patient.

Molecular genetic analysis has most recently been applied to investigate minimal residual disease in lymphomas. Minimal residual disease analysis has found a perfect partner in the PCR technique. This simple yet sensitive assay is replacing traditional restriction fragment analysis for routine clonal analysis, and is providing investigators with opportunities to detect and follow minimal disease at levels that were undetectable a few years ago. Using this technology, it is possible to identify a single tumor cell in a population of 10^6 normal cells or more. Although the application of PCR to the minimal disease setting is quite recent, it is already being used or being considered for use in initial

staging, for evaluating treatment, and for assessing the presence of tumor cells in purged marrow specimens earmarked for autologous reinfusion.

The purpose of this chapter is to present a general overview of the utility and molecular basis for lymphoma molecular diagnostics. The three major areas that will be discussed are the use and significance of molecular diagnostics in assessing clonality, its use and significance in assessing pathologic genetic changes, and finally its use in assessing minimal residual disease in the lymphomas.

Molecular basis for clonal analysis: rearranging genes

The ability to utilize antigen receptor genes as molecular targets for determining clonality resides in their unusual gene structure, and the unique rearrangement process that these genes undergo in developing B- and T-cells. Both the immunoglobulin (Ig) genes and the T-cell receptor (TCR) genes share the same basic germline structure (Figure 4.1). Rather than there being a single contiguous gene encoding each polypeptide chain, there are several smaller gene segments that must be joined to form a complete coding region. Two or three different gene segments called variable (V), diversity (D) and joining (J) segments encode the information for the variable region of each polypeptide chain, while a single segment encodes the constant region. What makes these genes truly unique is not that they are composed of discontinuous gene segments, but rather that these gene segments are brought together by a genetic recombination process. This is discussed in more detail below.

IMMUNOGLOBULIN GENES

All B-cells produce an Ig molecule that consists of two identical heavy chains and two identical light chains which may be of either the κ or λ isotype. Both the heavy and light chains are divided into variable and constant regions. The variable region contains the information for antigen binding, while the constant region contains information for orchestrating a number of different immune effector functions.

The genes that encode the three immunoglobulin polypeptide chains, IgH, Igκ, and Igλ are located at chromosome 14q32, 2p12 and 22q11, respectively [1–4]. The immunoglobulin heavy chain locus contains about 90 variable-region gene segments (V regions), of which about 50 are believed to be functional [5]. The V regions are divided into six families based on sequence homology, and are interspersed along one megabase of DNA. There are approximately 30 small diversity-region gene segments (D regions) located between the variable-region gene segments and six joining-region gene segments (J regions). These three sets of gene segments encode the components of the variable portion of the Ig heavy chain. Immediately following the joining regions are the nine constant-region gene segments (C regions) that encode the constant portion of the Ig heavy chain and define each of the heavy-chain subclasses ($C\mu$, $C\delta$, $C\gamma3$, $C\gamma1$, $C\gamma2$, $C\alpha1$, $C\gamma4$, $C\varepsilon$, and $C\alpha2$). It is the assembly of the variable regions, diversity regions and joining regions into a unique antibody-encoding gene that provides a tumor-specific target that is amenable to molecular analysis. The heavy chain is the major Ig target for clonal analysis.

The κ light chain locus has the simplest genomic structure of the Ig loci. It contains 76 germline V regions of which only 32 are believed to be functional [6]. Approximately 30 kb of intervening DNA separates the variable regions from five joining regions and a single constant region. In contrast to the Ig heavy chain locus, the κ light chain locus has no D regions. An interesting feature of the variable regions is that approximately half the V regions are located 3' to the constant-region gene segment with opposing polarity. The assembled κ light chain gene is a frequent target in the molecular analysis of B-cell tumors.

The λ light chain locus contains an undetermined number of variable region genes, although probably fewer than the κ light chain locus. The λ light chain locus, like the κ light chain locus, has no diversity regions. It contains seven separate, but homologous constant-region gene segments, $C\lambda 1$–7, each accompanied by its own single joining region. Of these seven, four are functional. The constant region contains unusual polymorphisms consisting of repeated sequences of 5.2 kb, located between $C\lambda 3$ and $C\lambda 4$ [7]. It is important to be aware of these constant-region polymorphisms when performing clonal analysis of this locus. The λ light chain gene is less frequently a target for molecular analysis, primarily because, in most cases, sufficient information can be acquired by analyzing the Ig heavy chain and κ light chain genes.

T-CELL RECEPTOR GENES

T-Cells express one of two types of antigen receptors. Approximately 95% of T-cells possess α/β

TCRs, while the remaining 5% possess γ/δ TCRs [8]. Like the Ig polypeptide chains, these four polypeptide chains are also divided into a variable and constant portions. Most T-cell leukemias and lymphomas express the α/β TCR, while only a small percentage express the γ/δ TCR, generally paralleling the percentages of α/β and γ/δ receptor-bearing cells in normal T-cell populations.

The TCR loci have the same basic segmental structure as the Ig genes, with subtle variations particular to each gene. The α-chain locus is located at chromosome 14q11 [9]. It is estimated to contain at least 50 V regions. It has an unusually large number (50 or more) of J segments and does not contain D segments. It has one constant region gene. The α-chain gene is rarely a target for molecular analysis, primarily due to the long stretch of joining segments that present technical problems for performing an analysis.

The β-chain locus is located at chromosome 7q35 [10,11]. It possesses 50–100 V regions and two separate, but homologous, constant regions, $C\beta 1$ and $C\beta 2$. Each constant region is preceded by a single D segment, and six or seven J regions. The β-chain gene and the γ-chain gene described below are the most frequently analyzed TCR genes.

The γ-chain locus is located at chromosome 7p11 [12]. Like the TCR β-chain locus, this locus also has two homologous constant regions, each preceded by two or three J regions. The γ-chain locus contains no D segments. An unusual feature of the γ-chain locus is the small number of V regions that it contains. The V regions are divided into four families, $V\gamma1$–4. Although there are nine $V\gamma$ genes within the $V\gamma1$ family, only five of the nine code for a functional V region, the other four being nonfunctional pseudogenes. The three remaining $V\gamma$ families each contain one functional gene and one pseudogene. The γ-chain gene is a frequent target for molecular analysis.

The δ-chain locus is located at chromosome 14q11 and has several unusual structural features [13,14]. First, it is located within the α-chain locus, between the α-chain V regions and the α-chain J regions. Second, like the γ-chain gene, it has a very restricted repertoire of V regions. The δ-locus has six known variable regions, of which two are primarily used [15]. The δ-chain gene is an infrequent target for molecular analysis in lymphomas.

ANTIGEN RECEPTOR GENE REARRANGEMENT

In their germline state, both the Ig and TCR coding sequences exist as widely dispersed, discontinuous gene segments as previously detailed. In this configuration, these gene segments are incapable of forming

IgH locus

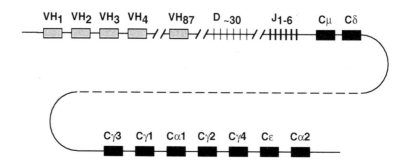

Igκ locus

Igλ locus

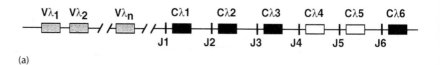

(a)

functional antigen receptor polypeptide chains. In developing B- and T-cells, a unique and complex process of gene rearrangement brings one of the tandemly arrayed V region gene segments into close proximity to a C region gene segment via one of several adjacent J region gene segments [16]. For the Ig heavy chain gene and the TCRβ- and δ-chain genes, an additional diversity or D region gene segment is also interposed between the V and J region gene segments during this recombination process. A continuous antigen receptor gene is formed, which is now capable of being transcribed and translated into a complete immunoglobulin or TCR polypeptide chain. This process is depicted in Figure 4.2 for the Ig heavy chain gene.

Additional modifications occur during the joining of the various gene segments. A small number of nucleotides may be lost or added to the free ends of the molecular intermediates that are formed during the strand breakage and rejoining reactions of the recombination process. Two types of added nucleotides occur at the junction regions, P nucleotides and N nucleotides [17–19]. P nucleotides are template-driven added nucleotides that inversely repeat the final one or two nucleotides at the breakpoint junction during the rearrangement process [17,18]. More important are the randomly added N nucleotides, which can account for as many as 20 additional nucleotides [19]. N region nucleotides contribute heavily to antibody diversity because of their location within the antigen binding sites of the antigen receptor molecules. Since junctional changes seldom account for more than 20 nucleotides of a rearranged antigen receptor gene, they do not affect traditional

TCRβ locus

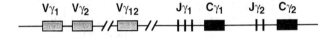

TCRγ locus

TCRα/δ locus

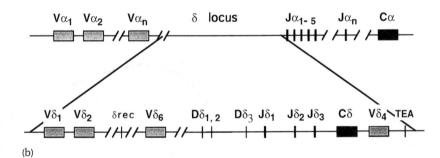

Figure 4.1 Antigen receptor gene loci. (a) Immunoglobulin heavy chain and κ and λ light chain gene loci. (b) T-cell receptor β, γ and α/δ gene loci.

(b)

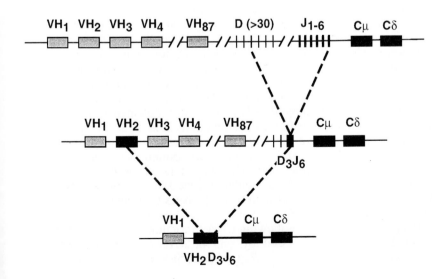

Figure 4.2 Immunoglobulin heavy chain gene rearrangement. Immunoglobulin heavy chain gene rearrangement occurs in two steps. In the first step, one of approximately 30 D segments rearranges to one of six J segments. In the second step, a single V region recombines to the rearranged D-J unit. In the example shown, D_3 is first joined to J_6, and is followed by the joining of VH_2 to the previously rearranged D_3-J_6 unit.

clonal analyses of lymphomas that rely on large restriction fragment analysis. They are, however, critical in molecular analyses of clonality that utilize PCR technology in which small fragments of 70–150 bases are analyzed. This will be discussed in more detail later.

The random assortment of V, D and J region gene segments, in combination with junctional alterations during the rearrangement process, allows a relatively small number of encoded DNA segments to generate most of the enormous diversity contained within the antigen receptor molecules. For the Ig heavy chain gene and the TCR α-chain gene, additional diversity is generated by somatic mutations that occur primarily during the subsequent maturation of the antibody response [20,21].

ONTOGENY AND ORDER OF GENE REARRANGEMENT

Antigen receptor gene rearrangement is a highly ordered developmental process. Rearrangement occurs very early during the differentiation of B- and T-cells from their progenitor stem cells. As a result, nearly all cells that are recognized phenotypically as B- or T-cells contain rearranged antigen receptor genes.

In B-cells, the Ig heavy chain locus rearranges prior to the light chain loci [22]. D to J joining occurs first, usually on both alleles, followed by V to D–J joining. κ light chain gene rearrangement follows. If the cell fails to generate a functional κ light chain gene, an unusual intramolecular deletional event occurs that eliminates a part of the κ light chain locus and brings a downstream element called the κde (kappa deleting element) into continuity with the κ locus [23]. This deletional event is followed by rearrangement of the λ light-chain genes [24]. The intracellular signaling that must occur to orchestrate this developmentally regulated rearrangement process is poorly understood. It has been suggested that the presence of an intact antigen receptor polypeptide chain may play a role in shutting down the rearrangement program.

T-cells also undergo a hierarchical rearrangement process. The TCRδ locus appears to be the first antigen receptor locus to undergo rearrangement [25]. This is followed shortly thereafter by rearrangement of both the γ- and β-chain gene loci. In cells that are destined to become α/β cells, an unusual intramolecular deletion of the δ-locus from within the α-locus must first occur [26]. This is reminiscent of the intramolecular deletion that affects the κ light chain locus prior to rearrangement of the λ-locus. A 5' locus designated the δ-recombination locus

(δ-Rec) recombines with a 3'-locus designated pseudo-Jα, deleting the entire intervening δ-chain locus [27]. Once this occurs, the α-locus is free to undergo rearrangement.

UTILITY OF MOLECULAR DIAGNOSTICS FOR ASSESSING CLONALITY

One of the practical outcomes of rearranging antigen receptor genes has been the ability to apply molecular biologic analyses to assess clonality in lymphoproliferative disorders. This analysis is possible because most lymphomas and lymphoid leukemias are derived from progenitor B- or T-cells that have undergone antigen receptor gene rearrangement *prior* to clonal expansion. As a result, all of the progeny tumor cells share the identical rearranged antigen receptor genes. This differs from a reactive polyclonal population in which the rearranged antigen receptor genes are different from one cell to the next. Thus, by assessing the status of the antigen receptor genes in a population of lymphoid cells, one can determine whether the population is composed of clonal tumor cells or polyclonal reactive cells. Furthermore, one can also obtain information concerning the lineage of the clonal population, since as a general rule, B-cell tumors contain rearranged Ig genes, while T-cell tumors have rearranged TCR genes.

Methods of assessing clonality-restriction fragment analysis

The traditional method for assessing clonality is through the use of restriction fragment analysis using Southern blotting. This technique involves several steps – extraction and digestion of genomic DNA, electrophoresis and Southern transfer of the resulting DNA fragments, and, finally, hybridization with appropriate antigen receptor gene probes.

A complete antigen receptor analysis requires about 50 μg of high molecular weight DNA. This is the amount of DNA in approximately 7.5 million diploid cells and is easily obtained from a surgical pathology specimen, as well as from the majority of fine-needle aspirations. Fresh or fresh-frozen tissue specimens are preferred for extraction of high molecular weight DNA. Attempts to extract high molecular weight DNA from formalin-fixed paraffin-embedded tissues have had limited success [28].

Following DNA extraction, 10–15 μg of DNA are digested by one of several restriction enzymes. These enzymes cut DNA at precise locations at specific palindromic nucleotide recognition sequences. For example, the restriction enzyme Hind III cuts at the sequence –AAGCTT–. The length of DNA defined by two adjacent restriction sequences (restriction sites) is called a restriction fragment. The sizes of the various restriction fragments generated by a particular enzyme are predetermined by the locations of the restriction sites in the DNA. Although no two genomes are exactly alike, owing to individual genetic polymorphisms, the location of many restriction sites are highly conserved, ensuring that many germline restriction fragments will be identical between individuals. For example, in the human genome, Bam H1 restriction sites located 5' and 3' to the Jκ gene segment define a germline restriction fragment 12 kb in length. This is true for all tissues, with the singular exception of B-lymphocytes and most tumors derived from B-lymphocytes. Because B-cells undergo V to J rearrangement of the κ light chain gene locus, the 12 kb Bam H1 germline restriction fragment will be altered by the loss of the 5' Bam H1 restriction site in the deleted intervening DNA, and the replacement of the deleted DNA segment by a V region sequence containing a new 5' Bam HI site (Figure 4.3).

Prior to detection of the altered restriction fragment, the cut fragments of DNA must be separated, on the basis of size, by electrophoresis through an agarose gel. The DNA fragments are subsequently transferred on to a nylon or nitrocellulose membrane according to the method of Southern [29]. The size of the Jκ-containing restriction fragment can now be determined according to its position in the gel.

The actual detection of rearranged restriction fragments is achieved through the use of previously cloned probes, which are fragments of the antigen receptor genes under investigation. When denatured, each strand of the probe will bind to the opposite strand of the same DNA region, which has been transferred to the nylon or nitrocellular membrane. To identify rearrangements of the κ light chain, a probe derived from the κ light chain locus is used. The probes are labeled either with radiochemicals or colorigens, and incubated with the membrane containing the size-separated DNA. These fragments anneal or hybridize to their corresponding fragments located on the membrane, and are detected by autoradiography or by color development. The location of the hybridized probe corresponds to the location of the restriction fragment containing either rearranged or germline antigen receptor DNA.

When one analyzes DNA from a *monoclonal* B-cell tumor by restriction fragment analysis using the Southern blot methodology, one finds either one or two *non*germline or 'rearranged' restriction fragments. If the progenitor B-cell that underwent the neoplastic event had one rearranged Jκ allele, then only one rearranged band would be seen; if both Jκ alleles were initially rearranged, then two rearranged bands would be seen. The assumption on which this reasoning is based – that lymphomas are clonal and derived from a single cell that underwent a neoplastic event – has been proven correct through the analysis in many laboratories, of many thousands of lymphoma samples that have been correlated with histology, phenotype and clinical outcome over the last 15 years [30–33].

In a *polyclonal* (e.g., reactive) population of B-

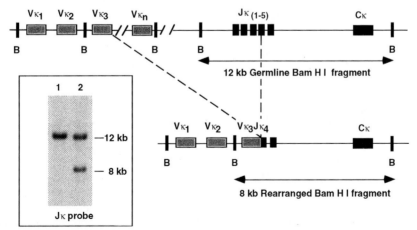

Figure 4.3   Restriction fragment analysis of the κ light chain locus. The germline structure of the κ locus is shown at the top of the figure. Bam H1 restriction enzyme sites (I) define a 12 kb restriction fragment that encompasses the entire κ light chain joining region and constant region. Rearrangement eliminates the 5' (on the left) Bam H1 site and contributes a new 5' Bam H1 site, changing the size of the restriction fragment, in this case, to 8 kb. A Southern blot of Bam H1-digested DNA probed with Jκ is shown in the inset. Lane 1 represents control placental DNA. Lane 2 shows a case with one allele rearranged and one allele remaining in the germline configuration.

cells, at least one Jκ allele in each B-cell within the population will be rearranged. However, since there are so many different V–J combinations in such a population, no single rearrangement predominates. In this case, restriction enzyme digestion of extracted DNA will result in a continuous ladder of rearranged DNA fragments containing the Jκ Ig gene segment. None of these rearranged fragments would be represented in large enough numbers to be detected.

The most commonly used diagnostic probes used for antigen receptor restriction fragment analysis are directed to either the constant regions or to the various joining regions. Ig gene rearrangements are generally assessed using probes to the heavy chain joining region (JH), the κ light chain joining region (Jκ), and the constant region of the λ light chain gene (Cλ). TCR gene rearrangements are usually assessed using probes to the TCR β-chain gene joining regions (Jβ1 and Jβ2) and/or to the TCR β-chain gene constant region. As a general rule, the most versatile probes are those that are located closest to the rearrangement breakpoints. Figure 4.4 is a restriction fragment analysis of DNA from a series of B-cell lymphomas analyzed with an Ig JH probe.

There are several problems and considerations one must take into account when analyzing antigen receptor gene rearrangements by this method. False-positive results can occur from incomplete digestion of DNA, which results in the appearance of a nongermline band of higher molecular weight. Even when DNA appears to be completely digested, there may still be some restriction sites that are par-

ticularly resistant to complete digestion. This phenomenon occurs frequently in TCRβ gene analyses. The TCRβ gene generally shows two germline bands when EcoR1-digested DNA is analyzed with a constant region probe, one of 12 kb containing the Cβ1 gene segment, and one of 4 kb, containing the Cβ2 gene segment. The EcoR1 restriction site located 5' to Cβ2 is frequently incompletely digested, yielding what may appear to be a nongermline band of approximately 8.5 kb [34].

Inherited polymorphisms are yet another potential source of false-positive interpretations. Polymorphisms result in restriction fragments of unexpected size. Fortunately there are only a few polymorphisms located in the regions of the antigen receptor genes that affect restriction fragment analyses. The most common polymorphism occurs in the Cλ locus and is due to the presence of repeated 5.2 kb sequences that result in polymorphic bands of either 13, 18, 23 or 28 kb [7]. Although the common polymorphisms of the antigen receptor gene loci have been well described, one must always be alert to the possibility that a 'rearranged' band may represent an uncommon polymorphism.

False-negative results may occur because a rearranged band happens to be the same size as, and therefore comigrates with, the germline band. The larger the germline restriction fragment of the locus under investigation, the more common is this problem. This is caused by the poorer resolution of separating higher molecular weight fragments. One can avoid this potential problem by studying each

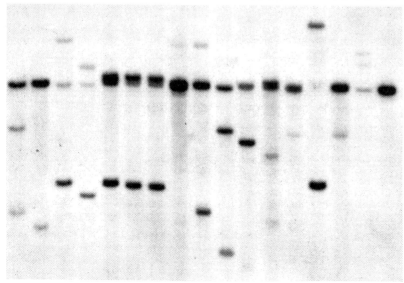

Figure 4.4 Immunoglobulin heavy chain gene rearrangements in a series of B-cell lymphomas. DNA was digested with the restriction enzyme Hind III, and a Southern blot prepared and hybridized with an immunoglobulin joining region probe. One or two rearranged bands can be identified in all lymphoma specimens. Lane 17 is placental control DNA.

gene locus with more than one restriction enzyme, as it is unlikely that several restriction enzymes will each generate rearranged fragments that comigrate with their respective germline bands.

There are some additional considerations that need to be mentioned with regard to analysis of the TCR gene loci. Since the majority of T-cell lymphomas are derived from α/β-bearing T-cells, the choices of genes to study are α, β or γ. As previously mentioned, α/β cells also have a rearranged γ-chain gene, but delete the δ-chain gene locus during rearrangement of the α-chain gene.

The TCR β-chain is the most commonly analyzed locus for assessing clonality of T-cell lymphomas in restriction fragment analysis. This locus is rearranged in most lymphomas and leukemias of T-cell phenotype. Rearrangements may be studied using probes to either the constant region (Cβ) or the joining region (Jβ1 and Jβ2). Probes to the constant region recognize both Cβ1 and Cβ2, while probes to the joining regions recognize only their respective joining region. The constant region probe has a disadvantage in that it can identify rearrangements involving Cβ1 in EcoR1 digests but not in Hind III digests, and Cβ2 rearrangements in Hind III digests but not in EcoR1 digests. This is due to the presence of a Hind III site between Jβ1 and Cβ1, and the presence of an EcoR1 site between Jβ2 and Cβ2.

The TCR α-chain gene is not commonly analyzed for rearrangement. The long stretch of J regions makes it unsuitable for analysis by traditional gel electrophoresis. Analysis of this locus can be achieved, however, by using either multiple-joining region probes and traditional gel electrophoresis, or by using rare restriction enzymes that cut DNA at infrequent intervals (i.e., generate large fragments) in combination with a constant region probe and pulse-field gel electrophoresis. The latter technique is used for separating large fragments of DNA from 30 kb to 2 megabases or more.

The TCR γ-chain gene is occasionally used to assess clonality, often as a confirmatory test in cases where TCRβ analysis has already been performed. Because of the small number of V regions in the γ-locus, the single D region and a biased use of J regions, only a limited number of potential V–D–J rearrangements can occur [35,36]. Nine different-sized rearrangements have been reported. This limited diversity presents two major problems for clonal analysis. The first is that polyclonal 'background' bands derived from normal T-lymphocytes in the population can obscure a small to moderate-sized clonal population [35]. The second problem is that, owing to the biased use of the V region gene segments, one may not always see all nine possible rearrangements in every polyclonal specimen examined [35]. In extreme cases, this could lead to an erroneous diagnosis of lymphoma.

The δ-gene locus is analyzed primarily in the setting of T-cell acute lymphoblastic lymphoma/leukemia [37], since this neoplasm appears to be arrested at an early stage of T-cell development in which T-cell rearrangements are still ongoing, and many cases will have partial rearrangements of the δ-chain locus. As previously mentioned, this gene has very few V region gene segments. However, since the majority of normal T-cells are α/β T-cells, which have deleted the δ gene, the identification of any δ-gene rearrangement is abnormal.

Restriction fragment analysis using the Southern blot technique has a reported sensitivity of 1–5%; that is, a detectable clone must comprise at least 1–5% of the total cellular population [30,31]. This is important to remember since most lymphomas are virtually never pure populations of tumor cells. Although the majority of lymphomas can be successfully studied by restriction fragment analysis, there are certain types of lymphomas such as the T-cell-rich B-cell lymphoma and pulmonary B-cell angiocentric lymphoma (formerly lymphomatoid granulomatosis) in which the percentage of tumor cells may fall below the limit of clonal detection. This 1–5% sensitivity limit should also be kept in mind when analyzing residual disease, and is the reason why more sensitive PCR methods are preferred in these circumstances. It is also important to recognize that the detection of a rearranged band implies only that some fraction of the cells belong to a single clone, not that the entire population is clonal. This has relevance to the determination of the clonality of lymphoproliferative processes arising, for example, in the posttransplant setting.

Methods of assessing clonality – PCR analysis of clonality

More recently, PCR has been used for the identification of clonal B- and T-cell proliferations. The PCR technique involves a series of linked reactions that result in an exponential increase in the copy number of a DNA sequence of interest. A single DNA target can be amplified over one million times. The reaction requires a pair of opposing oligonucleotide primers that flank the boundaries of the DNA target (template), a thermostable DNA polymerase, an excess of nucleotide triphosphates and the DNA template itself. The mixture is subjected to 25–40 cycles of heat denaturation, primer annealing and primer extension (DNA polymerization). With each cycle, a doubling of the target gene fragment occurs, as the newly synthesized copies can themselves serve as templates in the subsequent PCR cycles. The reaction is so robust that, in most cases, the presence of the target can be assessed by direct detection of the product in routine gel electrophoresis.

For a PCR reaction to occur, the primers must be located sufficiently close to each other so that the thermostable DNA polymerase can copy the entire length of the fragment defined by the two primers. The maximum fragment length in classical PCR is 1–2 kb. For clinical diagnostic studies, smaller

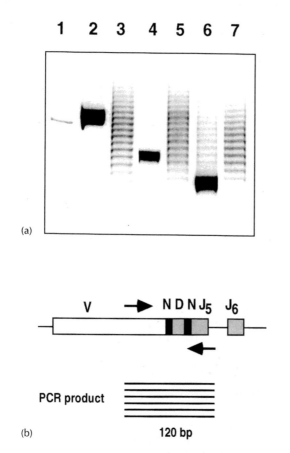

(a)

(b)   **120 bp**

Figure 4.5 Immunoglobulin VJ PCR. (a) PCR was performed using a V region framework 3 consensus primer and a consensus JH primer. The resulting product was run on a 20% acrylamide gel and stained with ethidium bromide. Lane 1 shows a 120 kb marker band. Lanes 3, 5 and 7 show a ladder of bands ranging in size from approximately 90 base pairs to 150 base pairs, diagnostic of a *polyclonal* B-cell population. Lanes 2 and 4 both show a single predominant band, diagnostic of a *monoclonal* B-cell population. Lane 6 illustrates a case containing a monoclonal population amidst a polyclonal background population. This sample came from a lymph node partially replaced by a monoclonal B-cell lymphoma, also containing normal polyclonal B-cells. (b) Schematic map of immunoglobulin VJ PCR showing position of consensus primers.

targets in the range of 100–300 base pairs are preferred. In antigen receptor PCR, V and J region primers of opposing orientation are used. In nonlymphoid DNA, PCR cannot occur because the V regions and J regions are located too far from each other. However, in B- and T-cells, the V and J segments are joined to each other by rearrangement, allowing the PCR reaction to occur. Thus, like restriction fragment analysis, antigen receptor PCR takes advantage of V–(D)–J rearrangement. However, in PCR analysis, it is the V–(D)–J junctional alterations that provide the critical clonal information, in contrast to the larger segmental changes that are evaluated by classical restriction fragment analysis.

For the detection of Ig gene rearrangements by PCR, consensus primers are generally designed that will span the V–D–J junction of the rearranged Ig heavy chain gene. A variety of V region primer sequences have been used, including family-specific V region primers [38,39], framework region two (FR2)-specific primers [40], and framework region three (FR3)-specific primers [41,42]. The most commonly used primer set is the FR3 primer, which lies at the most 3' portion of the V gene segment, in combination with a consensus JH region primer.

Amplification with a consensus FR3 primer and a consensus JH primer generates a product ranging in size from 70 to 150 base pairs. The variability of the PCR product is the result of junctional nucleotide additions and deletions that occur during V–D–J joining. Thus, a polyclonal B-cell population will generate a continuum of rearranged amplification products within this size range, reflecting the secondary junctional alterations that occur in individual B-cells during V–D–J joining. On the contrary, a clonal population will generate one or two single discrete products that are easily distinguished from the multiple products generated from a polyclonal population. The analysis of these small PCR products is best performed in acrylamide gels where the high resolution enhances interpretation of the result. An example of V–(D)–J PCR is shown in Figure 4.5.

PCR has also been applied to analysis of the TCR genes. The most commonly analyzed genes are TCRβ and TCRγ [43,44]. Analysis of the β-chain is complicated by the large number of V region families and the consequent difficulty in designing adequate consensus primers. The γ-chain, with its smaller number of variable regions, is more amenable to the design and construction of V region consensus primers and is preferred for the clonal analysis of T-cell tumors.

Clonal analysis using PCR has a higher false-negative detection rate than restriction fragment analysis. There are several reasons for this. Firstly, the detection of clonal populations using antigen receptor-targeted PCR is limited to complete V–(D)–J rearrangements, whereas restriction fragment analysis is not. Restriction fragment analysis will also detect incomplete rearrangements (i.e., D–J rearrangements without subsequent V–D joining) as well as rearrangements that result from chromosomal translocations involving the antigen receptor loci (not involving V–(D)–J joining). Secondly, although the variable region consensus regions are highly conserved, there may be rare or unknown variable regions that have sufficient sequence divergence to prevent primer annealing. If these variable regions are utilized in the clonal rearrangement primer/template annealing will not take place and a false-negative analysis will result. Finally, primer/template annealing may also not occur due to secondary somatic mutations, which may alter the primer target sequences in some lymphomas.

False-positive results occur primarily from carryover contamination of previously amplified products. Like any laboratory test, appropriate controls should always be run alongside the test specimens. There are several monographs that explain in great detail the quality-control procedures that should be followed in any laboratory performing PCR tests [45].

PCR methodology is rapid, cost effective and can identify clonal populations comprising about 1% of the total cell population. This sensitivity is slightly better than that achieved by restriction fragment analysis. Modifications using different detection methods, particularly denaturing gradient gel electrophoresis and single-strand conformation polymorphism (SSCP) analysis have been reported to increase detection sensitivity by as much as 5–10-fold [46–48]. The sensitivity of the PCR technique can be further increased several logs by making tumor-specific oligonucleotides and using these to probe Southern blots containing the V–(D)–J amplified fragments [49]. This modification of the basic technique, however, requires prior sequence analysis of the V–(D)–J junctional sequences, so that the tumor-specific oligonucleotide can be synthesized. The greatly increased sensitivity of this modification allows the use of V–(D)–J PCR to monitor patients for recurrent disease, response to chemotherapy and other minimal residual disease settings, and is discussed in more detail below.

PCR can be performed on minute amounts of tissue, requiring only 100 ng to 1 μg of DNA. Furthermore, the quality of the DNA is not as critical as that required for restriction fragment analysis, permitting the routine use of DNA extracted from formalin-fixed, paraffin-embedded tissue specimens. These advantages outweigh any disadvantages of PCR, and it should be regarded as the method of first choice for analyzing clonality. Restriction fragment analysis can be reserved for difficult cases in which PCR results are not definitive.

Significance of clonality

The detection of a clonal population is always abnormal and usually associated with a neoplastic proliferation. Using restriction fragment analysis and/or PCR, it can be demonstrated that 95% of lymphomas carry clonal rearrangements of their antigen receptor genes [33]. However, clonal populations may occasionally be found in lymphoid proliferations that are not clearly malignant. The most common setting where this has been reported is in the immunodeficiency syndromes (primary or secondary). Clonal B-cell populations have been reported in the lymphadenopathy syndrome associated with human immunodeficiency virus (HIV) infection [50], in patients with congenital immunodeficiencies, such as common variable immunodeficiency disease and the Wiscott–Aldrich syndrome [30,51], and in patients treated with cyclosporin following organ transplant [52,53]. In the latter case, some of these clinically aggressive lymphoproliferations have been considered benign because they may show partial or complete regression upon withdrawal of the immunosuppressive treatment. B-Cell clones have also been reported to occur in certain autoimmune diseases, such as Sjögren's syndrome [54]. Finally, benign monoclonal gammopathies, some associated with clonal proliferations, occur with increasing frequency in the aging population [55]. Perhaps the common problem in these conditions is a defect in the immune system's ability to regulate its response to antigenic stimulation. Excessive clonal proliferations result, which, if of sufficient magnitude, may be observed by one of the methods previously described.

Benign clonal T-cell proliferations are less commonly reported, but may be detected in a variety of cutaneous diseases, which have a benign course, including lymphomatoid papulosis [56], pagetoid reticulosis [57], pityriasis lichenoides et varioliformis acuta [58] and granulomatous slack skin disease [59]. Clonal T-cell rearrangements have also been reported in peripheral blood T-cells of patients with acute infectious mononucleosis [60], in synovial fluid T-cells in rheumatoid arthritis [61] and in cerebrospinal fluid T-cells in multiple sclerosis [62]. While the neoplastic nature of some of these conditions (e.g., lymphomatoid papulosis, pagetoid reticulosis and granulomatous slack skin disease) is controversial, it is still important to be aware breakpoint probes. PCR targeting of the two main breakpoint regions can result in the detection of about 70% of cases [100]. *bcl*-2 rearrangements, however, are also found in as many as 20–30% of diffuse large-cell lymphomas [101] and 20% or more of small noncleaved cell lymphomas of non-Burkitt's type (Burkitt-like lymphomas) [102]. It is possible that small noncleaved cell and large B-cell lymphomas that contain rearranged *bcl*-2 genes are transformed follicular lymphomas.

bcl-6 rearrangements

The *bcl*-6 gene was identified because of its location at the breakpoint of translocations involving chromosome 3q27 and one of the Ig gene loci [103–105]. *bcl*-6 rearrangements occur in 30–40% of diffuse large-cell lymphomas [106–109]. *bcl*-6 breakpoints usually occur between the first noncoding exon and the second exon of the gene, severing the coding region from its regulatory sequences. *bcl*-6 is homologous to several *Drosophila* transcription factors but, as yet, the function of this gene in humans is unknown.

bcl-6 translocations appear to be preferentially found in *de novo* large B-cell lymphomas, while the previously discussed *bcl*-2 rearrangements are preferentially found in large-cell lymphomas that have evolved from indolent follicular lymphomas [110]. This distinction is not absolute as transformed follicular lymphomas may contain *bcl*-6 rearrangements, while *de novo* large-cell lymphomas may contain *bcl*-2 rearrangements [111]. Patients with large B-cell lymphomas which contain *bcl*-6 rearrangements have been reported to have a favorable prognosis [109], but this finding has not been confirmed [108].

c-myc rearrangements

c-*myc* rearrangements are the hallmark of Burkitt's lymphoma. Nearly all of these aggressive lymphomas have translocations involving chromosome 8q24, although the site of translocation varies at the molecular level. Endemic Burkitt's lymphoma usually has chromosome 8 breakpoints far 5' to the c-*myc* gene, while their chromosome 14 breakpoints most often occur in the location of the Ig gene-joining segments. Because the chromosome 8 breakpoints are varied in location and far from the c-*myc* coding sequences in the endemic cases, it is usually not possible to demonstrate c-*myc* rearrangements with the commonly available probes. In contrast, sporadic cases frequently have c-*myc* breakpoints within noncoding introns and exons of the gene itself, typically in the first exon or intron, or in the 5'-flanking regions of the gene. This permits the

identification of c-*myc* rearrangements in most sporadic Burkitt's lymphoma.

PCR analysis of the breakpoints has been attempted for sporadic cases, which have breakpoints in or near the c-*myc* gene [112]. Nonetheless, because the breakpoints on chromosome 8 are not highly focused, this requires a large battery of primers. Consequently, PCR analysis is not commonly used diagnostically. PCR analysis for endemic breakpoints are even more limited, in this case, because only a few breakpoint sequences have been reported, and the breakpoints appear to be widely dispersed [113].

c-*myc* rearrangements also occur in about 10–20% of large-cell lymphomas of B-cell phenotype. They have also been reported in a small percentage of T-cell lymphomas, although in this case they involve T-cell receptor gene loci, rather than the Ig gene loci. They do not occur in low-grade lymphomas. c-*myc* rearrangements are also useful in differentiating Burkitt's lymphoma from Burkitt-like lymphomas, as the latter do not usually have molecularly identifiable c-*myc* rearrangements [102]. On the contrary, about 20–30% of the Burkitt-like lymphomas possess *bcl*-2 rearrangements, while *bcl*-2 rearrangements are never seen in Burkitt's lymphoma.

NPM/ALK rearrangements

Large-cell anaplastic lymphoma (ALCL) has recently been recognized as a distinct subset of large-cell lymphoma [114]. These tumors are composed of large cells with abundant amphophilic cytoplasm and have a predilection for involving lymph node sinuses. ALCL is characterized by a specific translocation involving chromosomes 2 and 5, which results in the juxtaposition of a novel tyrosine kinase gene (*ALK*) on chromosome 2p23 to the nucleophosmin gene (*NPM*) on chromosome 5q35 [77]. This leads to the inappropriate expression of an *NPM/ALK* fusion gene.

Both restriction fragment analysis and reverse transcription PCR (RT-PCR) (in which RNA is used as the starting material instead of DNA) have been used to identify the presence of this translocation through the presence of a chimeric mRNA. DNA PCR is not applicable yet as the breakpoint sequences have not been reported. The RT-PCR technique is currently the method of choice, owing to its speed and the ability to perform the assay on RNA extracted from formalin-fixed paraffin-embedded tissues. Using RT-PCR, about 40–60% of ALCL can be shown to possess the fusion transcript [115–117].

The specificity of *NPM/ALK* rearrangements for ALCL is controversial. *NPM/ALK* transcripts have also been reported in peripheral T-cell lymphomas

[116]. This may reflect differences in histopathologic diagnostic criteria. Regardless of the reason for these contradictory reports, it is possible that a molecular diagnosis may be more predictive of the tumor's biology, than a diagnosis on the basis of histology alone. This possibility is true not only for the *NPM/ALK* fusion transcript, but also for other genetic lesions found in lymphomas.

MOLECULAR CYTOGENETIC ANALYSIS AND PROGNOSTIC INFORMATION

Molecular analysis of abnormal genes has many other potential uses besides classification. By studying the molecular genetic profile of a tumor it is possible to obtain information about prognosis, drug sensitivity and the biologic behavior of an individual's tumor. This data may eventually be used to help tailor therapy, predict relapses and to counsel patients. For the lymphoid leukemias, cytogenetic and molecular cytogenetic profiles are routinely analyzed in major centers for these purposes, but, in the case of lymphomas, insufficient information presently exists to be of clinical value. One gene, however, that is being intensively examined with respect to the clinical utility of the detection of the presence of abnormalities is the p53 tumor suppressor gene. There is accumulating data that lymphomas which have acquired p53 abnormalities respond poorly to therapy and have a poor prognosis [78,79,81]. Studies in which possible correlations between molecular genetic abnormalities and clinical course are assessed, are likely to be increasingly frequent in the future.

Molecular analysis of minimal residual disease

Prior to the development of PCR the best sensitivity one could achieve using restriction fragment analysis was of the order of 1–5% of the total cellular population present. This level of sensitivity improved the ability to diagnose atypical lymphocytic infiltrates, but was generally insufficient for use in most minimal disease settings, such as monitoring residual disease following chemotherapy, analyzing autologous tissue transplants for the presence of tumor cells, or monitoring for early recurrences. The advent of PCR allowed for the development of much more sensitive tests that, for the first time, made it possible to analyze minimal residual disease. Both the antigen receptor genes and chromosomal translocations have been used as targets to detect minimal disease in a variety of settings.

The targeting of oncogene rearrangements by PCR for analysis of minimal residual disease is presently the most widely used method for detecting minimal disease. The conceptual basis for targeting the oncogene rearrangement was that translocations were believed to be a unique marker of the malignant cell. Therefore, any positive signal would indicate the presence of the malignant clone. Although it is now known that oncogene rearrangements can be found in nonlymphomatous, hyperplastic lymphoid tissues, at an operational level, these are rare and do not appear to affect minimal residual disease studies.

The first and most intensively studied target was the *bcl*-2 translocation. *bcl*-2/JH joining sequences were obvious targets for investigators, since the t(14;18) is the most common translocation in lymphomas, occurring in 85–95% of follicular lymphomas and in about 20–30% of diffuse large-cell lymphomas [118]. Furthermore, owing to variation of the *bcl*-2 breakpoints and the junctional alterations that occur in this translocation, the *bcl*-2/JH joining sequence is also tumor specific.

Several important studies have been reported using *bcl*-2/JH joining sequences as a molecular target to study. In the most comprehensive study to date, patients with *bcl*-2 translocated tumors were treated with ablative chemotherapy and autologous marrow transplantation [119]. These patients were subsequently followed by bone marrow and peripheral blood sampling and analysis for residual *bcl*-2/JH carrying tumor cells. There were no relapses among the 77 patients who achieved a complete molecular remission, while all 33 patients who subsequently relapsed had detectable *bcl*-2/JH-containing cells in multiple bone marrow biopsy specimens. Peripheral blood, however, was not as good a source for predicting relapse, primarily because of a high false-negative rate [120]. These promising data showed that failure to achieve complete molecular eradication of the *bcl*-2/JH clone in bone marrow samples was highly predictive of eventual relapse.

In a second study, 24 patients were treated with high-dose chemotherapy, transplanted with peripheral blood stem cells, and followed by PCR for *bcl*-2 or V–(D)–J rearrangements [121]. In this study, 13 of 14 patients who developed clinical relapse had positive PCR studies prior to or at the same time as clinical relapse, while 9 patients who never relapsed were negative for marker-carrying cells shortly after transplantation. Again, the failure to achieve a molecular remission was predictive of relapse.

These investigations suggest an important role for PCR in following minimal residual disease during and after treatment. They also imply that it may be desirable to continue treatment in patients who have not achieved complete molecular eradication of their clone.

Implications for gamma delta T cell lineages and for a novel intermediate of V–(D)–J joining. *Cell* 1989, **59**: 859–870.

18. Lewis SM. P nucleotides, hairpin DNA and V(D)J joining: Making the connection. *Semin. Immunol.* 1994, **6**: 131–141.

19. Desiderio SV, Yancopoulos GD, Paskind M, et al. Insertion of N regions into heavy-chain genes is correlated with expression of terminal deoxytransferase in B-cells. *Nature* 1984, **311**: 752–755.

20. Tonegawa S. Somatic generation of antibody diversity. *Nature* 1983, **302**: 575.

21. Zheng B, Xue W, Kelsoe G. Locus-specific somatic hypermutation in germinal centre T cells. *Nature* 1994, **372**: 556–559.

22. Korsmeyer SJ, Hieter PA, Ravetch JV, et al. Developmental hierarchy of immunoglobulin gene rearrangements in human leukemic pre-B-cells. *Proc. Natl Acad. Sci. USA* 1981, **78**: 7096–7100.

23. Siminovitch KA, Bakhshi A, Goldman P, et al. A uniform deleting element mediates the loss of kappa genes in human B-cells. *Nature* 1985, **316**: 260–262.

24. Korsmeyer SJ, Hieter PA, Sharrow SO, et al. Normal human B cells display ordered light chain gene rearrangements and deletions. *J. Exp. Med.* 1982, **156**: 975–985.

25. Chien YH, Iwashima M, Wettstein DA, et al. T-Cell receptor delta gene rearrangements in early thymocytes. *Nature* 1987, **330**: 722–727.

26. de Villartay JP, Lewis D, Hockett R, et al. Deletional rearrangement in the human T-cell receptor alpha-chain locus. *Proc. Natl Acad. Sci. USA* 1987, **84**: 8608–8612.

27. de Villartay JP, Hockett RD, Coran D, et al. Deletion of the human T-cell receptor delta-gene by a site-specific recombination. *Nature* 1988, **335**: 170–174.

28. Wu AM, Ben EJ, Winberg C, et al. Analysis of antigen receptor gene rearrangements in ethanol and formaldehyde-fixed, paraffin-embedded specimens. *Lab. Invest.* 1990, **63**: 107–114.

29. Southern EM. Detection of specific sequences among DNA fragments separated by gel electrophoresis. *J. Mol. Biol.* 1975, **98**: 503–517.

30. Arnold A, Cossman J, Bakhshi A, et al. Immunoglobulin-gene rearrangements as unique clonal markers in human lymphoid neoplasms. *N. Engl. J. Med.* 1983, **309**: 1593–1599.

31. Cleary ML, Chao J, Warnke R, et al. Immunoglobulin gene rearrangement as a diagnostic criterion of B-cell lymphoma. *Proc. Natl Acad. Sci. USA* 1984, **81**: 593–597.

32. Griesser H, Feller A, Lennert K, et al. Rearrangement of the beta chain of the T-cell antigen receptor and immunoglobulin genes in lymphoproliferative disorders. *J. Clin. Invest.* 1986, **78**: 1179–1184.

33. Cossman J, Zehnbauer B, Garrett CT, et al. Gene rearrangements in the diagnosis of lymphoma/leukemia. Guidelines for use based on a multiinstitutional study. *Am. J. Clin. Path.* 1991, **95**: 347–354.

34. Cossman J, Stetler-Stevenson M, Medeiros LJ, et al. Molecular genetics of lymphoproliferative processes. *Important Adv. Oncol.* 1990, **1990**: 101–113.

35. Uppenkamp M, Andrade R, Sundeen J, et al. Diagnostic interpretation of T gamma gene rearrangement: Effect of polyclonal T cells. *Hematol. Path.* 1988, **2**: 15–24.

36. Lefranc MP, Rabbitts TH. Genetic organization of the human T cell receptor gamma locus. *Curr. Top. Microbiol. Immunol.* 1991, **173**: 3–9.

37. van Dongen JJ, Wolvers-Tettero IL, Wassenaar F, et al. Rearrangement and expression of T-cell receptor delta genes in T-cell acute lymphoblastic leukemias. *Blood* 1989, **74**: 334–342.

38. Deane M, Norton JD. Immunoglobulin heavy chain variable region family usage is independent of tumor cell phenotype in human B lineage leukemias. *Eur. J. Immunol.* 1990, **20**: 2209–2217.

39. Campbell MJ, Zelenetz AD, Levy S, et al. Use of family specific leader region primers for PCR amplification of the human heavy chain variable region gene repertoire. *Mol. Immunol.* 1992, **29**: 193–203.

40. Ramasamy I, Brisco M, Morley A. Improved PCR method for detecting monoclonal immunoglobulin heavy chain rearrangement in B cell neoplasms. *J. Clin. Path.* 1992, **45**: 770–775.

41. McCarthy KP, Sloane JP, Wiedemann LM. Rapid method for distinguishing clonal from polyclonal B cell populations in surgical biopsy specimens. *J. Clin. Path.* 1990, **43**: 429–432.

42. Trainor KJ, Brisco MJ, Story CJ, et al. Monoclonality in B-lymphoproliferative disorders detected at the DNA level. *Blood* 1990, **75**: 2220–2222.

43. McCarthy KP, Sloane JP, Kabarowski JH, et al. The rapid detection of clonal T-cell proliferations in patients with lymphoid disorders. *Am. J. Path.* 1991, **138**: 821–828.

44. McCarthy KP, Sloane JP, Kabarowski JH, et al. A simplified method of detection of clonal rearrangements of the T-cell receptor-gamma chain gene. *Diagn. Mol. Path.* 1992, **1**: 173–179.

45. Innis MA, Gelfand DH, Sninsky JJ, et al. *PCR Protocols: A Guide to Methods and Applications.* San Diego: Academic Press, 1990, pp. 1–482.

46. Bourguin A, Tung R, Galili N, Sklar J. Rapid, nonradioactive detection of clonal T-cell receptor gene rearrangements in lymphoid neoplasms. *Proc. Natl Acad. Sci. USA* 1990, **87**: 8536–8540.

47. Greiner TC, Raffeld M, Lutz C, et al. Analysis of T cell receptor-gamma gene rearrangements by denaturing gradient gel electrophoresis of GC-clamped polymerase chain reaction products. Correlation with tumor-specific sequences. *Am. J. Path.* 1995, **146**: 46–55.

48. Baruchel A, Cayuela JM, MacIntyre E, et al. Assessment of clonal evolution at Ig/TCR loci in acute lymphoblastic leukaemia by single-strand conformation polymorphism studies and highly resolutive PCR derived methods: Implication for a general strategy of minimal residual disease detection. *Br. J. Haematol.* 1995, **90**: 85–93.

49. Yamada M, Hudson S, Tournay O, et al. Detection of minimal disease in hematopoietic malignancies of the B-cell lineage by using third-complementarity-determining region (CDR-III)-specific probes. *Proc. Natl Acad. Sci. USA* 1989, **86**: 5123–5127.

50. Pelicci PG, Knowles DM, Arlin ZA, et al. Multiple monoclonal B cell expansions and c-myc oncogene rearrangements in acquired immune deficiency syndrome-related lymphoproliferative disorders. Implications for lymphomagenesis. *J. Exp. Med.* 1986, **164**: 2049–2060.

51. Laszewski MJ, Kemp JD, Goeken JA, et al. Clonal immunoglobulin gene rearrangement in nodular lymphoid hyperplasia of the gastrointestinal tract associated with common variable immunodeficiency. *Am. J. Clin. Path.* 1990, **94**: 338–343.

52. Starzl TE, Nalesnik MA, Porter KA, et al. Reversibility of lymphomas and lymphoproliferative lesions developing under cyclosporin–steroid therapy. *Lancet* 1984, **1**: 583–587.

53. Nalesnik MA, Jaffe R, Starzl TE, et al. The pathology of posttransplant lymphoproliferative disorders occurring in the setting of cyclosporine A–prednisone immunosuppression. *Am. J. Path.* 1988, **133**: 173–192.

54. Fishleder A, Tubbs R, Hesse B, et al. Uniform detection of immunoglobulin-gene rearrangement in benign lymphoepithelial lesions. *N. Engl. J. Med.* 1987, **316**: 1118–1121.

55. Fend F, Weyrer K, Drach J, et al. Immunoglobulin gene rearrangement in plasma cell dyscrasias: Detection of small clonal cell populations in peripheral blood and bone marrow. *Leuk. Lymphoma* 1993, **10**: 223–229.

56. Weiss LM, Wood GS, Trela M, et al. Clonal T-cell populations in lymphomatoid papulosis. Evidence of a lymphoproliferative origin for a clinically benign disease. *N. Engl. J. Med.* 1986, **315**: 475–479.

57. Wood GS, Weiss LM, Hu CH, et al. T-Cell antigen deficiencies and clonal rearrangements of T-cell receptor genes in pagetoid reticulosis (Woringer–Kolopp disease). *N. Engl. J. Med.* 1988, **318**: 164–167.

58. Weiss LM, Wood GS, Ellisen LW, et al. Clonal T-cell populations in pityriasis lichenoides et varioliformis acuta (Mucha–Habermann disease). *Am. J. Path.* 1987, **126**: 417–421.

59. LeBoit PE, Beckstead JH, Bond B, et al. Granulomatous slack skin: Clonal rearrangement of the T-cell receptor beta gene is evidence for the lymphoproliferative nature of a cutaneous elastolytic disorder. *J. Invest. Dermatol.* 1987, **89**: 183–186.

60. Strickler JG, Movahed LA, Gajl-Peczalska KJ, et al. Oligoclonal T cell receptor gene rearrangements in blood lymphocytes of patients with acute Epstein–Barr virus-induced infectious mononucleosis. *J. Clin. Invest.* 1990, **86**: 1358–1363.

61. Savill CM, Delves PJ, Kioussis D, et al. A minority of patients with rheumatoid arthritis show a dominant rearrangement of T-cell receptor beta chain genes in synovial lymphocytes. *Scand. J. Immunol.* 1987, **25**: 629–635.

62. Hafler DA, Duby AD, Lee SJ, et al. Oligoclonal T lymphocytes in the cerebrospinal fluid of patients with multiple sclerosis. *J. Exp. Med.* 1988, **167**: 1313–1322.

63. Wood GS, Tung RM, Haeffner AC, et al. Detection of clonal T-cell receptor gamma gene rearrangements in early mycosis fungoides/Sezary syndrome by polymerase chain reaction and denaturing gradient gel electrophoresis (PCR/DGGE). *J. Invest. Dermatol.* 1994, **103**: 34–41.

64. Weiss LM, Arber DA, Strickler JG. Nasal T-cell lymphoma. *Ann. Oncol.* 1994, **5**(Suppl. 1): 39–42.

65. Ralfkiaer E, Delsol G, O'Connor NT, et al. Malignant lymphomas of true histiocytic origin. A clinical, histological, immunophenotypic and genotypic study. *J. Path.* 1990, **160**: 9–17.

66. Herbst H, Tippelmann G, Anagnostopoulos I, et al. Immunoglobulin and T-cell receptor gene rearrangements in Hodgkin's disease and Ki-1-positive anaplastic large cell lymphoma: Dissociation between phenotype and genotype. *Leuk. Res.* 1989, **13**: 103–116.

67. Pelicci PG, Knowles DM, Dalla-Favera R. Lymphoid tumors displaying rearrangements of both immunoglobulin and T-cell receptor genes. *J. Exp. Med.* 1985, **162**: 1015–1024.

68. Hollingsworth HC, Stetler-Stevenson M, Gagneten D, et al. Immunodeficiency-associated malignant lymphoma. Three cases showing genotypic evidence of both T- and B-cell lineages. *Am. J. Surg. Path.* 1994, **18**: 1092–1101.

69. van Dongen JJ, Wolvers-Tettero IL. Analysis of immunoglobulin and T cell receptor genes. Part II: Possibilities and limitations in the diagnosis and management of lymphoproliferative diseases and related disorders. *Clin. Chim. Acta.* 1991, **198**: 93–174.

70. Seremetis SV, Pelicci PG, Tabilio A, et al. High frequency of clonal immunoglobulin or T cell receptor gene rearrangements in acute myelogenous leukemia expressing terminal deoxyribonucleotidyltransferase. *J. Exp. Med.* 1987, **165**: 1703–1712.

71. Dalla-Favera R, Bregni M, Erikson J, et al. Human c-myc oncogene is located on the region of chromosome 8 that is translocated in Burkitt lymphoma cells. *Proc. Natl Acad. Sci. USA* 1982, **79**: 7824–7827.

72. Motokura T, Bloom T, Kim HG, et al. A novel cyclin encoded by a bcl1-linked candidate oncogene. *Nature* 1991, **350**: 512–515.

73. Withers DA, Harvey RC, Faust JB, et al. Characterization of a candidate bcl-1 gene. *Mol. Cell Biol.* 1991, **11**: 4846–4853.

74. Tsujimoto Y, Finger LR, Yunis J, et al. Cloning of the chromosome breakpoint of neoplastic B-cells with the t(14;18) chromosome translocation. *Science* 1984, **226**: 1097–1099.

75. Bakhshi A, Jensen JP, Goldman P, et al. Cloning the chromosomal breakpoint of t(14;18) human lymphomas: Clustering around JH on chromosome 14 and near a transcriptional unit on 18. *Cell* 1985, **41**: 899–906.

76. Korsmeyer SJ. Programmed cell death: Bcl-2. *Important Adv. Oncol.* 1993, 19–28.

77. Morris SW, Kirstein MN, Valentine MB, et al. Fusion of a kinase gene, ALK, to a nucleolar protein gene, NPM, in non-Hodgkin's lymphoma. *Science* 1994, **263**: 1281–1284.

78. Wattel E, Preudhomme C, Hecquet B, et al. p53 mutations are associated with resistance to chemotherapy and short survival in hematologic malignancies. *Blood* 1994, **84**: 3148–3157.

CHAPTER 5

Borderlands of pathological entities

KARL LENNERT

> Le plus bel artifice de l'esprit humain, qui consiste à creer des termes collectifs, a été le cause de presque toutes ses erreurs.*
>
> Antoine Rivarol
> (1753–1801)

Historical remarks

Thomas Hodgkin described the disease that was named after him in 1832 using only the naked eye; he had no microscope at his disposal. We cannot but admire his macroscopic ability, but in actuality the cases he published included a number of other diseases. The cases he examined have been restudied several times, by Fox in 1926 [1], Symmers in 1978 [2] and the author in 1987† (the tissues were fixed and stored in the Gordon Museum, Guy's Hospital, London). The results (Table 5.1) showed that some

*That finest device of the human mind, which consists in creating collective terms, has been the cause of almost all of his errors.
†I was kindly allowed to examine three of the cases histologically. For this I am very grateful to Dr R. N. Poston, London.

of the cases certainly fit the modern definition of Hodgkin's disease (HD), but that some would have to be classified as syphilis or what we know today as the non-Hodgkin's lymphomas (NHLs). Hence the borderline was fuzzy *ab initio*, and thus it has remained over the years.

Today we have reached a point at which the questions of whether HD really is an entity and not only a syndrome, and whether the distinction between HD and NHL is not much too arbitrary are being voiced more and more audibly. We shall discuss this point more in the next section. The reader will find that our concept largely corresponds to that of the International Lymphoma Study Group [2a], which was not published until after this chapter had been written (the author's original manuscript was completed in April 1994).

In the NHLs the situation is quite the reverse. Here one must ask which of the innumerable variants are

Table 5.1 Re-evaluation of Hodgkin's patients (1832) by Fox (1926), Symmers (1978) and Lennert (1987)

Patient	Diagnosis
1	Tuberculosis (+ HD?)
2	HD+
3	Syphilis
4	HD+
5	'Systemic lymphomatosis (lymphocytic)'
6	LP immunocytoma
7	HD?

HD, Hodgkin's disease; LP, lymphoplasmacytic/cytoid.

entities (see page 136). Then we must distinguish the NHLs from HD and the various NHLs from each other (see pages 140ff and 148ff). Further, we need to discuss the lymphoproliferative disorders that can develop into a frank malignant lymphoma (page 151ff) and the composite lymphomas (page 154ff).

What exactly do we mean by entity?

We define an entity today: (1) morphologically (cytologically, where possible corresponding to a definable normal cellular equivalent), verified and further specified by immunocytochemical methods and available genetic data; and (2) clinically. The morphological/immunocytochemical identification must be clear-cut and reproducible. The clinical definition includes the age (and sex) – there should be a recognizable age peak – the localization, the clinical course and response to treatment. Hence the term entity is tied to a clearly defined morphological and clinical *gestalt* (see footnote on page 157). Minor differences within an entity are called subentities or variants. They may have clinical significance, e.g., chronic lymphocytic leukemia of the B-cell type, the pseudofollicular versus the diffuse or tumor-forming subtype, centroblastic–centrocytic lymphoma, the follicular versus the purely diffuse subtype.

Our knowledge of virus etiology, molecular genetics and classical cytogenetics is not yet complete enough to use them as a basis for what we call entities, although it is interesting to learn that a good morphologically/immunocytochemically/clinically defined system of classification is increasingly being substantiated by new investigations in virology, classical cytogenetics and molecular genetics.

Is Hodgkin's disease an entity?

To establish a disease as an entity we require criteria that occur exclusively in this disease, as far as this is possible. Do we have such criteria for HD, and do they allow us to maintain that the morphologically and clinically different manifestations of HD are one single disease, and to distinguish HD from NHL?

Since Sternberg (1898) and Reed (1902) (see Chapter 2), a special kind of giant cell has been considered to be *the* criterion for HD. Today, however, we know that the Sternberg–Reed cell is not specific to HD. For instance, it occurs frequently in infectious mononucleosis [3–5], in malignant lymphomas of the mucosa-associated lymphoid tissue (MALT) type, for instance in the stomach [6] or in the salivary glands [7], in chronic lymphocytic leukemia of B-cell type [8,9], in T-cell lymphomas [10] (Plate 5.1) and even in nonspecific lymphadenitis [11] (Plate 5.2). Identification of a Sternberg–Reed cell is diagnostic of HD only if the histological setting is compatible. It should not be composed of a single cell type or show monoclonal Ig expression. Often the reticulin fiber pattern helps us with the diagnosis. Infiltrations of HD show more fibers and a different fiber pattern from that of chronic lymphocytic leukemia or immunocytoma. One also often finds some eosinophils and histiocytes in circumscribed areas, indicating a true composite lymphoma (see page 154).

The diagnostic evaluation of a giant cell requires subtle morphological techniques. On slides stained with Giemsa the chromatin and nuclear membranes of the Sternberg–Reed cells stain extremely weakly; the nucleolus is very large and slightly basophilic (grey–blue to greyish violet). In contrast, immunoblastic giant cells, for example, show strongly stainable chromatin and nuclear membranes and dark blue nucleoli.

The immunocytochemical analysis of giant cells does not reveal a homogeneous phenotype [12–14] and does not yield any absolute criteria for the existence of HD. Sternberg–Reed cells in HD are usually positive for CD30 (for overviews, see [15,16]), but definitely not always. Moreover, this antibody is by no means specific to HD. The situation is somewhat better with CD15. When positive, it is more meaningful diagnostically (see overview by Arber and Weiss 1993 [17]), but this antibody is negative in the nodular lymphocyte predominance type [18,19], which we call nodular paragranuloma [20,21]. In contrast, the Sternberg–Reed cells of this entity are positive for J chains, which seem to be lacking in all other types of HD [12,19]. The French groups of Delsol and Diebold [22] consider it particularly characteristic of nodular paragranuloma that the giant cells express epithelial membrane antigen (EMA), as do the large cell B-cell lymphomas that are associated with or transformed from paragranuloma. The Sternberg–Reed cells in nodular paragranuloma also differ morphologically (Lukes' 'L&H cells', 'popcorn cells') from the Sternberg–Reed cells of other HD types.

Further, nodular paragranuloma shows a clear peak in the fourth decade of life [20,23] and a 70% predominance of the male sex. Both of these points are at variance with all subtypes of the Rye classification. Finally, in about 3% of the cases, nodular paragranuloma shows a transformation to a high-grade lymphoma, usually of B-cell type, often of centroblastic type [24] (see page 150), whereas all other types of HD may develop into a high-grade lymphoma of the large-cell anaplastic lymphoma type (T- or null subtypes). Clinicians should reconsider their strategy of treating nodular paragranuloma in the same way as all variants of HD, as is done in most lymphoma treatment centers. This would be an unjustified overtreatment, for which there are no logical grounds. Unfortunately, a prospective study on the treatment of paragranuloma has yet to be done.

At the same time as the Rye classification was being created [25], McMahon [26] took a critical look at the bimodal age distribution in HD (all types included), with peaks in the third and seventh decades (Figure 5.1), and questioned whether there

really could be one single disease entity behind it. The histological analysis by Lukes et al. [27] and the epidemiological data showed that besides nodular paragranuloma there is another distinct type. It is the nodular sclerosing type with a high peak in the third decade (Figure 5.2) and a sex ratio of ≈ 1:1 [20]. In the mixed cellular type, however, the bimodal age distribution is even more pronounced, and a predominance of the male sex is still evident. Along with these epidemiological data more recent investigations on Epstein–Barr virus (EBV) infection of the Sternberg–Reed cells showed a difference between the nodular sclerosing type and the mixed cellular type. The mixed cellular type is much more frequently infected with EBV (80.9%) than the nodular sclerosing type (17.4% [28]).

Some of the types of HD classified together in the Rye classification as lymphocyte depleted should probably be considered peripheral T-cell lymphomas. Certainly the type of lymphoma known today as large-cell anaplastic lymphoma corresponds morphologically to the reticular type of Lukes and associates [27]. It can occur as a highly malignant evolution of

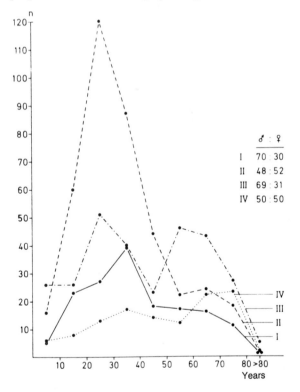

Figure 5.2 The same cases as in Figure 5.1 but classified as paragranuloma (nodular and diffuse) (= I), nodular sclerosing type (= II), mixed cellular type (= III) and lymphocyte depletion type (= IV). The nodular sclerosing type shows a peak in the third decade, the paragranuloma in the fourth decade. The mixed cellular type (III) shows the bimodal age distribution. The lymphocyte depletion type is most frequent in the higher age groups [20].

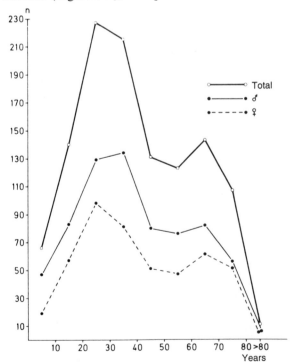

Figure 5.1 The typical bimodal age distribution in HD, without further specification. Based on 1181 patients diagnosed at the Lymph Node Registry in Kiel between 1965 and 1973 [20].

the other types of HD (except for nodular paragranu-loma), but is more often primary or occurs second-arily in peripheral T-cell lymphomas of virtually all subtypes. Although this large-cell tumor has mor-phologically much in common with what was formerly known as 'Hodgkin's sarcoma' [29], and although the HD characteristic marker CD30 is invariably positive and the more specific marker CD15 is occasionally positive, this tumor is clas-sified by general consent among the NHLs. Is this necessary or arbitrary?

After everything we have said there can no longer be any doubt that HD is not one uniform, discrete entity. Today clinicians also do not assume that it is. Many pathologists have energetically pronounced their skepticism, e.g., [30,31]. We too are of this opinion and therefore no longer speak of Hodgkin's disease, but of Hodgkin's lymphomas (HLs). Spector [33] proposed singing a requiem to HD. We agree, as does the International Lymphoma Study Group [2a], who have listed both HD and NHL in the Revised European–American Lymphoma (REAL) Classification.

Before we now proceed with the distinction between HL and the NHL, we need to first discuss the various types of NHL.

Which of the non-Hodgkin's lymphomas are proven entities?

Tumor entities are generally defined according to their normal counterparts, i.e., according to the cells and tissues from which they are derived. Usually they are further characterized (in subentities or variants) by specifying the degree or kind of dif-ferentiation. The same procedure was tried for the lymphomas [34], but without enough knowledge. At the time, the morphology of the normal counterparts was for the most part poorly defined and people did not yet realize that the term differentiation is not applicable to lymphocytes. Should one consider the small, apparently inactive lymphocyte or its transfor-mation form, the immunoblast, to be more highly differentiated? The phenomenon of the transfor-mability of lymphocytes [35] had to be taken into account. But in the late 1950s and the 1960s, it became clear that there are two main lineages of lym-phocytes, the B- and T-lymphocytic cells. Should they not also give rise to corresponding tumors?

In view of this situation, Lukes and Collins [36,37] and ourselves [38–40] sought to develop a classification of the NHLs that takes into account the new discoveries in the field of experimental immunology. Lukes and Collins photographed nor-mal reactive germinal centers and follicular lym-phomas at identical magnifications, and prepared camera lucida drawings of each process for com-parison. From this they arrived at the terms cleaved and noncleaved follicular center cells [41]. These they took as a preliminary basis for reclassifying the NHL.

We took a different route. In the 1950s we had studied normal and reactive lymph nodes with hematological and enzyme cytochemical methods in sections stained with Giemsa and in imprints stained with equivalent techniques. In the process we had recognized a number of special cells (e.g., centroblasts, immunoblasts, monocytoid B-cells), without being able to understand them correctly in the 'pre-immunological' era [42]. We then studied the same cells under the electron microscope [43]. In the process we encountered the first case of B-immunoblastic lymphoma [44]. We also recognized, purely cytologically, that the follicular lymphomas were composed of centrocytes and centroblasts (Lukes and Collins' cleaved and noncleaved fol-licular centre cells [41]) and not of the various cell types of Rappaport's classification [45]. However, the problem could not be solved with any of these methods, but they did provide a solid basis for immunological investigations of lymphomas that we began in 1972–1973 with Stein and Parwaresch [38–40,46]. These rapidly led to the Kiel clas-sification [8,47,48], which has quite a lot in common with that of Lukes and Collins [49]. The Kiel classification was updated in 1988 [10,50]. The updated Kiel classification (Table 5.2) is comparable to the newest version of the Lukes–Collins clas-sification [51]. The most recent detailed presentation of the updated Kiel classification in correlation with the underlying cell types was given by the author in 1994 and published in 1995 [51a].

After the first writing of this chapter, the Inter-national Lymphoma Study Group [2a] proposed a list of 24 lymphoma entities and called it the REAL Classification. The latter corresponds to the Kiel classification in many details. The REAL Classifi-cation includes extranodal lymphomas, however, whereas the Kiel classification covers only nodal lymphomas (with one exception).

MORPHOLOGY, VALIDATED BY IMMUNOCYTOCHEMISTRY, AS THE CURRENT BASIS FOR ESTABLISHING LYMPHOMA ENTITIES

The Kiel classification is based on a subtle assess-ment of morphology on slides stained with the

Table 5.2 Updated Kiel classification of non-Hodgkin's lymphomas (1988, modified in 1992, from [50a])

B	T
Low-grade malignant lymphomas	
Lymphocytic	Lymphocytic
Chronic lymphocytic leukemia	Chronic lymphocytic leukemia
Prolymphocytic leukemia	Prolymphocytic leukemia
Hairy cell leukemia	
	Small cell, cerebriform
	Mycosis fungoides, Sézary's syndrome
Lymphoplasmacytic/cytoid (immunocytoma)	Lymphoepithelioid (Lennert's lymphoma)
Plasmacytic	Angioimmunoblastic (AILD, LgX)
Centroblastic–centrocytic	T-zone lymphoma
Follicular ± diffuse	
Diffuse	
Centrocytic (mantle cell)	Pleomorphic, small cell (HTLV ±)
Monocytoid, including marginal zone cell	
High-grade malignant lymphomas	
Centroblastic	Pleomorphic, medium-sized and large cell (HTLV ±)
Immunoblastic	Immunoblastic (HTLV ±)
Burkitt's lymphoma	
Large-cell anaplastic (Ki-1+)	Large-cell anaplastic (Ki-1+)
Lymphoblastic	Lymphoblastic
Rare types	*Rare and ambiguous types*

hematological stain Giemsa and, where necessary, on the immunological characterization of the cells thus observed. Once certain cells had been characterized immunologically, it was often no longer necessary to apply immunological methods to recognize them again and to be certain that they represented a particular cell type and no other. Thus morphologists learned a great deal from immunology.

The objective of the Kiel classification was, from the very beginning, to define malignant lymphomas primarily according to the nature and appearance of the proliferating cells and secondarily according to their growth pattern [34,52]. We correlated the lymphoma cells with their normal and reactive counterparts in the lymphatic tissue. In so doing we were proceeding in the same manner as tumor pathologists in general. Since there are, however, cells that look the same or similar but differ greatly in nature (e.g., T- and B-lymphocytes, T- and B-immunoblasts), it is often necessary to apply immunocytochemical techniques in addition, especially when the slides are being evaluated for scientific purposes.

It was generally possible to define the B-cell lymphomas according to certain cell types. For the T-cell lymphomas this was not so simple, partly because no morphological correlates to the various functional and transforming variants of T-cells can

be recognized. We therefore included other criteria for the morphological classification, e.g., morphologically visible consequences of lymphokine production, such as epithelioid cells in lymphoepithelioid lymphoma or follicular dendritic cells in the angioimmunoblastic lymphadenopathy with dysproteinemia (AILD) type of T-cell lymphoma.

In addition to the cytology of the lymphoma, attention was also paid to the growth pattern and other histological criteria. A follicular growth pattern usually signifies centroblastic–centrocytic lymphoma, rarely centroblastic lymphoma; an intrasinusoidal growth pattern is indicative of large-cell anaplastic lymphoma. Staining reticulin fibers with silver impregnation gives some information on the nature of the tumor, because it reveals alteration of the lymph node architecture and the amount and type of fibers and vessels. T-Cell lymphomas, especially large-cell anaplastic lymphoma, often contain many fibers; in B-cell lymphomas, fibers are often scanty. Centroblastic–centrocytic lymphoma has a special sclerotic variant. A large number of high endothelial venules speaks in favor of a T-cell lymphoma. Angiocentricity and angiodestruction are observed in various malignant lymphomas, especially peripheral T-cell lymphomas and, in our experience, are not restricted to one entity [10,53], as Jaffe and her group state [54].

To determine the basic immunophenotype (B-cell versus T-cell) in day-to-day diagnostic work, the panel of monoclonal or polyclonal antibodies that can be applied to paraffin sections is usually sufficient. New techniques, e.g., heating by microwave [55,56], should soon yield results on paraffin sections with antibodies that presently can only be used in frozen sections.

With the aid of an exact morphological and, where necessary, immunocytochemical analysis in paraffin sections, one can today classify at least 90% of the malignant lymphomas unequivocally. Polyclonal and monoclonal pan-B-cell or pan-T-cell antibodies allow us to recognize not only the basic type of lymphoma cells (B- or T-cells), but also admixtures of nonneoplastic cells.

Determining the clonality plays an important role in the immunocytochemistry of B-cell lymphomas. T-Cell lymphomas can only be recognized as clonal T-cell proliferations by means of molecular genetics [57,58]. The monoclonality of a B-cell proliferation can be determined by demonstrating light chain restriction. For this, high-quality fixation and embedding are essential as well as an excellent staining technique that reveals subtle details, conditions that are often not met. It is very important to determine whether monoclonal cytoplasmic immunoglobulin (cIg) is present in the neoplastic B-cells, and it is nearly impossible to do so in cryostat sections. Therefore we need to use a good paraffin-embedding technique, so that, for instance, we may differentiate chronic lymphocytic leukemia of B-cell type containing reactive polyclonal plasma cells from immunocytoma with monoclonal plasma cells that are a part of the neoplasm. To avoid the technical difficulties of demonstrating cIg in paraffin sections and to analyze false-positive cases or cases with $\kappa + \lambda$ positivity, Lauder and his group introduced a method of *in situ* hybridization to light chain mRNA [59], which is very useful.

In addition to identifying B- and T-cell lymphomas as comprehensive categories, a large number of monoclonal and polyclonal antibodies can be applied to characterize subgroups and presumably to define entities (see page 1, and Chapter 10). A negative reaction for antigens that occur in normal counterpart cells is also of diagnostic significance, however, e.g., loss of CD3 in T-cell lymphomas [60].

Even after the immunocytochemical analysis is completed, there remain around 10% of cases which either cannot be placed in any of the categories of the classification – they remain unclassifiable – or that one can and would like to classify as B- or T-cell lymphomas with new techniques (see next section). Finally, there are true borderline cases in which it is difficult or impossible to distinguish between morphologically similar entities.

NEW TECHNIQUES FOR ANALYZING LYMPHOMAS

Flow cytometry

One method of establishing clonality for certain is flow cytometry [61,62]. It allows us to recognize not only clonality but also the immunophenotype of a lymphoproliferative disease very rapidly (and cheaply!). Its disadvantage is that it requires fresh material. However, it shows the direction in which modern lymphoma research is heading: morphological observations should be confirmed or replaced by highly sophisticated scientific methods – a development that has great advantages, but also dangers.

Molecular genetics

Rearrangements of Ig genes and T-cell receptor (TCR) genes are diagnostically very significant, because they are usually found in specific malignant lymphomas, provided these malignant lymphomas are diagnosed according to a biological classification, i.e., a classification defined by morphology assisted by immunocytochemistry. Both the Southern blot and polymerase chain reaction (PCR) techniques may be applied. The advantages and disadvantages of the two techniques are discussed by Griesser [63].

Clonal rearrangements of IgH genes speak in favor of a B-cell lymphoma; monoclonal rearrangements of TCRβ or γ are evaluated as strong hints of a T-cell lymphoma. There are, however, numerous exceptions and overlaps [63]. IgH gene rearrangement can also occur in T-cell lymphomas, especially those of AILD type [64,65].

Such unexpected Ig rearrangements may occur in so-called composite lymphomas due to the presence of a clonal B-cell population in addition to the clonal T-cell proliferation. In most instances, incomplete IgH rearrangements without clonal light chain gene recombinations represent aberrant rearrangements in the malignant T-cell clone. These cross-lineage rearrangements probably arise in activated or transformed lymphoid cells unrelated to the ontogenetic programme of lymphocyte development. This is rarely explained by chromosomal abnormalities involving Ig gene loci. More often an aberrant activation of the recombinase machinery, common to all immune receptor gene loci, may be the cause. This is supported by the observation that normal murine T-cells occasionally have D-J rearrangements of their IgH genes [66].

In a small proportion of T-cell lymphomas no rearrangement can be demonstrated by PCR. Thus even molecular genetic methods have their limitations.

Studies of the rearrangement of Ig genes and TCR genes allow us to classify a lymphoma as B-cell or T-cell derived (with limitations) and inform us about the monoclonality or polyclonality of a lymphoproliferation. They are of limited value for designating separate lymphoma entities. In the case of T-cell proliferation; monoclonality can only be proven by molecular genetics.

By contrast, deregulations of the expression of oncogenes demonstrate not only monoclonality, but also certain specificities: *bcl*-1 recombination appears to be specific to mantle cell lymphoma [67–71]. *bcl*-2 gene recombination occurs especially in centroblastic–centrocytic lymphoma, but also in centroblastic lymphoma (usually in cases that are secondary transformations of centroblastic–centrocytic lymphoma [72], and only rarely in primary cases [73]) and occasionally in Burkitt's lymphoma [72]. *bcl*-2 is of help immunocytochemically in distinguishing follicular hyperplasia, which is negative, from follicular centroblastic–centrocytic lymphoma, which shows an overexpression in the neoplastic germinal centers [74,75]. c-*myc* translocation, most frequently t(8;14), less frequently t(2;8),t(8;22), is characteristic for Burkitt's lymphoma, but also occurs in blastic transformations of low-grade B-cell lymphomas [63]. In addition, the identification of different breakpoints of the same recombination type may be of relevance, as is seen in Burkitt's lymphoma (see below). Woloschak et al. [76] reported on differences in oncogene expression in CD4+ and CD8+ T-cell lymphomas.

Classical cytogenetics

Major progress has been made in cytogenetics in the past few years, and in the process some entities of the Kiel classification have been confirmed (see Table 5.3), not to mention the scientific discoveries that have been made [77–80] (see Chapter 3). However, cytogenetic abnormalities have so far never been found in 100% of the cases of any entity of the Kiel classification. The reasons for this are probably partly technical. The cause may, however, be an inaccurate histological interpretation. Finally, other chromosomal abnormalities sometimes exist that differ from the usual ones. The application of the Working Formulation (WF) as a 'classification' [81,82], which its creators did not intend it to be, showed that most of the categories of the WF are not entities and therefore do not show specific chromosomal abnormalities.

The classical cytogenetic studies revealed a number of lymphoma-specific translocations, e.g., t(11;14), t(14;18), t(2;5) (see Table 5.3). By contrast, abnormalities involving extra chromosomes or chromosome deletions appear to be less specific. For instance, trisomy 3 is characteristic for low-grade T-cell lymphomas and occurs only rarely in high-grade T-cell lymphomas [83], but it is not at all specific to T-cell lymphomas (Table 5.3). Finn et al. [84] also found trisomy 3 in more than 50% of low-grade B-cell lymphomas of the MALT type.

The new cytogenetic techniques using routinely fixed paraffin sections and working with the DNA of interphase nuclei give us cause to hope that very soon a large amount of new data will appear, which will enhance the value of cytogenetic investigations considerably, e.g., nonisotopic *in situ* hybridization with chromosome-specific DNA probes, and comparative genomic hybridization to detect complete and partial chromosome gains and losses [85,86] or oncogene amplification. Simultaneous fluorescence immunophenotyping and interphase cytogenetics in tissue cultures will probably also prove to be very useful [87].

Table 5.3 Chromosomal abnormalities in some NHL entities

	Chromosome abnormality	Oncogene rearrangement
Chronic lymphocytic leukemia of B-cell type	trisomy 12, 13q abnormalities	
Mantle cell lymphoma ('centrocytic')	t(11;14)	*bcl*-1
Centroblastic–centrocytic lymphoma	t(14;18)	*bcl*-2
Centroblastic lymphoma	t(14;18), some cases	*bcl*-2
Burkitt's lymphoma	t(8;14)	c-*myc*
	t(8;22)	
	t(2;8)	
B-Lymphoblastic lymphoma	t(9;22)	c-*abl*
Chronic lymphocytic leukemia of T-cell type	Inv 14(q11;32), trisomy 8q	
Low-grade T-cell lymphomas	trisomy 3, 5 or +X	
Large-cell anaplastic lymphoma of T-cell type	t(2;5)(p23;35)	

THE PRACTICAL AND THEORETICAL IMPORTANCE OF MOLECULAR AND CLASSICAL GENETICS

So far molecular genetic techniques have only given us confirmation of entities that we had already recognized on the basis of morphology, with the assistance of immunocytochemistry where necessary. The same holds true for classical cytogenetics. But the question remains whether they will lead to confirmation of all of the defined entities, to differentiation of new ones or perhaps to combining of old entities. Examples of confirmation of entities defined by morphology with or without immunocytochemistry are shown in Table 5.3.

The methods of molecular genetics and cytogenetics have fulfilled another important function beyond that which we have just discussed. They opened our eyes to the fact, or confirmed our conjectures, that some lymphomas are closely connected with each other because they arise from the same compartment. Hence >30% of the cases of centroblastic lymphoma (mostly secondary centroblastic lymphoma arising after or together with centroblastic–centrocytic lymphoma) show a *bcl*-2 gene rearrangement ≈ t(14;18), while >80% of the cases of centroblastic–centrocytic lymphoma show the same findings. *bcl*-2 gene rearrangement is also occasionally seen in Burkitt's lymphomas. On the other hand, the c-*myc* rearrangement that is usually demonstrable in Burkitt's lymphoma can also be seen in <10% of the cases of centroblastic lymphoma [63]. This may point to a relationship between the two lymphomas (see page 150).

But how shall we deal with the handicap that usually not all malignant lymphomas of an entity show the specific abnormality? And what about the lymphomas of a certain entity that we have defined morphologically with or without the help of immunocytochemistry that show another abnormality? The future will teach us how many such 'fugitives' are the result of an inadequate cytological diagnosis, and how many negative cases are not yet recognized for technical reasons. Whether anomalies that deviate from the typical chromosome abnormality but have the same morphology and immunocytochemistry mean more than a variant of the entity in question will become clear in the future.

This also raises the fundamental question: which criterion really proves malignancy? As far as we can see none of the new methods is suitable for proving malignancy absolutely, neither the much-praised monoclonality nor some chromosome anomalies, such as t(14;18). Perhaps t(8;14) and t(2;5) define malignancy.

Monoclonality *per se* is no certain criterion of malignancy. Polyclonality, by contrast, points in all probability to a nonneoplastic lymphoproliferation. For some time, examples of monoclonal reactive and benign lymphoproliferative disorders have been being published, e.g., monoclonality in lymphomatoid papulosis [88,89,89a]. Reviews have been given by Goudie and Lee [90] and Slater [91]. Examples of our own experience are localized Castleman's tumor with monoclonal plasma cells [92], and TCR and IgH gene rearrangements in cutaneous, T-cell-rich pseudolymphomas [93].

In addition, early lymphomas or even prelymphomas may be monoclonal, e.g., Sjögren's syndrome in the salivary glands [94], plasma cells in the early phase of immunoproliferative small intestinal disease (IPSID) or early low-grade B-cell lymphomas of the MALT type, cured with an anti-*Helicobacter pylori* therapy ([95], Stolte, personal communication 1993). This has its equivalent in general tumor pathology. Preneoplastic liver cells grow clonally [96].

Theoretically, benign lymphomas would also have to be considered because benign tumors in general also show monoclonality, demonstrated, e.g., by a constant chromosomal abnormality in meningiomas [97]. However, so far no benign lymphoma has been recognized, except for localized Castleman's disease, and we may speculate about the true nature of low-grade B-cell lymphomas of the MALT type and certain skin lymphomas.

We can only agree with the dermatohistopathologist Slater [91], who still refers to morphology (with or without immunocytochemistry) together with the clinical picture as the gold standard of lymphoma diagnosis and thus the basis for establishing lymphoma entities. It would be too optimistic to assume that Aisenberg's [98] hope will be fulfilled within the foreseeable future, that 'molecular genetics will provide a classification superior to that provided by morphology'.

FURTHER POSSIBILITIES FOR ESTABLISHING PATHOLOGICAL LYMPHOMA ENTITIES

Generalizing concepts

The general terms low grade, intermediate grade, and high grade do not comprise entities, but rather groups of entities, which are defined either morphologically as low or high grade (Kiel classification) or according to survival rates as low, intermediate or high grade (WF).

The distinction between B- and T-cell lymphomas as a whole cannot be considered as delineating two entities, but, at the most, two superfamilies. It is a similar matter with the distinction between precursor and peripheral B- and T-cell lymphomas. Whereas one could view the B-cell and T-cell precursor cell lymphomas as two entities with multiple variants, the lymphomas of the peripheral lymphatic tissue consist of a large number of entities, some of them with subentities and variants. This must be stressed particularly for the peripheral T-cell lymphomas. The diagnosis 'malignant lymphoma of peripheral T-cell type' is merely a collective term and does not describe an entity [10,99]. This has been demonstrated by both clinicopathological [100,101], morphometric [102] and cytogenetic studies [83].

Lymphomas of the main groups of B- and T-cells

B-cells consist of the CD5+ CD23+ lymphocytes that predominate in the fetal period and the dominant CD5− CD23− lymphocytes of the postfetal period. There is a neoplasm of CD5+ CD23+ lymphocytes, chronic lymphocytic leukemia of B-cell type, which can be unequivocally distinguished from all other malignant lymphomas by its morphology, by its positive reactivity with CD5 and its negativity for all other T-cell markers. Lymphoplasmacytoid immunocytoma may be included in this entity, although it differs by the expression of cIg [103].

In the follicle mantle there is a population of CD5+, but CD23− cells ('follicle mantle cells'). Their neoplastic equivalent is mantle cell lymphoma [104], which we previously called centrocytic lymphoma [8,48]). Here, CD5 positivity and CD23 negativity help us to verify the morphological diagnosis. More important, where the morphology is appropriate, is to distinguish this lymphoma from low-grade B-cell lymphoma of the MALT type, which shows similar cells ('centrocyte-like cells'), but which is derived from CD5− cells, probably marginal zone cells, and is therefore CD5−. Here too the CD5 reaction pattern is a useful adjunctive diagnostic measure. The two entities that need to be distinguished here, however, had been defined as such morphologically prior to the use of CD5. All other B-cell lymphomas are CD5 negative. In our opinion it makes no sense to speak of two B-cell lymphoma entities, the CD5+ ones and the CD5− ones.

The situation is somewhat different with the T-cell lymphomas. Here also we distinguish two main cell types, which occur mainly fetally or postfetally: T-cells with the TCRγ/δ and T-cells with the TCRα/β. Whereas more than 95% of the T-cell lymphomas show a rearrangement of the TCRα/β gene, there are only very few TCRγ/δ+ malignant lymphomas. Some of these show a very characteristic clinical/pathological anatomical picture, e.g., the hepato-

splenic form of Gaulard et al. [105,106]. Only a few cases of lymphoblastic lymphoma [107], one case of subcutaneous lymphoma [108] and one case of 'midline granuloma' [109] γ/δ type have been described.

Demonstration of viral genomes and antigens

The innumerable studies on EBV in Burkitt's lymphomas (BL) have directed our attention to this virus. It has become apparent that sporadic EBV-negative cases cannot be distinguished morphologically and immunocytochemically from endemic EBV-positive cases, though there have turned out to be certain differences in the clinical picture [110,111] and in c-*myc* rearrangement [112,113]. The breakpoint on chromosome 14 differs in endemic and sporadic cases. In endemic Burkitt's lymphoma it involves the heavy chain joining region prior to gene rearrangement (corresponding to an early B-cell of the bone marrow?); in sporadic Burkitt's lymphoma it involves the heavy chain switch region (corresponding to a later B-cell stage of the germinal centre?). Thus one may speak of subentities or variants of BL that can be defined epidemiologically and by molecular genetics; the morphologically and immunocytochemically defined entity BL remains unaffected.

EBV-positive large-cell B-cell lymphomas were found in a large percentage of patients with congenital or acquired immunodeficiency [114,115], but only in around 5% of patients without immune defects [115,116]. EBV positivity is demonstrable in Burkitt's lymphomas in acquired immunodeficiency syndrome (AIDS) patients in 50% and more of the cases, compared with 10–15% positivity of Burkitt's lymphoma in nonendemic regions [116,117].

Jones et al. [118] were the first to find EBV in T-cell lymphomas. In the meantime a number of studies have been performed; EBV is found in 10–35% of the T-cell lymphomas [119], especially in pleomorphic medium-sized to large-cell types and in AILD types [120–122]. The percentage appears to be highest in China (62%) [119]. EBV is evidently found in 100% of the cases of pleomorphic or natural killer (NK) cell lymphoma of the nose ('midline granuloma') [53,109,123,124].

In cutaneous pleomorphic T-cell lymphomas EBV apparently does not occur [53]; however, de Bruin et al. [53] found EBV genome in one of 12 cases of gastrointestinal lymphoma and in two of six cases of pulmonary lymphoma. In contrast, de Bruin et al. [125] found EBV in only 15 of 46 cases of nodal T-cell lymphoma. Only eight of these showed a clustered or diffuse pattern of EBV positivity, which, in their opinion, speaks in favor of EBV association. In seven cases, only sporadic EBV-positive cells were found and EBV was probably not associated with the tumor. This means that T-cell lymphomas or NK cell lymphomas in different organs are associated with EBV with varying frequency. Only where viral genomes are positive in practically 100% of the lymphoma cells are we certain that there is an association between EBV and the tumor cells (e.g., nasal T-cell/NK cell lymphoma).

Human T-cell leukemia/lymphoma virus-1 (HTLV-1) is generally recognized as the pathogen that causes adult T-cell leukemia/lymphoma (ATLL), which is endemic in certain parts of Japan (for a review, see [126]). HTLV-1 does not cause a unique type of T-cell lymphoma, but rather an entire spectrum ranging from a T-cell chronic lymphocytic leukemia-like picture to large-cell anaplastic lymphoma (for large-cell anaplastic lymphoma, see [127]). Only a portion of the cases of ATLL can be suspected morphologically [128]. One cannot speak of a specific picture in any of the morphological variants of ATLL. One must therefore be content to affix the term HTLV-1 positive or negative to the morphological-immunocytochemical type of T-cell lymphoma. This need not preclude the possibility of also combining all HTLV-1 positive cases as one virologically (etiologically) defined entity called ATLL. This would not, however, be a pathological entity in the strict sense of the word.

The situation is quite similar in the T-cell lymphomas in baboons that are induced by simian T-cell leukemia virus 1 (STLV-1 [129], a retrovirus closely related to HTLV-1). Here too, one and the same virus triggers a spectrum of T-cell lymphomas ranging from T-cell chronic lymphocytic leukemia to large, cell anaplastic lymphoma [130]. There are various entities definable by morphology with or without immunocytochemistry, which appear to be one entity from a virological (etiological) standpoint.

An example of the importance of virus infection may be a CD30+ large-cell anaplastic lymphoma of T-cell type. When this lymphoma is localized primarily in the skin, it is described as HTLV-1 positive [131], has a relatively good prognosis and is said to lack the typical t(2;5) translocation of most nodal, often generalized large-cell anaplastic lymphomas. These also show a poorer clinical course [125] and may contain EBV genomes [132,133]. The viral findings are, however, controversial and by no means apply to all cases. In contrast, it does appear justified to distinguish two subentities of CD30+ large-cell anaplastic lymphoma of the T-cell type: the primary cutaneous type and the primary extracutaneous (nodal, etc.) type.

To sum things up, we can say that a pathological entity should be defined morphologically with or without immunocytochemistry, instead of by the demonstration of certain viral genomes. Virus demonstration may be important for epidemiological studies, but none of the viruses we have discussed define one 'morphological–immunological' entity with which a corresponding clinical behavior can be correlated. This can be shown particularly in ATLL.

Primary localization of the lymphoma

The primary localization of a lymphoma can tell us quite a bit about it, but it must always be defined by morphological with or without immunocytochemical data. Basically the question is one of distinguishing between nodal and extranodal lymphomas. For the nodal lymphomas the specific localization of the involved lymph nodes is of little importance – the exception being perhaps the sclerotic type of centroblastic–centrocytic lymphoma, which occurs primarily in the abdomen and the groin. It tends to occur as a localized disease process that can be managed therapeutically rather well, in contrast to the other types of centroblastic–centrocytic lymphoma, which often generalize at an early stage [8,134].

For the extranodal lymphomas the primary localization is very important, especially if we are dealing with one of the types that never have their primary sites in the lymph node.

Extranodal B-cell lymphomas

Of these the first type to think of is *low-grade B-cell lymphoma of the MALT type* [6,135,136], which is occurring with increasing frequency. This lymphoma occurs especially in the gastrointestinal tract, lung [137], salivary gland, thyroid gland, orbit, Waldeyer's ring and many other organs (see Table 5.4). It is linked to the existence of glandular epithelium (not only mucosa [138]), but there are exceptions (e.g., the thymus). This type of lymphoma has a characteristic morphology and immunocytochemistry. One finds polyclonal germinal centers. The actual – monoclonal – tumor cells are mostly 'centrocyte-like cells', probably marginal zone cells [139], often lymphocytes, or rarely monocytoid B-cells. They frequently contain plasma cells that belong to the same clone. In the lymphocytic variant this would correspond to lymphoplasmacytic immunocytoma of the lymph node. Further, large blasts are often interspersed, as are occasional Sternberg–Reed-like cells. In most cases the glandular epithelium is infiltrated and effaced by the tumor cells (lymphoepithelial lesions). *Helicobacter pylori* can frequently be detected in the stomach in the presence of such lymphomas; this finding is probably of etiological significance.

This lymphoma can develop into a large-cell high-grade lymphoma of extremely varied morphology. One can diagnose this without any doubt from the

Table 5.4 Primary localizations of B-cell lymphomas of MALT type

Conjunctiva, including orbit
Salivary glands
Waldeyer's ring
Larynx
Thyroid gland
Thymus
Breast
Lung
Stomach
Small and large intestine
Rectum
Gall bladder
Uterine tube
Uterus?
Prostate
Skin

remnants of a low-grade component. If this is not the case, it must remain open today whether all or some of the other high-grade B-cell lymphomas of the gastrointestinal tract (with the exception of BL) develop primarily or secondarily in a low-grade B-cell lymphoma of the MALT type. In the other organs in which low-grade B-cell lymphoma of MALT type occurs, the morphology is basically the same, but the lymphoepithelial lesions are sometimes difficult to find or are not present at all.

There is no doubt that the glandular organs in which B-cell lymphomas of MALT type (Table 5.4) occur must have something in common, e.g., special homing receptors. This would explain why in one and the same patient at intervals of several years different organs of the 'MALT system' are affected, e.g., first the stomach, then the lung or first the stomach, then the tonsils [140]. In one patient we observed low-grade B-cell lymphomas of the MALT type successively in the skin, orbit (both sides), Fallopian tube, skin (other localization), and finally, after 5 years, for the first time in a lymph node.

Primary lymphomas of this type apparently do not occur in lymph nodes, if we disregard lymphoplasmacytic lymphomas and monocytoid B-cell lymphoma. At any rate, primary marginal zone cell lymphomas of the lymph node have not yet been described, although marginal zone cells occur in the lymph node [141,142] (for further literature, see [10]). They may be hyperplastic and are then easily recognizable. In the spleen marginal zone cells are virtually always present in the outer part of the follicles [143–146] and may develop a special splenic lymphoma, marginal zone cell lymphoma of the spleen, which is, at least in the majority of the cases, the histological counterpart of Mulligan and

Catovsky's 'splenic lymphoma with villous lymphocytes' [147].

We consider it justifiable to speak of low-grade B-cell lymphoma of the MALT type as an entity if the primary site is the stomach or another organ that belongs to the 'MALT system', and if a marginal zone cell, lymphoplasmacytic or monocytoid B-cell morphology exists. Another point that would support this view is the particularly favorable prognosis of this lymphoma, which consequently often used to be considered a pseudolymphoma or a benign lymphoma.

Immunoproliferative small intestinal disease (IPSID) with and without α-chain secretion (α-chain disease) seems to be related to low-grade B-cell lymphoma of the stomach [148] (see Chapters 3 and 22). In the early phase, which is still curable with antibiotics [149], the mucosa is infiltrated by monotypic plasma cells that contain α-chain. Later a B-cell lymphoma of the MALT type develops, which is initially low grade and can later transform into a high-grade lymphoma. IPSID may be called an entity, whose peculiarity is that it has an epidemiological basis. It occurs only in the Mediterranean region.

The fact that malignant lymphomas whose primary localization is usually the lymph node also occur in the gastrointestinal tract and other organs of the 'MALT system' shows that the localization of the primary tumor *per se* does not justify establishing a pathological entity. The histological and immunocytochemical picture must also fit.

Of the malignant lymphomas that occur in the lymph node and in the intestine, we should mention *mantle cell lymphoma*, which gives rise to a characteristic clinical and pathological picture in the intestine: (multiple) lymphomatoid polyposis. This may be called a subentity of mantle cell lymphoma.

A further example of a malignant lymphoma whose primary localization can be either in lymph nodes or extranodal, especially the bone marrow, is *plasmacytoma*. Here too one must question whether these are subentities of a tumor or tumors of a different nature after all. At any rate the clinical course differs.

In *Burkitt's lymphoma* there are clinical differences depending on the primary localization (see above).

The primary malignant lymphomas of the *brain* deserve special consideration. It is remarkable that primary lymphomas of the brain are almost always B-cell lymphomas, sometimes with a large number of nonneoplastic T-cells and that they are usually of high-grade malignancy. They are often EBV-positive and then frequently show a polymorphic large-cell picture as polymorphic centroblastic lymphoma [150] or what has been named 'polymorphous high-grade B-cell lymphoma' [151]. It is difficult and sometimes impossible to differentiate from EBV-induced lymphoproliferative lesions in immunocompromised patients (see below).

Another special cerebral lymphoma is lymphoplasmacytic immunocytoma, which is discovered less often in biopsy specimens than at autopsy. It represents a part of the tumor called microglioma (tosis) [152]. It had been noticed long ago that this lymphoma, which was mistaken for a glioma, behaved peculiarly, i.e., it metastasized to extracerebral sites, which gliomas do not do.

Mediastinal large cell lymphoma of B-cell type with sclerosis [153–161] probably originates in the 'asteroid' CD23+ B-cells of the thymic medulla [162–164]. It is a high-grade lymphoma that is composed of medium-sized to large, slightly basophilic cells ('clear cells' according to Möller). The most important diagnostic criterion is sclerosis, which is occasionally overlooked, because it does not exist in all parts of the tumor. The tumor is localized in the anterior mediastinum and histologically it occasionally contains residual thymus. The immunophenotype is variable, the tumor cells are CD19+ CD20+, mostly CD22+ CD23+. They are often sIg-negative, and not cIg-positive [159,165]. They apparently show variable defects in MHC antigen expression [158]. Most frequently affected are relatively young adults, especially females between 30–40 years of age. Metastasis to lymph nodes does not occur, but extranodal metastasis is frequently observed, e.g., to the kidneys, adrenal glands, brain. Both morphology/immunology and the clinical picture speak in favor of a unique tumor, i.e., a well-defined lymphoma entity.

A last, exclusively extranodal B-cell lymphoma is *intravascular lymphomatosis* [166–168]. From our experience it is generally a large-cell B-cell lymphoma that looks very similar to a 'large-cell B-cell polymorphic lymphoma' of the brain (Plate 5.3). It grows as a primary tumor in the small blood vessels, especially of the lung, the skin, the bones and the brain. It runs a rapid course; aggressive therapy can be effective, however, if the diagnosis is made early enough.

Extranodal malignant lymphomas of T-cells and NK cells

In lymph nodes malignant lymphomas of T-cells and NK cells show the entities that are listed in the updated Kiel classification. In addition to these entities there are some extranodal lymphomas that can be differentiated as special types of lymphomas on the basis of their primary localization and often of their immunophenotype or molecular genetic characteristics.

'*Lethal midline granuloma*' ('midline polymorphic reticulosis') of the nose is mostly a lymphoma of CD3– CD56+ NK cells without TCRβ gene rearrangement. However, there are also some cases of true T-cell lymphoma (CD3+, mostly CD4– CD8–) and some CD3+ CD8+ cases [169] that show TCRβ gene rearrangement. Finally a T-cell lymphoma of γ/δ type has also been described in this location [109]. Angiocentricity and angiodestruction are often found [170] and may explain the occurrence of large areas of necrosis. Ho et al. [171] were often unable, however, to find such vascular lesions. Cytologically this is a pleomorphic lymphoma with cells ranging from small to large-sized. Sometimes a strong lymphocytic infiltration near the surface is seen (inflammatory?). Rarely monomorphic medium-sized cells are the dominating tumor cell type, especially in the γ/δ variant. In imprints azurophil granules may be seen (typical of CD3– NK cells and CD3+ CD8+ killer T-cells). All Hong Kong cases are evidently EBV-positive [123]. Jaffe et al. [123a] published the results of the Workshop on Nasal and Related Extranodal Angiocentric T/Natural Killer Cell Lymphomas in Hong Kong. A European collection of nasal T-cell lymphomas was studied by van Gorp et al. [123b]. Chan et al. [123c] proposed a classification of natural killer cell neoplasms. High-grade malignant extranasal NK cell-like T-cell lymphomas were described by Nakamura et al. [123d] and Macon et al. [123e].

The *skin* shows a specific type of lymphoma cell known as 'cerebriform' in the updated Kiel classification. It comprises mycosis fungoides and Sézary's syndrome. These must be considered two subentities with clear-cut differences in their clinical appearance, although the proliferating cell type looks identical. The cerebriform type occurs extracutaneously only as metastases, i.e., it appears to be of primary skin origin. Not only this type of lymphoma, but also a number of other lymphomas of the updated Kiel classification occur primarily in the skin. They are of TCRα/β type, usually CD4+ rarely CD8+. They characteristically express the homing receptor cutaneous lymphocyte antigen (CLA) $\approx$ HECA-452). Whether one should distinguish two main classes of skin lymphomas according to the outcome of the CLA reaction is not yet clear. Until we have concrete data we should classify skin lymphomas according to morphological criteria and note whether CLA is positive or negative. It might also be possible that irrespective of the morphology (pleomorphic or large-cell anaplastic) the clinical outcome is determined by CD30 positivity or negativity as such [172]. Willemze et al. [172a] recently suggested a special classification of cutaneous lymphomas; unfortunately, it is not possible to discuss this suggestion in more detail here.

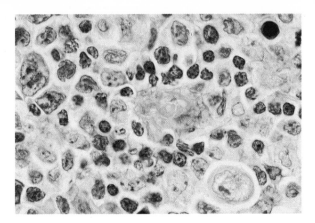

Plate 5.1 Adult T-cell leukemia/lymphoma. At the lower right is a Sternberg–Reed cell with a large violet nucleus and fine chromatin. At the upper left is a giant cell of Kikuchi type with basophilic nucleoli and coarse chromatin. Giemsa, x 723.

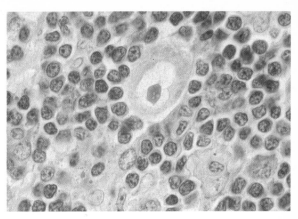

Plate 5.2 Mononuclear Sternberg–Reed cell in a reactive lymph node. No HD! Note the abundant grey cytoplasm, the fine chromatin and the very large vacuolated nucleolus. Giemsa, x 723.

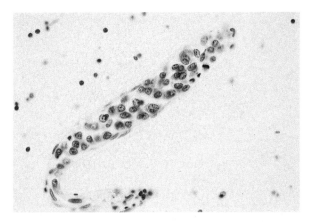

Plate 5.3 Intravascular lymphomatosis. Brain autopsy (therefore the basophilia of the cytoplasm is reduced) 'polymorphic B-cell lymphoma'. Giemsa, x 285.

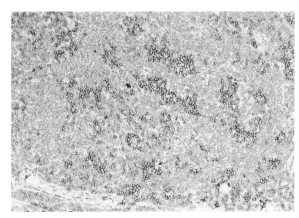

Plate 5.4 Nodular paragranuloma. Note the 'moth-eaten' appearance owing to focal accumulations of T-lymphocytes. CD2. x 68.

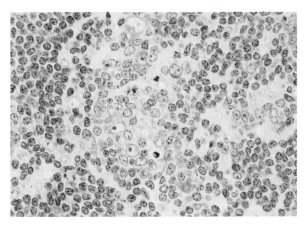

Plate 5.5 Nodular paragranuloma. A T-cell cluster with one mononuclear giant cell (L & H cell to the left of the middle of the upper edge) and a few very large basophilic cells with large solitary nucleolus (precursors of L & H cells). The T-cells are somewhat larger and lighter than the more distant B-lymphocytes. Giemsa, x 362.

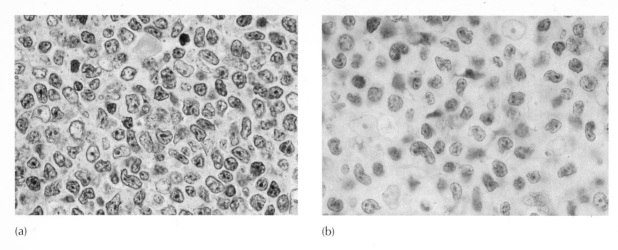

(a)   (b)

Plate 5.6   (a) Mantle cell lymphoma. No blast cells. The cytoplasm stains very weakly. Some follicular dendritic cells with very fine chromatin and solitary large nucleoli. Giemsa, x 723. (b) T-Cell lymphoma, pleomorphic small cell. Two histiocytes. No blast cells. Giemsa, x 723.

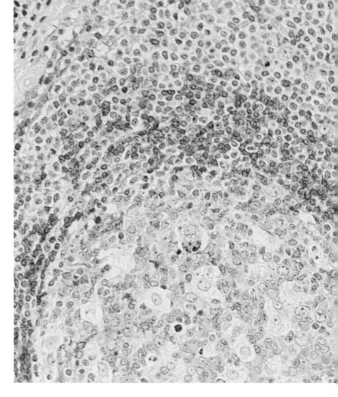

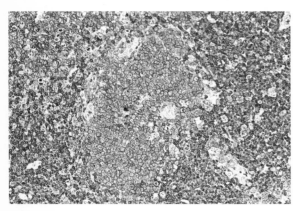

Plate 5.8   Monocytoid B-cell lymphoma growing in a dilated sinus. Strongly positive for Ki-B3, x 142.

Plate 5.7   Lymph node metastasis of a low-grade B-cell lymph They are negative for Ki-B3, x 347.

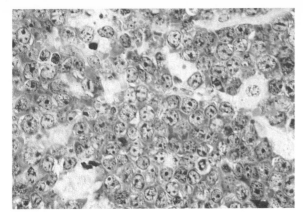

Plate 5.9 Burkitt's lymphoma. Multiple nucleoli in the center of the nuclei. Resin re-embedding. Giemsa, x 723.

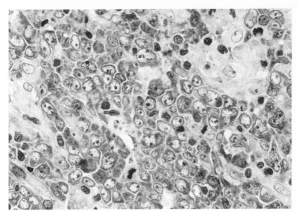

Plate 5.10 'Burkitt's lymphoma-like lymphoma'. There are some immunoblasts with large solitary central nucleoli and some centroblasts with medium-sized nucleoli at the nuclear membrane. Paraffin embedding, therefore not as 'cohesive' as in Figure 5.10. Giemsa, x 452.

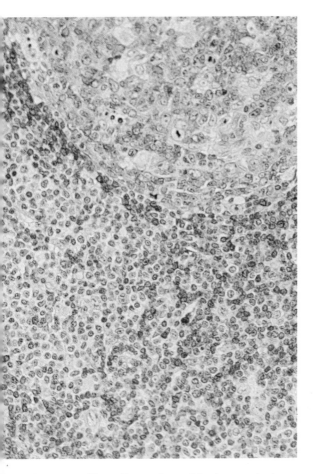

type. Centrocyte-like cells are situated in the marginal zone.

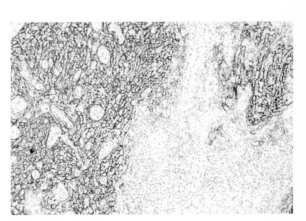

Plate 5.11 T-Cell lymphoma of AILD type. Staining of follicular dendritic cell networks (red). In between high endothelial venules. CD35 x 58.

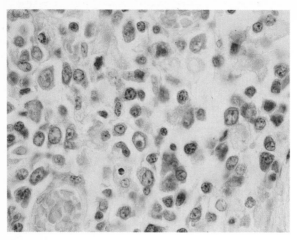

Plate 5.12 Polymorphic (nonneoplastic) EBV infection in kidney transplantation. Polyclonal. Testis. Case kindly provided by Dr J. Rosai. Giemsa, x 520.

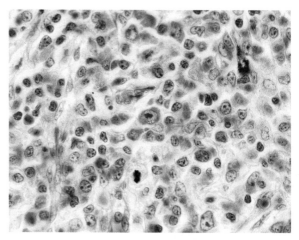

Plate 5.13 Polymorphic B-cell lymphoma in an HIV-positive patient. The tumor is EBV negative. IgH rearrangement in Southern blot. Case kindly provided by Dr J. Diebold. Giemsa, x 520.

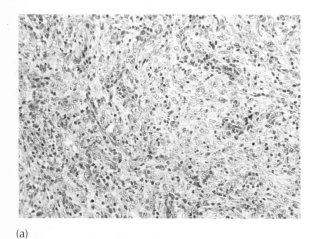

(a)

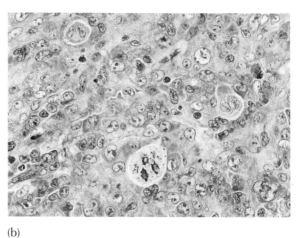

(b)

Plate 5.14 (a) T-Cell lymphoma of AILD type. Right of the center are follicular dendritic cells with clear nuclei. There are some high endothelial venules. The small cells are T-lymphocytes. Giemsa, x 147. (b) A different area of the same lymph node: large-cell anaplastic lymphoma with atypical mitotic figure. Giemsa, x 368.

The T-cell lymphomas of the *small intestine* are roughly divided into one type with enteropathy and one without [136,173]. The type with enteropathy is also observed following dermatitis herpetiformis. It is derived from the CD3+, CD7+, CD4–, CD8– ('double negative'), human mucosal lymphocyte-1 (HML-1)+ intraepithelial T-lymphocytes of the small intestine [174]. The immunophenotype is not absolutely specific, however. CD3 can be lacking, CD8 can be positive, and HML-1 positivity occasionally occurs in other peripheral T-cell lymphomas and in T-lymphoblastic lymphoma [6,175]. Even less homogeneous than the immunophenotype is the cytology of T-cell lymphoma with enteropathy. One finds small-cell, pleomorphic and large-cell pictures, the latter sometimes showing the typical features of CD30+ large-cell anaplastic lymphoma. Isaacson [6] considers the highly pleomorphic forms with numerous bizarre multinucleated cells to be the most characteristic appearance. In imprints azurophil granules are occasionally reported (e.g., [176]), as seen in about 25% of normal intraepithelial T-lymphocytes [177]. The tumors are not derived from TCRγ/δ cells, as initially speculated, but from TCRα/β cells.

There is much less information on T-cell lymphomas of the small intestine without enteropathy. The first major paper was by Shepherd et al. [178]. Cases with and without enteropathy were not distinguished, but Stansfeld later reported (personal communication) that 8 of 26 cases of intestinal lymphoma were enteropathy associated. The high content of eosinophils is stressed in this study. In a more recent paper, Chott et al. [179] assume, on the basis of 24 cases, that enteropathy-associated T-cell lymphomas of the small intestine are more frequent than those not associated with enteropathy.

It appears certain that the double negative T-cell lymphomas of the small intestine with enteropathy do represent an entity, even though not all immunocytological criteria are always fulfilled. A clear-cut definition of intestinal T-cell lymphomas without enteropathy is, however, a task that will have to be left to the future. How many are HLM-1 positive? Which types of nodal peripheral T-cell lymphomas also occur in the small intestine without enteropathy?

A special *hepatosplenic* T-cell lymphoma composed of TCRγ/δ cells was reported by a French group [105,106]. Wong et al. [179a] recently published another case and discussed it in relation to all previously published cases. The tumor appears to be very rare. Nonetheless, up to 1993 Gaulard had observed eight patients (personal communication). The tumor spreads especially in the sinus/sinusoids of the spleen and the liver, and does not affect lymph nodes, whereas the bone marrow shows discrete infiltrations. The tumor cells are medium-sized with relatively regular nuclei ('monomorphic medium-sized'). One

patient had a leukemic blood picture. There is no doubt that hepatosplenic lymphoma of TCRγ/δ type is an entity of its own.

Clinical data

The clinical picture should conform to the cytological–immunological diagnosis. This holds particularly for T-cell lymphomas of the skin. There are doubtless lesions which highly resemble T-cell lymphomas and fulfill all of the criteria of malignancy in their morphology, immunochemistry and molecular genetics (monoclonal), but which heal spontaneously. The most prominent example is lymphomatoid papulosis. As we know, in about 20% of cases it is wrongly considered to be a large-cell anaplastic lymphoma, but it heals spontaneously. The majority of cases can be distinguished from large-cell anaplastic lymphoma on the basis of defined morphological criteria [172a]. Clinically, multiple localizations point to a benign lesion, whereas large-cell anaplastic lymphoma generally occurs in a solitary localization.

Hence we must always compare the clinical picture with the morphological and immunocytochemical findings, and where they are in disagreement, we must re-examine, qualify or change the morphological/immunocytochemical diagnosis.

The clinical findings occasionally provide very important information, e.g., in T-cell lymphoma of the AILD type. Certain basic trends can be recognized in the survival curves: with the chemotherapy that is still customary today, some low-grade lymphomas, e.g., chronic lymphocytic leukemia, immunocytoma, mantle cell lymphoma, slowly but continuously take a fatal course, without being influenced very much. High-grade lymphomas and some of the low-grade lymphomas form a plateau, i.e., some of the patients are cured with the treatment usually given today, or at least remain free from relapse for many years.

Where there is a question whether two morphologically different lymphomas also represent two actual entities, survival curves from a large number of patients who have received standardized treatment can provide the required information. For instance, it has turned out that so-called 'large-cell lymphoma of B-type' is not one uniform disease. There are statistically significant differences in the survival curves between centroblastic lymphoma and immunoblastic lymphoma (Engelhard, personal communication).

SUMMING UP

The systematic scientific research of the past two decades on biological parameters of the lymphoid tissue and its malignancies, combining morphology and immunocytochemistry, permits us today to recognize most malignant lymphomas of the lymph nodes as clear-cut entities or subentities. Some of them have been further confirmed by molecular genetic and cytogenetic studies; some can only be recognized and defined as malignant lymphoproliferations on the basis of these studies – of course, in combination with the morphological and immunocytochemical picture. Other criteria, especially virological ones, may characterize etiologically defined groups of lymphomas, but they are morphologically and immunocytochemically nonuniform. Any data on viral infection should nevertheless be appended to the pathological entity, so that epidemiological connections will not be overlooked. The primary localization may, however, be of significance in extranodal lymphomas. Here too, though, the morphological definition with or without immunocytochemistry should take priority. However, the site of proliferation is occasionally so important that it must be listed in the diagnosis and thus becomes an integral part of the pathological entity (e.g., low-grade B-cell lymphoma of the MALT type). As far as the connection between nodal and extranodal lymphomas is concerned, we should point out that all nodal lymphomas can also originate in extranodal localizations, e.g., the MALT system. In contrast, the primary extranodal lymphomas have two possibilities: either they occur only extranodally, even as metastases (e.g., mediastinal B-cell lymphoma) or they also metastasize to the lymph nodes (e.g., classical low-grade lymphoma of the MALT type).

We must always remember that every morphological classification of malignant lymphomas is but a momentary inventory, including ours. We do not know what new studies, particularly in cytogenetics and molecular genetics, may have in store for us. This holds especially for the malignant lymphomas with proven chromosomal and molecular genetic abnormalities in which a remarkable percentage do not show these abnormalities. Do they represent subentities, or are there still unsolved technical problems or misdiagnoses? And what about morphological/immunocytochemical entities that have different cytogenetic/molecular genetic findings? How does the molecular genetic/cytogenetic diagnosis rank in comparison with the morphological/immunocytochemical diagnosis? To answer this question we shall have to refer to prospective studies.

Finally, it is possible that soon pathological entities that we now differentiate for morphological and/or immunocytochemical reasons may one day be combined on the basis of molecular genetic or cytogenetic findings. This is already being discussed for lymphohistiocytic lymphoma, which usually

develops into a (small-cell) CD30+ 'large-cell anaplastic lymphoma', and like a large-cell anaplastic lymphoma of T-cell and null cell type, can show a t(2;5)(p23;35) translocation [180, 180a].

Differentiating between Hodgkin's and non-Hodgkin's lymphomas

In the past few years the question of distinguishing between Hodgkin's and non-Hodgkin's lymphomas has shifted more and more into the limelight, especially since we have come to know the NHL of T-cell type better. T-Cell lymphomas are the most important entities that need to be differentiated.

T-CELL LYMPHOMAS

First we have *large-cell anaplastic lymphoma*, which documents its close relationship to HL by its positive CD30 reactivity [181] and by t(2;5)(p23;q35) translocation. The latter has been demonstrated by the team of Feller in Sternberg–Reed cells and has been found in a large percentage of cases of large-cell anaplastic lymphoma of T-cell or null-cell type [181a,181b]. To take it even further, large-cell anaplastic lymphoma can evolve from HL of the mixed cellularity and nodular sclerosing types. At times large-cell anaplastic lymphoma can totally infiltrate the lymph node, so that no remnants of the primary HL are left. Then the connection with the prior HL can no longer be verified. Frequently, however, remnants of the former HL can be recognized at the margins. Especially sclerosis and the presence of lacunar cells are helpful here. There may also be an increase in the number of eosinophils and neutrophils, but this is not a reliable criterion. Identification of Sternberg–Reed cells is irrelevant. They can occur in abundance in large-cell anaplastic lymphoma.

Certain resemblances to large-cell anaplastic lymphoma are also shown by nodular sclerosis type 2 [182], the 'syncytial variant' of nodular sclerosing HL of the American literature [183]. It is supposed to also occasionally reveal clonal bands with probes for the TCRβ region (Lukes and Labuguen, quoted in [184].) Here further morphological and molecular genetic studies are urgently needed.

The second type of T-cell lymphoma that is occasionally difficult to differentiate from HL, especially of mixed cellularity is the *AILD type*, which we used to call lymphogranulomatosis X (LgX) (see page 151). In our first series of 172 cases of LgX (now called T-cell lymphoma of AILD type), in 1979, we found five that 'developed' into an unmistakable HL. In two cases, development into HL and subsequent transformation back to LgX was diagnosed. This means that the borderline is not clear-cut. There are evidently cases of HL without diagnostic Sternberg–Reed cells and cases of T-cell lymphoma of AILD type with giant cells that cannot be distinguished from Sternberg–Reed cells. When we did our study of LgX (AILD), we were still limited in the procedures we could apply to the differential diagnosis. Today this can be done much more successfully with immunocytochemical techniques, but also with molecular genetic and cytogenetic methods (see page 152). Immunocytochemically one often finds predominantly CD4+ T lymphocytes in T-cell lymphomas of AILD type, but this is also true of many cases of HL. Thus such assays are not very useful. There is, however, a very stringent criterion that allows us to distinguish T-cell lymphomas of AILD type with certainty: increased numbers of follicular dendritic cells (FDC; Plates 5.11 and 5.14a) that accumulate in large sheets, often even outside of the lymph node capsule! This FDC hyperplasia is probably induced by lymphokines produced by the neoplastic T-cells, as can be concluded from *in vitro* experiments performed by Fliedner et al. [185]. The size of the B-cell fraction is highly variable (5–30%). This might additionally indicate that the FDC hyperplasia is most probably induced by the neoplastic T-cells. Molecular genetics usually shows a TCRβ rearrangement in T-cell lymphomas of the AILD type. In HL this is rare [186]. Classical cytogenetics reveals chromosomal abnormalities that increase quantitatively during the course of T-cell lymphomas of AILD type. Especially trisomy 3 and trisomy 5, and extra sex chromosomes can be found here (see page 152).

The third important entity is *lymphoepithelioid lymphoma* (Lennert's lymphoma). In a thorough study of almost 400 cases of lymphoma with focal epithelioid cell proliferation, Patsouris et al. [187,188] detailed the differences between lymphoepithelioid lymphoma and HL with a high content of epithelioid cells. The most important morphological criterion is the number of Sternberg–Reed cells. These giant cells rarely (in ≈ 2%) occur in lymphoepithelioid lymphoma and when they do, they are very sparse (never more than one or at the most two Sternberg–Reed cells per slide of at least 1 cm^2). There are also differences in the clinical pictures of lymphoepithelioid lymphoma and HL with a high content of epithelioid cells (see Table 5.5). Molecular genetic and cytogenetic studies have produced clear evidence of the difference between the two neoplasms. Lymphoepithelioid lymphoma always shows a rearrangement of TCRβb genes [189,190], and cyto-

Table 5.5 Clinical differences between the lymphomas with a high content of epithelioid cells

	LeL (%)	AILD (%)	HD (%)	LP-IC (%)
Generalized lymphadenopathy	71	84	57	73
Pruritis	18	46	12	17
Skin rash	7	38	3	9
Hemolytic anemia	—	18	—	14
Sjögren's syndrome	—	—	—	31
Other autoimmune diseases	2	16	3	15
Allergy to drugs	5	34	3	4
Monoclonal gammopathy	—	—	—	38
Transformation into high-grade ML	7	13	—	26
Carcinoma before or after ML	—	11	6	15
Male:female ratio	1.3:1	1.4:1	1.4:1	1:4

LeL, lymphoepithelioid lymphoma; AILD, angioimmunoblastic lymphadenopathy with dysproteinemia; HD, Hodgkin's disease; LP-IC, lymphoplasmacytic/cytoid immunocytoma; ML, malignant lymphoma.

genetic analyses almost always reveal trisomy 3. Both of these are findings that are rarely or never made in HL.

There is another entity that does not cause much difficulty in the differential diagnosis, although it can contain classical Sternberg–Reed cells: *adult T-cell leukemia/lymphoma*. Other features – the proliferating T-cells are usually extremely pleomorphic and there is no admixture of B-cells – almost always allow us to make a diagnosis. Furthermore, HTLV-1 is not found in HL.

One last entity only occasionally causes problems: *lymphohistiocytic lymphoma* [180,180a,191–193]. In addition to pleomorphic T-cells and large numbers of histiocytes, it often contains some or quite a few Ki-1+ cells that bear a certain resemblance to Sternberg–Reed cells. Molecular genetic analyses usually reveal a rearrangement of the TCRβ gene [180a] (rare in HL), and cytogenetically a t(2;5) (p23;35) translocation has been found in some cases (Delsol, personal communication) [180]). It would not be justifiable, in our opinion or that of Stansfeld [193], to simply call lymphohistiocytic lymphoma 'large-cell anaplastic lymphoma'. There are clear-cut cases which consist only of small to medium-sized nonbasophilic cells and histiocytes, some of which show the typical plasmacytoid appearance demonstrated, for instance, in Figure 159 in [10]. The CD30+ cells are also usually smaller than in large-cell anaplastic lymphoma, as was shown by Kinney et al. [180] and Böhm [180a].

B-CELL LYMPHOMAS

It is a B-cell lymphoma that has brought confusion into the diagnosis of T-cell lymphomas and HL: *T-cell-rich large B-cell lymphoma* [194–196]. The B-cells represent large blasts that can have a certain similarity to Sternberg–Reed cells. Between them are tremendous amounts of T-lymphocytes, which have been shown by molecular genetics to be polyclonal, whereas the B-cells belong to one clone [196]. The large cells are EMA+, like the Sternberg–Reed cells of nodular paragranuloma, which may be a hint that we should think of the diffuse lymphocyte predominance variant of HL [197]. But some T-cell-rich B-cell lymphomas express *bcl*-2 protein [198], whereas they do not show the large number of CD57+ T-cells that paragranuloma does [199,200]. Not all published cases will stand up to a critical examination; some at least should be considered composite (T-cell/B-cell type) lymphomas. Since in cases of HL (mixed cellularity type) a clonal IgH rearrangement has also been seen [201,202], the usefulness of demonstrating B-cell clonality is limited, especially because there are also cases of HL with Sternberg–Reed cells that react with B-cell markers and additionally may be CD30 and CD15 negative. Here the borderline between HL and NHL is extremely indistinct. We need additional methods, especially molecular genetic and cytogenetic ones. The currently used methods show mostly positive results in cases of NHL (rearrangements, cytogenetic abnormalities), whereas cases of HL are mostly negative.

Nodular paragranuloma is a type of HL that gives rise to a different set of problems than the nodular sclerosing and mixed cellular types of HL do. It is often confused with follicular lymphomas (centroblastic–centrocytic, follicular), especially of the so-called floral type [203,204], with mantle cell lymphoma and other low-grade B-cell lymphomas. When it has a high content of epithelioid cells, a lymphoepithelioid lymphoma may be misdiagnosed. If, in addition, the epithelioid cells are arranged in large granulomas (like tubercles), lymphoepithelioid lymphoma can be excluded. It is easy to recognize nodular paragranuloma if one knows the criteria: it has a nodular growth pattern arising from progressively transformed germinal centers. The nodularity can be recognized best with silver staining; with this method even rudimentary nodularity shows up well. The nodules often have a moth-eaten appearance (Plates 5.4 and 5.5), i.e., they are honeycombed with groups of cells that appear somewhat lighter at a low magnification and are negative when stained with pan-B antibodies. These groups of cells are T-cells, which are only slightly larger (slightly activated?) than the surrounding small B-lymphocytes. They are arranged around Sternberg–Reed cells of the L&H

type and give the appearance of rosettes. In slides stained with Ki-67 these T-cells show the greatest proliferative activity. They make it possible to understand the (rare) development of T-cell lymphomas from nodular paragranuloma [205].

Nodular paragranuloma can be recognized purely on the basis of morphology without any immunocytochemical or further techniques whatsoever. If one wants to be absolutely sure [206,207], one can determine the clonality of the B-lymphocytes. They are polyclonal; only the giant cells are often proven to be monoclonal [208]. Differentiation from progressively transformed germinal centers is sometimes difficult, and some time is required to search for L&H cells. They must be found at all events, to be certain that one is dealing with a case of paragranuloma. The existence of epithelioid cell clusters or large granulomas also speaks in favor of paragranuloma, but does not prove it. EBV is usually not found. The fact that *bcl*-2 and t(14;18) were demonstrated in HL [209,210] cannot yet be conclusively interpreted.

In conclusion, let us once more stress that Sternberg–Reed cells are not specific (see pages 134 and 147). Moreover, it is important to remember in all cases of doubt that the clinical picture helps to distinguish NHL from HL [211]. Finally, we should warn against overestimating the value of molecular genetics as a diagnostic tool at this moment in time [63,211].

Differentiating between different types of NHL

Problems arise with the borderlines between various non-Hodgkin's lymphomas particularly when tissue preparation is technically suboptimal. In such cases it is advisable to re-embed the specimen in resin [10]. Even then problematic cases may remain, and in such cases immunocytochemistry and molecular genetics (and cytogenetics) may be useful.

Chronic lymphocytic leukemia of B- and T-cell type can usually be differentiated purely on the basis of morphology: chronic lymphocytic leukemia of B-cell type often shows pseudofollicular proliferation centers and always contains some blast cells (para-immunoblasts) and only a moderate number of inconspicuous high endothelial venules. Chronic lymphocytic leukemia of T-cell type never shows proliferation centers and contains almost no blast cells, and many more high endothelial venules, which show evidence of migrating leukemic T-cells. Pan-B-cell and pan-T-cell markers definitively clarify whether a given case belongs to the B- or T-cell series.

Chronic lymphocytic leukemia of B-cell type and

immunocytoma can only be distinguished from each other for certain by demonstrating monotypic cIg in immunocytoma. Since chronic lymphocytic leukemia of B-cell type not infrequently contains polytypic (reactive) plasma cells, demonstration of Ig or the corresponding mRNA in paraffin sections is essential for the diagnosis. Inadequate fixation and embedding can, however, make it impossible to demonstrate light chain restriction. Other criteria are less specific. Immunocytoma often shows a significant increase in the number of mast cells, and considerable hemosiderosis is occasionally evident in the lymph node. Clinically, paraproteinemia often exists, usually of the IgM type. We distinguish between lymphoplasmacytoid and lymphoplasmacytic immunocytoma according to the type of plasma cells. The lymphoplasmacytoid cells are often difficult to recognize in sections stained with Giemsa, but they are clearly seen in immunostainings of paraffin sections. In contrast, the plasma cells of the lymphoplasmacytic type are typical Marschalkó-type plasma cells, which are easily found in Giemsa-stained sections. We put the question up for debate whether the lymphoplasmacytoid type should not be considered a variant of chronic lymphocytic leukemia of B-cell type, since the lymphocytes are CD5+ (in lymphoplasmacytic immunocytoma they are CD5−). As a matter of fact, the number of leukemic cases is greater and paraproteinemia is rarer in the lymphoplasmacytic type than in the lymphoplasmacytic type ([103], for further information on the clinical differences, see [212,213]).

Mantle cell lymphoma [104,214] and pleomorphic small-cell T-cell lymphoma are difficult to differentiate from each other (Plates 5.6a,b). Both are composed of more or less pleomorphic small cells and lack (basophilic) blasts. Immunostaining for CD20 (positive in mantle cell lymphoma, negative in pleomorphic small-cell T-cell lymphoma) and CD3 and βF1 (negative in mantle cell lymphoma and positive in pleomorphic T-cell lymphoma) immediately helps to clarify the diagnosis.

One can distinguish a relatively small cell from a relatively large cell mantle cell lymphoma, but they must not be considered two subentities. Satodate's nuclear measurements showed that the nuclear size distribution forms a continuum and does not show two peaks [8]. So-called 'centrocytoid centroblastic lymphoma', which contains atypical centrocytes and centroblast-like blast cells, appears to us to be clearly different. Feller (personal communication) and Weisenburger (personal communication) have each observed a case that had this morphology. It differs from typical mantle cell lymphoma in the existence of blast cells but, like other mantle zone lymphomas, shows a t(11;14) translocation. This finding needs to be related to the clinical behavior.

Monocytoid B-cell lymphoma [215–217] and *centrocyte-like (marginal zone cell?) lymphoma of MALT type* [218,219] are morphologically very similar. Actually there is an immunocytochemical distinction between reactive monocytoid B-cells and normal marginal zone cells. Marginal zone cells do not express Ki-B3 (CD45R-like) and DBA.44, whereas monocytoid B-cells do. There are, however, exceptions. The same holds for the two lymphomas. The centrocyte-like MALT-type lymphoma is negative, or only weakly positive, for both monoclonal antibodies, but a small number of cases show a definitely positive reaction for Ki-B3 and DBA.44. On the other hand, monocytoid B-cell lymphoma is generally strongly Ki-B3 and DBA.44 positive, though there are probably rare exceptions (Plates 5.7 and 5.8).

The assumption that monocytoid B-cell lymphoma is closely related to low-grade B-cell lymphoma of MALT type is based primarily on the findings of Nizze et al. [216]. In nine patients they found a monocytoid B-cell lymphoma in combination with a malignant lymphoma of the MALT. They also distinguished a small-cell and a medium-sized cell type. The small-cell type was Ki-B3 negative. A later analysis of the relationship between the cell types and the clinical behavior (by Paulsen, personal communication) showed that only the small-cell types were associated with a malignant lymphoma in the MALT. Thus it is likely that the small-cell 'monocytoid B-cell lymphomas' were in reality metastases of centrocyte-like Ki-B3 negative MALT-type lymphomas. This does not exclude the possibility, however, that medium-sized cell monocytoid B-cell lymphomas may occur as primary lymphomas in the MALT and metastasize to the lymph nodes.

The differential diagnosis of the large-cell B-cell lymphomas is very problematic, especially if one does not apply optimum histological techniques (see [220]). But it is important to recognize centroblastic lymphoma as such, because it has a better prognosis than the other large-cell B-cell lymphomas.

Centroblastic lymphomas can be monomorphic and are then composed of relatively monotonous medium-sized basophilic blasts, whose nuclei have predominantly marginal, medium-sized nucleoli. They are designated as polymorphic if they show a larger or smaller admixture of large basophilic cells with large central nucleoli. These can make up as much as 90% of the total. Nevertheless, the designation polymorphic centroblastic lymphoma is justified if at least 10% typical centroblasts are present or if centroblasts with multilobated nuclei are intermingled. The polymorphic variant has a worse prognosis than the monomorphic subtype. Large numbers of multilobated nuclei occur in a special form of centroblastic lymphoma called the multilobated subtype. *bcl*-2 positivity would point to a centroblastic lymphoma (see above). Immunostainings are not useful in the differential diagnosis of centroblastic lymphoma and immunoblastic lymphoma, which may look very much like polymorphic centroblastic lymphoma.

In any case one should apply a pan-B-cell and T-cell-specific antibodies, e.g., CD20, CD3 and βF1, to make certain that one is dealing with a B-cell lymphoma, since in very rare cases high-grade T-cell lymphomas, including the multilobated cell type, can show a centroblastic lymphoma-like picture.

If typical centroblasts or cells with multilobated nuclei are not present, we may speak of a 'polymorphic large-cell B-cell lymphoma', as typically occurs in the brain and the blood vessels. But it should be stressed here that this cannot automatically be equated morphologically with Frizzera's polymorphic large-cell B-cell lymphoma (see page 153). Among typical immunoblasts one finds small to medium-sized cells which do not fit into either the centroblastic or the plasmablastic category. They may be precursors of immunoblasts. Before trying to force a specific diagnosis at any price, one would do well to speak simply of an unclassified large-cell B-cell lymphoma.

Burkitt's lymphoma may be overdiagnosed or underdiagnosed in different laboratories. Where the diagnosis is made too frequently, it is often based on the unspecific starry sky pattern. The reason for too infrequent diagnoses can be that the two most important criteria are not recognized, for technical reasons. Burkitt's lymphoma cells generally have multiple, centrally located (i.e., not applied to the nuclear membrane) nucleoli and grow cohesively (Plates 5.9 and 5.10). In poorly embedded material, 'bubbling' can cause the nucleoli to seep to the nuclear membrane; the cells are misinterpreted as centroblasts. Cohesiveness cannot be seen in poorly embedded sections, or only in outer parts of the slide. Apart from these technical difficulties, there are, however, true borderline problems which can be made understandable through cytological knowledge of reactive germinal centers. MacLennan's so-called B-blast cells (with central multiple nucleoli [146, 221,222]), which we consider the normal equivalent of the Burkitt's lymphoma cells, lie in the dark zone of the germinal center and form centroblasts (with peripheral nucleoli), on the one hand, and probably also immunoblasts (with large solitary nucleoli).

This situation is reflected in some cases of Burkitt's lymphoma, i.e., there are cases of Burkitt's lymphoma with a certain degree of centroblastic 'differentiation', ones with immunoblast-like cells (with large central nucleoli) and ones with plasmablasts (cIg+), but in all variants the cohesiveness of the tumor cells remains an indispensable diagnostic criterion, which does not occur in either centro-

blastic lymphoma or immunoblastic lymphoma.

We do not need a special category 'Burkitt lymphoma-like lymphomas' (*cave* 'Burkitt-like lymphoma' – this would be rather embarrassing for D. Burkitt, who really did look quite different!). Molecular genetics should show the borderline between true Burkitt's lymphoma and centroblastic lymphoma.

Malignant lymphomas with strongly *focal epithelioid cell admixtures* need to be analyzed very carefully, to differentiate three types of NHL (HL with a high content of epithelioid cells is also in the differential diagnosis): *lymphoepithelioid lymphoma, T-cell lymphoma of AILD type with a high content of epithelioid cells* and *imunocytoma with a high content of epithelioid cells* [187,223,224], because the clinical aspects of these three lymphomas differ fundamentally. Immunocytoma with a high content of epithelioid cells differs clinically not only from the other lymphomas with a high content of epithelioid cells, but also from immunocytoma without an increased number of epithelioid cells. Immunocytomas with a high content of epithelioid cells are often connected with myoepithelial sialadenitis (Sjögren's syndrome). Histologically they mostly contain a large number of blast cells, and 26% of our cases developed into an immunoblastic lymphoma. Occasionally one finds groups of monocytoid B-cells. We cannot go into further detail here and refer the reader to Table 5.5. We would like to point out the two most prominent immunohistochemical findings: the AILD type shows extensive networks of FDC (Plate 5.11), while immunocytoma shows monotypic cIg. Neither of these findings are present in lymphoepithelioid lymphoma, which contains, in addition to epithelioid cells, many slightly pleomorphic or monomorphic T-lymphocytes and immunoblasts. (For further details, see [187,223,224].)

The majority of cases of *pleomorphic T-cell lymphoma* can be divided into small-cell and medium-sized to large-cell cases. But there are occasionally cases of predominantly small-cell T-cell lymphomas that also contain a few medium-sized or large T-cells. One will have to make the diagnosis according to the preponderant cell size. The borderline between pleomorphic large-cell T-cell lymphoma and immunoblastic lymphoma of T-cell type (monomorphic, with round to oval nuclei) is also not entirely clear-cut, although the consequences are not important. It remains to be seen whether the pleomorphic T-cell lymphomas, including immunoblastic lymphoma, do represent one entity, as Lukes' group wished to indicate when they used the term immunoblastic sarcoma [225], or whether one must assume that they are several entities. Immunoblastic lymphomas of B- and T-cell type can only be distinguished with certainty on the basis of immunocytochemistry or molecular genetics.

Distinguishing between immunoblastic lymphoma of T-cell type and *large-cell anaplastic lymphoma* [226] can occasionally cause difficulties. Large-cell anaplastic lymphoma often grows cohesively and in the sinus; immunoblastic lymphoma of T-cell type does not. CD30 can be positive in both types of lymphoma. The translocation t(2;5)(p23;q35) is restricted to large-cell anaplastic lymphoma of the T-cell and null cell type [227,228], but it is not found in every case.

There are certain limitations to how well precursor cell lymphomas – the *lymphoblastic lymphomas* – can be defined immunocytochemically in paraffin sections. T-Lymphoblastic lymphomas can be CD3+ in the mature forms; the same holds for CD20 in B-lymphoblastic lymphomas. Pre-pre-B acute lymphoblastic leukemia ('pro-B-ALL') is CD19+ and CD20– [229]. The vast majority of lymphoblastic lymphomas can, however, be defined immunocytochemically in cryostat sections, aspiration smears or blood smears. If one does not have the technical facilities to apply immunocytochemical or molecular genetic techniques, enzyme cytochemical staining for acid phosphatase allows one to recognize 90% of the cases of lymphoblastic lymphoma as T-cell derived by their focal positive reaction (in smears or frozen sections). That the difference in the shape of the nucleus, namely, convoluted versus non-convoluted, is significant, as Lukes initially assumed [230], has not been confirmed.

Lymphoproliferative disorders at the border of malignancy

ANGIOIMMUNOBLASTIC LYMPHADENOPATHY WITH DYSPROTEINAEMIA (AILD) AND T-CELL LYMPHOMA OF THE AILD TYPE

We are combining two seemingly different lesions here, which are still differentiated more or less sharply by other authors [231–233]. AILD ([234], now changed by Frizzera to AIL), also called immunoblastic lymphadenopathy (IBL [235]) or LgX [46,236], is considered to be a disease that has not yet evolved into a '*bona fide* T-cell lymphoma' [237] and was therefore classified by Frizzera [237] among the 'atypical lymphoproliferative disorders'. It is viewed as 'variable expressions of

an unstable lymphoproliferative state . . . characterized by the coexistence of a normal mitotic population and emerging, often multiple, unrelated clones' [238,239]. Shimoyama et al. [240] drew a line between AILD (IBL) and a T-cell lymphoma that they called IBL-like T-cell lymphoma. Frizzera [232,237] distinguishes three variants, which are not sharply differentiated from each other: (1) 'those without evidence of monoclonality by any of three parameters (immunophenotypic, immunogenotypic, and cytogenetic), for which only the term *AILD* or *AIL (IBL, LgX)* might be reserved; (2) those with evidence of clonality by all parameters, or *AIL (IBL, LgX)-like lymphomas*; and (3) those that, due to any discordance among the three parameters, do not fit into either of the above categories, and for which the term *AIL (IBL, LgX)-like dysplasias* is proposed'.

From our experience with more than 400 cases (2.7% of all NHL in the prospective lymphoma study by Brittinger et al. [212]), we see no possible way to draw a morphological line between 'reactive lymphoproliferation (AILD)' and the corresponding T-cell lymphoma ('T-cell lymphoma of AILD type'). We cannot even say that we suspect that a certain cytology speaks in favor of a not (yet) neoplastic lymphoproliferation. This also holds for the clear cells [241, 242], which according to Watanabe et al. [243] and Knecht [233] point to an AILD-like T-cell lymphoma.

For more than 20 years we have applied every method that was available to us, particularly cytogenetics and molecular genetics, and have also observed the clinical picture and studied the various therapeutic strategies and the course of a large number of cases. After the early cytogenetic investigations by Kaneko et al. [238] and Gödde-Salz et al. [244], the new data of Schlegelberger et al. [245] yielded further remarkable findings. Among 42 cases, chromosomal aberrations were found in 35 cases (83%). Of these 23 cases (56%) showed abnormalities that did not appear to be clonal and in 12 cases (29%) there were clonal chromosome abnormalities. Of the clonal abnormalities there were 10 cases with trisomy 3, six with trisomy 5, and two with trisomy 3 and trisomy 5. In addition to trisomy 3 and trisomy 5, an extra X chromosome was sometimes found. All but one case, however, showed TCRβ and some additional IgH gene rearrangement. This shows that a clonal T-cell proliferation is found more frequently (almost always) by molecular genetic techniques. Higher percentages of AILD cases without rearrangements mentioned in the literature [237] are probably due to a different histological definition of this entity and/or a less sensitive Southern blot technique. Germinal centers should not exist, and if they do exist, a second biopsy specimen taken a few weeks later should prove that they have disappeared. Recently, however, Feller (personal communication) observed a few cases in which follicular hyperplasia persisted for years. Hyperplastic follicular dendritic cells should also be demonstrated in AILD (Plates 5.11 and 5.14a). In later phases manifold chromosome anomalies develop, as is typical of high-grade T-cell lymphomas (Table 5.3). The morphology of later developmental phases is different; for example, some cases show evolvement of large-cell anaplastic lymphoma of T type (Plate 5.14b). Schlegelberger et al. [245] conclude from their initial findings that a step-wise development of chromosomal abnormalities takes place in AILD and speculate that the TCRβ chain rearrangement may precede the chromosomal abnormalities.

In a new study, Schlegelberger et al. [245a] report in detail on the fact that T-cell lymphoma of AILD type differs from all other T-cell lymphomas in that it 'shows a high frequency of unrelated clones and single cell aberrations with completely different karyotypes.... These cannot be derived from a common cell of origin'. It remained unclear from the first cytogenetic studies [239,245] 'whether single metaphases with a certain chromosome aberration are caused by increased chromosomal instability or whether they belong to an aberrant clone, which has not been detected due to the limited number of analysable metaphases'. This question Schlegelberger et al. were now able to answer by applying interphase cytogenetics. Using this method Schlegelberger et al. reanalyzed cells from 41 patients they had previously studied by metaphase cytogenetics. They found that aberrant clones are present in 89% of T-cell lymphomas of AILD type (including Frizzera's and Knechts's nonneoplastic AILD) and that clones with +3 or +X are substantially more frequent than hitherto assumed. When Schlegelberger et al. combined the results of metaphase and interphase cytogenetics, they found that 47% of AILD-type lymphomas had unrelated clones. 'This high frequency of oligoclonal proliferations may be due to increased genetic instability and an immune defect resulting in impaired elimination of aberrant cells'.

Some of our rearrangement studies that we mentioned above were already published in 1988 by Feller et al. [65]. They distinguished two groups, one consisting of 16 cases with TCRβ and γ gene rearrangements and the other of seven cases with additional IgH gene rearrangement. The cases in the first group showed exclusively CD4+ proliferating T-cells, a higher response to chemotherapy and a longer survival time. The patients in the second group had significantly elevated numbers of CD8+ proliferating T-cells, presented more often with hemolytic anemia and went into transient remission spontaneously or with steroid treatment.

Today 95% of the cases in our collection show a TCRβ rearrangement and, correspondingly, 89%

show chromosomal abnormalities. If an AILD-type lymphoma is or becomes hypercellular – in the early stages it is mostly relatively low in T-cells – and shows more atypical pleomorphic and polymorphic histological patterns, the chromosomal abnormalities change (see Table 5.3): we see a variety of other abnormalities and the tumor cells are often polyploid.

Hence AILD appears to us to be a dynamic process, possibly virus induced, which probably begins as one or very few small T-cell clones ('prelymphoma', 'early lymphoma') and ultimately develops into a T-cell clone that replaces all of the cells of the lymph node ('*bona fide* T-cell lymphoma'). EBV has even been detected in a clonal pattern in some cases [246–248]. The problem for the histopathologist is that he cannot foresee the expected course, unless a hypercellular pleomorphic variant has already developed.

For those concerned with therapy, this problem is less significant than it appears. In several prospective studies in all AILD/AILD-type lymphomas Siegert et al. treated patients with interferon-α [249] and achieved short-term complete remission in one-third of the patients. Later they also applied corticosteroids with or without COPBLAM/IMVP-16 [250], a chemotherapeutic regimen that has been successfully used in high-grade T-cell lymphomas. They proceeded pragmatically: all patients were initially treated with prednisone. Relapsing or refractory patients were treated with COPBLAM/IMVP-16. This treatment led to complete remission in about half of the patients and long-term disease-free survival in around one-third.

Recently, it has been shown that cytogenetic findings are of prognostic significance in AILD-type T-cell lymphoma. In particular, the presence of aberrant metaphases in unstimulated cultures, clones with additional X chromosomes, structural abnormalities of the short arm of chromosome 1 and complex aberrant clones are associated with a significantly shorter survival [250a]. The prognostic value of chromosome analysis appears to be equal to that of fluorescence *in situ* hybridization [250b].

LYMPHOPROLIFERATIVE DISORDERS IN IMMUNOCOMPROMISED PATIENTS

We encounter one of the most difficult borderline problems between nonneoplastic and neoplastic lymphoproliferation in cases of congenital and acquired immune deficiency. The final critical question is turning out to be the distinction between (EBV-induced) nonneoplastic 'polymorphic B-cell lymphoproliferative disorder' (Plate 5.12) and 'polymorphic B-cell lymphoma', two extremes of a spectrum that was described by Frizzera [251] in

EBV infections following kidney transplantation. They are said to form a continuum leading to monomorphic B-cell lymphomas, which are usually described as immunoblastic lymphoma with or without plasmacytic differentiation [251]. Nalesnik et al. [252] describe an EBV-induced spectrum of lymphoproliferation that leads from polymorphic clonal and nonclonal lesions to monomorphic clonal lesions. Even if the polymorphic lesions are clonal, half of the cases are supposed to be curable by reducing or eliminating the immunosuppression.

Later they put up a working model of four categories for discussion [253]. At the beginning is infectious mononucleosis consisting of a mixture of lymphocytes, plasmacytoid cells and immunoblasts; at the end large-cell, B-cell lymphoma. The border-line between the four categories is not sharp. As far as clinical treatment is concerned, monoclonal IgH appears to be most suitable for distinguishing non-neoplastic from neoplastic B-cell proliferations. Translocations near the c-*myc* gene, however, are not always observed in clonal proliferations. As far as clonality is concerned, there may be different clones in different localizations [253].

Hence this is a borderline situation, in which, so far, morphology, molecular genetics, immunocyto-chemistry (clonality) and cytogenetics have all been unable to decide the issue pro or contra malignancy. Perhaps, also, the new cytogenetic procedures in interphase cells will throw more light on this question. Perhaps the situation is similar to T-cell lymphomas of AILD type (see page 151).

Of the congenital immune deficiencies, Purtilo's X-linked lymphoproliferative (XLP) syndrome has been studied particularly well with respect to the role of EBV in the development of lymphomas because of the failure in immunological control of the EBV virus infection. In 161 patients Grierson and Purtilo [254] found 65% with severe to fatal lymphopro-liferations (fatal infectious mononucleosis) and 24% with malignant lymphomas.

The malignant lymphomas developing in human immunodeficiency virus (HIV) patients are mostly clear-cut, usually of high-grade B-cell type (BL, IBL, CBL), but rare cases of polymorphic B-cell lymphomas are seen (Plate 5.13, [255]). Hodgkin's lymphomas occur less frequently and are often difficult to recognize because of their unusual morphology (low content of lymphocytes).

MULTICENTRIC CASTLEMAN'S DISEASE

We have to distinguish between (1) localized Castle-man's disease and (2) multicentric Castleman's disease. Histologically there are two types: a hyaline vascular type and a plasma cell type. The hyaline vascular type is always localized and is, by nature, a hamartoma. It often contains atypical large vessels, and sinuses are lacking. The plasma cell type can be localized or multicentric (generalized, systemic). Here we are speaking only of the multicentric variant [256–262]. It is difficult to fit into a system. The plasma cells are predominantly polyclonal, but may sometimes be monoclonal (in localized and multi-centric types [263]), which does not affect the prognosis. If the plasma cells are monoclonal, κ+ plasma cells are always reported, and mostly γ chains are found. Occasionally, however, a B-cell lym-phoma evolves that is mostly κ+ [262]. The germinal centers are regressively transformed but their num-ber is increased. They contain CD5+ lymphocytes and increased numbers of follicular dendritic cells [264,265]. Autoimmune phenomena and other im-munological abnormalities are frequently associated with Castleman's disease, of either localized or multi-centric subtype. In three of four patients with the systemic plasma cell variant, Hanson et al. [266] found TCRβ gene rearrangements (twice) and IgH gene rearrangements (three times). In 29% of the cases the plasma cell type is associated with the POEMS (polyneuropathy, organomegaly, endocrino-pathy, monoclonal gammopathy with or without overt 'osteosclerotic' myeloma and skin abnor-malities) syndrome [264,267].

An excessive production of interleukin-6 (IL-6) is considered to play an important role in the patho-genesis of Castleman's disease [268]. It may be produced by follicular dendritic cells, of which there are large numbers in the 'regressively transformed germinal centers'. But according to Leger-Ravet et al. [269] only the localized form with systemic manifestations shows an overexpression of IL-6 in the follicular dendritic cells, whereas in the multi-centric form IL-6 production takes place in the interfollicular areas (in macrophages, interdigitating cells, lymphocytes?) outside the sinuses. Therefore they conclude that different immune mechanisms may be involved in the different forms of Castle-man's disease. Ultimately, the nature of Castleman's disease is still unclear and it may be heterogeneous.

So-called and true composite lymphomas

In 1954 Custer [270] introduced the term composite lymphoma for a lymphoma that is characterized by more than one histological pattern, irrespective of whether it is localized in the same organ or in two different organs. The term was adopted by Rappaport

Simultaneous occurrence of NHL and HL in different lymph nodes

Jaffe et al. [274] point out that there are also rare cases in which NHL of B- or T-cell type and HL can occur in different anatomic sites. They are referred to by Jaffe as 'coexistent', by Harris as 'discordant'. This is the case particularly for the combination of mycosis fungoides and HL [287], which we have also occasionally observed. According to Jaffe et al. [274] more than 20 well-documented cases of HL in patients with mycosis fungoides have been described since 1979.

SEQUENTIAL LYMPHOMAS OF NHL OR HL TYPE

Travis et al. [288] noted that NHL are the most frequent type of cancer following treatment of HL. The expected risk ratio was 4.16:1. Jaffe et al. [274] report on 22 such cases, which differ somewhat from the previous series [289]. Nine of them were follicular lymphoma, six diffuse large-cell or immunoblastic lymphoma, three chronic lymphocytic leukemia or small lymphocytic; most, if not all were B-cell lymphomas. Three cases of mycosis fungoides and one of ATLL are also listed; mycosis fungoides and ATLL were, however, the primary lesions.

The existence of paraproteinemia in Sézary's syndrome has been recognized for a long time [290]. The assumed cause is that the T-cells of the lymphoma stimulate monoclonal B-cell development. Similarly, paraproteinemia is found occasionally in T-cell lymphomas of AILD type [291,292].

The development of a T-cell lymphoma in a patient treated for HL has been reported several times in the past several years (e.g., [293] and was recently analyzed in an impressive cytogenetic/molecular genetic study of a single case [294]). The authors conclude from their findings that, despite the time lapse between the occurrence of the HL and the NHL, the case does represent a true composite lymphoma.

The occurrence of a pleomorphic medium-sized T-cell lymphoma after a high-grade B-cell lymphoma had been successfully treated, described by Shimizu et al. [295], is so far the only such case published and hence could be coincidental.

MECHANISMS OF DEVELOPMENT OF COMPOSITE LYMPHOMAS

The basic question is: are these combinations coincidental occurrences or are there pathogenetic relationships between the different types of lym-

phoma? The answer to this question will differ, depending on whether we are dealing with a true composite lymphoma or only a so-called composite lymphoma. In the so-called composite lymphoma designated as Richter's syndrome developing in chronic lymphocytic leukemia of B-cell type, the large-cell lymphoma is derived from the neoplastic clone of the chronic lymphocytic leukemia, even if this is not apparent at first sight [296]. Of course one must take great care to exclude the possibility of a combination with an HL (see [205]). Similar to Richter's syndrome, centroblastic lymphoma may develop in centroblastic–centrocytic lymphoma or immunoblastic lymphoma in immunocytoma.

For the true composite lymphomas there are three combinations that need to be particularly discussed: T-cell lymphomas developing from low-grade B-cell lymphoma, high-grade B-cell lymphoma developing out of low-grade T-cell lymphoma and the combination of NHL and HL.

In the development of T-cell lymphoma in follicular and small lymphocytic lymphoma, Medeiros and Stetler-Stevenson [296] consider it possible that the T-cell lymphoma is induced by cytokines secreted by the B-cell lymphoma cells. This is much more likely to be true of the many cases in which we saw high-grade B-cell lymphomas developing out of low-grade T-cell lymphomas. This holds particularly for T-cell lymphoma of AILD type, in which we can, in any case, assume that a large number of lymphokines are secreted. Points that speak in favor of this are the appearance of large numbers of newly formed FDC, the high content of venules, the frequent eosinophilia, etc. There have also been a number of reports in the literature of immunoblastic lymphoma of the B-cell type and of monoclonal gammopathy in T-cell lymphomas of the AILD type. A sophisticated analysis of the two clones (T-cell and B-cell) applying cytogenetic and molecular genetic methods should be carried out here similar to that performed by Wlodarska et al. [294].

For the development of HL in chronic lymphocytic leukemia of B-cell type, Jaffe and her group [9,297], like Tsang et al. [298], have suggested that EBV may play an important role in pathogenesis.

Conclusions

After applying all of the interesting and stimulating new techniques, we have come to the conclusion that a subtle assessment of morphology, validated by immunocytochemistry with or without genetic techniques, is still the *sine qua non* in the identification and differentiation of lymphoma entities. These entities are not artefacts, at least the vast majority of them are not, but biological entities, based on knowledge of the cytological variants observed in the development and functioning of lymphocytes. It is no wonder that more or less characteristic clinical syndromes can also be assigned to each of the entities. For morphology and clinical picture are but two aspects of the same *gestalt**. This high estimate of the diagnostic utility of immunocytochemically validated morphology presupposes that the fixation, processing and staining are technically of the highest quality. The importance of a high level of sample preparation is underestimated worldwide, and our special attention is required, so that we may raise the international standard.

When diagnosing borderline cases between reactive and neoplastic lymphoproliferation, we are aided to a certain extent by the new methods of molecular genetics and cytogenetics, but they too have their limitations. In particular, clonality must not be automatically equated with malignancy. We can expect that molecular genetics and classical cytogenetics will not only confirm or add precision to our understanding of lymphoma entities and correlations, but also open the horizon for further unexpected insights. The same holds for studies on the functional properties of the lymphoma cells, such as lymphokine formation and homing properties.

Our efforts continue to be directed towards the development of a biologically consistent system of classification of the malignant lymphomas, and one that is able to clearly differentiate malignant from reactive lesions.

Acknowledgments

This work was supported by the Deutsche Krebshilfe, Mildred Scheel Stiftung, project no. M33/91/Le2.

I am very grateful to Dr A. C. Feller, Department of Pathology of the Medical University of Lübeck, Dr H. Griesser, Department of Pathology, University of Toronto, and Dr P. Madarnas, Department of Pathology, University of Sherbrooke, Canada, for taking the time to critically read and discuss the manuscript. My thanks go to Mrs K. Dege, who translated and typed the manuscript and list of references, for her excellent cooperation.

References

1. Fox H. Remarks on the presentation of microscopical preparations made from some of the original tissue described by Thomas Hodgkin, 1832. *Ann. Med. History* 1926, **8**: 370–374.
2. Symmers WStC. The lymphoreticular system. In Symmers WStC (ed.) *Systemic Pathology*, Vol. 2. Edinburgh: Churchill Livingstone, 1978, pp. 504–892.
2a. Harris NL, Jaffe ES, Stein H, et al. A revised European–American classification of lymphoid neoplasms: A proposal from the International Lymphoma Study Group. *Blood* 1994, **84**: 1361–1392.
3. Strum SB, Park JK, Rappaport H. Observation of cells resembling Sternberg–Reed cells in conditions other than Hodgkin's disease. *Cancer* 1970, **26**: 176–190.
4. Tindle BH, Parker JW, Lukes RJ. 'Reed–Sternberg cells' in infectious mononucleosis? *Am. J. Clin. Pathol.* 1972, **58**: 607–617.
5. Fellbaum C, Hansmann M-L, Parwaresch MR, Lennert K. Monoclonal antibodies Ki-B3 and Leu-M1 discriminate giant cells of infectious mononucleosis and of Hodgkin's disease. *Hum. Pathol.* 1988, **19**: 1168–1173.
6. Isaacson PG. Gastrointestinal lymphomas and lymphoid hyperplasias. In Knowles DM (ed.) *Neoplastic Hematopathology*. Baltimore: Williams & Wilkins, 1992, pp. 953–978.
7. Schmid U, Helbron D, Lennert K. Development of malignant lymphoma in myoepithelial sialadenitis (Sjögren's syndrome). *Virchows Arch. A.* [*Pathol. Anat.*] 1982, **395**: 11–43.
8. Lennert K, in collaboration with Mohri N, Stein H, Kaiserling E, Müller-Hermelink HK. *Malignant Lymphomas other than Hodgkin's Disease*. Berlin, Heidelberg, New York: Springer, 1978.
9. Momose H, Jaffe ES, Shin SS, et al. Chronic lymphocytic leukemia/small lymphocytic lymphoma with Reed–Sternberg-like cells and possible transformation to Hodgkin's disease. Mediation by Epstein–Barr virus. *Am. J. Surg. Pathol.* 1992, **16**: 859–867.
10. Lennert K, Feller AC. *Histopathology of Non-Hodgkin's Lymphomas*. Berlin, Heidelberg, New York: Springer, 1992.
11. Lennert K. Die Beziehungen von Hodgkin- und Non-Hodgkin-Lymphomen. *Arzneim-Forsch./Drug Res.* 1987, **37**: 255–259.
12. Poppema S. The diversity of the immunohistological staining pattern of Sternberg–Reed cells. *J. Histochem. Cytochem.* 1980, **28**: 788–791.
13. Schwab U, Stein H, Gerdes J, et al. Production of a monoclonal antibody specific for Hodgkin and Sternberg–Reed cells of Hodgkin's disease and a subset of normal lymphoid cells. *Nature* 1982, **299**: 65–67.

---

*The use of the term *gestalt* in the sense we mean was initiated by Goethe. *Gestalt* denotes more than structure. It means the essence, the principle of a structure. Plato would presumably have called this principle 'idea'. *Gestalt* means the whole, which is always more than the sum of its parts (see [299] and further references cited there, including [300,301]).

rate and American–Japanese pathologists' comparability of a modified working formulation for non-Hodgkin's lymphomas. An analysis of the cases collected for the Fifth International Workshop on Chromosomes in Leukemia-lymphoma. *Cancer* 1987, **59**: 1463–1469.

83. Schlegelberger B, Himmler A, Gödde E, et al. Cytogenetic findings in peripheral T-cell lymphomas as a basis for distinguishing low-grade and high-grade lymphomas. *Blood* 1994, **83**: 505–511.

84. Finn T, Isaacson PG, Wotherspoon AC. Numerical abnormalities of chromosomes 3, 7, 12 and 18 in low-grade lymphomas of MALT-type and splenic marginal zone cell lymphomas detected by interphase cytogenetics on paraffin embedded tissue. *J. Pathol.* 1993, **170** (Suppl.): 335A.

85. Kallioniemi A, Kallioniemi O-P, Sudar D, et al. Comparative genomic hybridization for molecular cytogenetic analysis of solid tumors. *Science* 1992, **258**: 818–821.

86. Du Manoir S, Speicher MR, Joos S, et al. Detection of complete and partial chromosome gains and losses by comparative genomic in situ hybridization. *Hum. Genet.* 1993, **90**: 590–610.

87. Weber-Matthiesen K, Winkemann M, Müller-Hermelink A, et al. Simultaneous fluorescence immunophenotyping and interphase cytogenetics: A contribution to the characterization of tumor cells. *J. Histochem. Cytochem.* 1992, **40**: 171–175.

88. Weiss LM, Wood GS, Trela M, et al. Clonal T-cell populations in lymphomatoid papulosis. Evidence of a lymphoproliferative origin for a clinically benign disease. *N. Engl. J. Med.* 1986, **315**: 475–479.

89. Kadin ME, Vonderheid EC, Sako D, et al. Clonal composition of T-cells in lymphomatoid papulosis. *Am. J. Pathol.* 1987, **126**: 13–17.

89a. Zhang Y, Schlegelberger B, Plendl H, et al. Clonal t(8;14)(p11;q31) in a case of reactive lymphoproliferation. *Genes Chromosomes Cancer* 1993, **7**: 165–168.

90. Goudie RB, Lee FD. Does occult monoclonal proliferation of non-malignant T-cells cause secondary immunopathological disorders? [Editorial] *J. Pathol.* 1989, **158**: 91–92.

91. Slater D. Clonal dermatoses: A conceptual and diagnostic dilemma [Editorial]. *J. Pathol.* 1990, **162**: 1–3.

92. Radaszkiewicz T, Hansmann M-L, Lennert K. Monoclonality and polyclonality of plasma cells in Castleman's disease of the plasma cell variant. *Histopathology* 1989, **14**: 11–24.

93. Griesser H, Feller AC, Sterry W. T-cell receptor and immunoglobulin gene rearrangements in cutaneous T-cell-rich pseudolymphomas. *J. Invest. Dermatol.* 1990, **95**: 292–295.

94. Fishleder A, Tubbs R, Hesse B, Levine H. Uniform detection of immunoglobulin-gene rearrangement in benign lymphoepithelial lesions. *N. Engl. J. Med.* 1987, **316**: 1118–1121.

95. Wotherspoon AC, Doglioni C, Diss TC, et al. Regression of primary low-grade B-cell gastric lymphoma of mucosa associated lymphoid tissue type after eradication of *Helicobacter pylori. Lancet* 1993, **342**: 575–577.

96. Rabes HM, Bücher T, Hartmann A, et al. Clonal growth of carcinogen-induced enzyme-deficient preneoplastic cell populations in mouse liver. *Cancer Res.* 1982, **42**: 3220–3227.

97. Zankl H. *Der Karyotyp des Meningeoms. Veröffent. a.d. Pathol.*, Heft 111. Stuttgart: Fischer, 1979.

98. Aisenberg AC. *Malignant Lymphoma. Biology, Natural History and Treatment.* Philadelphia: Lea & Febiger, 1991.

99. Suchi T, Lennert K, Tu L-Y, et al. Histopathology and immunohistochemistry of peripheral T-cell lymphomas: A proposal for their classification. *J. Clin. Pathol.* 1987, **40**: 995–1015.

100. Caulet S, Delmer A, Audouin J, et al. Histopathological study of bone marrow biopsies in 30 cases of T-cell lymphoma with clinical, biological and survival correlations. *Hematol. Oncol.* 1990, **8**: 155–168.

101. Nakamura S, Suchi T, Koshikawa T, et al. Clinicopathologic study of 212 cases of peripheral T-cell lymphoma among the Japanese. *Cancer* 1993, **72**: 1762–1772.

102. Caulet S, Brousset P, Schoevaert D, et al. Quantitative study of Ki-67 antibody staining in 46 T-cell malignant lymphomas using image analysis. *Hematol. Oncol.* 1991, **9**: 323–335.

103. Lennert K, Tamm I, Wacker H-H. Histopathology and immunocytochemistry of lymph node biopsies in chronic lymphocytic leukemia and immunocytoma. *Leuk. Lymphoma* 1991, Suppl: 157–160.

104. Banks PM, Chan J, Cleary ML, et al. Mantle cell lymphoma. A proposal for unification of morphologic, immunologic, and molecular data. *Am. J. Surg. Pathol.* 1992, **16**: 637–640.

105. Farcet J-P, Gaulard P, Marolleau J-P, et al. Hepatosplenic T-cell lymphoma: sinusal/sinusoidal localization of malignant cells expressing the T-cell receptor γ/δ. *Blood* 1990, **11**: 1–7.

106. Gaulard P, Bourquelot P, Kanavaros P, et al. Expression of the alpha/beta and gamma/delta T-cell receptors in 57 cases of peripheral T-cell lymphomas. Identification of a subset of γ/δ T-cell lymphomas. *Am. J. Pathol.* 1990, **137**: 617–628.

107. Falini B, Flenghi L, Fagioli M, et al. T-lymphoblastic lymphomas expressing the non-disulfide-linked form of the T-cell receptor γ/δ: Characterization with monoclonal antibodies and genotypic analysis. *Blood* 1989, **74**: 2501–2507.

108. Burg G, Dummer R, Wilhelm M, et al. A subcutaneous delta-positive T-cell lymphoma that produces interferon gamma. *N. Engl. J. Med.* 1991, **325**: 1078–1081.

109. Kanavaros P, Lescs M-C, Brière J, et al. Nasal T-cell lymphoma: A clinicopathologic entity associated with peculiar phenotype and with Epstein–Barr virus. *Blood* 1993, **81**: 2688–2695.

110. Wright DH. Gross distribution and haematology. In Burkitt DP, Wright DH (eds) *Burkitt's Lymphoma.* Edinburgh: Livingstone, 1970, pp. 64–81.

111. Levine PH, Cho BR, Connelly RR, et al. The American Burkitt lymphoma registry: A progress report. *Ann. Intern. Med.* 1975, **83**: 31–36.

112. Pelicci PG, Knowles DM 2nd, Magrath I, Dalla-

Favera R. Chromosomal breakpoints and structural alterations of the c-myc locus differ in endemic and sporadic forms of Burkitt lymphoma. *Proc. Natl Acad. Sci. USA* 1986; **83**: 2984–2988.

113. Neri A, Barriga F, Knowles DM, et al. Different regions of the immunoglobulin heavy-chain locus are involved in chromosomal translocations in distinct pathogenetic forms of Burkitt lymphoma. *Proc. Natl Acad. Sci. USA* 1988, **85**: 2748–2752.

114. Hanto DW, Gajl-Peczalska KJ, Frizzera G, et al. Epstein–Barr virus (EBV) induced polyclonal and monoclonal B-cell lymphoproliferative diseases occurring after renal transplantation. Clinical, pathologic, and virologic findings and implications for therapy. *Ann. Surg.* 1983, **198**: 356–369.

115. Pallesen G, Hamilton-Dutoit S, Rowe M, et al. Expression of Epstein–Barr virus replicative proteins in AIDS-related non-Hodgkin's lymphoma cells. *J. Pathol.* 1991, **165**: 289–299.

116. Hamilton-Dutoit SJ, Pallesen G, Franzmann MB, et al. AIDS-related lymphoma. Histopathology, immunophenotype, and association with Epstein–Barr virus as demonstrated by in-situ nucleic acid hybridisation. *Am. J. Pathol.* 1991, **138**: 149–163.

117. Raphael MM, Audouin J, Lamine M, et al. Immunophenotypic and genotypic analysis of AIDS-related non-Hodgkin's lymphomas. Correlation with histologic features in 36 cases. *Am. J. Clin. Pathol.* 1994, **101**: 773–782.

118. Jones JF, Shurin S, Abramowsky C, et al. T-cell lymphomas containing Epstein–Barr viral DNA in patients with chronic Epstein–Barr virus infections. *N. Engl. J. Med.* 1988, **318**: 733–741.

119. Zhou XG, Hamilton-Dutoit SJ, Yan QH, Pallesen G. High frequency of Epstein–Barr virus in Chinese peripheral T-cell lymphoma. *Histopathology* 1994, **24**: 115–122.

120. Hamilton-Dutoit SJ, Pallesen G. A survey of Epstein–Barr virus gene expression in sporadic non-Hodgkin's lymphomas. Detection of Epstein–Barr virus in a subset of peripheral T-cell lymphomas. *Am. J. Pathol.* 1992, **140**: 1315–1325.

121. Anagnostopoulos I, Hummel M, Finn T, et al. Heterogeneous Epstein–Barr virus infection patterns in peripheral T-cell lymphoma of angioimmunoblastic lymphadenopathy type. *Blood* 1992, **80**: 1804–1812.

122. Borisch B, Caioni M, Hurwitz N, et al. Epstein–Barr virus subtype distribution in angioimmunoblastic lymphadenopathy. *Int. J. Cancer* 1993, **55**: 748–752.

123. Ho FCS, Srivasta G, Loke SL, et al. Presence of Epstein–Barr virus DNA in nasal lymphomas of B and 'T' cell type. *Hematol. Oncol.* 1990, **8**: 271–281.

123a. Jaffe ES, Chan JKC, Su I-J, et al. Report of the workshop on nasal and related extranodal angiocentric T/natural killer cell lymphomas. *Am. J. Surg. Pathol.* 1996, **20**: 103–111.

123b. Van Gorp J, De Bruin PC, Sie-Go DMDS, et al. Nasal T-cell lymphoma: A clinicopathological and immunophenotypic analysis of 13 cases. *Histopathology* 1995, **27**: 139–148.

123c. Chan JKC, Tsang WYW, Wong KF. Classification of natural killer cell neoplasms [Letter to the editor]. *Am. J. Surg. Pathol.* 1994, **18**: 1177–1178.

123d. Nakamura S, Koshikawa T, Koike K, et al. Clinicopathologic study of CD56 (NCAM)-positive angiocentric lymphoma occurring in sites other than the upper and lower respiratory tract. *Am. J. Surg. Pathol.* 1995, **19**: 284–296.

123e. Macon WR, Williams ME, Greer JP, et al. Natural killer-like T-cell lymphomas: Aggressive lymphomas of T-large granular lymphocytes. *Blood* 1996, **87**: 1474–1483.

124. Harabuchi Y, Yamanaka N, Kataura A, et al. Epstein–Barr virus in nasal T-cell lymphomas in patients with lethal midline granuloma. *Lancet* 1990, **335**: 128–130.

125. De Bruin PC, Jiwa NM, van der Valk P, et al. Detection of Epstein–Barr virus nucleic acid sequences and protein in nodal T-cell lymphomas: Relation between latent membrane protein-1 positivity and clinical course. *Histopathology* 1993, **23**: 509–518.

126. Tajima K, Tominaga S, Suchi T. Malignant lymphomas in Japan: Epidemiological analysis on adult T-cell leukemia/lymphoma. *Hematol. Oncol.* 1986, **4**: 31–44.

127. Uemura Y, Tokudome T, Tokunaga M, et al. Detection of HTLV-1 proviral DNA in Ki-1 positive lymphomas using PCR method. In Takahashi K, Kim S-H (eds) *Lymphoreticular Cells. Fundamentals and Pathology.* Kumamoto, Japan: Cell Foundation, 1991, pp. 264–273.

128. Lennert K, Kikuchi M, Sato E, et al. HTLV-positive and -negative T-cell lymphomas. Morphological and immunohistochemical differences between European and HTLV-positive Japanese T-cell lymphomas. *Int. J. Cancer* 1985, **35**: 65–72.

129. Saxinger WC, Lange-Wantzin G, Thomsen K, et al. Human T-cell leukemia virus: A diverse family of related exogenous retroviruses of human and old world primates. In Gallo RC, Essex ME, Gross L (eds) *Human T-Cell Leukemia/Lymphoma Viruses.* New York: Cold Spring Harbor Laboratory, 1984, pp. 323–330.

130. Yakovleva LA, Lennert K, Chikobava MG, et al. Morphological characteristics of malignant T-cell lymphomas in baboons. *Virchows Arch. A. [Pathol. Anat.]* 1993, **422**: 109–120.

131. Anagnostopoulos I, Hummel M, Kaudewitz P, et al. Detection of HTLV-1 proviral sequences in CD30-positive large cell cutaneous T-cell lymphomas. *Am. J. Pathol.* 1990, **137**: 1317–1322.

132. Anagnostopoulos I, Herbst H, Niedobitek G, Stein H. Demonstration of monoclonal EBV genomes in Hodgkin's disease and Ki-1-positive anaplastic large cell lymphoma by combined Southern blot and in situ hybridization. *Blood* 1989, **74**: 810–816.

133. Herbst H, Dallenbach F, Hummel M, et al. Epstein–Barr virus DNA and latent gene products in Ki-1 (CD30)-positive anaplastic large cell lymphoma. *Blood* 1991, **78**: 2666–2673.

134. Millett YL, Bennett MH, Jelliffe AM, Farrer-Brown G. Nodular sclerotic lymphosarcoma. A further review. *Br. J. Cancer* 1969, **23**: 683–692.

135. Isaacson PG, Wright DH. Extranodal malignant lymphoma arising from mucosa-associated lymphoid tissue. *Cancer* 1984, **53**: 2515–2524.

136. Isaacson PG, Spencer J. Malignant lymphoma of mucosa-associated lymphoid tissue. *Histopathology* 1987, **11**: 445–462.

137. Li G, Hansmann M-L, Zwingers T, Lennert K. Primary lymphomas of the lung: Morphological, immunohistochemical and clinical features. *Histopathology* 1990, **16**: 519–531.

138. Harris NL. Extranodal lymphoid infiltrates and mucosa-associated lymphoid tissue (MALT). A unifying concept. *Am. J. Surg. Pathol.* 1991, **15**: 879–884.

139. Spencer J, Finn T, Pulford KAF, et al. The human gut contains a novel population of B lymphocytes which resemble marginal zone cells. *Clin. Exp. Immunol.* 1985, **62**: 607–612.

140. Paulsen J, Lennert K. Low-grade B-cell lymphoma of mucosa-associated lymphoid tissue type in Waldeyer's ring. *Histopathology* 1994, **24**: 1–11.

141. Kaiserling E. Ultrastructure of non-Hodgkin's lymphomas. In Lennert K et al. (eds) *Malignant Lymphomas other than Hodgkin's Disease (Handbuch der speziellen pathologischen Anatomie und Histologie*, Vol. 1, Part 3B). Berlin: Springer, 1978, pp. 471–528.

142. Veldman JE, Keuning FJ, Molenaar I. Site of initiation of the plasma cell reaction in the rabbit lymph node. Ultrastructural evidence for two distinct antibody forming cell precursors. *Virchows Arch. B* 1978, **28**: 187–202.

143. Keuning FJ, van der Meer J, Nieuwenhuis P, Oudendijk P. The histophysiology of the antibody response. II. Antibody responses and splenic plasma cell reactions in sublethally X-irradiated rabbits. *Lab. Invest.* 1963, **12**: 156–170.

144. MacLennan ICM, Gray D, Kumararatne DS, Bazin H. The lymphocytes of splenic marginal zones. A distinct B-cell lineage. *Immunol. Today* 1982, **3**: 305–307.

145. Timens W, Poppema S. Lymphocyte compartments in human spleen. An immunohistologic study in normal spleens and noninvolved spleens in Hodgkin's disease. *Am. J. Pathol.* 1985, **120**: 443–454.

146. MacLennan ICM, Liu Y-J, Joshua DE, Gray D. The production and selection of memory B-cells in follicles. In Melchers F, et al (eds) *Progress in Immunology*. Berlin: Springer, 1989, pp. 443–447.

147. Mulligan SP, Catovsky D. Splenic lymphoma with villous lymphocytes. *Leukemia Lymphoma* 1992, **6**: 97–105.

148. Cammoun M, Jaafoura H, Tabbane F, et al. Immunoproliferative small intestinal disease without α-chain disease: A pathological study. *Gastroenterology* 1989, **96**: 750–763.

149. Rambaud J-C, Piel J-L, Galian A, et al. Rémission complète clinique, histologique et immunologique d'un cas de maladie des chaines alpha traité par antibiothérapie orale. *Gastroenterol. Clin. Biol.* 1978, **2**: 49–61.

150. Feiden W, Bise K, Steude U. Diagnosis of primary cerebral lymphoma with particular reference to CT-guided stereotactic biopsy. *Virchows Arch. A.* [Pathol. Anat.] 1990, **417**: 21–28.

151. Braus DF, Schwechheimer K, Müller-Hermelink HK, et al. Primary cerebral malignant non-Hodgkin's lymphomas: A retrospective clinical study. *J. Neurol.* 1992, **239**: 117–124.

152. Jellinger K, Radaszkiewicz T, Slowik F. Primary malignant lymphomas of the central nervous system in man. *Acta Neuropath.* 1975 (Suppl. VI): 95–102.

153. Lichtenstein AK, Levine A, Taylor CR, et al. Primary mediastinal lymphoma in adults. *Am. J. Med.* 1980, **68**: 509–514.

154. Trump DL, Mann RB. Diffuse large cell and undifferentiated lymphomas with prominent mediastinal involvement. A poor prognostic subset of patients with non-Hodgkin's lymphoma. *Cancer* 1982, **50**: 277–282.

155. Yousem SA, Weiss LM, Warnke RA. Primary mediastinal non-Hodgin's lymphomas: A morphologic and immunologic study of 19 cases. *Am. J. Clin. Pathol.* 1985, **83**: 676–680.

156. Menestrina F, Chilosi M, Bonetti F, et al. Mediastinal large-cell lymphoma of B-type, with sclerosis: Histopathological and immunohistochemical study of eight cases. *Histopathology* 1986, **10**: 589–600.

157. Peronne T, Frizzera G, Rosai J. Mediastinal diffuse large-cell lymphoma with sclerosis. A clinicopathologic study of 60 cases. *Am. J. Surg. Pathol.* 1986, **10**: 176–191.

158. Möller P, Lämmler B, Eberlein-Gonska M, et al. Primary mediastinal clear cell lymphoma of B-cell type. *Virchows Arch. A* [Pathol. Anat.] 1986, **409**: 79–92.

159. Möller P, Moldenhauer G, Momburg F, et al. Mediastinal lymphoma of clear cell type is a tumor corresponding to terminal steps of B-cell differentiation. *Blood* 1987, **69**: 1087–1095.

160. Jacobson JO, Aisenberg AC, Lamarre L, et al. Mediastinal large cell lymphoma. An uncommon subset of adult lymphoma curable with combined modality therapy. *Cancer* 1988, **62**: 1893–1898.

161. Nakagawa A, Nakamura S, Koshikawa T, et al. Clinicopathologic study of primary mediastinal non-lymphoblastic non-Hodgkin's lymphomas among the Japanese. *Acta Pathol. Jap.* 1993, **43**: 44–54.

162. Addis BJ, Isaacson PG. Large cell lymphoma of the mediastinum: a B-cell tumor of probable thymic origin. *Histopathology* 1986, **10**: 379–390.

163. Hofmann WJ, Momburg F, Möller P. Thymic medullary cells expressing B lymphocyte antigens. *Hum. Pathol.* 1988, **19**: 1280–1287.

164. Hofmann WJ, Momburg F, Möller P, Otto HF. Intra- and extrathymic B-cells in physiologic and pathologic conditions. Immunohistochemical study on normal thymus and lymphofollicular hyperplasia of the thymus. *Virchows Arch. A* [Pathol. Anat. Histopathol.] 1988, **412**: 431–442.

165. Lamarre L, Jacobson JO, Aisenberg AC, Harris NL. Primary large cell lymphoma of the mediastinum. A histologic and immunophenotypic study of 29 cases. *Am. J. Surg. Pathol.* 1989, **13**: 730–739.

166. Sheibani K, Battifora H, Winberg CD, et al. Further evidence that malignant angioendotheliomatosis is an angiotropic large cell lymphoma. *N. Engl. J. Med.* 1986, **314**: 943–948.

167. Ferry JA, Harris NL. Picker LJ, et al. Intravascular lymphomatosis (malignant angioendotheliomatosis): a B-cell neoplasm expressing surface homing receptors. *Mod. Pathol.* 1988, **1**: 444–452.

168. Stroup RM, Sheibani K, Moncada A, et al. Angiotropic (intravascular) large cell lymphoma. A clinicopathologic study of seven cases with unique clinical presentations. *Cancer* 1990, **66**: 1781–1788.

169. Chan JKC, Ng CS, Lau WH, Lo STH. Most nasal/nasopharyngeal lymphomas are peripheral T-cell neoplasms. *Am. J. Surg. Pathol.* 1987, **11**: 418–429.

170. Jaffe ES. Post-thymic lymphoid neoplasia. In Jaffe ES (ed.) *Surgical Pathology of the Lymph Nodes and Related Organs*. Philadelphia: W.B. Saunders Company, 1985, pp. 218–248.

171. Ho FCS, Choy D, Loke SL, et al. Polymorphic reticulosis and conventional lymphomas of the nose and upper aerodigestive tract: A clinicopathologic study of 70 cases, and immunophenotypic studies of 16 cases. *Hum. Pathol.* 1990, **21**: 1041–1050.

172. Beljaards RC, Kaudewitz P, Berti E, et al. Primary cutaneous CD30-positive large cell lymphoma: Definition of a new type of cutaneous lymphoma with a favorable prognosis: A European Multicenter Study of 47 patients. *Cancer* 1993, **71**: 2097–2104.

172a. Willemze R, Beljaards RC, Meijer CJLM. Classification of primary cutaneous T-cell lymphomas. *Histopathology* 1994, **24**: 405–415.

173. Isaacson PG, O'Connor NTJ, Spencer J, et al. Malignant histiocytosis of the intestine: A T-cell lymphoma. *Lancet* 1985, **ii**: 688–691.

174. Isaacson PG, Cerf-Bensussan N, Jarry A, et al. Enteropathy associated T-cell lymphoma (malignant histiocytosis of the intestine) is derived from intraepithelial T-cells. *J. Pathol.* 1987, **152**: 217A.

175. Pallesen G, Hamilton-Dutoit SJ. Monoclonal antibody (HML-1) labelling of T-cell lymphomas [Letter to the Editor]. *Lancet* 1989, **i**: 223.

176. Kanavaros P, Lavergne A, Galian A, et al. A primary immunoblastic T malignant lymphoma of the small bowel, with azurophilic intracytoplasmic granules. *Am. J. Surg. Pathol.* 1988, **12**: 641–647.

177. Cerf-Bensussan N, Schneeberger EE, Bhan AK. Immunohistologic and immunoelectron microscopic characterization of the mucosal lymphocytes of human small intestine by the use of monoclonal antibodies. *J. Immunol.* 1983, **130**: 2615–2622.

178. Shepherd NA, Blackshaw AJ, Hall PA, et al. Malignant lymphoma with eosinophilia of the gastrointestinal tract. *Histopathology* 1987, **11**: 115–130.

179. Chott A, Dragosics B, Radaszkiewicz T. Peripheral T-cell lymphomas of the intestine. *Am. J. Pathol.* 1992, **141**: 1361–1371.

179a. Wong KF, Chan JKC, Matutes E, et al. Hepatosplenic γδ T-cell lymphoma. A distinctive aggressive lymphoma type. *Am. J. Surg. Pathol.* 1995, **19**: 718–726.

180. Kinney MC, Collins RD, Greer JP, et al. A small-cell-predominant variant of primary Ki-1 (CD30)+ T-cell lymphoma. *Am. J. Surg. Pathol.* 1993, **17**: 859–868.

180a. Böhm M. Klinik und Zytologie des lymphohistiozytischen Lymphoms. Inauguraldissertation. Kiel: University of Kiel, 1996.

181. Kadin ME. Ki-1-positive anaplastic large-cell lymphoma: A clinicopathologic entity? [Editorial] *J. Clin. Oncol.* 1991, **9**: 533–536.

181a. Orscheschek K, Merz H, Hell J, et al. Large-cell anaplastic lymphoma-specific translocation (t[2;5] [p23;q35]) in Hodgkin's disease: Indication of a common pathogenesis? *Lancet* 1995, **345**: 87–90.

181b. Rimokh R, Magaud JP, Berger F, et al. A translocation involving a specific breakpoint (q35) on chromosome 5 is a characteristic of anaplastic large cell lymphoma ('Ki-1 lymphoma'). *Br. J. Haematol.* 1989, **71**: 31–36.

182. MacLennan KA, Bennett MH, Tu A, et al. Relationship of histopathologic features to survival and relapse in nodular sclerosing Hodgkin's disease. A study of 1659 patients. *Cancer* 1989, **64**: 1686–1693.

183. Strickler JG, Michie SA, Warnke RA, Dorfman RF. The 'syncytial variant' of nodular sclerosing Hodgkin's disease. *Am. J. Surg. Pathol.* 1986, **10**: 470–477.

184. Banks PM. The distinction of Hodgkin's disease from T-cell lymphoma. *Semin. Diagn. Pathol.* 1992, **9**: 279–283.

185. Fliedner A, Parwaresch MR, Feller AC. Induction of antigen expression of follicular dendritic cells in a monoblastic cell line. A contribution to its cellular origin. *J. Pathol.* 1990, **161**: 71–77.

186. Griesser H, Feller AC, Mak TW, Lennert K. Clonal rearrangements of T-cell receptor and immunoglobulin genes and immunophenotypic antigen expression in different subclasses of Hodgkin's disease. *Int. J. Cancer* 1987, **40**: 157–160.

187. Patsouris E, Noël H, Lennert K. Histological and immunohistological findings in lymphoepithelioid cell lymphoma (Lennert's lymphoma). *Am. J. Surg. Pathol.* 1988, **12**: 341–350.

188. Patsouris E, Noël H, Lennert K. Cytologic and immunohistochemical findings in Hodgkin's disease, mixed cellularity type, with a high content of epithelioid cells. *Am. J. Surg. Pathol.* 1989, **13**: 1014–1022.

189. Feller AC, Griesser GH, Mak TW, Lennert K. Lymphoepithelioid lymphoma (Lennert's lymphoma) is a monoclonal proliferation of helper/inducer T-cells. *Blood* 1986, **68**: 663–667.

190. O'Connor NTJ, Feller AC, Wainscoat JS, et al. T-cell origin of Lennert's lymphoma. *Br. J. Haematol.* 1986, **64**: 521–528.

191. Lennert K, Feller AC, Radzun HJ. Malignant histiocytosis/histiocytic sarcoma and related neoplasms. *Recent Adv. RES Res.* 1984, **24**: 1–16.

192. Pileri S, Falini B, Delsol G, et al. Lymphohistiocytic T-cell lymphoma (anaplastic large cell lymphoma CD30+/Ki-1+ with a high content of reactive histiocytes). *Histopathology* 1990, **16**: 383–391.

193. Stansfeld AG, D'Ardenne AJ. *Lymph Node Biopsy Interpretation*, 2nd edn. Edinburgh: Churchill Livingstone, 1992.

194. Ramsay AD, Smith WJ, Isaacson PG. T-cell-rich B-cell lymphoma. *Am. J. Surg. Pathol.* 1988, **12**: 433–443.

195. Ng CS, Chan JKC, Hui PK, Lau WH. Large B-cell

lymphomas with a high content of reactive T-cells. *Hum. Pathol.* 1989, **20**: 1145–1154.

196. Osborne BM, Butler JJ, Pugh WC. The value of immunophenotyping on paraffin sections in the identification of T-cell rich B-cell large-cell lymphomas: lineage confirmed by J_H rearrangement. *Am. J. Surg. Pathol.* 1990, **14**: 933–938.

197. Chittal SM, Brousset P, Voigt JJ, Delsol G. Large B-cell lymphoma rich in T-cells and simulating Hodgkin's disease. *Histopathology* 1991, **19**: 211–220.

198. Macon WR, Williams ME, Greer JP. T-cell-rich B-cell lymphomas. A clinicopathologic study of 19 cases. *Am. J. Surg. Pathol.* 1992, **16**: 351–363.

199. Hansmann M-L, Fellbaum C, Hui PK, Zwingers T. Correlation of content of B-cells and Leu7 positive cells with subtype and stage in lymphocyte predominance type Hodgkin's disease. *J. Cancer Res. Clin. Oncol.* 1988, **114**: 405–410.

200. Kamel OW, Gelb AB, Shibuya RB, Warnke RA. Leu 7 (CD57) reactivity distinguishes nodular lymphocyte predominance Hodgkin's disease from nodular sclerosing Hodgkin's disease, T-cell-rich B-cell lymphoma and follicular lymphoma. *Am. J. Pathol.* 1993, **142**: 541–546.

201. Herbst H, Tippelmann G, Anagnostopoulos I, et al. Immunoglobulin and T-cell receptor gene rearrangements in Hodgkin's and Ki-1-positive anaplastic large cell lymphoma: Dissociation between phenotype and genotype. *Leukemia Res.* 1989, **13**: 103–116.

202. Gledhill S, Krajewski AS, Dewar AE, et al. Analysis of T-cell receptor and immunoglobulin gene rearrangements in the diagnosis of Hodgkin's and non-Hodgkin's lymphoma. *J. Pathol.* 1990, **161**: 245–254.

203. Osborne BM, Butler JJ. Follicular lymphoma mimicking progressive transformation of germinal centers. *Am. J. Clin. Pathol.* 1987, **88**: 264–269.

204. Goates JJ, Kamel OW, LeBrun DP, et al. Floral variant of follicular lymphoma. Immunological and molecular studies support a neoplastic process. *Am. J. Surg. Pathol.* 1994, **18**: 37–47.

205. Harris NL. The relationship between Hodgkin's disease and non-Hodgkin's lymphoma. *Semin. Diagn. Pathol.* 1992, **9**: 304–310.

206. Algara P. Martinez P, Sanchez L, et al. Lymphocyte predominance Hodgkin's disease (nodular paragranuloma) – a bcl-2 negative germinal center lymphoma. *Histopathology* 1991, **19**: 69–75.

207. Said JW, Sassoon AF, Shintaku IP, et al. Absence of bcl-2 major breakpoint region and JH gene rearrangement in lymphocyte predominant Hodgkin's disease – results of Southern blot analysis and polymerase chain reaction. *Am. J. Pathol.* 1991, **138**: 261–264.

208. Hell K, Pringle JH, Hansmann M-L. et al. Demonstration of light chain mRNA in Hodgkin's disease. *J. Pathol.* 1993, **171**: 137–143.

209. Stetler-Stevenson M, Crush-Stanton S, Cossman J. Involvement of the bcl-2 gene in Hodgkin's disease. *J. Natl Cancer Inst.* 1990, **82**: 855–858.

210. Lorenzen J, Hansmann M-L, Pezzella F, et al.

Expression of the *bcl*-2 oncogene product and chromosomal translocation t(14;18) in Hodgkin's disease. *Hum. Pathol.* 1992, **23**: 1205–1209.

211. Banks PM. The pathology of Hodgkin's disease. *Semin. Oncol.* 1990, **17**: 683–695.

212. Brittinger G, Bartels H, Common H, et al. Clinical and prognostic relevance of the Kiel classification of non-Hodgkin lymphomas: Results of a prospective multicenter study by the Kiel lymphoma study group. *Hematol. Oncol.* 1984, **2**: 269–306.

213. Engelhard M, Brittinger G, Heinz R, et al. Chronic lymphocytic leukemia (B-CLL) and immunocytoma (LP-IC): Clinical and prognostic relevance of this distinction. *Leuk. Lymphoma* 1991 (Suppl.), 161–173.

214. Weisenburger DD. Mantle cell lymphoma. In Knowles DM (ed.) *Neoplastic Hematopathology*. Baltimore: Williams & Wilkins 1992, pp. 617–628.

215. Sheibani K, Sohn CS, Burke JS, et al. Monocytoid B-cell lymphoma. A novel B-cell neoplasm. *Am. J. Pathol.* 1986, **124**: 310–318.

216. Nizze H, Cogliatti SB, von Schilling C, et al. Monocytoid B-cell lymphoma: Morphological variants and relationship to low-grade B-cell lymphoma of the mucosa-associated lymphoid tissue. *Histopathology* 1991, **18**: 403–414.

217. Davis GG, York JC, Glick AD, et al. Plasmacytic differentiation in parafollicular (monocytoid) B-cell lymphoma. A study of 12 cases. *Am. J. Surg. Pathol.* 1992, **16**: 1066–1074.

218. Isaacson PG, Spencer J. Monocytoid B-cell lymphomas [letter to the editor]. *Am. J. Surg. Pathol.* 1990, **14**: 888–890.

219. Piris MA, Orradre JL, Rivas C. Monocytoid B-cell lymphoma – a MALT tumor [Letter to the editor]. *Histopathology* 1990, **17**: 287–288.

220. Hui PK, Feller AC, Lennert K. High-grade non-Hodgkin's lymphoma of B-cell type. I. Histopathology. *Histopathology* 1988, **12**: 127–143.

221. MacLennan ICM, Liu YL, Ling NR. B-cell proliferation in follicles, germinal center formation and the site of neoplastic transformation in Burkitt's lymphoma. *Curr. Top. Microbiol. Immunol.* 1988, **141**: 138–148.

222. Liu Y-J, Johnson GD, Gordon J, MacLennan ICM. Germinal centers in T-cell-dependent antibody responses. *Immunol. Today* 1992, **13**: 17–21.

223. Patsouris E, Noël H, Lennert K. Angioimmunoblastic lymphadenopathy-type of T-cell lymphoma with a high content of epithelioid cells. Histopathology and comparison with lymphoepithelioid cell lymphoma. *Am. J. Surg. Pathol.* 1989, **13**: 262–275.

224. Patsouris E, Noël H, Lennert K. Lymphoplasmacytic/lymphoplasmacytoid immunocytoma with a high content of epithelioid cells. Histologic and immunohistochemical findings. *Am. J. Surg. Pathol.* 1990, **14**: 660–670.

225. Schneider DR, Taylor CR, Parker JW, et al. Immunoblastic sarcoma of T- and B-cell types. *Hum. Pathol.* 1985, **16**: 885–900.

226. Stein H, Mason DY, Gerdes J, et al. The expression of the Hodgkin's disease associated antigen Ki-1 in reactive and neoplastic lymphoid tissue: Evidence

that Reed–Sternberg cells and histiocytic malignancies are derived from activated lymphoid cells. *Blood* 1985, **66**: 848–858.

227. Fischer P, Nacheva E, Mason DY, et al. A Ki-1 (CD30)-positive human cell line (Karpas 299) established from a high-grade non-Hodgkin's lymphoma, showing a 2;5 translocation and rearrangement of the T-cell receptor β-chain gene. *Blood* 1988, **72**: 234–240.

228. Mason DY, Bastard C, Rimokh R, et al. CD30-positive large cell lymphomas ('Ki-1 lymphoma') are associated with a chromosomal translocation involving 5q35. *Br. J. Haematol.* 1990, **74**: 161–168.

229. Nadler LM, Korsmeyer SJ, Anderson KC, et al. B-cell origin of non-T-cell acute lymphoblastic leukemia. A model for discrete stages of neoplastic and normal pre-B-cell differentiation. *J. Clin. Invest.* 1984, **74**: 332–340.

230. Barcos MP, Lukes RJ. Malignant lymphoma of convoluted lymphocytes: A new entity of possible T-cell type. In Sinks LF, Godden JE (eds) *Conflicts in Childhood Cancer: An Evaluation of Current Management*, Vol. 4. New York: Alan R. Liss, Inc. 1975, pp. 147–178.

231. Tobinai K, Minato K, Ohtsu T, et al. Clinicopathologic, immunophenotypic, and immunogenotypic analyses of immunoblastic lymphadenopathy-like T-cell lymphoma. *Blood* 1988, **72**: 1000–1006.

232. Frizzera G, Kaneko Y, Sakurai M. Angioimmunoblastic lymphadenopathy and related disorders: A retrospective look in search of definitions. *Leukemia* 1989, **3**: 1–5.

233. Knecht H. Angioimmunoblastic lymphadenopathy: Ten years' experience and state of current knowledge. *Semin. Hematol.* 1989, **26**: 208–215.

234. Frizzera G, Moran EM, Rappaport H. Angio-immunoblastic lymphadenopathy. Diagnosis and clinical course. *Am. J. Med.* 1975, **59**: 803–818.

235. Lukes RJ, Tindle BH. Immunoblastic lymphadenopathy. A hyperimmune entity resembling Hodgkin's disease. *N. Engl. J. Med.* 1975, **292**: 1–8.

236. Lennert K, Knecht H, Burkert M. Vorstadien maligner Lymphome. *Verh. Dtsch. Ges. Path.* 1979, **63**: 170–196.

237. Frizzera G. Atypical lymphoproliferative disorders. In Knowles DM (ed.) *Neoplastic Hematopathology*. Baltimore: Williams & Wilkins, 1992, pp. 459–495.

238. Kaneko Y, Larson RA, Variakojis D, et al. Nonrandom chromosome abnormalities in angioimmunoblastic lymphadenopathy. *Blood* 1982, **60**: 877–887.

239. Kaneko Y, Maseki N, Sakurai M, et al. Characteristic karyotypic pattern in T-cell lymphoproliferative disorders with reactive 'angioimmunoblastic lymphadenopathy with dysproteinemia-type' features. *Blood* 1988, **72**: 413–421.

240. Shimoyama M, Minato K, Saito H, et al. Immunoblastic lymphadenopathy (IBL)-like T-cell lymphoma. *Jpn. J. Clin. Oncol.* 1979, **9** (Suppl. 1): 347–356.

241. Suchi T. Atypical lymph node hyperplasia with fatal outcome – a report on the histopathological, immunological and clinical investigations of the cases. *Recent Adv. RES Res.* 1974, **14**: 13–34.

242. Knecht H, Lennert K. Ultrastructural findings in lymphogranulomatosis X ([angio-]immunoblastic lymphadenopathy). *Virchows Arch. [Cell. Pathol.]*. 1981, **37**: 29–47.

243. Watanabe S, Sato Y, Shimoyama M, et al. Immunoblastic lymphadenopathy, angioimmunoblastic lymphadenopathy, and IBL-like T-cell lymphoma. A spectrum of T-cell neoplasia. *Cancer* 1986, **58**: 2224–2232.

244. Gödde-Salz E, Feller AC, Lennert K. Chromosomal abnormalities in lymphogranulomatosis X (LgrX)/angioimmunoblastic lymphadenopathy (AILD). *Leukemia Res.* 1987, **11**: 181–190.

245. Schlegelberger B, Feller AC, Gödde E, et al. Stepwise development of chromosomal abnormalities in angioimmunoblastic lymphadenopathy. *Cancer Genet. Cytogenet.* 1990, **50**: 15–29.

245a. Schlegelberger B, Himmler A, Gödde E, et al. Cytogenetic findings in peripheral T-cell lymphomas as a basis for distinguishing low-grade and high-grade lymphomas. *Blood* 1994, **83**: 505–511.

246. Knecht H, Sahli R, Shaw P, et al. Detection of Epstein–Barr virus DNA by polymerase chain reaction in lymph node biopies from patients with angioimmunoblastic lymphadenopathy. *Br. J. Haematol..* 1990, **75**: 610–614.

247. Abruzzo LV, Schmidt K, Weiss LM, et al. B-cell lymphoma after angioimmunoblastic lymphadenopathy: A case with oligoclonal gene rearrangements associated with Epstein–Barr virus. *Blood* 1993, **82**: 241–246.

248. Borisch B, Caioni M, Hurwitz N, et al. Epstein–Barr virus subtype distribution in angioimmunoblastic lymphadenopathy. *Int. J. Cancer* 1993, **55**: 748–752.

249. Siegert W, Nerl C, Meuthen I, et al. Recombinant human interferon-α in the treatment of angioimmunoblastic lymphadenopathy: Results in 12 patients. *Leukemia* 1991, **5**: 892–895.

250. Siegert W, Agthe A, Griesser H, et al. Treatment of angioimmunoblastic lymphadenopathy (AILD)-type T-cell lymphoma using prednisone with or without the COPBLAM/IMVP-16 regimen. *Ann. Intern. Med.* 1992, **117**: 364–370.

250a. Schlegelberger B, Zwingers T, Hohenadel K, et al. Significance of cytogenetic findings for the clinical outcome in patients with T-cell lymphoma of angioimmunoblastic lymphadenopathy type. *J. Clin. Oncol.* 1996, **14**: 593–599.

250b. Younes A. Cytogenetic findings in T-cell lymphomas of angioimmunoblastic lymphadenopathy [Letter to the editor]. *J. Clin. Oncol.* 1996, **14**: 2188.

251. Hanto DW, Frizzera G, Gajl-Peczalska KJ, et al. Epstein–Barr virus-induced B-cell lymphoma after renal transplantation. Acyclovir therapy and transition from polyclonal to monoclonal B-cell proliferation. *N. Engl. J. Med.* 1982, **306**: 913–918.

252. Nalesnik MA, Jaffe R, Starzl TE, et al. The pathology of posttransplant lymphoproliferative disorders occurring in the setting of cyclosporine A–prednisone immunosuppression. *Am. J. Pathol.* 1988, **133**: 173–192.

253. Locker J, Nalesnik M. Molecular genetic analysis of lymphoid tumors arising after organ transplantation. *Am. J. Pathol.* 1989, **135**: 977–987.

254. Grierson H, Purtilo DT. Epstein–Barr virus infections in males with the X-linked lymphoproliferative syndrome. *Ann. Intern. Med.* 1987, **106**: 538–545.

255. Raphael MM, Audouin J, Lamine M, et al. Immunophenotypic and genotypic analysis of acquired immunodeficiency syndrome-related non-Hodgkin's lymphomas. *Am. J. Clin. Pathol.* 1994, **101**: 773–782.

256. Leibetseder F, Thurner J. Angiofollikuläre lymphknotenhyperplasie. *Med. Klin.* 1973, **68**: 817–820.

257. Diebold J, Tulliez M, Bernadou A, et al. Angiofollicular and plasmacytic polyadenopathy: a pseudotumorous syndrome with dysimmunity. *J. Clin. Pathol.* 1980, **33**: 1068–1076.

258. Frizzera G, Massarelli G, Banks PM, Rosai J. A systemic lymphoproliferative disorder with morphologic features of Castleman's disease. Pathological findings in 15 patients. *Am. J. Surg. Pathol.* 1983, **7**: 211–231.

259. Frizzera G. Castleman's disease: More questions than answers. *Hum. Pathol.* 1985, **16**: 202–205.

260. Weisenburger DD, Nathwani BN, Winberg CD, Rappaport H. Multicentric angiofollicular lymph node hyperplasia: A clinicopathologic study of 16 cases. *Hum. Pathol.* 1985, **16**: 162–172.

261. Hall PA, Donaghy M, Cotter FE, et al. An immunohistological and genotypic study of the plasma cell form of Castleman's disease. *Histopathology* 1989, **14**: 333–346.

262. Isaacson PG. Castleman's disease. Commentary. *Histopathology* 1989, **14**: 429–432.

263. Radaszkiewicz T, Hansmann M-L, Lennert K. Monoclonality and polyclonality of plasma cells in Castleman's disease of the plasma cell variant. *Histopathology* 1989, **14**: 11–24.

264. Kojima M, Sakuma H, Mori N. Histopathological features of plasma cell dyscrasia with polyneuropathy and endocrine disturbances, with special reference to germinal center lesions. *Jpn. J. Clin. Oncol.* 1983, **13**: 557–576.

265. Jones EL, Crocker J, Gregory J, et al. Angiofollicular lymph node hyperplasia (Castleman's disease): An immunohistochemical and enzyme-histochemical study of the hyaline-vascular form of lesion. *J. Pathol.* 1984, **144**: 131–147.

266. Hanson CA, Frizzera G, Patton DF, et al. Clonal rearrangement for immunoglobulin and T-cell receptor genes in systemic Castleman's disease. Association with Epstein–Barr virus. *Am. J. Pathol.* 1988, **131**: 84–91.

267. Takatsuki K, Sanada I. Plasma cell dyscrasia with polyneuropathy and endocrine disorder: Clinical and laboratory features of 109 reported cases. *Jpn. J. Clin. Oncol.* 1983, **13**: 543–556.

268. Yoshizaki K, Matsuda T, Nishimoto N, et al. Pathogenic significance of interleukin-6 (IL-6/BSF-2) in Castleman's disease. *Blood* 1989, **74**: 1360–1367.

269. Leger-Ravet MB, Peuchmaur M, Devergne O, et al. Interleukin-6 gene expression in Castleman's disease. *Blood* 1991, **78**: 2923–2930.

270. Custer RP. Pitfalls in the diagnosis of lymphoma and leukemia from the pathologist's point of view. Proceedings of the 2nd National Cancer Conference. New York: American Cancer Society, 1954, pp. 554–557.

271. The Non-Hodgkin's Lymphoma Pathologic Classification Project. National Cancer Institute sponsored study of classifications of non-Hodgkin's lymphomas. Summary and description of a Working Formulation for clinical usage. *Cancer* 1982, **49**: 2112–2135.

272. Kim H, Hendrickson MR, Dorfman RF. Composite lymphoma. *Cancer* 1977, **40**: 959–976.

273. Kim H. Composite lymphoma and related disorders. *Hematopathology* 1992, **99**: 445–451.

274. Jaffe ES, Zarate-Osorno A, Medeiros LJ. The interrelationship of Hodgkin's disease and non-Hodgkin's lymphomas – lessons learned from composite and sequential malignancies. *Semin. Diagn. Pathol.* 1992, **9**: 297–303.

275. York JC II, Cousar JB, Glick AD, et al. Morphologic and immunologic evidence of composite B- and T-cell lymphomas. *Am. J. Clin. Pathol.* 1985, **84**: 35–43.

275a. Bierwolf S. Cytomorphologische, immunhistologische und molekulargenetische Untersuchungen von T-zellreichen B-Zell-Lymphomen und composite Lymphomen. Inauguraldissertation. Kiel: Universtiy of Kiel, 1996.

276. Hansmann M-L, Fellbaum C, Hui PK, Lennert K. Morphological and immunohistochemical investigation of non-Hodgkin's lymphoma combined with Hodgkin's disease. *Histopathology* 1989, **15**: 35–48.

277. Lennert K, Stein H, Feller AC, Gerdes J. Morphology, cytochemistry and immunohistology of T cell lymphomas. In Vitetta ES (ed.) *B and T Cell Tumors* (*UCLA Symposia on Molecular and Cellular Biology*, Vol. XXIV). New York: Academic Press, 1982, pp. 9–28.

278. Kerrigan DP, Foucar K, Dressler L. High-grade non-Hodgkin lymphoma relapsing as low-grade follicular lymphoma: so-called downgraded lymphoma. *Am. J. Hematol.* 1989, **30**: 36–41.

279. Miettinen M, Franssila KO, Saxén E. Hodgkin's disease, lymphocytic predominance nodular. Increased risk for subsequent non-Hodgkin's lymphomas. *Cancer* 1983, **51**: 2293–2300.

280. Lennert K, Hansmann M-L. Progressive transformation of germinal centers: clinical significance and lymphocytic predominance Hodgkin's disease – the Kiel experience. *Am. J. Surg. Pathol.* 1987, **11**: 149–150A.

281. Bennett MH, MacLennan KA, Vaughan-Hudson G, Vaughan-Hudson B. Non-Hodgkin's lymphoma arising in patients treated for Hodgkin's disease in the BNLI: a 20-year experience. *Ann. Oncol.* 1991, **2** (Suppl. 2): 83–92.

282. Jennette JC, Reddick RL, Saunders AW, Wilkman AS. Diffuse T-cell lymphoma preceded by nodular lymphoma. *Am. J. Clin. Pathol.* 1982, **78**: 242–248.

283. Tokunaga M, Tokudome T, Shimizu S, et al. Biclonality of composite B- and T-cell lymphomas. A case report. *Acta Pathol. Jpn.* 1990, **40**: 522–530.

284. Strickler JG, Amsden TW, Kurtin PJ. Small B-cell lymphoid neoplasms with coexisting T-cell lymphomas. *Am. J. Clin. Pathol.* 1992, **98**: 424–429.

285. Hu E, Weiss LM, Warnke R, Sklar J. Non-Hodgkin's lymphoma containing both B and T-cell clones. *Blood* 1987, **70**: 287–292.

286. Gonzalez CL, Medeiros LJ, Jaffe ES. Composite lymphoma. A clinicopathologic analysis of nine patients with Hodgkin's disease and B-cell non-Hodgkin's lymphoma. *Am. J. Clin. Pathol.* 1991, **96**: 81–89.

287. Simrell CR, Boccia RV, Longo DL, Jaffe ES. Coexisting Hodgkin's disease and mycosis fungoides. Immunohistochemical proof of its existence. *Arch. Pathol. Lab. Med.* 1986, **110**: 1029–1034.

288. Travis LB, Curtis RE, Boice JD Jr, et al. Second cancers following non-Hodgkin's lymphoma. *Cancer* 1991, **67**: 2002–2009.

289. Zarate-Osorno A, Medeiros LJ, Longo DL, Jaffe ES. Non-Hodgkin's lymphomas arising in patients successfully treated for Hodgkin's disease. A clinical, histologic, and immunophenotypic study of 14 cases. *Am. J. Surg. Pathol.* 1992, **16**: 885–895.

290. Kövary PM, Niedorf H, Sommer G, et al. Paraproteinaemia in Sézary syndrome. *Dermatologica* 1977, **154**: 138–146.

291. Klajman A, Yaretzky A, Schneider M et al. Angioimmunoblastic lymphadenopathy with paraproteinemia: A T- and B-cell disorder. *Cancer* 1981, **48**: 2433–2437.

292. Knecht H, Lennert K. Vorgeschichte und klinisches Bild der Lymphogranulomatosis X (einschliesslich [angio]immunoblastischer Lymphadenopathie). *Schweiz med. Wschr.* 1981, **111**: 1108–1121.

293. Lowenthal RM, Harlow RWH, Mead AE, et al. T-cell non-Hodgkin's lymphoma after radiotherapy and chemotherapy for Hodgkin's disease. *Cancer* 1981, **48**: 1586–1589.

294. Wlodarska I, Delabie J, de Wolf-Peeters C, et al. T-cell lymphoma developing in Hodgkin's disease: evidence for two clones. *J. Pathol.* 1993, **170**: 239–248.

295. Shimizu K, Hirano M, Maruyama F, et al. T-cell malignancy following B-cell lymphoma in remission. *Am. J. Clin. Pathol.* 1989, **92**: 362–366.

296. Medeiros LJ, Stetler-Stevenson M. Composite B-cell and T-cell lymphoma. Coincidental occurrence or related neoplasms? *Am. J. Clin. Pathol.* 1992, **98**: 387–389.

297. Williams J, Schned A, Cotelingam JD, Jaffe ES. Chronic lymphocytic leukemia with coexistent Hodgkin's disease. Implications for the origin of the Reed–Sternberg cell. *Am. J. Surg. Pathol.* 1991, **15**: 33–42.

298. Tsang WYW. Chan JKC, Ng CS. Epstein–Barr virus and Reed–Sternberg-like cells in chronic lymphocytic leukemia [Letter to the editor]. *Am. J. Surg. Pathol.* 1993, **17**: 853–854.

299. Lennert K. Eröffnungsrede des Vorsitzenden [Opening address held by the Chairman]. *Verh. Dtsch. Ges. Path.* 1983, **67**: XXIII–XXXI.

300. Dudley HAF. Pay-off, heuristics, and pattern recognition in the diagnostic process. *Lancet* 1968, **ii**: 723–726.

301. Ackerman AB. *Histologic Diagnosis of Inflammatory Skin Diseases. A Method by Pattern Analysis.* Philadelphia: Lea & Febiger, 1978.

PART 3

Epidemiology and pathogenesis

CHAPTER 6

Epidemiology of non-Hodgkin's lymphomas

CHARLES S. RABKIN, MARY H. WARD, ANGELA MANNS
AND WILLIAM A. BLATTNER

Introduction

The non-Hodgkin's lymphomas (NHL) span a continuum of lymphoproliferative malignancies that vary in clinical behavior and morphologic appearance. The various types of NHL are thought to represent neoplastic lymphoid cells arrested at different stages of normal maturation [1]. Continual shifts in classification, owing to changing terminology and variation in diagnostic practice, tend to obscure epidemiologic distinctions among these malignancies. Nevertheless, their similarities and differences may reflect common mechanisms among their diverse etiologies.

Incidence rates

In 1995, an estimated 50 900 cases of NHL were diagnosed in the USA representing 4% of all cancers [2]. Approximately 22 700 people died from NHL in that year, which represents 4% of cancer deaths.

NHL incidence rates rise exponentially with age. Age-adjusted US rates for the years 1987–1991 were 8.5 annual cases per 100 000 under 65 years of age versus 68.8 per 100 000 for age 65 and over (Figure 6.1). There is a male predominance in incidence, which is more marked in younger than older individuals. The male:female rate ratio was 1.79 for age under 65 versus 1.33 for age 65 and over. Incidence also varies by race. Whites have 50% higher incidence than Blacks, and a roughly similar excess as compared to Japanese- and Chinese-Americans [3]. These differences are also reflected in international comparisons, in which US rates tend to exceed those of most other countries [4]. The difference is particularly striking for follicular lymphoma, which constitutes 20% of cases in Western countries, but is relatively rare in developing countries, China and Japan [5–7]. Racial genetic factors, as shown by the virtual absence of B-cell chronic lymphocytic leukemia in Asian populations and the excess occurrence of multiple myeloma in Blacks, may play a role in these international differences.

The incidence of NHL has been increasing much more rapidly than that of most other tumors [8]. Four large cancer registries in the USA – Atlanta, Detroit, San Francisco-Oakland and Connecticut – have incidence data available from the late 1940s to the present [9]. From the years 1947–1950 to the years 1984–1988, annual NHL incidence among Whites in these four areas rose by 150%; relative increases were similar in men and women. The respective incidence rates for those periods rose from 6.9 to 17.4 per 100 000 in men and from 4.7 to 11.6 per 100 000 in women. A consistent increasing trend is

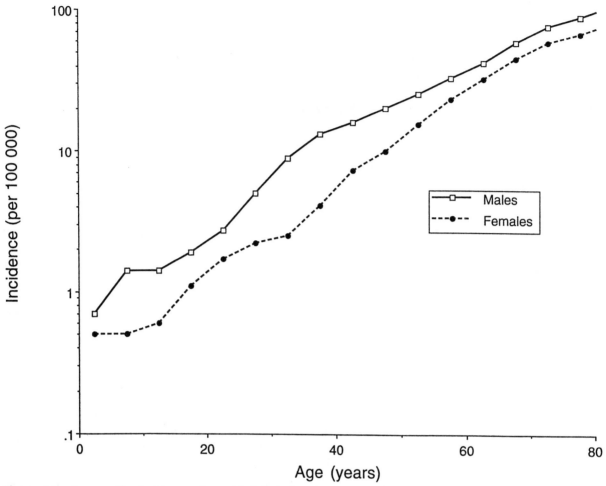

Figure 6.1 Age-specific incidence of non-Hodgkin's lymphoma in males and females in the US Surveillance, Epidemiology, and End Results Program, 1987–1991.

present throughout this period. As discussed below, there has also been a recent increase among men superimposed on the long-term trend coincident with the appearance of acquired immunodeficiency syndrome (AIDS)-associated NHL. Mortality from NHL has increased somewhat more slowly than incidence, presumably because of improvements in therapy (Figure 6.2).

Recorded NHL incidence varies between countries and age-adjusted rates in the USA are some of the highest in the world. However, time trends appear to be similar in most other countries. Data from more than 20 large registries worldwide indicate that NHL incidence has been increasing in nearly every registry [9]. Between 1970 and 1980, the average increase in these registries was 43% for both sexes combined, not dissimilar to the increases in the four US geographic areas.

Changes in NHL incidence vary by age. In the USA, increases have been most marked in the oldest age groups while relatively stable in younger groups. Among White men, an increase of at least 100% over the 40-year period was seen for each 10-year age group older than 45 years; incidence in those 75 years and older rose nearly 400%. However, lymphomas associated with the AIDS epidemic have introduced some deviations from linear trends: since the early 1980s, NHL incidence in men has increased abruptly in the age categories between 25 and 54.

Ecological analyses of county-level data have indicated a gradual diminution in the differences in NHL mortality rates by socioeconomic conditions, such as urbanization, household income and education. Apart from variation due to variation in prevalence of the human immunodeficiency virus (HIV), there is little differential in mortality rates based on socioeconomic status. Increases in NHL incidence have not been uniform for all histologies and sites. High-grade histologies have increased more than low-grade ones, and extranodal disease

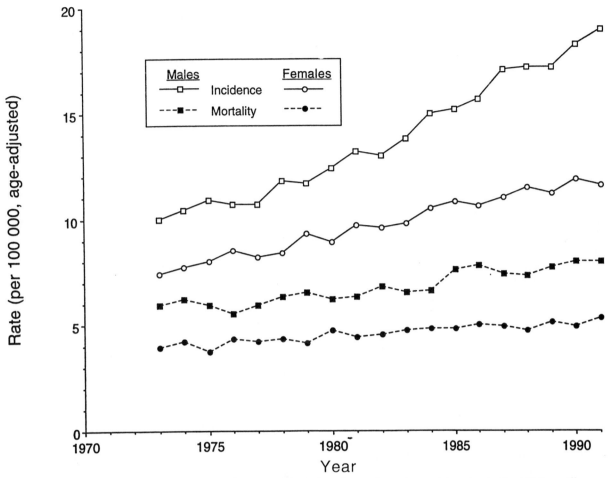

Figure 6.2 Incidence and mortality rates of non-Hodgkin's lymphoma in males and females in the US Surveillance, Epidemiology, and End Results Program, by year, 1973–1991.

has increased more rapidly than nodal disease [10].

The reasons for these increases are poorly understood. A recent analysis attempted to estimate the impact of changes in diagnosis and well-established risk factors on the trends in NHL incidence in the USA [11]. After accounting for these factors, there remained an unexplained increase in incidence of more than 40% over the past 40 years.

Etiologic factors

IMMUNODEFICIENCY

Several factors are known to increase NHL risk. The strongest association is with immunodeficiency. NHL is the most frequent malignancy in patients with some rare primary immunodeficiency disorders, including ataxia telangiectasia, Wiskott–Aldrich syndrome, subacute combined immunodeficiency, X-linked lymphoproliferative syndrome and common variable immunodeficiency [12]. Patients with secondary immunodeficiency, such as that owing to immunosuppressive therapy or HIV infection, have been observed to have up to 100 times more NHL than expected [13,14]. Immunodeficiency-associated tumors tend to be of higher-grade histology and frequently have extranodal primary sites, especially the brain. Some neoplasms occurring in the setting of immunodeficiency are actually polyclonal lymphoid proliferations, although they may be clinically and histologically indistinguishable from NHL [15].

The recent accelerating increases in NHL have been concentrated in populations at increased risk for AIDS. The rapid increase, since 1982, in NHL incidence among young men is probably the result of infection with HIV. About 3% of AIDS cases present with NHL as the AIDS-defining condition, and patients with other AIDS-defining conditions may subsequently develop NHL after their initial AIDS diagnosis [16]. Some of the largest increases in NHL incidence have been observed among single young men in the city of San Francisco, of whom an estimated one-fourth were infected with HIV-1 as of 1984. Cancer registration data indicate that NHL incidence for this high-risk group increased 20-fold between 1973–1979 and 1988–1990. The increases were most pronounced in tumors of higher-grade histology and extranodal (especially central nervous system) primary sites. Burkitt's and Burkitt-like tumors peaked in incidence in 1985–1987 whereas large-cell diffuse and immunoblastic lymphomas increased through 1990 (Figure 6.3) [17]. On the other hand, the incidence of low-grade NHL does not appear to be increased by HIV infection [18].

Other infectious agents may be involved in at least some AIDS-related lymphomas. In HIV-related primary central nervous system lymphomas, the Epstein–Barr virus (EBV) is consistently found both in tumors as well as in the cerebrospinal fluid [19,20]. EBV is also to be found in a fraction of systemic AIDS-related NHL, although its role is uncertain [21]. In contrast, with the exception of Burkitt's lymphoma and some T-cell neoplasms, EBV is rarely found in lymphomas unrelated to HIV (at least in the USA), including those originating in the central nervous system [22]. A direct role for HIV has been suggested in a report of four cases of AIDS-NHL with integrated HIV, although this work has not yet been confirmed [23].

INFECTIOUS AGENTS OTHER THAN HIV

HTLV-1 and adult T-cell leukemia/lymphoma

In 1976, Takatsuki and colleagues first identified cases of adult T-cell leukemia/lymphoma (ATLL) in Japan [24] and in the following year published a comprehensive description of this clinicopathological entity [25]. ATLL was characterized as a mature T-lymphocyte malignancy with: (1) adult onset; (2) acute or chronic leukemia with a rapidly progressive terminal course; (3) leukemic cells with deeply indented or lobulated nuclei, termed 'flower' cells; (4) typical skin involvement; and (5) frequent lymphadenopathy and hepatosplenomegaly. Hypercalcemia was later noted as a consistent feature of ATLL. An important epidemiological observation was the recognition that cases in Japan were geographically clustered in the southernmost islands of Kyushu, Shikoku and Okinawa. It was hypothesized that genetic and possibly viral factors might be important in the etiology of ATLL [24]. In 1978, human T-cell lymphotrophic virus-1 (HTLV-1), the etiologic agent, was isolated from cultured cells of a Black American patient whose diagnosis had originally been mycosis fungoides [26]. HTLV-1 was subsequently linked to ATLL clusters in Japan and the West Indies [27,28].

The prevalence of these HTLV-1-associated leukemia/lymphomas worldwide is unknown; the incidence in any population depends on the prevalence of viral infection. The highest incidences are found in

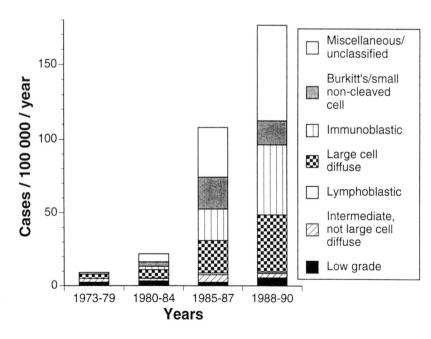

Figure 6.3 Standardized incidence rates of non-Hodgkin's lymphoma subtypes (classification by the Working Formulation for Clinical Usage [152]) in never-married San Francisco men aged 25–54 years, 1973–1979 to 1988–1990 (reprinted from Rabkin [17]).

southern Japan and the Caribbean basin, where HTLV-1 is highly endemic [29,30]. ATLL cases have been identified worldwide among migrants from viral endemic areas, as well as among aboriginal peoples in many parts of the world, including North and South America, Australia (associated with the Melanesian HTLV-1 variant), Africa and the Middle East [29,31]. In highly endemic areas, such as southern Japan and the Caribbean Basin, ATLL incidence is approximately 3/100 000 per year, accounting for one-half of all adult lymphoid malignancies. The lifetime cumulative risk for HTLV-1 carriers is estimated to be 1–5% [29,31]. Early life exposure to HTLV-1, as acquired in maternal–infant transmission via breastfeeding, has been postulated to be associated with the greatest risk of disease.

In contrast to the female predominance among HTLV-1 carriers [32], ATLL occurs with equal frequency among men and women (Figure 6.4). ATLL may also occur in children, albeit rarely, with reported cases as young as 5 and 6 years of age [33–35]. Age-specific incidence peaks in the sixth or seventh decade of life in Japan, and 10–20 years younger in Jamaica (Figure 6.4) [31]. A similar difference has been reported in the age distributions of Japanese-American and African-American ATLL patients in the USA [36], with median ages of disease onset 63 and 39 years, respectively. The two groups also differ in their clinical presentation, as classified according to criteria established by Shimoyama et al. [37]: African-Americans more commonly present with lymphoma-type ATLL, while Japanese-Americans more frequently present with the acute type. These differences may be a result of environmental or genetic modifiers of the disease.

In viral endemic areas, HTLV-1 is the chief cause of lymphoma in persons under 60 years of age. In Jamaica and Trinidad, for example, HTLV-1 exposure is estimated to account for more than 70% of T-cell lymphomas and over 50% of total lymphoid malig-

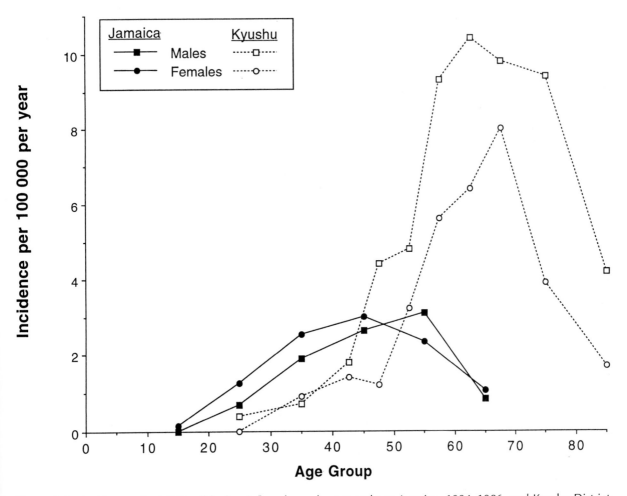

Figure 6.4 Incidence of adult T-cell leukemia/lymphoma by age and sex, Jamaica, 1984–1986, and Kyushu District, Japan, 1986–1987. Data from [31] and [33].

nancies [38]. NHL incidence rates in those who are infected with HTLV-1 in childhood are so dramatically high that exposure to HTLV-1 in some early critical period seems particularly important for lymphomagenesis [30]. As a corollary, most adult-acquired infection (which is usually through sexual exposure) is not relevant to NHL risk. These data indicate that prevention of early life infection with HTLV-1 would eliminate one-half of NHL cases in viral endemic areas.

The subsequent steps in HTLV-associated lymphomagenesis have yet to be elucidated but multiple insults are believed to be required for the final transformation to malignancy. Several factors have been implicated: host immune response associated with specific HLA haplotypes [39]; genetic abnormalities such as p53 mutations and cytogenetic changes [40,41]; farming occupation with possible pesticide exposure [42]; and co-infection with EBV [43]. Further epidemiologic and laboratory

investigations are necessary to clarify these relationships.

Burkitt's tumor and EBV

Burkitt's lymphoma (BL) is the most common malignant lymphoma of children, occurring in an endemic and sporadic form [44]. The disease is endemic in Africa and New Guinea, and occurs sporadically in the USA and other developed countries [45]. In the USA, the highest incidence used to be found in boys (Figure 6.5). However, since the advent of the AIDS epidemic and of AIDS-related cases, the peak incidence has shifted to older age groups. The endemic and sporadic BL are indistinguishable in histopathologic appearance, and both forms are characterized by similar chromosomal and oncogene abnormalities. However, the endemic form consistently has evidence of episomal EBV genome in tumor tissue, whereas less than 10–20% of

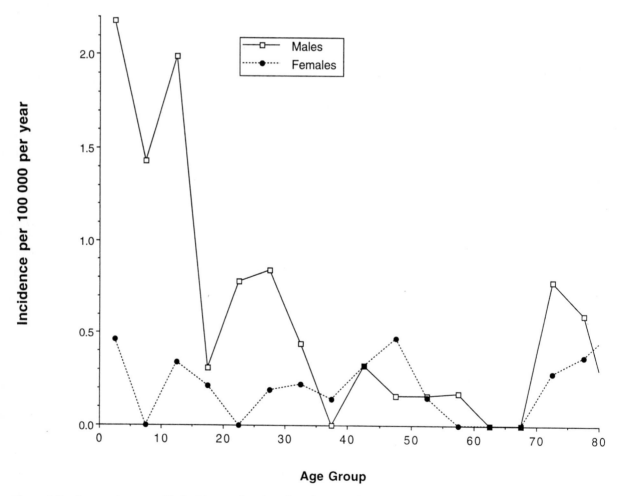

Figure 6.5 Age- and sex-specific incidence of Burkitt's lymphoma in the pre-AIDS period (1973–1979), US Surveillance and Epidemiology, and End Results Program. Data from [31] and [33].

sporadic cases have EBV in tumor tissue. Moreover, the endemic form, but not the sporadic form, characteristically presents in the jaw or orbit [44,46]. These differences suggest that the two forms may have different pathogenetic pathways, although few epidemiologic studies have focused on possible etiologic differences between them (Table 6.1) [47].

The endemic form of Burkitt's lymphoma was first recognized in Africa in 1958 [48]. African BL was intensively studied in the 1960s and 1970s and subsequently a great deal of progress has been made in understanding its pathogenesis, although there are still many unanswered questions. The early descriptive epidemiology suggested there were climatic determinants of the distribution of BL and an arthropod-borne virus was proposed as the possible etiology [49]. Although evidence never substantiated an arthropod vector, this thesis led to the discovery of EBV in 1964 [50]. EBV antigens and subsequently viral genome were identified in the tumor tissue of BL patients [51] and elevated EBV viral capsid antigen (VCA) antibody titers were shown to precede the development of BL in most instances [52]. The ability of EBV to transform lymphocytes and produce polyclonal tumors in subhuman primates and immunosuppressed subjects is indicative of its potential as an oncogenic virus. EBV, however, is ubiquitous. Nearly 99% of children in developing countries are infected by age 3 [53] and approximately 90% of individuals in developed countries are infected by adulthood. Therefore, EBV was suspected to be a necessary, but not sufficient, factor in the etiology of endemic BL.

It became evident that other cofactors must be involved in the pathogenesis of BL. Malaria was the most likely candidate, owing to epidemiologic evidence showing a parallel geographic distribution for BL and malaria. Malaria had the ability to cause immune suppression [54], which could potentiate the effects of EBV infection. Biggar et al. attempted to establish a correlation between malaria and EBV in Ghanaians living in urban versus rural areas; although rural residents had more prevalent malaria, there was no difference in EBV antibody titers [55]. Geser et al. [56] used another approach to examine whether the incidence of BL would decline if malaria was eradicated in a BL endemic area. A decline in BL incidence was observed, but it was not clear whether the decline was the result of the malaria intervention or other changes in the community.

In vitro laboratory studies have been performed in an attempt to elucidate the host response to malaria in the presence of EBV infection. One study evaluated cytotoxicity against EBV in EBV-seropositive controls and patients with acute malaria. The immunosuppressive effects of malaria were found to extend to defective control over EBV with resultant proliferation of B-lymphocytes, a decrease in the number and/or function of EB-virus specific T-cells, and a depressed CD4:CD8 ratio [57]. It has been suggested that the increase in number of EBV-genome positive cells during acute malaria increased the chance of cytogenetic abnormalities occurring in the B-lymphocyte, with consequent evolution to BL [58]. A multiple-hit model involving the interaction of EBV, malaria, and other events has been proposed.

Clearly, there is a potential role for host genetics or immunogenetics in BL causation. BL tumor tissue always has a chromosomal translocation at one of the regions coding for immunoglobulin (14q32, 22q11 or 2p11–12). However, the specific chromosomal breakpoints differ in different world regions [59]. Familial clusters of BL have been reported [60], which would be consistent with an inherited genetic susceptibility, although the specific lesion(s) is

Table 6.1   Characteristics of sporadic and endemic Burkitt's lymphoma

	Endemic	Sporadic
Average annual incidence Children < 15 years	$8.0/10^5$	$2/10^6$
Male:female ratio	2:1	2:1
Occurrence	Climatically and geographically influenced	Not climatically influenced
Association with EBV	100%	10–20%
Chromosome 8 breakpoints	Upstream of c-*myc*	Within c-*myc*
Common sites of tumor	Jaw, abdomen, orbit, paraspinal	Abdomen, bone marrow, nasopharynx

Adapted from [46].

unknown. Inherited mutations in the c-myc oncogene or p53 tumor suppressor gene are potential candidates, since both have been identified in BL tumors, but neither have been found abnormal in cases or their family members. Sickle cell trait, an inherited genetic abnormality of hemoglobin, is known to decrease the severity of malaria infection and it was hypothesized that this trait would also be protective against BL. However, no such protective effect was detected in a BL case-control study [61]. In an early study of BL patients and controls [62], there were no associations with HLA but HLA testing has subsequently undergone extensive refinements. A recent study using current techniques found that the class II antigen HLA-DR7 was more frequent among BL patients compared to controls, but the authors did not evaluate a possible correlation between malaria and BL [63].

Few environmental factors have been explored as potential causal factors in BL. Rural residence has frequently been reported in association with an elevated risk for BL [64]. It is unclear whether this association is caused by the social circumstance, increased malaria exposure, early age of EBV seroconversion or some life-style factor. Another potential practice, which may be more evident in the rural setting, is the more widespread use and availability of herbal medicines. Phorbol esters (particularly *Euphorbia triucalli*) are available in Africa and used to treat common ailments. Although no direct *in vivo* evidence exists to support a role for these plants in BL etiology, *in vitro* studies have provided some evidence of an interaction with EBV. Exposure to both *E. triucalli* and EBV induces chromosomal rearrangements affecting chromosome 8 with c-*myc* gene activation similar to that found in BL patients [65].

Infectious agents, genetic lesions, host factors and environmental factors have all been implicated in the etiology of BL. However, the relationship among these postulated factors is poorly understood. There are many unanswered questions, such as, why do some (but not all) EBV and/or malaria infected individuals develop BL? Though BL pathogenesis has been well characterized at the molecular level, it is still unclear what constellation of factors are important in triggering the specific events required for malignant transformation. Further epidemiologic investigation is necessary.

MALT lymphoma and Helicobacter pylori

An increasing body of evidence links chronic gastric infection with *Helicobacter pylori* to the development of low-grade gastric lymphoma arising from mucosa-associated lymphoid tissue (MALT). Con-

current *H. pylori* infection is common in patients with gastric lymphoma [66] and in a large prospective study seropositivity to *H. pylori* was associated with a six-fold increased risk of subsequent gastric lymphoma [67]. Furthermore, low-grade gastric MALT lymphoma may even regress and disappear with eradication of *H. pylori* [68]. *In vitro*, gastric MALT lymphoma tumor cells have been shown to proliferate in the presence of *H. pylori* antigens and *H. pylori*-specific T-cells [69]. These findings indicate that chronic antigenic stimulation and or inflammation may underlie this entity, and perhaps other forms of NHL as well.

PESTICIDES AND OTHER AGRICULTURAL EXPOSURES

Early evidence for an association of NHL and agriculture came from maps of US cancer mortality rates, by county, which showed higher rates of mortality from lymphoma in the highly agricultural central region of the country [70]. Initial analyses using death certificates indicated that mid-Western farmers have a higher risk of lymphoma than other occupations [71,72]. Subsequently, epidemiologic studies of various designs and populations have found an increased risk of NHL among farmers, although their risk for all cancers combined is lower than that among the general population [73].

A recent review of the descriptive and analytic studies concerning agriculture and cancer reported excess risks of NHL among farmers in 11 of the 21 cohort or occupational survey studies [73]. Of 19 analytic studies, which included case-control and cross-sectional studies, 12 reported excess risks of NHL, of which 8 showed statistically significant associations. These studies showed that farmers and agricultural workers in several states and countries have an elevated risk of NHL. However, specific exposures which may account for the increased risk, were not identified. Farmers and farm workers may come into contact with a wide variety of agents including pesticides, fertilizers, animal viruses, bacteria and fungi, solvents, fuels and dusts. In addition, nitrate contamination of groundwater from agricultural sources is a significant problem in some areas of the country, and affects both farmers and the general population of these areas.

Evidence for associations of NHL with agricultural exposure to pesticides comes primarily from interview-based case-control studies. Phenoxyacetic acid herbicides have been associated with an increased risk of NHL in studies in Sweden, Italy, Canada and the USA [74]. In particular, the herbicide 2,4-D has been associated with a 50–200% excess of NHL, with the most frequent and/or heaviest exposure associated with a relative risk of 3–8 [75–77]. Canine malignant lymphoma has also been associated with dog-owner use of 2,4-D and/or commercial lawn-pesticide treatments [78]. Organophosphate insecticides may also play a role in the development of NHL [76,79–81]. Farmers' use of protective equipment was shown to reduce pesticide-associated risks [75,76,79].

The amount of pesticides used in agriculture and around the home has increased dramatically over the past 40 years [82,83]. Although the fraction of agricultural workers in the population is small and has been decreasing over time, pesticide exposure of the general population has been increasing. Exposure to pesticides occurs through use in homes, gardens and lawns, as well as indirectly through food and water. The US Environmental Protection Agency (EPA) has estimated that 91% of households occupying single family dwellings use pesticides in the house (84%), garden (21%) and lawn (29%) [84]. The use of lawn-care pesticides is increasing by 5–8% annually [85]. Pesticides are applied to lawns at five times the application rate used on pesticide-treated agricultural lands [86]. General population exposures may be lower than those in occupational settings and associated with a smaller risk. However, assuming that over 90% of the population is exposed, a relative risk as small as 1.2 could explain 15% of current NHL cases.

An ecologic study in Nebraska found a correlation of county-specific incidence rates with fertilizer use and the proportion of wells exceeding 45 mg/liter of nitrate (equivalent to 10 mg NO_3-N/liter, the EPA regulatory limit) [87]. In a cluster of six counties in the Platte River Valley in central Nebraska, the incidence of lymphoma is twice the national average [88]. A case-control study of NHL in Nebraska found a 20% increase in risk associated with drinking private well water with ≥10 p.p.m. nitrate–nitrogen compared to drinking well water with <10 p.p.m. nitrate–nitrogen [89]. Long-term exposure to lower nitrate levels from community supplies was also associated with an elevated risk of NHL (M. H. Ward et al., unpublished data).

OCCUPATIONAL EXPOSURES

Besides farming, employment in other occupations has been linked with an increased risk of NHL. Occupational groups at increased risk as demonstrated by cohort studies include rubber workers [90–92], chemists [93,94], chemical workers [95–97], dry cleaners [98], petroleum refinery workers [99,100], printing workers [101,102], abattoir workers [103,104], workers exposed to ethylene oxide [105,

106], beauticians and cosmetologists [107,108], and wood workers, including carpenters [109], saw-mill workers [110], and pulp- and paper-mill workers [111]. Case-control studies of NHL that have evaluated occupation as a risk factor for NHL are summarized in Table 6.2. Consistent with the findings from the cohort studies, case-control studies found excess risks among rubber workers [112], beauticians and cosmetologists [113,114] and wood workers [112,115–117]. An increased risk of NHL was seen with exposure to phenoxyacetic acids [112,115,118], chlorophenols [118] and solvents [112,115,118,119].

Solvent exposure has been linked to increased NHL risk in various industrial settings, including chemical manufacturing [97], the rubber industry [90], aircraft maintenance [120] and dry cleaning [98]. Solvents may play a role in the elevated risk of NHL observed for some occupational groups with substantial exposure, including chemists [93,94], chemical workers [95–97], highway workers [121] and petroleum-refinery workers [100,122]. Exposure assessment for particular chemicals has been difficult owing to changing patterns of use over time in response to the latest toxicologic data, price or availability. Nevertheless, benzene has been associated with NHL risk in a few studies [97,123,124].

HAIR DYE

Hair dyes contain compounds which are mutagenic and carcinogenic in animals [125]. Cosmetologists and hair dressers have been reported to have excesses of hematopoietic and lymphatic cancers [107,108, 126], but their dermal exposure to hair dye may be less than that of persons whose hair is being colored [127]. Personal use of hair-coloring products has been associated with an increased risk of NHL in two case-control studies [127,128] and one cohort study [129], but not another cohort [130]. Increases in risk were observed in men [127] and women [128,129]. Among female users, risks were higher among permanent hair-coloring product users than among semi- or non-permanent product users and were higher for users of dark colors [128]. Permanent black hair-dye use was associated with a significantly elevated risk of NHL among women who were long-term users, but other colors showed no association [129]. Hair-coloring products were estimated to account for 20% of NHL in the study by Zahm, based on an exposure prevalence of 46% among the controls [128]. The use by men was much lower in both that study (7% of the controls) and in the study by Cantor [127] (3% of the controls), but both investigations were conducted in rural populations and urban men may be more heavily exposed [127].

Table 6.2   Occupations and exposures with significantly or ≥ 2.0-fold increased risk of non-Hodgkin's lymphoma in case-control studies

Study [ref.]	Occupation/ Industry	Exposures	No. of cases exposed	Odds ratio	95% CI
Hardell et al. [118]	NS*	Organic solvents	45	2.4	1.4–3.9
	NS	Phenoxyacetic acids	25	5.5	2.7–11.0
	NS	Chlorophenols	35	4.8	2.7–8.8
	Mechanic	NS	5	2.5	0.7–9.6
	Smelting-house worker	NS	4	2.3	0.5–9.5
Persson et al. [115]	Nursing	NS	3	5.6	1.0–30.0
	Lumberjacks	Fresh wood	9	6.0	1.1–31.0
	NS	Welding	15	2.3	1.0–5.1
	NS	Phenoxy herbicides	10	2.3	0.7–7.2
	NS	Solvents	3	2.9	0.3–22.0
Blair et al.† [113]	Barbers, cosmetologists	NS	7	2.1	0.7–5.9
	Tool makers	NS	8	2.6	0.8–8.8
	Domestic service	NS	4	4.6	0.5–42.0
	Pouring, casting	NS	3	3.2	0.3–33.0
	Metal working	NS	3	3.5	0.4–34.0
	Type setters	NS	3	2.7	0.3–27.0
	Pavers	NS	3	3.4	0.6–21.0
	NS	Metals	221	1.3	1.0–1.6
Scherr et al. [116]	Carpenter, plumber, stone mason, roofer	NS	NS	12.0	2.0–72.0
	Painters, plasterers	NS	NS	6.0	0.9–38.0
	Agriculture, fishing, forestry	NS	NS	3.0	1.0–8.8
	Construction	NS	NS	2.1	1.0–4.6
	Leather	NS	NS	2.1	0.9–4.8
Band et al. [117]	Pulp and paper workers‡	NS	5	10.0	1.2–86.0
	Furniture	NS	5	5.0	1.0–26.0
	Excavating, grading	NS	7	2.0	0.7–5.7
Persson et al.§ [112]	NS	Solvents	33	2.0	NS
	NS	Styrene	3	8.0	NS
	NS	Plastic/rubber chemicals	9	2.5	NS
	NS	Creosote	5	13.6	NS
	NS	Phenoxy acids	6	2.7	NS
	Carpenters, cabinet makers	NS	10	3.1	NS
Franceschi et al.¶ [150]					
Cartwright et al. [144]	NS	Wood dust‖	60	1.5	1.0–2.1
	NS	Glues	59	1.8	1.2–2.6
Olsson and Brandt [119]	NS	Solvents**	71	2.0	1.5–2.6
La Vecchia [151]	Agriculture, food processing	NS	38	1.9	1.2–3.0
Giles et al. [114]	Farmers, laborers	NS	NS	1.9	1.0–3.3
	Foundry workers	NS	NS	8.0	1.1–356
	Miners	NS	NS	3.0	NS
	Hairdressers	NS	5	Inf††	NS

*NS, not specified.
†Industries with OR ≥ 2.0 included agriculture, forestry, masonry, textile, metal working, barbershops, funeral service.
‡Occupation; OR = 3.5 for pulp and paper industry.
§Self-reported exposures >1 year, 5-year latency.
¶No occupations or exposures with significantly increased risk or odds ratio ≥ 2.0.
‖No occupational associations were significant; exposures from occupation or hobby > 3 months.
**Daily exposure for ≥ 1 year.
††Inf, infinite.

DIET

An international correlational study found a positive relationship between per capita animal protein consumption, and mortality from both NHL and Hodgkin's disease [131]. Associations between dietary factors and the risk of NHL have been further evaluated in a prospective study in Norway [132], and in case-control studies in Italy [133] and Nebraska (USA) [134]. Both the Norwegian prospective study [132] and the Italian case-control study [133] found two-fold greater risks of NHL with high milk consumption (>2 glasses/day). The Nebraskan case-control study [134] found a 60% elevated risk of NHL for high milk consumption among men but not women. The case-control studies found no association with animal protein [134] or the frequency of consumption of beef, fish and eggs [133,134]. Nitrite (found mainly in processed meats) was not associated with NHL risk in Nebraska [134].

High intakes of carotenes, vitamin C, carrots, dark green vegetables and citrus fruit were inversely associated with the risk of NHL among men in the Nebraska study [134]. Among women, there was little overall association with NHL. The Italian case-control study found risks below 1.0 for intermediate and high intake levels of carrots and green vegetables, but the trends in risks were not significant [133]. No association was observed with intake of fresh fruit in this study, but high consumption of whole-grain bread and pasta was protective.

The Italian case-control study reported elevated risk for high consumption of coffee, tea and methylxanthine containing beverages as a group. In contrast, the Nebraska case-control study found no association with tea consumption and a decreased risk of NHL among men with high-frequency coffee intake (>21 times/week).

On the whole, the strongest dietary associations of NHL is with consumption of milk. Epidemiologic studies to date do not support a role for animal protein consumption and NHL risk. The inverse associations seen for fruits and vegetables, vitamin C and carotenes in one study are consistent with findings for other cancer sites, and deserve consideration in future studies of NHL.

BLOOD TRANSFUSION RECIPIENTS

Several recent studies have examined the risk of lymphoma in recipients of blood transfusions. In a population-based survey and follow-up of women in Iowa, those who had ever received blood transfusion had a 2.2-fold (95% confidence interval, 1.4–3.6)

relative risk of NHL [135]. Blood recipients discharged from a hospital in Sweden had a 2.7–3.1-fold (95% confidence intervals, 1.4–4.6 and 1.6–6.2, respectively) relative risk [136]. A two-fold, but statistically insignificant, relative risk was detected in recipients of neonatal transfusions in Britain [137]. While these effects are small enough to represent confounding, their consistency suggests a blood-borne agent may be responsible for some cases of this disease.

RADIATION

Radiation exposure probably has little effect on NHL risk [138]. Although early analyses of the Japanese atomic bomb survivors suggested increased NHL risk, recent analyses based on improved dosimetry and case identification did not confirm this finding [139]. Most studies of medical radiation exposures do not indicate an increase in risk, although in one study high-dose X-irradiation (for therapy of ankylosing spondylitis) was associated with a 2.2-fold increase [140]. Occupationally exposed groups have generally had no excesses of NHL, with the exception of American radiologists who practiced in the 1920s and 1930s [141].

FAMILIAL

Relatives of patients with NHL may be at increased risk for NHL [142,143]. In some instances, the aggregation is associated with a familial immunodeficiency, although in many families no such abnormality can be discerned. In a large population-based case-control study, a family history of leukemia or lymphoma was associated with a statistically significant 3.3-fold risk ratio for low-grade lymphoma, whereas high-grade lymphoma was not significantly increased [144]. In any case, familial cases account for considerably less than 5% of total lymphoma incidence.

OTHER

Other environmental exposures and medical conditions that have been linked with NHL are generally either rare, only weakly associated or based on inconsistent reports. Some cancer chemotherapeutic agents modestly increase the risk of NHL [142]. In particular, NHL may be a late outcome of intensive chemotherapy for Hodgkin's disease [145]. Medical conditions which may confer a small increase in NHL risk include asthma, allergies, arthritis, rheumatic fever, tuberculosis and infectious mononucleosis

[144,146]. Phenytoin infrequently induces a drug reaction resembling a pseudolymphoma but was not associated with frank NHL in a large case-control study [147]. There are inconsistent reports of a weak association between NHL and use of corticosteroids [144,148].

Conclusions

The non-Hodgkin's lymphomas are a diverse group of disorders with a complex set of etiologic factors. Modern pathological diagnosis of these tumors includes immunophenotyping, cytogenetics and molecular analysis with consequent advances in the understanding of their pathogenesis. Specific groups of lymphomas can now be associated with identifiable etiologies, which tentatively delineates distinct syndromes. However, such syndromes usually include several histological entities and different etiological groups overlap [1,149]. This may signify true etiological relationships or could reflect defects in present histological classification systems. While it is necessary to continue to study groups of lymphomas in most epidemiologic settings for a variety of practical reasons, it will be important to characterize individual tumors in as detailed a fashion as possible to determine whether particularly strong etiological relationships exist with well-defined pathological entities.

Although immunodeficiency is the strongest risk factor for NHL, other risk factors do not seem to be explicable simply in terms of diminished immune function. It would appear that a variety of insults to the complex factors governing lymphocyte differentiation and function may be ultimately manifested as NHL.

References

1. Weisenburger DD. Pathological classification of non-Hodgkin's lymphoma for epidemiological studies. *Cancer Res.* 1992, **52**: 5456s–5462s.
2. Wingo PA, Tong T, Bolden S. Cancer statistics, 1995. *CA Cancer J. Clin.* 1995, **45**: 8–30.
3. Ries LAG, Miller BA, Hankey BF, et al. (eds). *SEER Cancer Statistics Review, 1973–1991: Tables and Graphs, Non-Hodgkin's Lymphoma* (NIH Publication no. 94–2789). Bethesda, MD: National Cancer Institute, 1994, pp. 313–332.
4. *Cancer Incidence in Five Continents*, Vol. VI (IARC Scientific Publications no. 120). Lyon: International Agency for Research on Cancer, 1992,
5. Wright DH, Magrath IT (eds). *The Non-Hodgkin's Lymphomas, Pathogenesis of Non-Hodgkin's Lymphomas: Clues from Geography*. London: Edward Arnold, 1990, pp. 122–134.
6. Ji X, Li W. Malignant lymphomas in Beijing. *J. Environ. Pathol. Toxicol. Oncol.* 1992, **11**: 327–329.
7. Nanba K. [Pathology of malignant lymphomas]. *Rinsho Ketsueki* 1994, **35**: 433–438.
8. Devesa SS, Silverman DT, Young JL, et al. Cancer incidence and mortality trends among whites in the United States, 1947–84. *J. Natl Cancer Inst.* 1987, **79**: 701–770.
9. Devesa SS, Fears T. Non-Hodgkin's lymphoma time trends: United States and international data. *Cancer Res.* 1992, **52**: 5432s–5440s.
10. Rabkin CS, Devesa SS, Zahm SH, et al. Increasing incidence of non-Hodgkin's lymphoma. *Semin. Hematol.* 1993, **30**: 286–296.
11. Hartge P, Devesa S. Quantitation of the impact of known risk factors on time trends in non-Hodgkin's lymphoma incidence. *Cancer Res.* 1992, **52**: 5566s–5569s.
12. Kersey JH, Shapiro RS, Filipovich AH. Relationship of immunodeficiency to lymphoid malignancy. *Pediatr. Infect. Dis. J.* 1988, **7**: S10–S12.
13. Hoover RH, Fraumeni JF Jr. Risk of cancer in renal-transplant recipients. *Lancet* 1973, **ii**: 55–57.
14. Rabkin CS, Hilgartner MW, Hedberg KW, et al. Incidence of lymphomas and other cancers in HIV-infected and HIV-uninfected patients with hemophilia. *JAMA* 1992, **267**: 1090–1094.
15. Cleary ML, Sklar J. Lymphoproliferative disorders in cardiac transplant recipients are multiclonal lymphomas. *Lancet* 1984, **ii**: 489–493.
16. Selik RM, Starcher ET, Curran JW. Opportunistic diseases reported in AIDS patients: Frequencies, associations, and trends. *AIDS* 1987, **1**: 175–182.
17. Rabkin CS, Yellin F. Cancer incidence in a population with a high prevalence of HIV-1 infection. *J. Natl Cancer Inst.* 1994, **86**(22): 1711–1716.
18. Rabkin CS, Biggar RJ, Horm JW. Increasing incidence of cancers associated with the human immunodeficiency virus epidemic. *Int. J. Cancer.* 1991, **47**: 692–696.
19. MacMahon EME, Glass JD, Hayward SD, et al. Epstein–Barr virus in AIDS-related primary central nervous system lymphoma. *Lancet* 1991, **338**: 969–974.
20. Cinque P, Brytting M, Vago L, et al. Epstein–Barr virus DNA in cerebrospinal fluid from patients with AIDS-related primary lymphoma of the central nervous system. *Lancet* 1993, **342**: 398–401.
21. Ballerini P, Gaidano G, Gong JZ, et al. Multiple genetic lesions in acquired immunodeficiency syndrome-related non-Hodgkin's lymphoma. *Blood* 1993, **81**: 166–176.
22. Hamilton-Dutoit SJ, Pallesen G. A survey of Epstein–Barr virus gene expression in sporadic non-Hodgkin's lymphomas. Detection of Epstein–Barr virus in a subset of peripheral T-cell lymphomas. *Am. J. Pathol.* 1992, **140**: 1315–1325.
23. Shiramizu B, Herndier BG, McGrath MS. Identification of a common clonal human immunodeficiency virus

integration site in human immunodeficiency virus-associated lymphomas. *Cancer Res.* 1994, **54**: 2069–2072.

24. Takatsuki K, Uchiyama T, Sagawa K, et al. In Seno S, Takaku F, Irino S (eds) *Topics in Hematology, Adult T Cell Leukemia in Japan.* Amsterdam: Excerpta Medica, 1976, pp. 73–78.

25. Uchiyama T, Yodoi J, Sagawa K, et al. Adult T-cell leukemia: Clinical and hematologic features of 16 cases. *Blood* 1977, **50**(3): 481–492.

26. Poiesz BJ, Ruscetti FW, Gazdar AF, et al. Detection and isolation of type-C retrovirus particles from fresh and cultured lymphocytes of a patient with cutaneous T-cell lymphoma. *Proc. Natl Acad. Sci. USA* 1980, **77**: 7415–7419.

27. Blattner WA, Kalyanaraman VS, Robert-Guroff M, et al. The human type-C retrovirus, HTLV, in blacks from the Caribbean region, and relationship to adult T-cell leukemia/lymphoma. *Int. J. Cancer* 1982, **30**: 257–264.

28. Catovsky D, Greaves MF, Rose M, et al. Adult T-cell lymphoma-leukaemia in Blacks from the West Indies. *Lancet* 1982, **1** (8273): 639–643.

29. Tajima K, Kuroishi T. Estimation of rate of incidence of ATLL among ATLLV (HTLV-1) carriers in Kyushu, Japan. *Jap. J. Clin. Oncol.* 1985, **15**: 423–430.

30. Cleghorn FR, Manns A, Falk R, et al. Effect of HTLV-1 infection on non-Hodgkin's lymphoma incidence. *J. Natl Cancer Inst.* 1995, **87**: 1009–1014.

31. Murphy EL, Hanchard B, Figueroa JP, et al. Modelling the risk of adult T-cell leukemia/lymphoma in persons infected with human T-lymphotropic virus type I. *Int. J. Cancer.* 1989, **43**: 250–253.

32. Murphy EL, Figueroa JP, Gibbs WN, et al. Human T-lymphotropic virus type I (HTLV-1) seroprevalence in Jamaica: I. Demographic determinants. *Am. J. Epidemiol.* 1991, **133**: 1114–1124.

33. Tajima K and the T- and B-Cell Malignancy Study Group. The 4th nation-wide study of adult T-cell leukemia/lymphoma (ATL) in Japan: Estimates of risk of ATL and its geographical and clinical features. *Int. J. Cancer* 1990, **45**: 237–243.

34. Matutes E, Dalgleish AG, Weiss RA, et al. Studies in healthy human T-cell-leukemia lymphoma virus (HTLV-1) carriers from the Caribbean. *Int. J. Cancer* 1986, **38**: 41–45.

35. De Oliveira MS, Matutes E, Famadas LC, et al. Adult T-cell leukaemia/lymphoma in Brazil and its relation to HTLV-1. *Lancet* 1990, **336** (8721): 987–990.

36. Levine PH, Manns A, Jaffe ES, et al. The effect of ethnic differences on the patterns of HTLV-1 associated T-cell leukemia/lymphoma (HATL) in the United States. *Int. J. Cancer* 1994, **56**: 177–181.

37. Shimoyama M. Diagnostic criteria and classification of clinical subtypes of adult T-cell leukaemia–lymphoma. *Br. J. Haematol.* 1991, **79**: 428–437.

38. Manns A, Cleghorn FR, Falk RT, et al. Role of HTLV-1 in development of non-Hodgkin's lymphoma in Jamaica and Trinidad and Tobago. *Lancet* 1993, **342**, 1447–1450.

39. Usuku K, Sonoda S, Osame M, et al. HLA haplotype-linked high immune responsiveness against HTLV-1 in HTLV-1-associated myelopathy: Comparison with adult T-cell leukemia/lymphoma. *Ann. Neurol.* 1988, **23**: S143–S150.

40. Kamada N, Sakurai M, Miyamoto K, et al. Chromosome abnormalities in adult T-cell leukemia/lymphoma: A karyotype review committee report. *Cancer Res.* 1992, **52**: 1481–1493.

41. Sakashita A, Hattori T, Miller C. Mutations of the p53 gene in adult T-cell leukemia. *Blood* 1992, **79**: 477–480.

42. Manns A, Falk R, Murphy EL, et al. Risk factors for development of non-Hodgkin's lymphoma in Jamaica (meeting abstract). *Proc. Annu. Meet. Am. Assoc. Cancer Res.* 1990, **31**: A1358.

43. Tokunaga M, Imai S, Uemura Y, et al. Epstein–Barr virus in adult T-cell leukemia/lymphoma. *Am. J. Pathol.* 1993, **143**: 1263–1269.

44. Poplack DG, Magrath IT, Kun LE, et al. Leukemia and lymphomas of childhood. In DeVita VT, Hellman S, Rosenberg SA (eds) *Cancer Principles and Practice of Oncology.* Philadelphia: J.B. Lippincott, 1993, pp. 1792–1808.

45. Stiller CA, Parkin DM. International variations in the incidence of childhood lymphomas. *Pediatr. Perinat. Epidemiol.* 1990, **4**: 303–324.

46. Levine PH, Blattner WA. The epidemiology of human virus-associated hematologic malignancies. *Leukemia* 1992, **6**: 54s–59s.

47. Levine PH, Kamaraju LS, Connelly RR, et al. The American Burkitt's Lymphoma Registry: Eight years' experience. *Cancer* 1982, **49**: 1016–1022.

48. Burkitt D. A sarcoma involving the jaws in African children. *Br. J. Surg.* 1958, **46**: 218–223.

49. Haddow AJ. An improved map for the study of Burkitt's lymphoma syndrome in Africa. *East Afr. J. Med.* 1963, **40**: 429–432.

50. Epstein MA, Achong BG, Bann YM. Virus particles in cultured lymphoblasts from Burkitt's lymphoma. *Lancet* 1964, **i**: 702–703.

51. Nadkarni JS, Nadkarni JJ, Klein G, et al. EB viral antigens in Burkitt tumor biopsies and early cultures. *Int. J. Cancer.* 1970, **6**: 10–17.

52. deThé G, Geser A, Day NE, et al. Epidemiological evidence for causal relationship between Epstein–Barr virus and Burkitt's lymphoma from Ugandan prospective study. *Nature* 1978, **274**: 756–761.

53. Biggar RJ, Henle N, Fleisher G, et al. Primary Epstein–Barr virus infections in African infants. I. Decline of maternal antibodies and time of infection. *Int. J. Cancer.* 1978, **22**: 239–243.

54. Morrow RH, Kisuule A, Pike MC, et al. Burkitt's lymphoma in the Mengo districts of Uganda: Epidemiologic features and their relationship to malaria. *J. Natl Cancer Inst.* 1976, **56**: 479–483.

55. Biggar RJ, Lennette ET, Nkrumah FK, et al. Malaria, sex, and place of residence as factors in antibody response to Epstein–Barr virus in Ghana, West Africa. *Lancet* 1981, **ii**: 115–118.

56. Geser A, Brubaker G, Drapen CC. Effect of a malaria suppression program on the incidence of African Burkitt's lymphoma. *Am. J. Epidemiol.* 1989, **129**: 740–752.

57. Gunapala DE, Facer CA, Davidson R, et al. In vitro analysis of Epstein–Barr virus: Lost balance in patients with acute Plasmodium falciparum malaria. I. Defective T-cell content. *Parasitol. Res.* 1990, **76**: 531–535.

58. Lam KM, Syed N, Whittle H, et al. Circulating Epstein–Barr virus carrying B-cells in acute malaria. *Lancet* 1991, **337**: 876–878.

59. Shiramizu B, Barriga F, Neequaye J, et al. Patterns of chromosomal breakpoint locations in Burkitt's lymphoma: Relevance to geography and Epstein–Barr virus association. *Blood* 1991, **77**: 1516–1526.

60. Brubaker G, Levin AG, Steel CM, et al. Multiple cases of Burkitt's lymphoma and other neoplasms in families in the North Mara District of Tanzania. *Int. J. Cancer.* 1980, **26**: 165–170.

61. Nkrumah FK, Perkins IV. Sickle cell trait, hemoglobin C trait, and Burkitt's lymphoma. *Am. J. Trop. Med. Hyg.* 1976, **25**: 633–636.

62. Bodmer JG, Bodmer WF, Pickbourne P, et al. Combined analysis of three studies of patients with Burkitt's lymphoma. *Tissue Antigens* 1975, **5**: 63–68.

63. Jones EH, Biggar RJ, Nkrumah FK, et al. HLA-DR7 association with African Burkitt's lymphoma. *Hum. Immunol.* 1985, **13**: 211–217.

64. Biggar RJ, Nkrumah FK. Burkitt's lymphoma in Ghana: Urban–rural distribution, time–space clustering and seasonality. *Int. J. Cancer.* 1979, **23**: 330–336.

65. Aya T, Kinoshita T, Imai S, et al. Chromosome translocation and c-myc activation by Epstein–Barr virus and *Euphorbia tirucalli* in B lymphocytes. *Lancet* 1991, **337**: 1190.

66. Wotherspoon AC, Ortiz-Hidalgo C, Falzon MR, et al. *Helicobacter pylori*-associated gastritis and primary B-cell gastric lymphoma. *Lancet* 1991, **338**: 1175–1176.

67. Parsonnet J, Hansen S, Rodriguez L, et al. *Helicobacter pylori* infection and gastric lymphoma. *N. Engl. J. Med.* 1994, **330**: 1267–1271.

68. Wotherspoon AC, Doglioni C, Diss TC, et al. Regression of primary low-grade B-cell gastric lymphoma of mucosa-associated lymphoid tissue type after eradication of *Helicobacter pylori*. *Lancet* 1993, **342**: 575–577.

69. Hussell T, Isaacson PG, Crabtree JE, et al. The response of cells from low-grade B-cell gastric lymphomas of mucosa-associated lymphoid tissue to *Helicobacter pylori*. *Lancet* 1993, **342**: 571–574.

70. Mason TJ, McKay FW, Hoover R, et al. *Atlas of Cancer Mortality for US Counties: 1950–1969*. DHEW Publication no. (NIH) 75–780. Bethesda, MD: US Department of Health, Education and Welfare, 1975.

71. Burmeister LF. Cancer mortality among Iowa farmers, 1971–1978. *J. Natl Cancer Inst.* 1981, **66**: 461–464.

72. Cantor KP. Farming and mortality from non-Hodgkin's lymphoma: A case-control study. *Int. J. Cancer.* 1982, **29**: 239–247.

73. Blair A, Zahm SH. Cancer among farmers. *Occup. Med. State Art Rev.* 1991, **6**: 335–354.

74. Zahm SH, Blair A. Pesticides and non-Hodgkin's lymphoma. *Cancer Res.* 1992, **52**: 5485s–5488s.

75. Hoar SK, Blair A, Holmes FF. Agricultural herbicide use and risk of lymphoma and soft-tissue sarcoma. *JAMA* 1986, **256**: 1141–1147.

76. Zahm SH, Weisenburger DD, Babbitt PA. A case-control study of non-Hodgkin's lymphoma and the herbicide 2,4-dichlorophenoxyacetic acid (2,4-D) in eastern Nebraska. *Epidemiol.* 1990, **1**: 349–356.

77. Wigle DT, Semenciw RM, Wilkins K, et al. Mortality study of Canadian male farm operators: non-Hodgkin's lymphoma mortality and agricultural practices in Saskatchewan. *J. Natl Cancer Inst.* 1990, **82**: 575–582.

78. Hayes HM, Tarone RE, Cantor KP. Case-control study of canine malignant lymphoma: Positive association with dog owner's use of 2,4-dichlorophenoxyacetic acid herbicides. *J. Natl Cancer Inst.* 1991, **83**: 1226–1231.

79. Cantor KP, Blair A, Everett G, et al. Pesticides and other agricultural risk factors for non-Hodgkin's lymphoma among men in Iowa and Minnesota. *Cancer Res.* 1992, **52**: 2447–2455.

80. Newcombe DS. Immune surveillance, organophosphorus exposure, and lymphomagenesis. *Lancet* 1992, **339**: 539–541.

81. Zahm SH, Weisenburger DD, Saal RC, et al. The role of agricultural pesticide use in the development of non-Hodgkin's lymphoma in women. *Arch. Environ. Health* 1993, **48**: 353–358.

82. Zilberman D, Schmitz A, Casterline G. The economics of pesticide use and regulation. *Science* 1991, **253**: 518–522.

83. Osteen CD, Szmedra PI. *Agricultural Pesticide Use Trends and Policy Issues*. Economic Research Service Agricultural Economic Report no. 622. Washington: US Department of Agriculture, 1989.

84. Savage EP, Keefe TJ, Wheeler HW, et al. Household pesticide usage in the United States. *Arch. Environ. Health* 1981, **36**: 304–309.

85. US Government Accounting Office. Lawn care pesticides: Risks remain uncertain while prohibited safety claims continue (US.GAO/RCED-90–134). Washington: US Government Printing Office, 1990.

86. Pimental D, McLaughlin L, Zepp A. Environmental and economic impacts of reducing US agricultural pesticide use. In Pimental D (ed.) *Handbook of Pest Management in Agriculture*, Vol. 1. Boca Raton: CRC Press, 1993, pp. 679–680.

87. Weisenburger DD, Bogarki I, Kuzelka RD (eds) Nitrate Contamination. *Potential Health Consequences of Ground-water Contamination by Nitrates in Nebraska*. NATO ASI Series, vol. G30. Berlin: Springer-Verlag, 1991, pp. 309–315.

88. Caldwell GG, Rosendof RC, Lemon HM, et al. Epidemiology of leukemia–lymphoma in mid-Nebraska. *Nebraska Med. J.* 1973, **58**: 233–237.

89. Ward MH, Zahm SH, Weisenburger DD, et al. Diet and drinking water source: Association with non-Hodgkin's lymphoma in eastern Nebraska. In McDuffie HH, Dosman JA, Semchuk K, et al. (eds) *Human Sustainability in agriculture: Health, Safety, Environment.* Chelsea, MI: Lewis Publishers, 1995,

90. Wilcosky TC, Checkoway H, Marshall EG, et al. Cancer mortality and solvent exposures in the rubber

industry. *Am. Ind. Hyg. Assoc. J.* 1984, **45**: 809–811.

91. McMichael AJ, Spirtas R, Kupper LL. An epidemiologic study of mortality within a cohort of rubber workers, 1964–72. *J. Occup. Med.* 1974, **16**: 458–464.

92. Monson RR, Fine LJ. Cancer mortality and morbidity among rubber workers. *J. Natl Cancer Inst.* 1978, **61**: 1047–1053.

93. Li FP, Fraumeni JF Jr, Mantel N, et al. Cancer mortality among chemists. *J. Natl Cancer Inst.* 1969, **43**: 1159–1164.

94. Olin R, Ahlbom A. The cancer mortality among Swedish chemists graduated during three decades. *Environ. Res.* 1980, **22**: 154–161.

95. Ott MG, Teta MJ, Greenberg HL. Lymphatic and hematopoietic tissue cancer in a chemical manufacturing environment. *Am. J. Indust. Med.* 1989, **16**: 631–643.

96. Rinsky RA, Ott G, Ward E, et al. Study of mortality among chemical workers in the Kanawha Valley of West Virginia. *Am. J. Indust. Med.* 1988, **13**: 429–438.

97. Wong O. An industry wide mortality study of chemical workers occupationally exposed to benzene. I. General results. *Br. J. Indust. Med.* 1987, **44**: 365–381.

98. Blair A, Stewart PA, Tolbert PE, et al. Cancer and other causes of death among a cohort of dry cleaners. *Br. J. Ind. Med.* 1990, **47**: 162–168.

99. Thomas TL, Waxweiler RJ, Moure-Eraso R, et al. Mortality patterns among workers in three Texas oil refineries. *J. Occup. Med.* 1982, **24**: 135–141.

100. Wong O, Morgan RW, Bailey WJ, et al. An epidemiological study of petroleum refinery employees. *Br. J. Indust. Med.* 1986, 43: 6–17.

101. Greene MH, Hoover RN, Eck RL, et al. Cancer mortality among printing plant workers. *Environ. Res.* 1979, **20**: 66–73.

102. Zoloth SR, Michaels DM, Villalbi JR, et al. Patterns of mortality among commercial pressmen. *J. Natl Cancer Inst.* 1986, **76**: 1047–1051.

103. Johnson ES, Fischman HR, Matanoski GM, et al. Cancer mortality among white males in the meat industry. *J. Occup. Med.* 1986, **28**: 23–32.

104. Pearce N, Smith AH, Reif JS. Increased risks of soft tissue sarcoma, malignant lymphoma, and acute myeloid leukemia in abattoir workers. *Am. J. Indust. Med.* 1988, **14**: 63–72.

105. Bisanti L, Maggini M, Raschetti R, et al. Cancer mortality in ethylene oxide workers. *Br. J. Indust. Med.* 1993, **50**: 317–324.

106. Wong O, Trent LS. An epidemiological study of workers potentially exposed to ethylene oxide. *Br. J. Indust. Med.* 1993, **50**: 308–316.

107. Kono S, Tokudome S, Ikeda M, et al. Cancer and other causes of death among female beauticians. *J. Natl Cancer Inst.* 1983, **70**: 443–446.

108. Teta JM, Walrath J, Meigs JW, et al. Cancer incidence among cosmetologists. *J. Natl Cancer Inst.* 1984, **72**: 1051–1057.

109. Kawachi I, Pearce NE, Fraser J. A New Zealand cancer registry-based study of cancer in wood workers. *Cancer* 1989, **64**: 2609–2613.

110. Jappinen P, Pukkala E, Tola S. Cancer incidence of workers in a Finnish sawmill. *Scand. J. Work Environ. Health* 1989, **15**: 18–23.

111. Kogevinas M, Boffetta P, Saracci R, et al. *Proceedings of the Dioxin '90 International Conference, Review of Carcinogenic Risks in the Pulp and Paper Industry.* Bayreuth: Germany, 1990,

112. Persson B, Dahlander AM, Fredriksson M, et al. Malignant lymphomas and occupational exposures. *Br. J. Indust. Med.* 1989, **46**: 516–520.

113. Blair A, Linos A, Stewart P, et al. Evaluation of risks for non-Hodgkin's lymphoma by occupation and industry exposures from a case-control study. *Am. J. Indust. Med.* 1993, **23**: 301–312.

114. Giles GG, Lickiss JN, Baikie MJ, et al. Myeloproliferative and lymphoproliferative disorders in Tasmania, 1972–1980: Occupational and familial aspects. *J. Natl Cancer Inst.* 1984, **72**: 1233–1240.

115. Persson B, Fredriksson M, Olsen K, et al. Some occupational exposures as risk factors for malignant lymphomas. *Cancer* 1993, **72**: 1773–1778.

116. Scherr PA, Hutchison GB, Neiman RS. Non-Hodgkin's lymphoma and occupational exposure. *Cancer Res.* 1992, **52**: 5503s–5509s.

117. Band PR, Spinelli JJ, Gallagher RP, et al. Identification of occupational cancer risks using a population-based cancer registry. *Rec. Results Cancer Res.* 1990, **120**: 106–121.

118. Hardell L, Eriksson M, Degerman A. Exposure to phenoxyacetic acids, chlorophenols, or organic solvents in relation to histopathology, stage, and anatomical localization of non-Hodgkin's lymphoma. *Cancer Res.* 1994, **54**: 2386–2389.

119. Olsson H, Brandt L. Risk of non-Hodgkin's lymphoma among men occupationally exposed to organic solvents. *Scand. J. Work Environ. Health* 1988, **14**: 246–251.

120. Spirtas R, Stewart PA, Lee JS. Retrospective cohort mortality study of workers at an aircraft maintenance facility. I. Epidemiologic results. *Br. J. Indust. Med.* 1991, **48**: 515–530.

121. Maizlish N, Beaumont JJ, Singleton J. Mortality among California highway workers. *Am. J. Indust. Med.* 1988, **13**: 363–379.

122. Delzell E, Austin H, Cole P. Epidemiologic studies of the petroleum industry. *Occup. Med. State Art Rev.* 1988, **3**: 455–474.

123. Vianna NJ, Polan A. Lymphomas and occupational benzene exposure. *Lancet* 1979, **1**: 1394–1395.

124. Li GL, Linet MS, Hayes RB, et al. Gender differences in hematopoietic and lymphoproliferative disorders and other cancer risks by major occupational group among workers exposed to benzene in China. *J. Occup. Med.* 1994, **36**: 875–881.

125. Monographs on the Evaluation of Carcinogenic Risks to Humans. *Some Aromatic Amines and Related Nitro Compounds – Hair Dyes, Colouring Agents and Miscellaneous Industrial Chemicals.* Monograph 16. Lyon, France: International Agency for Research on Cancer, 1978,

126. Boffetta P, Andersen A, Lynge E, et al. Employment as hairdresser and risk of ovarian cancer and non-Hodgkin's lymphomas among women. *J. Occup. Med.* 1994, **36**: 61–65.

127. Cantor KP, Blair A, Everett G. Hair dye use and risk of leukemia and lymphoma. *Am. J. Public Health* 1988, **78**: 570–571.

128. Zahm SH, Weisenburger DD, Babbitt PA, et al. Use of hair coloring products and the risk of lymphoma, multiple myeloma, and chronic lymphocytic leukemia. *Am. J. Public Health* 1992, **82**: 990–997.

129. Thun MJ, Altekruse SF, Namboodiri MM, et al. Hair dye use and risk of fatal cancers in US women. *J. Natl Cancer Inst.* 1994, **86**: 210–215.

130. Grodstein F, Hennekens CH, Colditz GA, et al. A prospective study of permanent hair dye use and hematopoietic cancer. *J. Natl Cancer Inst.* 1994, **86**: 1466–1470.

131. Cunningham AS. Lymphomas and animal-protein consumption. *Lancet* 1976, **ii**: 1184–1186.

132. Ursin G, Bjelke E, Heuch I, et al. Milk consumption and cancer incidence: A Norwegian prospective study. *Br. J. Cancer* 1990, **61**: 456–459.

133. Franceschi S, Serraino D, Carbone A. Dietary factors and non-Hodgkin's lymphoma: A case-control study in the northeastern part of Italy. *Nutr. Cancer* 1989, **12**: 333–341.

134. Ward MH, Zahm SH, Weisenburger DD, et al. Dietary factors and non-Hodgkin's lymphoma in Nebraska (United States). *Cancer Causes Control* 1994, **5**: 422–432.

135. Cerhan JR, Wallace RB, Folsom AR, et al. Transfusion history and cancer risk in older women. *Ann. Intern. Med.* 1993, **119**: 8–15.

136. Blomberg J, Moller T, Olsson H, et al. Cancer morbidity in blood recipients – results of a cohort study. *Eur. J. Cancer* 1993, **29A**: 2101–2105.

137. Memon A, Doll R. A search for unknown blood-borne oncogenic viruses. A search for unknown blood-borne oncogenic viruses. *Int. J. Cancer.* 1994, **58**: 366–368.

138. Boice JD Jr. Radiation and non-Hodgkin's lymphoma. *Cancer Res.* 1992, **52**: 5489s–5491s.

139. Shimizu Y, Kato H, Schull WJ. Studies of the mortality of A-bomb survivors. 9. Mortality, 1950–1985: Part 2. Cancer mortality based on the recently revised doses (DS86). *Radiat. Res.* 1990, **121**: 120–141.

140. Darby SC, Doll R, Gill SK, et al. Long term mortality after a single treatment course with X-rays in patients treated for ankylosing spondylitis. *Br. J. Cancer* 1987, **55**: 179–190.

141. Matanoski GM, Sartwell PE, Elliott EA, et al. Cancer risks in radiologists and radiation workers. In Boice JD Jr, Fraumeni JF Jr (eds) *Radiation Carcinogenesis: Epidemiology and Biological Significance.* New York: Raven Press, 1984, pp. 83–96.

142. Greene MH. Schottenfeld D, Fraumeni JF Jr (eds) *Cancer Epidemiology and Prevention, Non-Hodgkin's Lymphoma and Mycosis Fungoides.* Philadelphia: W.B. Saunders Company, 1982.

143. Linet MS, Pottern LM. Familial aggregation of hematopoietic malignancies and risk of non-Hodgkin's lymphoma. *Cancer Res.* 1992, **52**: 5468s–5473s.

144. Cartwright RA, McKinney PA, O'Brien C, et al. Non-Hodgkin's lymphoma: Case control epidemiologic study in Yorkshire. *Leuk. Res.* 1988, **12**: 81–88.

145. Sont JK, van Stiphout WA, Noordijk EM, et al. Increased risk of second cancers in managing Hodgkin's disease: The 20-year Leiden experience. *Ann. Hematol.* 1992, **65**: 213–218.

146. Tielsch JM, Linet MS, Szklo M. Acquired disorders affecting the immune system and non-Hodgkin's lymphoma. *Prev. Med.* 1987, **16**: 96–106.

147. Bernstein L, Ross RK. Prior medication use and health history as risk factors for non-Hodgkin's lymphoma: Preliminary results from a case-control study in Los Angeles County. *Cancer Res.* 1992, **52**: 5510s–5515s.

148. Bernard SM, Cartwright RA, Bird CC, et al. Aetological factors in lymphoid malignancies: A case-control epidemiologic study. *Leuk. Res.* 1984, **8**: 681–688.

149. Banks P. Non-Hodgkin lymphoma time trends: Changes in pathologic classification over time. *Cancer Res.* 1992, **52**: 5453s–5455s.

150. Franceschi S, Serraino D, Bidoli E, et al. The epidemiology of non-Hodgkin's lymphoma in the north-east of Italy: A hospital-based case-control study. *Leuk. Res.* 1989, **13**: 465–472.

151. LaVecchia C, Negri E, D'Avanzo B, et al. Occupation and lymphoid neoplasms. *Br. J. Cancer* 1989, **60**: 385–388.

152. National Cancer Institute Sponsored Study of Classifications of Non-Hodgkin's Lymphomas. Summary and description of a working formulation for clinical usage. *Cancer* 1982, **49**: 2112–2135.

CHAPTER 7

Ontogeny, distribution and functions of T-lymphocytes

HENRIK GRIESSER AND TAK W. MAK

Introduction

T-lymphocytes are generated throughout life in the thymus after its colonization by lymphopoietic precursor cells. The survivors of radical intrathymic selection processes carry antigen-recognition molecules, the T-cell receptors for antigen (TCRs), on the cell surface. These receptors make T-cells react specifically with antigens from outside (such as microorganisms) or from within the host organism (e.g., malignant tumor cells). Unlike immunoglobulin molecules, TCRs do not recognize soluble antigens. They commonly interact with antigens bound to special presentation molecules encoded by the major histocompatibility complex (MHC) [1]. TCR binding is of low avidity; antigenic binding and subsequent T-cell activation therefore require additional coreceptors. TCR molecules are physically associated with a variety of surface molecules including CD3, CD4 or CD8, CD2, integrin receptors, CD45, or CD28 molecules. Such molecular ensembles elicit the complete response of a T-cell that specifically recognizes an antigen. Specific antigen binding transforms T-lymphocytes into blast cells and initiates their clonal expansion.

Different lineages of lymphocytes have different effector functions: destruction of virus-infected cells is mainly mediated by cytotoxic T-cells, and T-helper cells secrete hormone-like lymphokines that support antibody production by B-cells or expansion of cytotoxic T-cells. Helper cells typically express CD4 and interact with cells displaying MHC class II molecules. CD8 lymphocytes are primarily cytotoxic and recognize MHC class I molecules.

In this chapter we shall review the current knowledge and understanding of the TCR structure, the role of coreceptors, and the signal transduction events induced by activation of the receptor molecules. In addition, the various mechanisms that shape the TCR repertoire and regulate T-cell maturation will be discussed. Results from experiments in mice with designed germline mutations have greatly contributed to our understanding of thymic ontogeny and selection of the T-cell repertoire [2]. They will be referred to throughout this chapter to the extent that they provide clues for T-cell ontogeny and function in man.

The T-cell receptor, its coreceptors and ligands

THE T-CELL RECEPTOR

TCRs are disulfide-linked heterodimeric polypeptide molecules consisting mainly of α/β chains. In 5–10% of mature T-lymphocytes an alternative TCR is found composed of γ/δ chains [3–5]. Depending on glycosylation patterns and individual allelic variations, TCRα chains are 40–50 kD and TCRβ chains are 40–45 kD glycoproteins. Human TCR Cγ1 and Cγ2 encoded proteins are 35–55 kD and δ chains 40–60 kD. TCR chains attain a large diversity by the random rearrangement of multiple V, D and J genes, and by nucleotide sequence alterations at the V-D, D-D and D-J junctions. Together these rearranged gene segments encode the extracellular variable domain. TCRs interact through their V domains with antigens and MHC molecules. TCR C regions can be subdivided into four functional domains. The first distal extracellular domains of all four TCR polypeptides probably fold structurally like immunoglobulin C1 regions. Between these domains and the transmembrane spanning regions resides a third cystein residue encoded by a separate exon. The cystein residue is covalently bound to the equivalent cystein on the corresponding partner chain (α–β, γ–δ) by sulfhydral groups. This region is designated the connecting peptide or hinge region. The human Cγ2-encoded protein does not have a cystein residue at the hinge region and interacts with the δ chain noncovalently [6]. The third C region is hydrophobic, appears to span the membrane, and comprises positively charged amino acids at conserved sites. Finally, all TCR polypeptides have a very short intracellular cytoplasmic region with unknown function.

T-CELL CORECEPTOR MOLECULES

CD3

TCRs noncovalently associate with the CD3 complex, which consists of the invariant CD3γ, δ, ε, and the homodimeric ζ–ζ or, in mice, heterodimeric ζ–η chains. The η chain represents an alternatively spliced protein product of the ζ chain [7]. It remains to be shown whether an equivalent alternative splicing form of the human η chain exists at the protein level.

CD3 molecules transduce T-cell activation signals [8]. CD3 peptides have long cytoplasmic domains as compared to the short intracellular portions of TCR chains. These domains contain conserved amino acid motifs (Y-L) that are important for the communication with other molecules involved in signal transduction, such as ZAP-70 and its associated kinases [9,10]. CD3γ, CD3δ and CD3ε genes are tightly linked with genes encoding Thy-1 and the neural cell adhesion molecule (NCAM) on chromosome 11q23 [11]. Similarly, the CD2 and LFA-1 encoding genes closely map to chromosome 1p13 implying that this receptor/ligand pair has evolved from one ancestor gene [12,13]. Recent structural and functional data intimate very different roles for CD3γ, δ, ε on the one hand, and the ζ–ζ and ζ–η dimers on the other. ζ Chains are not members of the Ig superfamily and have important roles in the signal transduction of NK cells. Both chain compositions form two parallel signal transducing units, both being able to elicit interleukin-2 (IL-2) production [9].

CD4 and CD8

Mature T-cells express either the CD4 or the CD8 receptor on the surface which bind to nonpolymorphic regions of the MHC class II or class I molecules, respectively. These coreceptors stabilize the binding of the TCR complex to antigen and participate in signal transduction [14,15]. Recent experiments using CD4- and CD8-deficient mice confirmed that CD4 molecules are mainly responsible for helper activity. Mice without CD8 cells have severely impaired MHC I-dependent responses against viruses. However, mice lacking CD4 and mice without CD8 molecules still have rudimentary helper and cytotoxic responses [16,17].

CD4 molecules are expressed as monomers on the cell surface of T-cells, some monocytes and macrophages, follicular dendritic reticulum cells, Langerhans cells of the skin, thymic dendritic cells, some B-cells and microglial cells in the brain [18,19]. CD4 molecules probably interact with nonpolymorphic sites within MHC II domains [20]. CD4 contacts MHC II along a surface that includes one side of the CDR1-like and CDR3-like loops of the N-terminal domain, and a part of the second immunoglobulin-like domain [21]. After CD3 stimulation, CD4 molecules move in close association with the TCR/CD3 complex. Up to 90% of cellular protein tyrosine kinase (PTK) p56^{lck} is noncovalently bound to CD4 [22]. CD4-TCR/CD3 association and consequently antigen-specific signal transduction depends on the physical interaction between p56^{lck} and CD4 molecules [23,24].

CD8 molecules are transmembrane glycoproteins. They predominantly exist as disulfide-linked heterodimers of an α and a β chain. Sometimes two CD8α chains form a homodimer. A subset of human CD8+ intraepithelial lymphocytes (IEL) expresses such homodimers rather than the more usual CD8$\alpha\beta$ heterodimers [25]. Human T-cells can alter the relative number of CD8$\alpha\alpha$ and CD8$\alpha\beta$ dimers on the cell surface upon stimulation [26]. Heterodimers composed of CD8α and of the MHC I-like molecule, CD1a, have been described. CD8 molecules interact with a nonpolymorphic region on MHC I molecules [27]. The short cytoplasmic portion of only the CD8α chain (but not the CDβ chain) contains conserved cystein motifs at basic amino acid residues which mediate physical association with the tyrosine kinase, p56^{lck} [28,29]. Only 10–25% of p56^{lck} is associated with CD8α, and cross-linking of CD8 and p56^{lck} does not increase TCR-mediated signals. This differs from the functional findings for the CD4 – p56^{lck} association.

CD2

The CD2 glycoprotein is a member of the immunoglobulin superfamily. It is expressed at early stages of thymic T-cell differentiation and maintained on almost all peripheral T-cells [30]. CD2 binds with very high affinity to its ligand LFA-3 which is expressed on the surface of nearly all nucleated cells. The major role of CD2 molecules is the enhancement of the CD3/TCR-mediated response, particularly in resting and naive T-cells [30,31]. It is a major factor in stabilizing initial cell–cell interactions and adhesion before specific TCR activation. TCR activation on the other hand leads to increased CD2 surface expression. This interaction may be important for initial functional binding of T-helper (T$_H$) cells to antigen presenting cells, of cytotoxic T-cells to their targets, and of immature thymocytes to epithelial or bone marrow-derived stromal cells. CD2 molecules are physically associated with the transmembrane phosphatase CD45 which may mediate signalling through its associated kinases.

CD45

As discussed later in more detail, CD45 phosphatase activity is essential for CD2-mediated tyrosine kinase activation, phospholipase Cγ-1 (PLCγ-1) phosphorylation and IL-2 production [26,32]. CD45 is a major transmembrane glycoprotein making up about 10% of all surface molecules on leukocytes and hematopoietic progenitor cells [33]. The intracellular CD45 region comprises two subdomains, repeated in tandem, that contain protein tyrosine phosphatase activity. T- and B-cells express different isoforms of CD45 with a molecular weight ranging from 180 to 235 kD because of differential splicing of the four variable exons 4,5,6 and 7 in the NH$_2$-terminal domain of the molecule. Expression of different isoforms is specific for the cell type, differentiation stage and activation stage. Immature CD4+ CD8+ thymocytes, memory T-cells and macrophages mainly express the lowest molecular weight form of 180 kD, and B-cells express the highest molecular weight form of 220 kD. Other mature peripheral T-cells and CD4 or CD8 single positive thymocytes express multiple isoforms and can express more than one isoform on the surface [34,35]. Activated T-cells express low molecular weight, and resting T-cells, high molecular weight forms. Several different antibodies are able to detect the expression of variable exons or restricted epitopes of CD45. The CD45 isoforms, identifiable by anti-exon 4, anti-exon-5, and anti-exon 6 specific monoclonal antibodies, are also known as CD45RA, CD45RB and CD45RC, respectively. The antibody CD45RO recognizes the 180 kD low molecular weight form of CD45. Different isoforms of CD45 display major differences in glycosylation patterns and thus differences in negatively charged sugar residues on the cell surface. High molecular weight (HMW) forms might interfere with physical contacts of specific ligand/receptor pairs. Low molecular weight (LMW) CD45 isoforms which carry fewer sialic acid residues and less negative charge, may allow increased cell–cell interactions such as is found in activated and memory T-cells. Exon switching of CD45 molecules upon T-cell activation may also influence the interaction of CD45 with intercellular receptors present on other cells and/or lateral ligands expressed on the same cell [33]. Besides the association of CD45 with the TCR/CD3 complex, interaction also occurs with T-cell accessory molecules [36]. The integrin receptor LFA-1 preferentially associates with the HMW CD45 isoforms, whereas CD2 aggregates with LMW isoforms. CD4 and CD8 accessory molecules presumably interact with CD45RC.

T-CELL RECEPTOR LIGANDS

Major histocompatibility complexes

The TCR α/β receptors recognize antigen under physiological conditions only when it is presented on a cell surface in the context of a self-MHC molecule. This phenomenon is termed MHC-restriction [1]. TCR γ/δ cells, in contrast, can function as cytotoxic T-cells, without the need to recognize classical MHC class I or II molecules [3]. Although the tissue distribution and receptor gene usage of γ/δ T-cells is well known, the physiological role and the potential ligands of these lymphocytes are still unclear. Class I molecules are expressed on cells of almost all somatic tissues. Class II molecules are normally restricted to certain cell types such as macrophages, dendritic cells, B-cells and activated T-cells. The expression of MHC molecules is specifically regulated at the transcriptional level and can be influenced by cytokines (i.e., interferons). Peptides destined for presentation on MHC I molecules are generated from proteins degraded in the cytosol ('endogeneous antigens') and transported into the endoplasmic reticulum (ER) where they are complexed to MHC I [37,38]. These complexes then move to the plasma membrane via the Golgi complex and post-Golgi vesicles. MHC II molecules can also present peptides derived from proteins entering the cell from an outside milieu ('exogenous antigens') via mechanisms such as phagocytosis, endocytosis or internalization of membrane molecules.

MHC class I molecules contain an MHC-encoded α or heavy chain of 44 kD, and a non-MHC encoded, noncovalently associated 12 kD β or light chain known as β_2-microglobulin. Class II molecules are composed of a 32–34 kD α and a smaller 29–32 kD β chain. Class II α and β heterodimers complex with an invariant peptide chain in the ER and are then routed to an acidic endosomal/endolysosomal compartment. Class II heterodimers are loaded with peptides in phagolysosomes after degradation of the invariant chain. Ii chain is not required for initial folding or dimer formation but it may be required to complete the formation of class II molecules that are recognized in the ER as completely folded, properly assembled protein complexes [39]. Peptide/class II complexes are shuttled to the cell surface and corecognized by CD4+ T-lymphocytes. The number of naturally processed peptides bound to MHC I after infection of cells with live influenza virus probably ranges between 220 and 540 copies [40]. It has been suggested that MHC molecules are constitutively occupied by peptides and that different MHC alleles 'select' for different motifs ('anchors') out of the supply of foreign extra- and intracellular proteins [41].

Generation of V region diversity of the T-cell receptors

As members of the immunoglobulin gene superfamily, TCR molecules are structurally similar to immunoglobulin chains [42]. TCR molecules have a large extracellular portion consisting of a constant (C) and a variable (V) domain. The V region is assembled from two or three gene segments: a V segment, a short joining (J) gene segment, and (in TCRβ or TCRδ genes) a diversity (D) segment. An estimated 10^{19} different combinations occur for the TCR$\alpha\beta$ molecules [5]. The combinatorial diversity of the TCR$\gamma\delta$ molecules is lower (around 10^{13} combinations) [43] since at most 8 functional Vγ, 5 Jγ, 10 Vδ, 3 Dδ and 3 Jδ^- segments can be rearranged to form functional TCRγ and δ chain genes [44]. However, actual recombination frequencies might differ: the repertoire can be greatly shaped by genomic deletions of long stretches of V gene segments [45–47] and positive or negative selection of T-cells expressing certain TCR VDJ combinations during thymic maturation or post-thymic circulation. The momentary activation of lymphocyte subsets by environmental antigens, e.g., bacterial or retroviral superantigens, may also influence recombinatorial diversity [48–52]. The V region diversity of TCR$\delta\gamma$ molecules is likely to be much larger than estimated because of the extensive junctional diversity at the joining sites of V-D, D-D and J-D gene segments.

Germline V, D and J gene segments are flanked by a set of conserved nucleotides arranged as heptamers and nonamers. They function as recombination signal sequences for V-D, D-J or V-J joining, and as recognition elements for a recombinase enzyme system [53]. These signal sequences are separated by a nonconserved 'spacer'. The spacer situated 3' of the V or D gene segment is 21–23 bp long (about two turns of the DNA helix), while that located 5' of the D or J gene segment is 11–12 bp long (about one turn of the double helix). Flanking sequences with a one-turn spacer signal can only rearrange to a two-turn signal. This probably ensures joining of appropriate gene segments. Thus, only one V and one J can recombine, but more than one D segment can join. Dδ1-Dδ2, Dδ1-Dδ3 and Dδ1-Dδ2-Dδ3 joinings frequently occur [54]. Intervening DNA stretches are either deleted or retained, if the two segments are joined in an opposite transcriptional orientation (conversion). At the coding ends, the joining is commonly imprecise. Differential trimming of recombining gene termini by exonucleases and duplication of one or two nucleotides at the recombination cleavage sites (P-nucleotides) contribute to this phenomenon [55]. Introduction of up to six (in TCRδ gene recombinations even more) nucleotides between V-D, D-D, D-J or V-J junctions in every possible random sequence generates N diversity. The enzyme terminal deoxynucleotidyl transferase (TdT) mediates the addition of nontemplate N-nucleotides [56]. This process contributes most significantly the potential diversity of the immune receptor but it may also result in the generation of stop codons at the coding junctions [57]. Distinct regions of the TCR may interact separately with peptide antigens or with polymorphic epitopes of the surrounding MHC molecule [5]. TCR molecules, very similar to immunoglobulin receptor molecules, contain three hypervariable regions or so-called complementarity-determining regions (CDR) in the V domain. These hypervariable loops are clustered together to form the antigen/MHC binding site. The CDR1 and/or CDR2 regions of TCRα chains, encoded by V region genes, seem to play a role critical to the fine specificity of MHC recognition [58]. The β VDJ and α VJ joints encode the most variable portions of TCR (CD3) which may be mainly involved in T-cell antigen specificity [5,59]. Somatic hypermutation, one major mechanism for Ig V region diversity, has not been documented for TCR genes [5,44]. Lack of somatic mutation in TCR after completion of the thymic selection is an advantage. Secondary alterations of V regions could result in a loss of recognition of polymorphic self-MHC determinants or in the formation of high-affinity self-reactive T-cell clones.

Recombinase activity is at least in part initiated by products of two recombinase activating genes, RAG1 and RAG2. Expression of these genes strictly correlates with V(D)J recombinase activity. Their transcripts occur in pre-B- and pre-T-cells but not in later stages of lymphocyte development [60]. During T-cell development, RAG-1 gene expression does not seem to occur in prothymocytes or mature thymocytes either [61]. It is expressed in two waves in DN (CD4 and CD8 double negative) and DP (CD4 and CD8 double positive) thymocytes reflecting the start of TCRβ rearrangement and the transcription of the TCRα chain, respectively [62]. RAG1-deficient mice have small lymphoid organs because of a lack of mature B- and T-cells. The maturational arrest occurs at an early developmental stage in these animals. Development and function of natural killer (NK) cells (in which TCR homologues are postulated for antigen recognition) and development of macrophages and granulocytes is not impaired [63,64].

Genomic organization of the T-cell receptors

TCR polypeptides generally form mutually exclusive pairs of TCRαβ or TCRγδ heterodimers. Rarely, however, TCRδ chains can bind to a β chain in place of an α chain [65]. Because of allelic exclusion, each T-cell usually expresses only one TCR product [66].

T-CELL RECEPTOR α CHAIN GENES

The human TCRα chain gene maps to the long arm of chromosome 14 (14q11–12) [67] and harbors the TCRδ genes between its V and J region gene sequences (Figure 7.1). An estimated number of 44 Vα genes belonging to 32 subfamilies [68,69] are spread out over more than 750 kb [70]. An area of at least 50 kb of DNA contains 61 Jα gene segments [71–73]. D region coding sequences have not been identified but N region diversification seems to exist in the V-J junctional regions [74]. The α chain locus contains only one C region gene composed of four exons [71].

T-CELL RECEPTOR β CHAIN GENES

The TCRβ chain locus spans about 600 kb on chromosome 7q35 [75]. The 65 different V region genes belong to 26 subfamilies [69,76]. They map to the 5' end of the two D-J-C clusters [77]. All Vβ genes rearrange to both Jβ clusters with similar frequency [5,78]. The two constant region genes of the β chain are separated by approximately 8 kb from each other. Their amino acid sequences are highly homologous [79]. Two J gene clusters, Jβ1 and Jβ2, are each located 2–5 kb 5' to the constant region genes (Figure 7.1). They contain six and seven J gene segments, respectively. Rearrangements in the TCRβ locus more frequently involve D-Jβ2 than D-Jβ1 joinings, which results in the deletion of the DJCβ1 gene segments [80].

T-CELL RECEPTOR γ CHAIN GENES

The human TCRγ chain gene maps to the short arm of chromosome 7 (7p15) where it spans a distance of approximately 160 kb [81]. Only 10 of the 15 known Vγ segments undergo rearrangement, and only eight are functional (V2–5, V8–11) [82,83]. The other V genes are pseudogenes that are not expressed at the protein level due to transcriptional or translational defects. The five joining segments identified in the TCRγ locus so far belong to two groups comprising Jγ1.1, Jγ1.2 and Jγ1.3, residing upstream of Cγ1, and Jγ2.1 and Jγ2.3, located upstream of Cγ2 [84] (Figure 7.1). Both Cγ segments are structurally similar to the Cα and Cβ genes, but have three instead of four exons [85]. The first exon codes for the immunoglobulin-like domain, the second for the connector peptide that includes a cystein residue, and the third exon codes for the transmembrane and intracytoplasmic portions of the polypeptide. Exon II sequences in Cγ1 and Cγ2 are different. Cγ2 contains

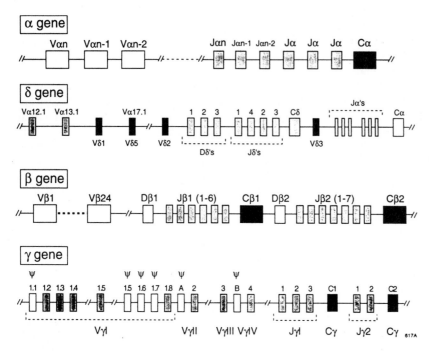

Figure 7.1 Organization of the human T-cell receptor (TCR) genes. All four TCR gene loci contain multiple variable (V) region genes and several joining (J) gene segments 5' to the one (TCRα and δ) or two (TCRβ and γ) constant (C) genes. Diversity (D) segments have been detected in the TCRδ and the TCRβ loci. The TCRδ genes are nested between the Vα and Jα gene clusters. Some of the Vγ genes have been mapped and their genomic localization is indicated. The TCRγ locus contains V pseudogenes (ψ). 5'–3', left to right.

two or three copies of the second exon but none of these code for the cysteine residue thought to be important for interchain disulfide linkage [86]. Thus, depending upon whether Cγ1 or Cγ2 is used, the TCRγ chain may associate with the TCRδ chain either covalently, forming disulfide bonds, or noncovalently [87].

T-CELL RECEPTOR δ CHAIN GENES

The TCRδ chain gene sequences are nested between the Vα and the Jα gene cluster. Only one Cδ region gene exists (Figure 7.1). The three joining gene segments (Jδ 1–3) are localized 3.4, 5.7 and 12 kb upstream of the first Cδ exon [88]. Most early fetal δ rearrangements involve C-proximal Jδ segments (Jδ3) while most δ chains at a later developmental stage and in peripheral T-cells use C-distal Jδ segments (Jδ1). Until now, six different functional Vδ genes have been characterized [69]. Vδ3 maps 3' to Cδ and upstream of Jα genes in an inverse orientation. Most of the $\gamma\delta$ T-cells use Vδ1 or Vδ2 [89], and T-cells of early ontogenic origin use predominantly Vδ2 segments [90]. The TCR α and δ locus can share these V region segments [3,91]. Four D gene segments have been characterized [92, 92a]. Since joining of several D segments can occur during recombination, variability of γ/δ heterodimers might be higher than one would expect from their limited number of functional V genes [54]. α/β TCR-bearing cells usually delete both alleles of the δ locus.

Regulatory genes for T-cell receptor rearrangements

Despite the use of a common recombinase [53], rearrangement processes are under tight regulation in both Ig and TCR genes. After V-(D)-J rearrangement a promoter 5' to the recombined V segment initiates transcription, which results in a primary RNA message. The sequences between V-D-J and C exons are excised by splicing and the final, processed mRNA is translated into a TCR polypeptide.

Promoters at the transcriptional start sites of V genes control the initiation of TCR transcription. TCR promotors are active in cells of both TCR$\alpha\beta$ and TCR$\gamma\delta$ lineage [93]. The promoter regions contain a binding site for leucine zipper transcription factors (TFs) belonging to the cyclic-AMP-responsive element binding protein/activating transcription factor (CREB/ATF) family [94]. Though the promoter itself is not T-cell specific, it may potentiate the activity of the 3' enhancer. Promoter genes are additionally controlled by multiple upstream regulatory sequences comprising regulatory binding sites for tissue specific and promiscuous, *trans*-acting TFs. Enhancers can increase transcriptional activity (after initiation by a promoter) independent of their genomic orientation and location. The enhancers for the different TCRs contain similar binding sites for TFs such as GATA-3, TCF-1, CREB proteins, core binding factors (CBFs), and *ets* [95]. Ets expression becomes detectable late in murine thymic ontogeny, coinciding with TCRα gene expression [96]. It thus represents a candidate trigger factor for TCRα gene expression [97]. GATA-3, a zinc finger protein, is expressed very early in T-cell development and may be one factor that determines T-lineage commitment in lymphoid precursor cells [95]. Promoters located in the 5' flanking region of the Vβ genes (Vβ promoters) interact with a potent transcriptional enhancer located 3' of the Cβ2 gene segment [98,99]. This, the 3' enhancer is not deleted during the recombinational events and its activation is required for significant transcriptional activity of the TCR promoters [94]. TCRβ gene expression may be limited to αβ T-cells because only in αβ T-cells are Vβ promoters brought, by gene rearrangement, into proximity with the enhancer [95]. The presence of silencers that limit enhancer activity has been postulated. A *cis*-regulatory element located between Cα and the TCRα enhancer in murine TCRγδ cells silences the TCRα enhancer independent of distance and orientation [100]. Downregulation of this silencer activates the TCRα enhancer and may initiate deletion of the TCRδ genes as circular DNAs during TCRα rearrangement. This could be one of the mechanisms responsible for lineage determination in TCRαβ lymphocytes. Negative transcriptional regulation of the TCRγ locus occurs in murine αβ T-cells. This is probably exerted by a putative silencer located 3' of the murine Cγ1 gene segment [101]. This could explain the absence of TCRγ mRNA in freshly isolated αβ T-cells with productive VDJ TCRγ rearrangement [102].

The human TCRα enhancer maps 4.5 kb downstream of the Cα gene and consists of two small TF binding sequences (Tα1 and Tα2). Tα2 functions as a potent transcriptional activator in the context of the TCRα enhancer. Depending on its physical relationship to other regulatory elements, it has also been shown in Jurkat cells to function as an effective transcriptional repressor, e.g., when positioned upstream or downstream of several promoter and enhancer elements [103]. In addition, a regulatory sequence designated TEA (T early alpha) located between Vδ2 and the Jα gene cluster has been described [104]. Cells of the αβ lineage delete TEA along with the complete DJCδ locus on both chromosomes, but TEA is present in TCRγδ cells, and may regulate lineage determination in this T-cell subset. Similar structural relationships in the promoter/enhancer regions is found in TCRα and γ genes.

T-Cell ontogeny and thymic selection

The progress of stem cell migration begins at the seventh week of gestation in the human embryo. The origin of these cells from sites in which hematopoiesis occurs, such as fetal liver and adult bone marrow, is well established. Proliferation of lymphocytes in the thymus depends upon the interaction of various interleukins and possibly other unknown growth signals. Thymocyte proliferation precedes TCR expression and is independent of the pathways involved in antigen-driven proliferation of mature peripheral T-cells; indeed, stem cells that enter the thymus have not yet initiated the process of gene rearrangement required for the production of functional T-cell receptors for antigens. Thymocytes develop along either the γδ or αβ T-cell lineage, undergoing TCR gene recombination that generates a large repertoire of individual TCR V gene combinations. The variable regions are approximated to their respective C region genes by RNA splicing [66].

T-CELL ONTOGENY

From gestational week 7 onwards, putative prothymocytes with cytoplasmic CD3 (cCD3) positivity have been identified in the fetal liver. These immature cells are TdT− and express no class II molecules, but do express CD7 and CD45 [105]. Once they have entered the thymus, immature thymocytes are committed to the T-cell lineage, and express cCD3 and TdT. These most immature thymocytes are large blasts and intermediate-sized cells, and have the highest TdT expression level and the highest proliferative activity of all thymocytes. They are CD4− and CD8− double negative (DN), CD2+, CD1−, and TCRβ−, since the rearrangement of β genes probably takes place at this stage and the β genes are therefore not yet functional. More than 90% of cCD3+ cells also express IL-2 receptor (IL-2R) at 8.5 weeks [106]. In the next stage of differentiation, common thymocytes are cCD3+ and TdT−. They have a medium level of proliferative activity and are distinguished by the appearance of cytoplasmic TCRβ expression. Since these cortical thymocytes are beginning to rearrange their α genes, TCRαβ is not yet expressed. Typically, these cells are CD4 and CD8 double positive (DP), CD1+ and CD2+. Mature thymocytes characterize the last stage of thymic development. They are either CD4 or CD8 single positive (SP), TdT−, CD1−, membrane CD3+ (mCD3+, CD2+ and TCRαβ+) (Figure 7.2).

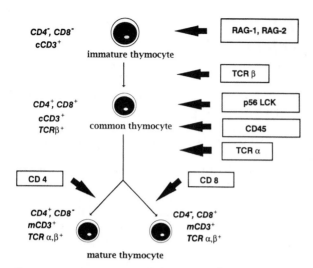

Figure 7.2 Impairment of thymocyte development by gene inactivation. Designed germline mutations in mice show that deficiency of recombinase activating gene (RAG) products, TCRβ and γ molecules, p56*lck*, CD45, CD4 and CD8 leads to arrests at distinct stages of thymocyte development (arrow heads). The main thymocyte subpopulations are depicted, and their expression profiles of CD4, CD8, cytoplasmic (c) or membrane-bound (m) CD3, and TCRα/β are indicated.

The exact order in which the various TCR chain genes rearrange, is unknown. What data there are on this issue are derived mainly from studies in the murine system and molecular analyses of thymic T-cell leukemias, which are presumed to have been arrested at different developmental stages. In mice, rearrangements in the TCRδ locus appear to precede recombination of the other TCR genes [80,107,108]. The TCRγ genes rearrange before the TCRβ genes. Productive TCRβ rearrangement on one allele leads to receptor protein translation. This blocks recombination of the TCRβ locus on the other chromosome, a phenomenon termed allelic exclusion [109]. Rearrangement at the TCRβ locus occurs at the DN stage and precedes rearrangement at the TCRα locus [52,105,110]. Unlike the TCRβ protein, the TCRα protein does not feedback and prevent further TCRα rearrangement. Thus, mature T-cells can have two productive TCRα genes as has been observed in human T-lymphocytes [111]. After expression of a functional TCR and following positive and negative selection, remaining thymocytes differentiate into mature SP cells [112].

From 9.5 weeks to birth TCRβ+ cells expand until they comprise more than 90% of all CD7+ cells. At the same time, the proportion of TCRδ+ cells fall from a peak of 11% of CD7+ cells at 9.5 weeks to 1% of CD7+ cells at birth. These data suggest that CD7+, CD2+, cCD3+ T-cell precursors in man produce

TCRδ T-cells as well as T-cells expressing αβ. Furthermore, DN and mCD3– thymocytes differentiate in culture into mature γδ T-cells [113]. The division between αβ and γδ lineages can probably occur during or after TCRβ rearrangement since the TCRβ gene is frequently rearranged in γδ T-cells [114].

IDENTIFICATION OF PIVOTAL EVENTS IN THYMOCYTE DIFFERENTIATION THROUGH GENE DELETION

More detailed knowledge about molecules involved in rearrangement events, accessory T-cell receptor molecules and signal transducing molecules has come from investigations in mice carrying germline mutations in the genes encoding these proteins [2]. Central to this approach is the introduction of a so-called 'targeting vector' – a DNA construct which contains a disrupted version of the gene of interest – into totipotent embryonic stem (ES) cells. Occasionally, homologous recombination occurs with one of the two normal copies of the gene and renders this copy inactive. Cloned cells containing the disrupted gene are injected into blastocysts of an appropriate mouse strain which are then implanted into a foster mother. If the mutant gene contributes to the germline in the mosaic mice that develop from these blastocyts, progeny animals will be heterozygous at the targeted locus. Cross-breeding of heterozygotes will then produce homozygotes. The latter 'knock-out' mice can be examined for the consequences of gene deprivation (Figure 7.2).

Inactivation of the RAG-1 or the RAG-2 gene leads to an absence of any V(D)J rearrangements. Thymocyte maturation stops at a very early DN stage and mature T- and B-cells are missing [63,64].

In mice with a genomic deletion in the TCRβ locus spanning a region between Dβ1 and downstream Cβ2 thymocytes are arrested at an early developmental stage prior to massive cell proliferation [115], demonstrating the importance of TCRβ rearrangement to the DP cell expansion. TCRβ–/– thymocytes lack any detectable TCR expression. However, substantial recombination of the TCRα has been detected suggesting that TCRβ rearrangement is not a prerequisite for TCRα rearrangement. Maturation of γδ cells does not depend on a functional TCRβ locus either. These data suggest that expression of TCRβ is necessary to drive DN IL-2R+ thymocytes to the DP stage.

A targeted disruption of the TCRδ gene causes the complete absence of γδ T-cells. This mutation, however, does not affect the development of thymocytes expressing TCRαβ receptors [116]. The thymocyte populations from TCRβ/TCRδ double knock-out mice, however, contain only DN thymocytes and the number of thymocytes is lower than in TCRβ-deficient mice [115]. This suggests that the DP thymocytes in TCRβ–/– mice are committed to the γδ lineage.

The arrest in TCRα chain disrupted mice occurs later in thymocyte ontogeny than in TCRβ-deficient mice [115,117]; maturation ceases at the DP stage and SP thymocytes are not detectable. The numbers of DN and DP thymocytes are normal but CD4 and CD8 SP cells are virtually absent. Thus, TCRα chain expression is not limiting for the progression of thymocytes from the DN to the DP stage and for the expansion of DP cells. TCRα and possibly the expression of functional αβ heterodimers is, however, required for the transition to the SP stage. Rearrangement of TCRα is observed in TCR Cα disrupted thymocytes at reduced levels, but rearrangement of TCRβ in these mice occurs as extensively as in normal mice. This suggests that a functional TCRα locus is not necessary for TCRα or TCRβ rearrangement. Maturation of γδ T-cells appears to proceed normally in these mice.

Mice lacking CD3ζ chains are almost devoid of DP thymocytes and have greatly reduced numbers of peripheral T-cells [118]. The few αβ T-cells express only low levels of TCR and their proliferation is impaired. TCRγδ IEL are not obviously affected by this germline deletion [119]. These results support the importance of the ζ chain for thymocyte differentiation. But they also show that this molecule is not absolutely required for the generation of SP T-cells and might be dispensable for γδ T-cell development.

CD4–/– mutant mice have markedly decreased helper cell activity but CD8+ T-cells develop and function normally. Thus, the expression of CD4 on progenitor cells and DP thymocytes may not be obligatory for development [16]. Normal mice have an extremely small proportion of DN T-cells in the periphery, but in CD4-deficient mice up to 15% of peripheral T-cells are DN. Cytotoxic T-cell (CTL) activity against virus-infected cells is undetectable in CD8 knockout mice. Clearance of the virus from the host organism is strongly impaired and virus titers stay high after infection. Development and function of the CD4+ T-lymphocytes, however, are not affected [17,120]. The introduction of specific TCR transgenes into CD8–/– mice showed that CD8 expression is necessary for positive selection of thymocytes carrying the transgenes [121].

CD2 is expressed very early in thymic ontogeny, but thymocyte development and selection are not affected in CD2–/– mice [122].

CD45 isoform expression is known to correlate with thymic selection events [35]. Recently, there-fore, mice were generated with a targeted deletion of exon 6 of the CD45 molecule to determine the effect of this on thymocyte differentiation [123]. The phosphotyrosine phosphatase (PTPase) domain of CD45 probably interacts with the tyrosine kinases $p56^{lck}$ and $p59^{fyn}$ leading to dephosphorylation of the negative regulatory sites of these *src* family members [124,125]. Disruption of exon 6 of the CD45 gene results in an impairment of thymocyte differentiation at the transition from DP to SP cells. Expression of all CD45 isoforms is almost undetectable. Thus, CD45 PTPase activity has a pivotal role at the transition of the DP to SP stage of the thymocyte developmental program. This may at least be partially due to a lack of dephosphorylation of the tyrosine kinase $p56^{lck}$. In CD45 exon 6–/– mice, DP thymocytes have upregulated levels of CD4 and CD8. The maturational block of CD45 exon 6–/– thymocytes may be at a later stage than the block in $p56^{lck}$–/– thymocytes. This suggests that in CD45 exon 6–/– mice, so far unidentified PTPases mediate the activation of $p56^{lck}$ required in early thymic differentiation. As in $p56^{lck}$–/– mice, very few T-cells are present in the periphery of CD45 exon 6–/– animals and CD8+ cytotoxic T-cells are undetectable after infection with LCM virus. However, in contrast to $p56^{lck}$–/– T-cells, mitogen activation and TCR cross-linking cannot induce a proliferative response in T-cells derived from CD45 exon 6–/– mice.

Targeted mutation of the $p56^{lck}$ gene results in a dramatic reduction of thymocytes in the resultant knockout mice (8×10^6) [126]. The number of DP cells is drastically reduced, thymocyte maturation is blocked at the early DP stage and mature SP lymphocytes are almost undetectable, but CD4 and CD8 expression levels on DP thymocytes are comparable to wild-type levels. In contrast, the development of intestinal γδ TCR-positive extrathymic IEL seems not to be affected by the absence of $p56^{lck}$, suggesting a differential dependency of $p56^{lck}$ for the thymus-derived and thymus-independent T-cells. CD4–8– thymocytes bearing a transgenic γδ TCR, however, remain severely impaired in their development in $p56^{lck}$-deficient mice [127]. Taken together these findings suggest that $p56^{lck}$ has an essential function in early thymocyte development that is independent from its association with CD4 and CD8.

Thymocytes upregulate their IL-2R during ontogeny suggesting a role for IL-2 in thymic maturation [128]. In humans, a congenital defect in IL-2Rγ chain leads to a severe combined immunodeficiency (SCID) syndrome. The absence or marked reduction of T-cells in association with thymic hypoplasia suggests an essential role for IL-2Rγ in thymocyte maturation [129]. Mice deficient for IL-2, however, have an apparently normal thymocyte development and normal peripheral T-cell populations, although *in vitro*, proliferative responses after polyclonal T-cell stimulation are impaired. The addition of exogenous IL-2 restores this defect [130]. At a younger age, the *in vivo* immunoresponsiveness of IL-2–/– mice is surprisingly normal. Ig production of B-cells is reduced but still efficient and NK cell activity remains detectable [131]. Thus, other mediators may be able to substitute for IL-2, at least in part. IL-2 binds to a cell surface receptor complex comprising at least three components (α, β, γ) [128], and it is possible, therefore, that IL-2R has additional ligands, or that individual components of the IL-2R also contribute to other receptor complexes.

THYMIC SELECTION

Thymocytes of the TCR$\alpha\beta$ lineage are subject to thymic selection that shapes the TCR repertoire of the peripheral T-lymphocyte population for self-MHC restriction, self-tolerance and immunocompetence. This ensures that only the most useful lymphocytes enter the peripheral pool.

Two main processes contribute to thymic selection. The intrathymic process that generates differentiated functional T-cells competent to interact with antigen bound to MHC molecules is termed positive selection. Positive selection occurs when the $\alpha\beta$ TCR binds to an MHC molecule in the absence of the specific peptide which would be recognized by the TCR of mature T-cells. Developing CD4+8+ thymocytes continue to express new $\alpha\beta$ TCRs until they are positively selected and the receptor is fixed, or until the cells die. Negative selection possibly eliminates thymocytes with high affinity to self-antigens. T-Cells with no affinity to self-MHC and associated antigen probably perish by programmed cell death as well [132].

Two obvious candidates for cells that actually present TCR-reactive peptides or epitopes to the developing T-cells are known: epithelial cells that form the nonlymphoid framework of the thymus, and specialized antigen presenting cells known as dendritic cells, which invade the thymic rudiment from the bone marrow about half way through intrauterine life. Bone marrow-derived accessory cells, mainly dendritic cells, can deliver the lethal signal in many but not necessarily all models [133]. Thymic epithelial cells are largely responsible for positive selection, but studies from thymic epithelial cell lines suggest that they can participate in negative selection of thymocytes as well [134]. Recent results from transgenic mice suggest that a single thymocyte clone can either be negatively or positively selected by the same peptide–MHC complexes depending on

the avidity of the interaction between the TCRs and the peptide–MHC complexes [135,136]. In the so-called differential avidity model positive selection occurs when the avidity is relatively low. When the avidity exceeds this low range, the thymocytes undergo negative selection [137].

Two models have been proposed to account for CD4 and CD8 lineage commitment. In a stochastic/selective model, SP T-cells are generated irrespective of TCR specificity; rescue from cell death requires co-engagement of TCR and the matched coreceptor (either CD4 or CD8), i.e., one capable of binding to the same MHC molecule as the TCR. The instruction model postulates that co-engagement of TCR, CD8 and MHC class I on DP thymocytes leads to generation of a signal distinct from that generated by co-engagement of TCR, CD4 and MHC class II, resulting in a downregulation of the unengaged coreceptor (either CD4 or CD8) and selection [50]. The instruction model predicts that CD4 SP and CD8 SP thymocytes always have TCRs and coreceptors that recognize the same MHC molecule. The stochastic/selection model predicts instead that some SP cells will have mismatched TCRs and coreceptors and therefore fail to mature.

Recently, analysis of thymocyte commitment of MHC class II β chain–/– and MHC class I-associated β_2-microglobulin–/– mice has provided evidence for the stochastic/selective model [138,139]. Cells from mutant animals lacking the Ii chain show aberrant transport of class II molecules resulting in a moderately reduced level of class II heterodimer expression at the cell surface [140]. This suggests that without the Ii chain, MHC class II molecules are not delivered to compartments that generate the appropriate antigenic peptides. This predictably affects the CD4+ T-cell compartment in these mutant mice. Thymocyte development of SP CD4+ cells is disturbed and negative selection appears impaired. β_2-microglobulin-deficient mice express little if any functional MHC class I antigen on the cell surface. Strikingly, CD8+ T-cells are absent showing that MHC class I molecules are critical in a positive selection of CD8+ T-lymphocytes [141]. These MHC class I knockout mice displayed similar functional losses in cytotoxicity as the CD8–/– mutant mice. This confirms that CD8 is essential for the maturation and positive selection of MHC class I-restricted cytotoxic T-lymphocytes but is unnecessary for the MHC class II restricted T-helper cells [17].

The concept of positive and negative thymic selection has been confirmed by experiments with TCR transgenic mice [142]. The nature of the ligands presented by thymic epithelial cells to induce positive selection and the requirements for the selection processes are still under investigation. Studies in MHC class I transgenic mice and in mice with mutant CD8 genes introduced in the germline emphasize the importance of corecognizing MHC class I molecules by the TCR and the CD8 receptor during thymic selection [17,143].

Positively selected cells eventually leave the thymus and patrol the body as long-lived resting lymphocytes. Reactivation can occur as a rule only by foreign peptides presented by self-MHC. Immune activation normally involves T-cells leaving the G_0 state, entering the cell cycle and creating a clone of progressively more differentiated immunological effector cells, e.g., cytokine-secreting T-cells. This is called clonal selection. By analogy, deletion of a self-reactive lymphocyte is termed clonal deletion. However, lymphocytes can be functionally silenced by antigen without being killed. The term clonal anergy describes this state of unresponsiveness [144]. Pre-activated effector T-cells undergo apoptosis when they encounter self-antigen presented in context with self-MHC but in the absence of 'professional' antigen presenting cells (APC) [145,146]. Anergy induction or apoptosis of activated T-lymphocytes also happens in the periphery as part of extrathymic negative selection events.

The selective processes acting on TCR $\gamma\delta$ cells probably differ from those known for TCR $\alpha\beta$ cells.

They apparently belong to separate intrathymic lineages [115]. There is evidence for intrathymic selection of cells expressing certain $\gamma\delta$ heterodimers in mice [147,148], but the repertoire of this T-cell population also can be influenced by extrathymic expression of MHC or MHC-like molecules [149, 150]. The nonrandom pairing of protein products of the γ-δ chains could thus result from thymic or peripheral selection [44].

Signal transduction in T-cells

Specific TCR-mediated interactions have to signal the lymphocyte into proliferation and nonproliferative effector functions, such as production of cytokines or cytotoxic substances. Cellular stimulation prompts a signal transduction from the cell surface to the cytoplasm and nucleus, inducing gene transcription and a response. Signalling is organized in cascades and ultimately results in activation or inactivation of other regulatory molecules and transcription factors. TCR molecules are physically associated with a variety of other surface molecules including CD3, CD4 or CD8, CD2, integrin receptors, CD45 or CD28 molecules. All of these molecules cooperate

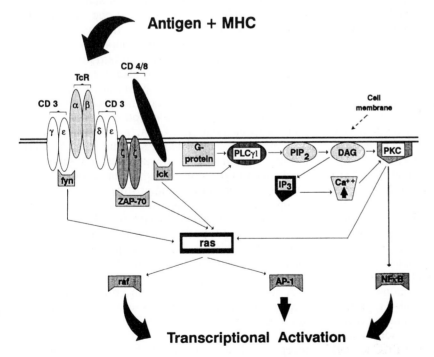

Figure 7.3 Signal transduction in $\alpha\beta$ T-cells following antigen stimulation. The cytoplasmic domains of the TCR coreceptors CD8 and CD4 are associated with the protein tyrosine kinase p56[lck]. The CD3 complex signals through the hematopoietic form of the PTK p59[fyn]; the ζ-chain homodimer interacts with the PTK ZAP-70. Following ligation of the TCR complex signalling can occur either through a protein kinase C (PKC)-independent PTK-induced p21[ras] activation or through a PKC-dependent pathway.

Tyrosine phosphorylation and/or GTP-binding (G-) proteins induce phospholipase Cγ1 (PLCγ) activity. PLCγ hydrolyzes phosphatidylinositol-4,5-biphosphate (PIP$_2$) into inositol-1,4,5-triphosphate (IP$_3$) and diacylglycerol (DAG). IP$_3$ mobilizes calcium ions that together with DAG activate PKC. This recruits among others transcription factors such as NFκB and activates p21[ras]. Direct PTK-mediated *ras* activation as well controls transcription factors (TFs) such as c-*jun*/c-*fos*, which together form the AP-1 complex, and p74[raf]. Cytoplasmic *raf* may then translocate to the nucleus and phosphorylate nuclear TFs.

with respect to their receptor and signal transducer functions and induce a response in a T-cell upon antigen recognition (Figure 7.3). Activation of T-lymphocytes through the T-cell receptor results in the progression of cells into the cell cycle (G_0–G_1) and the production of the growth factor IL-2 and its receptor [151]. The interaction of IL-2 with its receptor is essential for cell cycle progression from G_1 to S phase, and its commitment event in triggering T-cell proliferation. Induction of proliferative T-cell response should ultimately result in the expression of the genes encoding IL-2, and the IL-2R. Cytokines made by APC or other T-cells also influence signalling cascades. Antigen-capturing cells such as dendritic cells or macrophages ('professional APC') have stimulatory capabilities not shared by other tissue cells even though the latter may possess adequate amounts of the MHC molecules harboring the T-cell epitope in question. Recent work has suggested that one important molecular mechanism of co-stimulation results from the B7 activation molecule expressed on APC. B7 binds CD28 or its homolog CTLA-4 on the T-cell surface. In the absence of co-stimulatory signals the engagement of TCR with MHC may deliver a downregulatory signal to the T-cell [152].

TCR stimulation activates at least two signal transduction pathways, the inositol-phospholipide second messenger pathway and a tyrosine kinase pathway (Figure 7.3). Stimulation of T-cells by antigen activates the intracellular enzyme, phospholipase Cγ1 (PLC γ1), a process which is probably mediated by intramembrane guanine nucleotide-binding proteins (G proteins). Tyrosine phosphorylation may also directly activate PLCγ1 [153]. Activation of PLCγ1 by tyrosine phosphorylation and/or through GTP binding proteins results in the activation of protein kinase C (PKC). This serine/threonine kinase, when activated, results in enhanced cell growth rates and can lead to tumor formation, suggesting that it functions upstream of positive growth effector molecules [154,155]. PLC-γ1 hydrolyzes phosphatidylinositol-4,5-biphosphate (PIP$_2$) into inositol-1,4,5-trisphosphate (IP$_3$) and a minor membrane phospholipid termed diacylglycerol (DAG). These two second messengers are responsible for the rapid mobilization of intracellular Ca^{2+}. This is followed by further Ca^{2+} accumulation due to an altered calcium influx across the plasma membrane and the activation of PKC [156]. DAG in turn translocates the cytosolic PKC to the plasma membrane where it acquires its calcium-dependent active form. Both the activation of PKC (the PKC signal) and the elevation of the intracellular calcium ion concentration (calcium signal) may play central roles in the signal transduction that leads to cytokine gene induction [157]. The balance between the

activities of the two signals could contribute to cytokine expression. Active PKC was shown to phosphorylate the inhibitory subunit, IκB, of the pleiotropic transcription factor, NF-κB, *in vitro* which then translocates to the nucleus to act as a transactivating factor for many genes including the IL-2 gene [158].

PKC can also function as an upstream activator of p21^{ras}, a role which appears unique to T-cells [159]. Activation commonly occurs after TCR/CD3, CD2 or IL-2 stimulation [160]. p21^{ras}, a GTP binding protein, exists either as the activated, GTP-bound form, or the inactive, GDP-bound form after GTP hydrolysis. In unactivated lymphocytes almost all p21^{ras} is complexed to GDP. The state of activation of p21^{ras} is controlled by molecules which regulate the GTPase-mediated turnover of Ras-GTP to Ras-GDP. One candidate for a GTPase activating enzyme is p21^{ras}-GTPase activating protein, GAP [161]. In fibroblasts, p21^{ras} has been shown to control transcription factors such as c-*jun* and c-*fos*, which together form the AP-1 complex that is involved in the regulation of IL-2 gene transcription [151,162, 163]. Mice lacking c-*fos* as a result of homologous recombination have reduced numbers of peripheral T- and B-lymphocytes but increased numbers of macrophages [164]. Ras alone cannot activate IL-2 expression but can do so in the presence of additional signals, requiring at least a calcium signal [159]. It seems possible that NF-AT is one target, but probably not the only target, for the ras-dependent pathway. In T-cells, PKC phosphorylates a serine residue in the serine/threonine protein kinase p74^{raf} [165]. Cytoplasmic p74^{raf} may also translocate to the nucleus, presumably to phosphorylate nuclear transcription factors, and thus links cell membrane activation events with transcriptional activity [162, 166]. It appears that p74^{raf} functions downstream of protein tyrosine-activated PKC and p21^{ras} [160]. Possibly, raf binding to activated ras may serve as a mechanism to translocate to the membrane where it can act as a substrate for an upstream kinase and/or phosphorylate downstream targets. These complexes may then activate MEK (MAP kinase kinase) which activates mitogen-activated protein (MAP) kinase [167]. MAP kinase closes the pathway between membrane and genome by activating various transcription factors.

A second signal transduction group operates via tyrosine kinase pathways. Protein tyrosine kinases are not intrinsic to the TCR but linked to the intracytoplasmic portion of the CD3, 4 and 8 receptors. TCR stimulation by antigen leads to phosphorylation of tyrosine residues in several proteins, including the CD3ζ chain. An activation signal from TCR to PLCγ is believed to be mediated mainly through interactions between the TCRζ chain and members of the src family of PTKs such as p59^{fyn} and/or p56^{lck} [168]. Furthermore, PTKs induce PKC-independent p21^{ras} activation. IL-2Rβ and TCR/CD3 or CD2 triggered activation probably use this alternative pathway [160,169]. Two tyrosine kinases of the src family have been well characterized: p56^{lck} and p59^{fyn}. src family genes encode proteins about 500 amino acids in length with similar structure. They contain two noncatalytic, regulatory regions, known as *src* homology 2 and 3 (SH2, SH3) and the kinase domain which contains an autophosphorylation site. This site is next to a short carboxy-terminal region that negatively affects the kinase domain when the tyrosine residue is phosphorylated. Thus, src proteins are themselves regulated by tyrosine kinases and phosphatases [170]. Dephosphorylation at their regulatory residues activates both kinases during mitosis. This increased kinase activity during M phase presumably promotes proliferation [162]. Membrane phosphotyrosine phosphatase CD45 activity represents 90% of the PTPase activity in lymphocyte membranes which suggests that CD45 is likely to be responsible for p56^{lck} and p59^{fyn} activation. Moreover, the importance of intracellular CD45 domains for signaling events has been shown in CD45-deficient cells [171]. TCR signaling in these cells is restored by a chimeric protein in which the extracellular and transmembrane domains of CD45 are replaced with those of the epidermal growth factor receptor (EGF-R). Thus, the cytoplasmic domain of CD45 is necessary and sufficient for TCR signal transduction. Moreover, EGF-R ligands functionally inactivate the EGF-R/CD45 chimera through a process which involves dimerization of chimeric protein. Inactivation of EGF-R/CD45 chimera function results in the loss of TCR signaling, showing that the CD45 function is continuously required for TCR-mediated proximal signal events. However, although CD45 may positively regulate signaling by dephosphorylating the carboxy-terminal tyrosine of p56^{lck} and p59^{fyn}, cross-linking of TCR/CD3 or CD2 with different CD45 isoforms may result in very different signaling events, including inhibition of signaling.

p56^{lck} is recruited via the CD4 or CD8 molecules. As much as 90% of membrane associated p56^{lck} interacts with CD4 [172]. T-lymphocytes cannot be activated by specific antigen bound to class II molecules if they express mutant CD4 molecules, which either lack the carboxy tail or contain mutations at the intracellular cystein residues shown to mediate CD4-p56^{lck} interaction [23,24]. Some substrates of p56^{lck} have been identified by specific association after TCR stimulation including PLCγ1 and GAP [173,174]. p56^{lck} probably also phosphorylates MAP-2 kinases in T-cells directly [175]. Expression of the ζ chain is required for functional

synergy of the TCR with CD4 in the activation of PLCγ1. This may reflect an interaction between p56^{lck} and ζ-associated kinase ZAP-70. ZAP-70 is a 70 kD PTK expressed exclusively in T-cells and NK cells [176]. It is not associated with the TCR in the basal state but rapidly recruited to the ζ and CD3 chains following TCR stimulation. ZAP-70 only associates with the tyrosine phosphorylated forms of ζ that are found within the stimulated fraction of receptors. In patients with a selective T-cell defect due to a ZAP-70 gene mutation, CD8 T-cell development in the thymus is abolished and peripheral CD4 T-cells have impaired signal transduction and function [177].

p56^{lck} can also act independently from CD4 and CD8 molecules and its association with CD4/8 might only be relevant in MHC I or II restricted TCR cells. In other cell types such as double negative TCR$\gamma\delta$ cells, NK cells and possibly B-cells, p56^{lck} may act independently or it could be associated with yet undefined surface molecules [22].

PTK p59^{fyn} has two isoforms resulting from alternative splicing of exon 7. T-Cells express the p59^{fynT} isoform and brain cells use the second isoform, p59^{fynB}. p59^{fyn} is required for TCR signaling, and overexpression of *fyn* in transgenic mice results in enhanced TCR response [178]. The stochiometry of p59^{fynT} association with the TCR, however, is very low. Less than 1% of the membrane-bound p59^{fynT} may bind to TCR/CD3 complexes [172]. *Fyn* kinase associates with CD3ε and the ζ chain in T-cells [179]. Based on experimental data, the ζ chain appears to represent a novel guanosine nucleotide binding protein [180]. Since the GTP-binding of ζ has been found in functionally active TCR/CD3 complexes as well as in intracellular ζ-ζ homodimers, an energetically driven conformational change of ζ probably plays a role in cell signal transduction.

Tissue distribution and recirculation of peripheral T-lymphocytes

T-cells, which have a longer life span than B-cells, are the major lymphocyte population in peripheral blood and in the lymphatic circulation. They recirculate and migrate to the secondary lymphoid organs such as spleen, lymph nodes, and the gut- and lung-associated lymphoid tissue. Lymphocyte recirculation through the spleen is predominantly from blood to blood. CD4+ T-cells predominate over CD8+ cells in the white pulp, whereas an inverse relationship of the two lymphocyte subsets is found in the red pulp. Many T-cells reach the lymph nodes in the afferent lymphatics that drain into the subcapsular sinus. Most lymphocytes enter the nodes from the blood across a specialized vascular endothelium in post-capillary venules, termed high endothelial venules (HEV). These are mainly at the junction of the cortical and paracortical regions. T-Cells home to the paracortical regions of the lymph node and are also found in the medulla mixed with B lymphocytes and plasma cells. In these areas, CD4+ T-cells predominate over CD8+ lymphocytes and cluster around interdigitating reticulum cells (IDC). Scattered T-cells with a helper phenotype also occur within germinal centers. All cells which have entered the node from either blood or lymph, and those produced because of clonal expansion within the node, leave the node in the efferent lymph via the medullary sinuses. Efferent lymphocytes are responsible for the establishment of immunological memory and distribution of the immune response to other lymphoid organs. Efferent lymph T-cells are predominantly CD4+ rather than CD8+, implying that there is a preferential recirculation of the CD4+ cells into lymph node tissue [181]. Peripheral lymph nodes have a lower afferent input of T-cells than central nodes which receive all the efferent lymphocytes from the previous node in the chain. Both T- and B-cell areas are readily identified within the small intestinal Peyer's patches, with the T-cell area underlying the epithelial cells. High endothelial venules are present in these areas. Nearly all T-cells in tissues such as skin, gut lamina propria, and on bronchial surfaces are of the memory phenotype (CD45RO^{high}). Memory cells migrate into both normal and inflamed nonlymphoid tissue, and they preferentially return to the tissue in which they were originally stimulated [182]. Conversely, naive T-cells account for most of the cells entering the lymph node. T-Cells within the gut epithelium are predominantly CD8+, CD3+, $\alpha\beta$+ and CD45RO−.

In man, TCR$\gamma\delta$ cells account for approximately 5% of the CD3+ cells in all organized lymphoid organs, and in the skin- and gut-associated lymphoid tissues [183]. Lymphocytes expressing the $\gamma\delta$ TCR represent a small subpopulation of the CD3+ T-cells in the human gut where they are randomly distributed within both the epithelium and the lamina propria [184]. TCR$\gamma\delta$ T-cells preferentially reside in the splenic sinusoids while TCR$\alpha\beta$-bearing lymphocytes mostly occupy the periarteriolar sheets of penicillary arteries [185]. The preferential homing of $\gamma\delta$ T-cells to the epidermis seen in the mouse, does not occur in man. However, the percentage of $\gamma\delta$ T-cells in epidermis is on average higher than in papillary dermis. Therefore, there may be a difference in migration of $\gamma\delta$ versus $\alpha\beta$ T-cells [186].

Circulatory and migratory properties of T-lymphocytes are determined by interaction with either specialized endothelium in lymphoid organs, called HEVs, or activated endothelial cells. Adhesion molecules mediate this interaction (Figure 7.4). They play a role in signal transduction and T-cell activation, incrementally increasing the avidity of the TCR-ligand interactions [187]. The adhesion of T-cells to endothelium precedes lymphocyte emigration into lymphoid or inflamed nonlymphoid tissue sites. Adhesion molecule expression profiles differ between naive, activated and memory T-cells. Differential expression is observed, as well, among flat and high endothelial venules, and inflamed vessel walls. Three general principles apply to T-cell trafficking [182]: (1) naive T-cells migrate into lymph nodes while memory T-cells preferentially home to extranodal locations; (2) memory cells become biased to recirculate to the tissue type where they were previously stimulated; (3) inflammation augments the influx of T-cells and reduces the selectivity that governs physiological homing properties (Figure 7.4).

Three known, unrelated molecular families influence the association of lymphocytes with endothelia: the selectins, the CD44 family and the integrins. Lymphocyte binding to lymph node HEV is thought to be mediated principally by L-selectin (also called LECAM-1, MEL-14, LAM-1) which is expressed on virtually all CD45RO+ T-cells. Following activation, L-selectin is downregulated and other adhesion molecules are upregulated. Activated lymphocytes may bind less avidly to lymph node HEV, but more strongly to other endothelial surfaces [188]. E-Selectin (also designated ELAM-1) is induced on vascular endothelial cells by cytokines and mediates attachment of a subpopulation of resting CD4+ memory T-cells. The ligands for selectins are specific sialylated carbohydrates [182].

CD44 binds to the glycosaminoglycan, hyaluronic acid and additional ligands, such as the mucosal vascular addressin defined by the monoclonal antibody MECA-367. Integrins are a family of $\alpha\beta$ heterodimeric cell surface proteins binding to adhesion molecules that belong to the immunoglobulin gene superfamily. They play a major role in T-cell adhesion to activated endothelium. The integrin leukocyte function-associated antigen 1 (LFA-1) binds to intercellular adhesion molecules 1 and 2 (ICAM-1,-2) on HEVs. LFA-1 is expressed on all T-cells but in higher levels on memory than on naive T-cells. Very late antigen 4 (VLA-4) expression is weak on most naive T-cells and increased on memory T-cells. The ligand for this integrin is vascular cell adhesion molecule 1 (VCAM-1). ICAM-2 shows a constitutively high expression on resting endothelial cells and is not augmented by endothelial

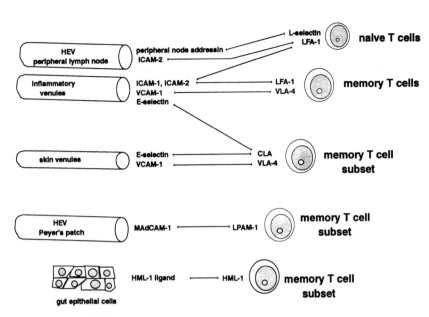

Figure 7.4 Regulation of T-lymphocyte-endothelial and gut epithelial interactions by adhesion molecules. Differential expression of integrins (such as LFA-1, VLA-4, LPAM-1, HML-1) and selectins on naive or memory T-cells, or specific memory T-cell subsets promotes binding to ligands on different types of high endothelial venules (HEV) and venules with activated endothelial cells in the skin or at inflammatory sites. These ligands mainly belong to the selectin or to the immunoglobulin gene super-family (such as ICAM-1, ICAM-2, VCAM-1, MAdCAM-1). HML-1 ligand probably redirects a memory T-cell subset with HML-1 expression to the basement membrane of intestinal epithelial cells.

cell activation. ICAM-1, which is weakly expressed, and VCAM-1, which is absent from resting endothelium, are both strongly and rapidly expressed following endothelial cell activation [182].

Memory T-cells express increased levels of adhesion molecules, including CD2, LFA-1, LFA-3, CD44, ICAM-1, and VLA-4, 5, and 6.

Molecules that are important for adhesion to normal flat endothelium or to inflamed endothelium include VLA-4, binding to VCAM-1, CD44, binding to hyaluronate, and LFA-1, binding to ICAM-1. VLA-4, CD44 and LFA-1 are upregulated on activated and memory T-cells. T-Lymphocytes localized in the skin, but not those present in the gut, express a carbohydrate termed cutaneous lymphocyte-associated antigen (CLA) that can bind to E-selectin. Delayed-type hypersensitivity and chronic inflammation of the skin leads to selectin induction on dermal endothelial cells. The interaction between E-selectin and CLA may thus contribute to skin tropism of T-cell subsets [189]. Gut afferent lymphocytes, in contrast to T-cells localized in the skin, express the integrin lymphocyte Peyer's patch adhesion molecule (LPAM-1). This molecule may be important for the interaction with mucosal addressin cell adhesion molecule 1 (MAdCAM-1) found on Peyer's patch HEVs and postcapillary venules in the lamina propria [190]. The subpopulation of intra-epithelial gut lymphocytes expresses the human mucosal lymphocyte 1 (HML-1) integrin [191] but is negative for CLA. These differential homing patterns, however, may be abrogated under pathologic conditions. Inflammatory processes and the production of soluble factors by activated leukocytes may lead to activation of integrin functions, increase

receptor-ligand expression, and induce conformational changes in adhesion receptors through increased local divalent cation concentrations [192].

T-Cell functions

T-Lymphocytes are functionally heterogenous. Their activation results in cell-mediated immunity dependent on effector cell clones that exert their influence, e.g., lymphokine secretion or cytotoxic killing, over a short range. The classic effector functions include delayed hypersensitivity, allograft rejections, graft-versus-host reactions and cytotoxic reactions against virus-infected target cells. T-Cells also regulate the clonal expansion of both T- and B-cells, the responsible regulatory lymphocyte subset consisting mainly of TCRαβ+, CD3+, and CD4+ T-helper cells. MHC-restricted cytotoxic activity is mainly exerted by peripheral CD8+ T-cells. Antigenic peptides encountered by CD4 T-cells on MHC class II molecules are predominantly derived from extracellular sources. MHC class I molecules, which present antigens to CD8 T-cells and are expressed on essentially all nucleated cells, obtain their peptides primarily from the intracellular protein pool. It is advantageous that CD8+ cytotoxic T-cells eliminate virally infected cells with endogenously produced foreign proteins in the context of their MHC class I molecules. It would be inappropriate, however, to generate CTLs against cells that have endocytosed nonreplicating foreign proteins. In this case, the proteins are expressed in the context of MHC class II molecules and the T_H response, mainly mediated by CD4 T-cells, is more suitable: it induces a humoral response against the extracellular antigen. Helper (T_H) T-lymphocytes carry out their activities mostly by secreting an array of cytokines. They amplify specific immune responses by supporting the proliferation of small numbers of lymphocytes specific for a given antigen and by recruiting the multiple effector mechanisms to eliminate foreign antigens [157]. Naive CD4+ T-cells represent a set of relatively recent thymic emigrants that have not yet encountered or not yet responded to antigen. Naive CD4+ T-cells produce IL-2, but little or no IL-4 or interferon-γ(IFNγ) when stimulated by receptor engagement in the context of a co-stimulatory signal. They have been called precursors of T_H cells, or pT_H cells, and express CD45RA [193]. Compared with CD45RA+ naive T-cells, CD45RO+ memory cells are functionally much more potent and are stimulated by much lower amounts of antigen or anti-CD3 monoclonal antibodies. In the mouse, CD4, CD45 and the TCR complex are physically associated on memory T-cells, whereas on naive T-cells they are separate [194]. This physical association allows for a much greater efficiency in T-cell triggering, and forms the molecular basis for T-cell memory. Memory T-cells have many similarities to activated T-cells or T-cell clones: both are CD45RO+ and express increased levels of adhesion molecules, MHC class II molecules and IL-2 receptors. CD45RO+ T-cells, although not as large as activated T-cells, are larger than CD45RA+ T-cells [195]. Activated helper cells can differentiate into T_{H1}-cells that secrete predominantly tumor necrosis factor (TNF) and IFNγ, or T_{H2}-cells that release mainly IL-4, IL-5, IL-6 and IL-10. The T_{H1}-clones, through their production of IFNγ and TNFβ, are well suited to induce enhanced microbicidal activity in macrophages (enhanced cellular immunity) while the T_{H2}-clones synthesize molecules that effectively interact with B-cells.

T_{H2}-cells express CD40 ligand that binds to CD40 on the B-cell surface. The binding of CD40 and the effect of cytokines secreted by the T_{H2}-cells lead to B-cell proliferation, class switching and the development of memory B-cells [196]. T_{H2}-like responses oppose the effects of IFNγ on macrophages through the actions of IL-10 and IL-4, and possibly suppress the production of IFNγ and other cytokines by T_{H1} cells. These negative regulatory effects may be important in the control of self-inflicted injury.

Cytotoxic T-cells contain lytic granules that can destroy the integrity of most cell membranes. In addition, it appears that serine proteases in the granules may initiate apoptosis when they gain access into target cells, possibly via a perforin pore.

Cytotoxicity may also involve contact-dependent signals from the killer to the target cells. Thus, one of the mechanisms a T-cell uses to kill, which is not dependent on extracellular calcium, requires the expression of Fas on the target cell surface [196]. CD8+ T-cells can also be subdivided into CD45RA- and CD45RO-positive subsets which may reflect a functional dichotomy similar to the CD4+ T-lymphocyte subsets. The recognition process in the cytotoxic reaction against nonself-MHC antigens differs from the corecognition of self-MHC class I molecules and endogenous antigen in virus-infected T-cells. T-cells bearing TCR$\alpha\beta$ show a high frequency of reactivity to allelic variants of MHC class I and II molecules, a phenomenon called 'alloreactivity'. CD4+ T-cells are both necessary and sufficient to initiate allograft rejection even without CD8+ lymphocytes. The host T-cells probably recognize the differently shaped and charged grooves of the MHC complexes and the different peptide composition of the minor histocompatibility antigens on the allograft as numerous novel antigens.

DN $\alpha\beta$ T-cells make up about 0.5% of peripheral T-cells and may use antigen presenting cells, restriction molecules, and selection routes different from those used by antigen-specific CD4+ T-cells. They can recognize bacterial antigens, are often oligoclonal and the expanded clones may persist for several years [197,198]. Nearly all $\gamma\delta$ T-cells lack expression of CD4 and most lack CD8 or express it at relatively low levels. In contrast to the SP $\alpha\beta$ T-cells, no common restriction element such as MHC is presently known for $\gamma\delta$ T-cells. TCR$\gamma\delta$ can potentially interact with MHC molecules but this may be the exception rather than the rule. Recent studies with murine $\gamma\delta$ T-cell clones have shown that their activation requires neither class I nor class II antigen processing and that peptides do not confer specificity [199]. These T-lymphocytes could be more flexible than $\alpha\beta$ T-cells in their immune response since they might recognize antigens directly without the requirement for APC. Obvious candidates for other antigen presenting molecules are the products of so-called nonclassical MHC class I genes. Human CD1 molecules represent perhaps the best characterized candidates for non-MHC-encoded antigen presenting molecules for $\gamma\delta$ T-cells. Genes for CD1 molecules show a domain organization similar to that of MHC class I genes. Another notable similarity between CD1 and MHC class I molecules is the association of the heavy chain with β_2-microglobulin which is, in both cases, required for cell surface expression. TCR$\gamma\delta$ lymphocytes, which accumulate in reactive granulomatous lesions of leprosy and cutaneous leishmaniasis, appear genetically restricted and require self-antigen presentation [200]. Upon stimulation with antigen they secrete lymphokines that cause macrophage adhesion, aggregation and proliferation [201]. Comparison of cytokine secretion profiles for a series of $\gamma\delta$ T-cell clones with a series of $\alpha\beta$ T-cell clones reveals evidence of quantitative rather than qualitative differences. Many $\gamma\delta$ T-cell clones secrete lower or undetectable amounts of IL-2 and IL-4. These cells either have a greater requirement for exogenous growth factors than do their $\alpha\beta$ bearing counterparts, or they produce and respond to different autocrine growth factors.

Conclusion

We have outlined the establishment of the TCR repertoire by developmentally regulated TCR gene rearrangements and predominantly intrathymic selection processes. On the one hand, delicate and redundant control mechanisms keep the immune system alert for the presence of foreign proteins, neo-antigens and microorganisms. On the other hand, the immune response has to be under tight control and self-limited in order to avoid self-destruction of the host. Autoimmune disease or malignant lymphoproliferations may develop if the system fails to maintain this delicate balance. Antigenic stimulation generates a polyclonal or oligoclonal lymphoproliferation. Clonal populations can emerge if immune surveillance fails to control the lymphoproliferation. These clonal populations, if sufficiently deregulated, may become autonomously growing tumor cells. Clonality is an important, though not absolutely diagnostic, criterion for malignant lymphomas. Aberrant activation of PTKs and nuclear transcription factors during thymic ontogeny or antigenic T-cell stimulation may lead to an altered signaling cascade which interferes with ordered T-cell development, differentiation and proliferation.

We are beginning to understand the pleiotropic effects of cytokines on T-cells. Various cell lineages of the immune system express cytokine receptors clustered with other transmembrane molecules. Abnormal activation of these receptors or unbalanced cytokine secretion profiles may contribute to the highly variable cytomorphological features seen in peripheral T-cell lymphomas. Results emerging from the investigation of homing receptors and adhesion molecules on T-lymphocytes are about to help us understand the recirculation pathways of malignant T-cells to lymphoid organs and to extranodal sites.

A more detailed knowledge of T-cell development, requirements for TCR receptor interactions, and intracellular signal transduction pathways will eventually improve our understanding of the pathobiology in reactive and malignant immune disorders. This in turn will provide us with new diagnostic capabilities and will profoundly influence the specific therapy of T-cell disorders in the future.

References

1. Zinkernagel RM, Doherty PC. MHC-restricted cytotoxic T-cells: Studies on the biological role of a polymorphic major transplantation antigen determining T-cell restriction-specificity, function, and responsiveness. *Adv. Immunol.* 1979, **27**: 52–142.
2. Pfeffer K, Mak TW. Lymphocyte ontogeny and activation in gene targeted mutant mice. *Annu. Rev. Immunol.* 1994, **12**: 367–411.
3. Brenner MB, Strominger JL, Krangel MS. The $\gamma\delta$ T cell receptor. *Adv. Immunol.* 1988, **43**: 133–192.
4. Meuer SC, Fitzgerald KA, Hussey RE, et al. Clonotypic structures involved in antigen-specific human T-cell function. Relationship to the T3 molecular complex. *J. Exp. Med.* 1983, **157**: 705–719.
5. Davis MM, Bjorkman PJ. T-cell antigen receptor genes and T-cell recognition. *Nature* 1988, **334**: 395–402.
6. Lefranc M-P, Rabbitts TH. The human T-cell receptor γ (TRG) genes. *TIBS* 1989, **14**: 214–218.
7. Jin Y-J, Clayton LK, Howard FD, et al. Molecular cloning of the CD3ε subunit identifies a CD3ζ-related product in thymus-derived cells. *Proc. Natl Acad. Sci. USA* 1990, **87**: 3319–3323.
8. Klausner RD, Samelson LE. T cell antigen receptor activation pathways: The tyrosine kinase connection. *Cell* 1991, **64**: 875–878.
9. Wegener A-MK, Letourneur F, Hoeveler A, et al. The T-cell receptor/CD3 complex is composed of at least two autonomous transduction modules. *Cell* 1992, **68**: 83–95.
10. Frank SJ, Niklinska BB, Orloff DG, et al. Structural mutations of the T cell receptor zeta chain and its role in T cell activation. *Science* 1990, **249**: 174–177.
11. Clevers H, Alarcon B, Wileman T, et al. The T cell receptor/CD3 complex: A dynamic protein ensemble. *Annu. Rev. Immunol.* 1988, **6**: 629–662.
12. Springer TA, Dustin TH, Kishimoto TK, et al. The lymphocyte function associated LFA-1, CD2, and LFA-3 molecules: Cell adhesion receptors of the immune system. *Annu. Rev. Immunol.* 1987, **5**: 223–252.
13. Williams AF, Barclay AN. The immunoglobulin superfamily-domains for cell surface recognition. *Annu. Rev. Immunol.* 1988, **6**: 381–405.
14. Doyle C, Strominger JL. Interaction between CD4 and class II MHC molecules mediates cell adhesion. *Nature* 1988, **330**: 256–258.
15. Norment AM, Salter RD, Parham P, et al. Cell–cell adhesion mediated by CD8 and MHC class I molecules. *Nature* 1988, **336**: 79–81.

16. Rahemtulla A, Fung-Leung W-P, Schilham MW, et al. Normal development and function of CD8+ cells but markedly decreased helper cell activity in mice lacking CD4. *Nature* 1991, **353**: 180–184.

17. Fung-Leung W-P, Schilham M, Rahemtulla A, et al. CD8 is needed for development of cytotoxic T-cells but not helper T-cells. *Cell* 1991, **65**: 443–449.

18. Parnes JR. Molecular biology and function of CD4 and CD8. *Adv. Immunol.* 1988, **44**: 265–311.

19. Janeway CA. The role of CD4 in T-cell activation: accessory molecule or coreceptor. *Immunol. Today* 1989, **10**: 234–238.

20. Robey E, Axel R. CD4: Collaborateur in immune recognition and HIV infection. *Cell* 1990, **60**: 697–700.

21. Fleury S, Lamarre D, Meloche S, et al. Mutational analysis of the interaction between CD4 and class II MHC: Class II antigens contact CD4 on a surface opposite the gp120 binding site. *Cell* 1991, **66**: 1037–1049.

22. Veillette A, Davidson D. Src-related protein tyrosine kinases and T-cell receptor signalling. *TIBS* 1992, **8**: 61–66.

23. Glaichenhaus N, Shastri N, Littman DR, et al. Requirement for association of p56lck with CD4 in antigen-specific signal transduction in T-cells. *Cell* 1991, **64**: 511–520.

24. Collins TL, Uniyal S, Shin J, et al. p56lck association with CD4 is required for the interaction between and the TCR/CD3 complex and for optimal antigen stimulation. *J. Immunol.* 1992, **148**: 2159–2162.

25. van Kerckhove C, Russell GJ, Deusch K, et al. Oligoclonality of human intestinal intraepithelial T-cells. *J. Exp. Med.* 1992, **175**: 57–63.

26. Terry LA, DiSanto JP, Small TN, et al. Differential expression and regulation of the human CD8α and CD8β chains. *Tissue Antigens* 1990, **35**: 82–91.

27. Salter RD, Benjamin RJ, Wesley PK, et al. A binding site for the T-cell co-receptor CD8 on the a3 domain of HLA-2. *Nature* 1990, **345**: 41–46.

28. Pingel JT, Thomas ML. Evidence that the leukocyte-common antigen is required for antigen-induced T lymphocyte proliferation. *Cell* 1989, **58**: 1055–1065.

29. Klausner RD, Lippincott-Schwartz J, Bonifacino JS. The T-cell antigen receptor: Insights into organelle biology. *Annu. Rev. Cell Biol.* 1990, **6**: 403–431.

30. Springer TA. Adhesion receptors and the immune system. *Nature* 1990, **346**: 425–434.

31. Meuer S, Resch K. Cellular signalling in T-lymphocytes. *Immunol. Today* 1989, **10**: 22–25.

32. Kanner SB, Damle NK, Blake J, et al. CD2/LFA-3 ligation induces phospholipase Cγl tyrosine phosphorylation and regulates CD3 signalling. *J. Immunol.* 1992, **148**: 2023–2029.

33. Thomas ML. The leukocyte common antigen family. *Annu. Rev. Immunol.* 1989, **7**: 339–369.

34. Hathcock KS, Lazlo G, Dickler HB, et al. Expression of variable exon A-, B-, and C-specific CD45 determinants on peripheral and thymic T-cell populations. *J. Immunol.* 1992, **148**: 19–28.

35. Wallace VA, Fung-Leung WP, Gray D, et al. CD45RA and CD45RB high expression induced by thymic selection events. *J. Exp. Med.* 1992, **176**: 1657–1663.

36. Dianziani U, Redoglia V, Malavasi F, et al. Isoform-specific association of CD45 with accessory molecules in human T lymphocytes. *Eur. J. Immunol.* 1992, **22**: 365–371.

37. Townsend A, Bodmer H. Antigen-recognition by class I-restricted T lymphocytes. *Annu. Rev. Immunol.* 1989, **7**: 601–624.

38. Rothbard JB, Gefter ML. Interactions between immunogenic peptides and MHC proteins. *Annu. Rev. Immunol.* 1991, **9**: 527–565.

39. Elliott EA, Drake JR, Amigorena S, et al. The invariant chain is required for intracellular transport and function of major histocompatibility complex class II molecules. *J. Exp. Med.* 1994, **179**: 681–694.

40. Falk K, Rotzschke O, Deres K, et al. Identification of naturally processed viral nonapeptides allows their quantification in infected cells and suggests an allele-specific T-cell epitope forecast. *J. Exp. Med.* 1991, **174**: 425–434.

41. Falk K, Rotzschke O, Rammensee HG. Cellular peptide composition governed by major histocompatibility complex class I molecules. *Nature* 1990, **348**: 248–251.

42. Hood L, Kronenberg M, Hunkapiller T. T-cell antigen receptors and the immunoglobulin supergene family. *Cell* 1985, **40**: 225–229.

43. Elliott JF, Rock EP, Patten PA, et al. The adult T-cell receptor δ chain is diverse and distinct of that of fetal thymocytes. *Nature* 1988, **331**: 627–631.

44. Raulet DH. The structure, function and molecular genetics of the gamma/delta T-cell receptor. *Annu. Rev. Immunol.* 1989, **7**: 175–208.

45. Kotzin BL, Barr VL, Palmer E. A large deletion within the T cell receptor beta-chain gene complex in New Zealand white mice. *Science* 1985, **229**: 167–171.

46. Behlke MA, Chou HS, Huppi K, et al. Murine T-cell receptor mutants with deletions of β-chain variable region genes. *Proc. Natl Acad. Sci. USA* 1986, **83**: 767–771.

47. Noonan DJJ, Kofler R, Singer PA, et al. Delineation of a defect in T-cell receptor β genes of NZW mice predisposed to autoimmunity. *J. Exp. Med.* 1986, **163**: 644–653.

48. Kappler JW, Roehm N, Marrack P. T-cell tolerance by clonal elimination in the thymus. *Cell* 1987, **49**: 273–280.

49. Kappler JW, Staerz U, White J, et al. Self-tolerance eliminates T-cells specific for mls-modified products of the major histocompatibility complex. *Nature* 1988, **332**: 35–40.

50. von Boehmer H, Teh HS, Kisielow P. The thymus selects the useful, neglects the useless and destroys the harmful. *Immunol. Today* 1989, **10**: 57–61.

51. Schwartz RH. Acquisition of immunological self-tolerance. *Cell* 1989, **57**: 1073–1081.

52. Ferrick DA, Ohashi PS, Wallace V, et al. Thymic ontogeny and selection of $\alpha\beta$ and $\gamma\delta$ T-cells. *Immunol. Today* 1989, **10**: 403–407.

53. Yancopoulos GD, Blackwell TK, Suh H, et al. Introduced T cell receptor variable region gene segments recombine in pre-B-cells: evidence that B and

T cells use a common recombinase. *Cell* 1986, **44**: 251–259.

54. Boehm T, Rabbitts TH. A chromosomal basis of lymphoid malignancy in man. *Eur. J. Biochem.* 1989, **185**: 1–17.

55. Lafaille JJ, DeCloux A, Bonneville M, et al. Junctional sequences of T-cell receptor γδ genes: implications for γδ T-cell lineages and for a novel intermediate of V-(D)-J joining. *Cell* 1989, **59**: 859–870.

56. Landau NR, Schatz PG, Rosa M, et al. Increased frequency of N-region insertion in a murine pre-B-cell line infected with a terminal deoxynucleotidyl transferase retroviral expression vector. *Mol. Cell. Biol.* 1987, **7**: 3237–3243.

57. Alt FW, Oltz EM, Young F, et al. VDJ recombination. *Immunol. Today* 1992, **13**: 306–314.

58. Hong S-C, Chelouche A, Lin R-H, et al. An MHC interaction site maps to the amino-terminal half of the T-cell receptor α chain variable domain. *Cell* 1992, **69**: 999–1009.

59. Bjorkman PJ, Saper MA, Samraoui B, et al. The foreign antigen binding site and T cell recognition regions of class I histocompatibility antigens. *Nature* 1987, **329**: 512–518.

60. Schatz DG, Oettinger MA, Schlissel MS. V(D)J recombination: molecular biology and regulation. *Annu. Rev. Immunol.* 1992, **10**: 359–383.

61. Yoneda N, Tatsumi E, Kawano S, et al. Human recombination activating gene-1 in leukemia/lymphoma cells: Expression depends on stage of lymphoid differentiation defined by phenotype and genotype. *Blood* 1993, **82**: 207–216.

62. Ezine S, Ceredig R. Haemopoiesis and early T-cell differentiation. *Immunol. Today* 1994, **15**: 151–154.

63. Mombaerts P, Iacomini J, Johnson RS, et al. RAG-1 deficient mice have no mature B and T lymphocytes. *Cell* 1992, **68**: 869–877.

64. Shinkai Y, Rathbun G, Lam K-P, et al. RAG-2 deficient mice lack mature lymphocytes owing to inability to V(D)J rearrangement. *Cell* 1992, **68**: 855–867.

65. Hochstenbach F, Brenner MB. T-cell receptor δ-chain can substitue for α to form a βδ heterodimer. *Nature* 1989, **340**: 562–565.

66. Kronenberg M, Siu G, Hood L, et al. The molecular genetics of the T cell antigen receptor and T cell antigen recognition. *Annu. Rev. Immunol.* 1986, **4**: 529–591.

67. Caccia N, Bruns GAP, Kirsch IR, et al. T-cell receptor α chain genes are located on chromosome 14 at 14q11–14q12 in humans. *J. Exp. Med.* 1985, **161**: 1255–1260.

68. Yoshikai Y, Kimura N, Toyonaga B, et al. Sequences and repertoire of human T cell receptor alpha chain variable region genes in mature lymphocytes. *J. Exp. Med.* 1986, **164**: 90–103.

69. Arden B, Clark SP, Mak TW. Human T-cell receptor variable gene segment families. *Immunogenetics* 1994, **42**: 455–500.

70. Griesser H, Champagne E, Tkachuk D, et al. Mapping of the human α–δ region: A locus with a new constant region gene and prone to multiple chromosomal translocations. *Eur. J. Immunol.* 1988, **18**: 641–644.

71. Hayday AC, Diamond DJ, Tanigawa G, et al. Unusual organization and diversity of T-cell receptor α-chain genes. *Nature* 1985, **316**: 828–832.

72. Champagne E, Sagman U, Biondi A, et al. Structure and rearrangement of the T-cell receptor J α locus in T cells and leukemia T-cell lines. *Eur. J. Immunol.* 1988, **18**: 1033–1036.

73. Baer R, Boehm T, Yssel H, et al. Complex rearrangements within the human Jδ-Cδ/Jα-Cα locus and aberrant recombination between Jα segments. *EMBO J.* 1988, **7**: 1661–1668.

74. Klein MH, Concannon P, Everett M, et al. Diversity and structure of human T-cell receptor α-chain variable region genes. *Proc. Natl Acad. Sci. USA* 1987, **84**: 6884–6888.

75. Caccia N, Kronenberg M, Saxe D, et al. The T cell receptor β chain genes are located on chromosome 6 in mice and chromosome 7 in humans. *Cell* 1984, **37**: 1091–1099.

76. Kimura N, Toyonaga B, Yoshikai Y, et al. Sequences and diversity of human T cell receptor β chain variable region genes. *J. Exp. Med.* 1986, **164**: 739–750.

77. Lai E, Concannon P, Hood L. Conserved organization of the human and murine T-cell receptor β-gene families. *Nature* 1988, **331**: 543–546.

78. Yusuki H, Yoshikai Y, Kishihara K, et al. The expression and sequences of the T cell antigen receptor β-chain genes in the thymus at an early stage after sublethal irradiation. *J. Immunol.* 1989, **142**: 3683–3691.

79. Toyonaga B, Yoshikai Y, Vadasz V, et al. Organization and sequences of the diversity, joining, constant region genes of the human T-cell receptor β chain. *Proc. Natl Acad. Sci. USA* 1985, **82**: 8624–8628.

80. Leiden JM, Strominger JL. Generation of diversity of the β chain of the human T-lymphocyte receptor for antigen. *Proc. Natl Acad. Sci. USA* 1986, **83**: 4456–4460.

81. Strauss WM, Quertermous T, Seidman JG. Measuring the human T cell receptor γ-chain locus. *Science* 1987, **237**: 1217–1219.

82. Chen Z, Font MP, Loiseau P, et al. The human T-cell Vγ gene locus: cloning of new segments and study of Vγ rearrangements in neoplastic T and B cells. *Blood* 1988, **72**: 776–783.

83. Forster A, Huck S, Ghanem N, et al. New subgroups in the human T cell rearranging Vγ gene locus. *EMBO J.* 1987, **6**: 1945–1950.

84. Quertermous T, Murre C, Dialynas D, et al. Human T-cell γ chain genes: Organization, diversity, and rearrangement. *Science* 1986, **231**: 252–255.

85. LeFranc M-P, Forster A, Baer R, et al. Diversity and rearrangement of the human T cell rearranging γ genes: Nine germ-line variable genes belonging to two subgroups. *Cell* 1986, **45**: 237–246.

86. Krangel MS, Band H, Hata S, et al. Structurally divergent human T cell receptor γ proteins encoded by distinct Cγ genes. *Science* 1987, **237**: 64–67.

87. Hochstenbach F, Parker C, McLean J, et al. Characterization of a third form of the human T cell receptor γ/δ. *J. Exp. Med.* 1988, **168**: 761–776.

88. Takihara Y, Tkachuk D, Michalopoulos E, et al. Sequence and organization of the diversity, joining, and constant region genes of the human T-cell δ-chain locus. *Proc. Natl Acad. Sci. USA* 1988, **85**: 6097–6101.

89. Takihara Y, Reimann J, Michalopoulos E, et al. Diversity and structure of human T cell receptor δ chain genes in peripheral blood γ/δ-bearing T lymphocytes. *J. Exp. Med.* 1989, **169**: 393–405.

90. Krangel MS, Yssel H, Brocklehurst C, et al. A distinct wave of human T cell receptor γδ lymphocytes in the early fetal thymus: Evidence for controlled gene rearrange ments and cytokine production. *J. Exp. Med.* 1990, **172**: 847–859.

91. Guglielmi P, Davi F, D'Auriol L, et al. Use of a variable α region to create a functional T-cell receptor δ chain. *Proc. Natl Acad. Sci. USA* 1988, **85**: 5634–5638.

92. Loh EY, Cwirla S, Serafini AT, et al. Human T-cell-receptor δ chain: genomic organization, diversity, and expression in populations of cells. *Proc. Natl Acad. Sci. USA* 1988, **85**: 9714–9718.

92a. Davodeau F, Peyrat MA, Hallet MM, et al. Characterization of a new functional TCR Jδ segment in humans. *J. Immunol.* 1994, **153**: 137–142.

93. Clevers HC, Owen MJ. Towards a molecular understanding of T-cell differentiation. *Immunol. Today* 1991, **12**: 167–173.

94. Gottschalk LR, Leiden JM. Identification and functional characterization of the human T-cell receptor β gene transcriptional enhancer: Common nuclear proteins interact with the transcriptional regulatory elements of the T-cell receptor α and β genes. *Mol. Cell. Biol.* 1990, **10**: 5486–5495.

95. Leiden JM. Transcriptional regulation of T cell receptor genes. *Annu. Rev. Immunol.* 1993, **11**: 539–570.

96. Bhat NK, Komschlies KL, Fisher RJ, et al. Expression of ets genes in mouse thymocyte subsets and T-cells. *J. Immunol.* 1989, **142**: 672–678.

97. Ho I-C, Bhat NK, Gottschalk LR, et al. Sequence-specific binding of human ets-1 to the T-cell receptor α gene enhancer. *Science* 1990, **250**: 814–818.

98. McDougall S, Peterson CL, Calame K. A transcriptional enhancer 3' of Cβ2 in the T cell receptor β locus. *Science* 1988, **241**: 205–208.

99. Anderson SJ, Miyake S, Loh DY. Transcription from amurine T-cell receptor Vβ promoter depends on a conserved decamer motif similar to the cyclic AMP response element. *Mol. Cell. Biol.* 1989, **9**: 4835–4845.

100. Winoto A, Baltimore D. αβ lineage-specific expression of the T-cell receptor gene by nearby silencers. *Cell* 1989, **59**: 649–655.

101. Ishida I, Verbeek S, Bonneville M, et al. T-cell receptor gamma delta and gamma transgenic mice suggest a role of a gamma gene silencer in the generation of alpha beta T cells. *Proc. Natl Acad. Sci. USA* 1990, **87**: 3067–3071.

102. Garman RD, Doherty PJ, Raulet DH. Diversity, rearrangement, and expression of murine T cell gamma genes. *Cell* 1986, **45**: 733–742.

103. Ho IC, Leiden ML. The Tα2 nuclear protein binding site from the human T cell receptor α enhancer functions as both a T cell-specific transcriptional activator and repressor. *J. Exp. Med.* 1990, **172**: 1443–1449.

104. de Villartay JP, Hockett RD, Coran D, et al. Deletion of the human T-cell receptor δ-gene by a site-specific recombination. *Nature* 1988, **335**: 170–174.

105. Campana D, Janossy G, Coustan-Smith E, et al. The expression of T cell receptor-associated proteins during T-cell ontogeny in man. *J. Immunol.* 1989, **142**: 57–66.

106. Haynes BF, Singer KH, Denning SM, et al. Analysis of expression of CD2, CD3, and T cell antigen receptor molecules during early human fetal thymic development. *J. Immunol.* 1988, **141**: 3776–3784.

107. Bories JC, Loiseau P, d'Auriol L, et al. Regulation of the transcription of the human T cell antigen receptor δ chain gene: A T-lineage specific enhancer element is located in the Jδ3-Cδ intron. *J. Exp. Med.* 1990, **171**: 75–83.

108. De Villartay J-P, Pullmann AB, Anrade R, et al. γ/δ lineage relationship within a consecutive series of human precursor T-cell neoplasms. *Blood* 1989, **74**: 2508–2518.

109. Uematsu Y, Ryser S, Dembic Z, et al. In transgenic mice the introduced functional T cell receptor β gene prevents expression of endogeneous β genes. *Cell* 1988, **52**: 831–841.

110. Raulet DM, Garman RD, Saito H, et al. Developmental regulation of T-cell receptor gene expression. *Nature* 1985, **314**: 103–107.

111. Padovan E, Casorati G, Dellabona P, et al. Frequent expression of two TCRα chains in human αβ lymphocytes creates dual receptor cells. *Science* 1993, **262**: 422–424.

112. Shortman K. Cellular aspects of early T-cell development. *Curr. Opin. Immunol.* 1992, **4**: 140–146.

113. Haas W, Kaufman S, Martinez-A C. The development and function of γδ T cells. *Immunol. Today* 1990, **11**: 340–343.

114. Borst J, Brouns GS, de Vries E, et al. Antigen receptors on T and B lymphocytes: Parallels in organization and function. Immunol. Rev. 1993, **132**: 49–84.

115. Mombaerts P, Clarke AR, Rudnicki MA, et al. Mutations in T-cell antigen receptor genes α and β block thymocyte development at different stages. *Nature* 1992, **360**: 225–231.

116. Itohara S, Mombaerts P, Lafaille J, et al. T cell receptor delta gene mutant mice: Independent generation of alpha beta T cells and programmed rearrangements of gamma delta TCR genes. *Cell* 1993, **72**: 337–348.

117. Philcott KL, Viney JL, Kay G, et al. Lymphoid development in mice congenitally lacking T cell receptor alpha-beta-expressing cells. *Science* 1992, **256**: 1448–1452.

118. Love PE, Shores EW, Johnson MD, et al. T cell development in mice that lack the zeta chain of the T cell antigen receptor complex. *Science* 1993, **261**: 918–921.

119. Ohno H, Aoe T, Taki S, et al. Development and functional impairment of T cells in mice lacking CD3 zeta chains. *EMBO J.* 1993, **12**: 4357–4366.

120. Fung-Leung WP, Kündig TM, Zinkernagel RM, et al. Immune response against lymphocytic choriomeningitis virus infection in mice without CD8 expression. *J. Exp. Med.* 1991, **174**: 1425–1429.

121. Fung-Leung WP, Wallace VA, Gray D, et al. CD8 is needed for positive selection but differentially required for negative selection of T cells during thymic ontogeny. *Eur. J. Immunol.* 1993, **23**: 212–216.

122. Killeen N, Stuart SG, Littman DR. Development and function of T cells in mice with a disrupted CD2 gene. *EMBO J.* 1992, **11**: 4329–4336.

123. Kishihara K, Penninger J, Wallace VA, et al. Normal B lymphocyte development but impaired T cell maturation in CD45-Exon6 protein tyrosine phosphatase-deficient mice. *Cell* 1993, **74**: 143–156.

124. Hurley TR, Hyman R, Sefton BM. Differential effects of expression of the CD45 tyrosine protein phosphatase on the tyrosine phosphorylation of lck, fyn, and c-src tyrosine protein kinases. *Mol. Cell. Biol.* 1993, **13**: 1651–1656.

125. Janeway CA. The T-cell receptor as a multicomponent signalling machine: CD4/CD8 and CD45 in T-cell activation. *Annu. Rev. Immunol.* 1992, **10**: 645–674.

126. Molina TJ, Kishihara K, Siderovski DP, et al. Profound block in thymocyte development in mice lacking p56lck. *Nature* 1992, **357**: 161–164.

127. Penninger J, Kishihara K, Molina T, et al. Requirement for tyrosine kinase p56 lck for thymic development of transgenic γδ T cells. *Science* 1993, **260**: 358–361.

128. Taniguchi T, Minami Y. The IL-2/IL-2 receptor system: a current overview. *Cell* 1993, **73**: 5–8.

129. Griscelli C, Lisowska-Grospierre B. Combined immunodeficiency with defective expression in MHC class II genes. *Immunodeficiency Rev.* 1989, **1**: 135–153.

130. Schorle H, Holtschke T, Hünig T, et al. Development and function of T cells in mice rendered interleukin-2 deficient by gene targeting. *Nature* 1991, **352**: 621–624.

131. Kündig TM, Schorle H, Bachmann MF, et al. Immune responses in interleukin-2 deficient mice. *Science* 1993, **262**: 1059–1061.

132. Kappler J, Wade T, White J, et al. A T cell receptor Vβ segment that imparts rectivity to a class II major histocompatibility complex product. *Cell* 1987, **49**: 263–271.

133. Miller JFAP, Heath WR. Self-ignorance in the peripheral T cell pool. *Immunol. Rev.* 1993, **133**: 131–150.

134. Hugo P, Kappler JW, Godfrey DI, et al. Thymic epithelial cell lines that mediate positive selection can also induce thymocyte clonal deletion. *J. Immunol.* 1994, **152**: 1022–1031.

135. Hogquist KA, Jameson SC, Heath WR, et al. T cell receptor antagonist peptides induce positive selection. *Cell* 1994, **76**: 17–27.

136. Ashton-Rickardt PG, Bandeira A, Delaney JR, et al. Evidence for a differential avidity model of T cell selection in the thymus. *Cell* 1994, **76**: 651–663.

137. Sebzda E, Wallace VA, Mayer J, et al. Positive and negative thymocyte selection induced by different concentrations of a single peptide. *Science* 1994, **263**: 1615–1618.

138. Chan SH, Cosgrove D, Waltzinger C, et al. Another view of the selective model of thymocyte selection. *Cell* 1993, **73**: 225–236.

139. Davis CB, Killeen N, Crooks MEC, et al. Evidence for a stochastic mechanism in the differentiation of mature subsets of T lymphocytes. *Cell* 1993, **73**: 237–247.

140. Viville S, Neefjes J, Lotteau V, et al. Mice lacking the MHC class II-associated invariant chain. *Cell* 1993, **72**: 635–648.

141. Zijlstra M, Li E, Sajjadi F, et al. Germ-line transmission of a disrupted beta 2-microglobulin gene produced by homologous recombination in embryonic stem cells. *Nature* 1989, **342**: 435–438.

142. von Boehmer H. Developmental biology of T cells in T-cell receptor transgenic mice. *Annu. Rev. Immunol.* 1990, **8**: 531–556.

143. Aldrich CJ, Hammer RE, Jones-Youngblood S, et al. Negative and positive selection of antigen-specific cytotoxic T lymphocytes affected by the α3 domain of MHC I molecules. *Nature* 1991, **352**: 718–721.

144. Nossal GJV, Pike BL. Clonal anergy: Persistence in tolerant mice of antigen-binding B lymphocytes incapable of responding to antigen or mitogen. *Proc. Natl Acad. Sci. USA* 1980, **77**: 1602–1606.

145. Liu Y, Janeway CA. Interferone γ plays a critical role in induced cell death of effector T-cells: A possible third mechanism of self tolerance. *J. Exp. Med.* 1990, **172**: 1735–1739.

146. Walden PR, Eisen HN. Cognate peptides induce self-destruction of CD8+ cytolytic T lymphocytes. *Proc. Natl Acad. Sci. USA* 1990, **87**: 9015–9019.

147. Dent AL, Matis LA, Hooshmand F, et al. Self-reactive γδ T cells are eliminated in the thymus. *Nature* 1990, **343**: 714–719.

148. Bonneville M, Ishida I, Itohara S, et al. Self-tolerance to transgenic γδ T-cells by intrathymic inactivation. *Nature* 1990, **344**: 163–165.

149. Sim GK, Augustin A. Extrathymic positive selection of γδ T-cells. *J. Immunol.* 1991, **146**: 2439–2445.

150. Lefrancois L, LeCorre R, Mayo J, et al. Extrathymic selection of TCRγδ+ T-cells by class II major histocompatibility complex molecules. *Cell* 1990, **63**: 333–340.

151. Crabtree G. Contingent genetic regulatory events in T lymphocyte activation. *Science* 1989, **243**: 355–361.

152. Linsley PS, Brady W, Grosmaire L, et al. Binding of the B cell activation antigen B7 to CD28 costimulates T cell proliferation and interleukin-2 mRNA accumulation. *J. Exp. Med.* 1991, **173**: 721–730.

153. Weiss A, Koretzky G, Schatzman RC, et al. Functional activation of the T-cell antigen receptor induces tyrosine phosphorylation of PLCγ-1. *Proc. Natl Acad. Sci. USA* 1991, **88**: 5484–5488.

154. Cantley LC, Auger KR, Carpenter C, et al. Oncogenes and signal transduction. *Cell* 1991, **64**: 281–302.

155. Gschwendt M, Kittstein W, Marks F. Protein kinase C activation by phorbol esters: Do cystein-rich regions and pseudosubstrate motifs play a role? *TIBS* 1991, **16**: 167–169.

156. Weiss A, Imboden J, Hardy K, et al. The role of the T3/antigen receptor complex in T cell activation. *Annu. Rev. Immunol.* 1986, **4**: 593–679.

157. Arai KI, Lee F, Miyajima A, et al. Cytokines: Coordinators of immune and inflammatory responses. *Annu. Rev. Biochem.* 1990, **59**: 783–836.

158. Ghosh S, Baltimore D. Activation in vitro of NF-κB by phosphorylation of the inhibitor IκB. *Nature* 1990, **344**: 678–682.

159. Rayter SI, Woodrow M, Lucas SC, et al. p21ras mediates control of IL-2 gene promoter function in T cell activation. *EMBO J.* 1992, **11**: 4549–4556.

160. Downward J, Graves JD, Cantrell DA. The regulation and function of p21ras in T-cells. *Immunol. Today* 1992, **13**: 89–92.

161. Hanley MR, Jackson TJ. The ras gene, transformer and transducer. *Nature* 1987, **328**: 668–669.

162. Hunter T. Cooperation between oncogenes. *Cell* 1991, **64**: 249–270.

163. Jamal S, Ziff E. Transactivation of c-fos and β-actin genes by raf as a step in early response transmembrane signals. *Nature* 1990, **344**: 463–466.

164. Wang Z-Q, Ovitt C, Grigoriadis AE, et al. Bone and hematopoietic defects in mice lacking c-fos. *Nature* 1992, **360**: 741–745.

165. Siegel JN, Klausner RD, Rapp UR, et al. T-cell antigen receptor engagement stimulates c-raf phosphorylation and induces c-raf associated kinase activity via a protein kinase dependent pathway. *J. Biol. Chem.* 1990, **265**: 18472–18480.

166. Bruder JT, Heidecker G, Rapp UR. Serum TPA- and ras-induced expression from AP1/ets-driven promoters requires raf-1 kinase. *Genes Develop.* 1992, **6**: 545–556.

167. Crews CM, Erikson RL. Extracellular signals and reversible protein phosphorylation: what to mek of it all. *Cell* 1993, **74**: 215–217.

168. Perlmutter RM, Levin SD, Appleby MW, et al. Regulation of lymphocyte function by protein phosphorylation. *Annu. Rev. Immunol.* 1993, **11**: 451–499.

169. Izquierdo M, Downward J, Otani H, et al. Interleukin 2 activation of p21ras in murine myeloid cells transfected with the human IL-2 receptor α-chain. *Eur. J. Immunol.* 1992, **22**: 817–821.

170. Varmus HE, Lowell CA. Cancer genes and hematopoiesis. *Blood* 1994, **83**: 5–9.

171. Desai DM, Sap J, Schlessinger J, et al. Ligand-mediated negative regulation of a chimeric transmembrane receptor tyrosine phosphatase. *Cell* 1993, **73**: 541–554.

172. Rudd CE. CD4, CD8, and the TCR-CD3 complex: A novel class of protein-tyrosine kinase receptor. *Immunol. Today* 1990, **11**: 400–410.

173. Weber JR, Bell GM, Han MY, et al. Association of the tyrosine kinase lck with phospholipase C-γ1 after stimulation of the T cell antigen receptor. *J. Exp. Med.* 1992, **176**: 373–379.

174. Amrein KE, Flint N, Panholzer B, et al. Ras GTPase-activating protein: A substrate and a potential binding protein of the protein-tyrosine kinase p56lck. *Proc. Natl Acad. Sci. USA* 1992, **89**: 3343–3346.

175. Ettehadieh E, Sanghera JS, Pelech SL, et al. Tyrosyl phosphorylation and activation of MAP kinases by p56lck. *Science* 1992, **255**: 853–856.

176. Chan AC, Iwashima M, Turck CW, et al. ZAP-70 kd protein-tyrosine kinase that associates with the TCRζ chain. *Cell* 1992, **71**: 649–662.

177. Arpaia E, Shahar M, Dadi H, et al. Defective T cell receptor signaling and CD8+ thymic selection in humans lacking Zap-70 kinase. *Cell* 1994, **76**: 947–958.

178. Cooke MP, Abraham KM, Forbush KA, et al. Regulation of T-cell receptor signalling by the src family protein-tyrosine kinase p59fyn. *Cell* 1991, **65**: 281–291.

179. Sancho J, Choi MS, Dasgupta JD, et al. Stimulation of T cells through the TCR/CD3-complex induces tyrosine phosphorylation of a 70 kDa polypeptide chain associated with the CD3-zeta chain. *J. Biol. Chem.* 1992, **267**: 7871–7879.

180. Peter ME, Hall C, Ruhlmann A, et al. The T cell receptor zeta chain contains a GTP/GDP binding site. *EMBO J.* 1992, **11**: 933–941.

181. Mackay CR, Kimpton WG, Brandom MR, et al. Lymphocyte subsets show marked differences in their distribution between blood and the afferent and efferent lymph of peripheral lymph nodes. *J. Exp. Med.* 1988, **167**: 1755–1756.

182. Shimizu Y, Newman W, Tanaka Y, et al. Lymphocyte interactions with endothelial cells. *Immunol. Today* 1992, **13**: 106–112.

183. Groh V, Porcelli S, Fabbi M, et al. Human lymphocytes bearing T cell receptor γ/δ are phenotypically diverse and evenly distributed throughout the lymphoid system. *J. Exp. Med.* 1989, **169**: 1277–1294.

184. Inghirami G, Zhu BY, Chess L, et al. Flow cytometric and immunohistochemical characterization of the γ/δ T-lymphocyte population in normal human lymphoid tissue and peripheral blood. *Am. J. Pathol.* 1990, **136**: 357–367.

185. Falini B, Flenghi L, Pileri S, et al. Distribution of T cells bearing different forms of the T cell receptor γ/δ in normal and pathological human tissues. *J. Immunol.* 1989, **143**: 2480–2488.

186. Bos JD, Kapsenberg ML. The skin immune system: Progress in cutaneous biology. *Immunol. Today* 1993, **14**: 75–78.

187. Matsui K, Boniface JJ, Reay PA, et al. Low affinity interaction of peptide-MHC complexes with T-cell receptors. *Science* 1991, **254**: 1788–1791.

188. Mackay CR. T-Cell memory: The connection between function, phenotype and migration pathways. *Immunol. Today* 1991, **12**: 189–192.

189. Picker LJ, Butcher EC. Physiological and molecular mechanisms of lymphocyte homing. *Annu. Rev. Immunol.* 1992, **10**: 561–591.

190. Springer TA. Traffic signals for lymphocyte recirculation and leukocyte emigration: The multistep paradigm. *Cell* 1994, **76**: 301–314.

191. Cerff-Bensussan N, Jarry A, Brousse N, et al. A monoclonal antibody (HML-1) defining a novel membrane molecule present on human intestinal lymphocytes. *Eur. J. Immunol.* 1987, **17**: 1279–1285.

192. Pardi R, Inverardi L, Bender JR. Regulatory mechanisms in leukocyte adhesion: flexible receptors for

sophisticated travelers. *Immunol. Today* 1992, **13**: 224–230.

193. Paul WE, Seder RA. Lymphocyte responses and cytokines. *Cell* 1994, **76**: 241–251.

194. Dianzani U, Luqman M, Rojo J, et al. Molecular associations on the T cell surface correlate with immunological memory. *Eur. J. Immunol.* 1990, **20**: 2249–2257.

195. Beverley PCL. Human T-cell memory. *Curr. Topics Microbiol. Immunol.* 1990, **159**: 111–122.

196. Janeway CA, Golstein P. Lymphocyte activation and effector functions. *Curr. Opinion Immunol.* 1993, **5**: 313–323.

197. Dellabona P, Casorati G, Friedli B, et al. In vivo persistence of expanded clones specific for bacterial antigens within the human T-cell receptor α/β CD4–8–

subset. *J. Exp. Med.* 1993, **177**: 1763–1771.

198. Porcelli S, Yockey CE, Brenner MB, et al. Analysis of T cell antigen receptor (TCR) expression by human peripheral blood CD4–8– α/β+ T cells demonstrates a preferential use of several Vβ genes and an invariant TCRα chain. *J. Exp. Med.* 1993, **178**: 1–16.

199. Schild H, Mavaddat N, Litzenberger C, et al. The nature of major histocompatibility complex recognition by $\gamma\delta$ T-cells. *Cell* 1994, **76**: 29–37.

200. Uyemura K, Deans RJ, Band H, et al. Evidence for clonal selection of γ/γ T-cells in response to a human pathogen. *J. Exp. Med.* 1991, **174**: 683–692.

201. Modlin RL, Pirmez C, Hofman FM, et al. Lymphocytes bearing antigen-specific $\gamma\delta$ T-cell receptors accumulate in human infectious disease lesions. *Nature* 1989, **339**: 544–548.

can be expressed on the cell surface even in the absence of μH expression, that is, in pro-B-cells and early pre-B-cells [85–87]. Transport to the cell surface at this stage presumably involves association with a complex of glycoproteins (p130, p65), which may act as forerunners of $D_H J_H C_\mu$ proteins and μH chains [85,86]. Cross-linking of λ_5 proteins on μH–pre-B-cells induces an increase of intracellular free calcium, suggesting that the surrogate L-chain–early protein complex could function as a signal transducing receptor and that binding to ligands (which have not yet been discovered) in the fetal liver or bone marrow environment might transduce signals to the pro- and pre-B-cells, which control differentiation [61–63,75,85]. Indeed, inactivation of the λ_5 gene by targeted integration of a defective gene

has provided evidence for an important role of surrogate L-chain in B-lymphopoiesis. Mice with such a defective λ_5 gene show a severe disruption of normal B-cell development [60,61,77,85–87]: while they have a pre-BI-cell compartment of approximately normal size they show a 40-fold reduced bone marrow pre-BII compartment, a drastic reduction of the number of sIg+ immature B-cells and severely delayed filling of the peripheral mature B-cell compartment. Since mice with a disrupted transmembrane portion of the μH chain show similar defects in B-cell differentiation, surface expression of μH chain in association with surrogate light chain presumably controls the entry of B-cell into the pre-BII compartment [62,76]. The finding that the normal pre-BII compartment contains cells mainly

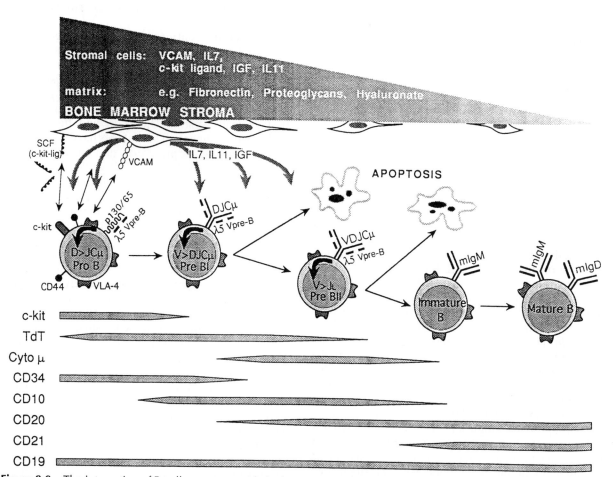

Figure 8.9 The interaction of B-cell precursors with the hematopoietic microenvironment. Differentiation from a pro-B- to a mature B-cell is marked by successive rearrangements of the immunoglobulin heavy and light chain genes, and by sequential expression of the surrogate light chain (λ_5 Vpre-B) with its different partners, followed by membrane expression of IgM and IgM plus IgD. During differentiation, the B-cell precursors physically interact with bone marrow stromal cells and with the extracellular matrix (ECM) via c-kit–SCF (c-kit ligand), VLA-4–VCAM-1, VLA-4–fibronectin and CD44–hyaluronate. In addition, their growth and differentiation depends on a number of cytokines including the soluble form of c-kit-ligand, IL-7, IL-11, and IGF. These cytokines may either be present in soluble form or may be immobilized by proteoglycans in the ECM and on cells.

with productively $V_HD_HJ_H$-rearranged H-chain loci expressing μH-chains, and hence is depleted of cells with nonproductively rearranged H-chain loci, also favors a role of the μH/surrogate L-chain complex in B-cell selection into the pre-BII pool [85]. The pre-B-cell receptor presumably delivers a signal required for cell survival. The nonproductively rearranged cells die *in situ*, probably by apoptosis.

THE HEMATOPOIETIC MICROENVIRONMENT IN LYMPHOPOIESIS

Hematopoietic cell development is dependent on contact with a variety of cells, matrix molecules and growth factors that make up the hematopoietic microenvironment (Figure 8.9). Ultrastructural studies have provided a general picture of the structure of the bone marrow and of areas of hematopoiesis [88, 89]. Part of the space within the bones is occupied by fat (yellow marrow) and is not engaged in blood cell production. In conditions of unusual demand, active hematopoietic marrow (red marrow) can expand into such areas. Newly formed blood cells leave the marrow after traversing the endothelium of venous sinuses.

The different blood cell types are made in specialized locations in the bone marrow. Stem cells and hematopoietic progenitor cells are in the extravascular areas and tend to be concentrated in the subendosteal area, i.e., in the vicinity of bone cortex [90]. Myelopoiesis is also mainly localized subendosteally, but platelet formation from megakaryocytes and erythropoiesis takes place in the more central areas of the bone marrow. Although the exact topography of the different steps of B-lymphopoiesis is unknown, early B-lineage lymphocytes are more abundant in the subendosteal area of the marrow [91–93]. However, areas of focal proliferation comparable to follicles in the avian bursa of Fabricius are not apparent, suggesting that differentiating cells move away continuously from the site of replication.

Most of our knowledge of the role of the microenvironment in hematopoiesis is derived from studies using *in vitro* culture systems. These studies were pioneered by Dexter and colleagues [94,95], who were the first to describe *in vitro* conditions for sustaining hematopoiesis. The adaption of this system for the selective growth of B-lymphocytes by Whitlock and Witte [96], has allowed characterization of the macrophages, endothelial cells, fibroblasts and adipocytes that are key cellular elements of the lymphopoietic microenvironment, as well as many of the growth factors they produce. Although many questions still remain, it is currently believed that the microenvironment provides direct cell–cell contact and anchorage for both growth factor-producing cells and B-cell precursors, and that it also supplies specific positive and negative regulatory factors required for growth and differentiation. Thus, B-lymphopoiesis takes place in a complex network involving multiple interactions of B-cell precursors with stromal cells, matrix molecules, and growth factors (Figure 8.9) [63,93]. In the following paragraphs some examples of these interactions will be discussed in more detail.

Soluble mediators involved in lymphopoiesis

A variety of stromal cells and cell lines have been shown to support *in vitro* proliferation of precursor B-cells in mice [61,63,74,97]. Interleukin-7 (IL-7), a stromal cell derived factor, co-stimulates this proliferation and promotes preferential expansion of pre-B-cells from bone marrow and fetal liver [98]. These IL-7 expanded pre-B-cells are capable of differentiation into sIg+ B-cells *in vitro* and *in vivo*. Hence, they have properties of B-lineage committed progenitors. In addition to IL-7, other growth factors contribute to the proliferation and differentiation of B-cell progenitors. Stem cell factor (SCF) (also known as mast cell growth factor, steel factor, or c-kit ligand) has been reported to play an important role in early B-lymphopoiesis. SCF is an early acting hematopoietic factor that was first identified by the fact that mice deficient in expression of this gene show anemia and stem cell deficiency [99]. In B-lymphopoiesis it synergizes with IL-7 in inducing proliferation [97, 100]. This increase in IL-7-induced proliferation can largely be accounted for by an increased frequency of responding cells, suggesting that SCF promotes the transition of IL-7 unresponsive progenitors to the stage of IL-7 responsiveness [97,101]. IL-11, a stromal cell derived cytokine [102,103] that influences the cycling time of multilineage progenitor cells [104], can, in combination with SCF and IL-7, induce differentiation in early B-cell progenitors and renders this differentiation stromal cell independent [97]. Early pro-B-cells can differentiate into Cμ positive cells in the presence of IL-7 and insulin-like growth factor 1 (IGF-1) [105]. Although still far from providing a complete understanding, these studies clearly show that multiple growth factors are involved in B-lymphopoiesis and that these factors act at distinct steps of differentiation.

Cell adhesion in lymphopoiesis

Like other developmental processes, lymphopoiesis is highly dependent on cell adhesion molecules. These molecules mediate direct cell contact with the microenvironment of stromal cells in the primary organs where B-cells develop. Furthermore, they play a key role in the egress of mature virgin B-cells from the bone marrow and in their subsequent homing to the lymph nodes, MALT and spleen [93,106,107]. In analogy with their role in other systems, adhesion molecules presumably function not only as anchors that bind the precursor cells to stromal cells, extracellular matrix molecules or endothelium [106,108–110], but also function as important signal transducers that contribute to the regulation of B-cell growth and differentiation. Also, adhesive interactions have been shown to be important in preventing cells from entering apoptosis [111,112]. As in the germinal center [112], adhesion molecules or their ligands may, hence, contribute to the B-cell selection that takes place in the bone marrow. In conjunction with locally produced growth factors, adhesion ligands exposed in circumscribed areas of the bone marrow may create a microenvironmental niche where specific differentiation steps take place (Figure 8.9).

Lymphohematopoietic progenitors have been shown to express $\beta1$ (very late antigen (VLA), CD29) and $\beta2$ (LFA-1, CD18) integrins, members of the large family of integrin adhesion molecules, consisting of α- and β-chains, that function in multiple cell–cell and cell–matrix interactions [113–118]. Of these molecules, the $\beta1$ integrins $\alpha4\beta1$ and $\alpha5\beta1$ particularly appear to have an important role in early B-cell development. $\alpha4\beta1$, expressed on stem cells and lymphoid progenitors, interacts with vascular cell adhesion molecule-1 (VCAM-1, CD106), a transmembrane molecule and member of the immunoglobulin superfamily, that is expressed on bone marrow stromal cells (Figure 8.9) [116–118]. Antibodies that disrupt this interaction completely block lymphopoiesis in long term bone marrow cultures [119]. Apart from binding VCAM-1, lymphohematopoietic cells interact with fibronectin exposed on stromal cells or deposited in the extracellular matrix through both $\alpha4\beta1$ and $\alpha5\beta1$, an interaction resulting in cell adhesion as well as in migration [118,120].

CD44, a family of molecules encoded by a single gene [121,122], is also believed to be involved in lymphopoiesis. CD44 molecules are expressed on both hematopoietic progenitor and on bone marrow stromal cells [123–126]. Antibodies against CD44 block the early phases of development of myeloid and lymphoid precursor cells in long-term culture [125,126] presumably by preventing interaction with hyaluronate, collagen and/or fibronectin, known ligands of CD44. CD44 can undergo extensive alternative splicing and posttranslational modification and is converted to proteoglycan by certain tissues [121,125]. Proteoglycan-bearing forms of CD44 have unique functions which include recogni-

tion and migration through the extracellular matrix [127,128]. Interestingly, proteoglycans in bone marrow have been shown to be involved in immobilizing cytokines [129]. Heparan sulfate forms of CD44 might function in this way. In support of this, it was demonstrated, in a recent study, that CD44 can bind MIP-1ß, a member of the chemokine family [130]. In lymphocytes which contact this CD44-immobilized proadhesive cytokine this leads to an increase in the avidity of the integrin $\alpha4\beta7$ for its ligand VCAM-1 [130].

Other adhesion molecules are presumably also involved in lymphopoiesis. Syndecan, like some forms of CD44, a heparan sulfate proteoglycan, is expressed on pre-B-cells but lost as these cells mature [131,132]. There is evidence that this molecule is involved in cell adhesion and can immobilize regulatory cytokines [131,133]. Expression of members of the selectin family as well as of heavily glycosylated proteins like CD34 and CD43, which may function as scaffolds for selectin ligands, is closely regulated during hematopoiesis and lymphopoiesis [134–139]. These molecules may have a role in lymphocyte stromal cell interaction but certainly play a key role in interactions with the vasculature during lymphocyte migration and homing. Furthermore, certain growth factors may function as adhesion ligands, either because they are made in both soluble and transmembrane forms or because they are immobilized by extracellular matrix components. For example, alternative splicing of transcripts for SCF (c-kit ligand, steel factor) results in secreted or transmembrane forms of the protein [140]. The transmembrane form may both facilitate physical interaction of precursors with stromal cells and provide an important co-stimulus for survival and growth. Granulocyte–macrophage colony-stimulating factor (GM-CSF), IL-3 and IL-7 can attach to the matrix, presumably through heparan sulfate proteoglycans [129,141]. This immobilization not only contributes to effective stimulation, but the immobilized growth factors are also recognized as adhesion ligands by hematopoietic progenitors [142]. The immobilization of soluble mediators by proteoglycans on hematopoietic precursor and stromal cells, and on matrix components spatially limits the inductive microenvironment since only the cells in the direct vicinity of the immobilized factors can respond to them.

CD5 B-cells: a distinct developmental lineage

In the model described in the preceding paragraphs, B-lymphopoiesis is looked upon as a linear process in which all B-cells descend in line from a common progenitor population whose developmental potential remains constant throughout life. Although presumably valid for the vast majority of developing B-cells in the adult, studies of the ontogeny of CD5+ B-cells have challenged the general validity of this 'single progenitor' model for B-lymphopoiesis. These studies have provided evidence for the generation of CD5+ and CD5− B-cells from distinctive progenitors and suggest that they belong to separate B-cell lineages [143,144]. Several important classes of non-Hodgkin's lymphomas in the human, including lymphocytic lymphoma/B-CLL and mantle cell lymphoma, express CD5 and thus presumably are related to the CD5 B-cell lineage. In this section some of the specific features of the CD5 B-cell lineage are discussed.

ORIGINS OF CD5 B-CELLS

B-cells expressing CD5, a 67 kD glycoprotein originally described as a T-cell differentiation antigen, are present in both mouse and human. The function of the CD5 molecule, which can bind to CD72, is presently unknown [143,144]. In mice, B-cells expressing CD5 are present in low frequencies in the spleen and peripheral blood, but are normally undetectable in bone marrow, lymph nodes and Peyer's patches. However, they are present in high frequency in the peritoneal cavity [144]. Apart from this specific anatomical location, CD5+ B-cells have a number of features that distinguish them from conventional CD5− B-cells. Thus, CD5+ B-cells were shown to be associated with self-reactivity, particularly with the production of 'natural' (non-pathogenic) autoantibodies and mount only low-affinity responses against typical haptens [144,145]. Furthermore, both normal and neoplastic CD5+ B-cells display a remarkably biased V_H and V_L gene usage and show no or only few N-region additions. The repeated utilization of distinctive V genes is believed to result from antigenic selection, but a role of preferential V gene rearrangement has not been ruled out [143,144].

Several studies have yielded compelling evidence for a distinctive origin of CD5+ and conventional (CD5−) B-cells. Cell transfer experiments using mixtures of fetal liver and bone marrow, in which an allotype difference allowed discrimination of their progeny, showed that CD5+ B-cells are only efficiently generated from fetal liver, but not from bone marrow [143,144,146]. Similar results were obtained in experiments in which sorted pro-B-cells from fetal liver and bone marrow were transferred to SCID mice [147]. Hence, CD5 B-cells appear to represent a 'fetal' B-cell lineage the progenitors of which are only (or mainly) residing in fetal hematopoietic tissues. Since transferred mature CD5-positive B-cells can self-reconstitute the CD5 B-cell pool and hence have self-renewal activity, it has been suggested that the reservoir of CD5+ B-cells present in the adult is generated during fetal life and maintained lifelong through this self-renewal activity [143,144].

CD5 B-CELLS IN THE HUMAN

In the human, CD5+ B-cells constitute a large fraction of early lymph node B-cells after 17 weeks of gestation. Furthermore, fluorescence-activated cell sorting (FACS) analysis of umbilical cord blood has shown that the majority (50–95%) of B-cells at birth are CD5+, whereas only 10–20% of B-cells in the adult peripheral blood and a small minority of B-cells in the lymphoid tissues are CD5+ [144]. As in the mouse, autoreactivity has been associated with CD5+ B-cells in the human. Thus, increased levels of these cells were found in patients with rheumatoid arthritis and Sjögren's syndrome, and EBV-transformed CD5+ B-cells were show to have a high frequency of rheumatoid factor specificity [148,149]. Furthermore, like murine CD5 B-cells, both normal and malignantly transformed (chronic lymphoytic leukemia (CLL)) human CD5 B-cells show preferential usage of particular V genes, which is probably caused by antigen-driven selection and expansion. This selection does not, however, appear to lead to affinity maturation: analysis of CD5+ and CD5− B-lymphocytic lymphomas has shown that those that express CD5 have unmutated germline genes, whereas tumors lacking CD5 often show extensive somatic hypermutation [144,150–152].

Immunopoiesis: antigen-dependent B-cell differentiation

The term 'immunopoiesis' refers to the lymphocyte differentiation and maturation events that follow contact of mature 'virgin' lymphocytes with their cognate antigen. Following this antigenic contact an immune response is generated, which involves activation and subsequently differentiation of naive T- and B-lymphocytes into effector cells and memory cells. The effector T-cells interact with and lyse antigen-bearing cells, whereas the effector B-cells (plasma cells) release immunoglobulins that specifically interact with the antigen. Only those T- and B-lymphocytes that specifically bind to the antigen via their T-cell receptor (TCR) and surface immunoglobulin molecules, become activated. A subsequent encounter with the same antigen will lead to an amplified immune response, that is, a faster response of higher magnitude and of higher avidity than the primary response, a phenomenon called memory. The primary and memory B-cell responses are generated in specialized microenvironments within the secondary lymphoid organs, i.e., in the interfollicular areas and the germinal centers, respectively. Each microenvironment is composed of several distinct cell types, soluble factors (cytokines) and extracellular matrix molecules. Importantly, the generation of an effective immune response depends on the coordinated interaction between all these components. In this section we describe the structural organization of the secondary lymphoid organs. Subsequently, the primary and memory B-cell responses will be described in more detail and in relationship to their respective microenvironments.

SECONDARY LYMPHOID ORGANS

The major secondary lymphoid organs are the well-organized and encapsulated spleen and lymph nodes, and the nonencapsulated accumulations of lymphoid tissue that are localized along mucosal surfaces, the MALTs [153,154]. Within the secondary lymphoid organs separate areas are populated by T- and B-cells. In the spleen, the lymphoid tissue, called the white pulp, is organized around central arterioles (Figure 8.10). The T-cells are located directly adjacent to the central arterioles and form the periarteriolar lymphoid sheath (PALS). B-Lymphocytes are found in separate follicles that may consist entirely of naive B-cells, the primary follicles, or, during an ongoing immune response, can contain a germinal center in which memory B-cells are formed. PALS and follicles are surrounded by the marginal zone, consisting of B-cells. The white pulp is

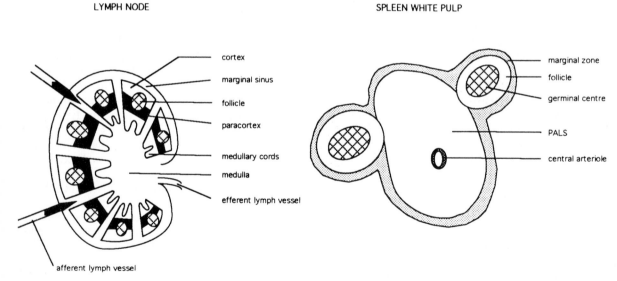

LYMPH NODE   SPLEEN WHITE PULP

cortex
marginal sinus
follicle
paracortex
medullary cords
medulla
efferent lymph vessel

afferent lymph vessel

marginal zone
follicle
germinal centre
PALS
central arteriole

Figure 8.10 The basic architecture of the lymph node and spleen. The lymph that enters the lymph node via the afferent lymphatic vessels first passes through the marginal sinus, which is lined by phagocytic cells. Antigens and lymphoid cells in the lymph then pass through the cortex and medulla, and leave the lymph node through the efferent lymphatic vessel. The cortex contains aggregates of B-cells organized in follicles, while the paracortex contains mainly T-cells, which closely interact with antigen presenting, interdigitating cells. In the medulla, lymphoid cells are mainly found in the medullary cords, which are surrounded by sinuses. Lymphocytes in the blood enter the lymph node via specialized high endothelial venules in the paracortex.

In the spleen the white pulp contains the lymphoid tissue. The bulk of the lymphoid tissue is arranged around a central arteriole, the periarteriolar lymphoid sheath (PALS). The area directly adjacent to the central arteriole contains T-cells, while the more outward part of the PALS contains T- as well as B-cells. B-Cells are also found in follicles. PALS and follicles are surrounded by the marginal zone.

surrounded by the red pulp, where macrophages are involved in the destruction of aged erythrocytes and the removal of antigens from the blood.

In the lymph nodes, which form part of the meshwork of lymphatic vessels draining the tissues, most of the lymphoid cells are found in the cortex (Figure 8.10) while some lymphoid tissue extends into the medulla where it forms the medullary cords. These cords are separated by large sinuses that contain many plasma cells and macrophages, the latter capable of removing antigens from the lymph while it is flowing from the afferent lymphatic vessels to the efferent lymphatic vessels. The cortex can be subdivided into separate subregions that differ in T- and B-lymphocyte composition. The paracortex, which lies adjacent to the medulla, primarily contains T-lymphocytes, while the B-lymphocytes are organized into primary or secondary (containing a germinal center) follicles and also predominate in the areas bordering the marginal sinus. The afferent lymphatics enter the lymph node in the marginal sinus, which is located under the collagenous capsule that encompasses the lymph node.

MALTs are found in the lamina propria and submucosal areas of the gastrointestinal, nasopharyngeal, respiratory and urogenital tracts. Besides diffusely distributed lymphoid tissue of the lamina propria, the intestinal wall also contains nodular accumulations of lymphoid tissue containing distinctive T- and B-cell areas, for example, in Peyer's patches.

Besides lymphocytes, the lymphoid organs contain many other cell types that play an important role in immune function, like macrophages, interdigitating cells and follicular dendritic cells. The function of these cells and their interaction with the lymphocytes will be further discussed below.

LYMPHOCYTE TRAFFIC

Lymphocytes continuously migrate from one lymphoid organ to another via the blood and the lymph [155]. This migration process is essential for effective immunosurveillance, as it increases the probability that lymphocytes with a particular antigenic specificity, but present in low numbers, will meet their cognate antigen. In the spleen, lymphocytes simply leave the blood and enter the white pulp through the capillary branches of the central arterioles that end in the marginal zone. In the other secondary lymphoid organs, lymphocytes extravasate via specialized venules lined by high endothelial cells (HEV) [156]. These HEV are located in the T-areas of lymph nodes and MALT. Lymphocytes may also enter the lymph nodes through the afferent lymph

vessels that drain the tissues or are connected to other lymph nodes. Lymphocytes leave the lymph node through the efferent lymphatics and finally re-enter the blood via the thoracic duct.

Transendothelial migration is a complex process, involving adhesion receptors on both lymphocyte and endothelium, whose function and expression is regulated by cytokines [157–160]. A four-step model has been proposed in which lymphocytes first interact with endothelial cells through adhesion molecules of the selectin family [106,161,162]. This initial interaction, which is reversible, leads to margination of the lymphocytes and rolling (movement) over the endothelial lining. Subsequently, lymphocytes can become activated by local cytokines, which results in activation of adhesion receptors of the integrin family. These then mediate strong binding to the endothelium followed by transmigration. It has been proposed that this complex series of events forms the basis for the selective homing of lymphocytes into specific anatomical sites; for example, T-lymphocyte migration to the skin, peripheral lymph nodes, MALT and chronically inflamed tissue, like synovium in rheumatoid arthritis patients, involves distinct combinations of adhesion receptors and cytokines [157,163–166]. However, few data are available concerning site-specific homing of B-lymphocytes.

THE PRIMARY B-CELL RESPONSE

As previously described (see section on the B-cell receptor complex on page 217) binding of antigen to the mIg receptor results in B-cell activation. Some multivalent antigens that contain multiple identical epitopes placed at a regular distance can extensively cross-link the Ig receptor. These antigens, known as thymus-independent (TI) antigens, can directly induce B-cell proliferation. For the thymus-dependent (TD) antigens, however, the induction of B-cell proliferation and differentiation requires co-stimulatory signals (help) provided by the T-cell. The initial activation of B-cells is thought to take place in the T-cell regions of the lymphoid organs, i.e., paracortical areas of lymph nodes and MALT and in the PALS of the spleen [167,168]. At these sites, the B-cells interact with T-cells, which have been activated by antigen presented on specialized antigen presenting (interdigitating, dendritic) cells (Figure 8.11a,b) [169,170]. T-Cells that have been activated (artificially) by CD3–TCR cross-linking can also provide signals for B-cell activation [171,172]. Studies using these T-cells have revealed that they provide at least two activation signals to the B-cell, i.e., (1) a cell contact-dependent activation signal, and (2) a cytokine signal. Thus, cell membranes of activated T-cells cell antigen receptor complex: Association of Igα and Igβ with distinct cytoplasmic effectors. *Science* 1992, **258**: 123–126.

49. Noesel CJM, Brouns G, Schijndel GMW van, et al. Comparison of the human B cell antigen receptor complexes: Membrane-expressed forms of immunoglobulin (Ig)M, IgD, and IgA, are associated with structurally related heterodimers. *J. Exp. Med.* 1992, **175**: 1511–1519.

50. Campbell KS, Hager EJ, Friedrich RJ, et al. IgM antigen receptor complex contains phosphoprotein products of B29 and mb-1 genes. *Proc. Natl Acad. Sci. USA* 1991, **88**: 3982–3986.

51. Hombach J, Tsubata T, Leclercq L, et al. Molecular components of the B-cell antigen receptor complex of the IgM class. *Nature* 1990, **343**: 760–762.

52. Yamanashi Y, Fukui Y, Wongsasant W, et al. Activation of Src-like protein-tyrosine kinase Lyn and its association with phosphatidylinositol 3-kinase upon B-cell antigen receptor-mediated signaling. *Proc. Natl Acad. Sci. USA* 1992, **89**: 1118–1122.

53. Burkhardt AL, Brunswick M, Bolen JB, et al. Anti-immunoglobulin stimulation of B lymphocytes activates src-related protein-tyrosine kinase. *Proc. Natl Acad. Sci. USA* 1991, **88**: 7410–7414.

54. Hutchcroft JE, Harrison ML, Geahlen RL. B lymphocyte activation is accompanied by phosphorylation of a 72 kDa protein-tyrosine kinase. *J. Biol. Chem.* 1991, **266**: 14846–14849.

55. Campbell MA, Sefton BM. Protein tyrosine phosphorylation is induced in murine B lymphocytes in response to stimulation with anti-immunoglobulin. *EMBO J.* 1990, **9**: 2125–2131.

56. Hutchcroft JE, Harrison ML, Geahlen RL. Association of the 72-kDa protein-tyrosine kinase PTK72 with the B cell antigen receptor. *J. Biol. Chem.* 1992, **267**: 8613–8619.

57. Taniguchi T, Kobayashi T, Kondo J, et al. Molecular cloning of a porcine gene syk that encodes a 72-kDa protein-tyrosine kinase showing high susceptibility to proteolysis. *J. Biol. Chem.* 1991, **266**: 15790–15796.

58. Gold MR, Crowley MT, Martin GA, et al. Targets of B lymphocyte antigen receptor signal transduction include the p21[ras] GTPase-activating protein (GAP) and two GAP-associated proteins. *J. Immunol.* 1992, **150**: 377–386.

59. Casillas A, Hanekom C, Williams K, et al. Stimulation of B-cells via the membrane immunoglobulin receptor or with phorbol myristate 13-acetate induces tyrosine phosphorylation and activation of a 42-kDa microtubule-associated protein-2-kinase. *J. Biol. Chem.* 1991, **266**: 19088–19091.

60. Coggeshall KM, McHugh JC, Altman A. Predominant expression and activation-induced tyrosine phosphorylation of phospholipase C-γ2 in B lymphocytes. *Proc. Natl Acad. Sci. USA* 1992, **89**: 5660–5664.

61. Rolink A, Melchers F. B lymphopoiesis in the mouse. *Adv. Immunol.* 1993, **53**: 123–156.

62. Löffert D, Schaal S, Ehlich A et al. Early B-cell development in the mouse: Insight from mutations introduced by gene targeting. *Immunol. Rev.* 1994, **137**: 133–153.

63. Kincade PW, Lee G, Pietrageli CG, et al. Cells and molecules that regulate B lymphopoiesis in the bone marrow. *Annu. Rev. Immunol.* 1989, **7**: 1111–1143.

64. Uckun F. The regulation of human B-cell ontogeny. *Blood* 1990, **76**: 1908–1923.

65. Gutierrez-Ramos JC, Palacios R. In vitro differentiation of embryonic stem cells into lymphocyte precursors able to generate T and B lymphocytes in vivo. *Proc. Natl Acad. Sci. USA* 1992, **89**: 9171–9175.

66. Chen U, Kosco M, Staerz U. Establishment and characterization of lymphoid and myeloid mixed-cell populations from mouse late embryoid bodies, 'embryonic-stem-cell fetuses'. *Proc. Natl Acad. Sci. USA* 1992, **89**: 2541–2545.

67. Civin CI, Strauss LC, Brovall C, et al. A haematopoietic progenitor cell surface antigen defined by a monoclonal antibody raised against KG-1a cells. *J. Immunol.* 1984, **133**: 157–165.

68. Loken MR, Shah VO, Dattillio KL, et al. Flow cytometric analysis of human bone marrow: II. Normal B lymphocyte development. *Blood* 1987, **70**: 1316–1324.

69. Simmons PJ, Torok-Storb B. CD34 expression by stromal precursors in the normal human adult bone marrow. *Blood* 1991, **78**: 2848–2853.

70. Andrews RG, Singer JW, Bernstein ID. Precursors of colony-forming cells in humans can be distinguished from colony-forming cells by expression of the CD33 and CD34 antigens and light scatter properties. *J. Exp. Med.* 1989, **169**: 1721–1731.

71. Huang S, Terstappen LWMM. Lymphoid and myeloid differentiation of single human CD34+, HLA-DR+, CD38-haematopoietic cells. *Blood* 1994, **83**: 1515–1526.

72. Huang S, Terstappen LWMM. Formation of both haematopoietic microenvironment and haematopoietic stem cells from single human marrow stem cells. *Nature* 1992, **360**: 745–749.

73. Osmond DG. B cell development in bone marrow. *Semin. Immunol.* 1990, **2**: 173–180.

74. Dorshkind K. Regulation of haematopoiesis by bone marrow stromal cells and their products. *Annu. Rev. Immunol.* 1990, **8**: 111–137.

75. Rolink A, Melchers F. Molecular and cellular origins of B lymphocyte diversity. *Cell* 1991, **66**: 1081–1094.

76. Kitamura D, Roes J, Kuhn R, et al. A B-cell deficient mouse generated through targeted disruption of the membrane exon of immunoglobulin μ chain. *Nature* 1991, **350**: 423–426.

77. Kitamura D, Kudo A, Schaal S. A critical role for λ5 protein in B-cell development. *Cell* 1992, **69**: 823–831.

78. Lassoued K, Nunez CA, Billips L, et al. Expression of surrogate light chains is restricted to a late stage in pre-B-cell differentiation. *Cell* 1993, **73**: 73–86.

79. Alt FW, Blackwell TK, Yancopoulos GD. Development of the primary antibody repertoire. *Science* 1987, **238**: 1079–1087.

80. Sakaguchi N, Melchers F. λ5, a new light-chain related locus selectively expressed in pre-B lymphocytes. *Nature* 1986, **324**: 579–582.

81. Kudo A, Melchers F. A second gene V pre-B in the λ5 locus of the mouse, which appears selectively expressed in pre-B lymphocytes. *EMBO J.* 1987, **6**: 2267–2272.

81a. Chang H, Dmitrovsky E, Hieter PA, Mitchell K, Leder P, Turoczi L, Kirsch IR, Hollis GF. Identification of three new Ig λ-like genes in man. *J. Exp. Med.* 1986, **163**: 425–435.

81b. Hollis GF, Evans RJ, Stafford-Hollis JM, Korsmeyer SJ, McKearn JP. Immunoglobulin λ light-chain-related genes 14.1 and 16.1 are expressed in pre-B cells and may encode the human immunoglobulin α light-chain protein. *Proc. Natl Acad. Sci. USA* 1989, **86**: 5552–5556.

81c. Schiff C, Bensmana M, Guglielmi P, Milili M, Lefranc MP, Fougereau M. The immunoglobulin λ-like gene cluster (14.1, 16.1 and Fλ1) contains gene(s) selectively expressed in pre-B cells and is the human counterpart of the mouse λ5 gene. *Int. Immunol.* 1990, **2**: 201–207.

82. Tsubata T, Reth M. The products of the pre-B cell-specific genes (λ5 and Vpre-B) and the immunoglobulin μ chain form a complex that is transported onto the cell surface. *J. Exp. Med.* 1990, **172**: 973–976.

83. Karasuyama H, Kudo A, Melchers F. The proteins encoded by the Vpre-B and λ5 pre-B cell specific genes can associate with each other and with the μ heavy chain. *J. Exp. Med.* 1990, **172**: 969–972.

84. Tsubata T, Tsubata R, Reth M. Cell surface expression of the short immunoglobulin μ chain (Dμ protein) in murine pre-B cells is differently regulated from that of intact μ chain. *Eur. J. Immunol.* 1991, **21**: 1359–1363.

85. Melchers F, Karasuyama H, Haasner D, et al. The surrogate light chain in B-cell development. *Immunol. Today* 1993, **14**: 60–68.

86. Rolink A, Karasuyama H, Haasner D, et al. Two pathways of B-lymphocyte development in the mouse bone marrow and roles of surrogate L chain in this development. *Immunol. Rev.* 1994, **137**: 185–201.

87. Karasuyama H, Rolink A, Shinkai Y, et al. The expression of Vpre-B/λ5 surrogate light chain in early bone marrow precursor B cells of normal and B cell deficient mutant mice. *Cell* 1994, **77**: 133–143.

88. Weiss L, Chen LT. The organisation of haematopoietic cords and vascular sinuses in bone marrow. *Blood Cells* 1975, **1**: 617–688.

89. Lichtman MA. The ultrastructure of the haematopoietic microenvironment of the marrow: A review. *Exp. Hematol.* 1981, **9**: 391–410.

90. Lord BI, Testa NG, Hendry JH. The relative spatial distribution of CFU-s and CFU-c in the normal mouse femur. *Blood* 1975, **46**: 65–72.

91. Hermans MHA, Hartsuiker H, Opstelten D. An in situ study of B-lymphopoiesis in rat bone marrow: Topographical arrangement of terminal deoxynucleotidyl transferase-positive cells and pre-B cells. *J. Immunol.* 1989, **142**: 67–73.

92. Jacobsen K, Osmond DG. Microenvironmental organization and stromal cell associations of B lymphocyte precursor cells in mouse bone marrow. *Eur. J. Immunol.* 1990, **20**: 2395–2404.

93. Kincade PW. Cell adhesion mechanisms utilized for lymphohaematopoiesis. In: Shimizu Y (ed.) *Lymphocyte Adhesion Molecules.* Austin, TX: R. G. Landes Company, 1993, pp. 249–279.

94. Dexter TM, Lajta LG. Proliferation of haematopoietic stem cells in vitro. *Br. J. Haematol.* 1974, **28**: 525–530.

95. Dexter TM, Allan TD, Lajta LG. Condition controlling the proliferation of haematopoietic stem cells in vitro. *J. Cell Physiol.* 1977, **91**: 335–344.

96. Whitlock CA, Witte ON. Long-term culture of B lymphocytes and their precursors from murine bone marrow. *Proc. Natl Acad. Sci. USA* 1982, **79**: 3608–3612.

97. Cuomo A, Kee BL, Ramsden RA. Development of B-lymphocytes from lymphoid committed and uncommitted progenitors. *Immunol. Rev.* 1994, **137**: 4–33.

98. Namen AE, Lupton S, Hjerrild K, et al. Stimulation of B-cell progenitors by cloned murine IL-7. *Nature* 1988, **333**: 571–573.

99. Sarveila PA, Russell LB. Steel a new dominant gene in the mouse. *J. Hered.* 1956, **47**: 123–133.

100. Billips LG, Petitte D, Dorshkind K. Differential roles of stromal cells, interleukin 7, and kit-ligand in the regulation of B lymphopoiesis. *Blood* 1992, **79**: 1185–1192.

101. Narendran A, Ramsden D, Cumano A, et al. The stromal cell line S17 supports the growth of LPS stimulated CBA/N B-cell colonies in vitro. *Eur. J. Immunol.* 1992, **22**: 1001–1006.

102. Paul SR, Bennet F, Calvetti JA, et al. Molecular cloning of a cDNA encoding interleukin 11, a stromal cell-derived lymphopoietic and haematopoietic cytokine. *Proc. Natl Acad. Sci. USA.* 1990, **87**: 7512–7516.

103. Du XX, Williams DA. Interleukin 11, a multifunctional growth factor derived from the haematopoietic microenvironment. *Blood* 1994, **83**: 2023–2030.

104. Schibler KR, Yany YC, Christensen RD. Effect of interleukin 11 on cycling status and clonogenic maturation of fetal and adult haematopoietic progenitors. *Blood* 1992, **80**: 900–903.

105. Landreth KS, Narayanan R, Dorshkind K. Insulin like growth factor-1 regulates pro-B-cell differentiation. *Blood* 1992, **80**: 1207–1212.

106. Springer TA. Traffic signals for lymphocyte recirculation and leucocyte emigration: The multistep paradigm. *Cell* 1994, **76**: 301–314.

107. Picker LJ, Butcher EC. Physiological and molecular mechanisms of lymphocyte homing. *Annu. Rev. Immunol.* 1992, **10**: 561–591.

108. Maguire JE, van Seventer GA. Adhesion molecules as signal transducers in T-cell activation. In: Shimizu Y (ed.) *Lymphocyte Adhesion Molecules.* Austin, TX: R. G. Landes Company, 1993, pp. 313–331.

109. Noesel C van, Miedema F, Brouwer M, et al. Regulatory properties of LFA-1 alpha and beta chains in lymphocyte activation. *Nature* 1988, **333**: 850–852.

110. Tedder TF, Engel P, Wagner N, et al. Adhesion receptors of B lymphocytes: Expression and function on normal and malignant cells. In: Shimizu Y (ed.) *Lymphocyte Adhesion Molecules.* Austin, TX: R. G. Landes Company, 1993, pp. 280–312.

111. Frisch SM, Francis H. Disruption of epithelial cell-matrix interactions induces apoptosis. *J. Cell Biol.* 1994, **124**: 619–626.

CD11a/CD18-CD54 interactions in human T cell dependent B cell activation. *J. Immunol.* 1991, **146**: 492–499.

179. Altman A, Coggeshall KM, Mustelin T. Molecular events mediating T cell activation. *Adv. Immunol.* 1990, **48**: 227–360.

180. Clark EA, Ledbetter JA. How B and T cells talk to each other. *Nature* 1994, **367**: 425–428.

181. Rock KL, Benacerraf B, Abbas AK. Antigen presentation by hapten specific B lymphocytes. I. Role of surface immunoglobulin receptors. *J. Exp. Med.* 1984, **160**: 1102–1113.

182. Sanders VM, Snyder JM, Uhr JW, et al. Characterization of the physical interaction between antigen-specific B and T cells. *J. Immunol.* 1986, **137**: 2395–2404.

183. Stein H, Gerdes J, Mason DY. The normal and malignant germinal center. *Clin. Haematol.* 1982, **11**: 531–559.

184. Butcher EC, Rouse RV, Coffman RL, et al. Surface phenotype of Peyer's patch germinal center cells: Implications for the role of germinal centers in B cell differentiation. *J. Immunol.* 1982, **129**: 2698–2707.

185. Rouse VR, Ledbetter JA, Weissman IL. Mouse lymph node germinal centers contain a selected subset of T cells – the helper phenotype. *J. Immunol.* 1982, **128**: 2243–2246.

186. Nossal GJ, Abbot AP, Mitchell J, et al. Antigens in immunity. XV. Ultrastructural features of antigen capture in primary and secondary lymphoid follicles. *J. Exp. Med.* 1968, **127**: 277–279.

187. Szakal AK, Hanna MG Jr. The ultrastructure of antigen localization and virus-like particles in mouse spleen germinal centers. *Exp. Mol. Pathol.* 1968, **8**: 75–89.

188. Gerdes J, Stein H, Mason DY, et al. Human dendritic reticulum cells of lymphoid follicles: Their antigenic profile and their identification as multi-nucleated giant cells. *Virchows Arch. B* 1983, **42**: 161–172.

189. Humphrey JH, Grennan D, Sundram V. The origin of follicular dendritic cells in the mouse and the mechanism of trapping of immune complexes on them. *Eur. J. Immunol.* 1984, **14**: 859–864.

190. Kapasi ZF, Burton GF, Shultz LD, et al. Cellular requirements for functional reconstitution of follicular dendritic cells in SCID mice. *Adv. Exp. Med. Biol.* 1993, **329**: 383–386.

191. Schriever F, Freedman AS, Freeman G, et al. Isolated human follicular dendritic cells display a unique antigenic phenotype. *J. Exp. Med.* 1989, **169**: 2043–2058.

192. Sellheyer K, Schwarting R, Stein H. Isolation and antigenic profile of follicular dendritic cells. *Clin. Exp. Immunol.* 1989, **78**: 431–436.

193. Petrasch S, Perez-Alvarez C, Schmitz J, et al. Antigenic phenotyping of human follicular dendritic cells isolated from non-malignant and malignant lymphatic tissue. *Eur. J. Immunol.* 1990, **20**: 1013–1018.

194. Tew JG, Mandel TE. Prolonged antigen half-life in the lymphoid follicles of specifically immunized mice. *Immunology* 1979, **37**: 69–76.

195. Klaus GGB, Humphrey JH, Kunkl A, et al. The follicular dendritic cell: Its role in antigen presentation in the generation of immunological memory. *Immunol. Rev.* 1980, **53**: 3–28.

196. Szakal AK, Kosco MH, Tew JG. A novel in vivo follicular dendritic cell-dependent iccosome mediated mechanism for delivery of antigen to antigen processing cells. *J. Immunol.* 1988, **140**: 341–353.

197. Szakal AK, Kosco MH, Tew JG. Microanatomy of lymphoid tissue during humoral immune responses. Structure function relationships. *Annu. Rev. Immunol.* 1989, **7**: 91–109.

198. Gray D, Kosco M, Stockinger B. Novel pathways of antigen presentation for the maintenance of memory. *Int. Immunol.* 1991, **3**: 141–148.

199. Freedman AS, Munro JM, Rice GE, et al. Adhesion of human B cells to germinal centers in vitro involves VLA-4 and INCAM-110. *Science* 1990, **249**: 1030–1033.

200. Koopman G, Parmentier HK, Schuurman HJ, et al. Adhesion of human B cells to follicular dendritic cells involves both the lymphocyte function-associated antigen 1/intercellular adhesion molecule 1 and very late antigen 4/vascular cell adhesion molecule 1 pathways. *J. Exp. Med.* 1991, **173**: 1297–1304.

201. Rice GE, Munro JM, Corless C, et al. Vascular and nonvascular expression of INCAM-110. A target for mononuclear leucocyte adhesion in normal and inflamed human tissues. *Am. J. Pathol.* 1991, **138**: 385–394.

202. Bowen MB, Butch AW, Parvin CA, et al. Germinal center T cells are distinct helper-inducer T cells. *Hum. Immunol.* 1991, **31**: 67–75.

203. Kroese FGM, Wubenna AS, Seijen HG, et al. Germinal centers develop oligoclonally. *Eur. J. Immunol.* 1987, **17**: 1069–1072.

204. Kraal G, Weissman IL, Butcher EC. Germinal center B cells: Antigen specificity and changes in heavy chain class expression. *Nature* 1982, **298**: 377–379.

205. Mangeney M, Richard Y, Coulaud D, et al. CD77: An antigen of germinal center B cells entering apoptosis. *Eur. J. Immunol.* 1991, **21**: 1131–1140.

206. Ling NR, MacLennan ICM, Mason DY. B-Cell and plasma cell antigens: New and previously defined clusters. In McMichael A, et al. (eds) *Leucocyte Typing III*. Oxford: Oxford University Press, 1987, pp. 302–335.

207. Zutter M, Hockenbery D, Silverman GA, et al. Immunolocalization of the Bcl-2 protein within haematopoietic neoplasms. *Blood* 1991, **78**: 1062–1068.

208. Hockenbery D, Nunez G, Milliman C, et al. Bcl-2 is an inner mitochondrial membrane protein that blocks programmed cell death. *Nature* 1990, **348**: 334–336.

209. Levine EG, Arthur DC, Frizzera G, et al. There are differences in cytogenetic abnormalities among histologic subtypes of the non-Hodgkin's lymphomas. *Blood* 1985, **66**: 1414–1422.

210. Yunis JJ, Frizzera G, Oken MM, et al. Multiple recurrent genomic defects in follicular lymphoma: A possible model for cancer. *N. Engl. J. Med.* 1987, **316**: 79–84.

211. Tsujimoto Y, Gorham G, Cossman J, et al. The t(14;18) chromosome translocations involved in B cell neoplasms result from mistakes in VDJ joining. *Science* 1985, **229**: 1390–1393.

212. Bakhshi A, Wright JJ, Graninger W, et al. Mechanism of the t(14;18) chromosomal translocation: Structural analysis of both derivative 14 and 18 reciprocal partners. *Proc. Natl Acad. Sci. USA* 1987, **84**: 2396–2400.

213. McDonnell TJ, Deane N, Platt FM, et al. Bcl-2-immunoglobulin transgenic mice demonstrate extended B cell survival and follicular lymphoproliferation. *Cell* 1989, **57**: 79–88.

214. McDonnell TJ, Nunez G, Platt FM, et al. Deregulated Bcl-2-Ig transgene expands a resting but responsive immunoglobulin M and D-expressing B-cell population. *Mol. Cell Biol.* 1990, **10**: 1901–1907.

215. McDonnell TJM, Korsmeyer SJ. Progression from lymphoid hyperplasia to high-grade malignant lymphoma in mice transgenic for the t(14;18). *Nature* 1991, **349**: 254–256.

216. Lagresle C, Bella C, DeFrance T. Phenotypic and functional heterogeneity of the IgD⁻B cell compartment: Identification of two major tonsillar B cell subsets. *Int. Immunol.* 1993, **5**: 1259–1268.

217. Liu Y-J, Johnson GD, Gordon J, et al. Germinal centers in T-cell-dependent antibody responses. *Immunol. Today* 1992, **13**: 17–21.

218. MacLennan ICM, Liu Y-L, Johnson GD. Maturation and dispersal of B-cell clones during T cell-dependent antibody responses. *Immunol. Rev.* 1992, **126**: 143–161.

219. Berek C, Griffiths GM, Milstein C. Molecular events during maturation of the immune response to oxazolone. *Nature* 1984, **312**: 271–275.

220. Griffiths GM, Berek C, Kaartinen M, et al. Somatic mutation and maturation of the immune response to 2-phenyloxazolone. *Nature* 1984, **312**: 271–275.

221. Liu JY, Joshua DE, Williams GT, et al. Mechanisms of antigen-driven selection in germinal centres. *Nature* 1989, **342**: 929–931.

222. Liu JY, Cairns JA, Holder MJ, et al. Recombinant 25 kDa CD23 and interleukin-1α promote the survival of germinal center B cells: Evidence for bifurcation in the development of centrocytes rescued from apoptosis. *Eur. J. Immunol.* 1991, **21**: 1107–1114.

223. Roy M, Waldschmidt T, Aruffo A, et al. The regulation of the expression of gp39, the CD40 ligand, on normal and cloned CD4⁺ T cells. *J. Immunol.* 1993, **151**: 2497–2510.

224. Arpin C, Déchanet J, van Kooten C, et al. Generation of memory B cells and plasma cells in vitro. *Science* 1995, **268**: 720–722.

225. Casamayor-Palleja M, Khan M, MacLennan ICM. A subset of CD4+ memory T cells contain preformed CD40 ligand that is rapidly but transiently expressed on their surface after activation through the T cell receptor complex. *J. Exp. Med.* 1995, **181**: 1293–1301.

226. Tew JG, DiLosa RM, Burton GF, et al. Germinal centers and antibody production in bone marrow. *Immunol. Rev.* 1992, **126**: 99–112.

227. Armitage R, Fanslow W, Strockbine L, et al. Molecular and biological characterization of a murine ligand for CD40. *Nature* 1992, **357**: 80–82.

228. Spriggs MK, Armitage RJ, Strockbine L, et al. Recombinant human CD40 ligand stimulates B cell proliferation and immunoglobulin E secretion. *J. Exp. Med.* 1992, **176**: 1543–1550.

229. Jabara HH, Fu SM, Geha RS, et al. CD40 and IgE: Synergism between anti-CD40 monoclonal antibody and interleukin 4 in the induction of IgE synthesis by highly purified human B cells. *J. Exp. Med.* 1990, **172**: 1861–1864.

230. Rousset F, Garcia E, Banchereau J. Cytokine-induced proliferation and immunoglobulin production of human B lymphocytes triggered through the CD40 antigen. *J. Exp. Med.* 1991, **173**: 705–710.

231. Allen RC, Armitage RJ, Conley ME, et al. CD40 ligand gene defects responsible for X-linked hyper-IgM syndrome. *Science* 1993, **259**: 990–993.

232. Calland RE, Armitage RJ, Fanslow WC, et al. CD40 ligand and its role in X-linked hyper IgM syndrome. *Immunol. Today* 1993, **14**: 559–564.

233. Pene J, Rousset F, Briere F, et al. IgE production by normal human B cells induced by alloreactive T cell clones is mediated by IL-4 and suppressed by IFN gamma. *J. Immunol.* 1988, **141**: 1218–1224.

234. Pene J, Rousset F, Briere F, et al. IgE production by normal human lymphocytes is induced by interleukin 4 and suppressed by interferons gamma and alpha and prostaglandin E2. *Proc. Natl Acad. Sci. USA* 1988, **85**: 6880–6884.

235. DeFrance T, Vanbervliet B, Briere F, et al. Interleukin 10 and transforming growth factor beta cooperate to induce anti-CD40 activated naive human B cells to secrete immunoglobulin A. *J. Exp. Med.* 1992, **175**: 671–682.

236. Jabara HH, Ahern DJ, Vercelli D, et al. Hydrocortisone and IL-4 induce IgE isotype switching in human B cells. *J. Immunol.* 1991, **147**: 1557–1560.

237. Shapira SK, Vercelli D, Jabara HH, et al. Molecular analysis of immunoglobulin E synthesis in human B cells by interleukin 4 and engagement of CD40 antigen. *J. Exp. Med.* 1992, **175**: 289–292.

238. Zan-Bar I, Strober S, Vitetta ES. The relationship between surface immunoglobulin isotype and immune function of murine B lymphocytes. IV. Role of IgD-bearing cells in the propagation of immunologic memory. *J. Immunol.* 1979, **123**: 925–930.

239. Black SJ, Tokuhisa T, Herzenberg LA, et al. Memory B cells at successive stages of differentiation: expression of surface IgD and capacity of self renewal. *Eur. J. Immunol.* 1980, **10**: 846–851.

240. Herzenberg LA, Black SJ, Tokuhisa, et al. Memory B cells at successive stages of differentiation. Affinity maturation and the role of IgD receptors. *J. Exp. Med.* 1980, **151**: 1071–1087.

241. Teale JM, Lafrenz D, Klinman NR, et al. Immunoglobulin class commitment exhibited by B lymphocytes separated according to surface isotype. *J. Immunol.* 1981, **126**: 1952–1957.

242. Yaoita Y, Kumagai Y, Okumura K, et al. Expression of lymphocyte surface IgE does not require switch recombination. *Nature* 1982, **297**: 697–699.

243. Perlmutter AP, Gilbert W. Antibodies of the secondary response can be expressed without switch recombination in normal mouse B cells. *Proc. Natl Acad. Sci. USA* 1984, **81**: 7189–7193.

244. Chen Y-W, Word C, Dev V, et al. Double isotype production by a neoplastic B cell line. II. Allelically excluded production of μ and $\gamma 1$ heavy chains without CH gene rearrangement. *J. Exp. Med.* 1986, **164**: 562–579.

245. Gray D. Immunological memory. *Annu. Rev. Immunol.* 1993, **11**: 49–77.

246. Linton PJ, Decker D, Klinman NR. Primary antibody-forming cells and secondary B cells are generated from separate precursor populations. *Cell* 1989, **59**: 1049–1059.

247. Linton PJ, Klinman NR. The generation of memory B cells. *Semin. Immunol.* 1992, **4**: 3–9.

248. Linton PJ, Lo D, Lai L, et al. Among naive precursor cell subpopulations only progenitors of memory B cells originate in germinal centers. *Eur. J. Immunol.* 1992, **22**: 1293–1297.

CHAPTER 9

Lymphokines and interleukins

HARUO SUGIYAMA AND TADAMITSU KISHIMOTO

Introduction

Lymphokines and interleukins play important roles in the pathogenesis of lymphomas. The cytokines that are produced from lymphoma cells and/or from the reactive cells surrounding the tumors (Table 9.1) provide growth advantages for lymphoma cells in either an autocrine or a paracrine fashion. The cytokines also contribute to the systemic symptoms experienced by patients and to the characteristic histopathologic appearances of lymphomas. The elucidation of the roles of cytokines in the histopathogenesis of malignant lymphomas will provide us with new ideas and strategies directed towards the treatments of lymphomas. In this chapter, we provide an overview of the potential importance of the cytokines in the pathogenesis of the non-Hodgkin's lymphomas (NHLs).

Interleukin-1

Interleukin-1 (IL-1) refers to a group of three polypeptide hormones, interleukin-1α(IL-1α), inter-

leukin-1β (IL-1β), and interleukin-1 receptor antagonist (IL-1ra), which play a central role in the regulation of immune and inflammatory responses [1]. IL-1α and IL-1β appear to be agonists for both types of IL-1 receptor (type I and type II), whereas IL-1ra is an antagonist for both IL-1 receptors. IL-1 affects a wide variety of cells *in vitro*: tumor cells (e.g., k562), fibroblasts, smooth muscle cells, keratinocytes, endothelial cells, osteoclasts, chondrocytes, hepatocytes, bone marrow cells, pre-B-cells, mature B-cells, thymocytes, mature T-cells, natural killer (NK) cells, macrophages, and islet cells/insulinomas [1]. IL-1 also plays a central role in a wide variety of immune and inflammatory responses *in vivo*.

IL-1α and IL-1β are produced from monocytes and myeloid cell lines, keratinocytes, B-cells, B-lymphoma cell lines, astrocytes, kidney mesangial cells, and endothelial cells. IL-1ra is produced from activated macrophages.

Ruco et al. immunohistochemically examined IL-1 expression in Hodgkin's disease and NHLs (16 B-cell lymphomas and four T-cell lymphomas) using antibodies directed to IL-1 and tumor necrosis factor α (TNFα) [2]. Cells containing IL-1 and/or TNFα were detected mainly in pathologic conditions characterized by reactive or neoplastic expansion of the lymph node paracortex. Cells positive for IL-1 were

Table 9.1   Possible involvement of cytokines in non-Hodgkin's lymphomas

	Autocrine		Paracrine
	Proliferation	Histopathological effect	Proliferation
HTLV-1+ T-cell lymphoma	IL-2		
Follicular lymphoma			IL-3
T-cell-rich B-cell lymphoma		IL-4	
AILD-like T-cell lymphoma		IL-4, IL-6	
B-cell and T-cell lymphoma with eosinophilia		IL-5	
Ki-positive large-cell anaplastic lymphoma	IL-6, IL-9		
Lennert's lymphoma			?IL-6
Immunoblastic lymphoma	IL-6		
Small lymphocytic lymphoma	IL-6		
Sézary syndrome			IL-7
AIDS lymphoma containing EBV	IL-10		

detected in 16 out of 21 cases of Hodgkin's disease, in four of four cases of T-cell NHL (T-NHL), and in five cases of diffuse or mixed lymphadenitis. IL-1α was detected in macrophages, interdigitating reticulum cells, endothelial cells, and neoplastic Hodgkin's and Reed–Sternberg cells. Cells positive for IL-1β were far fewer and consisted mainly of macrophages. Thus, although IL-1 was detected in neoplastic Hodgkin's and Reed–Sternberg cells and a variety of normal cells infiltrating NHL, it was not detected in the neoplastic B- or T-NHL cells.

Takeshita et al. also examined IL-1 expression by immunohistochemistry in 68 patients with malignant lymphomas (10 patients with Hodgkin's disease and 58 patients with NHL) [3]. In only two cases of T-cell lymphoma (lymphoblastic and angioimmunoblastic lymphadenopathy) and one case of follicular B-cell lymphoma IL-1α was detectable (and in all three cases, weakly) in the neoplastic cells.

Taken together, these two reports suggest that IL-1 is rarely expressed in the neoplastic cells of NHLs.

Interleukin-2

Interleukin-2 (IL-2) is produced by activated T-lymphocytes following antigen or mitogen stimulation and exerts various biological effects. The effects of IL-2 are mediated by its interaction with the IL-2 receptor (IL-2R) that is expressed on T-lymphocytes, and on some B-lymphocytes and monocytes after activation. Three distinct forms of the IL-2R have been identified: a high-affinity IL-2R composed of IL-2Rα and IL-2Rβ subunits, an intermediate IL-2R composed of IL-2Rβ alone, and a low-affinity IL-2R

corresponding to IL-2Rα alone [4]. Only high-affinity and intermediate-affinity IL-2R appear to have functional significance.

Twenty-one low-grade follicular lymphomas were examined for the production of IL-2 using *in situ* hybridization with specific RNA radiolabeled probes [5]. All of the 21 follicular lymphomas tested contained IL-2-synthesizing cells in the interfollicular and follicular areas. Enumeration of lymphokine-synthesizing cells indicated heterogenous IL-2 production among the lymph nodes tested; two of the 21 had much higher densities of IL-2-producing cells (855 and 570/cm^2) than did the remaining 19 (mean, 92 ± 15/cm^2). The detailed distribution of lymphokine-producing cells showed that IL-2-producing cells were located mainly in the follicular areas. The mean follicular/interfollicular ratio was 1.82 ± 0.16. The results showed that T-cell activation, defined as lymphokine production, occurs in lymph nodes containing follicular lymphoma – apparently by T-cells in direct contact with malignant B-cells. Thus, lymphokine production may play an important role in tumor growth, which is the result of an interaction between tumor cells and normal immune cells [5].

A T-cell line, IARC 301, was established from the lymph nodes of a patient with high-grade non-Hodgkin's T-cell lymphoma [6]. This cell line constitutively expresses biologically functional, high-affinity cell surface receptors for IL-2 and synthesizes IL-2, which is bound to cell surface receptors. Monoclonal antibodies directed against either IL-2 or the IL-2R block cell growth. The results demonstrate that the proliferation of this tumor cell line is mediated by an autocrine pathway involving endogenous IL-2 production and its binding to cell surface receptors. These results may imply that IL-2 plays a role in pathogenesis of some T-cell lymphomas.

Adult T-cell leukemia/lymphoma (ATLL) is a disseminated malignancy of T-lymphocytes infected by the human T-lymphotropic virus type 1 (HTLV-1), and is endemic in southern Japan, the Caribbean basin, the southeastern United States and central Africa. The malignant cells are activated T-helper cells that have suppressor function [7]. ATLL cells consistently express a high level of the p55 or IL-2α (Tac) component of the IL-2R. When plasmid vectors p1319βcat and pRPXβcat, each of which contains a chloramphenicol acetyl transferase (CAT) gene and the upstream sequences of the IL-2 and IL-2R genes, respectively, were each cotransfected with Tax genes into a human T4+ cell line, Jurkat, expression of the CAT gene was clearly demonstrated whereas cotransfection with pBR322 control DNA did not result in CAT expression [8]. Thus, a model was proposed whereby the Tax gene of HTLV-1 transactivates transcription of Tac and (weakly) IL-2 [8]. Mitogenic stimulation of a HTLV-1-infected, Tax-expressing T-cells is known to result in synergistic activation of IL-2 transcription, and it has therefore been proposed that antigen receptor triggering of an HTLV-1-infected T-cell could lead to autocrine growth stimulation by IL-2 and subsequent progression to ATLL. However, autonomous growth in the *in vitro* system does not appear to be due to autocrine production because IL-2 is not usually detectable in cell supernatants, and IL-2 mRNA is not usually detectable by Northern blot analysis in primary and short-term cultured ATLL cells. However, analysis of HTLV-1-infected cell lines by *in situ* hybridization identified IL-2 mRNA expressing cells, occurring at a frequency of approximately 1/100 cells, raising the possibility of paracrine growth simulation by IL-2. Thus, it would appear that if autocrine growth simulation by IL-2 is involved in the malignant transformation of T-cells, secretion of IL-2 either ceases or is dramatically diminished during disease progression. The explanation for this apparent discrepancy may be that secretion of IL-2 by potentially immunogenic tumor cells will enhance their rejection by the host immune system [8].

While tumor cells may not secrete IL-2, a soluble form of IL-2Rα that is released by activated normal peripheral blood mononuclear cells and synthesized in large amounts *in vitro* by HTLV-1-infected leukemic cell lines has been detected by Rubin et al., using monoclonal antibodies directed against different epitopes of human IL-2R [9]. The soluble IL-2R is smaller than its cellular counterpart but retains the ability to bind IL-2. Subsequent studies disclosed comparable levels of soluble IL-2R in cord blood and peripheral blood from normal adults. Increased serum levels of IL-2R have been found in patients with certain B- or T-cell malignancies, including HTLV-1-associated adult T-cell leukemia, Sézary syndrome, Hodgkin's disease, chronic lymphocytic leukemia and hairy cell leukemia [10].

The serum levels of a soluble receptor for interleukin-2 (sIL-2R) were determined in patients with NHL. Increased sIL-2R levels were found in most cases, when compared with levels observed in healthy controls [10–14]. The serum levels of sIL-2R correlated with poor prognosis and related to tumor burden, disease progression and B-symptoms. In mycosis fungoides, a close and significant correlation was found between sIL-2R levels and stage of disease [4]. The biological significance of the presence of high concentrations of sIL-2R in patients with NHL remains unclear. Soluble IL-2R molecules still retain an efficient capacity to bind IL-2 [15,16]. Natural killer cells are particularly sensitive to IL-2 starvation because they express low-affinity membrane IL-2R. For this reason, the triggering of NK cell proliferation requires a much higher concentration of IL-2 than that required for proliferation of normal phytohemaglutinin (PHA)-stimulated T-cells [12]. Elevation of sIL-2R and the resulting reduction of IL-2 concentration by the binding of IL-2 with sIL-2R might impair NK activity, allowing tumor growth in patients with NHL.

Interleukin-3

Interleukin-3 (IL-3) stimulates the growth and differentiation of pluripotent hematopoietic stem cells and of progenitors of neutrophils, macrophages, megakaryocytes, erythrocytes, eosinophils, basophils and mast cells [1]. IL-3 also stimulates the functions of mature mast cells, basophils, eosinophils and macrophages. *In vivo* administration of IL-3 increases the numbers of pluripotential hematopoietic stem cells and hematopoietic progenitor cells, of mast cells in skin, spleen and liver, and of basophils, eosinophils, monocytes and neutrophils in the peripheral blood [1]. The major source of IL-3 is activated T-lymphocytes [1], but activated NK and mast cells also produce IL-3.

IL-3 does not have any effects on the proliferation of B-cell tumor cells of diffuse large cell type, but has been reported to stimulate the *in vitro* proliferation of both the follicular lymphoma cell line BLT and fresh follicular lymphoma cells [17]. This proliferation could be completely abrogated by the addition of anti-IL-3 antibodies to the cultures. IL-1, -2, -4, -5 and -6 did not induce proliferation nor did various combinations of these cytokines. All samples of primary follicular lymphomas tested, in one

yielded an easily identifiable, EBV-specific amplification product. From one of these cases they were also able to extract mRNA and used PCR to demonstrate the presence of mRNA coding for IL-5. Thus, they concluded that some acquired immunodeficiency syndrome (AIDS)-related lymphomas are associated with eosinophilia, and that the eosinophilia may be related to EBV infection and transcriptional activation of the IL-5 gene.

Samoszuk et al. also detected an IL-5-specific amplification product in three cases of T-cell lymphoma with eosinophilia, unassociated with HIV infection, by using RNA PCR, and speculated that the eosinophilia in certain T-cell lymphomas is attributable to expression of IL-5 [29].

Interleukin-6

Interleukin-6 (IL-6) is a growth factor with diverse biological activity, which was originally described as a T-cell product that induces the terminal differentiation of B-cells to plasma cells. IL-6 also acts on a variety of cells including T-cells, myeloma cells, megakaryocytes, hematopoietic stem cells, hepatocytes, nerve cells, mesangial cells and epidermal keratinocytes [30]. *In vivo* administration of IL-6 induces the increase in platelet count. IL-6 is produced by variety of cells including T-cells, B-cells, monocytes, macrophages, syncytiotrophoblast, mesangial cells, fibroblasts, endothelial cells and epidermal keratinocytes.

CARDIAC MYXOMA

The first evidence concerning the participation of IL-6 in human diseases was obtained from cardiac myxoma. Cardiac myxoma is a rare primary cardiac tumor. Patients with cardiac myxoma present various clinical manifestations, such as easy fatiguability, weight loss, arthralgia and low-grade fever (collagen disease-like symptoms). It is well known that various clinical manifestations in patients with cardiac myxoma disappear after the resection of the myxoma. However, the reason that myxoma produces collagen disease-like symptoms remained unknown until recently. Shimizu et al. demonstrated that cardiac myxoma produces IL-6, which produces the typical symptom complex associated with myxoma [31].

MYELOMA

Kawano et al. showed that myeloma cells freshly isolated from patients produce IL-6 and express its receptors, and that anti-IL-6 antibody inhibits *in vitro* growth of myeloma cells [32].

CASTLEMAN'S DISEASE

Castleman's disease (plasma cell type) is a syndrome characterized by fever, anemia, hypergammaglobulinemia, an increase in plasma level of acute phase proteins and giant lymph node hyperplasia with plasma cell infiltration [33]. It was known that the clinical abnormalities disappear after the resection of the affected lymph nodes, suggesting that products of the lymph nodes may cause the associated clinical abnormalities. Yoshizaki et al. clearly demonstrated the production of IL-6 by B-cells in the germinal centers of hyperplastic lymph nodes in Castleman's disease [34]. Lymph node cells in two patients with Castleman's disease were cultured without any stimulant and the culture supernatant was examined for the IL-6 activity. The culture supernatants induced production of IgM in SKW6-CL-4, an EBV-transformed B-cell line, in a dose-dependent manner and amounts of IL-6 in the culture supernatants in two patients were estimated to be equivalent to 69.2 ng/ml and 1.16 ng/ml, respectively (IL-6 activity in culture supernatant of normal lymph nodes was equivalent to 0.02–0.04 ng/ml). The IL-6 activity in the culture supernatants was neutralized by anti-IL-6 antibody. In order to examine which cells in the affected lymph nodes produce IL-6, immunohistochemical analysis was performed using monoclonal mouse anti-IL-6 antibody. The cells in the germinal center were stained positively with anti-IL-6 antibody, and the staining was inhibited in the presence of excess IL-6. Moreover, the lymph nodes of the patients were stained with anti-Leu-4 (anti-pan-T), anti-Leu-14 (anti-pan-B), anti-DRC1 (dendritic cells), anti-IgD (mature resting B-cells) and anti-Leu M5 (macrophage). Leu-14+ cells (B-cells) were found in the follicular region including the germinal center, whereas Leu-4+ (T-cells) were mainly seen in interfollicular area and rarely in the germinal center. Anti-DRC1 also stained the germinal center. However, the staining patterns of anti-IL-6 and anti-DRC1 were different; the cells stained with anti-IL-6 antibody were localized in the germinal center whereas the staining with anti-DRC1 was much wider and included the mantle zone of lymphoid follicles. Anti-IgD antibody stained the mantle zone but not the germinal center of lymph follicles and anti-Leu-M5-positive cells were observed scattered through the germinal center. These histochemical findings indicate that the IgD-negative B-cells may produce IL-6 and that the production of IL-6 by B-cells in the germinal centers of hyperplastic lymph nodes in Castleman's disease may be the key element responsible for the variety of clinical symptoms in this disease. Very recently, it has been confirmed that this hypothesis is correct. Beck et al. treated a man who had Castleman's disease and an elevated serum IL-6 concentration with a prolonged course of monoclonal anti-IL-6 antibody [35]. The symptoms and signs of disease resolved and most of the abnormal laboratory values improved dramatically within a few days, but the abnormalities returned on cessation of therapy.

Ki-1 POSITIVE LARGE-CELL ANAPLASTIC LYMPHOMA

Ki-1(CD30) positive large-cell anaplastic lymphoma is a newly recognized clinicopathologic syndrome with fever, cutaneous involvement and peripheral lymphadenopathy, occurring more often in children and adolescents. A patient with Ki-1 positive large-cell anaplastic lymphoma of T-cell origin was examined for the production of IL-6 [36]. Culture supernatant of the unstimulated neoplastic cells in suspension contained large amounts of IL-6. The neoplastic cells survived *in vitro* for 4 weeks and the culture supernatant contained extremely large amounts of IL-6, which were comparable to those in the culture supernatant of the lymph node cells from Castleman's disease.

OTHER NON-HODGKIN'S LYMPHOMAS

Yee et al. tested the production of growth factors in many lymphoma cell lines established from patients with NHLs [37]. Two lymphoma cell lines, one of B-cell origin and one of T-cell origin, secreted and responded to IL-6. Addition of recombinant IL-6 stimulated their growth, whereas addition of polyclonal anti-IL-6 antibody had a marked inhibitory effect on proliferation. These results suggested an autocrine role for IL-6 in the growth of these lymphoma cells in culture. Thus, for lymphoma, IL-6 may be an important growth factor. In these two cell lines, IL-6 is being produced by the cell itself. However, in other cases, IL-6 may be produced by other cells that constitute the cellular environment of the malignant growth.

Lennert's lymphoma is a special form of T-cell lymphoma. The lymph node lesion is characterized by complete effacement of the normal lymph node architecture by a massive proliferation of epithelioid cell (histiocyte) clusters intermingled with many, mostly small, lymphoma cells. It has been suggested that the characteristic histology is a consequence of the effects of cytokines secreted by lymphoma cells or epithelioid histiocytes. A T-lymphoma cell line (KT-3) established from a patient with Lennert's lymphoma showed macrophage-dependent growth [38]. This macrophage's functions could be replaced with IL-6. Anti-IL-6 antibody almost completely neutralized the activity of IL-6. Scatchard plot analysis demonstrated that KT-3 cells indeed express IL-6 receptors. These results indicated that the macrophage-derived factor that supports the growth of KT-3 was IL-6, suggesting that macrophage-derived IL-6 may play an important role in the histopathogenesis of Lennert's lymphoma. However, Merz et al. reported that IL-6 mRNA was not readily detectable in a patient with Lennert's lymphoma [39]. The role of IL-6 in the *in vivo* growth of Lennert's T-lymphoma cells awaits further confirmation [18].

Freeman et al. examined the expression of IL-6 mRNA in B-cell lymphomas using Northern blotting analysis. Eleven of 25 non-Hodgkin's B-cell lymphomas expressed IL-6 mRNA (nodular poor differentiated lymphoma, 4/8; diffuse large cell lymphoma, 4/9; diffuse poorly differentiated lymphoma, 2/6; Burkitt's lymphoma, 1/2) [40].

Using *in situ* hybridization, Merz et al. examined 29 patients with B-cell lymphoma for IL-6 production [22]. Twenty cases were classified as low-grade and nine cases as high-grade malignant lymphoma. Strong signals were found for IL-6 in five cases, whereas the majority of the remaining cases did not show any detectable mRNA-signals for IL-6. Comparison with immunohistochemistry demonstrated low numbers of infiltrating T-cells and monocytes in these strongly positive cases. *In situ* hybridization in four of the five cases clearly demonstrated a positive IL-6 mRNA signal in 20–60% of cells in the specimen, two of which had a T-cell content of less than 10%. It could therefore be concluded that the IL-6 signal was produced at least in part by the tumor cells themselves. The most striking result of this investigation is the fact that some well-defined malignant B-cell lymphomas express high amounts of IL-6, whereas in other histologically identical cases, no IL-6 message was detected. It is tempting to speculate that, in a subset of B-cell lymphomas, IL-6 may influence tumor cell proliferation and accessory cell activity [22].

Emilie et al. analyzed the *in situ* production of IL-6 in lymphoma samples taken from 24 patients (11 Burkitt's lymphomas, seven diffuse large-cell lymphomas, and six immunoblastic lymphomas), 18 of which were obtained from patients infected with HIV [41]. The level of expression of the IL-6 gene was highly heterogenous among these lymphomas, but there was a correlation with pathologic findings. Ten of the 11 Burkitt's lymphomas did not express the IL-6 gene at a higher level than control lymph nodes. The six immunoblastic lymphomas all contained particularly large numbers of IL-6 gene-expressing cells. Three of the seven diffuse large-cell lymphomas also contained numerous cells expressing IL-6. The number of cells expressing IL-6 was seven times higher in the non-Burkitt's lymphomas than in the Burkitt's lymphomas, and it was 17 times higher than that of 14 control lymph nodes displaying a benign follicular hyperplasia. Analysis of individual cases indicated that the level of IL-6 gene expression was strongly correlated with the presence of immunoblasts within the malignant clone. The presence of immunoblasts in the lymphomatous tissue may thus be an important pathologic parameter associated with an increase in IL-6 gene expression. In contrast, IL-6 gene expression was not correlated with the presence of EBV genome in the lymphoma or with the HIV status of patients. Immunohistochemical studies with an anti-IL-6 monoclonal antibody showed that IL-6 was produced in non-Burkitt's lymphomas, but not in Burkitt's lymphomas. In the former, IL-6 was produced mainly if not exclusively by reactive cells, and several cell populations (including endothelial cells, macrophages and normal lymphoid cells) were involved in this production. Immunohistochemical analyses of non-Burkitt's lymphomas also showed that malignant cells produced the IL-6 receptor. Taken together, these results suggested that IL-6 produced by tumor-infiltrating reactive cells may act as a growth factor in some forms of high-grade B-lymphomas (immunoblastic lymphomas) [41].

Hsu et al. immunohistochemically examined 55 non-Hodgkin's B-cell lymphomas, including polymorphic immunocytoma (PI), small lymphocytic lymphoma (SLL), and immunoblastic lymphoma (IBL) with or without plasmacytoid differentiation [42]. In PI and in IBL with plasmacytoid differentiation, IL-6 was detected only in immunoglobulin-containing plasmacytoid cells, and it was absent from proliferating lymphoma cells. In SLL, IL-6 was not observed in lymphoplasmacytoid cells; instead, IL-6 was observed in transformed tumor cells in proliferation centers. In IBL without obvious plasmacytoid differentiation, IL-6 was detected in most tumor cells that were highly proliferative. In this study, IL-6 was undetectable in most lymphomas related to follicular centers, in lymphoblastic lymphoma, in small non-cleaved cell lymphomas of the Burkitt's and non-Burkitt types, and in diffuse large-cell lymphoma. This finding is compatible with

previous findings that IL-6 mRNA was absent from follicular center cells in reactive lymphoid tissues. The function of IL-6 in these lymphomas may be quite diverse. It appears that IL-6, as an autocrine factor, is responsible for the plasmacytoid differentiation of lymphoma cells in PI and some IBL. The differentiation of lymphoplasmacytoid lymphoma cells in SLL, however, may not be mediated by an autocrine IL-6 mechanism. IL-6 may provide a growth signal, rather than acting as a differentiation factor, for some IBL cells and for some transformed tumor cells in proliferative centers in SLL [42].

AILD-TYPE T-CELL LYMPHOMA

Hsu et al. also examined IL-6 expression by immunohistochemistry in four patients with AILD-type T-cell lymphoma [43]. They detected a correlation between the number of plasma cells in tissue and the extent of IL-6 expression in lymphoma cells. In one patient they observed an abundant IL-6 production by lymphoma cells, which accounted for a B-cell plasmacytic tissue response and for hypergammaglobulinemia. The pathogenic significance of IL-6 was substantiated by changes that occurred immediately after chemotherapy. There was a concomitant decrease in the serum IL-6 level, measurable tumor mass and immunoglobulin levels, as well as a decline in the proportion of plasmacytoid cells in peripheral blood. Plasmacytoid B-cells could be maintained in culture in the presence of IL-6, but viability was lost on co-incubation with anti-IL-6. IL-1 and tumor necrosis factor were not produced by T-lymphoma cells and were incapable of sustaining plasmacytoid B-cell viability *in vitro*. Small amounts of IL-4 were noted in T-lymphoma cells. Thus, in this case of AILD-type T-cell lymphoma, tumor cells with a T-cell phenotype produced IL-6 in large quantities, explaining the accompanying B-cell and plasmacytic histologic changes and humoral disease manifestation, including marked hypergammaglobulinemia. However, there was no evidence that IL-6 contributed to autocrine growth of the lymphoma cells in this case.

HODGKIN'S DISEASE

Hodgkin's disease is a neoplastic disease that is characterized by unbalanced and/or unregulated cytokine production [44]. Information accumulated indicates that the cytokines IL-1, IL-5, IL-9, TNFα, G-CSF, M-CSF and TGFβ are secreted by Hodgkin's and Reed–Sternberg (H-RS) cells. These and additional cytokines are likely to be responsible for the unique histopathologic and clinical findings in patients with Hodgkin's disease. Hsu et al. confirmed that IL-6 was produced by cultured H-RS cells as well as by H-RS cells in tissues. In tissues, they were able to immunolocalize IL-6 in the cytoplasm in 10–30% of H-RS cells by using anti-IL-6 antibody. In three of 17 cases studied, a large number (60%) of H-RS cells were positive for IL-6. In one patient, the involved lymph node also showed histologic features similar to those of Castleman's disease. In this patient, they noted abundant IL-6 expression not only in H-RS cells but also in most reactive histiocytes. The cultured H-RS cells did not express functional receptors for IL-6 and exogenously added IL-6 did not induce proliferation of these cells. Thus, these studies demonstrated that adequate amounts of IL-6 are required for an abundant plasma cell reaction, and that an additional source of IL-6 from histiocytes is essential for the formation of Castleman's disease-like changes in lymph nodes involved by Hodgkin's disease [44].

SINUS HISTIOCYTOSIS

Kuroki et al. reported a very rare case of cardiac myxoma with mediastinal lymphadenopathy [45]. A 60-year-old woman with cardiac myxoma had a high level of IL-6 activity in serum and typical clinical manifestations for this disease. This patient also had numerous enlarged mediastinal lymph nodes, although this is a very rare clinical manifestation. Surgery was performed, and the cardiac tumor and a mediastinal lymph node were resected. Interestingly, after the removal of the cardiac tumor, the level of serum IL-6 decreased and the mediastinal lymphadenopathy disappeared on chest computed tomography. Histology of the cardiac tumor and resected lymph node showed a typical appearance of cardiac myxoma and accumulation of sinus histiocytes, which phagocytosed coal pigment and hemosiderin. There were enlarged germinal centers and a small number of plasma cells in the interfollicular area, respectively. Immunohistochemical analysis using monoclonal antibody (CD45RD and CD20) revealed that the distribution of T- and B-cells was almost normal. These findings were compatible with sinus histiocytosis. Taken together, these findings suggest that IL-6, probably produced from cardiac myxoma, may have played an important role in the development of sinus histiocytosis.

EBV-POSITVE LYMPHOMAS IN SCID MICE

Nadal et al. inoculated intraperitoneally 50 × 10^6

human tonsillar mononuclear cells (hu-TMCs) from EBV-seropositive or seronegative human subjects into mice with severe combined immunodeficiency (SCID) [46]. Between 5 and 11 weeks later, 29.4% (10/34) of mice injected with hu-TMCs from EBV-seropositive donors, but none of 34 animals receiving hu-TMCs from EBV-seronegative donors, developed intra-abdominal and/or intrathoracic tumors (P = 0.002). By means of *in situ* hybridization using alpha satellite DNA from human chromosome 17, all tumors produced after cell transfer from EBV-seropositive donors were identified to be of human origin. Histologically the tumors resembled large-cell lymphomas although they are generally believed to represent *in vivo* proliferation of genetically normal EBV-transformed B-cells (see Chapter 12). The EBV genome was detected by *in situ* hybridization and EBV nuclear antigen by immunofluorescence in these tumors. The tumors were polyclonal or oligoclonal, and stained for human IgG and IgM, and less frequently IgA and IgD. Serum levels of human immunoglobulin in animals developing human tumors were significantly higher than in reconstituted mice without tumors and the sera exhibited poly-, oligo- or monoclonality in immunoelectrophoresis. Human IL-6 was detected in the serum of six of 10 animals with human lymhomas, but not in any animals without human lymphoma. The authors suggested that IL-6 potentiates EBV-associated lymphomagenesis but is unlikely to be a prerequisite for such virus-induced lymphoproliferation.

Interleukin-7

Although interleukin-7 (IL-7) was originally characterized on the basis of its ability to promote the proliferation of precursor B-lymphocytes in mice (B220+, sIgG–), it has now been shown that IL-7 can also induce the proliferation of both thymocytes and mature T-cells. IL-7 stimulates the proliferation of murine B-cell progenitors (both pre-B and pro-B) and CD4–, CD8– T-cell progenitors (murine and human), but not the proliferation of sIgM+ B-cells (murine and human) [47]. IL-7 is produced from human spleen and thymus, and from murine spleen, thymus, kidney and bone marrow [1].

Sézary syndrome is a lymphoproliferative disorder characterized by infiltration of the skin by malignant T-cells, and associated with erythroderma, generalized lymphadenopathy and circulating neoplastic cells containing convoluted cerebriform nuclei [48]. Sézary cells are of mature T-helper phenotype, although a lack of CD7 antigen expression is a general feature of these cells. In contrast to ATLL, an aggressive disorder that has been shown to be associated with infection by HTLV-1, Sézary syndrome is a relatively indolent disorder of unknown etiology. Dalloul et al. studied the action of IL-1, IL-2, IL3, IL-4, IL-6 and IL-7 on the proliferation of Sézary cells from 12 patients [48]. Peripheral blood mononuclear cells from these patients did not respond to IL-1β, IL-3, and IL-4 (only one patient responded to IL-2). In contrast, IL-7 generated a very substantial (3–40-fold increase) proliferative response in all patients, whereas IL-2 had only a low proliferative effect (2–3-fold increase) on peripheral blood mononuclear cells. IL-7 was used successfully to generate cell lines in three of eight cases. The growth of Sézary cell lines was shown to be strictly dependent upon IL-7. When compared to normal T-cells, the IL-7 response peaked on days 2–3 in Sézary peripheral blood mononuclear cells, while normal cells showed maximal proliferation on days 6–7. Based on these data, IL-7 was the best of the cytokines tested with respect to their ability to induce Sézary cell proliferation. Interestingly, IL-7 may also be involved in the propensity of Sézary cells to proliferate in the skin. Sézary syndrome is associated with hyperkeratosis, and it has been shown that keratinocytes produce a factor that can induce the proliferation of lymphoma cells and that can be blocked by anti-IL-7 antibody, i.e., presumably IL-7. In conclusion, it has been demonstrated that IL-7 is a potent growth factor for Sézary cells, and may be an important paracrine cytokine in the pathophysiology of cutaneous T-cell lymphoma [48].

Interleukin-8

Human interleukin-8 (IL-8) was originally identified, isolated and purified by virtue of its neutrophil chemotactic or activating capacity [1]. IL-8 exerts an effect *in vitro* on neutrophils (release of chemoattractant and change of shape), T-lymphocytes (release of chemoattractant) and basophils (release of chemoattractant and histamine). *In vivo*, IL-8 induces infiltration of neutrophils and lymphocytes. IL-8 is generally not produced constitutively, but only in response to specific stimuli, such as lipopolysaccharide stimulation of human monocytes–macrophages, and endothelial cells, or tumor necrosis factor-α and interleukin-1 stimulation of fibroblasts, epithelial cells, synovial cells and mesothelial cells [49].

Srivastava et al. have recently reported for the first time, constitutive production of IL-8 by normal B-cells, and by several human B-cell lines of normal and malignant origin. The culture supernatants from 43 human cell lines were examined for IL-8 production using an enzyme-linked immunosorbent assay (ELISA). Constitutive IL-8 production was found in 14/15 B-cell lines (5 derived from normal persons and 2 from acute myelogenous leukemia patients, 1 pre-B-acute lymphoblastic leukemia cell line, 2 chronic lymphocytic leukemia with trisomy 12, 2 HTLV-1+, 1 HTLV-2+, 1/2 Burkitt's lymphoma), 4/16 T-cell lines (3/6 HTLV-1+, 1 HTLV-2+, 0/9 T-ALL), a myeloid line, HL-60, a monocytoid line, U937, 3/3 ovarian carcinomas, 1/1 endometrial cells, 2/2 normal fibroblasts, 0/2 c-ALL cell lines, 0/1 pre-erythroid line, K562, as well as in normal B-lymphocytes. At the present time, however, the role of IL-8 in the pathogenesis of NHLs remains obscure and further studies are awaited.

Interleukin-9

Interleukin-9 (IL-9) has been shown to cause antigen-independent proliferation as well as prolonged survival of some murine T-cell clones [50]. IL-9 has growth factor activity for mouse mast cells in combination with IL-3 and IL-4, as well as for murine immature thymocytes in combination with IL-2. IL-9 also supports the growth of human erythroid blast-forming units, suggesting that responsiveness to IL-9 might appear in an early progenitor cell population before erythroid commitment. IL-9 is produced from anti-CD3 or mitogen-activated normal CD4+ T-cells.

Merz et al. examined IL-9 expression in a variety of tumors both by Northern blot analysis and by *in situ* hybridization [50]. Of 18 B-cell lymphomas and 11 peripheral T-cell lymphomas, none expressed IL-9 mRNA. By contrast, IL-9 mRNA was found in two of six cases of large-cell anaplastic lymphoma (LCAL) and in six of 13 cases of Hodgkin's disease (HD). In HD the strongest signals were observed in H-RS cells, but IL-9 mRNA was also detected in small lymphocytic cells. A search for IL-9 mRNA in a panel of 20 cell lines derived both from hematopoietic and nonhematopoietic tumors confirmed the unique association of IL-9 expression with HD and LCAL. These results suggest that IL-9 is not involved as an autocrine growth factor in the pathogenesis of most B- and T-cell lymphomas, but that it may play a role in HD and LCAL [50].

Interleukin-10

Interleukin-10 (IL-10) was first characterized as a T-cell-derived cytokine able to block interferon gamma production by T_{H1} helper cell clones and as a B-cell-derived thymocyte growth factor [51]. The murine and human IL-10 genes have extensive homology with the BCRF1 gene, an open reading frame of the EBV. The product of the BCRF1 gene, viral IL-10, exhibits partial IL-10 activity *in vitro* and could play an important role during EBV infection. EBV may have captured this mammalian gene to confer some survival advantage upon itself. IL-10 acts on hematopoietic cell lineages, including monocytes, T- and B-lymphocytes. It is a growth and differentiation factor for B-cells in humans and a growth factor for T-cells in the mouse model. Moreover, IL-10 inhibits antigen-specific T-cell activation and blocks cytokine production by monocytes and macrophages in both human and mouse models. IL-10 is produced under different conditions of immune activation by the T_{H0} and T_{H2} subsets of helper T-cells, as well as by monocytes, macrophages and B-cells [52].

Emilie et al. undertook to document the *in situ* production of IL-10 in human lymphomas, with particular attention to lymphomas developing in HIV-infected patients [53]. *In situ* hybridization experiments were performed in frozen tissue sections from 15 AIDS lymphomas using an IL-10/BCRF1 RNA probe. This probe, which is a fragment of the BCRF1 gene, is very similar to human IL-10 cDNA. Hybridization was detected in eight of 15 lymphomas (in three of seven Burkitt's lymphomas, in two of five diffuse large-cell lymphomas, in both of the immunoblastic lymphomas and in the only anaplastic large-cell lymphoma, i.e., there was no correlation with histology). In these eight positive samples, most cells of the lymphomatous tissue were labeled; the vast majority of cells present in these tissues are neoplastic. Presumably therefore, lymphoma cells in AIDS lymphomas express the IL-10 and/or BCRF1 genes. No hybridization was detected in the seven other AIDS lymphomas. In contrast, IL-10/BCRF1 gene expression was detected in only one of 11 lymphomas from HIV-seronegative patients. (The only lymphoma which scored positive with the IL-10/BCRF1 probe was from a transplanted patient. The number of labeled cells in this case was extremely low, contrasting with the large number of positive cells detected in the eight positive AIDS lymphomas.) In AIDS lymphomas, the number of cells labeled with a BCRF1-specific probe was dramatically lower than that of cells labeled with the IL-10/BCRF1 probe. Thus, the cellular IL-10 gene rather than the EBV

BCRF1 gene was expressed. Production of IL-10 was associated with IL-10 mRNA, as shown by immunodetection of the protein in numerous cells. In contrast, BCRF1-producing cells were rarely detected. Thus, both *in situ* hybridization and immunochemical experiments indicated that IL-10 is produced by the malignant cells themselves in AIDS lymphomas. The EBV genome is detected in about 40% of AIDS lymphomas. Thus, an association between IL-10 expression and the presence of EBV was sought. Of the eight AIDS lymphomas in which the IL-10 gene was expressed, EBV was detected in the tumor cells in seven cases. In contrast, it was detected in only one of the AIDS lymphomas which did not express the IL-10 gene. Thus, IL-10 production in AIDS lymphomas is mainly detected in those lymphomas which contain EBV. Overall, these results indicate that diffuse expression of IL-10 by lymphoma cells is related to both the presence of EBV in lymphomas and the HIV status of the patient. EBV is clearly able to trigger IL-10 production by human B-lymphocytes: several EBV-negative Burkitt's cell lines do not express the IL-10 gene, even when analyzed using reverse PCR, but IL-10 production can be detected in these same cell lines following infection with EBV [52,53].

Benjamin et al. also sought to determine whether human B-cells express IL-10 and, if so, its correlation with the presence of EBV [54]. They studied 21 EBV-positive B-cell lines derived from patients with AIDS and Burkitt's lymphoma (of American and African origin), and normal lymphoblastoid cell lines, in comparison with seven EBV-negative Burkitt's lymphoma cell lines. EBV-positive cell lines derived from patients with American Burkitt's lymphoma, and especially those from patients with AIDS, constitutively expressed large quantities of IL-10 by Northern blot analysis and ELISA, and both teleocidin and phorbol myristate acetate (PMA) induced IL-10 in these cell lines. In contrast, six of the seven EBV-negative cell lines did not express IL-10, even by RT-PCR, and IL-10 was not triggered by PMA or teleocidin. The detection of large quantities of IL-10 in B-cell lines derived from AIDS patients, the close association between EBV and IL-10, and the ability of BCRF1 to mimic IL-10 activities, make IL-10/BCRF1 an attractive candidate as a factor causing B-cell growth and immortalization in patients with AIDS and B-cell lymphomas. As IL-10 is a potent growth factor for human B-lymphocytes, these results suggest that IL-10 may stimulate the proliferation of malignant cells in an autocrine pathway in a number of AIDS lymphomas, and that EBV and HIV may synergistically trigger its production [53,55].

Blay et al. measured serum levels of IL-10 in 153 patients with NHL using an ELISA [51]. IL-10 was

CHAPTER 10

Molecular genetics of lymphomagenesis: an overview*

ILAN R. KIRSCH

Introduction

Cancer is a genetic disease that results from a subversion, alteration or dysregulation of the normal genes that govern cell growth and development. Much of what a cancer cell does was also carried out at times prior to its malignant transformation. With transformation comes a loss of control of its growth and developmental pathway(s), rather than a fundamental change in course.

This is not to say that a cancer cell is no different from the 'normal' cells from which it arises. In every tumor cell that has been studied in sufficient depth, molecular genetic analyses have demonstrated that DNA is altered compared to the nonmalignant 'normal' counterpart. The mechanistic consequences of many (if not all) of the point mutations, deletions, transpositions, amplifications, insertions, and translocations that can comprise these DNA alteration(s) (Figure 10.1) represent the gene disruption/dysregulation that contributes to malignant transformation.

The study of lymphomagenesis underscores these concepts. A step in malignant transformation of lymphocytes very frequently occurs by the juxtaposition of a primary differentiated product of a lymphocyte, an immunoglobulin or T-cell antigen receptor gene, with a gene that helps govern growth or a differentiative program. Moreover, the mechanism of this juxtaposition involves a structural reconfiguration of genomic DNA that is, at least in part, mediated by other lymphocyte-specific functions, namely, V(D)J and 'switch' recombination. Thus, normal lymphocyte-specific mechanisms of gene rearrangement and normal lymphocyte-specific differentiated products contribute to lymphocyte transformation.

*This chapter is a modification of a chapter that was originally written for the book *Clinical Immunology* (edited by R. Rich, Mosby Year Book, Inc., St Louis).

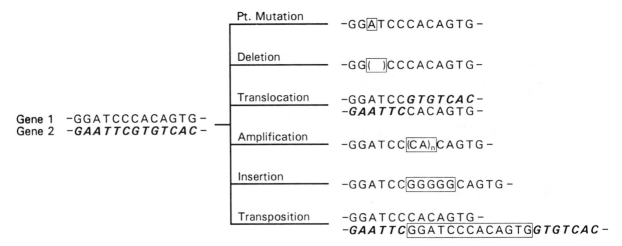

Figure 10.1 Examples of different types of genetic instability. Two hypothetical segments of DNA corresponding to two genetic loci are shown (one in plain text, one bold and italicized). Alterations in the primary sequence caused by point mutation, deletion, translocation, amplification, insertion and transposition are demonstrated. While the example of amplification shown consists of amplification of a dinucleotide repeat, much larger segments of the genome can also be part of an amplified unit (amplicon).

Genetic instability

The fact that cancer is not a rare event underscores the point that DNA is not a static and immutable structure. It is the inherent instability of DNA that accounts for evolutionary development and this same inherent instability that is the basis of cancer. The instability of DNA has two components, one that is inherited and represents the physiologic 'program' with which an organism is born. This is a function of the the specific nucleotide sequence, the structure and level of various histones and other chromatin covering proteins, repair enzymes, recombinases, nuclear matrix components, etc. The other aspect of genetic instability is acquired, a function of stabilizing or destabilizing influences from the environment, diet, medication and other sources. These influences act in combination with the underlying 'baseline' level of genetic instability to make DNA alteration more or less likely at any given point in time. Corresponding to this level of DNA instability, there is an accompanying level of risk for the development of a particular malignancy.

Genetic instability in lymphocytes

It is not just in evolution and cancer that the force of genetic instability dominates. Normal development requires that DNA be able to change, to reconfigure itself. The classic example of this in higher organisms is the rearrangement of DNA that is required for the generation of the immune response. The role of lymphocytes in the generation of the immune response depends on the elaboration of a group of particular 'destabilizing' enzymes, and probably also requires the organization of chromatin (at least in certain regions) into a state that makes it particularly amenable to DNA breakage and rejoining events. This 'lymphocyte-specific' genetic instability becomes an important factor in consideration of the process of malignant transformation of these cells.

Immune receptor rearrangement

The DNA that will eventually code for a functional immune receptor (immunoglobulin (Ig) or T-cell antigen receptor (TCR)) initially exists in germline DNA as a series of discrete noncontiguous segments (Figure 10.2). Within a prototypical immune receptor locus there are multiple variable (V) segments separated by one to hundreds of kilobases (kb) of intervening DNA from multiple joining (J) segments. These, in turn, are located a few thousand nucleotides upstream of one or a small number of constant (C) segments (for an additional review of immune receptor rearrangement, see [1]). For the Ig heavy chain (H) locus and the TCRβ and TCRδ

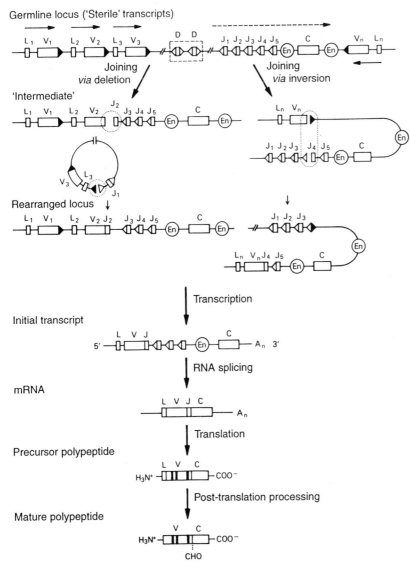

Germline locus ('Sterile' transcripts)

'Intermediate'

Rearranged locus

Initial transcript

Transcription

mRNA

RNA splicing

Precursor polypeptide

Translation

Mature polypeptide

Post-translation processing

Figure 10.2 V(D)J recombination. A generalized schematic illustrating the structural reconfigurations of immune receptor loci that are a prerequisite to the formation of a functional polypeptide and therefore to the generation of immune diversity. The gene that will eventually constitute the immune receptor exists initially in germline DNA as a set of discrete, noncontiguous segments. There are multiple variable (V) segments with their upstream leader (L) exons that mediate transport of the polypeptide into or through a membrane. For certain of the immune receptor loci (IgH, TCRβ, TCRδ) there are diversity (D) segments. For all the loci, one finds joining (J) segments upstream from constant (C) segments. Prior to gene rearrangement, 'sterile' transcription (solid and dashed arrows over the first line of the schematic) of the loci about to be rearranged occurs, probably indicative of a change in the status and 'accessibility' of the chromatin at these sites (see text). Structural and irreversible rearrangement of the DNA occurs either by deletion of the DNA between the rearranging segments or by inversion. The reaction is essentially site specific, mediated by a recombinase enzyme complex that recognizes heterologous signal sequences (solid and open triangles) that flank the rearranging segments. Following recombination, a now contiguous V(D)J region is formed, which can still begin from the promoter located 5' of the rearranged V segment, with transcriptional activity 'enhanced' by enhancer elements (En) that are found around the DNA flanking the C segment. A precursor RNA is transcribed up to the point where addition of a run of adenosine residues (A_n) is sited. RNA intervening between coding segments is spliced out, yielding the mature messenger RNA (mRNA). The mRNA is translated into protein and transported to its position in the membrane. The mature polypeptide is finished after additional processing, which includes cleavage of the leader peptide and possible glycosylation (CHO) of certain sites within the peptide. From Kirsch [1a].

(B and Dl) loci there are also diversity (D) segments interposed between the V and J segments. As a prerequisite to the formation of a functional Ig or TCR, one of the V segments undergoes a site-specific rearrangement with a J (or previously site-specifically rearranged DJ) segment to form a now contiguous VJ (VDJ) region still upstream from the C segment. The segments appear to be targeted for rearrangement because they are flanked by particular signal sequences consisting of a heptamer nucleotide with consensus CACAGTG separated by 12 or 23 nucleotides from a nonamer with consensus ACAAAAACC. In most cases the rearrangement is accompanied by deletion of the intervening DNA between the rearranging segments. The DNA in the rearranged cell is therefore fundamentally different from the unrearranged cell. The reaction is irreversible.

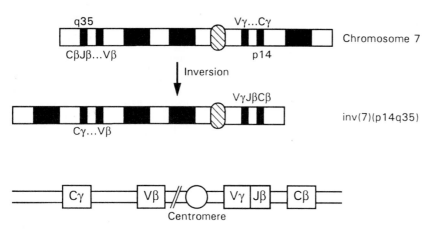

Figure 10.3 A model for the mechanism of inversion of chromosome 7 via TCRγV-TCRβJ site-specific recombination. Idiograms of normal and inverted chromosomes 7 are depicted. Orientations and locations of TCRγ and TCRβ chain loci in both germline and inverted states are illustrated. A schematic representation of the interlocus rearrangment and hybrid gene formation is shown below. From Stern et al. [9a] with permission of Grune and Stratton.

This rearrangement reaction is catalyzed by a complex of enzymes (recombinase complex) that includes the products of the *rag*1 [2] and *rag*2 [3] genes, the *scid* gene [4, 4a], other recombination signal sequence (RSS) binding proteins [5], DNA breakage and rejoining enzymes, and, in some cases terminal deoxynucleotidyl transferase (TdT) [6]. This complex of enzymes targets the specific signal sequences that flank the rearranging segments. The presence of the recombinase complex in a cell is not, by itself, sufficient for V(D)J rearrangement. The segments to be rearranged must be accessible to the complex. Within nonlymphoid cells it appears that, in general, the immune receptor loci are not accessible [7]. The accessibility of these segments within lymphocytes is observed as a change in chromatin status heralded by an increased DNAse sensitivity, alteration in pattern of methylation and the production of 'sterile' transcripts (transcripts that do not appear to encode a protein) [8] from the locus about to be rearranged. These transcripts are not believed to be necessary for the recombination event itself [9]. Rather their presence suggests that accessibility to an RNA polymerase is accompanied by accessibility to the recombinase complex. In addition to V(D)J recombination, the IgH locus is also subject to 'switch' recombination (see below and Chapter 8) in which the immunoglobulin isotype changes from μ to γ, ε, or α. The switch recombination event is believed to be mediated by a different set of enzymes. Accessibility of the loci undergoing rearrangement is also critical for switch recombination.

OTHER V(D)J RECOMBINASE-MEDIATED GENOMIC REARRANGEMENTS

Interlocus rearrangements

Classically, the V(D)J recombination process has been viewed as occurring *within* a given immune receptor locus. However, the process can also occur between two distinct immune receptor loci leading to the formation of a 'hybrid' immune receptor with a V segment from one locus and (D)J and C segments from another (Figure 10.3). Formation of such hybrids is not a freak event but rather is a routine occurrence. All normal humans that have been studied carry such hybrid genes in a small fraction of their peripheral blood lymphocyte population [10,11].

The finding of these hybrid genes has a number of implications. First, from a strictly mechanistic point of view, it demonstrates that the V(D)J recombinase complex (or complexes, when more than one is involved) does not require linear contiguous DNA in order to mediate recombination. Second, the formation of hybrid genes raises certain issues from the standpoint of development and immunology. Based on the study of intralocus rearrangement, the finding of hybrid genes strongly suggests that two disparate immune receptors must have been simultaneously accessible both temporally and topologically. In addition, the occurrence of such hybrids is of interest in terms of clonal selection of immune receptor-bearing lymphocytes (see earlier chapters). In the peripheral blood, 30–50% (or higher depending on the loci involved) of these hybrid immune receptor genes are in-frame at the level of genomic DNA, and over 90% are in-frame at the detectable mRNA level. This is similar to the situation for normal intralocus rearrangements and suggests that hybrid genes are capable of being functional and positively selected. One might speculate that combinations of Vs and Js that were routinely beneficial to an organism would lead to their being brought together within the same locus and thus be favored for recombinatorial joining. The actual role that interlocus hybrids play in the normal immune response remains to be determined.

HYBRID IMMUNE RECEPTORS AS MARKERS OF GENETIC INSTABILITY AND POSSIBLE CANCER RISK

The hybrid genes that we carry are a polyclonal population. Multiple independent interlocus rearrangements have occurred in each individual. The sum total of all these clones defines the frequency of these genes in the peripheral blood. For example, for a hybrid involving the recombination of a V segment from the TCRγ locus with a J segment from the TCRβ locus, the frequency in normal individuals is in the range of 0.001–0.0001% of circulating T-cells. In the autosomal recessive disease ataxia telangiectasia (AT) there is an approximately 100-fold increase in the frequency of interlocus hybrid genes found in the peripheral blood lymphocyte population [11]. AT is a complex disease with the homozygotes demonstrating oculocutaneous telangiectasia, progressive cerebellar degeneration, premature aging, radiosensitivity, immunodeficiency and a predisposition to the development of cancer, particularly lymphoid malignancies [12]. Coincidentally or not, the risk to an AT patient of developing lymphoma is approximately 100 times that of the unaffected population. Interestingly, the V(D)J recombination machinery and process appears normal in an AT patient [12a]. At the nucleotide sequence level, the hybrid genes formed in an AT patient are indistinguishable from the hybrids found in an unaffected individual. Thus, the increased frequency of these hybrids in AT might reflect an increased accessibility of these loci to the recombinase complex. This implies a difference in chromatin structure or organization between AT patients and unaffected individuals. Such a qualitative difference in chromatin has also been suggested based on an increased frequency in the conversion of double-strand DNA breaks into chromosome breaks following irradiation of AT patient-derived cell lines [13].

An increase in the frequency of hybrid gene formation can be acquired as well as inherited. In a pilot study, agriculture workers exposed to pesticides, fumigants and herbicides were shown, as a group, to have an increased incidence of hybrid genes in their peripheral blood lymphocytes compared to a control population. Interestingly, these agriculture workers were representative of a population which has also demonstrated an increased risk for the development of lymphoid malignancy [14].

At any point in time we have a finite risk of developing lymphoid malignancy and a certain level of genetic instability as measured by, among other things, a particular frequency of hybrid gene formation. The level of these hybrids at any moment seems to be a function of the inherent propensity for the interlocus recombination event to occur. This propensity is a summation of chromatin accessibility, topographic (the relative positions of genes in the nucleus), and topologic (the configuration of one locus *vis-à-vis* another) organization of DNA in the interphase nucleus, and exposure to stabilizing or destabilizing agents which can alter these reaction prerequisites. Thus, the frequency of hybrid gene formation may be a marker for the risk of developing lymphoid malignancy. As an event, moreover, hybrid gene formation may not simply be a fortuitous marker. The mechanism that mediates the formation of hybrid genes, V(D)J recombination, is, at least in part, the same mechanism that mediates the formation of many of the malevolent translocations associated with the development of lymphoid malignancy [15]. An increased level of hybrid genes does not mean that a person has leukemia or lymphoma, or that he or she will develop one of these diseases. It only means that the conditions are more favorable than usual for the generation of the kind of chromosomal rearrangements which appear to facilitate, contribute to, or mediate lymphocyte transformation.

Chromosomal aberrations associated with lymphoid malignancy

Table 10.1 lists chromosomal aberrations that have been specifically associated with the development of lymphoid malignancy. Only those chromosomal aberrations that have been cloned and analyzed at the level of the DNA are included while purely descriptive cytogenetic data are not included. The list is extensive, but it is not all inclusive and other chapters in this section focus on some of the disease-specific aberrations that are listed. Throughout the remainder of this chapter various entries will be taken from this list to provide examples of the particular phenomenon or mechanism being described.

V(D)J RECOMBINASE-MEDIATED REARRANGEMENTS

Immunoglobulins and T-cell receptors as oncogenes

Immunoglobulins and T-cell receptors are cell surface receptors which transduce ligand-dependent part of the V(D)J recombinase, permitting ligation in the absence of recognizable signals (at least on rare occasions) or that a different set or subset of recombinase enzymes is involved in this DNA breakage. In certain cases, the DNA found at the sites of chromosomal breakage is notable for containing alternating stretches of purine and pyrimidine nucleotides compatible with the model for formation of 'Z' (left-handed helical turn) DNA [21]. Perhaps this conformational change is recombinogenic under certain circumstances, in the presence of certain enzyme systems. Even in the setting of an endonuclease-generated break in the nonimmune receptor chromosome, an explanation of how the disparate ends are brought into the same nuclear location and ligated together is still required.

It is still possible that the occurrence of chromosomal aberrations is a random event. In this model, DNA breaks would occur anywhere in the genome and selection would be based on the fortuitous juxtaposition of particular DNA sequences that confer a growth advantage on the cell. While formally a possibility, certain observations seem to make this less likely as a dominant mechanism. There are stringent requirements for chromosomal accessibility allowing for routine immune receptor rearrangements. Chromosomal aberration in lymphocytes appears to be a variation on this theme. Furthermore, the translocations are often reciprocal; that is to say that a t(1;14) generates a derivative chromosome 1 and a complementary derivative chromosome 14. The fact that so many of the chromosomal aberrations are reciprocal makes a random and chaotic model problematic. If a chromosome breaks and its ends are 'floating free', a random model would suggest that one end could religate to the end of a subsequently disrupted chromosome, while the other end might be lost or united with a completely different, fortuitously disrupted, part of the genome. The reciprocity actually observed implies that the breakage and rejoining event occurs specifically at a point in time and space. This would seem to favor the concept that certain parts of the genome are more predisposed to undergo chromosomal aberration in specific cell lineages at certain times during lineage development or differentiation.

It has been speculated that a single V(D)J recombinase cluster is capable of holding only four DNA ends at a time. The structure and end products of many of the translocations listed in Table 10.1 – t(1;14) is one well-characterized example [22] – would require that at least six DNA ends be involved. The t(1;14) seems to occur during D-D rearrangement in the TCRδ locus. Thus at the time of translocation there would be the two coding D ends, the two signal sequence ends flanking the D segments, and the two ends of the *scl* locus at the site of

translocation. Explanation for this event may require more than one recombinase complex.

In review, the overall structure and specificity of these various translocations, their association with distinctive malignant phenotypes representing particular stages of lymphocyte development, and their overall structural consistency, suggests that these events are not random. These findings imply that in a given cell type, certain parts of the genome, because of structure, function and differential accessibility are more likely to undergo chromosomal translocation than other parts of the genome. This concept is reinforced and strengthened by an understanding of the constraints and prerequisites for normal immune receptor rearrangement previously discussed. Perhaps the V(D)J (and switch) recombinase complexes are sequestered or matrix bound in a particular part of the lymphocyte nucleus and DNA of a particular transcriptional state and chromatin structure is more likely to encounter this recombinational site in the cell (Figure 10.4).

V(D)J recombinase-mediated rearrangements that do not involve immune receptors

While many of the chromosomal translocations in lymphocytes involve an immune receptor locus and a nonimmune receptor locus, recent cloning studies have identified significant chromosomal aberrations associated with lymphoid malignancy that appear to involve V(D)J recombinase mediation, where *neither* locus is an immune receptor (Figure 10.5). Analyses of the variable rearrangements involving chromosome 11, band q23, provide one example of this phenomenon. The mixed lineage leukemia (MLL) gene, identified within this region [23,24], is disrupted in a variety of lymphoid and nonlymphoid leukemias, probably leading to the generation of a novel protein with transforming potential (see below). The t(4;11) involving the gene AF4 on chromosome 4, band q21, is the most common translocation. Other partners for the many translocations involving this locus include sites on chromosomes 1, 6, 9, 10 and 19. An analysis of the regions of breakage and rejoining for the t(4;11) and several other translocations reveal possible heptamer/nonamer recombinase targeted signal sequences proximate to the sites of chromosomal breakage and rejoining [25]. In some of these cases the sequences show only a rough fit with the heptamer/nonamer consensus. However, it has been proposed that many of these sequences are, indeed, cryptic heptamer/nonamer signals, particularly in consideration of the 12/23 nucleotide spacing that appears to be present. Exonucleolytic 'nibbling'

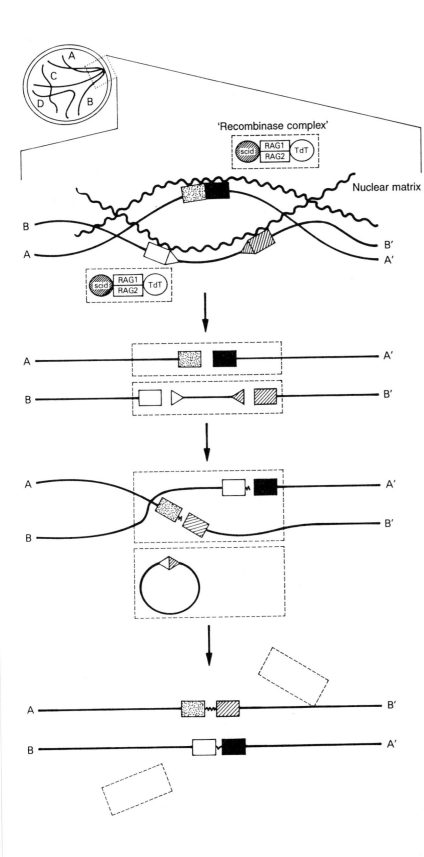

Figure 10.4 Postulated nuclear localization of the recombinase complex and targets of recombinase-mediated translocation. The circle at the very top of the figure represents a cell – for example, a lymphocyte – in which a part of chromosome A and a part of chromosome B are sequestered in a part of the nucleus, perhaps attached to the nuclear matrix (wavy line) because of their particular structure, function, chromatin status or accessibility . . . or by chance. The recombinase complexes are operative in this part of the nucleus and act on the two chromosomes to cause breakage and rejoining events. The complex (dashed line box) consists of targeting, nucleolytic and repair enzymes, including RAG-1, RAG-2, the *scid* gene product, and TdT. The hatched and open boxes delineate 'coding' segments and the triangle 'signal' sequences. The structure shown on chromosome B in the upper part of the figure is consistent with an immune receptor locus. Part of the recombination reaction proceeds normally; the ends of the intervening sequence carrying the signal segments are joined together in an extrachromosomal circle. However, the topography and topology of chromosomes A and B cause an interchromosomal rather than an intralocus rearrangment, which results in a chromosomal translocation. From Kirsch [1a] with permission.

defy current concepts of mutational frequencies in eukaryotic cells. Part of the solution to this paradox is suggested by the finding that mutation of certain genes (e.g., p53, [39]) seems to result in loss of a checkpoint control at the cell cycle transition from G_1 to S phase. This checkpoint is a conjectured interval during which the cell can repair DNA damage or alteration and restore genomic integrity [40]. With its loss the ability to accumulate additional mutations may increase substantially [41–44]. A second type of destabilizing event in solid tumors has recently been appreciated with the realization that a subset of malignancies are mutated in one of a few genes which confer the ability to repair nucleotide mismatches that occur during replication [45,46]. Thus, in many solid tumors there appears to be a step specifically required to destabilize the genome after which follows a series of additional mutational events that in combination contribute to cellular transformation. Whether this is true for every solid tumor is not clear. The question of whether there is a programmed sequence of mutational events which must, more or less, be followed in order to transform a cell is still under investigation. Whether there is a fundamental difference between leukemias, lymphomas and other solid tumors with regard to this destabilization step deserves further discussion.

Certainly there are examples of hematopoietic malignancies in which multiple mutational events have occurred. In Table 10.1 it is noted that for HIV-related lymphomas carrying translocations of the c-*myc* proto-oncogene several other gene mutations have been observed at variable (high in the case of p53) frequency. It is equally striking that, for a number of hematopoietic malignancies (particularly certain lymphoid malignancies), a vast accumulation of mutations has not been observed at the time of first presentation. These observations are not consistent with a multistep model of carcinogenesis. In many cases of lymphoid malignancy there is often one predominant genetic alteration, frequently consisting of a specific chromosomal aberration, which can be a diagnostic and subclassifying marker for that type of malignancy. There are examples of similar diagnostic chromosomal changes that allow identification of certain pediatric sarcomas and occasional adult cancers, but the general picture in carcinomas is not as simple as that of the hematopoietic malignancies [47]. Perhaps the inherent targeted mechanisms of genetic instability in lymphocytes (see the discussion of V(D)J and switch recombinases above) makes the *de novo* generation of early destabilizing mutations unnecessary in the progression to malignancy. This would somewhat limit the average number of alterations that are required to initiate transformation in lymphocytes compared to other types of cancer. In this regard the lymphoid

neoplasms that do manifest diffuse and multiple karyotypic abnormalities and multiple mutations are intriguing for what they may be demonstrating with regard to etiology and requirements for tranformation. Certain correlations between types of mutations have been noted suggesting distinct interactions among tranformation promoting pathways. For example, p53 mutation in lymphoid malignancies seems closely correlated with those malignancies in which the c-*myc* proto-oncogene is also dysregulated [48,49].

The apparent (perhaps deceptive) simplicity suggested by distinct chromosomal aberrations that correlate with specific subtypes of lymphoid malignancies has provided an obvious target for studying genes critical to lymphoid growth and development. Strategically, numerous investigators have viewed the cloning and characterization of the genes flanking various leukemia or lymphoma-associated chromosomal aberrations as a way to examine malignant transformation as well as normal lymphoid proliferation and development. The validity of this strategy has been borne out numerous times over the past 14 years. Table 10.2 offers a partial list of the genes that have been found flanking the chromosomal breakpoints of specific leukemia or lymphoma subtypes. This represents a slightly different way of looking at the data in Table 10.1. The existence of some of these genes was determined prior to identifying their involvement in a particular chromosomal aberration. However, the majority of genes on this list were first discovered because of their proximity to and disruption by the chromosomal rearrangement event.

About half of the genes discovered at the junctions of chromosomal aberrations associated with the development of lymphoid malignancy are transcription factors. In many cases these transcription factors are members of families of genes that not only bind to DNA to activate a particular genetic program but also are capable of direct protein–protein interaction with other transcription factors within the cell. This protein interaction effect can either increase or decrease the affinity of these other factors for their target DNA sequences (Figure 10.6). The net result of this interplay can be the inhibition or activation of entire programs and cascades of gene expression. The DNA binding and protein–protein interaction capabilities enable these genes to play a role in a complex dynamic equilibrium of forces governing cellular developmental programs, proliferation and differentiative decisions. The other genes listed in Table 10.2 cover almost all other facets of a growth regulatory cascade including growth factors, growth factor receptors transducing, factors and apoptosis-preventing factors.

Table 10.2 Functional classification of genes found at or proximate to translocation junctions. The author thanks Dr Janet Rowley for her efforts and guidance in the preparation of this table

Homeodomain			
PBX	1q23	t(1;19)	Pre-B-ALL
HOX11	10q24	t(10;14),t(7;10)	T-ALL
Helix–loop–helix			
LYL1	19p13	t(7;19)	T-ALL
MYC	8q24	t(8;14),t(2;8), t(8;22)	B-ALL, T-ALL, NHL
SCL(TAL1)	1p32-1p34	t(1;14), del(1p)	T-ALL
TAL2	9q32	t(7;9)	T-ALL
TCF3(E2A)	19p13	t(1;19)	Pre-B-ALL
NFkB/rel			
BCL3	19q13	t(14;19)	B-CLL
NFkB2/Lyt10	10q24	t(10;14) and others	B-NHL peripheral T-cell
Zn finger			
BCL6	3q27	t(3;14)and t(3;others)	DLCL
ETO	8q24	t(8;21)	AML-M2
MLL	11q23	t(11;many)	ALL/AML
PLZF	11q23.1	t(11;17)	APL
PML	15q22	t(15;17)	APL
RARA	17q12	t(15;17)	APL
LIM			
RBTN1(TTG1)	11p15	t(11;14)	T-ALL
RBTN2(TTG2)	11p13	t(11;14)	T-ALL
Leucine zipper			
CAN	9q34	t(6;9)	AML
HLF	17q22	t(17;19)	Pre-B-ALL
Other transcription factor			
CBFa(AML1)	21q22	t(8;21)	AML-M2
CBFb	16q22	inv(16)	AML-M4eo
SRC family (Tyr protein kinases)			
ABL	9q34	t(9;22)	CML/ALL
LCK	1p34	t(1;7)	T-ALL
ALK	2p23	t(2;5)	T-NHL (Ki-1)
Serine protein kinase			
BCR	22q11	t(9;22)	CML/ALL
Cell surface receptor			
TAN1	9q34	t(7;9)	T-ALL
Growth factor			
IL3	5q31	t(5;14)	Pre-B-ALL
Nuclear/endoplasmic reticulum/mitochondrial membranes			
BCL2	18q21	t(14;18)	NHL
Cell cycle regulatory			
Cyclin D (BCL1)	11q13	t(11;14)	CLL/NHL
Unknown			
DEK	6p23	t(6;9)	AML-M2/M4
NPM	5q35	t(2;5)	T-NHL (Ki-1)

from within the first exon into the first intron appears to be targeted for mutation accompanying or shortly following the translocation event [54–56]. Within this region are sites that are normally involved in blocking the elongation of the *myc* transcript, one mechanism of control of c-*myc* during normal growth and development [57,58]. This same mutational 'hotspot' also contains a potential binding site of a c-*myc* regulatory protein, *myc* inhibitory factor (MIF) [59]. Mutations of this region, therefore, could be at least partly responsible for c-*myc* dysregulation [60]. In addition, somatic mutation of the second exon of the translocated c-*myc* gene within regions that encode the transactivational domain of the protein have been reported [61]. The mechanism by which these regions of the c-*myc* gene become targets for somatic hypermutation has not been determined, but, of course, somatic hypermutation of Ig variable segments is a recognized phenomenon and it is tempting to speculate that placing the c-*myc* gene in the context of the IgH locus might lead to these mutational events. In that light it is relevant that in a small number of sequence analyses of c-*myc* genes translocated in T-cell malignancies, these mutational events were not noted (R. Dalla-Favera, personal communication). T-Cell antigen receptors are *not* subject to somatic hypermutation [62].

The direct connection has not yet been made between c-*myc* dysregulation by chromosomal translocation and transformation of the cell in which the translocation occurs. However, a great deal of circumstantial information is accumulating regarding the role of c-*myc* in lymphoid transformation. *myc* is one of those transcription factors with both DNA binding and protein–protein interactive capabilities, complex function and complex regulation [63]. The c-*myc* gene encodes a protein with both a basic DNA binding domain (b) as well as two distinct motifs mediating protein dimerization, a helix-loop-helix (HLH) [64] and a leucine zipper (LZ) [65]. The presence of these two dimerization motifs suggests a complex panoply of interactions of this gene product with numerous other transcription factors within the cell. A dimerization partner of c-Myc, called Max, has now been identified [66]. The half-lives of these two proteins in the cell are quite different, Myc having a very short half-life ($\approx$20 min), Max having a half-life closer to 24 h. In addition two partners that dimerize with Max (but not Myc) have also been identified, Mad [67] and Mxi1 [68]. Depending on the dynamic equilibrium among all these proteins, transcriptional activation or inhibition is the result. Clearly, constitutive expression of c-*myc* occurring secondary to its placement under the control of an immune receptor locus would have a substantial effect on this dynamic equilibrium.

What genes under the control of c-*myc* might contribute to malignant transformation? It is not yet possible to answer this question definitively but certain potentially relevant genes are beginning to be identified. These include heat shock proteins, class I major histocompatibility complex (MHC) cell surface components, plasminogen activator, and α-prothymosin. Among the more interesting candidates in terms of B-cell transformation is the α-chain of the leukocyte adhesion protein, leukocyte function-associated molecule (LFA-1), the expression of which appears to be suppressed by c-*myc* [69]. The role of LFA-1 in B-cells appears to be relevant for cell–cell interactions that are required for cytotoxic T-cell killing, vascular endothelial adhesion and lymph node organization. It is tempting to speculate that downregulation of this member of the integrin receptor family might promote growth independence, abrogation of T-cell killing, and increased vascular permeability of these cells, all consistent with more virulent transformed behavior.

Although c-*myc* is a particularly dramatic example of promoter disruption and enhancer insertion as a mechanism of dysregulation, it is not unique in this regard. The majority of genes listed in Tables 10.1 and 10.2 show altered patterns of expression on this same basis. The enhancer sequence may be introduced upstream of the gene, for example, in translocations involving c-*myc*, *bcl*-2, *bcl*-3 and *lyl*-1. Alternatively, the enhancer may be introduced downstream of the gene, for example, in translocations involving c-*myc*, *bcl*-2 and *scl*. In addition, the promoter region may be truncated or mutated, for example, with translocations involving *scl*, c-*myc*, *ttg*-1 and *ttg*-2.

Some of the dysregulated genes are not felt to be classic transcription factors. Study of their dysregulation has, in some cases, revealed or supported novel and fundamental principles of growth and development. *bcl*-2 is a prime example of this. This gene is dysregulated by its translocation to the IgH locus coincident with the t(14;18) translocation associated with the development of follicular lymphoma [70]. The *bcl*-2 gene product appears to abrogate the 'programmed cell death' (apoptosis) pathway normally occurring in B-lymphocytes that are not positively selected [71,72]. The Bcl-2 protein is found associated with mitochondrial, nuclear and endoplasmic reticulum membrane structures. Among the stimuli for which the activity of Bcl-2 is essential is prevention of cell death following ionizing radiation. The actions of other agents whose lethality may be more complexly orchestrated are also counteracted by Bcl-2. In experimental systems it has been suggested that Bcl-2 may regulate and promote an antioxidant pathway that protects the cell from apoptotic cell death [73]. As in the case of the transcription factors mentioned above, the action of Bcl-2 appears to be mediated through its interaction with a variety of dimerizing partners [74,75]. Depending on the relative levels of the various proteins apoptosis is favored or suppressed. Thus, constitutive expression of the Bcl-2 protein may be a mechanism by which the program is directed toward the maintenance of cells that would normally be destined to die. Less is known about the Bcl-1 (PRAD-1) and Bcl-3 proteins but there are suggestions as to how their dysregulated expression might contribute to malignant transformation in B-cells carrying the t(11;14) or t(10;14) in which these two genes are involved. Bcl-1 is a member of the cyclin family of proteins and is likely to exert its effect at the G_1/S checkpoint in the cell cycle [76,77]. Bcl-3 also shares a motif characteristic of cell cycle-relevant genes [78].

Accessibility

Earlier in this chapter the role of accessibility in promoting chromosomal translocations was discussed. It is relevant to consider this issue once again when considering the mechanism of transcriptional dysregulation. The implication of the 'accessibility argument' is that loci that are being transcribed will be more likely to undergo chromosomal recombination events. Thus, it would be reasonable to predict that genes involved in the various characteristic cell-type and leukemia/lymphoma specific translocations (Tables 10.1 and 10.2) are actively expressed in these cell types at the time of their translocation. c-*myc* fits this hypothesis since it is rather ubiquitously expressed in actively dividing lymphocytes. This fact leads to the premise that the translocation is not turning on the c-*myc* gene but rather making it impossible to turn the c-*myc* gene off (as noted, the normal c-*myc* on the untranslocated allele is subject to the usual regulation and is turned off). However, other examples taken from Tables 10.1 and 10.2 do not fit this hypothesis nearly as well. Scl is expressed in cells of the hematopoietic lineage but has not been shown to be expressed in normal T-cells that are phenotypically analogous to the blasts carrying scl translocations [27]. Lyl-1 is also expressed in the hematopoietic lineage, but not primarily in T-cells [79]. Hox-11 expression is noted in liver [80], and an analogous murine gene is expressed in pre-B, myeloid and macrophage lineages, but not primarily in T-cells [81]. Ttg 1 [82] and Ttg 2 [83] are most clearly expressed in neural tissue, although there is also expression in T-cells and a possible role in hematopoiesis. All five of these genes are implicated in the development of T-cell leukemia despite the fact that,

unlike c-*myc*, their normal roles appear to lie outside the T-cell lineage. However, this does not necessarily infer that they are not 'accessible' in the T-cell or T-cell progenitor lineage. Instead it supports a *random translocation with subsequent selection* model. At present this paradox is unresolved. It may be that the pre-T-cells involved in these various translocation events do express these genes but have not yet been identified. Alternatively the level of transcription in T-cells or hematopoietic progenitors that has been observed for these five genes may be an indication of sufficient locus accessibility. It may be that even though these loci are transcriptionally silent they are nonetheless 'accessible' in terms of chromatin configuration, methylation, hypersensitivity to DNAse, replication timing, etc. [84–87]. Their position in the genome might make them passive recipients of chromatin changes occurring because of other loci located upstream or downstream that are differentially activated [88,89]. An example of such regulation would include the effect of the locus control region (LCR) on regulation of β-globin expression during red cell development [90–92]. Translocations involving the five loci named above may also occur in other cell types where they are more highly expressed, but without malignant consequence because of the particular developmental and proliferative controls active in these particular cells.

THE FORMATION OF FUSION PROTEINS

Transcriptional dysregulation routinely leads to the expression of a normal gene product, but at the 'wrong' time. Another mechanism of gene disruption by chromosomal translocation is alteration in the gene product (Figure 10.8). Examples of this mechanism of gene alteration that are associated with leukemia development include: (1) the E2a-Pbx1 hybrid formed by the t(1;19) translocation and associated with pre-B-ALL [93]; (2) the E2a-Hlf hybrid formed by the t(17;19) translocation and associated with pre-B-ALL [94]; (3) the MLL (HTRX, ALL1) gene fusions with partners on a variety of other chromosomes in various lymphoid and myeloid lineage leukemias [95–100]; (4) the acute myelogenous 1 (AML1)–ETO fusion associated with the t(8;21) translocation in AML French American British (FAB) subtype M2 [101–103]; (5) the Dek-Can and Set-Can fusions associated with the t(6;9) and del(9q) in AML subtype M2 or M4 and acute undifferentiated leukemia (AUL) [104]; (6) the promyelocytic leukemia–retinoic acid receptorα (Pml–Rarα) fusion in the t(15;17) associated with AML subtype M3 (APL) [105,106] ; and, of course, (7) the Bcr–Abl fusion [107,108] associated with the

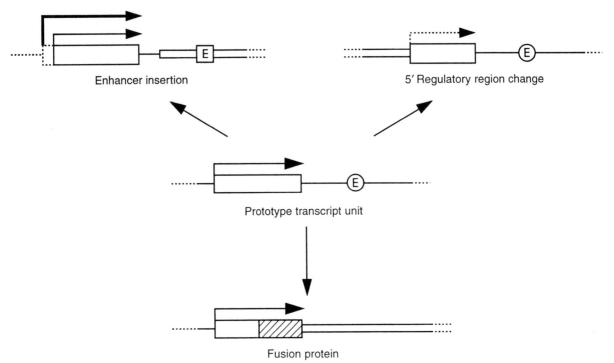

Enhancer insertion

5′ Regulatory region change

Prototype transcript unit

Fusion protein

Figure 10.8 Mechanisms of gene disruption caused by chromosomal translocations. A prototype transcript unit is disrupted in its 3′ region (upper left) by a translocation that removes one and substitutes a different enhancer sequence. This enhancer causes transcription to start upstream of its usual position and also increases the quantity of transcript emanating from the locus. A different kind of translocation (upper right) removes the normal 5′ regulatory region and substitutes a different region, which changes the transcriptional regulation of the locus. Yet another way in which chromsomal translocation can alter a gene is by structurally changing it so as to create a novel protein composed of segments from the two loci formerly separate, but now contiguous.

t(9;22) in chronic myelogenous leukemia and a particularly virulent form of ALL. In many cases it is not just gene fusion, but also fusion gene dysregulation which leads to malignant transformation. Thus, a novel protein is made and its expression is also altered compared to the expression of the native proteins from which it was formed.

Transcription factors, generically, contain specific domains that mediate aspects of their complex function. They must bind to DNA often via a domain rich in basic amino acids. They often interact with other proteins forming homodimers, heterodimers or more complex structures. These protein–protein interactions can occur at various points along the primary amino acid sequence, but frequently occur within domains characterized by primary amino acid sequences that are conjectured to form amphipathic helices or interdigitating leucine residues. Additionally these factors seem to carry transactivation domains which, once the factors are bound, mediate the enhancing or inhibiting effects on the RNA PolII complex. The E2a-Pbx1 and E2a–Hlf fusions are transcriptionally provocative fusions of genes, each one of which is likely to function normally in its own

transcription regulating pathway. E2a is a member of the basic domain, helix-loop-helix (bHLH) family of transcription factors. Pbx1 is a member of the homeodomain family. Hlf is a member of the basic domain (b) LZ family. In the t(1;19) translocation associated with pre-B-ALL, the breakage and rejoining of E2a and Pbx1 results in the replacement of the bHLH motif of E2a by the homeodomain of Pbx1. An LZ-like containing portion of E2a is retained with this fusion. Thus, the fusion protein carries a DNA binding segment from Pbx1 but an interactive (and presumably activating segment) from a completely different transcription factor. The mixing together of different DNA binding and protein dimerization capabilities could result in abnormal activation or repression of a variety of growth and proliferative pathways. This suggestion is supported by the E2a–Hlf hybrid in which, analogously, the bHLH portion of E2a is again removed from the fusion protein, replaced by the zipper region of Hlf – leading, again, to a putative mixing of DNA binding, protein interacting and transcriptional activation regions of two different proteins.

In the Bcr–Abl fusion the contribution of the *abl* gene is relatively constant, whereas the contribution of the *bcr* gene is somewhat variable. This variability results in the production of two varieties of fusion proteins, p210 (containing more *bcr* exons), seen in CML and ALL, and p190 (containing fewer *bcr* exons) noted in juvenile and adult Philadelphia chromosome-positive ALL [109,110]. *abl* is a well-established proto-oncogene which has been noted to have tyrosine phosphorylation capability. The Bcr–Abl fusion protein shows increased activity and is capable of autophosphorylation. There is some evidence that a critical upstream exon of *bcr* is capable of interacting with a src homology regulatory domain (SH2) of the Abl protein [111]. The construction of transgenic mice carrying expressed *bcr–abl* fusion genes has been accomplished and these mice frequently succumb to hematopoietic malignancies [112,113]. However, the fusion gene does not appear to be highly oncogenic in non-hematopoietic tissues.

Gene rearrangements as tumor-specific markers

(see Chapter 4)

As is clear from the preceding discussion, the DNA in a malignant lymphocyte is not the same as that in other tissues nor in nontransformed lymphocytes. Irreversible reconfigurations of the DNA have occurred, reconfigurations which are unique to the transformed cell. One class of these rearrangements is the specific Ig and TCR locus rearrangements which the cell has elaborated in the process of generating a functional antigen binding moiety. The other class is the rearrangements of growth-affecting genes whose disruption has contributed to the process of malignant transformation. Both kinds of rearrangements provide unique 'molecular fingerprints' of the transformed cell. Recognition of these molecular fingerprints is finding increased use in the diagnosis, classification and staging of individual patient's malignancies. Furthermore, the high sensitivity and specificity of the molecular genetic tests now being used is promoting the application of tumor-specific gene rearrangements as a means of following a given patient's response to therapy, residual tumor burden during or after therapy, and early diagnosis of relapse.

Summary

The primary differentiated and expressed products of lymphocytes are immunoglobulins and T-cell antigen receptors. When considering the molecular genetics of lymphoid malignancies, it is often observed that the transformation event includes the juxtaposition of one of these immune receptors with a growth-affecting gene. This may lead to the constitutive expression of a growth stimulatory protein. In certain cases there may also be a requirement for the elaboration of a functional immune receptor whose antigen reactivity may provide an additional essential proliferative stimulus. The mechanism by which these transformation events occur are diverse, but often reflect the genome destabilizing and gene rearranging enzymes present during normal lymphocyte development. Whether this inherent genetic instability of lymphocytes distinguishes the etiology of lymphoid malignancies from that of solid tumors, or rather focuses attention on universal prerequisites of transformation, is an issue that continues to provoke thought and experimentation. The DNA in a transformed lymphocyte is not the same as that of its normal counterpart. The recognition of this fact provides a ready tool for leukemia and lymphoma diagnosis, staging, classification, minimal residual disease determination and gene discovery.

References

1. Kirsch IR, Kuehl WM. Gene rearrangements in lymphoid cells. In Stamatoyannopoulos, G, et al. (eds) *The Molecular Basis of Blood Diseases*, Philadelphia, PA: WB Saunders Co., 1993, pp. 381–419.
1a. Kirsch IR. Genetics of pediatric tumors: The causes and consequences of chromosomal aberrations. In Pizzo, P, Poplack D (eds) *Principles and Practice of Pediatric Oncology*, 2nd edn. Philadelphia: JB Lippincott, 1993.
2. Schatz DG, Oettinger MA, Baltimore D. The V(D)J recombination activating gene, RAG-1. *Cell* 1989, **59**: 1035–1048.
3. Oettinger MA, Schatz DG, Gorka C, et al. RAG-1 and RAG-2, adjacent genes that synergistically activate V(D)J recombination. *Science* 1990, **248**: 1517–1523.
4. Lieber MR, Hesse JE, Lewis S, et al. The defect in murine severe combined immune deficiency: Joining of signal sequences but not coding segments in V(D)J recombination. *Cell* 1988, **55**: 7–16.
4a. Kirchgessner CV, Patil CK, Evans JW, et al. DNA-dependent kinase (p350) as a candidate gene for the murine SCID defect. *Science* 1995, **267**: 1178–1183.

5. Matsunami N, Hamaguchi Y, Yamamoto Y. A protein binding to the Jκ recombination sequence of immunoglobulin genes contains a sequence related to the integrase motif. *Nature* 1989, **342**: 934.

6. Landau NR, Schatz DG, Rosa M, et al. Increased frequency of N-region insertion in a murine pre-B-cell line infected with a terminal deoxynucleotidyl transferase retroviral expression vector. *Mol. Cell. Biol.* 1987, **7**: 3237–3243.

7. Yancopoulos GD, Alt FW. Developmentally controlled and tissue-specific expression of unrearranged VH gene segments. *Cell* 1985, **40**: 271–281.

8. Blackwell TK, Moore MW, Yancopoulos GD, et al. Recombination between immunoglobulin variable region gene segments is enhanced by transcription. *Nature* 1986, **324**: 585–589.

9. Hsieh CL, McCloskey RP, Lieber MR. V(D)J recombination on minichromosomes is not affected by transcription. *J. Biol. Chem.* 1992, **267**: 15613–15619.

9a. Stern MH, Lipkowitz S, Aurias A, et al. Inversion of chromosome 7 in ataxia telangiectasia is generated by a rearrangement between T-cell receptor beta and T-cell receptor gamma genes. *Blood*, **74**: 2076–2080.

10. Tycko B, Palmer JD, Sklar J. T-cell receptor gene trans-rearrangements: Chimeric g δ genes in normal lymphoid tissues. *Science* 1989, **245**: 1242–1246.

11. Lipkowitz S, Stern MH, Kirsch IR. Hybrid T cell receptor genes formed by interlocus recombination in normal and ataxia-telangiectasia lymphocytes. *J. Exp. Med.* 1990, **172**: 409–418.

12. Boder E. Ataxia-telangiectasia: An overview. In Gatti RA, Swift M (eds) *Ataxia-Telangiectasia: Genetics, Neuropathology, and Immunology of a Degenerative Disease of Childhood*, New York: Alan R. Liss, 1985, pp. 1–63.

12a. Hsieh C-L, Arlett CF, Lieber MR. V(D)J recombination in ataxia telangiectasia, Bloom's syndrome, and a DNA ligase 1-associated immunodeficiency disorder. *J. Biol. Chem.* 1993, **27**: 20105–20109.

13. Pandita TK, Hittelman WN. Initial chromosome damage but not DNA damage is greater in ataxia telangiectasia cells. *Radiat. Res.* 1992, **130**: 94–103.

14. Lipkowitz S, Garry VF, Kirsch IR. Interlocus V-J recombination measures genomic instability in agriculture workers at risk for lymphoid malignancies. *Proc. Natl Acad. Sci. USA* 1992, **89**: 5301–5305.

15. Lieber MR. The role of site-directed recombinases in physiologic and pathologic chromosomal rearrangements. In Kirsch IR (ed.) *The Causes and Consequences of Chromosomal Aberrations*, Boca Raton, FL: CRC Press, Inc., 1993, pp. 239–275.

16. Bahler DW, Levy R. Clonal evolution of a follicular lymphoma: Evidence for antigen selection. *Proc. Natl Acad. Sci. USA* 1992, **89**: 6770–6774.

17. Shen-Ong GL, Keath EJ, Piccoli SP, et al. Novel myc oncogene RNA from abortive immunoglobulin-gene recombination in mouse plasmacytomas. *Cell* 1982, **31**: 443–452.

18. Dalla-Favera R, Bregni M, Erickson J, et al. Human c-myc oncogene is located on the region of chromosome 8 that is translocated in Burkitt lymphoma cells. *Proc. Natl Acad. Sci. USA* 1982, **79**: 7824–7827.

19. Taub R, Kirsch I, Morton C, et al. Translocation of the c-myc gene into the immunoglobulin heavy chain locus in human Burkitt lymphoma and murine plasmacytoma cells. *Proc. Natl Acad. Sci. USA* 1982, **79**: 7837–7841.

20. Hesse JE, Lieber MR, Mizuuchi K, et al. V(D)J recombination: A functional definition of the joining signals. *Genes Dev.* 1989, **3**: 1053–1061.

21. Boehm T, Mengle-Gaw L, Kees UR, et al. Alternating purine-pyrimidine tracts may promote chomosomal translocation seen in a variety of human lymphoid tumors. *EMBO J.* 1989, **8**: 2621–2631.

22. Begley CG, Aplan PD, Davey MP, et al. Chromosomal translocation in a human leukemic stem-cell line disrupts the T-cell antigen receptor δ chain diversity region and results in a previously unreported fusion transcript. *Proc. Natl Acad. Sci. USA* 1989, **86**: 2031–2035.

23. Cimino G, Mopir DT, Canaani O, et al. Cloning of ALL-1, the locus involved in leukemias with the t(4;11)(q21;q23), t(9;11)(p22;q23), and t(11;19)(q23; p13) chromosome translocations. *Cancer Res.* 1991, **51**: 6712–6714.

24. Ziemin-van der Poel S, McCabe NR, Gill HJ, et al. Identification of a gene, MLL, that spans the breakpoint in 11q23 translocations associated with human leukemias. *Proc. Natl Acad. Sci. USA* 1991, **86**: 10735–10739.

25. Gu Y, Cimino G, Alder H, et al. The (4;11)(q21;q23) chromosome translocations in acute leukemias involve the VDJ recombinase. *Proc. Natl Acad. Sci. USA* 1992, **89**: 10464–10468.

25a. Aplan PD, Chervinsky DS, Stanulla M, Burhams WC. Site-specific DNA cleavage within the MLL breakpoint cluster region induced by topoisomerase II inhibitors. *Blood* 1996, **87**: 2649–2658.

26. Aplan PD, Lombardi DP, Reaman GH, et al. Involvement of the putative hematopoietic transcription factor SCL in T-cell acute lymphoblastic leukemia. *Blood* 1992, **79**: 1327–1333.

27. Aplan PD, Begley CG, Bertness V, et al. The SCL gene is formed from a transcriptionally complex locus. *Mol. Cell Biol.* 1990, **10**: 6426–6435.

28. Aplan PD, Lombardi DP, Kirsch IR. Structural characterization of SIL, a gene frequently disrupted in T-cell acute lymphoblastic leukemia. *Mol. Cell Biol.* 1991, **11**: 5462–5469.

29. Haluska FG, Tsujimoto Y, Croce CM. Mechanisms of chromosome translocation in B- and T-cell neoplasia. *Trends Genet.* 1987, **3**: 11–15.

30. Neri A, Barriga F, Knowles DM, et al. Different regions of the immunoglobulin heavy-chain locus are involved in chromosomal translocations in distinct pathogenetic forms of Burkitt's lymphoma. *Proc. Natl Acad. Sci. USA* 1988, **85**: 2748–2752.

30a. Chesi M, Bergsagel PL, Brents LA, Smith CM, Gerhard DS and Kuehl WM. Dysregulation of cyclin D₁ by translocation into an IgH gamma switch region in two multiple myeloma cell lines. *Blood* 1996, **88**: 674–681.

31. Nowell P, Hungerford D. A minute chromosome in human chronic granulocytic leukemia. *Science* 1960, **132**: 1497.

32. Rowley JD. A new and consistent chromosomal abnormality in chronic myelogenous leukemia identified by quinacrine fluorescence and Giemsa staining. *Nature* 1973, **243**: 290–293.

33. de Klein A, Geurts van Kessel A, Grosveld G, et al. A cellular oncogene is translocated to the Philadelphia chromosome in chronic myelocytic leukemia. *Nature* 1982, **300**: 765.

34. Groffen J, Stephenson JR, Heisterkamp N, et al. Philadelphia chromosomal breakpoints are clustered within a limited region, bcr, on chromosome 22. *Cell* 1984, **36**: 93.

35. Denny CT, Shah N, Ogden S, et al. Localization of preferential sites of rearrangement within the BCR gene in Philadelphia chromosome positive acute lymphoblastic leukemia. *Proc. Natl Acad. Sci. USA* 1989, **86**: 4254.

36. Vogelstein B. A deadly inheritance. *Nature* 1990, **348**: 681.

37. Fearon ER, Vogelstein B. A genetic model for colorectal tumorigenesis. *Cell* 1990, **61**: 759.

38. Sandberg AA. Chromosome changes in leukemia and cancer and their molecular limning. In Kirsch IR (ed.) *The Causes and Consequences of Chromosomal Aberrations*, Boca Raton, FL: CRC Press, Inc., 1993, pp. 141–163.

39. Kuerbitz SJ, Plunkett BS, Walsh WV, et al. Wild-type p53 is a cell cycle checkpoint determinant following irradiation. *Proc. Natl Acad. Sci. USA* 1992, **89**: 7491–7495.

40. Hartwell LH, Weinert TA. Checkpoints: Controls that ensure the order of cell cycle events. *Science* 1989, **246**: 629–634.

41. Livingstone LR, White A, Sprouse J, et al. Altered cell cycle arrest and gene amplification potential accompany loss of wild-type p53. *Cell* 1992, **70**: 923–935.

42. Yin Y, Tainsky MA, Bischoff FZ, et al. Wild-type p53 restores cell cycle control and inhibits gene amplification in cells with mutant p53 alleles. *Cell* 1992, **70**: 937–948.

43. Hartwell L. Defects in a cell cycle checkpoint may be responsible for the genomic instability of cancer cells. *Cell* 1992, **71**: 543–546.

44. Kastan MB, Zhan Q, El-Deiry WS, et al. A mammalian cell cycle checkpoint pathway utilizing p53 and GADD45 is defective in ataxia-telangiectasia. *Cell* 1992, **71**: 587–597.

45. Parsons R, Li GL, Longley MJ, et al. Hypermutability and mismatch repair deficiency in RER+ tumor cells. *Cell* 1993, **75**: 1227–1236.

46. Aaltonen LA, Peltomaki P, Mecklin JP, et al. Replication errors in benign and malignant tumors from hereditary nonpolyposis colorectal cancer patients. *Cancer Res.* 1994, **54**: 1645–1648.

47. Sandberg AA. *The Chromosomes in Human Cancer and Leukemia*, 2nd edn., Amsterdam: Elsevier Science, 1990.

48. Gaidano G, Ballerini P, Gong J, et al. p53 mutations in human lymphoid malignancies: Association with Burkitt lymphoma and chronic lymphocytic leukemia. *Proc. Natl Acad. Sci. USA* 1991, **88**: 5413–5417.

49. Ballerini P, Gaidano G, Gong JZ, et al. Multiple genetic lesions in acquired immunodeficiency syndrome-related non-Hodgkin's lymphoma. *Blood* 1993, **81**: 166–176.

50. Dalla-Favera R. Chromosomal translocations involving the c-myc oncogene in lymphoid neoplasia. In Kirsch IR (ed.) *The Causes and Consequences of Chromosomal Aberrations*, Boca Raton, FL: CRC Press, Inc., 1993.

51. Haluska FG, Tsujimoto Y, Croce CM. Oncogene activation by chromosomal translocation in human malignancy. *Annu. Rev. Genet.* 1987, **21**: 313–332.

52. Eick D, Bornkamm GW. Expression of normal and translocated c-myc alleles in Burkitt's lymphoma cells: Evidence for different regulation. *EMBO J.* 1989, **8**: 1965.

53. Grignani F, Lombardi L, Inghirami G, et al. Negative autoregulation of c-myc gene expression is inactivated in transformed cells. *EMBO J.* 1990, **9**: 3913.

54. Leder P, Battey J, Lenoir G, et al. Translocations among antibody genes in human cancer. *Science* 1983, **222**: 765–771.

55. Taub R, Moulding C, Battey J, et al. Activation and somatic mutation of the translocated c-myc gene in Burkitt lymphoma cells. *Cell* 1984, **36**: 339–348.

56. Pelicci PG, Knowles DK, Magrath I, et al., Chromosomal breakpoints and structural alterations of the c-myc locus differ in endemic and sporadic forms of Burkitt lymphoma. *Proc. Natl Acad. Sci. USA* 1986, **83**: 2984.

57. Bentley DL, Groudine M. A block to elongation is largely responsible for decreased transcription of c-myc in differentiated HL-60 cells. *Nature* 1986, **321**: 702.

58. Nepveu A, Marcu KB. Intragenic pausing and antisense transcription within the murine c-myc locus. *EMBO J.* 1986, **5**: 2859.

59. Zajac-Kaye M, Gelmann EP, Levens S. A point mutation in the c-myc locus of a Burkitt lymphoma abolishes binding of a nuclear protein. *Science* 1988, **240**: 1776.

60. Cesarman E, Dalla-Favera RBD, Groudine M. Mutations in the first exon are associated with altered transcription of c-myc in Burkitt lymphoma. *Science* 1987, **238**: 1272.

61. Bhatia K, Huppi K, Spangler G, et al. Point mutations in the c-myc transactivation domain are common in Burkitt's lymphoma and mouse plasmacytomas. *Nature Genet.* 1993, **5**: 56–61.

62. Caccia N, Toyonaga B, Kimura N, et al. The α and β chains of the T cell receptor. In Mak TW (ed.) *The T-Cell Receptors*, New York: Plenum Press, 1988, pp. 9–52.

63. Marcu KB, Bossone SA, Patel AS. Myc function and regulation. *Annu. Rev. Biochem.* 1992, **61**: 809–860.

64. Murre C, McCaw PS, Baltimore D. A new DNA binding and dimerization motif in immunoglobulin enhancer binding, daughterless, MyoD, and myc proteins. *Cell* 1989, **56**: 777–783.

65. Landshulz WH, Johnson PF, McKnight SL. The leucine zipper: A hypothetical structure common to a new class of DNA binding proteins. *Science* 1988, **240**: 1759–1764.

66. Blackwood EM, Eisenman RN. Max: A helix-loop-helix zipper protein that forms a sequence-specific DNA-binding complex with Myc. *Science* 1991, **251**: 1211–1217.

67. Ayer DD, Kretzner L, Eisenman RN. Mad: A heterodimeric partner for Max that antagonizes myc transcriptional activity. *Cell* 1993, **72**: 211–222.

68. Zervos AS, Gyuris J, Brent R. Mxi1, a protein that specifically interacts with Max to bind Myc-Max recognition sites. *Cell* 1993, **72**: 223–232.

69. Inghirami G, Grignani F, Sternas L, et al. Downregulation of LFA-1 adhesion receptors by c-myc oncogene in human B lymphoblastoid cells. *Science* 1990, **250**: 682–686.

70. Tsujimoto Y, Finger LR, Yunis J, et al. Cloning of the chromosome breakpoint of neoplastic B cells with the t(14;18) chromosome translocation. *Science* 1984, **266**: 1097–1099.

71. McDonnell TJ, Deane N, Platt F, et al. Bcl-2 immunoglobulin transgenic mice demonstrate extended B cell survival and follicular lymphoproliferation. *Cell* 1989, **57**: 79–88.

72. Hockenbery D, Zutter M, Hickey W, et al. Bcl-2 protein is topographically restricted in tissues characterized by apoptotoic cell death. *Proc. Natl Acad. Sci. USA* 1991, **88**: 6961–6965.

73. Hockenbery DM, Oltvai ZN, Yin XM, et al. Bcl-2 functions in an antioxidant pathway to prevent apoptosis. *Cell* 1993, **75**: 241–252.

74. Boise LH, Gonzalez-Garcia M, Postema CE, et al. bcl-x, a bcl-2-related gene that functions as a dominant regulator of apoptotic cell death. *Cell* 1993, **74**: 597–608.

75. Oltvai ZN, Milliman CL, Korsmeyer SJ. Bcl-2 heterodimerizes in vivo with a conserved homolog, Bax, that accelerates programmed cell death. *Cell* 1993, **74**: 609–620.

76. Motokura T, Bloom T, Kim HG, et al. A novel cyclin encoded by a bcl1 linked candidate oncogene. *Nature* 1991, **350**: 512–515.

77. Matsushime HR MF, Ashmun RA, Sherr CJ. Colony-stimulating factor 1 regulates novel cyclins during the G1 phase of the cell cycle. *Cell* 1991, **65**: 691–699.

78. Ohno H, Takimoto G, McKeithan T. The candidate proto-oncogene bcl-3 is related to genes implicated in cell lineage determination and cell cycle control. *Cell* 1990, **60**: 991–997.

79. Visvader J, Begley CG, Adams JM. Differential expression of the LYL, SCL, and E2A helix-loop-helix genes within the hemopoietic system. *Oncogene* 1991, **6**: 187–194.

80. Hatano M, Roberts CWM, Minden M, et al. Deregulation of a homeobox gene HOX11, by the t(10;14) in T cell leukemia. *Science* 1991, **253**: 79–82.

81. Allen JD, Lints T, Jenkins NA, et al. Novel murine homeo box gene on chromosome 1 expressed in specific hematopoietic lineages and during embryogenesis. *Genes Dev.* 1991, **5**: 509–520.

82. Boehm T, Spillantini MG, Sofroniew MV, et al. Developmentally regulated and tissue specific expression of mRNAs encoding the two alternative forms of the LIM domain oncogene rhombotin: Evidence for thymus expression. *Oncogene* 1991, **6**: 695–704.

83. Royer-Pokora B, Loos U, Ludwig WD. TTG-2, a new gene encoding a cystein-rich protein with the LIM motif, is overexpressed in acute T-cell leukaemia with the t(11;14)(p13;q11). *Oncogene* 1991, **6**: 1887–1894.

84. Tauchi T, Ohyashili JH, Ohyashili K, et al. Methylation status of T-cell receptor β-chain gene in B precursor acute lymphoblastic leukemia: Correlation with hypomethylation and gene rearrangement. *Cancer Res.* 1991, **52**: 2917.

85. Ohyashiki JH, Ohyashiki K, Kawakubo K, et al. T-cell receptor β chain gene rearrangement in acute myeloid leukemia always occurs at the allele that contains the undermethylated Jβ1 region. *Cancer Res.* 1992, **52**: 6598.

86. Ohyashiki JJ, Ohyashiki K, Kawakubo K, et al. The methylation status of the major breakpoint cluster region in human leukemia cells, including Philadelphia chromosome-positive cells, is linked to the lineage of hematopoietic cells. *Leukemia* 1993, **7**: 801.

87. Engler P, Weng A, Storb U. Influence of CpG methylation and target spacing on V(D)J recombination in a transgeneic substrate. *Mol. Cell. Biol.* 1993, **13**: 571.

88. Burger C, Radbruch A. Protective methylation of immunoglobulin and T cell receptor (TcR) gene loci prior to induction of class switch and TcR recombination. *Eur. J. Immunol.* 1990, **20**: 2285.

89. Bird A. The essentials of DNA methylation. *Cell* 1992, **70**: 5.

90. Kioussis D, Vanin E, deLange T, et al. β-Globin gene inactivation by DNA translocation in γβ-thalassemia. *Nature* 1983, **306**: 662.

91. Forrester WC, Epner E, Driscoll MC, et al. A deletion of the human β-globin locus activation region causes a major alteration in chromatin structure and replication across the entire β-globin locus. *Genes Dev.* 1990, **4**: 1637.

92. Kim CG, Epner EM, Forrester WC, et al. Inactivation of the human β-globin gene by targeted insertion into the β-globin locus control region. *Genes Dev.* 1992, **6**: 928–938.

93. Hunger SP, Galili NG, Carroll AJ, et al. The t(1;19)(q23;p13) results in consistent fusion of E2A and PBX1 coding sequences in acute lymphoblastic leukemias. *Blood* 1991, **77**: 687–693.

94. Hunger SP, Ohyashiki K, Toyoma K, et al. HLF, a novel hepatic bZIP protein, shows altered DNA-binding properties following fusion to E2A in t(17;19)-ALL. *Genes Dev.* 1992, **6**: 1608–1620.

95. Tkachuk DC, Kohler S, Cleary ML. Involvement of a homolog of Drosophila trithorax by 11q23 chromosomal translocations in acute leukemias. *Cell* 1992, **71**: 691–700.

96. Gu Y, Nakamura H, Alder H, et al. The t(4;11) chromosome translocation of human acute leukemias fuses the ALL-1 gene, related to Drosophila trithorax, to the AF-4 gene. *Cell* 1992, **71**: 701–708.

97. Corral J, Forster A, Thompson SP, et al. Acute leukemias of different lineages have similar MLL gene fusions encoding related chimeric proteins resulting from chromsomal translocation. *Proc. Natl Acad. Sci. USA* 1993, **90**: 8538–8542.

98. Domer PH, Fakharzadeh SS, Chen CS, et al. Acute mixed-lineage leukemia t(4;11)(q21;q23) generates an MLL-AF4 fusion product. *Proc. Natl Acad. Sci. USA* 1993, **90**: 7884–7888.

99. Morrissey J, Tkachuk DC, Milatovich A, et al. A serine/proline-rich protein is fused to HRX in t(4;11) acute leukemias. *Blood* 1993, **81**: 1124–1131.

100. Nakamura T, Alder H, Gu Y, et al. Genes on chromosomes 4, 9, and 19 involved in 11q23 abnormalities in acute leukemia share sequence homology and/or common motifs. *Proc. Natl Acad. Sci. USA* 1993, **90**: 4631–4635.

101. Miyoshi H, Shimizu K, Kozu T, et al. t(8;21) breakpoints on chromosome 21 in acute myeloid leukemia are clustered within a limited region of a single gene, AML1. *Proc. Natl Acad. Sci. USA* 1991, **88**: 10431–10434.

102. Erickson P, Gao J, Chang KS, et al. Identification of breakpoints in t(8;21) acute myelogenous leukemia and isolation of a fusion transcript, AML1/ETO, with similarity to *Drosophila* segmentation gene, runt. *Blood* 1992, **80**: 1825–1831.

103. Miyoshi H, Kozu T, Shimizu K, et al. The t(8;21) translocation in acute myeloid leukemia results in production of an AML1-MTG8 fusion transcript. *EMBO J.* 1993, **12**: 2715–2721.

104. von Lindern M, Breems D, van Baal S, et al. Characterization of the translocation breakpoint sequences of two DEK-CAN fusion genes present in t(6;9) acute myeloid leukemia and a SET-CAN fusion gene found in a case of acute undifferentiated leukemia. *Genes Chrom. Cancer* 1992, **5**: 227–234.

105. Kakizuka A, Miller WH Jr, Umesono K, et al. Chromosomal translocation t(15;17) in human acute promyelocytic leukemia fuses RARα with a novel putative transcription factor, PML. *Cell* 1991, **66**: 663–674.

106. de The H, Lavau C, Marchio A, Chomienne C, et al. The PML-RARα fusion mRNA generated by the t(15;17) translocation in acute promyelocytic leukemia encodes a functionally altered RAR. *Cell* 1991, **66**: 675–684.

107. Shtivelman E, Lifshitz B, Gale RP, et al. Fused transcript of abl and bcr genes in chronic in chronic myelogenous leukaemia. *Nature* 1985, **315**: 550.

108. Konopka JB, Watanabe SM, Witte ON. An alteration of the human c-abl protein in K562 leukemia cells unmask associated tyrosine kinase activity. *Cell* 1984, **37**: 1035.

109. Hermans A, Heisterkamp N, von Lindern M, et al. Unique fusion of bcr and c-abl genes in Philadelphia chromosome positive acute lymphoblastic leukemia. *Cell* 1987, **51**: 33.

110. Clark SS, McLaughlin J, Crist WM, et al. Unique forms of the abl tyrosine kinase distinguish Ph-1 positive CML from Ph1-positive ALL. *Science* 1987, **235**: 85.

111. Pendergast AM, Muller AJ, Havlik MH, et al. BCR sequences essential for transformation by the BCR/ABL oncogene bind to the ABL SH2 regulatory domain in a non-phosphotyrosine-dependent manner. *Cell* 1991, **66**: 1.

112. Kelliher MA, McLaughlin J, Witte ON, et al. Induction of a chronic myelogenous leukmia-like syndrome in mice with v-abl and BCR/ABL. *Proc. Natl Acad. Sci. USA* 1990, **87**: 6649.

113. Elefanty AG, Hariharan IK, Cory S. bcr-abl, the hallmark of chronic myeloid leukaemia in man, induces multiple haemopoietic neoplasms in mice. *EMBO J.* 1990, **9**: 1069.

CHAPTER 11

Cytogenetics of non-Hodgkin's lymphomas

JACQUELINE WHANG-PENG AND TURID KNUTSEN

Introduction

In contrast to Hodgkin's disease, the non-Hodgkin's lymphomas (NHLs) are composed of a wide range of tumors with histological, immunological, and cytogenetic heterogeneity [1,2]. The various subtypes have diverse etiologies and differ in both their clinical presentations and response to treatment. Classification is generally based on cytologic characteristics, growth patterns, and immunophenotype (B or T). Although cytogenetic analysis of more than 2000 cases of lymphoma has been reported in the medical literature and at least 90% of lymphomas exhibit chromosomal abnormalities (most, multiple abnormalities) [3–7], some of which can be correlated with specific histologic and immunologic phenotypes, the existence of various classification systems has made it difficult in the past to compare cytogenetic data with histopathologic features. Nevertheless, and despite the fact that lymphomas are generally cytogenetically more complex then leukemias, cytogenetic analysis has become a useful diagnostic and prognostic aid in lymphoma, as well as leading to the identification of the molecular changes associated with this heterogenous group of diseases.

Materials and methods

Successful cytogenetic studies of neoplastic disorders depend upon obtaining a good sample of tumor cells and upon the availability of dividing cells. Then it must be determined whether the anticipated chromosomal abnormalities are readily visible using standard harvesting techniques, or high-resolution techniques may be required to detect very subtle aberrations.

LYMPH NODES

Lymphomas usually present in the lymph node, which is consequently the most convenient and most frequent choice for cytogenetic studies. When biopsies are not available, fine-needle aspiration of a lymph node may also provide sufficient material for study [8]. Aspirates have the advantage of being easy to obtain and are useful for studying the evolution of the disease over time and at different sites; the disadvantage is the limited number of cells obtained, which is usually only enough for a single culture.

Table 11.2   Most frequent chromosomal abnormalities found in the non-Hodgkin's lymphomas

Low Grade

A.   Malignant lymphoma, small lymphocytic (29 patients)

Numerical: +12(7x), −9(2x)

Structural:

14q32(8x)	**14q22(2x)**	**11q(7x)**	**6q(5x)**	**12p13(3x)**
t(1;14)(p32;q32)	del(14)(q22)	dup(11)(q13;q25)	del(6)(q15)(2x)	t(12;?)(p13;?)
t(11;14)(p11;q32)	t(7;14)(p22;q22)	del(11q)(2x)	t(X;6)(q27;?)	t(12;13)(p13;q22)
t(11;14)(q22;q32)		del(11)(q21)	t(6;12)(q21;p13)	(see 6q)
t(11;14)(q13;q32)		inv ins(11)(q14.2q23)	t(6;?)(q27;?)	
t(14;?)(q32;?)		(see14q)		
t(14;19)(q32;813)				

B.   Malignant lymphoma, follicular, predominantly small cleaved cell (36 patients)

Numerical: +3(4x), +2(3x), +7(2x), −8(2x), −9(3x), +12(2x), +X(2x)

Structural:

18q(25x)	**14q32(32x)**	**6q(11x)**	**i(17q)(3x)**
t(14;18)(q32;q21)(22x)	t(14;?)(q32;?)	del(6)(q)	
t(6;18)(q21;q23)	t(1;14)(q42;q32)	del(6)(q21)(3x)	
t(18;?)(q23;?)	t(11;14)(q23;q32)	del(6)(q22)(2x)	
t(4;18)(p15;q21)	t(7;14)(q34;q32)	del(6)(23)(2x)	
	t(5;14)(q23;q32)	del(6)(q15)	
	t(6;14)(q21;q32)	t(6;17)(q15;p13)	
	t(8;14)(q22;q32)	i(6p)	
	t(3;14)(p21;q32)		
	(see 18q)		

C.   Malignant lymphoma, follicular, mixed, small cleaved and large cell (14 patients)

Numerical: +3(4x), +7(4x), +12(3x), +X(3x), +2(2x)m +8(3x), +16(2x)

Structural:

14q32(8x)	**18q(6x)**	**13p13(2x)**
t(14;18)(q32;q21)(5x)	18q−	t(5;13)(q15;p13)
14q+	(see 14q32)	t(13;?)(p13;?)
t(1;14)(q42;q32)		
t(14;?)(32;?)		

Intermediate

D.   Malignant lymphoma, follicular, predominantly large cell (11 patients)

Numerical: +7(3x), +10(3x), +12(3x), +21(3x)

Structural:

14q32(10x)	**17q(4x)**
t(14;18)(q32;q21)(6x)	t(1;17)(q25;q24)
t(2;14)(q23;q32)	dup 17(q22–24)
t(1;14)(q42;q32)	i(17q)
t(14;16)(q32;q21)	t(17;?)(q25;?)
t(14;17)(q32;q21)	

E.   Malignant lymphoma, diffuse cleaved cell (12 patients)

Numerical: −9(4x), +3(4x), +4(3x), +7(3x), +10(3x), +12(3x), +14(3x) +17(3x), +20(3x)

Table 11.2 (continued)

Structural:

14q32(5x)	1q(5x)	6q(5x)	3q(3x)
t(14;18)(q32;q21)	del(1)(q23)(2x)	del(6)(q21)(2x)	t(3q9q)
t(14;?)(q32;?;q13)	inv ins(X;1)(p22;q31qter)	del(6)(q)(2x)	t(3q9p)
t(14;14)(q32;q24)	dup(1)(q21;q32)	i(6p)	
t(2;14)(q21;q24)	der(1)t(1;1)(pter-->)		
14q+	q32::q21-->qter)		

F. Malignant lymphoma, diffuse mixed small and large cell (15 patients)

Numerical: +12(3x), +18(3x), +1(2x)

Structural:

14q+(8x)	1p(4x)	1q(3x)
t(8;14)(q24;q32)	t(1;2)(p11;q11)	del(1)(q32)(2x)
t(14;18)(q32;q21)(?)(2x)	t(1;6)(p22;q24)	t(1;18)(q25;q23)
t(11;14)(q23;q32)	t(1;?)(p36;?)(2x)	t(1;10)(q42;q22)
t(10;14)(q22;q32)		
t(14;19)(q32;q13)		
t(14;?)(q32;?)(2x)		

G. Malignant lymphoma, diffuse large cell (23 patients)

Numerical: +7(8x), +12(7x), +2(5x), +3(5x), +21(5x), +10(3x), +13(3x), +19(3x), +20(3x)

Structural:

14q32(15x)	6q(13x)	t(3;)(7x)	18q(8x)	1q(5x)
t(8;14)(q24;q32)(5x)	t(2;6)(q37;q21)	t(3;22)(q21;q11)(2x)	t(X;18)(p22;q12)	t(1;3)(q32;q27)
t(14;18)(q32;q21)(4x)	t(3;6)(q27;q21)	t(3;9)(p21;q34)	del(18)(q12)(3x)	dup(1)(q22-44)
t(11;14)	t(3;6)(p25;q21)	t(3;11)(p21;q23)	t(18;?)(q23;?)	dup(1)(q)
t(14;?)(q32;?)(3x)	del(6)(q21)(5x)	(see1q)	t(2;18)(q14;q23)	t(1;3)(q23;p26)
t(1;14)(q23;q32)	del(6)(q15)(3x)		(see14q32)	(see14q)
t(3;14)(p21;q32)	t(5;6)(q15;q27)			

High Grade

H. Malignant lymphoma, large cell, immunoblastic (11 patients)

Numerical: +12(3x), −6(2x), −21(2x), +11(2x)

Structural:

8q(3x)	6q21(3x or 4x)
t(8;14)(2x)	del(6)(q21)(2x or 3x)
t(8;13)(q22;q32)	t(6;11)(q21;p14)

I. Malignant lymphoma, lymphoblastic (9 patients)

Structural:

14q(4x)	14q11(3x)
t(8;14)(q11;q32)	del(14)(q11)
inv(14)(q11;q32)	t(9;14)(q34;q11)
t(14;15)(q;q)	t(11;14)(p11 or 13;q11)
14q+	

J. Malignant lymphoma, small noncleaved cell, Burkitt's and non-Burkitt's (7 patients)

Structural:

t(8;14)(q24;q32)(7x)   dup(1q)(2x)

The number of patients with each abnormality is indicated in parentheses, e.g., +12(7x) indicates seven patients with an additional chromosome 12.

CORRELATION WITH THE WORKING FORMULATION

Tables 11.1 and 11.2 summarize the cytogenetic findings in a total of 167 patients collected from the literature in 1987. Although more cases are now available, the relative proportions of both the number of cells and types of chromosome abnormalities in each subtype of NHL have not changed significantly since that time. Six (3.6%) of patients had a normal karyotype with the remaining 96.4% exhibiting cytogenetic abnormalities. Specific changes reported for each type of lymphoma, according to the Working Formulation [22], are described. It should be borne in mind that these histological categories often encompass multiple pathological entitites (see Chapters 1 and 3).

PLOIDY AND CHROMOSOME ABNORMALITIES

There are no clear-cut differences in modal chromosome number between the three main subgroups of lymphoma in the Working Formulation (low-, intermediate- or high-grade tumors). However, when individual histologies are considered, there are differences in ploidy. Tumors of the small-cell type tend to be pseudodiploid or hyperdiploid, as do the small noncleaved and mixed-cell types, while large-cell lymphomas tend to be hyperdiploid or tetraploid. The most common chromosomal abnormalities in NHL are listed in Table 11.3.

NUMERICAL AND STRUCTURAL ABNORMALITIES

Low grade

Malignant lymphoma, small lymphocytic

Eighty-six per cent of the 29 tumors examined were pseudodiploid or hyperdiploid and 21% had more than five structural rearrangements. The most frequent numerical abnormality was +12 (24% patients), followed by loss of chromosome 9.

The most frequent structural abnormalities were translocations involving chromosome 14 with the breakpoint in the q32 region (28% patients). Translocations with chromosome 11 were found in three cases, with chromosome 1 and with chromosome 19 in one case each, and with an unknown chromosome in three cases. In two instances a higher breakpoint on chromosome 14, at q22, was noted with t(7;14) occurring in one case and del(14)(q22) in the second.

Abnormalities of 11q and 6q were the next most frequent structural abnormalities.

Malignant lymphoma, follicular, predominantly small cleaved cell

Eighty-nine percent of the 36 tumors were pseudo- or hyperdiploid, and 58% had more than five chromosomal rearrangements.

Numerical abnormalities included +3(4x), +2(3x), −9(3x), +7(2x), −8(2x), +12(2x) and +X(2x).

Again, translocations involving chromosome 14 at band q32 were the most frequent structural abnormalities, occurring in 32 of 36 patients (89%). Twenty-two of 36 patients (61%) had t(14;18)(q32; q21) (Figure 11.1), and the remainder had translocations with other chromosomes including 1, 3, 5, 6, 7, 8, 11, or, in three instances, with unidentified chromosomes. In addition to the 18q21 breakpoint associated with t(14;18), there was one patient with t(4;18)(p15;q21), and there were translocations involving 18q23 in two patients. One had a translocation with chromosome 6 and one with an unknown chromosome. Structural abnormalities of chromosome 6 were also frequent in this group (30%). Many of these were deletions that consisted of breaks at q15, q21, q23 and q33; in one instance there was absence of the entire long arm, i(6p). In one patient there was a translocation t(6;17)(q15;p13) (Figure 11.1).

Malignant lymphoma, follicular, mixed, small cleaved and large cell

Sixty-four per cent of these 14 tumors were either pseudo- or hyperdiploid, and 50% had more than five structural abnormalities.

Numerical abnormalities included +3(4x), +7(4x), +8(3x), +12(3x) and +X(3x). Eight of the patients (57%) had chromosomal rearrangements involving chromosome 14 at band q32; five had t(14;18)(q32; q21) and one each had 14q+, t(1;14)(q42;q32), or t(14;?)(q32;?). There were two cases with a rare change, the involvement of 13p13.

Intermediate

Malignant lymphoma, follicular, predominantly large cell

The majority of these 11 tumors (82%) were hyperdiploid or near tetraploid, and 73% had five or more chromosomal abnormalities.

Numerical changes seen included +7(3x), +10(3x), +12(3x), and +21(3x).

Structural changes occurred mostly in the 14q32

Table 11.3 Most common chromosome abnormalities in non-Hodgkin's lymphoma

Abnormality	Related abnormalities	Association	Immuno-phenotype	Grade
Structural				
A. Translocations, inversions				
t(2;5)(p23;q35)		Ki-positive anaplastic large cell	T	High
(3;14)(q27;q32)	t(2;3)(p11–12;q27) t(3;22)(q27;q11)	Diffuse cleaved diffuse large cell	B	High
t(8;14)(q24;q32)	t(2;8)(p12;q24) t(8;22)(q24;q11)	Burkitt's lymphoma	B	High
t(9;14)(p13;q32)		Small lymphocytic lymphoma		
9q11–13,q31–32		Diffuse lymphoma		
10q22–26		Diffuse large-cell cleaved lymphoma	B	
t(11;14)(q13;q32)		Small lymphocytic lymphoma; mantle cell lymphoma	B	Low/Intermed
inv(14)(q11q32)		ATLL	T	
t(14:18)(q32;q21)	t(2;18)(p11–12;q21) t(18;22)(q21;q11)	Follicular lymphoma		Low/Intermed
B. Deletions				
del(6)(q13–14,q21–27) (q21 most common)		All types NHL; usually secondary change; poor survival in non-t(14;18)	B	
del(11)(q14–q23)		Diffuse mixed small and large cell	B	Low
del(14)(q11–24,q22–32)		Adult T-cell leukemia/lymphoma	T	
C. Other structural				
1p36		Associated with t(14;18)		
1q, including dup(1q)		Diffuse large cell; usually secondary change		
D. Isochromosome				
i(1q)		All types of NHL; secondary change		
i(6p)		Associated with t(14;18); secondary change	B	
i(17q)		Associated with loss of 6q		
Numerical				
+3		ATL; Diffuse mixed large- and small-cell lymphoma		
+7		Follicular large-cell lymphoma; secondary change (most frequent)		All grades
+12		Small lymphocytic lymphoma (usually primary change) Diffuse large-cell lymphoma and usually secondary change	B	Low
+18 (partial or complete)		Disease progression; usually secondary change		

region (91%). Sixty per cent of these were t(14;18) (q32;q21), and the others involved translocations with chromosomes 1, 2, 16 and 17.

Malignant lymphoma, diffuse cleaved cell

Either hyperdiploidy or near tetraploidy was found in the majority of these 12 tumors (75%) and 67% of

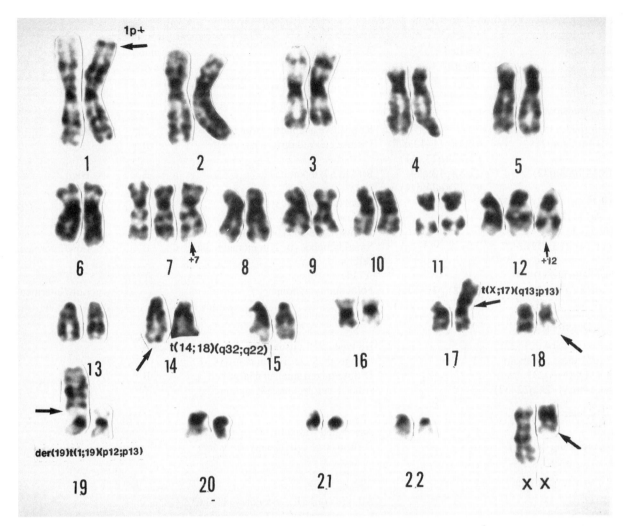

Figure 11.1   A karyotype prepared from a one-day culture of pleural fluid obtained from an NIH patient with malignant lymphoma, follicular small cleaved cell type showing 48,X,t(X;7)(q13;p13),add(1)(p36),+7,+12,t(14;18)(q32;q22), der(19)t(1;19)(p12;p13).

the patients had more than five structural abnormalities.

The most frequent changes in chromosome number were −9(4x), +3(4x), +4(3x), +7(3x), +10(3x), +12(3x), +14(3x), +17(3x) and +20(3x).

Chromosome 14 at band q32 was again the chromosome most frequently involved in structural abnormalities. There was one patient with t(14;18) (q32;q21), one with a translocation involving a second 14, one with a three-way translocation involving a second 14 and an unknown chromosome, one with a translocation involving chromosome 2 and one with a translocation involving an unknown chromosome. Abnormalities of the long arm of chromosome 1, either as a duplication or translocation, and deletions of 6q also occurred frequently. Since these data were collected, the importance of

t(11;14) in mantle cell lymphoma, formerly included in the category of diffuse, small cleaved cell lymphoma, has been recognized. This translocation is discussed below.

Malignant lymphoma, diffuse mixed small and large cell

Eighty-seven per cent of these 15 tumors were pseudo- or hyperdiploid, and 53% had more than five structural abnormalities.

The most frequent numerical abnormalities were +12(3x), +18(3x) and +1(2x).

Structural abnormalities of 14q32 were once again the most frequently found and occurred in 60% of the patients. Two, or possibly three, patients had t(14;18)(q32;q21), in two the identify of the second chromosome was not known, one had t(8;14)(q24; q32), and the remaining three had translocations with chromosome 10, 11 or 19. Involvement of 1p occurred in four tumors and of 1q in three tumors.

Malignant lymphoma, diffuse large cell

The majority of these 23 tumors were hyperdiploid (75%) and 91% had more than five structural abnormalities. The most common numerical changes were associated with +7(8x), +12(7x), +2(5x), +3(5x) and +21(5x). Other changes included +10(3x), +13(3x), +19(3x) and +20(3x).

Sixty-five per cent of the patients had structural abnormalities of 14q32. In five instances, there was a translocation t(8;14)(q24;q32) and in four instances a translocation t(14;18)(q32;q21). The rest had translocations with chromosomes 1, 3, 11 or, in three cases, with unidentified chromosomes. Abnormalities of 6q were also very frequently described in this group, occurring in 35% of the patients. The most frequent finding was del(6)(q21) followed by deletions at q15. In 17% of the cases there was a translocation involving chromosomes 2, 3 and 5. Deletion 18q12 was noted in three instances and a translocation with an unknown chromosome involving a breakpoint at 18q23 was also reported. Duplication, deletion or translocations of chromosome 1q involving bands q22, q23, q26 and q32 were found in four cases, and a duplication was reported in a fifth case, although the breakpoints were not identified.

High grade

Malignant lymphoma, large cell, immunoblastic

Fifty-five per cent of the 11 tumors had chromosome numbers in the hyperdiploid range and 73% had more than five structural abnormalities.

Trisomy 12(3x) was the most frequent numerical change; translocations involving chromosome 8q were the most frequent structural abnormality; two patients had t(8;14) and one had t(8;13)(q22;q32). Three, and possibly four, patients had abnormalities of 6q21; these occurred as deletions or translocations.

Malignant lymphoma, lymphoblastic

Chromosome numbers in these tumors clustered in the pseudodiploid or hyperdiploid region (78%) and most of the nine tumors had one to four structural abnormalities (78%). The most frequent structural abnormalities again occurred on 14q (78%), although not usually at band q32. In one case each there was t(8;14)(q11;q32) and t(14;15). There were four

instances in which 14q11 was involved either as a deletion or as a translocation with chromosome 9 or 11, or was associated with inv(14)(q11q32).

Malignant lymphoma, small noncleaved cell

Most of these patients have been reported as single cases; only seven are included here. Six patients were pseudodiploid and one was hyperdiploid. The majority had fewer than three structural abnormalities and only one case had five. All of these tumors had t(8;14)(q24;q32) and in two cases there was duplication of 1q.

The Burkitt's lymphomas and the non-Burkitt's lymphomas are included in this category. Many cytogenetic studies have been carried out on these patients and the findings may have important implications for the etiology of all lymphomas.

Burkitt's lymphoma, which is endemic in Africa and New Guinea, is closely associated with EBV. Approximately 95–98% of these tumors contain the EBV genome; in contrast a much lower percentage of EBV positivity (15–20%) is found in the sporadic or nonendemic tumors occurring in other areas [39].

In a review of 36 published reports of both endemic and sporadic cases, Berger and Bernheim [40] described cytogenetic findings in 121 patients with Burkitt's lymphoma and 65 cell lines. The most common specific translocation was t(8;14)(q24;q32) found in almost 80% of the tumors. Variants included t(8;22)(q24;q11) found in about 15% of the patients and t(2;8)(p12;q24) in approximately 5% of the patients. In other cases there was a 14q+ or 8q–, although the presence of t(8;14) could not be determined. These abnormalities are similar to those described in B-cell acute lymphoblastic leukemia (ALL) of the FAB L3 type (French–American–British classification). Sporadic tumors usually have additional chromosomal abnormalities, such as duplication of 1q and deletion of 6q as well as abnormalities involving chromosomes 3, 4, 7, 9, 13, 22, X, and Y (Figures 11.2 and 11.3).

Other chromosomal abnormalities have also been reported. Cytogenetic studies in a 44-year-old white male with Burkitt's lymphoma/leukemia revealed a variant translocation t(8;22)(q24;q11), t(3;17)(q27; q12–21) and del(15)(q22) [41]. The breakpoints of chromosomes 17 and 15 are similar to those found in acute promyelocytic leukemia (APL).

Miscellaneous lymphomas

Cutaneous T-cell lymphoma

The criteria for diagnosis of a cutaneous T-cell

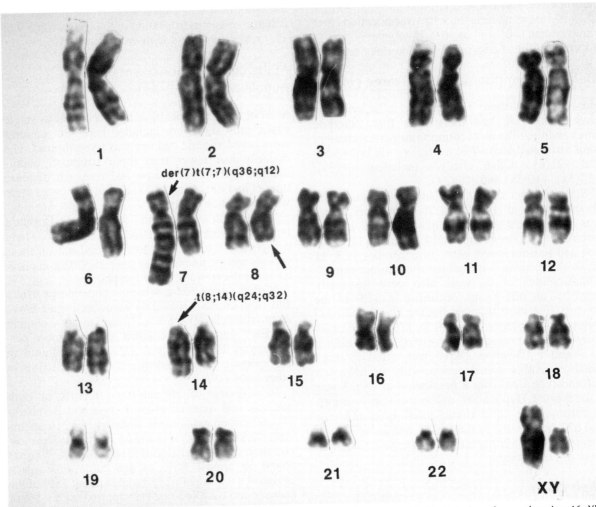

Figure 11.2   A karyotype from a one-day culture of peripheral blood of a patient with Burkitt's lymphoma showing 46, XY, der(7) t(7;7)(q36;q12),t(8;14)(q24;q32).

lymphoma (CTCL) were established by the National CTCL Workshop [42] and four clinical stages were established: IA, limited plaques; IB, generalized plaques; IIA, generalized plaques with adenopathy; IIB, cutaneous tumors with or without adenopathy; III, erythroderma; IVA, any skin involvement with histologically positive nodes; and IVB, any skin stage with visceral involvement.

In our study of 41 CTCL patients [43], there were four patients with limited plaques, 13 with generalized plaques, 8 with cutaneous tumors and 16 with generalized erythroderma. Cytogenetic abnormalities were found in many of these patients in specimens of peripheral blood and lymph nodes, although these tissues were histologically negative: 62% of the peripheral blood samples were cytogenetically positive; 80% of the lymph nodes were cytogenetically positive versus 45% morphologically positive; 6% of the bone marrow samples were cytogenetically

positive versus 3% morphologically positive. No specific chromosomal abnormalities were found in CTCL. Structural abnormalities of chromosome 1, and numerical abnormalities of chromosomes 11, 21 and 22 were the most frequent. Extensive cytogenetic abnormalities and lack of clone formation are two characteristics seen in the early stages. Clone formation is seen only in advanced disease (eight patients) along with hyperdiploidy and near tetraploidy, and is associated with poor prognosis and short survival. Other investigators have confirmed that cytogenetic abnormalities parallel clinical symptoms and that there are fewer changes in the early stages. In a study of 124 patients with CTCL, Vonderheid et al. [44] found that a total cerebriform count above 15% on a blood smear obtained at the time of cytogenetic study strongly correlated with the presence of chromosomally abnormal malignant clones, and that the appearance of polyploid cells reflected poor

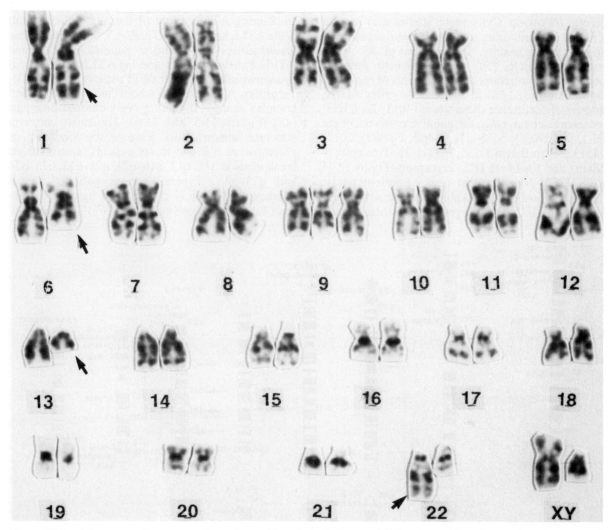

Figure 11.3 A karyotype from a one-day culture of lymph node from an NIH patient with malignant lymphoma, small noncleaved cell type showing 47,XY, der(1)t(1;13)(q32;q14),del(6)(q21),+9,der(22) t(1;22)(q21;q13).

survival. Other reports of cytogenetic studies include a study by Gamperl [45] of a 66-year-old male in the tumor phase of mycosis fungoides who had a clone with a karyotype of 49,XY,+8,11p–,+17,int del (14)(q22q24) in PHA-stimulated peripheral blood cells, and a study by Barbieri et al. [46] of a 62-year-old female with mycosis fungoides (stage IIB) who had cytogenetic abnormalities including 45–46,X, –X,t(4:16)(q34;q21),inv(12)(q15q24),+12,–18,del(21) (q11q21),±21.

Adult T-cell lymphoma/leukemia

Human T-cell lymphotrophic virus (HTLV-1) was the first exogenous retrovirus to be demonstrated in a human cancer: adult T-cell lymphoma/leukemia (ATLL) [47]. Affected patients are geographically clustered in southwestern Japan, the Caribbean basin and southeastern USA. The virus is endemic in these areas, although only a small portion of those with antibodies to the virus will develop leukemia. The clinical course includes acute onset, rapidly developing skin lesions, widespread infiltration of lymph nodes and other organs, development of opportunistic infections, and a syndrome of increased bone turnover that leads to bone lesions and hypercalcemia [48].

Cytogenetic findings in patients with ATLL suggest that more complex numerical and structural abnormalities are found in those patients with a more aggressive clinical course. Cytogenetic studies of five healthy adults who were seropositive showed that three had clonal abnormalities [49]. One had rearrangements of chromosomes 7 and 14, one had a minute chromosome of unknown origin and one had a few cells with clonal abnormalities. The determination of the significance of these findings will require careful follow-up. Cytogenetic studies may provide a means of monitoring seropositive individuals who appear to be healthy. In a review of 85 ATLL patients, Pandolfi [50] related relevant genes or oncogenes to structural rearrangements of regions of eight chromosomes. In descending order of frequency of occurrence these were: 14q11–12, q32(T-receptor α-chain, c-*fos*, the putative proto-oncogene tcl-1, IgH chain); 6q15–q21 (c-*myb*, c-*yes*-2); 2q11–24, 13q21, 1p(B-lym-1), 3q; 7q32 or 35 (T-receptor β-chain); and 10p14–15 I (IL-2 receptor) (Figure 11.4). Both HTLV-1-positive and -negative patients tend to have chromosomal breakpoints at the same band locations. ATLL was categorized into three clinical

stages by Sanada et al. [51]: acute, chronic and smoldering ATLL. Eight of the nine patients with acute ATLL had trisomy 3 and/or 7, but none of these abnormalities was found in patients with chronic ATLL. Patients with smoldering ATLL were normal cytogenetically. We studied 11 patients with HTLV-1-positive ATLL, 10 of whom had numerous and complex changes involving every chromosome pair [48] (Figues 11.5 and 11.6). The most common structural abnormalities were of the long arm of chromosome 6 found in six patients, and involved breakpoints at q11, q13, q16–q23, q21–q23, q22–q24 and q23–q24. Typically these patients had a characteristic clinical course with aggressive disease, high white blood cell count (WBC), hypercalc-

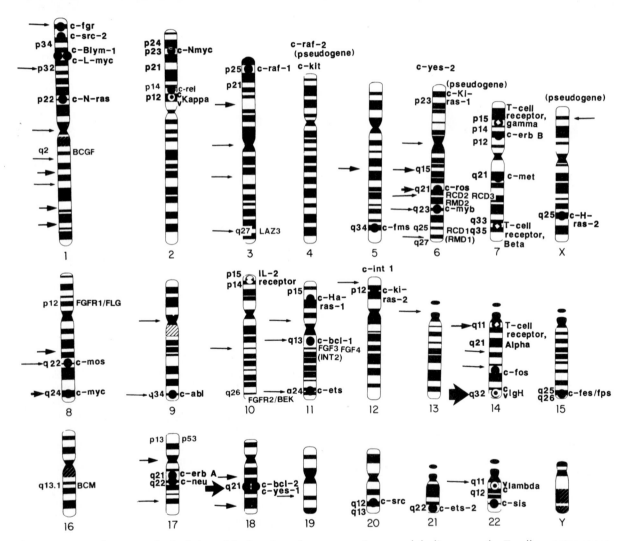

Figure 11.4 A diagrammatic depiction of the location of oncogenes, immunoglobulin genes, the T-cell receptor genes, and the most frequently occurring chromosomal breakpoints in patients with non-Hodgkin's lymphomas as shown. ●, Oncogenes (for those oncogenes placed on top of the chromosomes, the precise location on the chromosomes has not been determined); ◉, immunoglobulin genes; ◯, T-cell receptor genes; ◔, IL-2 receptor; ▸, most frequently occurring breakpoints. Size of arrow indicates frequency of breakpoints, with the largest indicating the most frequent.

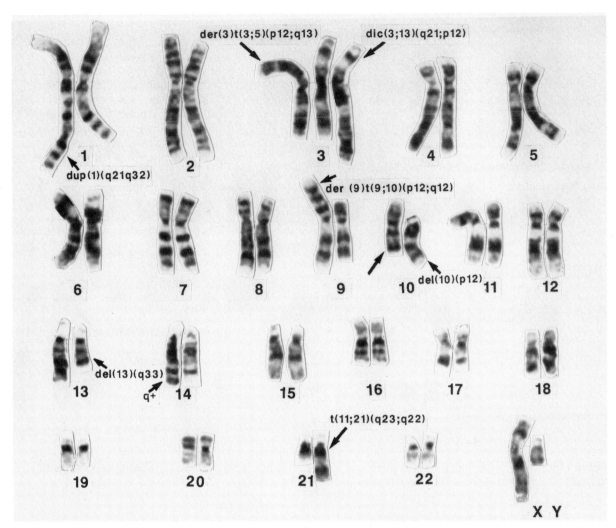

Figure 11.5 A karyotype from a one-day culture of ascites fluid from a patient with ATLL showing 46,XY, dup(1)(q21;q32), der(3)t(3;5)(p12;q13),+dic(3;13)(q21;p12),der(9)t(9;10)(p12;q12),del(10)(p12),del(13)(q33),add(14)(q32),t(11;21) (q23;q22).

emia with bony lesions as well as poor response to chemotherapy and short survival, while those patients without abnormalities of 6q tended to have a more indolent course.

Lymphoepithelioid cell lymphoma (Lennert's lymphoma)

In the late 1960s, a special variant of Hodgkin's disease that was characterized by clusters of epithelioid cells and only sporadic Sternberg–Reed cells was described [52]. Later it was determined that this disease was not a variant of Hodgkin's disease, and it was designated lymphoepithelioid cell lymphoma (LEL) or Lennert's lymphoma [53]. It was also determined, by immunohistochemical means, that the proliferating cells were of T-cell origin. Cytogenetic studies have been reported in a total of eight

patients. Seven of these had numerical or structural abnormalities of chromosome 3; three had +3 as the sole abnormality, two had multiple abnormalities in addition to +3, and two had structural abnormalities: one had der(3)t(3;9)(q22;p13) and the other had der(3)(pter->q24::q22-->pter). The remaining patient had a normal karyotype. Other structural abnormalities involved chromosomes 1, 7, 18 and 19. The structural abnormalities of chromosome 1 appeared to be random with the exception of one patient with duplication of 1q at q32 and two other patients who had breakpoints at 1q13.2 (abnormalities that occur in other lymphomas).

Angioimmunoblastic lymphadenopathy

Angioimmunoblastic lymphadenopathy (AILD) has been considered by some to be a benign proliferative

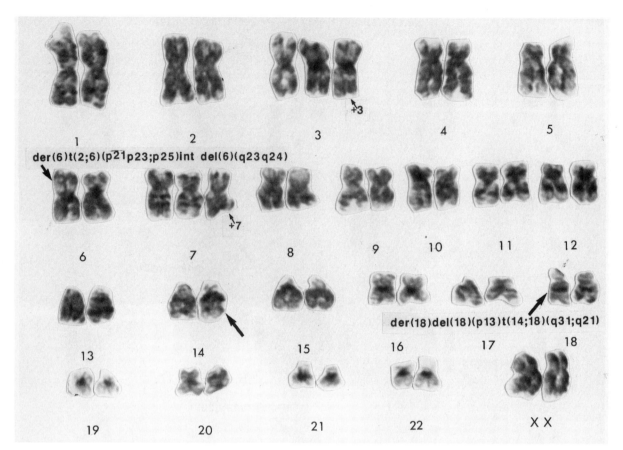

Figure 11.6   A karyotype from a one-day peripheral blood culture of a patient with ATLL showing 48,XX+3,der(6)t(2;6)
(p21p23;p25),del(6)(q23q24),+7,der(18)(del)(18)(p13)t(14;18)(q31;q21).

process. The architecture of the lymph nodes shows
loss of germinal centers as a result of infiltration by a
wide spectrum of polymorphic cells, lymphocytes,
immunoblasts, histiocytes, plasma cells and eosinophils. Cytogenetic findings have been reported in
14 patients. Kaneko et al. [54] studied six patients
and reviewed seven published cases. Although the
karyotypes of the bone marrow were normal, there
were chromosomal abnormalities, both numerical
and structural, in the lymph nodes. Nonrandom
abnormalities included +3 (six patients), +5 (five
patients) and 14q+ (four patients). These findings led
the authors to suggest that, although this disease is
not necessarily monoclonal in the early stages, one
clone may become dominant in later stages. They
also felt that AILD should be considered a malignant
disease that requires aggressive chemotherapy. In a
case studied by Whang-Peng et al. [55], three
consecutive lymph nodes were studied over 14
months: the first was cytogenetically normal and the
following two both showed del(8)(p21) as the sole
chromosomal abnormality.

Richter's syndrome

Richter's syndrome is a term that has been applied to
a small group of patients with chronic lymphocytic
leukemia (CLL) who develop diffuse large-cell
lymphoma (DLC). Nowell et al. [56] performed
sequential chromosome studies in a patient with
untreated T-cell CLL who later developed subcutaneous and abdominal DLC. In the early, indolent
phase, the karyotype of the lymphocytes was pseudodiploid with 3q+ and 14q+ chromosome markers.
After development of DLC, the lymphocytes became
hypertriploid (70–74 chromosomes), and had the
same 3q+ and 14q+ markers. This study indicates
that in this patient the DLC evolved from the
leukemic T-cells.

Malignant lymphoma of mucosa-associated lymphoid tissue

Malignant lymphoma of mucosa-associated lymphoid tissue (MALT) is a recently recognized
subtype of NHL. It is a low-grade B-cell lymphoma

of extranodal origin, which occurs most commonly in the stomach; other sites include the small intestine, lung, thyroid and salivary gland [57]. A lack of *bcl*-l, *bcl*-2, and c-*myc* rearrangements helps to distinguish MALT lymphomas from other B-cell malignancies [58,59].

Clonal cytogenetic abnormalities have been reported in about 20 cases [60–64], which have been reviewed by Whang-Peng et al. [64]. Although no unique or specific aberrations have been reported, several recurring abnormalities have been observed, including trisomies of chromosomes 3 (nine cases), 7 (four cases) and 12 (four cases) (Figure 11.7). Trisomy 3, one of the most common numerical abnormalities in lymphoma, has been reported in

several different subtypes of NHL. Trisomy 7 occurs in several other types of malignancies, including melanoma and renal cell carcinoma, and trisomy 12 is most frequently associated with CLL; both have also been observed in various subtypes of lymphoma. The majority of MALT lymphoma cases have had structural abnormalities, with involvement of chromosomes 1, 2, 6, 8, 10, 11, 12, 14, 15 and 18. The only recurring abnormality was t(11;18)(q21; q21.1), seen in one case identified as MALT lymphoma [60], and two cases reported as small lymphocytic lymphoma of extranodal origin [61]; none of these cases had rearrangement of the *bcl*-2 oncogene, located at 18q21.3. Although no specific abnormality marks this subtype of NHL, cytogenetic studies can be

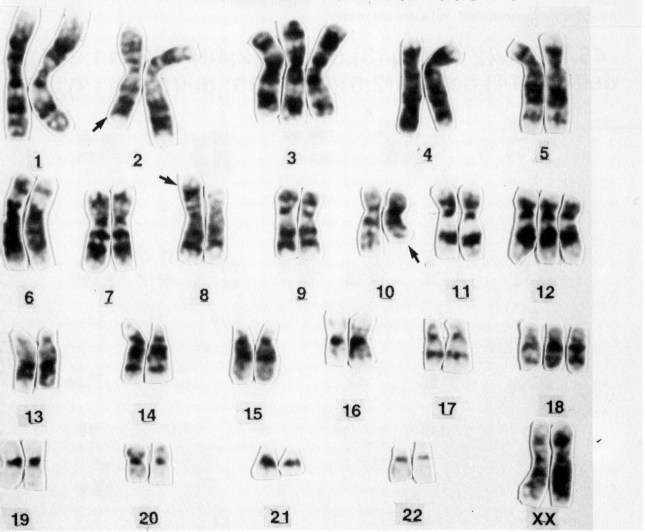

49,XX,+3,t(2;8)(q33;p23),del(10)(q23),+12,+18

Figure 11.7 A karyotype from a four-day stimulated culture of salivary gland from a patient with MALT showing 49,XX,t(2;8)(q33;p23),+3,del(10)(q23),+12,+18.

helpful in establishing a diagnosis when the differential diagnosis includes reactive hyperplasia.

Ki-1 lymphoma

Ki-1 lymphoma is a specific subset of pleomorphic diffuse large-cell NHL, which expresses the Ki-1 (CD30) antigen [65,66], an activation-associated lymphoid differentiation marker often accompanied by the epithelial membrane antigen (EMA). Histologically relatively uniform, these lymphomas exhibit immunophenotypic and immunogenotypic heterogeneity, and are predominantly of T-cell lineage, with less than 10% showing B-cell markers or uncertain lineage. Approximately 40% [67] of cases show a specific translocation, t(2;5)(p23;q35) (Figure 11.8), which is now considered a marker for Ki-1 lymphoma. Several reports [68,69] have indicated that the translocation was characteristic of malignant histiocytosis (MH) but additional studies

have revealed that those MH cases that displayed t(2;5) also expressed the CD30 (Ki-1) antigen, and phenotypic and genotypic analysis indicated that these cases were lymphoid malignancies of T-cell and not histiocytic origin [70–72].

In a study of ten non-B-cell NHLs identified from 278 cytogenetically abnormal NHLs, Ebrahim et al. [67] identified 12 Ki-1-positive lymphomas, 8 of T-cell and 4 of uncertain lineage; 5 of the 12 (42%) had translocations involving 5q35, and there was no histologic difference between those with and those without the translocation. Several of the cases showed unusual patterns of rearrangements of antigen receptor genes (TCRβ, TCRγ, and IgH), suggesting that the Ki-1-positive NHL represents 'malignant transformation of an uncommitted lymphoid cell with subsequent disruption of ordered lineage commitment and aberrant expression of late activation related antigens'.

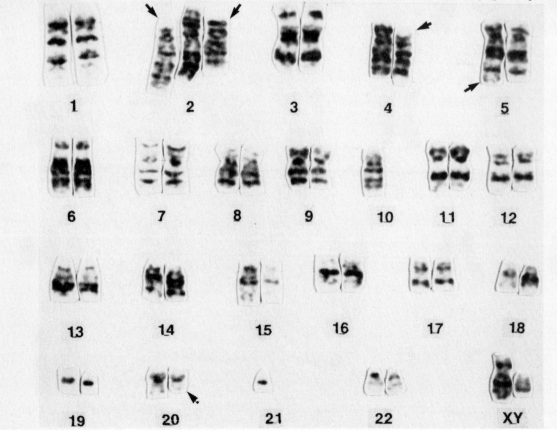

45,XY,inv(2)(p25q13),der(2)t(2;10)(p23q11;q11), del(4)(p14),der(5)t(2;5)(p23;q35),del(20)(q13),−21

Figure 11.8 A karyotype from a two-day pleural fluid culture of a patient with Ki-1 lymphoma showing 45,XY,inv(2)(p25q13),der(2)t(2;10)(p23q11;q11),del(4)(p14),der(5)t(2;5)(p23;q35),del(20)(q13),−21.

Primary intravascular (angiotropic) lymphoma

Primary intravascular (angiotropic) lymphoma or malignant angioendotheliomatosis is a rare malignant lymphoproliferative disorder, which originates in the intravascular compartments with the proliferation of atypical mononuclear cells. First described in 1959, and known by various synonyms, this disorder is characterized by unexplained fever, cutaneous lesions, dementia, neurologic abnormalities and multisystem failure [73,74]. Immunologic and Southern blot analysis have demonstrated that the malignant cells are lymphoid in origin, of either B- or T-cell lineage. Cytogenetic studies have been performed in two cases; Molina et al. [74], found a composite karyotype of 53,XY,+X,+5q,−6,i(6p), +7,−10,+11,−12,+12p−x2,+18,+marl,+mar2,+mar3, t(1;3)(p22;p21),3q+,8p+ in the peripheral blood cells of a 76-year-old male. The second case was an 80-year-old male with a near-tetraploid line in the bone marrow: 94(90–97),XY,del(1)(q21),del(1)(p34), intdel(2)(q22),4p+,i(6p),t(3;6)(p11;q11),t(3;6) (q21;p21),t(7;8)(p22;q22),del(7)(q22),t(1;10) (q21;q13),t(14;18)(q32;q21)x2,t(1;16)(q21;q24),

+20x3,+21 (Figure 11.9). The only common chromosomal aberration in the two cases is i(6p). Within the hematologic malignancies, deletion of 6q is usually confined to lymphoid malignancies such as ALL, CLL and NHL. i(6p) is the second most common isochromosome in NHL; it is not specific to any particular subtype and is considered to be a secondary change in these diseases. With only two reported cases, the significance of chromosome abnormalities in this rare disorder remains to be determined.

AIDS-associated lymphoma

It has been recognized for some time that immunodeficiency, regardless of cause, confers an increased risk for the development of neoplastic disease, particularly Karposi's sarcoma and NHL [75], which account for more than half of all tumors seen in these patients. NHL has been observed in patients with congenital immunodeficiency disorders such as Wiscott–Aldrich syndrome [76] and common variable hypogammaglobulinemia, in iatrogenically immunosuppressive organ transplant recipients [77], and in patients infected with the human immunodeficiency virus (HIV) [78].

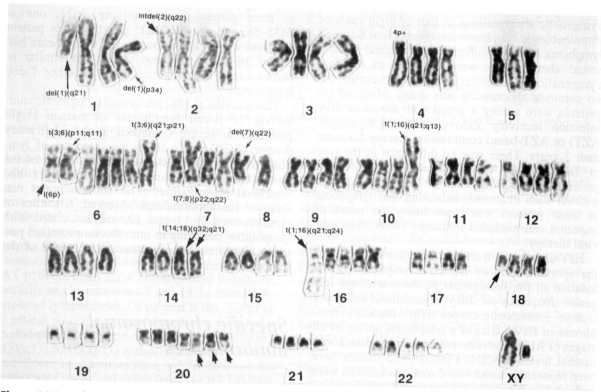

Figure 11.9 A karyotype from a direct bone marrow preparation of a patient with primary intravascular (angiotropic) lymphoma showing 95,XY,del(1)(q21),del(1)(p34),intdel(2)(q22),add(4)(p16),5,+i(6p),+der(6)t(3;6)(p11;q11),+der(6) t(3;6)(q21;p21),der(7)t(7;8)(p22;q22),+del(7)(q22)−8x3,(1;10)(q21;q13),t(14;18)(q32;q21)x2,+t(1;16)(q21;q24),+20x3, +22t.

evolution, presaging a poor outcome. The p53 gene is located at 17p and in a study of p53 abnormalities in lymphoma, Rodriguez et al. [140] observed allelic loss in two out of four lymphoma cell lines and one out of four tumors with -17 or del(17p), and no p53 loss in 21 tumor samples without 17 abnormalities. However, p53 mutations may be observed in lymphomas without karyotypic changes, being most often present in small noncleaved cell lymphomas (30–40%) followed by CLL (6%) [141].

TRISOMY 7

Trisomy 7, in addition to other chromosomal abnormalities, has been reported in about 30% of intermediate-grade lymphomas. Trisomy 7 has also been reported in four of ten previously published patients with γ heavy chain disease, a rare B-cell lymphoproliferative disorder characterized by the production of a monoclonal IgG heavy chain fragment in the absence of light chain [28]. In somatic cell hybrids between murine and SV40-transformed human cells, human chromosome 7 was shown to be carrying the SV40 genome, and to be responsible for the malignant phenotype [142]. The occurrence of i(7q) seems to be specific for acute lymphoblastic leukemia and lymphoma [38].

ABNORMALITIES OF CHROMOSOME 1

Structural abnormalities of chromosome 1, especially duplication of part or all of 1q, are found in many different malignancies and are also frequently found in intermediate-grade NHL. Fukuhara et al. [35] described duplication of 1q in a case of histiocytic lymphoma. This abnormality, dup(1)(q12q;31), in addition to dup(1)(q21;q31), has also been observed in BL (both endemic and nonendemic types and in some patients with HIV-associated BL) as a nonrandom marker, and indicates a poor prognosis [143,144].

ISOCHROMOSOMES

According to a review of isochromosomes in neoplasia by Mertens et al. [145], who succinctly defined isochromsomeas as '. . . monocentric or dicentric chromsomes with homologous arms that are mirror images of one another', approximately 10% of all tumors display isochromosome formation, including 10% (191 out of 1903) of lymphoma patients. The most common isochromosomes in NHL, in decreasing order of frequency, are i(17q) (55 cases), i(6p) (40 cases) and i(1q) (29 cases). Isochromosome for-

mation may be important in the neoplastic process, since it can lead to both the loss and gain of genetic material, resulting in either loss of tumor suppressor genes or amplification of oncogenes.

i(17q), for example, which is also by far the most common isochromosome found in neoplasia, has been associated with loss of p53 on 17p, and is usually found in cells showing both 17p loss and 17q gain. In NHL, it appears to be associated with loss of 6q material. i(6p) and i(1q) are both considered to be secondary changes in NHL. i(6p) is associated with t(14;18) and a B-cell phenotype and it appears that it is loss of 6q that is important rather than gain of 6p. i(1q), which is a recurrent abnormality in almost all tumor types, results in both 1p loss and 1q gain in NHL.

HOMOGENEOUSLY STAINING REGIONS AND DOUBLE MINUTES

Four cases of follicular or diffuse large-cell lymphoma [146,147] and one case of BL [55] exhibiting homogeneously staining regions (hsrs) in their lymphoma cells have been reported. The chromosomal location of the hsr was variable, and little or no clinical data were available, except in the BL patient, who achieved only partial remission and survived for 6 months. This patient exhibited both t(8;14) and t(11;hsr;2)(q11;hsr;q23) (Figure 11.11). In addition to their single case of hsr, Yunis et al. [99] reported three cases with double minutes (dmin); all had follicular large-cell lymphoma, which evolved into diffuse large-cell lymphoma in three cases, and all had short (<6.5 months) survivals. Judging from the available data, hsrs and dmin appear to be terminal events associated with poor survival.

Correlation between chromosomal abnormalities and immunophenotype

In 1986, Levine et al. [148] correlated immunological phenotype with karyotype in 118 patients with malignant lymphoma. Patients with T-cell lymphomas had more normal metaphases and more frequent abnormalities, including trisomy 19, and translocations or deletions involving breakpoints at 1q21, 2q21, 3q27, 4q21 and 17q21. In patients with B-cell lymphomas, certain chromosome abnormalities were associated with the expression of specific immunoglobulin heavy chains. Breakpoints at 14q22

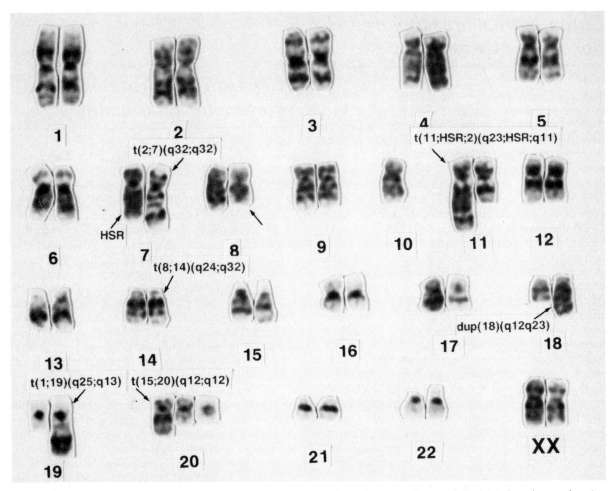

Figure 11.11 A karyotype from a two-hour peripheral blood culture from a patient with Burkitt's lymphoma showing 46,XY,der(7)t(2;7)(q32;q32),−10,der(11)+(11;hsr;q11),t(8;14)(q24;q32),dup(18)(q12q23),der(19)t(1;19)(q25;q13),+der (20)t(15;20)(q12;q12).

or q24 were associated with surface $\delta\mu$ immunoglobulin ($P = 0.02$), trisomy 22 or breaks at 22q12 and a break at 2q32 were associated with surface immunoglobulins ($P \leq 0.01$), and trisomy 12 and breaks at 2p13 with cytoplasmic immunoglobulins ($P \leq 0.01$). Among B-cell lymphomas, lack of CD24 surface antigen was associated with breaks in 2p25, 5q15–34, 6q21, while lack of CD9 occurred in patients with del(6)(q15).

In a study of immunological markers found in Burkitt's lymphoma, Preud'homme et al. [149] demonstrated a correlation between variant chromosomal translocations and the expression of light chain immunoglobulins. In normal cells the gene for the light chain κ is located on 2p12 and λ is located on 22q11. In the variant translocations, these genes are split, with the sequences encoding the variable (V_κ or V_λ) portion of the immunoglobulin molecule

remaining on chromosome 2 and 22, respectively, and the constant regions, either C_κ (from 2) or C_λ (from 22) are translocated to 8q. In general, tumors with t(2;8) express κ, and those with t(8;22) express λ chains. If the tumor has t(8;14), the cells may express either κ or λ chains. However, Magrath et al. [150] and Denny et al. [151] have reported cases with t(8;22) in which synthesis of the κ chain was seen, and the relationship between the type of variant translocation and light chain expression is presently rather weak.

Chromosomal breakpoints and oncogene expression

There is clearly pathogenetic significance to some of the breakpoints associated with translocations in the aneuploid cells of the 167 lymphoma patients listed in Tables 11.1 and 11.2 since some of them occur at very high frequency. The most frequently occurring breakpoint was at 14q32, found in 60% of the patients. Breakpoints at 18q21 occurred in 28% of the patients, and 6q21 and 8q24 in about 10% of the patients. Breakpoints occurring four to five times were at 1q32, 5q15, 8q21, 18q23, 14q11, 1q23, 3p21, at the centromere of 17 and 8q12. The remainder of the translocation breakpoints were present in only two or three patients. The translocation breakpoints are shown in Figure 11.4 (breakpoints occurring in only one patient are not shown). Chromosomal breakage may be the initial step for chromosomal translocation, deletion or inversion. Many of these breakpoints are either located close to or even within important constitutional genes or oncogenes (see Figure 11.4). It is highly probable that the consequences of chromosomal rearrangement provide essential steps in the development of malignant transformation. Careful examination, using DNA probes, etc., of the breakpoints involved in chromosomal rearrangements has led to the identification of numerous genes involved in oncogenesis (*bcl*-2, *lyt*10, *bcl*-1, etc.), and continued studies of this kind will doubtless lead to the discovery of additional cancer-related genes.

In a very thorough review of the possible role of oncogenes in the etiology of the NHL, Chenevix-Trench [152] lists those oncogenes that are found at frequently occurring chromosomal breakpoints in NHL; these are c-*myc*, *bcl*-1, *bcl*-2, c-*yes*-1, c-*ets*-1 and c-*abl* (Figure 11.4). The oncogenes found by transfection assays to be activated include c-*abl*, N-*ras*, *Blym*-1 and *Tlym*-1, while those that are expressed include c-*abl*, c-*erb* B, c-*ets*-1, c-*fos*, H-*ras*, K-*ras*, c-*myb* and c-*myc*. There is no consistent relationship between the expression of specific oncogenes and specific subtypes of NHL. This is, however, hardly surprising, since these genes are involved in the normal processes of cell growth and differentiation, and so may be expressed either because the normal counterpart cell would express them, or because they have been switched on along with the relevant pathway, e.g., c-*myc* with proliferation, and *ras* and *abl* as elements of intracellular signalling. In some cases, however, the chromosomal abnormalities are directly responsible for oncogene activation, or for the production of abnormal hybrid proteins, which interfere with the normal processes of cell growth and differentiation.

Prognostic implications of cytogenetic abnormalities

Bauer et al. [153] in a study of 50 patients with diffuse large-cell lymphoma, noted that the single most important pretreatment adverse prognostic factor was high proliferative activity, which they defined to be less than 80% of the cells in G_0 or G_1 as measured by flow cytometry. However, they could not demonstrate that DNA aneuploidy, detected in 62% of the patients, was of prognostic significance.

One hundred and six patients with NHL were classified by Kristoffersson et al. [3] according to cytogenetic findings, and then analyzed for the prognostic significance of the chromosomal abnormalities. The authors came to the following conclusions. There was significant difference in survival between those with abnormal metaphases (AA) and those with all normal (NN) metaphases, irrespective of whether the sample was taken at diagnosis or during relapse. Survival was significantly shorter for patients with ten or more clonal aberrations than for those with no or only one to four aberrations. This applied to patients with either high-grade lymphomas or low-grade lymphomas. There were no differences in survival between patients with reciprocal translocations and patients with other abnormalities, but both groups had a significantly shorter survival than those who had NN tumors. The survival was significantly shorter in patients with either completely or partially unidentified marker chromosomes. Survival was also significantly shorter in patients who were hypodiploid than in those with NN karyotypes. When patients were categorized according to the chromosome involved in numerical or structural abnormalities, those with 1p+ had a significantly shorter survival. In those who had an additional chromosome 7, there was a borderline significantly decreased survival.

In a report by Bloomfield et al. [25] of 73 patients who were examined cytogenetically at the time of diagnosis (prior to treatment), 65% of the patients achieved a complete remission, but there was no significant correlation between achieving a remission and cytogenetic findings. Survival in these patients varied with the percentage of normal karotypes as well as with the modal chromosome number. Patients who had more than 20% normal metaphases had significantly longer survival and patients who had a modal number of 46 survived longer than those who were either hypo- or hyperdiploid.

References

1. Jones SE, Butler JJ, Bryne GE Jr, et al. Histopathologic review of lymphoma cases from the Southwest Oncology Group. *Cancer* 1977, **39**: 1071–1076.
2. DeVita VT, Jaffe ES, Hellmann S. Hodgkin's disease and the non-Hodgkin's lymphomas. In DeVita VT, Hellman S, Rosenberg SA (eds) *Cancer. Principles and Practice of Oncology.* Philadelphia: JB Lippincott Company, 1985, pp. 1623–1709.
3. Kristoffersson U, Heim S, Mandahl N, et al. Prognostic implication of cytogenetic findings in 106 patients with non-Hodgkin's lymphoma. *Cancer Genet. Cytogenet.* 1987, **25**: 55–64.
4. Rowley JD, Fukuhara S. Chromosome studies in non-Hodgkin's lymphomas. *Semin. Oncol.* 1980, **7**: 255–266.
5. Yunis JJ, Oken MM, Theologides A, et al. Recurrent chromosomal defects are found in most patients with non-Hodgkin's lymphoma. *Cancer Genet. Cytogenet.* 1984, **13**: 17–28.
6. Levine EG, Arthur DC, Frizzera G, et al. There are differences in cytogenetic abnormalities among histologic subtypes of the non-Hodgkin's lymphomas. *Blood* 1985, **66**: 1414–1422.
7. Koduru PR, Filippa DA, Richardson ME. Cytogenetic and histologic correlations in malignant lymphoma. *Blood* 1987, **69**: 97–102.
8. Kristoffersson U, Olsson H, Mark-Vendel E, et al. Fine needle aspiration biopsy: A useful tool in tumor cytogenetics. *Cancer Genet. Cytogenet.* 1981, **4**: 53–60.
9. Harrison CJ. The lymphomas and chronic lymphoproliferative disorders. In Rooney DE, Czepulkowski BH (eds) *Human Cytogenetics.* Vol. II. *Malignancy and Acquired Abnormalities.* Oxford: Oxford University Press, 1991, pp. 97–120.
10. ISCN. 1995. Mitelman F (ed.) *An International System for Human Cytogenetics Nomenclature.* Basel: S. Karger, 1995.
11. Cremer T, Lichter P, Borden J, et al. Detection of chromosome aberrations in metaphase and interphase tumor cells by *in situ* hybridization using chromosome-specific library probes. *Hum. Genet.* 1988, **80**: 235–246.
12. Ferguson-Smith MA. Putting the genetics back into cytogenetics [editorial]. *Am. J. Humn. Genet.* 1991, **48**: 179–182.
13. Hopman AH, Ramaekers FC, Rapp AK, et al. *In situ* hybridization as a tool to study numerical chromosome aberrations in solid bladder tumors. *Histochemistry* 1988, **89**: 307–316.
14. Nederlof PM, van der Flier S, Raap AK, et al. Detection of chromosome aberrations in interphase tumor nuclei by nonradioactive *in situ* hybridization. *Cancer Genet. Cytogenet.* 1989, **42**: 87–98.
15. Nederlof PM, van der Flier S, Wiegant J, et al. Multiple fluorescence in situ hybridization. *Cytometry* 1990, **11**: 126–131.
16. Bajalica S, Brondum-Nielsen K, Sorensen AG, et al. Identification of a whole-arm translocation by *in situ* hybridization with directly fluorochrome-labeled probes in a myelodysplastic syndrome. *Genes Chromosom. Cancer* 1992, **5**: 128–131.
17. Bajalica S, Sorensen AG, Pedersen N, et al. Chromosome painting as a supplement to cytogenetic banding analysis in non-Hodgkin's lymphoma. *Genes Chromosom. Cancer* 1993, **7**: 231–239.
18. Younes A, Pugh W, Goodacre A, et al. Polysomy of chromosome 12 in 60 patients with non-Hodgkin's lymphoma assessed by fluorescence *in situ* hybridization: Differences between follicular and diffuse large cell lymphoma. *Genes Chromosom. Cancer* 1994, **9**: 161–167.
19. Kallioniemi A, Kallioniemi OP, Sudar D, et al. Comparative genomic hybridization for molecular cytogenetic analysis of solid tumors. *Science* 1992, **258**: 818–821.
20. Bentz M, Dohner H, Huck K, et al. Comparative genomic hybridization reveals a high incidence of chromosomal imbalances and gene amplifications in low grade lymphoproliferative disorders. *Blood* 1994, **84**: 142a.
21. Goodacre A, Ford R, Andreeff M. Comparative genomic hybridization resolves karyotypic heterogeneity and complexity in high grade non-Hodgkin's lymphoma. *Blood* 1994, **84**: 143a.
22. National Cancer Institute sponsored study of classification of non-Hodgkin's lymphomas. Summary and descriptions of a working formulation for clinical usage. *Cancer* 1982, **49**: 2112–2135.
23. Gaunt KL, Callaghan J, Roberts DF. Karyotype abnormalities in non-Hodgkin's lymphomas. *Ann. Genet.* 1986, **29**: 82–87.
24. Yunis JJ, Oken MM, Kaplan ME, et al. Distinctive chromosomal abnormalities in histologic subtypes of non-Hodgkin's lymphoma. *N. Engl. J. Med.* 1982, **307**, 1231–1236.
25. Bloomfield CD, Arthur DC, Frizzera G, et al. Nonrandom chromosome abnormalities in lymphoma. *Cancer Res.* 1983, **43**: 2975–2984.
26. Mark J, Dahlenfors R, Ekedahl C. Recurrent chromosomal aberrations in non-Hodgkin's and non-Burkitt lymphomas. *Cancer Genet. Cytogenet.* 1979, **1**: 39–56.
27. Takeuchi J, Ochi H, Minowada J, et al. Cytogenetic studies of a diffuse mixed cell lymphoma of T cell origin. *Cancer Genet. Cytogenet.* 1985, **14**: 257–266.
28. O'Conor GT, Wyandt HE, Innes DJ, et al. Gamma heavy chain disease: Report of a case associated with trisomy of chromosome 7. *Cancer Genet. Cytogenet.* 1985, **15**: 1–5.
29. Brusamolino E, Bernasconi P, Pasquali F, et al. Trisomy 12 in a case of large cell, immunoblastic, polymorphous non-Hodgkin's lymphoma with IgG kappa monoclonal paraprotein [letter]. *Cancer Genet. Cytogenet.* 1984, **13**: 279–280.
30. Slavutsky I, de Vinuesa ML, Dupont J, et al. Abnormalities of chromosome no. 1: Two cases with lymphocytic lymphomas. *Cancer Genet. Cytogenet.* 1981, **3**: 341–346.
31. Panani A, Ferti-Passantonopoulou A, Dervenoulas J. Partial duplication of 1q in a malignant lymphoma. *Cancer Genet. Cytogenet.* 1984, **11**: 87–90.

32. Clare N, Boldt D, Messerschmidt G, et al. Lymphocyte malignancy and chromosome 14: Structural aberrations involving band q11. *Blood* 1986, **67**: 704–709.

33. Rovigatti U, Watson DK, Yunis JJ. Amplification and rearrangement of Hu-ets-1 in leukemia and lymphoma with involvement of 11q23. *Science* 1986, **232**: 398–400.

34. Kaneko Y, Abe R, Sampi K, et al. An analysis of chromosome findings in non-Hodgkin's lymphomas. *Cancer Genet. Cytogenet.* 1982, **5**: 107–121.

35. Fukuhara S, Rowley JD, Variakojis D, et al. Banding studies on chromosomes in diffuse histiocytic lymphomas: Correlation of 14q+ marker chromosome with cytology. *Blood* 1978, **52**: 989–1002.

36. Ohyashiki K, Yoshida MA, Ohyashiki J, et al. Two 14q+ chromosomes in malignant lymphoma: Crucial cytogenetic changes on 14q. *Cancer Genet. Cytogenet.* 1985, **17**: 325–331.

37. Oshimura M, Ohyashiki K, Tonomura A, et al. A 14q+ chromosome in a malignant lymphoma in a patient with Down's syndrome. *Cancer Genet. Cytogenet.* 1981, **4**: 245–250.

38. De Braekeleer M. Acute lymphoblastic leukemia and lymphoma associated with an isochromosome 7q. *Leukemia Res.* 1985, **9**: 1571–1572.

39. Klein G. The Epstein–Barr virus and neoplasia. *N. Engl. J. Med.* 1975, **293**: 1353–1357.

40. Berger R, Bernheim A. Cytogenetics of Burkitt's lymphoma–leukaemia: A review. *IARC Sci. Publ.* 1985, **60**: 65–80.

41. Daly P, Brito-Babapulle V, Lawlor E, et al. Variant translocation t(8;22) and abnormalities of chromosome 15(q22) and 17(q12–21) in a Burkitt's lymphoma/leukaemia with disseminated intravascular coagulation. *Br. J. Haematol.* 1986, **64**: 561–569.

42. Bunn PA Jr, Lamberg SI. Report of the committee on staging and classification of cutaneous T-cell lymphomas. *Cancer Treatment Rep.* 1979, **63**: 725–728.

43. Whang-Peng J, Bunn PA Jr., Knutsen T, et al. Clinical implications of cytogenetic Studies in cutaneous T-cell lymphoma (CTCL). *Cancer* 1982, **50**: 1539–1553.

44. Vonderheid EC, Sobel EL, Nowell PC, et al. Diagnostic and prognostic significance of Sézary cells in peripheral blood smears from patients with cutaneous T cell lymphoma. *Blood* 1985, **66**: 358–366.

45. Gamperl R. Clonal chromosome aberrations in a case of cutaneous T-cell lymphoma. *Cancer Genet. Cytogenet.* 1986, **19**: 341–344.

46. Barbieri D, Spanedda R, Castoldi GL. Involvement of chromosomes 12 and 14 in the cutaneous stage of mycosis fungoides: Cytogenetic evidence for a multistep pathogenesis of the disease. *Cancer Genet. Cytogenet.* 1986, **20**: 287–292.

47. Gallo RC, de-The GB, Ito Y. Meeting report: Kyoto workshop on some specific recent advances in human tumor virology. *Cancer Res.* 1981, **41**: 4738–4739.

48. Whang-Peng J, Bunn PA, Knutsen T, et al. Cytogenetic studies in human T-cell lymphoma virus (HTLV)-positive leukemia–lymphoma in the United States. *J. Natl Cancer Inst.* 1985, **74**: 357–369.

49. Fukuhara S, Hinuma Y, Gotoh Y, et al. Chromosome aberrations in T lymphocytes carrying adult T-cell leukemia-associated antigens (ATLA) from healthy adults. *Blood* 1983, **61**: 205–207.

50. Pandolfi F. T-CLL and allied diseases: New insights into classification and pathogenesis. *Diagn. Immunol.* 1986, **4**: 61–74.

51. Sanada I, Tanaka R, Kumagai E, et al. Chromosomal aberrations in adult T-cell leukemia: Relationship to the clinical severity. *Blood* 1984, **65**: 649–654.

52. Lennert K, Mestadagh J. Lymphogranulomatose mit konstant hohem epitheloidzellgehalt. *Virchows Arch. Pathol. Anat. Physiol. Klin. Med.* 1968, **344**: 1–20.

53. Godde-Salz E, Feller AC, Lennert K. Cytogenetic and immunohistochemical analysis of lymphoepitheloid cell lymphoma (Lennert's lymphoma): Further substantiation of its T-cell nature. *Leuk. Res.* 1986, **10**: 313–323.

54. Kaneko Y, Larson RA, Variakojis D, et al. Nonrandom chromosome abnormalities in angioimmunoblastic lymphadenopathy. *Blood* 1982, **60**: 877–887.

55. Whang-Peng J, Knutsen T, Jaffe E, et al. Sequential analysis of 43 patients with non-Hodgkin's lymphoma: Clinical correlations with cytogenetic, histologic, immunophenotyping and molecular studies. *Blood* 1995, **85**: 203–216.

56. Nowell P, Finan J, Glover D, et al. Cytogenetic evidence for the clonal nature of Richter's syndrome. *Blood* 1981, **58**: 183–186.

57. Isaacson PG, Wright DH. Extranodal lymphomas. In Anthony PP, MacSween RNM (eds) *Recent Advances in Histopathology*. Edinburgh: Churchill Livingstone, 1987, pp. 159–184.

58. Wotherspoon AC, Pan LX, Diss TC, et al. A genotypic study of low grade B-cell lymphomas, including lymphomas of mucosa associated lymphoid tissue (MALT). *J. Pathol.* 1990, **162**: 135–140.

59. Weiss LM, Warnke RA, Sklar J, et al. Molecular analysis of the t(14;18) chromosomal translocation in malignant lymphomas. *N. Engl. J. Med.* 1987, **317**: 1185–1189.

60. Horsman D, Gascoyne R, Klasa R, et al. t(11;18)(q21;q21.1): A recurring translocation in lymphomas of mucosa-associated lymphoid tissue (MALT)? *Genes Chromosom. Cancer* 1992, **4**: 183–187.

61. Griffin CA, Zehnbauer BA, Beschorner WE, et al. t(11;18)(q21;q21) is A recurrent chromosome abnormality in small lymphocytic lymphoma. *Genes Chromosom. Cancer* 1992, **4**: 153–157.

62. Wotherspoon AC, Pan LX, Diss TC, et al. Cytogenetic study of B-cell lymphoma of mucosa-associated lymphoid tissue. *Cancer Genet. Cytogenet.* 1992, **58**: 35–38.

63. Clark HM, Jones DB, Wright DH. Cytogenetic and molecular studies of t(14;18) and t(14;19) in nodal and extranodal B-cell lymphoma. *J. Pathol.* 1992, **166**: 129–137.

64. Whang-Peng J, Knutsen T, Jaffe E, et al. Cytogenetic study of two cases with lymphoma of mucosa-associated lymphoid tissue. *Cancer Genet. Cytogenet.* 1994, **77**: 74–80.

65. Schwab U, Stein H, Gerdes J, et al. Production of a monoclonal antibody specific for Hodgkin and

Sternberg–Reed cells of Hodgkin's disease and a subset of normal lymphoid cells. *Nature* 1982, **299**: 65–67.

66. Froese P, Lemke H, Gerdes J, et al. Biochemical characterization and biosynthesis of the Ki-1 antigen in Hodgkin-derived and virus-transformed human B and T lymphoid cell lines. *J. Immunol.* 1987, **139**: 2081–2087.

67. Ebrahim SAD, Ladanyi M, Desai SB, et al. Immunohistochemical, molecular, and cytogenetic analysis of a consecutive series of 20 peripheral T-cell lymphomas and lymphomas of uncertain lineage, including 12 Ki-1 positive lymphomas. *Genes Chromosom. Cancer* 1990, **2**: 27–35.

68. Nezelof C, Barbey S, Gogusev J, et al. Malignant histiocytosis in childhood: A distinctive CD30-positive clincopathological entity associated with a chromosomal translocation involving 5q35. *Semin. Diagn. Pathol.* 1992, **9**: 75–89.

69. Morgan R, Smith SD, Hecht BF, et al. Lack of involvement of the c-fms and N-myc genes by chromosomal translocation t(2;5) (p23;q35) common to malignancies with features of so-called malignant histiocytosis. *Blood* 1989, **73**: 2155–2164.

70. Mason DY, Bastard C, Rimokh R, et al. CD30-positive large cell lymphomas ('Ki-1 lymphoma') are associated with a chromosomal translocation involving 5q35. *Br. J. Haematol.* 1990, **74**: 161–168.

71. Kaneko Y, Frizzera G, Edamura S, et al. A novel translocation, t(2;5) (p23;q35), in childhood phagocytic large T-cell lymphoma mimicking malignant histiocytosis. *Blood* 1989, **73**: 806–813.

72. Fischer P, Nacheva E, Mason DY, et al. A Ki-1 (CD30)-positive human cell line (Karpas 299) established from a high-grade non-Hodgkin's lymphoma, showing a 2;5 translocation and rearrangement of the T-cell receptor beta-chain gene. *Blood* 1988, **72**: 234–240.

73. Pfeger L, Tappeiner J. Zur kenntnis der systemi sierten endotheliomatose der cutanen blutgefusse (reticulo endotheliose?). *Hautarzt.* 1959, **10**: 359–363.

74. Molina A, Lombard C, Donlon T, et al. Immunohistochemical and cytogenetic studies indicate that malignant angioendotheliomatosis is a primary intravascular (angiotropic) lymphoma. *Cancer* 1990, **66**: 474–479.

75. Filipovich AH, Heinitz KJ, Robison LL, et al. The immunodeficiency cancer registry. A research resource. *Am. J. Pediatr. Hematol. Oncol.* 1987, **9**: 183–184.

76. Cotelingam JD, Witebsky FG, Hsu SM, et al. Malignant lymphoma in patients with the Wiskott–Aldrich syndrome. *Cancer Invest.* 1985, **3**: 515–522.

77. Penn I. Kaposi's sarcoma in organ transplant recipients: Report of 20 cases. *Transplantation* 1979, **27**: 8–11.

78. Bower M. The biology of HIV-associated lymphomas. *Br. J. Cancer* 1992, **66**: 421–423.

79. Pluda JM, Brawley OW, Yarchoan R, et al. Neoplasms associated with AIDS. In Calebresi P, Schein PS (eds) *Medical Oncology Basic Principles and Clinical Management of Cancer.* New York: McGraw Hill, 1993, pp. 1174–1201.

80. Ziegler JL, Drew WL, Miner RC, et al. Outbreak of Burkitt's-like lymphoma in homosexual men. *Lancet* 1982, **2**: 631–633.

81. Ladanyi M, Offit K, Jhanwar SC. MYC rearrangement and translocations involving band 8q24 in diffuse large cell lymphomas. *Blood* 1991, **77**: 1057–1063.

82. Whang-Peng J, Raffeld M, Knutsen T. (In preparation.)

83. Bernheim A, Berger R. Cytogenetic studies of Burkitt lymphoma–leukemia in patients with acquired immunodeficiency syndrome. *Genes Chromosom. Cancer* 1988, **32**: 67–74.

84. Kornblau SM, Goodacre A, Cabanillas F. Chromosomal abnormalities in adult non-endemic Burkitt's lymphoma and leukemia: 22 new reports and a review of 148 cases from the literature. *Hematol. Oncol.* 1991, **9**: 63–78.

85. Berman M, Minowada J, Loew JM, et al. Burkitt cell acute lymphoblastic leukemia with partial expression of T-cell markers and subclonal chromosome abnormalities in a man with acquired immunodeficiency syndrome. *Cancer Genet. Cytogenet.* 1985, **16**: 341–347.

86. Jones JF, Shurin S, Abramowsky C, et al. T-cell lymphomas containing Epstein–Barr viral DNA in patients with chronic Epstein–Barr virus infections. *N. Engl. J. Med.* 1988, **318**: 733–741.

87. Tien HF, Su IJ, Chuang SM, et al. Cytogenetic characterization of Epstein–Barr virus-associated T-cell malignancies. *Cancer Genet. Cytogenet.* 1993, **69**: 25–30.

88. Thangavelu M, Snyder L, Anastasi J. Cytogenetic chracterization of B-cell lymphomas from severe combined immunodeficiency disease mice given injections of lymphocytes from Epstein–Barr virus-positive donors. *Cancer Res.* 1992, **52**: 4678–4681.

89. Becher R. Klinefelter's syndrome and malignant lymphoma. *Cancer Genet. Cytogenet.* 1986, **21**: 271–273.

90. Petkovic I, Ligutic I, Dominis M, et al. Cytogenetic analysis in ataxia telangiectasia with malignant lymphoma. *Cancer Gent. Cytogenet.* 1992, **60**: 158–163.

91. Egeler RM, de Kraker J, Slater R, et al. Documentation of Burkitt lymphoma with t(8;14) (q24;q32) in X-linked lymphoproliferative disease. *Cancer* 1992, **70**: 683–687.

92. Miyanishi S, Ohno H. Characterization of a novel T-cell lymphoma cell line established from a patient with systemic lupus erythematosus associated lymphoma. *Cancer Genet. Cytogenet.* 1992, **59**: 199–205.

93. Salles MT, Neyra O, Taja L, et al. Constitutional translocation (8;13) in a patient with non-Hodgkin's lymphoma. *Cancer Genet. Cytogenet.* 1992, **59**: 80–83.

94. Masik P, Nakanine H, Sanger W. Oncogene rearrangement in non-Hodgkin's lymphomas with a 14q+ chromosome of unknown origin. *Proceedings of the Annual Meeting of the American Association for Cancer Research*, 1991, Vol. 32, p. A180.

95. Fukuhara S, Ueshima Y, Shirakawa S, et al. 14q translocations, having a breakpoint at 14q13 in lymphoid malignancy. *Int. J. Cancer* 1979, **23**: 739–743.

96. Kennaugh AA, Butterworth SV, Hollis R, et al. The chromosome breakpoint at 14q32 in an ataxia telangiectasia t(14;14) T cell clone is different from the 14q32 breakpoint in Burkitts and an inv(14) T cell lymphoma. *Hum. Genet.* 1986, **73**: 254–259.

97. McCaw BK, Hecht F, Harnden DG, et al. Somatic rearrangement of chromosome 14 in human lymphocytes. *Proc. Natl Acad. Sci. USA* 1975, **72**: 2071–2075.

98. Ueshima Y, Rowley JD, Variakojis D, et al. Cytogenetic studies on patients with chronic T cell leukemia/lymphoma. *Blood* 1984, **63**: 1028–1038.

99. Yunis JJ, Frizzera G, Oken MM, et al. Multiple recurrent genomic defects in follicular lymphoma. *N. Engl. J. Med.* 1987, **316**: 79–84.

100. Kaneko Y, Rowley JD, Variakojis D, et al. Prognostic implications of karyotype and morphology in patients with non-Hodgkin's lymphoma. Int. J. Cancer 1983, **32**: 683–692.

101. Baer R, Chen KC, Smith SD, et al. Fusion of an immunoglobulin variable gene and a T cell receptor constant gene in the chromosome 14 inversion associated with T-cell tumors. *Cell* 1985, **43**: 705–713.

102. Bakhshi A, Jensen JP, Goldman P, et al. Cloning the chromosomal breakpoint of t(14;18) human lymphomas: Clustering around JH on chromosome 14 and near a transcriptional unit on 18. *Cell* 1985, **41**: 899–906.

103. Raffeld M, Wright JJ, Lipford E, et al. Clonal evolution of t(14;18) follicular lymphomas demonstrated by immunoglobulin genes and the 18q21 major breakpoint region. *Cancer Res.* 1987, **47**: 2537–2542.

104. Tsujimoto Y, Cossman J, Jaffe E, et al. Involvement of the bcl-2 gene in human follicular lymphoma. *Science* 1985, **228**: 1440–1443.

105. Lipford E, Wright JJ, Urba W, et al. Refinement of lymphoma cytogenetics by the chromosome 18q21 major breakpoint region. *Blood* 1987, **70**: 1816–1823.

106. Offit K, Parsa NZ, Gaidano G, et al. 6q deletions define distinct clinico-pathologic subsets of non-Hodgkin's lymphoma. *Blood* 1993, **82**: 2157–2162.

107. Gaidano G, Hauptschein RS, Parsa NZ, et al. Deletions involving two distinct regions of 6q in B-cell non-Hodgkin's lymphoma. *Blood* 1992, **80**: 1781–1787.

108. Menasce LP, Orphanos V, Santibanej-Korf M, et al. Common region of deletion on the long arm of chromosome 6 in non-Hodgkin's lymphoma and acute lymphoblastic leukaemia. *Genes Chromosom. Cancer* 1994, **10**: 286–288.

109. Schouten HC, Sangar WG, Weisenburger DD, et al. Abnormalities involving chromosome 6 in newly diagnosed patients with non-Hodgkin's lymphoma. Nebraska Lymphoma Study Group. *Cancer Genet. Cytogenet* 1990, **47**: 73–82.

110. Raffeld M, Jaffe ES. Bcl-1, t(11;14), and mantle cell-derived lymphomas. *Blood* 1991, **78**: 259–263.

111. Vandenberghe E, DeWolfe Peeters C, Wlodarska I, et al. Chromosome 11q rearrangements in B non-Hodgkin's lymphoma. *Br. J. Haematol.* 1992, **81**: 212–217.

112. Leroux D, Le Marc'Hadour F, Gressin R, et al. Non-Hodgkin's lymphomas with t(11;14) (q13;q32): A

subset of mantle zone/intermediate lymphocytic lymphoma? *Br. J. Haematol.* 1991, **77**: 346–353.

113. Van den Berghe H, Parloir C, David G, et al. A new characteristic karyotypic anomaly in lymphoproliferative disorders. *Cancer* 1979, **44**: 188–195.

114. Tsujimoto Y, Jaffe E, Cossman J, et al. Clustering of breakpoints on chromosome 11 in human B-cell neoplasms with the t(11;14) chromosome translocation. *Nature* 1985, **315**: 340–343.

115. Rosenberg CL, Wong E, Petty EM, et al. PRAD1, a candidate BCL1 oncogene: Mapping and expression in centrocytic lymphoma. *Proc. Natl Acad. Sci. USA* 1991, **88**: 9638–9642.

116. Leroux D, Monteil M. Diagnosis of t(11;14)(q13;q32) using interphase fluorescent in situ hybridization. *Blood* 1994, **84**: 608a.

117. Correlation of chromosome abnormalities with histologic and immunologic characteristics in non-Hodgkin's lymphoma and adult T cell leukemia–lymphoma. Fifth International Workshop on Chromosomes in Leukemia–Lymphoma. *Blood* 1987, **70**: 1554–1564.

118. Fleischman E, Prigogina EL, Ilynskaya CW, et al. Chromosomal characteristics of malignant lymphoma. *Hum. Genet.* 1989, **82**: 343–348.

119. Armitage JO, Sanger WG, Weisenburger DD, et al. Correlation of secondary cytogenetic abnormalities with histologic appearance in non-Hodgkin's lymphomas bearing t(14;18)(q32;q21). *J. Natl Cancer Inst.* 1988, **80**: 576–580.

120. Offit K, Jhanwar SC, Ladanyi M, et al. Cytogenetic analysis of 434 consecutively ascertained specimens of non-Hodgkin's lymphoma: Correlations between recurrent aberrations, histology, and exposure to cytotoxic treatment. *Genes Chromosom. Cancer* 1991, **3**: 189–201.

121. Jonveaux P, Le Coniat M, Derre J, et al. Loss of genetic material from the short arm of chromosome 12 is a frequent secondary abnormality in non-Hodgkin's lymphoma. *Hematol. Pathol.* 1991, **5**: 21–26.

122. Cabanillas F, Pathak S, Trujillo J. Frequent nonrandom chromosome abnormalities in 27 patients with untreated large cell lymphoma and immunoblastic lymphoma. *Cancer Res.* 1988, **48**: 5557–5564.

123. Berger R, Le Coniat M, Derre J. Partial deletion of chromosome 2 in non-Hodgkin lymphoma. *Cancer Genet. Cytogenet.* 1991, **53**: 113–117.

124. Lu D, Thompson JD, Gorski GK, et al. Alterations at the REL locus in human lymphoma. *Oncogene* 1991; 1235–1241.

125. Offit K, Jhanwar S, Ebrahim SAD, et al. t(3;22) (q27;q11): A novel translocation associated with diffuse non-Hodgkin's lymphoma. *Blood* 1989, **74**: 1876–1879.

126. Bastard C, Tilly H, Lenormand B, et al. Translocations involving band 3q27 and Ig gene regions in non-Hodgkin's lymphoma. *Blood* 1992, **79**: 2527–2531.

127. Slavutsky I, de Vinuesa ML, Larripa I, et al. Translocation (2;3) in hematologic malignancies. *Cancer Genet. Cytogenet.* 1986, **21**: 335–342.

128. Ye BH, Rao PH, Chaganti RS, et al. Cloning of bcl-6,

the locus involved in chromosome translocations affecting band 3q27 in B-cell lymphoma. *Cancer Res.* 1993, **53**: 2732–2735.

129. Deweindt C, Kerchaert J-P, Tilly H, et al. Cloning of a breakpoint cluster region at band 3127 involved in human non-Hodgkin's lymphoma. *Genes Chromosom. Cancer* 1993, **8**: 149–154.

130. Otsuki T, Yano T, Clark H, et al. Analysis of LAZ3 (BCL-6) status in B-cell Hodgkin's lymphomas: Results of rearrangement and gene expression studies and a mutational analysis of coding region sequences. *Blood* 1995, **85**: 2877–2884.

131. Offit K, Parsa NZ, Jhanwar S, et al. Clusters of chromosome 9 aberrations are associated with clinico-pathologic subsets of non-Hodgkin's lymphoma. *Genes Chromosom. Cancer* 1993, **7**: 1–7.

132. Chaganti SR, Gaidano G, Louie DC, et al. Diffuse large cell lymphomas exhibit frequent deletions in 9p21–22 and 9q31–34 regions. *Genes Chromosom. Cancer* 1995, **12**: 32–36.

133. Juneja CD, Lukeis R, Tan L, et al. Cytogenetic analysis of 147 cases of non-Hodgkin's lymphoma: Non-random chromosomal abnormalities and his-tological correlations. *Br. J. Haematol.* 1990, **76**: 231–237.

134. Speaks S, Sanger WS, Masih AS, et al. Recurrent abnormalities of chromosome bands 10q23–25 in non-Hodgkin's lymphoma. *Genes Chromosom. Cancer* 1992, **5**: 239–243.

135. Neri A, Chang CC, Lombardi L, et al. B cell lymphoma-associated chromosomal translocation in-volves candidate oncogene lyt-10, homologous to Nfkappa B p50. *Cell* 1991, **67**: 1075–1087.

136. Levine EG, Arthur DC, Frizzera G, et al. Cyto-genetic abnormalities predict clinical outcome in non-Hodgkin's lymphoma. *Ann. Int. Med.* 1988, **108**: 14–20.

137. Cabanillas F, Pathak S, Grant G, et al. Refractoriness to chemotherapy and poor survival related to abnor-malities of chromosomes 17 and 7 in lymphoma. *Am. J. Med.* 1989, **87**: 167–172.

138. Schouten HC, Sanger WG, Weisenburger DD, et al. Chromosomal abnormalities in untreated patients with non-Hodgkin's lymphoma: Associations with histology, clinical characteristics, and treatment out-come. The Nebraska Study Group. *Blood* 1990, **75**: 1841–1847.

139. Levine EG, Juneja S, Arthur D, et al. Sequential karyotypes in non-Hodgkin lymphoma: Their nature and significance. *Genes Chromosom. Cancer* 1990, **1**: 270–280.

140. Rodriguez MA, Ford RJ, Goodacre A. Chromosome

17- and p53 changes in lymphoma. *Br. J. Haematol.* 1991, **79**: 575–582.

141. Gaidano G, Ballerini P, Gong JZ, et al. P53 muta-tions in human lymphoid malignancies: Association with Burkitt's lymphoma and chronic lymphocytic leukemia. *Proc. Natl Acad. Sci. USA* 1991, **88**: 5413–5417.

142. Croce CM. Assignment of gene(s) for cell transfor-mation and malignancy to human chromosome 7 carrying the SV40 genome. In Crowell RL, Friedman H, Prier JE (eds) *Tumor Virus Infections and Immunity.* Baltimore: University Park Press, 1976, pp. 223–230.

143. Whang-Peng J, Lee EC, Sieverts H, et al. Burkitt's lymphoma in AIDS: Cytogenetic study. *Blood* 1984, **63**: 818–822.

144. Douglass EC, Magrath IT, Lee EC, et al. Cytogenetic studies in non-African Burkitt lympoma. *Blood* 1980, **55**: 148–155.

145. Mertens F, Johansson B, Mitelman F. Isochromo-somes in neoplasia. *Genes Chromosom. Cancer* 1994, **10**: 221–230.

146. Mitelman F (ed.). *Catalog of Chromosome Aber-rations in Cancer.* 4th edn. New York, Wiley-Liss, 1991.

147. Cabanillas F, Trujillo JM, Barlogie B, et al. Chromo-somal abnormalities in lymphoma and their correla-tions with nucleic acid flow cytometry. *Cancer Genet. Cytogenet.* 1986, **21**: 99–106.

148. Levine EG, Arthur DC, Gaji-Peczalska K, et al. Correlations between immunological phenotype and karyotype in malignant lymphoma. *Cancer Res.* 1986, **46**: 6481–6488.

149. Preud'homme JL, Dellagi K, Guglielmi P, et al. Immunologic markers of Burkitt's lymphoma cells. *IARC Sci. Publ.* 1985, **60**: 47–64.

150. Magrath I, Erikson J, Whang-Peng J, et al. Synthesis of kappa light chains by cell lines containing an 8;22 chromosomal translocation derived from a male homosexual with Burkitt's lymphoma. *Science* 1983, **222**: 1094–1098.

151. Denny CT, Hollis GF, Magrath IT, et al. Burkitt lymphoma cell line carrying a variant translocation creates new DNA at the breakpoint and violates the hierarchy of immunoglobulin gene rearrangement. *Mol. Cell. Biol.* 1985, **5**: 3199–3207.

152. Chenevix-Trench G. The molecular genetics of human non-Hodgkin's lymphoma. *Cancer Genet. Cytogenet.* 1987, **27**: 191–213.

153. Bauer KO, Merkel DE, Winter JN, et al. Prognostic implications of ploidy and proliferative activity in diffuse large cell lymphomas. *Cancer Res.* 1986, **46**: 3173–3178.

CHAPTER 12

Epstein–Barr virus and non-Hodgkin's lymphomas

GERALD NIEDOBITEK AND LAWRENCE S. YOUNG

Introduction

Epstein–Barr virus (EBV) is a human herpesvirus which is found as a widespread and largely asymptomatic infection in all human communities. Primary infection with EBV usually occurs in childhood and, once infected, individuals become lifelong virus carriers. The virus is the causative agent of infectious mononucleosis (IM), a self-limiting lymphoproliferative disease resulting from delayed primary EBV infection, and is also associated with a number of malignant tumors, including Burkitt's lymphoma (BL) and immunoblastic lymphomas arising in immunocompromised patients [1]. The B-lymphotropic nature of EBV is evidenced by its association with these lymphoproliferations and by the ability of the virus to immortalize normal resting B-lymphocytes *in vitro*, converting them into permanently growing lymphoblastoid cell lines (LCLs) [2]. When peripheral blood lymphocytes from chronic virus carriers are placed in culture, the few virus-infected B-cells that are present regularly give rise to spontaneous outgrowth of EBV-transformed LCLs provided that immune T-cells are either removed or inhibited by

addition of cyclosporin A to the culture [3]. This phenomenon highlights the importance of EBV-specific cytotoxic T-lymphocytes (CTLs) in controlling EBV-induced B-cell transformation.

EBV is an orally transmitted and infectious virus, measured by its ability to immortalize B-cells *in vitro*, can be detected in oropharyngeal secretions from IM patients, from patients who are immunosuppressed and, at lower levels, from healthy EBV-seropositive individuals [4–6].

The ability of EBV to infect epithelial cells is illustrated by the regular detection of the virus in the tumor cells of undifferentiated nasopharyngeal carcinomas (NPCs) [1]. More recently, replicating EBV has been demonstrated in desquamated oropharyngeal epithelial cells from IM patients [7] and in the AIDS-associated epithelial lesion, oral hairy leukoplakia (HL) [8]. These findings have been used to argue that oropharyngeal epithelial cells are the target of primary EBV infection and that epithelial cells are the site of viral persistence and replication in normal virus carriers [9]. In this scenario, EBV infection of B-lymphocytes would be a secondary event. However, this concept has been challenged recently by several lines of evidence all pointing to

B-lymphocytes as mediators of primary and persistent EBV infection [10]. Thus, in IM, EBV genomes and gene products are readily identified in the extrafollicular B-lymphoid blasts and there is no evidence of epithelial cell infection by EBV in IM tonsils [11,12] suggesting that tonsillar B-cells rather than epithelial cells are the primary target of EBV infection. In chronic virus carriers, variable numbers of EBV-harboring lymphoid cells are detectable in lymphoreticular tissues [12]. The number of these cells appears to correlate with the degree of lymphoid hyperplasia and with any underlying immunodeficiency [12]. Thus, only rare EBV-positive lymphoid cells are observed in nonactivated lymph nodes from immunocompetent individuals whilst larger numbers are seen in hyperplastic lymph nodes from human immunodeficiency virus (HIV)-infected individuals [12]. Importantly, in a few cases, expansion of EBV-positive cells has been observed in isolated germinal centers, indicating that EBV-carrying B-cells may participate in physiological germinal center reactions [12]. The earlier model of EBV persistence in epithelial cells is also challenged by other lines of evidence. In bone marrow transplant recipients whose resident hematopoietic tissue has been destroyed, eradication of EBV has been demonstrated in some cases [13]. Treatment of IM patients or EBV-seropositive individuals with antiviral therapy led to a reduction of oropharyngeal virus shedding whilst the number of EBV-carrying circulating B-cells remained constant [14,15]. Recent studies suggest that HL represents a focus of EBV replication in the absence of a truly latent infection [16,17]. Thus, there is as yet no direct evidence to suggest that latent EBV infection of epithelial cells is a frequent event *in vivo*. By contrast, latent EBV infection of B-lymphocytes is readily demonstrated in chronic virus carriers and participation of these cells in germinal center cell reactions could provide a mechanism ensuring the long-term survival of such cells in the human host. These studies, therefore, challenge earlier models of EBV persistence and point to the lymphoid system as the site of EBV persistence [10]. The potential interactions between lymphocytes and epithelial cells are illustrated in Figure 12.1. In the present chapter, we discuss the role of EBV in the development of non-Hodgkin's lymphomas.

EBV biology

MODELS OF EBV LATENCY

In vitro models of latent EBV infection have provided an opportunity to examine how different patterns of viral gene expression influence cellular phenotype. The best characterized *in vitro* model of latency is provided by LCLs generated by infecting primary, resting B-cells with EBV [18]. Every cell in an LCL carries multiple copies of the viral episome and constitutively expresses a limited set of viral gene products, the so-called latent proteins (Table 12.1), consisting of six nuclear antigens (EBNAs 1, 2, 3A, 3B, 3C and -LP) and three latent membrane proteins (LMPs 1, 2A and 2B). The relative positions and orientations of these latent genes on the large (172 kb), covalently closed EBV episome are shown schematically in Figure 12.2. The different EBNAs are encoded by individual mRNAs generated by differential splicing of the same long 'rightward' primary transcript expressed from one of two promotors (Cp and Wp) located close together in the BamHI C and W region of the genome (Figure 12.2) [19]. The LMP transcripts are expressed from separate promoters in the BamHI N region of the EBV genome, with the leftward latent membrane protein (LMP)1 and rightward LMP2B mRNAs apparently controlled by the same bidirectional promoter sequence (Figure 12.2) [19,20]. LMP1 is oncogenic in rodent fibroblasts [21] and a mutant EBV strain lacking the EBNA2 gene is unable to immortalize B-cells [22,23], suggesting that these two latent proteins are particularly important in the immortalization process. However, the general consensus is that immortalization of B-cells by EBV involves the coordinated action of several latent gene functions since no single immortalizing gene has been identified. In addition to the latent proteins, LCLs also show abundant expression of the small non-polyadenylated (and therefore noncoding) RNAs, EBV-encoded RNA (EBER)1 and 2 (Figure 12.2), whose function is not clear but whose expression is a constant feature of all types of latent EBV infection [18].

The consistent pattern of EBV latent protein expression in LCLs is matched by an equally consistent and characteristic cellular phenotype (Figure 12.3) with high-level expression of the activation markers CD23, CD30, CD39 and CD70 and of the cellular adhesion molecules leukocyte function-associated molecule (LFA)-1 (CD11a/18), LFA-3 (CD58) and intracellular adhesion molecule (ICAM)-1 (CD54) [24,25]. That these markers are either absent or expressed at low levels on resting B-cells, but are transiently induced to high levels when these cells are activated into short-term growth by antigenic or mitogenic stimulation, suggests that EBV-induced immortalization may be elicited through the constitutive activation of the same cellular pathways that drive physiological B-cell proliferation. The ability of EBNA2, EBNA3C and

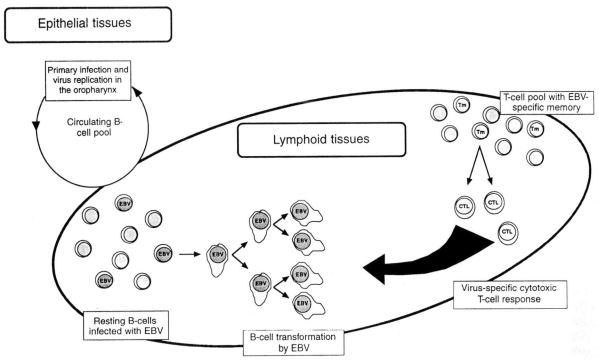

Figure 12.1 EBV infection in normal healthy virus carriers. Virus infection involves two cellular compartments: (i) B-lymphocytes, where infection is predominantly latent and has the potential to induce growth-transformation of infected cells and (ii) epithelial cells, where infection is predominantly replicative. Whilst the exact mode of primary and persistent EBV infection and the relative contributions of B-cells and epithelial cells are uncertain, recent data point to the B-cell compartment as the main mediator of primary as well as persistent infection. Following primary infection of B-lymphocytes, a chronic virus carrier state is established in which the outgrowth of EBV growth-transformed B-cells is controlled by an EBV-specific cytotoxic T-cell (CTL) response reactivated from a pool of virus-specific memory T-cells. At certain sites, presumably in the oropharynx, latently infected B-cells may become permissive for lytic EBV infection. Infectious virus released from these cells may be shed directly into the saliva or may infect other epithelial cells and B-cells. In this way a virus-carrier state is established, which is characterized by persistent, latent infection in circulating B-cells, and occasional EBV replication in B-cells and epithelial cells.

LMP1 to induce LCL-like phenotypic changes when expressed individually in human B-cell lines implicates these viral proteins as key effectors of the immortalization process [26,27].

The pattern of latent EBV gene expression in LCLs is referred to as the 'latency III' (Lat III) form of EBV infection. A second form of EBV infection in

Table 12.1 Viral gene expression in different types of EBV latency

Latency	EBERs	EBNAs 1	2	3A,B,C	LP	LMP1	LMP2A/B
Lat I	+	+	—	—	—	—	—
Lat II	+	+	—	—	—	+	+
Lat III	+	+	+	+	+	+	+

For details, see text.

B-cells, referred to as 'latency I' (Lat I, Table 12.1), has been identified in BL tumor biopsy cells and in early passage BL cell lines where abundant EBER transcription is found and EBNA1 is selectively expressed in the absence of the other EBNA and LMP proteins [28,29]. The selective expression of EBNA1 involves a different mRNA expressed from a novel EBNA1 promoter (Fp) in the BamHI F region of the viral genome which is independent of Cp or Wp promoter (Figure 12.2) [30,31]. In culture, BL cells grow as a carpet of dispersed cells, in contrast to the multicellular aggregates that are observed in LCL cultures. Furthermore, BL cells display a distinct cell surface marker phenotype characterized by expression of CD10 (CALLA) and CD77 (BLA), but no or little expression of the cellular activation antigens and adhesion molecules that are regularly expressed at high levels in LCLs [28,29]. The Lat I form of latency observed in BL cell lines is not always stably maintained *in vitro*, and

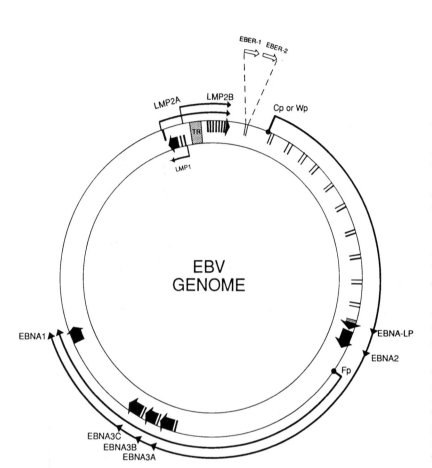

Figure 12.2 Location and transcription of the EBV latent genes on the double-stranded viral DNA episome. The large solid arrows represent coding exons for each of the latent proteins and the direction in which they are transcribed. EBNA-LP is transcribed from variable numbers of repetitive exons in the BamHI W fragments. LMP2 is composed of multiple exons located either side of the terminal repeat (TR) region, which is formed during the circularization of the linear DNA to produce the viral episome. The open arrows represent the highly transcribed nonpolyadenylated RNAs, EBER1 and EBER2, which are a consistent feature of latent EBV infection. The outer long-arrowed line represents EBV transcription in Lat III, where all the EBNAs are transcribed from either the Cp or Wp promoter; the different EBNAs are encoded by individual mRNAs generated by differential splicing of the same long primary transcript. The inner shorter arrowed line represents the EBNA1 transcript originating from the Fp promoter located in the BamHI F region; this is transcribed in latency types I and II.

on serial passage a drift to a Lat III pattern of gene expression can be observed concomitant with a change in the cellular phenotype towards that seen in LCLs (Figure 12.3) [24,29].

Another form of EBV latency, Lat II (Table 12.1), is characterized by selective expression of the Fp-driven EBNA1 mRNA, of the LMP1, 2A and 2B transcripts, and of the EBERs. This form of infection was first identified in biopsies of nasopharyngeal carcinoma [32], but is clearly not restricted to epithelial cells, since it is also observed in EBV-positive cases of Hodgkin's disease (HD) [33] and can under some circumstances be experimentally induced in BL cells *in vitro* [34]. All three forms of EBV latency can be interconverted in somatic cell hybrids between LCLs and either BL cells or certain nonlymphoid lines [35]. These transitions are influenced by the cell phenotype of the resultant hybrids, thus emphasizing the complex interplay between cellular factors and the resident pattern of EBV latent gene expression.

EBV TYPES 1 AND 2

There are two major types of EBV isolates, originally referred to as A and B and now called types 1 and 2, which appear to be identical over the bulk of the EBV genome but show polymorphisms (with 50–80% sequence homology depending on the locus) in a subset of latent genes, namely those encoding EBNA-LP, EBNA2, EBNA3A, EBNA3B and EBNA3C [36–38]. A combination of virus isolation and sero-epidemiological studies suggest that type 1 virus isolates are predominant (but not exclusively so) in many Western countries, whereas both types are widespread in equatorial Africa, New Guinea and perhaps certain other regions [39–42]. The balance of evidence to date suggests that healthy individuals are only infected with one virus type [42], although this may well change in immunologically compromised patients [41].

Work in the cell culture model systems described above indicates that both types of EBV can establish the same spectrum of latent infections. Interestingly,

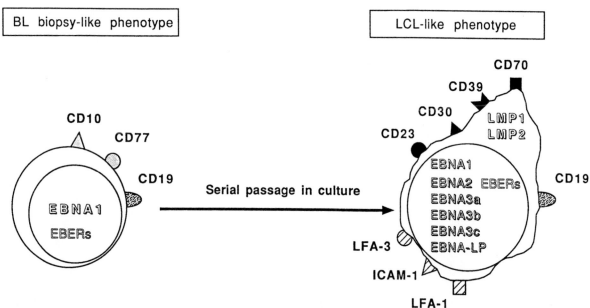

Figure 12.3 Correlation between cellular phenotype and EBV gene expression during 'phenotypic drift' of BL cell lines in culture. Serial passage of BL biopsy cells with a Lat I pattern of EBV latent gene expression can result in the generation of LCL-like cell lines expressing all the EBNAs (Lat III) and an activated B-cell phenotype. Such observations originally suggested that individual EBV latent proteins may influence the expression of certain phenotypic markers.

however, type 1 isolates are more potent than type 2 in achieving B-cell immortalization *in vitro*; the type 2 virus-transformed LCLs characteristically showing much slower growth especially in early passage [43]. In view of this biological difference in experimental systems, it is important to determine the relative contributions of the two virus types to lymphoid malignancies. This question is by no means fully resolved at present. The available evidence suggests that both virus types are equally represented amongst BL tumors in Africa and New Guinea, consistent with the relative incidence of the two virus types in the healthy populations in these areas [39,40]. More interesting is the relative association of the two types of EBV with lymphomas in the immunosuppressed. Surprisingly, recent reports suggest that type 2 virus isolates can be detected with unusually high frequency amongst immunologically compromised patients and also in their accompanying lymphomas [41,44]. Parallel studies on EBV-positive HD in different geographical areas are likewise now an important priority.

EBV-associated non-Hodgkin's lymphomas

In the three decades since EBV was discovered, a vast

body of literature has accumulated implicating the virus in a variety of lymphoproliferative disorders. The application of different molecular biological techniques to the detection of EBV reflects the development of new methodologies over this period. Thus, studies in the 1970s were largely performed using nucleic acid reassociation kinetics; in the 1980s Southern blot hybridization and later DNA *in situ* hybridization (ISH) were applied; in the 1990s the polymerase chain reaction (PCR) and ISH for the detection of the EBERs have been employed. Recently, monoclonal antibodies suitable for immunohistochemical analysis of EBV infection have become available. The methods based on the extraction of nucleic acids from tissues containing a mixture of cells do not provide information as to the cellular source of any viral nucleic acids detected. This is a particular problem with the highly sensitive PCR, as EBV-carrying nonneoplastic lymphoid cells are present in many tissues, including EBV-negative and EBV-positive tumors [12,45]. This problem can be overcome by employing techniques that allow the microscopic analysis of the distribution of viral genomes or gene products at the cellular level in tissue sections. Whilst DNA ISH has been used with some success [11,46], the sensitivity of this method is limited. In recent years, ISH for the detection of the EBERs has been established as the standard method for examining the association of EBV with human tumors. Studies of a variety of EBV-positive tumors and cell lines have indicated that the EBERs

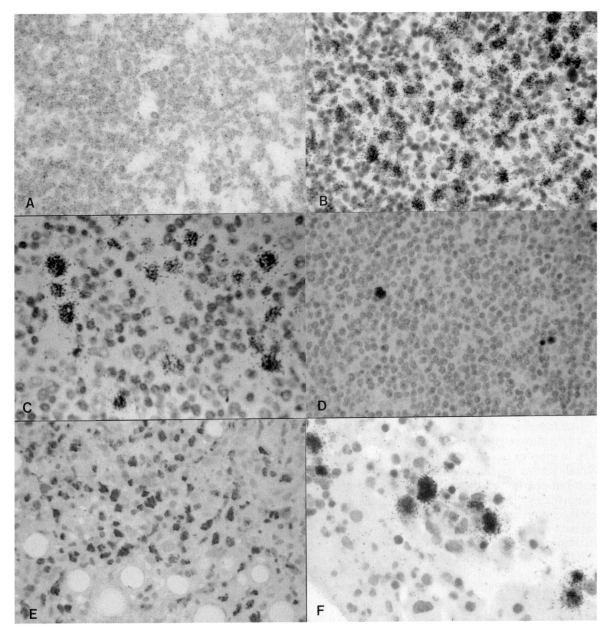

Figure 12.4   Expression of the EBERs is demonstrated in (A) a Burkitt's lymphoma, (B) a posttransplant lymphoma, (C) an anaplastic large-cell lymphoma, (D) isolated tumor cells of a chronic lymphocytic leukemia, (E) a peripheral pleomorphic T-cell lymphoma, and (F) T-cells in an EBV-associated hemophagocytic syndrome using *in situ* hybridization (ISH) with ^{35}S (A–C and F) or digoxigenin-labelled (D and E) probes. (F) shows double-staining ISH with ^{35}S-labelled EBER-specific probes and immunohistology with a T-cell-specific monoclonal antibody and the APAAP technique.

are expressed in all states of viral latency, and their high-level expression allows reliable detection with radioactive or nonradioactive probes (Figure 12.4) [12,47]. Furthermore, EBER ISH is readily combined with immunohistology allowing the phenotypic characterization of EBV-infected cells (Figure 12.4F) [12,45]. Immunohistology with monoclonal antibodies allows further characterization of EBV

gene expression and thus complements EBER ISH [48–50]. It has been shown recently that some of these antibodies can be applied to paraffin sections following antigen retrieval by microwave irradiation, allowing their use on a wide range of archival material (Figure 12.5).

Southern blot hybridization may be used to gain additional information about the clonality of EBV

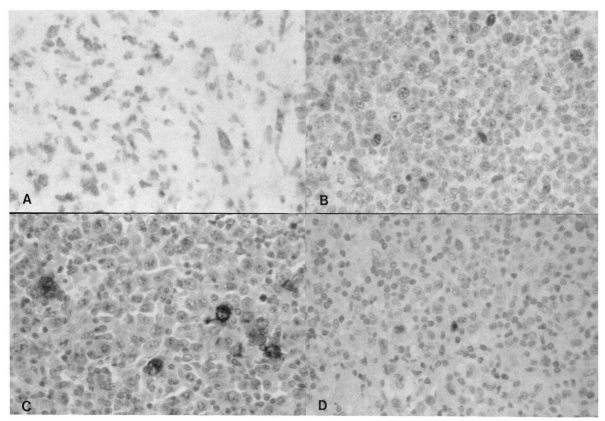

Figure 12.5   Immunohistochemical detection of EBV-encoded proteins in paraffin sections; (A) EBNA1 in a peripheral pleomorphic T-cell lymphoma, (B) EBNA2 in an EBV-induced lymphoma from a cottontop tamarin, (C) LMP1 in a posttransplant lymphoma, and (D) BZLF1 in a posttransplant lymphoma.

genomes in virus-associated tumors [51]. The formation of viral episomes in the nuclei of infected cells is mediated by the terminal repeat (TR) sequences at either end of the linear viral genome. The number of these TRs is variable, resulting in variable configurations of the fused termini in cells infected with different virions. Progeny of a single EBV-infected cell, by contrast, harbour viral episomes with identical fused termini. According to this model, Southern blot hybridization with a probe specific for unique sequences adjacent to the TRs reveals a single band in cases with monoclonal viral genomes and multiple bands in cases with viral episomes derived from more than one infection event [51]. This method has been used to infer the clonality of the cell population harbouring the virus.

NON-HODGKIN'S LYMPHOMAS ARISING IN PATIENTS WITH IMMUNE DEFECTS

Given the importance of T-cell immunosurveillance in the control of EBV infection, it is not surprising that an increased frequency of EBV-associated lymphoproliferative disorders has been observed in patients with either primary or secondary immune defects. However, the spectrum of lymphoproliferations developing in these patients varies and not all cases are associated with EBV, demonstrating that the nature and severity of the underlying immune defect is important, and raising the possibility that other factors, possibly other viruses, may contribute to the development of lymphomas in this group. Moreover, some EBV-negative non-Hodgkin's lymphomas (NHLs) developing in immunocompromised individuals may well reflect sporadic lymphomas arising in the general population.

Primary immune defects

An increased frequency of lymphoproliferative disorders has been demonstrated in several primary immune defects such as X-linked lymphoproliferative disease (XLPD), Wiskott–Aldrich syndrome (WAS), common variable immunodeficiency (CVID), and ataxia telangiectasia (AT) [52–56]. Lymphoproliferative disorders in these patients are diverse and include lymphoid hyperplasia, atypical lymphoid hyperplasia and overtly malignant lymphomas including BLs and other high-grade NHLs [53,54]. Most NHL cases are of B-cell phenotype and are EBV-positive [53,54]. Nakanishi et al. [52] recently reported a case of WAS with disseminated high-grade B-cell NHL. Multiple tumor foci were analyzed but immunoglobulin (Ig) heavy chain gene rearrangement could only be demonstrated in one tissue sample while most of the specimens showed germline configuration suggesting polyclonality of the resident B-cell population in most samples [52]. Conversely, analysis of the fused terminal repeat region of the EBV episome suggested monoclonality of the viral genomes in each individual tumor focus; the configuration of the fused terminal repeat fragments varied between different sites, suggesting a multiclonal origin [52]. Lymphoproliferative lesions arising in XLPD appear to be largely polyclonal with an LCL-like pattern of EBV gene expression [56]. However, some cases show monoclonal EBV episomes associated with a more restricted pattern of viral gene expression [56], and it has been suggested that there is a progression from polyclonal LCL-like lesions to monoclonal lymphomas.

Transplant patients

The risk of developing posttransplant lymphoproliferative disorders (PTLDs) is largely associated with degree, duration and type of immunosuppression [57–60]. The highest risk appears to be associated with the use of anti-CD3 antibodies as immunsuppressive agents [58,59]. However, the frequent primary occurrence of PTLD lesions in the transplanted organ seems to suggest that other factors are also important [59]. Furthermore, the risk seems to be higher in patients undergoing primary EBV infection following transplantation [61,62], an observation which may account for the higher incidence of PTLDs in pediatric transplant recipients [63].

PTLDs represent a spectrum of lesions ranging from an IM-like benign lymphoproliferation to monomorphous high-grade B-cell lymphomas [58]. Numerous studies have demonstrated an association of PTLDs with EBV by detecting viral nucleic acids or viral gene products in PTLD lesions. This close association seems to hold regardless of the morphology of the individual PTLD lesion [46,48,58,60,64–69]. Several authors have analyzed the configuration of the fused termini of the EBV episomes using Southern blot hybridization. Katz et al. [69] found monoclonal EBV episomes in 11 PTLD cases and a polyclonal pattern in six cases. Cleary et al. [64] identified a single band in most specimens analyzed, indicating monoclonality. In some cases with multiple specimens, a monoclonal pattern was observed

in the individual lesions but the configuration of the termini varied between lesions suggesting that different clones had given rise to PTLD at different sites [64]. In other cases, a polyclonal pattern of viral termini was present [64]. Patton et al. [66] reported a monoclonal pattern of viral termini in seven cases, a biclonal pattern in two and a polyclonal configuration in one case. In a detailed molecular genetic study, Locker and Nalesnik [65] identified heterogenous patterns of clonality as identified by analysis of Ig gene rearrangement and configuration of EBV termini. Monomorphic large-cell NHL proved to be monoclonal by both parameters. Some polymorphic lymphoproliferations were either monoclonal or polyclonal by both parameters and some cases showed a polyclonal Ig gene configuration but clonal viral episomes [65]. Based on these studies it has been proposed that EBV-positive PTLD progress from early polyclonal polymorphic lesions to monoclonal lymphomas. It has been suggested that antiviral therapy may be of use in the early stages of the disease [66]. Regression of some PTLDs upon reduction of the immunosuppressive therapy is well documented [70] and it appears that a polymorphic morphology together with polyclonal configuration of viral termini and/or Ig genes are favorable prognostic indicators in this respect whilst monomorphic and monoclonal lymphomas tend to progress [65].

In some EBV-positive PTLDs, virus replication has been demonstrated, possibly reflecting the reduced immune control over the infection. Most of the lesions in the study by Cen et al. [71] contained linear (replicating) viral genomes indicating replicative infection. In the study by Patton et al. [66], four cases, including two biclonal and two monoclonal PTLDs, showed linear viral DNA. Katz et al. [69] detected replicative forms of viral DNA in three of six PTLDs with polyclonal episomes but only in two of 11 cases with monoclonal episomes. Similarly, Locker and Nalesnik detected replicative viral DNA only in cases showing nonclonal viral episomes [65]. Viral gene expression patterns in EBV-positive PTLDs have been studied by several groups. Young et al. [48] demonstrated the expression of EBNA2 and LMP1 in five PTLD cases suggesting a Lat III form of infection as seen in LCLs. Similar results were obtained by Thomas et al. and Gratama et al. [68,72]. However, Cen et al. [71] found a more restricted pattern of EBV gene expression. In 23 lesions analyzed by immunoblotting, these authors found LMP1 expression in 22 cases but EBNA2 was detected in only three cases [71]. Whilst these results raise the possibility that some PTLDs sustain a Lat II or even Lat I-type infection, it should be noted that immunoblotting is not the most appropriate technique for such analysis. For instance, LMP1 expression has been observed only in a proportion of tumor cells in cases analyzed by immunohistology [48,68] (Figure 12.4C) and such cases may be missed by the relatively insensitive immunoblotting technique. In some cases, expression of the BZLF1 transactivator protein is observed in a few cells (unpublished observation, Figure 12.4D) further indicating that replicative infection may be possible in PTLD lesions.

Borisch et al. [73] recently reported two cases of CD30-positive anaplastic large-cell (ALC) lymphomas arising in transplant patients. Both were of B-cell phenotype and showed a clonal configuration of EBV termini [73]. Kumar et al. [74] reported a single case of CD30-positive T-immunoblastic NHL with monoclonal EBV genomes in a renal transplant recipient. Waller et al. [75] recently reported two cases of PTLD, both of which were EBV DNA positive, and were phenotypically and genotypically derived from T-cells. These cases further illustrate the wide spectrum of EBV-positive lymphomas which can arise in transplant patients. However, some lymphomas arising in transplant recipients are EBV-negative. Euvrard et al. [76] recently reported the occurrence of an EBV-positive nodal B-cell NHL and an EBV-negative cutaneous T-cell NHL in the same renal transplant patient and EBV-negative PTLD cases have also been reported by others [61,63].

Acquired immunodeficiency syndrome (AIDS)

HIV-infected individuals have an increased risk of developing malignant lymphomas. Most of these AIDS-related lymphomas (ARLs) are high-grade B-cell NHLs with a notable tendency to present at extranodal sites, e.g., the central nervous system (CNS). It has been proposed that on morphological grounds AIDS-associated NHL can be divided into two large groups, Burkitt-type lymphomas and large-cell lymphomas with a prominent immunoblast component [77]. A few cases of T-cell NHL have also been reported [78,79].

A large proportion of NHLs arising in AIDS patients have been associated with EBV and it appears that detectable EBV infection in non-neoplastic lymph nodes from HIV-infected patients is associated with an increased risk of developing EBV-associated NHLs [80]. Hamilton-Dutoit et al. [77] detected EBV DNA in 12 of 24 ARLs using DNA ISH. Borisch et al. [78] identified EBV DNA in 7 of 14 NHLs, including one T-immunoblastic NHL. Boyle et al. [44] found EBV in 10 of 20 cases. In a large study using EBER ISH, Hamilton-Dutoit et al. [47] found EBV in 46 of 60 (77%) immunoblast-rich NHLs but only in 12 of 35 (34%) Burkitt-type

lymphomas. These authors also reported that patients with immunoblast-rich NHLs had a more severely impaired immune system in comparison to AIDS patients with Burkitt-type lymphomas [81]. Recently, Thomas et al. [79] described three cases of EBV-associated oral T-cell NHLs in AIDS patients. ARLs arising in the CNS have been studied in detail and it appears that most or all of these cases are EBV-positive [47,82,83]. Analysis of the configuration of viral termini in EBV-positive ARLs invariably indicated monoclonality of viral episomes [44,82,84, 85]. Determination of the virus type prevalent in ARLs has revealed type 1 EBV in the majority of cases but the incidence of type 2 EBV was surprisingly high [69,82,84–86]. A recent study suggested the possibility of a greater heterogeneity of ARLs [87]. These authors identified EBV DNA in only 15 of 40 ARLs including six primary CNS lymphomas. Fourteen of the EBV-negative lymphomas in this study proved to be polyclonal in gene rearrangement studies [87].

The pattern of EBV gene expression in ARLs appears to be heterogeneous. MacMahon et al. detected LMP1 expression in nine of 21 EBV-positive primary CNS lymphomas [83]. By PCR analysis of mRNA transcripts, Shibata et al. [88] identified Fp promoter-driven EBNA1 mRNA in four ARLs, but no Cp- or Wp-derived transcripts. LMP1 transcripts were also detectable in these cases. In an immunohistological study, LMP1 expression was detected in 16 of 22 EBV-positive immunoblast-rich large-cell lymphomas, with EBNA2 expression in nine of the LMP1-positive cases [89]. Thus, most of these cases appeared to show either a Lat II or III pattern of EBV gene expression. By contrast, Burkitt-type lymphomas displayed a more restricted pattern of viral gene expression. Three of 11 EBV-positive Burkitt-type lymphomas showed LMP1 expression in a proportion of tumor cells whilst immunostaining for EBNA2 was consistently negative, suggesting a Lat I form of infection in most and Lat II in a few cases [89].

Thus, it appears that there are two main groups of ARLs. Large-cell lymphomas with prominent immunoblasts are largely EBV-positive and display either Lat II or Lat III form of EBV infection. These tumors are associated with a more severe impairment of the immune system and may be similar to PTLDs. Primary CNS lymphomas probably belong in this group [47]. Burkitt-type lymphomas are associated with EBV in a smaller proportion of cases and the virus latency established in these tumors is more restricted. These tumors may be comparable to sporadic BL arising in immunocompetent individuals.

demonstrated proliferation of EBV-positive T-lymphocytes in various tissues. The T-lymphocytes were small and not obviously atypical. T-Cell receptor genes were in germline configuration but analysis of the terminal repeat region of the EBV episomes suggested monoclonality [126]. Monoclonal, and in one case biclonal, EBV episomes were also reported in three other EBV-AHS cases by Kikuta et al. [127]. However, these authors did not localize the virus to T-cells. Craig et al. [128] reported a single case of EBV-AHS associated with primary EBV infection. In this case, a T-cell NHL with monoclonal T-cell receptor β gene rearrangement and clonal EBV genomes developed. A case of EBV-positive T-immunoblastic lymphoma with hemophagocytic syndrome was reported by Gaffey et al. [129]. Thus, EBV-AHS appears to comprise a spectrum of T-cell lymphoproliferations ranging from preneoplastic to overtly neoplastic conditions. Further studies are required to assess the part played by EBV in these cases. In particular, it will be important to analyze the pattern of viral gene expression in EBV-AHS lesions.

EBV was first identified in peripheral T-cell lymphomas (PTLs) in three patients with chronic active EBV infection [130]. Subsequently, an increasing number of EBV-positive PTLs have been described while T-lymphoblastic lymphomas have proved to be consistently EBV-negative (for review, see [131]). In a survey of NHLs, Hamilton-Dutoit and Pallesen [108] found expression of LMP1 in eight of 82 PTLs but only in about 4% of high-grade B-cell NHLs, suggesting for the first time that T-cell NHL may be more frequently EBV-associated than B-cell NHL. Since then a growing number of publications have confirmed this observation.

When assessing the possible role of EBV in the development of PTL, two problems have to be considered. Firstly, the morphological classification of PTL is difficult and the differential diagnosis of some cases from HD may be problematic. This is important because a significant proportion of HD cases are associated with EBV. Secondly, it appears that the proportion of EBV-carrying cells in PTLs varies greatly [131]. Whilst in some cases most or all tumor cells are EBV infected, others may only harbor the virus in a small fraction of cells. The significance of EBV infection in a subclone of a tumor cell population will be considered later. Another problem arising from this observation is the difficulty in identifying, on purely morphological grounds, whether an EBV-positive cell is a tumor cell, particularly in lesions composed of a mixture of different cell types.

In a recently published ISH study, a high incidence (47%) of EBV infection in 81 European peripheral pleomorphic T-cell NHLs was reported [132]. However, in only eight of these cases (10%) was the virus detectable in a significant proportion of tumor cells (>20%). In most cases, either only a small proportion of tumor cells EBV-positive or the virus was detected in nonneoplastic 'bystander' cells [132]. Similar results were reported by others [131,133]. However, all of these studies were carried out using nonradioactive EBER-specific probes and, in view of the limited sensitivity of this approach, it is possible that the proportion of EBV-positive tumor cells may have been underestimated. Further studies using more sensitive radioactive probes are required to clarify this issue.

Both Korbjuhn et al. [132] and Pallesen et al. [131] observed a higher rate of EBV infection in nodal and nasal PTL than in PTL arising at other extranodal sites. Interest has focused particularly on two types of PTL, angiocentric lymphoma (also termed lethal midline granuloma, angiocentric immunoproliferative lesion, lymphomatoid granulomatosis) and PTL of the angioimmunoblastic lymphadenopathy type (AILD). Angiocentric sinonasal PTLs arise more frequently in Asian patients than in Western populations but they appear to be invariably EBV associated. Ho et al. [134] demonstrated monoclonal EBV DNA in eight of eight cases of sinonasal PTL arising in Chinese patients. Harabuchi et al. [135] detected the presence of EBV in five cases of sinonasal PTL. A case of sinonasal PTL in a Caucasian patient was also found to be EBV-positive by EBER ISH [136]. Medeiros et al. [137] described five EBV-positive angiocentric PTL, all involving the respiratory tract. Borisch et al. [138] studied six cases of EBV-positive sinonasal PTL and identified type 1 EBV in three cases and type 2 EBV in the other three cases. The authors speculated that the relatively frequent detection of type 2 EBV may point to an underlying immune defect in these patients [138].

Based on PCR studies it had been suggested that most cases of AILD may be associated with EBV [139]. In support of this finding, Su et al. [140] demonstrated monoclonal viral episomes in four cases of AILD-like PTL and Ott et al. [141] detected EBV DNA in eight of 14 AILD cases. However, analysis of morphology, distribution and phenotype of EBV-infected cells in AILD revealed a heterogenous pattern. Anagnostopoulos et al. [142] studied 31 cases of AILD and found EBV in the neoplastic T-cells of 13 cases (42%). Eight cases (26%) showed nodular aggregates of EBV-positive B-lymphoid cells within the remnants of follicles and a further ten cases (32%) revealed occasional EBV-positive small lymphoid cells. Expression of LMP1 was frequently detected in those cases showing either numerous EBV-infected neoplastic T-cells or many EBV-positive B-lymphoid blasts [142]. Weiss et al. [143]

detected EBER-positive cells in 96% of their AILD cases but, in contrast to the results of Anagnostopoulos et al., found the virus almost exclusively in B-cells and not in neoplastic T-cells [143]. The same authors also described a case of an EBV-negative AILD with subsequent occurrence of an EBV-positive high-grade B-cell NHL in the same patient [144]. Taken together, these findings suggest that AILD represents a heterogenous group of lymphoproliferations. Whilst EBV may be causally involved in the proliferation of neoplastic T-cells in some cases, in others the expansion of EBV-positive B-cells and the occurrence of occasional EBV-positive high-grade B-cell NHL may simply reflect an underlying immune defect.

Pan et al. [145] detected monoclonal EBV genomes in four of 11 enteropathy-associated T-cell lymphomas (EATL). LMP1 expression was observed in two of these cases. However, we were unable to find evidence of EBV infection in seven EATLs whilst one of two cases of intestinal B-cell lymphomas arising in this clinical setting was EBV-positive [145a].

The association of human T-cell leukemia/lymphoma virus (HTLV)-1 with adult T-cell lymphoma (ATL) in Japan is well documented. Recently, Tokunaya et al. [146] demonstrated the presence of EBV in the neoplastic T-cells in 16 of 96 ATL cases. Expression of LMP1 and EBNA2 was reported in the majority of these cases [146]. The significance of this observation is at present unclear, but it raises the intriguing possibility that EBV and HTLV-1 may be cofactors in the pathogenesis of a proportion of ATLs.

Viral gene expression has been studied in five EBV-positive PTLs by Chen et al. [147]. These authors observed LMP1 expression by immunofluorescence in one case and in three of four cases studied by PCR, suggesting low levels of LMP1 expression. LMP2 expression was also frequently detected by PCR whilst EBNA2 expression was absent [147]. These findings together with immunohistological results obtained by others indicate that in most PTLs, a Lat II from of infection is sustained. However, in some sinonasal PTLs and in EBV-positive ATL cases, LMP1 and EBNA2 expression were observed, suggesting that a Lat III form of infection may be possible in some cases [135,146].

Anaplastic large-cell (ALC) lymphomas

CD30-positive ALC lymphomas are in several aspects related to HD [33]. Because an association of a significant proportion of HD cases with EBV has now been established [33,105] ALC lymphomas have also been studied for EBV infection. EBV DNA has been identified in approximately 32% of cases by PCR analysis and EBER ISH has confirmed the presence of the virus in the tumor cell population in most of these cases [148]. EBV was identified in a higher proportion of B-cell ALC lymphomas (67%) than in T-cell ALC lymphomas (28%) [148]. In a study confined to T-cell ALC lyphomas, Pallesen et al. [131] demonstrated EBV infection in only one of 21 cases from Denmark. Different patterns of viral gene expression have been identified in ALC lymphomas. Herbst et al. [148] found that six of 11 EBV DNA-positive cases did not express either LMP1 or EBNA2, suggesting a type I latency; five cases displayed LMP1 expression in the tumor cells and in two of these EBNA2 expression was also observed. Whilst LMP1 expression was detected in ALC lymphomas of B- and of T-cell phenotype, EBNA2 expression was seen only in two cases with B-cell phenotype [148]. The single EBV-positive case reported by Pallesen et al. was also LMP1-positive and EBNA2-negative [131]. Thus, it appears that virus infection in ALC lyphomas may encompass all three known patterns of latency. The significance of this observation is as yet uncertain. However, in this respect ALC lymphomas are different from HD, where a Lat II form of infection is consistently observed [33].

Animal models

The increasing number of EBV-associated human malignancies emphasizes the need for novel approaches aimed at the prevention and treatment of EBV infection. In this context, animal models in which EBV can induce lymphoproliferative diseases are vital. Cottontop tamarins (*Saguinus oedipus oedipus*) have been used in EBV vaccine studies because, following challenge with a tumorigenic dose of EBV, these animals consistently develop oligoclonal or monoclonal large-cell lymphomas, which in many respects resemble the PTLDs arising in humans [149,150]. These lymphomas harbor EBV in all tumor cells and express an LCL-like (Lat III) spectrum of latent viral genes [151] and thus are the simplest example of an EBV-driven tumor. Several vaccines based on the major envelope glycoprotein gp340/220 have been generated, which prevent the development of EBV-associated lymphomas in cottontop tamarins [152,153]. Whilst EBV infection in common marmosets has also been described [154], cottontop tamarins are the only primates which develop a well-documented and reproducible EBV-associated tumor with similarity to human disease. Surprisingly, we have recently found variable numbers of EBV-carrying lymphoid cells in immunized animals protected against the development of EBV-associated lymphomas 70 days following challenge with a tumorigenic dose of the virus. Immunohistology and PCR analysis showed a restricted pattern of EBV gene expression in these cells, consistent with a type I latency [154a]. It is presently not clear if a long-term latency can be established in cottontop tamarins. It has been shown that in some cases, EBV-induced lymphomas in cottontop tamarins may regress spontaneously and that this phenomenon is associated with the development of cell-mediated immunity to EBV [155]. Furthermore, it has been demonstrated that vaccine-induced protection against EBV-driven lymphomas is at least partially cell-mediated [155]. This suggests that T-cell-controlled long-term persistence of EBV in cottontop tamarins may be possible. Further studies are necessary to establish whether cottontop tamarins protected against the immediate and lethal effects of EBV infection may be a useful model for virus-associated diseases in humans.

Another animal which has been used as a model of EBV-induced lymphoma is the severe combined immunodeficiency (SCID) mouse. In these animals inoculation with peripheral blood lymphocytes (PBLs) from healthy EBV-carrying individuals or with PBLs from EBV seronegatives followed by injection of EBV results in the rapid development of EBV-positive large-cell (immunoblastic) lymphomas [156–159]. These tumors resemble those that develop in immunosuppressed individuals with regard to their LCL-like phenotype, Lat III pattern of EBV gene expression, and their presentation at multiple sites as individual monoclonal or oligoclonal foci [156–159]. More recent studies in which LCLs have been grown in SCID mice suggest that the resulting tumors may not be truly LCL-like but predominantly plasmacytoid with reduced expression of certain phenotypic markers (CD20, CD23) and of EBV genes (EBNA2, LMP1) relative to LCLs grown *in vitro* [160]. It therefore appears that the type of lymphoma developing in SCID mice depends on the experimental approach employed.

Interestingly, a requirement for activated T-cells in the generation of B-cell lymphomas in SCID mice has been demonstrated [157]. Thus, inoculation of purified B-cells from EBV seropositives or treatment of PBL-injected animals with cyclosporin A prevented the outgrowth of B-cell tumors [157]. These data raise the possibility that chronic T-cell activation may be important in the pathogenesis of EBV-positive lymphomas in the immunocompromised host.

The remarkable efficiency of tumor development in both the marmoset and SCID mouse models is strong circumstantial evidence that the development of immunoblastic lymphomas in an immunosuppressed setting in man need only require EBV-induced B-cell immortalization with no necessity for secondary genetic change. This clearly sets these particular lesions apart from all other EBV-positive malignancies where viral infection is but one event in a complex multistep lymphomagenic process.

Conclusions

The association of EBV with an ever-increasing number of different types of NHLs suggests that the natural history of EBV infection is more complex than originally anticipated. One of the most surprising observations is that EBV appears to be more frequently associated with T-cell lymphoproliferations than with B-cell tumors. Whilst C3d/EBV receptor expression has been demonstrated in T-cells at certain stages of differentiation [161], the susceptibility of these cells to EBV infection in the normal host and the extent to which such infected cells might contribute to virus persistence remain unknown. The frequent detection of EBV in atypical T-cell proliferations and in T-cell NHLs may indicate that T-lymphocytes are less well adapted than B-lymphocytes to EBV and are therefore not able to sustain a nontransforming latent infection.

The part played by EBV in the development of these diverse virus-associated neoplasms is still only poorly understood. EBV is detectable in virtually all endemic BL cases, suggesting that the virus is an essential requirement in the oncogenic process. By contrast, only a proportion of sporadic BL cases is EBV-associated. Recent studies on other NHLs have identified a few entities which appear to be invariably EBV-positive, e.g., sinonasal T-cell lymphoma. However, in the majority of entities, EBV is detected only in a proportion of cases and, thus, it appears that EBV infection is only one step in the oncogenic process, the functional consequences of which can be substituted for by other factors.

The detection of monoclonal EBV episomes together with the detection of the virus in virtually all tumor cells of EBV-associated NHLs has been taken as evidence that virus infection occurs before the clonal expansion of the neoplastic cells. The virus would therefore be present during a time frame relevant to the oncogenic process. Anecdotal evidence, however, indicates that in some EBV-positive lymphomas only a subclone of tumor cells carries the virus, suggesting that EBV infection may occur in established malignant tumors [47,115,132,133]. EBV infection at this late stage may not alter the behavior of the tumor or alternatively may confer a growth advantage, leading to the outgrowth of one or more EBV-positive clones. The latter scenario could then lead to the detection of monoclonal viral episomes in Southern blots, falsely suggesting EBV infection early in the neoplastic process.

The EBV-encoded protein, LMP1, is oncogenic in rodent fibroblasts and expression of LMP1 is associated with a range of phenotypic changes in several *in vitro* models. Thus, detection of LMP1 expression in virus-associated tumors has been interpreted as further evidence for an etiological role of the virus in these cases. However, EBV-positive NHLs of B- or T-cell phenotype are heterogeneous with regard to EBV gene expression and cellular phenotype. Morphologically identical cases of EBV-associated NHLs may display variable patterns of EBV gene expression. Moreover, it is now clear that EBV gene expression within any one lymphoma may be heterogenous, implying that different forms of viral latency are present in different tumor cells and at different stages of tumor growth. This serves to emphasize that the operational definitions of EBV latency which have been used to categorize cell lines do not rigidly apply in the 'real life' *in vivo* situation. Moreover, an association of tumor cell phenotype with EBV gene expression *in vivo* is not as readily discernible as would be expected from the data generated *in vitro*. Recent reports have indicated that in NHLs expression of LMP1 may be associated with the expression of the CD30 antigen [89,162]. Studies on epithelial cells and nasopharyngeal carcinomas have suggested that LMP1 may be able to trigger the expression of another lymphocyte activation antigen, CD70 [163,164]. However, for most other antigens which are induced or upregulated by LMP1 *in vitro*, clear-cut correlations have not been observed *in vivo*.

The ability of EBV to induce lymphoproliferative diseases *in vivo* is best illustrated by the remarkably efficient development of EBV-associated tumors in cottontop tamarins and SCID mice, and by the increased frequency of virus-associated tumors in humans with overt primary or secondary immune defects. By contrast, endemic BL develops in the face of apparently normal EBV immunity leading to the suggestion that expression of only a very limited set of EBV genes together with the downregulation of certain cellular antigens may allow BL cells to escape virus-specific CTL responses. Some virus-associated NHLs arising in patients without overt immune defects show a Lat II or even Lat III form of EBV infection. This observation together with the frequent detection of EBV type 2 in some entities points to an underlying, specific immune defect in some of these patients. There is thus the possibility that subclinical immune disturbances affecting aspects

of EBV-specific immunosurveillance mechanisms may contribute to the development of EBV-associated NHLs. This could help to explain the apparently paradoxical expression of LMP1, a known target of EBV-specific CTL response, in the absence of clinically overt immune defects.

Thus, an ever more complex picture of virus-associated malignancies is emerging. EBV is detected in a far greater spectrum of human tumors than anticipated, including B- and T-cell NHLs, Hodgkin's disease and various carcinomas. In most entities, EBV is identified only in a proportion of cases and EBV infection appears to be a late event in the oncogenic process in at least some of these cases. It is therefore likely that the contribution of EBV in the oncogenic processes of these diverse entities is variable. For a better understanding of the role of EBV in the development of virus-associated tumors, knowledge of the mode of EBV persistence and identification of the step in the carcinogenic process at which EBV infection occurs are essential. It is hoped that such an understanding will facilitate the development of novel approaches aimed at the prevention and treatment of EBV-associated lymphomas.

Acknowledgments

Work in the authors' laboratory was supported by the Cancer Research Campaign, the Medical Research Council, and the United Birmingham Hospitals Endowment Fund. We are very grateful to Professor George Klein for providing a tissue sample, and to Dr Hermann Herbst for providing illustrative material. We would also like to thank Dr Herbst, Dr N. Rooney and Professor E. L. Jones for critical reading of the manuscript.

References

1. Miller G. Epstein–Barr virus. Biology, pathogenesis, and medical aspects. In Fields BN, Knipe DM (eds) *Fields' Virology.* New York: Raven Press, 1990, pp. 1921–1958.
2. Nilsson K, Klein G, Henle W, et al. The establishment of lymphoblastoid cell lines from adult and from foetal human lymphoid tissue and its dependence on EBV. *Int. J. Cancer* 1971, **8**: 443–450.
3. Rickinson AB, Rowe M, Hart IJ, et al. T-cell-mediated regression of 'spontaneous' and of Epstein–Barr virus-induced B-cell transformation in vitro: Studies with cyclosporin A. *Cell. Immunol.* 1984, **87**: 646–658.

4. Gerber P, Nonoyama M, Lucas S, et al. Oral excretion of Epstein–Barr virus by healthy subjects and patients with infectious mononucleosis. *Lancet.* 1972, ii: 988–989.

5. Strauch B, Andrews L-L, Siegel N, et al. Oropharyngeal excretion of Epstein–Barr virus by renal transplant recipients and other patients with immunosuppressive drugs. *Lancet* 1974, **i**: 234–237.

6. Yao QY, Rickinson AB, Epstein MA. A re-examination of the Epstein–Barr virus carrier state in healthy seropositive individuals. *Int. J. Cancer.* 1985, **35**: 35–42.

7. Sixbey JW, Nedrud JG, Raab-Traub N, et al. Epstein–Barr virus replication in oropharyngeal epithelial cells. *N. Engl. J. Med.* 1984, **310**: 1225–1230.

8. Greenspan JS, Greenspan D, Lennette ET, et al. Replication of Epstein–Barr virus within the epithelial cells of oral hairy leukoplakia, an AIDS-associated lesion. *N. Engl. J. Med.* 1985, **313**: 1564–1571.

9. Allday MJ, Crawford DH. Role of epithelium in EBV persistence and pathogenesis of B-cell tumors. *Lancet* 1988, **i**: 855–857.

10. Niedobitek G, Young LS. Persistence of Epstein–Barr virus and the pathogenesis of virus-associated tumors. *Lancet* 1994, **343**: 333–335.

11. Niedobitek G, Hamilton-Dutoit S, Herbst H, et al. Identification of Epstein–Barr virus infected cells in tonsils of acute infectious mononucleosis by in situ hybridisation. *Hum. Pathol.* 1989, **20**: 796–799.

12. Niedobitek G, Herbst H, Young LS, et al. Patterns of Epstein–Barr virus infection in nonneoplastic lymphoid tissue. *Blood* 1992, **79**: 2520–2526.

13. Gratama JW, Oosterveer MAP, Zwaan FE, et al. Eradication of Epstein–Barr virus by allogeneic bone marrow transplantation: Implications for the site of viral latency. *Proc. Natl Acad. Sci. USA* 1988, **85**: 8693–8699.

14. Yao QY, Ogan P, Rowe M, et al. The Epstein–Barr virus: Host balance in acute infectious mononucleosis patients receiving Acyclovir anti-viral therapy. *Int. J. Cancer* 1989, **43**: 61–66.

15. Yao QY, Ogan P, Rowe M, et al. Epstein–Barr virus-infected B cells persist in the circulation of Acyclovir-treated virus carriers. *Int. J. Cancer* 1989, **43**: 67–71.

16. Niedobitek G, Young LS, Lau R, et al. Epstein–Barr virus infection in oral hairy leukoplakia: Virus replication in the absence of a detectable latent phase. *J. Gen. Virol.* 1991, **72**: 3035–3046.

17. Thomas JA, Felix DH, Wray D, et al. Epstein–Barr virus gene expression and epithelial cell differentiation in oral hairy leukoplakia. *Am. J. Pathol.* 1991, **139**: 1369–1380.

18. Kieff E, Leibowitz D. Epstein–Barr virus and its replication. In Fields BN, Knipe DM (eds) *Fields' Virology.* New York: Raven Press, 1990, pp. 1889–1920.

19. Speck SH, Strominger JL. Transcription of Epstein–Barr virus in latently infected, growth-transformed lymphocytes. *Adv. Viral Oncol.* 1989, **8**: 133–150.

20. Laux G, Economou A, Farrell P. The terminal protein gene 2 of Epstein–Barr virus is transcribed from a bidirectional latent promoter region. *J. Gen. Virol.* 1989, **70**: 3079–3084.

21. Wang D, Liebowitz D, Kieff E. An EBV membrane protein expressed in immortalized lymphocytes transforms established rodent cells. *Cell* 1985, **43**: 831–840.

22. Bornkamm GW, Hudewentz J, Freese UK, et al. Deletion of the non-transforming Epstein–Barr virus strain P3HR-1 causes fusion of the large internal repeat to the DSL region. *J. Virol.* 1982, **43**: 952–968.

23. Rabson M, Gradoville L, Heston L, et al. Non-immortalizing P3J-HR-1 Epstein–Barr virus: A deletion mutant of its transforming parent. *J. Virol.* 1982, **44**: 834–844.

24. Rowe M, Rooney CM, Rickinson AB, et al. Distinctions between endemic and sporadic forms of Epstein–Barr virus-positive Burkitt's lymphoma. *Int. J. Cancer* 1985, **35**: 435–441.

25. Gregory CD, Murray RJ, Edwards CF, et al. Down regulation of cell adhesion molecules LFA-3 and ICAM-1 in Epstein–Barr virus-positive Burkitt's lymphoma underlies tumor cell escape from virus-specific T-cell surveillance. *J. Exp. Med.* 1988, **167**: 1811–1824.

26. Wang F, Gregory CD, Rowe M, et al. Epstein–Barr virus nuclear protein 2 specifically induces expression of the B-cell activation antigen CD23. *Proc. Natl Acad. Sci. USA* 1987, **84**: 3452–3456.

27. Wang F, Gregory CD, Sample C, et al. Epstein–Barr virus latent membrane protein (LMP-1) and nuclear proteins 2 and 3C are effectors of phenotypic changes in B lymphocytes: EBNA2 and LMP-1 cooperatively induce CD23. *J. Virol.* 1990, **64**: 2309–2318.

28. Rowe M, Rowe DT, Gregory CD, et al. Differences in B cell growth phenotype reflect novel patterns of Epstein–Barr virus latent gene expression in Burkitt's lymphoma. *EMBO J.* 1987, **6**: 2743–2751.

29. Gregory CD, Rowe M, Rickinson AB. Different Epstein–Barr virus (EBV)-B cell interactions in phenotypically distinct clones of a Burkitt lymphoma cell line. *J. Gen. Virol.* 1990, **71**: 1481–1495.

30. Sample J, Brooks L, Sample C, et al. Restricted Epstein–Barr virus protein expression in Burkitt lymphoma is due to a different Epstein–Barr Nuclear Antigen-1 transcriptional initiation site. *Proc. Natl Acad. Sci. USA* 1991, **88**: 6343–6347.

31. Schaeffer BC, Woisetschlaeger M, Strominger JL, et al. Exclusive expression of Epstein–Barr virus nuclear antigen 1 in Burkitt lymphoma arises from a third promoter, distinct from the promoters used in latently infected lymphocytes. *Proc. Natl Acad. Sci. USA* 1991, **88**: 6550–6554.

32. Brooks L, Yao QY, Rickinson AB, et al. Epstein–Barr virus latent gene transcription in nasopharyngeal carcinoma cells: Coexpression of EBNA1, LMP1, and LMP2 transcripts. *J. Virol.* 1992, **66**: 2689–2697.

33. Herbst H, Stein H, Niedobitek G. Epstein–Barr virus and CD30+ malignant lymphomas. *CRC Crit. Rev. Oncogenesis* 1993, **4**: 191–239.

34. Rowe M, Lear A, Croom-Carter D, et al. Three pathways of Epstein–Barr virus (EBV) gene activation from EBNA1-positive latency in B lymphocytes. *J. Virol.* 1992, **66**: 122–131.

35. Kerr BM, Lear AL, Rowe M, et al. Three transcriptionally distinct forms of Epstein–Barr virus latency in somatic cell hybrids: Cell phenotype dependence of virus promotor usage. *Virology* 1992, **187**: 189–201.

36. Dambaugh T, Hennessy K, Chamnankit L, et al. U2 region of Epstein–Barr virus DNA may encode Epstein–Barr nuclear antigen 2. *Proc. Natl Acad. Sci. USA* 1984, **81**: 7632–7636.

37. Rowe M, Young LS, Cadwallader K, et al. Distinction between Epstein–Barr virus type A (EBNA 2A) and type B (EBNA 2B) isolates extends to the EBNA 3 family of nuclear proteins. *J. Virol.* 1989, **63**: 1031–1039.

38. Sample J, Young L, Martin B, et al. Epstein–Barr virus type-1 (EBV-1) and 2 (EBV-2) differ in their EBNA 3A, EBNA 3B, and EBNA 3C genes. *J. Virol.* 1990, **64**: 4084–4092.

39. Zimber U, Adldinger HK, Lenior GM, et al. Geographical prevalence of two Epstein–Barr virus types. *Virology* 1986, **154**: 56–66.

40. Young LS, Yao QY, Rooney CM, et al. New type B isolates of Epstein–Barr virus from Burkitt's lymphoma and from normal individuals in endemic areas. *J. Gen. Virol.* 1987, **68**: 2853–2862.

41. Sixbey JW, Shirley P, Chesney PJ, et al. Detection of a second widespread strain of Epstein–Barr virus. *Lancet* 1989, **ii**: 761–765.

42. Yao QY, Rowe M, Martin B, et al. The Epstein–Barr virus carrier state: Dominance of a single growth-transforming isolate in the blood and in the oropharynx of healthy virus carriers. *J. Gen. Virol.* 1991, **72**: 1579–1590.

43. Rickinson AB, Young LS, Rowe M. Influence of the Epstein–Barr virus nuclear antigen EBNA 2 on the growth phenotype of virus-transformed B cells. *J. Virol.* 1987, **61**: 1310–1317.

44. Boyle MJ, Sewell WA, Sculley TB, et al. Subtypes of Epstein–Barr virus in human immunodeficiency virus-associated non-Hodgkin lymphomas. *Blood* 1991, **78**: 3004–3011.

45. Herbst H, Steinbrecher E, Niedobitek G, et al. Distribution and phenotype of Epstein–Barr virus-harboring cells in Hodgkin's disease. *Blood* 1992, **80**: 484–491.

46. Weiss LM, Movahed LA. In situ demonstration of Epstein–Barr viral genomes in viral-associated B cell lymphoproliferations. *Am. J. Pathol.* 1989, **134**: 651–659.

47. Hamilton-Dutoit SJ, Raphael M, Audouin J, et al. In situ demonstration of Epstein–Barr virus small RNAs (EBER1) in acquired immunodeficiency syndrome-related lymphomas: Correlation with tumor morphology and primary site. *Blood* 1993, **82**: 619–624.

48. Young L, Alfieri C, Hennessy K, et al. Expression of Epstein–Barr virus transformation-associated genes in tissues of patients with EBV lymphoproliferative disease. *N. Engl J. Med.* 1989, **321**: 1080–1085.

49. Young LS, Lau R, Rowe M, et al. Differentiation-associated expression of the Epstein–Barr virus BZLF1 transactivator protein in oral hairy leukoplakia. *J. Virol.* 1991, **65**: 2868–2874.

50. Pallesen G, Hamilton-Dutoit SJ, Rowe M, et al. Expression of Epstein–Barr virus replicative proteins in AIDS-related non-Hodgkin's lymphoma cells. *J. Pathol.* 1991, **165**: 289–299.

51. Raab-Traub N, Flynn K. The structure of the termini of the Epstein–Barr virus as a marker of clonal cellular proliferation. *Cell* 1986, **47**: 883–889.

52. Nakanishi M, Kikuta H, Tomizawa K, et al. Distinct clonotypic Epstein–Barr virus-induced fatal lymphoproliferative disorder in a patient with Wiskott–Aldrich syndrome. *Cancer* 1993, **72**: 1376–1381.

53. Purtilo DT, Luka J, Brichacek B, et al. Non-Hodgkin's lymphomas in X-linked lymphoproliferative disease. In Tursz T, Pagano JS, Ablashi DV et al. (eds) *The Epstein–Barr Virus and Associated Diseases.* Colloque INSERM/John Libbey Eurotext 1993, Vol. 225, pp. 411–414.

54. Purtilo DT. Malignant lymphomas in children with primary immunodeficiency disease. *Clin. Transplantation* 1992, **6**: 223–226.

55. Sander CA, Medeiros LJ, Weiss LM, et al. Lymphoproliferative lesions in patients with common variable immunodeficiency syndrome. *Am. J. Surg. Pathol.* 1992, **16**: 1170–1182.

56. Falk K, Ernberg I, Sakthivel R, et al. Expression of Epstein–Barr virus-encoded proteins and B-cell markers in fatal infectious mononucleosis. *Int. J. Cancer* 1990, **46**: 976–984.

57. Alfrey EJ, Friedman AL, Grossman RA, et al. Two distinct patterns of post-transplantation lymphoproliferative disorder (PTLD): Early and late onset. *Clin. Transplantation* 1992, **6**: 246–248.

58. Swerdlow SH. Post-transplant lymphoproliferative disorders: A morphologic, phenotypic and genotypic spectrum of disease. *Histopathology* 1992, **20**: 373–385.

59. Opelz G, Henderson R. Incidence of non-Hodgkin lymphoma in kidney and heart transplant recipients. *Lancet* 1993, **342**: 1512–1516.

60. Zutter MM, Martin PJ, Sale GE, et al. Epstein–Barr virus lymphoproliferation after bone marrow transplantation. *Blood* 1988, **72**: 520–529.

61. Ho M, Miller G, Atchison RW, et al. Epstein–Barr virus infection and DNA hybridization studies in posttransplantation lymphoma and lymphoproliferative lesions: The role of primary infection. *J. Infect. Dis.* 1985, **152**: 876–886.

62. Randhawa PS, Yousem SA, Paradis IL, et al. The clinical spectrum, pathology, and clonal analysis of Epstein–Barr virus-associated lymphoproliferative disorders in heart–lung transplant recipients. *Am. J. Clin. Pathol.* 1989, **92**: 177–185.

63. Ho M, Jaffe R, Miller G, et al. The frequency of Epstein–Barr virus infection and associated lymphoproliferative syndrome after transplantation and its manifestations in children. *Transplantation* 1988, **45**: 719–727.

64. Cleary ML, Nalesnik MA, Shearer WT, et al. Clonal analysis of transplant-associated lymphoproliferations based on the structure of genomic termini of the Epstein–Barr virus. *Blood* 1988, **72**: 349–352.

65. Locker J, Nalesnik M. Molecular genetic analysis of lymphoid tumors arising after organ transplantation. *Am. J. Pathol.* 1989, **135**: 977–987.

66. Patton DF, Wilkowski CW, Hanson CA, et al. Epstein–Barr virus-determined clonality in posttransplant lymphoproliferative disease. *Transplantation* 1990, **49**: 1080–1084.

67. Randhawa PS, Yousem SA. Epstein–Barr virus-associated lymphoproliferative disease in heart-lung allograft. *Transplantation* 1990, **49**: 126–130.

68. Thomas JA, Hotchin NA, Allday MJ, et al. Immunohistology of Epstein–Barr virus-associated antigens in B cell disorders from immunocompromised individuals. *Transplantation* 1990, **49**: 944–953.

69. Katz BZ, Raab-Traub N, Miller G. Latent and replicating forms of Epstein–Barr virus DNA in lymphomas and lymphoproliferative diseases. *J. Infect. Dis.* 1989, **160**: 589–598.

70. Starzl TE, Nalesnik MA, Porter KA, et al. Reversibility of lymphomas and lymphoproliferative lesions developing under cyclosporin-steroid therapy. *Lancet* 1984, **i**: 583–587.

71. Cen H, Williams PA, McWilliams HP, et al. Evidence for restricted Epstein–Barr virus latent gene expression and anti-EBNA antibody response in solid organ transplant recipients with post-transplant lymphoproliferative disorders. *Blood* 1993, **81**: 1393–1403.

72. Gratama JW, Zutter MM, Minarovits J, et al. Expression of Epstein–Barr virus-encoded growth-transformation-associated proteins in lymphoproliferations of bone-marrow transplant recipients. *Int. J. Cancer* 1991, **47**: 188–192.

73. Borisch B, Gatter KC, Tobler A, et al. Epstein–Barr virus-associated anaplastic large cell lymphoma in renal transplant patients. *Am. J. Clin. Pathol.* 1992, **98**: 312–318.

74. Kumar S, Kumar D, Kingma DW, et al. Epstein–Barr virus-associated T-cell lymphoma in a renal transplant patient. *Am. J. Surg. Pathol.* 1993, **17**: 1046–1053.

75. Waller EK, Ziemianska M, Bangs CD, et al. Characterization of posttransplant lymphomas that express T-cell-associated markers: Immunophenotypes, molecular genetics, cytogenetics, and heterotransplantation in severe combined immunodeficient mice. *Blood* 1993, **82**: 247–261.

76. Euvrard S, Pouteil Noble C, Kanitakis J, et al. Successive occurrence of T-cell and B-cell lymphomas after renal transplantation in a patient with multiple cutaneous squamous cell carcinomas. *N. Engl. J. Med.* 1992, **327**: 1924–1926.

77. Hamilton-Dutoit SJ, Pallesen G, Franzmann MB, et al. AIDS-related lymphoma. Histopathology, immunophenotype, and association with Epstein–Barr virus as demonstrated by in situ nucleic acid hybridization. *Am. J. Pathol.* 1991, **138**: 149–163.

78. Borisch Chappuis B, Müller H, Stutte J, et al. Identification of EBV-DNA in lymph nodes from patients with lymphadenopathy and lymphomas associated with AIDS. *Virchows Arch. B.* 1990, **58**: 199–205.

79. Thomas JA, Cotter F, Hanby AM, et al. Epstein–Barr virus-related oral T-cell lymphoma associated with human immunodeficiency virus immunosuppression. *Blood* 1993, **81**: 3350–3356.

80. Shibata D, Weiss LM, Nathwani BN, et al. Epstein–Barr virus in benign lymph node biopsies from individuals infected with the human immunodeficiency virus is associated with concurrent or subsequent development of non-Hodgkin's lymphoma. *Blood* 1991, **77**: 1527–1533.

81. Pedersen C, Gerstoft J, Lundgren JO, et al. HIV-associated lymphoma: Histopathology and association with Epstein–Barr virus genome related to clinical, immunological and prognostic factors. *Eur. J. Cancer* 1991, **27**: 1416–1423.

82. Herndier BG, Shiramizu BT, McGrath MS. AIDS associated non-Hodgkin's lymphomas represent a broad spectrum of monoclonal and polyclonal lymphoproliferative processes. *Curr. Topics Microbiol. Immunol.* 1992, **182**: 385–394.

83. MacMahon EM, Glass JD, Hayward DS, et al. Epstein–Barr virus in AIDS-related primary central nervous system lymphoma. *Lancet* 1991, **338**: 969–973.

84. Ballerini P, Gaidano G, Gong JZ, et al. Multiple genetic lesions in acquired immunodeficiency syndrome-related non-Hodgkin's lymphoma. *Blood* 1993, **81**: 166–176.

85. Neri A, Barriga F, Inghirami G, et al. Epstein–Barr virus infection precedes clonal expansion in Burkitt's and acquired immunodeficiency syndrome-associated lymphoma. *Blood* 1991, **77**: 1092–1095.

86. Borisch B, Finke J, Hennig I, et al. Distribution and localization of Epstein–Barr virus subtypes A and B in AIDS-related lymphomas and lymphatic tissue of HIV-positive patients. *J. Pathol.* 1992, **168**: 229–236.

87. Shiramizu B, Herndier B, Meeker T, et al. Molecular and immunophenotypic characterization of AIDS-associated, Epstein–Barr virus-negative, polyclonal lymphoma. *J. Clin. Oncol.* 1992, **10**: 383–389.

88. Shibata D, Weiss LM, Hernandez AM, et al. Epstein–Barr virus-associated non-Hodgkin's lymphoma in patients infected with the human immunodeficiency virus. *Blood* 1993, **81**: 2102–2109.

89. Hamilton-Dutoit SJ, Rea D, Raphael M, et al. Epstein–Barr virus-latent gene expression and tumor cell phenotype in acquired immunodeficiency syndrome-related non-Hodgkin's lymphomas. Correlation of lymphoma phenotype with three distinct patterns of viral latency. *Am. J. Pathol.* 1993, **143**: 1072–1085.

90. Zur Hausen H, Schulte-Holthausen H, Klein G, et al. EBV DNA in biopsies of Burkitt tumors and anaplastic carcinomas of the nasopharynx. *Nature* 1970, **228**: 1056–1058.

91. Lindahl T, Klein G, Reedman B, et al. Relationship between Epstein–Barr virus (EBV) DNA and the EBV-determined nuclear antigen (EBNA) in Burkitt lymphoma biopsies and other lymphoproliferative malignancies. *Int. J. Cancer* 1974, **13**: 764–772.

92. Ziegler JL, Andersson M, Klein G, et al. Detection of Epstein–Barr virus DNA in American Burkitt's lymphoma. *Int. J. Cancer* 1976, **17**: 701–706.

93. Hummel H, Anagnostopoulos I, Korbjuhn P, et al. Epstein–Barr virus infection patterns in malignant lymphomas. In Tursz T, Pagano JS, Ablashi DV et al (eds) *The Epstein–Barr Virus and Associated Diseases.* Colloque INSERM/John Libbey Eurotext 1993, Vol. 225, pp. 433–441.

94. Gutierrez MI, Bhatia K, Barriga F, et al. Molecular epidemiology of Burkitt's lymphoma from South America: Differences in breakpoint location and Epstein–Barr virus association from tumors in other world regions. *Blood* 1992, **79**: 3261–3266.

95. Henle W, Henle G. Seroepidemiology of the virus. In Epstein MA, Achong BG (eds) *The Epstein–Barr Virus.* Berlin: Springer Verlag 1979, pp. 61–78.

96. Gutierrez MI, Bhatia K, Magrath I. Replicative viral DNA in Epstein–Barr virus associated Burkitt's lymphoma biopsies. *Leukemia Res.* 1993, **17**: 285–289.

96a. Niedobitek G, Agathanggelou A, Rowe M, et al. Heterogeneous expression of EBV latent proteins in endemic Burkitt's lymphoma. *Blood* 1995, **86**: 659–665.

97. Magrath I, Jain V, Bhatia, K. Molecular epidemiology of Burkitt's lymphoma. In Tursz T, Pagano JS, Ablashi DV et al (eds) *The Epstein–Barr Virus and Associated Diseases.* Colloque INSERM/John Libbey Eurotext 1993, Vol. 225, pp. 377–396.

98. Wilson JB, Levine AJ. The oncogenic potential of Epstein–Barr virus nuclear antigen 1 in transgenic mice. *Curr. Topics Microbiol. Immunol.* 1992, **182**: 375–384.

99. Rickinson AB, Murray RJ, Brooks J, et al. T-cell recognition of Epstein–Barr virus associated lymphomas. *Cancer Surveys* 1992, **13**: 53–80.

100. Murray RJ, Kurilla MG, Griffin HM, et al. Human cytotoxic T-cell responses against Epstein–Barr virus nuclear antigens demonstrated using recombinant vaccinia viruses. *Proc. Natl Acad. Sci. USA* 1990, **87**: 2906–2910.

101. Khanna R, Burrows SR, Kurilla MG, et al. Localisation of Epstein–Barr virus cytotoxic T-cell epitopes using recombinant vaccinia: Implications for vaccine development. *J. Exp. Med.* 1992, **176**: 169–176.

102. Murray RJ, Kurilla MG, Brooks JM, et al. Identification of target antigens for the human cytotoxic T-cell response to Epstein–Barr virus (EBV): Implications for the immune control of EBV-positive malignancies. *J. Exp. Med.* 1992, **176**: 157–168.

103. Torsteinsdottir S, Brautbar C, Ben Bassat H, et al. Differential expression of HLA antigens on human B-cell lines of normal and malignant origin: A consequence of immune surveillance or a phenotype vestige of the progenitor cells? *Int. J. Cancer* 1988, **41**: 913–919.

104. Andersson ML, Stam NJ, Klein G, et al. Aberrant expression of HLA Class-I antigens in Burkitt lymphoma cells. *Int. J. Cancer* 1991, **47**: 544–550.

105. Herbst H, Niedobitek G, Kneba M, et al. High incidence of Epstein–Barr virus genomes in Hodgkin's disease. *Am. J. Pathol.* 1990, **137**: 13–18.

106. Prevot S, Hamilton-Dutoit S, Audouin J, et al. Analysis of African Burkitt's and high grade B cell non-Burkitt's lymphoma for Epstein–Barr virus genomes using in situ hybridization. *Br. J. Haematol.* 1992, **80**: 27–32.

107. Weiss LM, Gaffey MJ, Chen YY, et al. Frequency of Epstein–Barr viral DNA in 'Western' sinonasal and Waldeyer's ring non-Hodgkin's lymphomas. *Am. J. Surg. Pathol.* 1992, **16**: 156–162.

108. Hamilton-Dutoit SJ, Pallesen G. A survey of Epstein–Barr virus gene expression in sporadic non-Hodgkin's lymphomas. Detection of Epstein–Barr virus in a subset of peripheral T-cell lymphomas. *Am. J. Pathol.* 1992, **140**: 1315–1325.

109. Hochberg FH, Miller G, Schooley RT, et al. Central-nervous-system lymphoma related to Epstein–Barr virus. *N. Engl J. Med.* 1983, **309**: 745–748.

110. Geddes JF, Bhattacharjee MB, Savage K, et al. Primary cerebral lymphoma: A study of 47 cases probed for Epstein–Barr virus genome *J. Clin. Pathol.* 1992, **45**: 587–590.

111. Wolf BC, Martin AW, Neiman RS, et al. The detection of Epstein–Barr virus in hairy cell leukemia cells by in situ hybridization. *Am. J. Pathol.* 1990, **136**: 717–723.

112. Schiller JH, Bittner G, Meisner LF, et al. Establishment and characterization of an Epstein–Barr virus spontaneously transformed lymphocytic cell line derived from a hairy cell leukemia patient. *Leukemia* 1991, **5**: 399–407.

113. Chang K, Chen YY, Weiss LM. Lack of evidence of Epstein–Barr virus in hairy cell leukemia and monocytoid B-cell lymphoma. *Hum. Pathol.* 1993, **24**: 58–61.

114. Momose H, Jaffe ES, Shin SS, et al. Chronic lymphocytic leukemia/small lymphocytic lymphoma with Reed–Sternberg-like cells and possible transformation to Hodgkin's disease. *Am. J. Surg. Pathol.* 1992, **16**: 859–867.

115. Lewin N, Aman P, Mellstedt H, et al. Direct outgrowth of in vivo Epstein–Barr virus (EBV)-infected chronic lymphocytic leukemia (CLL) cells into permanent lines. *Int. J. Cancer* 1988, **41**: 892–895.

116. Ramsay AD, Smith WJ, Isaacson PG. T-cell-rich B-cell lymphoma. *Am. J. Surg. Pathol.* 1988, **12**: 433–443.

117. Loke SL, Ho F, Srivastava G, et al. Clonal Epstein–Barr virus genome in T-cell-rich lymphomas of B or probable B lineage. *Am. J. Pathol.* 1992, **140**: 981–989.

118. Dolcetti R, Carbone A, Zagonel V, et al. Type 2 Epstein–Barr virus genome and latent membrane protein-1 expression in a T-cell-rich lymphoma of probable B-cell lineage. *Am. J. Clin. Pathol.* 1993, **100**: 541–549.

119. Khan G, Norton AJ, Slavin G. Epstein–Barr virus in Reed–Sternberg-like cells in non-Hodgkin's lymphoma. *J. Pathol.* 1993, **169**: 9–14.

120. Fukayama M, Ibuka T, Hayashi Y, et al. Epstein–Barr virus in pyothorax-associated pleural lymphomas. *Am. J. Pathol.* 1993, **14**: 1044–1049.

121. Sasajima Y, Yamabe H, Kobashi Y, et al. High expression of the Epstein–Barr virus latent protein EB nuclear antigen-2 on pyothorax-associated lymphomas. *Am. J. Pathol.* 1993, **143**: 1280–1285.

122. Kikuta H, Taguchi Y, Tomizawa K, et al. Epstein–Barr virus genome-positive T lymphocytes in a boy with chronic active EBV infection associated with Kawasaki-like disease. *Nature* 1988, **333**: 455–457.

123. Mori M, Kurozumi H, Akagi K, et al. Monoclonal proliferation of T-cells containing Epstein–Barr virus in fatal infectious mononucleosis. *N. Engl J. Med.* 1992, **327**: 58.

124. Yoneda N, Tatsumi E, Kawanishi M, et al. Detection of Epstein–Barr virus genome in benign polyclonal proliferative T-cells of a young male patient. *Blood* 1990, **76**: 172–177.

125. Gaillard F, Mechinaud-Lacroix F, Papin S, et al. Primary Epstein–Barr virus infection with clonal T-cell proliferation. *Am. J. Clin. Pathol.* 1992, **98**: 324–333.

126. Kawaguchi H, Miyashita T, Herbst H, et al. Subclinical proliferation of Epstein–Barr virus infected T-lymphocytes in Epstein–Barr virus associated hemophagocytic syndrome (EBV-AHS). *J. Clin. Invest.* 1993, **92**: 1444–1450.

127. Kikuta H, Sakiyama Y, Matsumoto S, et al. Fatal Epstein–Barr virus-associated hemophagocytic syndrome. *Blood* 1993, **82**: 3259–3264.

128. Craig FE, Clare CN, Sklar JL, et al. T-cell lymphoma and the virus-associated hemophagocytic syndrome. *Am. J. Clin. Pathol.* 1992, **97**: 189–194.

129. Gaffey MJ, Frierson HF, Medeiros LJ, et al. The relationship of Epstein–Barr virus to infection-related (sporadic) and familial hemophagocytic syndrome and secondary (lymphoma-related) hemophagocytosis: An in situ hybridization study. *Hum. Pathol.* 1993, **24**: 657–667.

130. Jones JF, Shurin S, Abramowsky C, et al. T-cell lymphomas containing Epstein–Barr viral DNA in patients with chronic Epstein–Barr virus infections. *N. Engl J. Med.* 1988, **318**: 733–741.

131. Pallesen G, Hamilton-Dutoit SJ, Zhou X. The association of Epstein–Barr virus (EBV) with T-cell lymphoproliferations and Hodgkin's disease: Two new developments in the EBV field. *Adv. Cancer Res.* 1994, **62**: 179–239.

132. Korbjuhn P, Anagnostopoulos I, Hummel M, et al. Frequent latent Epstein–Barr virus infection of neoplastic T cells and bystander B cells in human immunodeficiency virus-negative European peripheral pleomorphic T-cell lymphomas. *Blood* 1993, **82**: 217–223.

133. de Bruin PC, Jiwa NM, van der Valk P, et al. Detection of Epstein–Barr virus nucleic acid sequences and protein in nodal T-cell lymphomas: Relation between latent membrane protein-1 positivity and clinical course. *Histopathology* 1993, **23**: 509–518.

134. Ho FCS, Srivastava G, Loke SL, et al. Presence of Epstein–Barr virus DNA in nasal lymphomas of B and 'T' cell type. *Hematol. Oncol.* 1990, **8**: 271–281.

135. Harabuchi Y, Yamanaka N, Kataura A, et al. Epstein–Barr virus in nasal T-cell lymphomas in patients with midline granuloma. *Lancet* 1990, **335**: 128–130.

136. Dhaliwal J, Rowlands DC, Niedobitek G, et al. Nasal T-cell lymphoma associated with Epstein–Barr virus infection. *J. Laryngol. Otol.* 1993, **107**: 468–470.

137. Medeiros LJ, Jaffe ES, Chen YY, et al. Localization of Epstein–Barr viral genomes in angiocentric immunoproliferative lesions. *Am. J. Surg. Pathol.* 1992, **16**: 439–447.

138. Borisch B, Hennig I, Laeng RH, et al. Association of the subtype 2 of the Epstein–Barr virus with T-cell non-Hodgkin lymphoma of the midline granuloma type. *Blood* 1993, **82**: 858–864.

139. Knecht H, Sahli R, Shaw P, et al. Detection of Epstein–Barr virus DNA by polymerase chain reaction in lymph node biopsies from patients with angioimmunoblastic lymphadenopathy. *Br. J. Haematol.* 1990, **75**: 610–614.

140. Su IJ, Hsieh HC, Lin KH, et al. Aggressive peripheral T-cell lymphomas containing Epstein–Barr viral DNA: A clinicopathologic and molecular analysis. *Blood* 1991, **77**: 799–808.

141. Ott G, Ott MM, Feller AC, et al. Prevalence of Epstein–Barr virus DNA in different T-cell lymphoma entities in a European population. *Int. J. Cancer* 1992, **51**: 562–567.

142. Anagnostopoulos I, Hummel M, Finn T, et al. Heterogeneous Epstein–Barr virus infection patterns in peripheral T-cell lymphoma of angioimmunoblastic lymphadenopathy type. *Blood* 1992, **80**: 1804–1812.

143. Weiss LM, Jaffe ES, Liu XF, et al. Detection and localization of Epstein–Barr viral genomes in angioimmunoblastic lymphadenopathy and angioimmunoblastic lymphadenopathy-like lymphoma. *Blood* 1992, **79**: 1789–1795.

144. Abruzzo LV, Schmidt K, Weiss LM, et al. B-cell lymphoma after angioimmunoblastic lymphadenopathy: A case with oligoclonal gene rearrangements associated with Epstein–Barr virus. *Blood* 1993, **82**: 241–246.

145. Pan L, Diss TC, Peng H, et al. Epstein–Barr virus (EBV) in enteropathy-associated T-cell lymphoma (EATL). *J. Pathol.* 1993, **170**: 137–143.

145a. Ilyas M, Niedobitek G, Agathanggelou A, et al. Nonhodgkin's lymphoma, celiac disease and Epstein–Barr virus: A study of 13 cases of enteropathy-associated T- and B-cell lymphoma. *J. Pathol.* 1995, **177**: 115–122.

146. Tokunaga M, Imai S, Uemura Y, et al. Epstein–Barr virus in adult T-cell leukemia/lymphoma. *Am. J. Pathol.* 1993, **143**: 1263–1269.

147. Chen CL, Sadler RH, Walling DM, et al. Epstein–Barr virus (EBV) gene expression in EBV-positive peripheral T-cell lymphomas. *J. Virol.* 1993, **67**: 6303–6308.

148. Herbst H, Dallenbach F, Hummel M, et al. Epstein–Barr virus DNA and latent gene products in Ki-1 (CD30)-positive anaplastic large cell lymphomas. *Blood* 1991, **78**: 2666–2673.

149. Shope T, Dechairo D, Miller G. Malignant lymphoma in cotton-top marmosets after inoculation with Epstein–Barr virus. *Proc. Natl Acad. Sci. USA.* 1973, **70**: 2487–2491.

150. Cleary ML, Epstein MA, Finerty S, et al. Individual tumors of multifocal EB virus-induced malignant lymphomas in tamarins arise from different B-cell clones. *Science* 1985, **228**: 722–724.

151. Young LS, Finerty S, Brooks L, et al. Epstein–Barr virus gene expression in malignant lymphomas induced by experimental virus infection of cottontop tamarins. *J. Virol.* 1989, **63**: 1967–1974.

152. Morgan AJ, Finerty S, Lovgren K, et al. Prevention of Epstein–Barr (EB) virus-induced lymphoma in cotton-top tamarins by vaccination with the EB virus envelope glycoprotein gp340 incorporated into immune-stimulat-

ing complexes. *J. Gen. Virol.* 1988, **69**: 2093–2096.

153. Ragot T, Finerty S, Watkins PE, et al. Replication-defective recombinant adenovirus expressing the Epstein–Barr virus (EBV) envelope glycoprotein gp340/220 induces protective immunity against EBV-induced lymphomas in cottontop tamarins. *J. Gen. Virol.* 1993, **74**: 501–507.

154. Wedderburn N, Edwards JMB, Desgranges C, et al. Infectious mononucleosis-like response in common marmosets infected with Epstein–Barr virus. *J. Infect. Dis.* 1984, **150**: 878–882.

154a. Niedobitek G, Agathanggelou A, Finerty S, et al. Latent Epstein–Barr virus infection in cottontop tamarins. A possible model for Epstein–Barr virus infection in humans. *Am. J. Pathol.* 1994, **145**: 969–978.

155. Finerty S, Scullion FT, Morgan AJ. Demonstration in vitro of cell mediated immunity to Epstein–Barr virus in cotton-top tamarins. *Clin. Exp. Immunol.* 1988, **73**: 181–185.

156. Rowe M, Young LS, Crocker J, et al. Epstein–Barr virus (EBV)-associated lymphoproliferative disease in the SCID mouse model: Implications for the pathogenesis of EBV-positive lymphomas in man. *J. Exp. Med.* 1991, **173**: 147–158.

157. Veronese ML, Veronesi A, D'Andrea E, et al. Lymphoproliferative disease in human peripheral blood mononuclear cell-injected SCID mice. I. T lymphocyte requirement for B-cell tumor generation. *J. Exp. Med.* 1992, **176**: 1763–1767.

158. Boyle TJ, Tamburini M, Berend KR, et al. Human B-cell lymphoma in severe combined immunodeficient mice after active infection with Epstein–Barr virus. *Surgery* 1992, **112**: 378–386.

159. Okano M, Taguchi Y, Nakamine H, et al. Characterization of Epstein–Barr virus-induced lymphoproliferation derived from human peripheral blood mononuclear cells transferred to severe combined immunodeficient mice. *Am. J. Pathol.* 1990, **137**: 517–522.

160. Rochford R, Hobbs MV, Garnier JL, et al. Plasmacytoid differentiation of Epstein–Barr virus-transformed B cells in vivo is associated with reduced expression of viral latent genes. *Proc. Natl Acad. Sci. USA* 1993, **90**: 352–356.

161. Fischer E, Delibrias C, Kazatchkine MD. Expression of CR2 (the C3dg/EBV receptor, CD21) on normal human peripheral blood T lymphocytes. *J. Immunol.* 1991, **146**: 865–869.

162. Kanavaros P, Jiwa M, van der Valk P, et al. Expression of Epstein–Barr virus latent gene products and related cellular activation and adhesion molecules in Hodgkin's disease and non-Hodgkin's lymphomas arising in patients without overt pre-existing immunodeficiency. *Hum. Pathol.* 1993, **24**: 725–729.

163. Niedobitek G, Fahraeus R, Herbst H, et al. The Epstein–Barr virus encoded membrane protein (LMP) induces phenotypic changes in epithelial cells. *Virchows Arch. B.* 1992, **62**: 55–59.

164. Niedobitek G, Young LS, Sam CK, et al. Expression of Epstein–Barr virus genes and of lymphocyte activation molecules in undifferentiated nasopharyngeal carcinomas. *Am. J. Pathol.* 1992, **140**: 879–887.

NOTE ADDED IN PROOF

Since the preparation of this chapter, work has been published suggesting possible mechanisms for the function of LMP1. The transcriptional regulation of EBNA1 expression has also been further characterized [for review see 165,166].

165. Kieff E. Epstein–Barr virus and its replication. In Fields BN, Knipe DM, Howley PM (eds) *Fields' Virology*. 2nd edn. Philadelphia: Lippincot–Raven, 1996, pp. 2343–2396.

166. Rickinson AB, Kieff E. Epstein–Barr virus. In Fields BN, Knipe DM, Howley PM (eds) *Fields' Virology*. 2nd edn. Philadelphia: Lippincot–Raven, 1996, pp. 2397–2446.

species exhibit common features which include a similar genetic structure, the existence of defective viruses, the importance for pathogenesis of the mode, dose and time of infection, the ubiquity/endemicity of these viruses, their low infection/pathogenic ratio, and the role of environmental and genetic factors in determining susceptibility or resistance to retrovirus associated malignancies.

Molecular virology and biology of HTLV-1 and HTLV-2

Members of the oncoretroviridae subfamily, the human T-cell leukemia–lymphoma viruses (HTLVs), together with the bovine leukemia virus (BLV) and the simian T-cell leukemia viruses (STLVs), are distinct from avian and murine oncoretroviruses, inasmuch as they do not harbor oncogene sequences of cellular origin, but rather possess specific genes encoding regulatory proteins (tax and rex), which both regulate viral replication and interact with the host genes involved in cell cycle.

The genetic organization of HTLV-1 is shown in Figure 13.1. This virus, as is the case for all retroviruses, contains genes that encode three major virion proteins 5'-gag-pol-env-3' and are flanked by long terminal repeats (LTR) on either side. The LTRs are 755 nucleotides long and divided into U3, R and U5 regions. The U3 region contains a TATA box, three imperfect 21 nucleotide repeats called tax-responsive elements, a polyadenylation signal AATAAA and a polyadenylation site. The R region contains the first spliced donor site at position 119 for the mRNAs. The function of the U5 region has not been clearly determined.

The gag (or group antigen) region, initially translated as a polyprotein precursor p55, is subsequently cleaved into a 19 kD matrix protein (MA), the major capsid 24 kD protein (CA) and a 15 kD product. While the major p24 proteins of HTLV-1 and HTLV-2 are 83% homologous, the p19 matrix (MA) proteins of their viruses share only 56% of their nucleotide sequences [6].

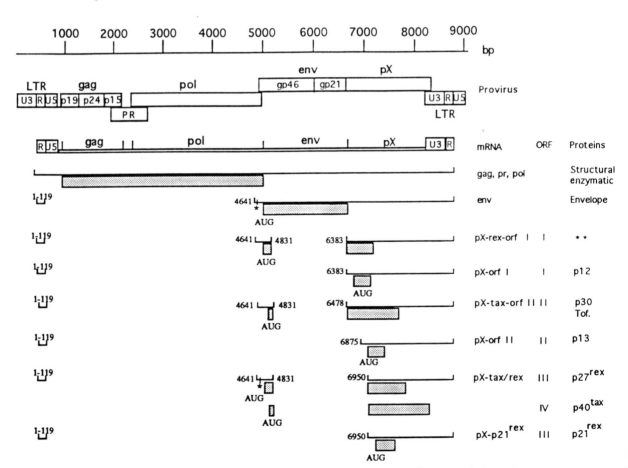

Figure 13.1 Genomic structure of HTLV-I provirus and mRNAs with corresponding encoded proteins.

The pol region contains the largest open reading frame of the HTLV genome, encoding polymerases of 896 or 982 amino acids, respectively, in HTLV-1 and HTLV-2 and overlapping the protease gene at the 5' end.

The envelope proteins are synthesized from a 4.2 kb singly spliced mRNA as a 488 amino acid glycosylated precursor of 62 kD. This precursor is cleaved into the mature 46 kD surface glycoprotein of 312 amino acids and the 21 kD transmembrane glycoprotein of 176 amino acids.

In addition to these structural genes, there is a region at the 3' end of the genome, not found in other replicating animal retroviruses, which was initially referred to as the 'X' region, because of its unknown function [5–8]. This region contains at least four open reading frames (ORF). The ORF III and IV are expressed through a single polycistronic, doubly spliced mRNA, which encodes two major regulatory proteins: the tax protein and the rex protein [9]. The p40 tax is a 40 kD nuclear phosphoprotein of 353 amino acids. It is a transactivator protein that binds to the level of the tax-responsive elements located in the U3 portion of the viral 5' LTR, thereby increasing viral transcription. In addition, tax indirectly interacts with numerous heterologous cellular promotors by upregulating the nuclear transcription factor (NF-kB), which in turn increases the expression of interleukin-2, interleukin-2 receptor α and granulocyte–macrophage colony-stimulating factor (GM-CSF). These genes play a crucial role in the growth and functions of T-lymphocytes. A number of additional cellular genes are transactivated by the tax protein, including c-sis, c-jun, interleukin-6 (IL-6), tumor necrosis factor-β (TNFβ), transforming growth factor-β (TGFβ) nerve growth factor (NGF), the globin and vimentin genes and the parathyroid hormone-related protein.

The p27 rex protein is a 27 kD nucleolar phosphoprotein of 189 amino acids [9]. In contrast to tax, rex has no influence on viral transcription but acts at the posttranscriptional level to regulate viral gene expression. Rex increases the expression of viral structural proteins and enzymes by facilitating the passage from nucleus to cytoplasm of unspliced or singly spliced mRNAs coding for gag, pol and env proteins. Rex is itself regulated through a specific *cis*-acting sequence located in the R region of the 3' LTR, upstream from the polyadenylation sites. This 255 nucleotide long, energetically stable stem loop RNA structure is called the rex-responsive element. In addition to p27 rex, the ORF III encodes a second rex 21 kD protein of 111 amino acids called p21 rex. The function of this protein remains unknown.

Novel, alternatively spliced mRNAs encoded by ORF I and II of the pX region have recently been discovered [9–12] using the very sensitive technique of reverse transcriptase – polymerase chain reaction (PCR) in HTLV-1-infected cell lines, peripheral blood lymphocytes from ATLL, from tropical spastic paraparesis/HTLV-1-associated myelopathy (TSP/HAM) patients and from healthy carriers as well as in a human fibroblast cell line transfected with an HTLV-1 molecular clone (Table 13.1). These mRNAs code for three new proteins named p12$^\mathrm{I}$, p13$^\mathrm{II}$ and p30$^\mathrm{II}$. The p12$^\mathrm{I}$ is a proline- and leucine-rich, hydrophobic protein of 99 amino acids, which localizes in endoplasmic membranes and bears a structural and functional similarity to the E5 oncoprotein of bovine papilloma virus [12]. Furthermore, the p12$^\mathrm{I}$ specifically interacts with the interleukin-2 (IL-2) receptor β and γ but not α-chains, suggesting its possible involvement in IL-2 signaling and T-cell transformation. The functions of the p13$^\mathrm{II}$ and p30$^\mathrm{II}$ are currently unknown.

CELL–VIRUS RELATIONSHIP [6,13,14]

Infection by cell-free HTLV virions *in vitro* is very inefficient and direct cell-to-cell contact is usually required. While many cell types can be infected by HTLV-1 *in vitro*, including B-cells, fibroblasts, epithelial, endothelial cells as well as macrophages, *in vivo*, HTLV-1 mainly infects CD4 T-cells while HTLV-2 predominantly infects CD8 T-cells.

The receptor for HTLV-1 and 2 remains unknown [13].

T-Cell transformation by HTLV-1 results in continuous polyclonal CD4+ cell proliferation, calling to mind the Epstein–Barr virus (EBV)-induced B-cell immortalization, and possibly involving an autocrine IL-2/IL-2 receptor (IL-2R) loop mentioned above [5,7,9].

Mitogenic stimulation of CD4 and CD8 cells seems to be not dependent upon viral infection but to result directly from the interaction between the gp46 of the viral envelope and the as yet unknown T-cell surface receptor [6,13]. Persistent cell proliferation, however, is mediated by tax gene transactivation of IL-2 and IL-2R [5].

Epidemiological characteristics of HTLV-1 and 2

HTLV-1 infection was found to be endemic in the South Western islands of the Nippon Archipelago (Kyushu-Shikoku), then in large parts of the Caribbean area, in tropical Africa, and in Central and South America [15–18]. It is estimated that between

Table 13.1 Characteristics of the proteins encoded by the pX region of HTLV-1

Name	Size*	ORF†	Localization	Function
p12^{I}	99	I	Cytoplasm	Binds 16 kD IL-2 receptor
p13^{II}	87	II	Nulear matrix	Unknown
p30^{II}	241	II	Nucleoli	Unknown
p27^{Rex}	189	III	Nucleoli	Posttranscriptional regulation
p21^{Rex}	111	III	Cytoplasm	Unknown
p40^{Tax}	353	IV	Nuclear matrix	Transactivator

* Number of amino acids.
† Open reading frame of the pX region.
Adapted from Koralnik [9].

15 and 20 million individuals are infected by HTLV-1 throughout the world today [18]. HTLV-1 antibody prevalence rates among adults vary from 0.5% to 10% in different geographical areas [15,18]. Furthermore, significant variations in prevalence exist within endemic areas, the microepidemiology of high prevalence nests reflecting either a founder effect in certain ethnic groups, or strong environmental and cultural influences facilitating transmission. In Japan, where nationwide surveys were carried out in early 1980, the prevalence rate in blood donors varies from 0.1–1% in Central Japan to 2–10% in Kyushu island. Even in these islands, foci of higher prevalence were repeatedly observed.

In every HTLV-1 endemic area, a female preponderance has been observed starting around age 20–30 years. Prevalence increases with age, and eventually reaches 20–40% of the female population aged 60 and above in Okinawa island [15–19]. Such a female and age dependence may be the result either of the continual addition of infected individuals by sexual contacts, or a cohort effect, which seems possible in Japan, or else the existence of immuno-silent viral infection in a large proportion of the population with an age-dependant natural immunodeficiency leading to viral reactivation.

Table 13.2 Diseases associated with HTLV-1 infection. The strength of association is based on epidemiological studies as well as molecular data, animal models and intervention trials

Disease	Association
Adult	
Adult T-cell leukemia/lymphoma	++++
Tropical spastic paraparesis/HTLV-1-associated myelopathy	++++
Intermediate uveitis (frequent in Japan)	+++
Infective dermatitis (rare)	+++
Polymyositis	++
HTLV-1-associated arthritis	++
Pulmonary infiltrative pneumonitis	++
Invasive cervical cancer	+
Small cell carcinoma of lung	+
Sjögren's disease	+
Childhood	
Infective dermatitis (frequent in Jamaica)	++++
Tropical spastic paraparesis/HTLV-1-associated myelopathy (rare)	++++
Adult T-cell leukemia/lymphoma (very rare)	++++
Persistent lymphadenopathy	++

++++, proven association; +++, probable association; ++, likely association; +, possible association.
Adapted from Blattner [18].

In every endemic area, the two major diseases associated with HTLV-1, namely ATLL and TSP/HAM (Table 13.2) are both present, but with significant differences in incidence and prevalence. While the incidence of ATLL exhibits minor variations (1–5 per 100 000 per year) in high HTLV-1 endemic areas (including Japan, the Caribbean area and South America) [20–23], the incidence of TSP/HAM seems to be high in the Caribbean islands and in some countries of South America and low in Japan [15,18].

Three modes of infection are recognized for HTLV-1. Mother to child transmission appears to be a major mode in endemic areas with a transmission rate of 10–20% [24–26]. Thus, postnatal infection by HTLV-1 is predominantly through breast feeding (milk lymphocytes contain HTLV-1 provirus), after the decline of the protective immunoglobulin G (IgG) maternal antibody around 6–9 months after birth. Advice to HTLV-1-seropositive mothers in Japan not to breast feed their babies led to a significant decrease in mother to child transmission of the virus, but with variable results in different areas, for unknown reasons [24–26].

Since the risk of developing ATLL late in life seems linked to infection early in life, i.e., through mother to child transmission, it is important to avoid such transmission. The excess of non-Hodgkin's T-cell lymphomas (NHL) in Caribbean adults, especially in Jamaica, appears to be directly related to HTLV-1, and specifically to early infection [18–22]. Prevention of vertical transmission could therefore result in a 70–80% reduction in NHL among adults in these areas.

The second most important mode of transmission for HTLV-1 is the sexual route [15,17,18]. Studies in Japan clearly showed a much higher efficiency of transmission from male to female than from female to male [17]. Such differences could account for the HTLV-1 female prevalence increasing with age, but observations in African prostitutes indicate a low sexual transmission rate of HTLV-1, as compared to HIV.

The intravenous route of infection, either by blood or by needle sharing, appears to be the most efficient mode of transmission with a 15–60% risk of infection for persons transfused with contaminated blood products [27,28]. Infection via blood carries a much higher risk of developing TSP/HAM (see below) than does vertical transmission [29]. In Japan and in Martinique, up to 20% of TSP/HAM patients have had a blood transfusion in the previous 5 years. We reported the first evidence for a causal relationship in describing a seronegative cardiac graft recipient who became HTLV-1-seropositive 14 weeks after an HTLV-1-positive blood transfusion, and 4 weeks later exhibited a severe pyramidal tract syndrome

identical to TSP/HAM. HTLV-1 was isolated from the cerebrospinal fluid (CSF). In contrast, the development of ATLL after HTLV-1 contamination by blood transfusion seems extremely rare, if it exists at all [30]. Screening of blood donations was implemented in Japan in 1986, in the French Caribbean in 1989, in the USA in 1989 [27,28], in Canada in 1990, in France in 1991, and in Denmark and the Netherlands in 1994.

HTLV-2 is highly endemic in some Indian tribes living in North, Central and South America, and is becoming endemic among American and European intravenous drug users (IVDU). The preferential transmission of HTLV-2 rather than HTLV-1 among IVDU is unexplained. The risk of an epidemic in the general population from this reservoir exists and preventive measures may need to be considered. In the US IVDU population, between 1% and 30% of IVDU were infected with HTLV-2 in 1993. In Europe, between 1% and 5% of the IVDU are HTLV-2-seropositive in Italy and in Spain, but HTLV-2 is quite rare in other European countries, although it is slowly spreading in this high-risk population.

Hematological manifestations of HTLV-1 infection: ATLL

ATLL is a lymphoproliferation of T-cells, mostly CD4-activated T-cells, characterized by clonal integration (complete or defective) of HTLV-1 provirus(es) in the tumor cells. Present in every HTLV-1 endemic area, ATLL has a wide range of clinical presentations, sometimes making the diagnosis difficult at the onset of the disease.

EPIDEMIOLOGY

ATLL was first discovered and reported by Takatsuki et al. in 1977 in Japan [4], where it has a high incidence in South Western regions of the country [16,17,31,32]. It was subsequently recognized in Caribbean immigrants living in United Kingdom by Catowski et al. in 1982 [32] and was later found to be present in most of the HTLV-1 endemic areas including intertropical Africa, South and Central America and Iran [33–39]. Sporadic cases of ATLL have also been described in areas of low HTLV-1 endemicity such as Europe and the USA, mostly in immigrant patients originating from high HTLV-1 endemic regions. Nationwide studies in Japan revealed that 50% of ATLL patients were from Kyushyu and 25% from large metropolitan areas [16,17,31]. However, 80% of the latter had been born in Kyushyu. The sex ratio (male/female) is around 1.4 in Japan. Age- and sex-specific incidence rates of ATLL in Japan show a steep increase with age after 40, reaching a plateau at the age of 50 in males but continuing to increase in females up to the age of 70. The average age of ATLL patients in Japan is 57 years [16,17,31], while in the Caribbean and in Africa the mean age at ATLL onset is around 40–45 years (Table 13.3) [32], suggesting the presence of yet unknown cofactors in the pathogenesis of this disease in different environmental and cultural areas. In Japan, the average annual case rate of ATLL and the number of HTLV-1 carriers have been estimated at 700 and 1.2 million, respectively, giving an estimated yearly incidence rate of ATLL in the range of 0.6–1.5 per 1000 adult HTLV-1 carriers aged 30–40. In Jamaica, the estimated incidence rate was similar [22]. The cumulative lifetime risk of ATLL among carriers was calculated to be in the range of 1–5% in both sexes in Japan and Jamaica. A higher incidence was observed in the noir marron population in French Guyana [33].

Recent studies performed in Brazil [34,37], Gabon [35] and French Guyana [33] demonstrated that the prevalence of ATLL is greatly underestimated until a specific search for the disease is performed. This is mainly due to the acuteness and rapid evolution of the disease, but also to the fact that patients die before a diagnosis can be made, and to confusion of ATLL with pathologically similar diseases [40], such as Sézary syndrome, mycosis fungoides or other types of NHL [34]. Furthermore, HTLV-1 serological confirmatory tests such as Western blot and/or molecular investigations are not readily available in most tropical countries in which HTLV-1 is endemic.

DIAGNOSIS AND CLASSIFICATION OF ATLL

The diagnostic criteria for HTLV-1-associated ATLL have been defined by Takatsuki et al. [41,42] and Shimoyama [43,44] (Table 13.4). These are: (1) a histologically and/or cytologically proven lymphoid malignancy with T-cell surface antigens (usually CD2, CD3 and CD4 positive); (2) abnormal T-lymphocytes present in the peripheral blood (not present in the lymphoma type), including not only typical ATLL cells, the so-called 'flower' cells (Figure 13.2), but also small, mature T-lymphocytes with incised or lobulated nuclei, which are characteristic of the chronic or smoldering type of disease; and (3) specific antibodies to HTLV-1 detected in the sera at diagnosis. The main clinical features of ATLL are summarized in Table 13.3.

Table 13.3 Main clinical features of ATLL

	Japan*	Caribbean†
Age at onset	58 years (range 27–82)	47 years
Sex ratio male/female	1.4	0.6
Lymphadenopathy	60%	70%
Hepatomegaly	26%	27%
Splenomegaly	22%	31%
Specific skin lesion	39%	41%
Hypercalcemia	32%	51%

* From Takatsuki [41,42], based on a series of 187 patients.
† Matutes and Catovsky [32] on a series of 57 patients seen in the United Kingdom with 46 of Caribbean origin.

Because of the diversity of the clinical presentations, and the evolution of the disease, a classification of ATLL into four major subtypes has been recently proposed by Shimoyama and the members of the lymphoma study group in Japan [43] (Tables 13.4 and 13.5). The main features of these four groups, which include a smoldering type, a chronic type, a lymphoma type and an acute type, are summarized in Table 13.4. Both chronic and smoldering types can evolve into an acute form of leukemia or lymphoma following a progressive acceleration of the clinical picture [44,45]. This classification is very useful in discriminating ATLL from other types of lymphomas or leukemias (other non-Hodgkin's lymphomas, or cutaneous T-cell lymphomas). An accurate classification of the ATLL subtype is critical to making therapeutic decisions because, based on Japanese studies, patients with the smoldering type and about 30% of those with chronic ATLL have a relatively good prognosis, even without chemotherapy [43,44]. A new classification of the clinical stages of ATLL, which is relevant to the prognosis of the disease, has been proposed recently by Shiroro et al. [46]. This is based on the expression of Ki-67 antigen in the peripheral blood T-lymphocytes. Aggressive ATLL (with death occurring within one year and a mean survival of 105 days) is defined by the presence of greater than 18% Ki-67-positive peripheral blood T-lymphocytes. Stable ATLL (with a mean survival of 750 days) is defined by a percentage of Ki-67-positive T-cells less than 18%. Criteria for determining the diagnosis of ATLL for epidemiological studies have also been proposed recently by Levine et al. [47] (Table 13.6). This would greatly help the comparison of the epidemiological characteristics of ATLL in the Caribbean, Central and South America and tropical Africa.

Table 13.4 Diagnostic criteria for clinical subtypes of HTLV-1-associated ATLL

	Smoldering	Chronic	Lymphoma	Acute
Anti-HTLV-1 antibody	+	+	+	+
Lymphocyte ($\times 10^3/\mu$l)	<4	≥4‡	<4	*
Abnormal T-lymphocytes	≥5%¶	+§	≤1%	+§
Flower cells of T-cell marker	†≤	†	No	+
LDH	≤1.5N	≤2N	*	*
Corrected Ca (mEq/l)	<5.5	<5.5	*	*
Histology-proven lymphadenopathy	No	*	+	*
Tumor lesion				
Skin and/or lung	*¶	*	*	*
Lymph node	No	*	Yes	*
Liver	No	*	*	*
Spleen	No	*	*	*
Central nervous system	No	No	*	*
Bone	No	No	*	*
Ascites	No	No	*	*
Pleural effusion	No	No	*	*
Gastrointestinal tract	No	No	*	*

N, normal upper limit.
* No essential qualification except terms required for other subtype(s).
† Typical flower cells seen occasionally.
‡ Accompanied by T-lymphoctosis ($3.5\times10^3/\mu$l or more).
§ If abnormal T-lymphocytes are less than 5% in peripheral blood, histology-proven tumor lesion is required.
¶ Histology-proven skin and/or pulmonary lesion(s) is required if abnormal T-lymphocytes are less than 5% in peripheral blood.

Adapted with permission from Shimoyama [43,44].

CYTOLOGICAL, IMMUNO-VIROLOGICAL AND MOLECULAR FEATURES OF ATLL

All ATLL are, by definition, associated with HTLV-1, the patients being HTLV-1-seropositive by Western blot (Table 13.5). Particle agglutination, ELISA and immunofluorescence can also be used to titrate these antibodies. The cytological aspects of ATLL [32, 41,42,48] cells vary according to the subtype: in the typical acute leukemia subtype, most of the abnormal lymphoid cells exhibit multilobulated nuclei (flower cells) as seen in Figure 13.2. In terminal crisis, the cells often vary greatly in size (between 10 and 40 μm) as well as with respect to the degree of cytoplasmic basophilia and nuclear lobulation (which is more marked) [48]. Some cells may resemble Sézary cells. In more chronic ATLL, cells are generally small and uniform with minor nuclear abnormalities, such as indentation or convolutions, while in smoldering cases the ATLL cells are often relatively large with a bi- or trifoliate nucleus [41,42].

In typical cases [41,42,49,50], ATLL cells express the immunophenotypic characteristics of mature T-cells of helper/inducer phenotype (CD2+, CD3+, CD4+, CD7−, CD8−) with activation markers (CD25+, HLA, DP+, DQ+, DR+). Double negative ATLL cells (CD4−, CD8−) are exceptional [51]. A characteristic feature is a decrease in CD3/T-cell receptor expression on the ATLL cell surface. Antigenic stimulation of ATLL cells *in vitro* results in a downregulation of the CD3/TCR complex, suggesting that antigenic stimulation plays a pathogenetic role in ATLL [51].

Lymph-node histology usually shows an infiltration by medium and large T-cells with irregular nuclei, which efface the nodal architecture, a pattern consistent with the diagnosis of pleomorphic large T-cell lymphoma [45]. However, there is no specific histological pattern for ATLL [32,34].

The cytogenetic abnormalities found in ATLL are not specific, but are more frequent in acute and lymphoma types than in the chronic or smoldering type [52–53]. They include various karyotypic abnormalities of chromosome 14, especially translocations involving 14q32 and 14q11, and deletion of 6q, but numerical abnormalities such as trisomy of 3,7 and 21 have been described.

Mutations in the p53 tumor suppressor gene have been detected in 30% of ATLL patients, mostly in

Table 13.5 Biological features of HTLV-1-associated syndromes

| | ATLL | | | | |
	Leukemic form	'Smoldering' form	TSP/HAM	Intermediate state	Healthy carriers
Lymphocytosis/mm³	10^4–5×10^5	Normal	Normal	Normal	Normal
ATLL cells (%)	10–99	0.5–5.0	0–20	0–2	Absent – rare
CD4/CD8 ratio	↑++	↑±	↑+	Normal	Normal
CD25 (TAC) +ve cells	↑++	↑±	↑+	↑±	Normal
HLA.DR, DP, DQ +ve cells	↑++	↑±	↑++	↑±	Normal
Hypercalcemia (% of cases)	50	—	—	—	—
Specific cutaneous lesions	Frequent	Very frequent	Absent	Absent	Absent
Immunodeficiency	++	+	+	+	±
Clinical severity	++	+	++	±	–
Anti-HTLV-1 antibodies					
Serum	+	+	++ (high titer)	+	+
CSF	—	—	+	—	—
Intrathecal synthesis of IgG	—	—	+	—	—
CSF IgG oligoclonal bands	—	—	+	—	—
Soluble serum IL2 receptor	++++	+++	++	+	+
HTLV-1* proviral integration { Mode	Monoclonal	Monoclonal	Polyclonal†	Polyclonal	Nondetectable
Site	leukemic, lymph node Pleural, ascitic fluid cells	leukemic cells, cutaneous infiltrate	PBMCs	PBMCs	PBMCs
% of cases	100	100	85	100	0
PCR HTLV-1	+++	++	++	++	+
Viral load in PBMC		High	High	High	Low
T-Cell receptor (α, β, γ)	Clonal, rearranged	Clonal, rearranged	Non-rearranged	Non-rearranged	Non-rearranged

* Determined by Southern blot analysis.
† In 10–20% of cases a clonal integration of HTLV-1 is present in the PBMCs.
PBMCs, peripheral blood mononuclear cells.
PCR, polymerase chain reaction.

advanced cases, suggesting the involvement of p53 mutation in a late stage of leukemogenesis, or in tumor progression [54,55].

Using different sets of HTLV-1-specific primers, PCR permits the amplification of HTLV-1 proviruses from DNA extracted from tumor cells [56] (Table 13.5). These amplified products can be cloned and sequenced, permitting the determination of the viral genotype. However, PCR positivity does not prove that HTLV-1 has a causal role in ATLL. Since proviral DNA can be regularly amplified from peripheral blood mononuclear cells (PBMCs) of HTLV-1-seropositive individuals, it is highly probably that additional genetic changes are essential to the pathogenesis of ATLL. The demonstration by Southern blot analysis, using EcoRI and/or PstI digestion to detect clonal integration of HTLV-1 provirus in the tumor cells (from leukemic cell, lymph nodes, skin infiltrate, pleural or ascitic fluid) provides

the best means of defining ATLL [57–61] (Figure 13.3a,b). These proviruses are defective in 5–20% of cases (a band of less than 9 kb is detected on Southern blot), but the pX region is always conserved (the deletion occurs mainly in gag, pol, and/or env sequences). These data strongly suggest that the pX region plays a critical role in leukemogenesis [5, 62]. Recent studies demonstrate, however, that HTLV-1 monoclonality is not synonymous with malignant proliferation [63–66]: by Southern blot analysis 10–20% of TSP/HAM exhibit a clonal integration of HTLV-1 in their PBMCs [63]. Furthermore monoclonal or oligoclonal proliferation of T-cells infected by HTLV-1 can be detected by sensitive PCR techniques (inverse PCR) in most TSP/HAM and healthy seropositive carriers [65,66]. The detection of clonal (but not malignant) proliferation of HTLV-1-infected cells could prove useful in following high-risk groups and could also be used to

Table 13.6 Registry criteria for definition of ATLL

Definition of ATLL	
Clinical/routine laboratory criteria	
Hypercalcemia	1 point
Skin lesions*	1 point
Leukemic phase†	1 point
Research laboratory criteria	
T-Cell lymphoma or leukemia	2 points
HTLV-1 antibody	2 points
TAC-positive tumor cells	1 point
HTLV-1-positive tumors‡	2 points
ATLL classification	
Classical	≥3–7 points
Probable	5 or 6 points
Possible	3 or 4 points
Inconsistent with ATLL	<3 points
Exclusion criteria	
B-Cell positivity, nodular or follicular lymphoma lymphoblastic lymphoma, small lymphocytic lymphoma	

* Lymphomatous cells documented morphologically.
† More than 2% abnormal lymphocytes.
‡ Determined by PCR or Southern blot analysis of the DNA of tumoral cells and indicating a monoclonal integration of HTLV-1 provirus(es).

Adapted from Levine [47].

detect residual ATLL cells in the bone marrow after transplantation [65]. Worth noting here, some studies indicated that or three copies of HTLV-1 provirus, rather than a single copy per cell, were in a small proportion of patients with ATLL [57–59]. Other unusual patterns have been observed. For example, in a recent study performed on 89 ATLL

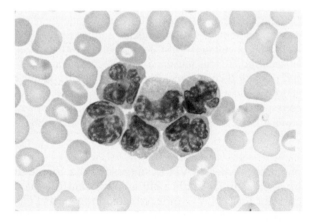

Figure 13.2 Peripheral blood smear from a Caribbean ATLL leukemic patient showing a cluster of atypical lymphoid cells with multilobulated nuclei (May Grunwald Giemsa).

cases [67], a single clear band greater than 9 kb was detected in Southern blots from 83 patients, while 'unusual' integration patterns of HTLV-1 proviral DNA were detected in six patients: three showed two bands and three exhibited one band smaller than 9 kb. The patients with such 'unusual' integration pattern had clinical characteristics different from those of the other 83 patients. Thus, viral integration patterns may be related to the heterogeneous clinical behavior of this disease [67].

MAIN CLINICAL FEATURES AND COMPLICATIONS

Hypercalcemia

Hypercalcemia is a very frequent and quite specific biological feature of ATLL with a prevalence of 20–30% at admission and of more than 50% at some time in the clinical course [41,42,68,69] (Table 13.5). Hypercalcemia may be mediated by the parathyroid hormone-related protein (PTHrP) in conjunction with IL-1 and TGFβ. Interestingly, the tax protein has been shown to transactivate the PTHrP gene, providing a possible pathway whereby the virus may mediate this effect [70].

Cutaneous lesions

Skin infiltration by specific lymphoid tumor cells clonally infected by HTLV-1 represents a frequent clinical feature of ATLL, being present in 20–40% of all ATLL types and in more than 50% of smoldering types [41,42,71] (Table 13.5). Various cutaneous lesions have been described including papules, nodules, erythroderma, plaques, tumors and ulcerative lesions. ATLL cells densely infiltrate both dermis and epidermis forming Pautrier's microabscesses [72,73] (Figures 13.4 and 13.5). When skin lesions dominate the clinical picture, the disease is often refered to as cutaneous ATLL [71]. In such cases, clinicopathological differentiation of these lesions from other cutaneous T-cell lymphomas (CTCL) might be difficult and requires molecular studies to detect the presence of viral sequences [72,73] (Figure 13.3).

Infectious complications

HTLV-1 induces a mild T-cell immune deficiency state and opportunistic infections have been reported in HTLV-1-seropositive carriers not suffering from ATLL [15–18]. Infestation by *Strongyloides stercoralis* is quite frequent in HTLV-1-seropositive carriers and *S. stercoralis*-infected individuals are

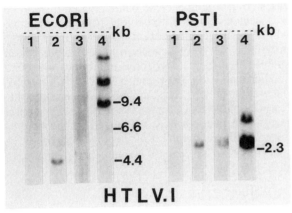

(a)

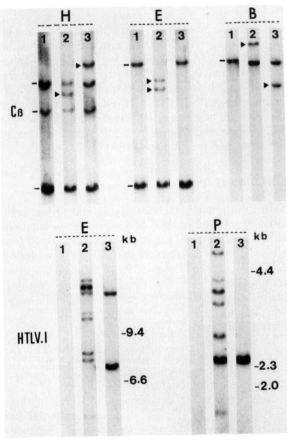

(b)

Figure 13.3 (a) Southern blot analysis. High molecular weight DNA was extracted from control peripheral blood mononuclear cells (1), PBMC of an ATLL with a defective HTLV-I provirus (2), PBMC of a patient with skin tumor (3) and cutaneous tumor biopsy of the same patient (4). Because there is no one EcoRI site in HTLV-I provirus, the observation of three bands in lane 4 denotes a clonal integration of three proviral genomes in the DNA of the cutaneous lesions. Pst I digestion generates three internal bands; one of them (2.4 kb) can be detected with the HTLV-I probe used. This observation indicates a polyclonal integration of the HTLV-I provirus in the PBMC of this patient. (b) Southern blot analysis of DNA from uncultured PBMC. High molecular weight DNA was extracted from uncultured PBMC of a patient with an ATLL, digested with Hind III, EcoRI, BamH I and PstI restriction enzymes, and transferred to nylon filters using the method of Southern. Digests were analyzed under high stringency conditions using probes recognizing the constant regions of the T-cell receptor β-chain gene and the env region of HTLV-I genome. Left lane: uncultured PBMC from a healthy blood donor. Middle lane: HTLV-I-infected cell line, HUT 102. Right lane: uncultured PMNC from a patient with an acute leukemic adult T-cell leukemia. Top: Rearrangement of T-cell receptor β-chain gene. Bottom: clonal integration of HTLV-I provirus. Two distinct bands on EcoRI digests correspond to one complete and one defective copy of proviral DNA. B, BamH I; E, Ecor I; H, Hind III; P, PstI.

often infected by HTLV-1 in highly endemic areas such as the Okinawa islands [76] and the Caribbean region [77]. This association could be explained either by HTLV-1-induced immunosuppression, allowing proliferation of *S. stercoralis,* or by the promotion of the growth of HTLV-1 by chronic *S. stercoralis* infestation. Numerous studies have shown the presence of *S. stercoralis* in acute or lym-

phomatous types of ATLL, suggesting that infection by *S. stercoralis* might play a significant role as a cofactor for HTLV-1-induced leukemogenesis [77]. Monoclonal integration of HTLV-1 proviral DNA has been found by Southern blot analysis in some patients with *S. stecoralis* infestation who do not have overt ATLL [78,79].

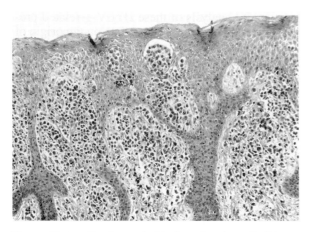

Figure 13.4 Histology of skin invasion in a Caribbean patient with a cutaneous ATLL showing an infiltration of the dermis and epidermis with presence of Pautrier abscess. These tumoral cells were CD2+, CD3+, CD4+, CD8– and CD25+.

DIFFERENTIAL DIAGNOSIS

In most cases, the clinical and biological diagnosis of ATLL can be made easily. However, the differential diagnosis between smoldering or chronic forms of ATLL, and other postthymic T-cell malignancies, including cutaneous T-cell lymphoma, may be difficult. In the case of cutaneous lesions, only molecular studies of biopsied tumor can separate HTLV-1-related malignancies from cutaneous lesions of other etiologies (which could well occur in HTLV-1-seropositive individuals [71–75]).

The histopathologic findings in ATLL may closely resemble those of cutaneous localizations of T-cell lymphomas unrelated to HTLV-1. Similarly, the presence of the T-cell activation antigens CD25, HLA-DR and HLA-DP can be found in some cases

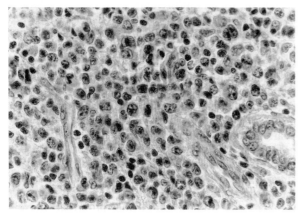

Figure 13.5 Diffuse infiltration of the dermis by medium-sized atypical lymphoid cells (original magnification, x 200).

of CTCL. Positive HTLV-1 serology, the presence of circulating ATLL-like cells, the detection of HTLV-1 by a PCR test performed on PBMC and/or tumor cell DNA, together with the release of viral particles by cultured PBMC expressing HTLV-1 antigens, provide important evidence favoring a diagnosis of ATLL. Nevertheless, such findings do not prove a direct etiologic link between the virus and the cutaneous lesions manifested by the patients. Since these features can be seen in healthy seropositive individuals, and represent stigmata of an HTLV-1 viral infection, the only available evidence for a causal link between HTLV-1 and a T-cell tumoral proliferation is the demonstration of the clonal integration of a HTLV-1 provirus in the tumor cells of the skin infiltrate by Southern blot analysis [72,73]. Even this has its limitations, as described above.

According to Matutes and Catovsky [32], the only features that can be considered specific for ATLL are: hypercalcemia, the peripheral blood cell morphology and the presence of clonally integrated HTLV-1 in the neoplastic cells. Features such as skin and lymph node histology, immunological markers and certain chromosome abnormalities can be found in other T-cell leukemias or lymphomas and thus they do not distinguish them from ATLL [32,80].

THERAPEUTIC ASPECTS OF ATLL

ATLL remains, despite the employment of a number of treatment strategies, a lymphoid neoplasm with a very poor prognosis. In a Japanese study coordinated by Shimoyama, which included 818 ATLL cases, the median survival time was 9 months, with survival rate at 2 and 4 years being only 27% and 10%, respectively [44,81]. However, differences in survival rates among the subtypes are marked, 4-year survival being 66% for the smoldering type, 27% for the chronic type and 5–6% for the lymphoma and acute types [44,81,82]. Furthermore, spontaneous regression can very occasionally be observed in ATLL [83,84]. The major prognosis factors associated with a poor response and survival rates in ATLL are a high lactate dehydrogenase (LDH) value, high peripheral blood tumor cell counts (both reflecting a high tumor burden) and a poor clinical performance. The main obstacles to a good outcome of therapy are infectious complications (*Pneumocystis carinii*, *Cryptococcus* meningitis, disseminated *Herpes zoster*), hypercalcemia, and liver or kidney dysfunctions. Various strategies [44,81,85–87], including classical combination chemotherapy, the use of newer drugs (deoxycoformycin), leukocytopheresis, photochemotherapy, low-dose total body irradiation, interferon

mediated immunity directed against EBV-specific antigens expressed at the cell surface.

In the HTLV model, T-cell-mediated immunity, recognizing the env 99–109 epitope of the gp46 surface glycoprotein, is thought to control the circulating CD4 cells population infected by HTLV-1 [103–105] in a manner comparable to the EBV/B-cell model mentioned above.

A very early primary viral infection of babies through mother to child exchange of body fluids (saliva for EBV or breast milk for HTLV-1) [24,25] appears to be the most likely event that triggers development of a polyclonal proliferation of virally infected cells in an immunologically intact host. This step can be compared to that of 'initiation' in multistep chemical carcinogenesis.

The second critical step in ATLL pathogenesis was believed, until recently, to be linked to a monoclonal expansion of such 'immortalized' HTLV-1-infected CD4 cells. However, the confirmed observation of monoclonal integration of HTLV-1 provirus in PBMCs of TSP/HAM patients, and even in HTLV-1 healthy carriers [63,66] suggests that it is not the monoclonality of provirus integration, nor CD4 cell proliferation *per se* that is important but additional genetic changes that occur in the proliferating cells. The proliferating CD4 clones in HTLV-1-carrying individuals express both tax and rex, as well as env-encoded glycoproteins and IL-2α receptor at their surface. Subsequently, owing to internal control by rex of tax expression and to the T-cell-mediated immune control of proliferating cells [103–105], selection of silently infected clones takes place. In this context, the possibility that infected individuals remain seronegative should be considered.

Owing to a yet unknown cause, a second genetic event presumably takes place in some infected individuals, with decreased expression of IL-2 and increased expression of IL-2Rα at the surface of HTLV-1-infected emerging clones. This progressive autonomy is likely to be a critical step in the progress toward leukemia [5,103].

Molecular epidemiology of HTLV-1. Are there leukemogenic HTLV-1 strains?

After the discovery of TSP/HAM a question arose as to whether the same virus could induce two different diseases or whether, as in the case of murine leukemia viruses, specific mutations in structural and/or regulatory viral genes would direct HTLV-1 tissue tropism and pathogenesis.

Sequence analysis of the LTR and env gene of HTLV-1 isolated from TSP/HAM patients were found to be similar to the viruses isolated from ATLL patients or from healthy carriers [106–108], with, however, some slight nucleotide differences (mainly substitutions). Studies are currently underway to determine whether or not the TSP/HAM and ATLL viruses are functionally identical, or whether these slight differences reflect only intrastrain variability or variation in the geographical origin of these patients [102].

The use of PCR since 1988 has led to rapid progress in understanding the molecular epidemiology of HTLV-1. Furthermore, PCR represents a powerful tool to study directly the *ex vivo* genomic variability of HTLV-1 with the possibility of detecting a rare event in the genomic DNA of an infected individual without having to use cell culture, thus eliminating the possibility of an *in vitro* viral selection as demonstrated in the human immunodeficiency virus (HIV)/simian immunodeficiency virus (SIV) system. PCR is also an efficient way of searching for the presence of different viral strains within an individual at different times (intrastrain variability, quasi species), since multiple clones can be recognized by sequencing from a single amplified product. Another technique, well suited to molecular epidemiology, is a study of the restriction fragment length polymorphism (RFLP) of amplified PCR product. This technique has been applied in our laboratory to the study of the LTR in 180 HTLV specimens from various geographical areas, including ATLL, TSP/HAM patients or asymptomatic HTLV-1 healthy carriers [108]. This study showed the presence of 12 different RFLP profiles with five major molecular subtypes (Cosmopolitan, Central and Western African, Japanese and Melanesian) [108]. Thus, we and other groups have demonstrated without ambiguity that, while no mutation could be specifically linked to a specific hematological or neurological disorder, the nucleotidic changes observed in some genomic regions of the HTLV-1 provirus were specific to the geographical origin of the specimens [106–108].

Assuming similar mutation rates and constant selective forces among the different geographical HTLV-1 subtypes, the topology of the phylogenetic trees should reflect the duration of HTLV's evolution and the migrations of HTLV-infected populations in the recent and distant past [106,107]. Recently, the existence of five major molecular geographic subtypes has been confirmed by sequence analysis of the LTR (see Figure 13.6). The first, the cosmopolitan subtype, is the most homogenous HTLV-1 molecular strain. Its dissemination from a common ancestor

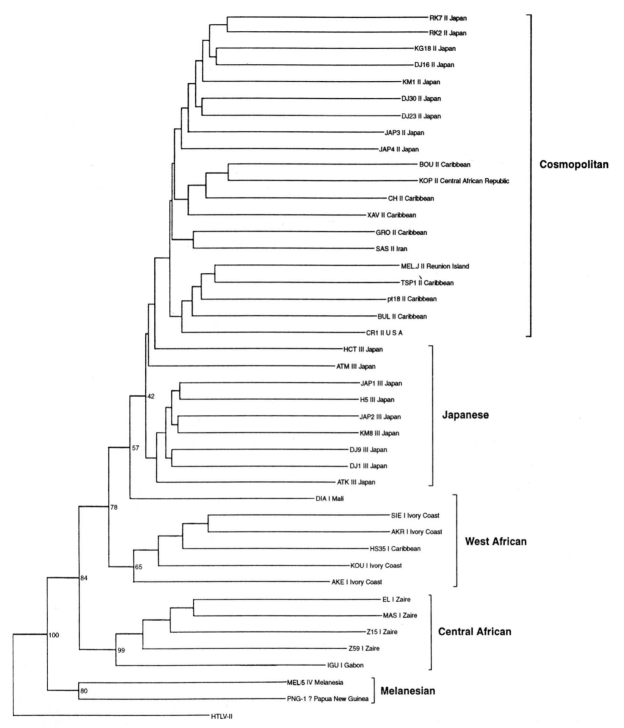

Figure 13.6 Phylogenetic tree obtained, after sequence alignment and bootstrapping, by the maximum parsimony method. The compared sequences correspond to a 315 base pairs fragment of the LTR region encompassing most of the U3 and the R region. The number indicated at some nodes represents their frequency of occurrence out of 100 trees and is therefore a measure of the robustness of the proposed tree. The length of the branches is not proportional to nucleotide substitutions. The topology of the tree demonstrates the existence of five molecular clusters of HTLV-I genotypes related to the geographical origin of the studied specimens and not to the disease of the patient (ATLL, TSP/HAM). Adapted from Ureta Vidal [108].

towards many regions of the world can be associated with recent migrations of HTLV-1-infected individuals, including involuntary displacement from Africa to the Americas (the slave trade). The second is the Japanese subtype, closely related to the cosmopolitan subtype and mainly found in Japan, but also present in few other places of Asia. The Japanese subtype is present in 75% of HTLV-1 carriers in Japan, the cosmopolitan subtype accounting for the remaining 25%, which is exclusively located in the southernmost Japanese islands. The third subtype is the West African subtype and the fourth, the Central African cluster. The latter exhibits a great diversity of HTLV-1 strains scattered among the different countries of Central Africa. This diversity may reflect genetic drift that has occurred over a long period of evolution in remote areas but is also probably a consequence of interspecies transmission among primates including the infection of humans by simian T-cell leukemia virus type 1 (STLV-1) [107,108]. The latter possibility has been recently suggested by the finding of a high degree of similarity (98%) between HTLV-1 present in individuals living in the Equatorial region of Zaire and some STLV-1 from chimpanzees [107,108]. The fifth subtype of HTLV-1 is represented by the Australo-Melanesian strain, which is molecularly quite distant from the four other subtypes. The presence of a distinct molecular variant of HTLV-1 in Papua–New Guineans, Solomon Islanders and Australian aboriginals has almost certainly resulted from genetic drift over several millennia occurring in remote populations, which migrated some 10000 to 40000 years ago from the Indo-Malay region [107]. Further molecular genetic studies from different isolated African and Amerindian populations, but also mongoloid populations from Asian regions including China, India and Siberia, will be crucial to the development of new insights into the origin and pathways of global dissemination of this human oncoretrovirus whose low degree of genetic drift *in vivo* may be a useful marker for charting the migrations of infected human populations in the recent or distant past [106–108].

Epidemiology, biology and clinical manifestation of HTLV-2 infection

HTLV-2, the second human oncoretrovirus, was isolated in 1982 from a T-cell line established from the splenic cells of a White American with a hairy cell leukemia of T-cell type [109,110]. A number of further isolates have been made from CD8 lymphoproliferative diseases, chronic myelopathies, intravenous drug abusers and healthy seropositive HTLV-2 carriers. This virus, now becoming epidemic in the intravenous drug abuser population (often also HIV-1 infected) of most American cities, is also being identified in some European countries, including the United Kingdom, Italy and Spain. Furthermore, the virus is naturally endemic in some Amerindian populations in which the HTLV-2 seroprevalence can reach 50% [109]. From a molecular point of view, most of the available data relate to the American continent, and predominantly involve isolates from different Amerindian groups and intravenous drug abusers. These recent studies have clearly demonstrated the existence of two molecular subtypes (called A and B) with a nucleotide divergence of 4–7%, depending on the gene studied. In contrast to HTLV-1, molecular clusters related to the geographical origin of the specimens have not been observed. It is worth noting that in all except one case, HTLV-2 associated with a clinical disease has always been subtype A.

The origin and the routes of the worldwide dissemination of the human and simian T-cell lymphotropic oncoretroviruses (HTLV-1, HTLV-2 and STLV-1) remain a matter of active research and debate. Based on epidemiological and phylogenetic analysis, HTLV-1 and STLV-1 can be considered as 'Old World' viruses, present in Africa and Asia, probably for millennia, whereas HTLV-2, endemic in some native Amerindian tribes, appears to be a 'New World' virus brought from Asia into the Americas by population migrations through the Bering Strait some 10000 to 40000 years ago. Recent serological evidence of sporadic infection with HTLV-2 A and B in West Africa, Guinea, Ghana and Central Africa (Gabon, Cameroon and Zaire), raised the possibility that HTLV-2 has also been present in Africa over a long period of time. Imported infection, especially HTLV-2 A in prostitutes (in Cameroon, Zaire and Ghana) cannot be excluded, but familial clusters of genuine HTLV-2 B virus do exist in Central Africa [111].

In HIV/HTLV-2-co-infected individuals, HTLV-2 is mainly present in T-CD8 lymphocyte subpopulations [112] and there is often an overall increase of T-CD8 cells in such individuals [113]. Moreover, *in vitro* cultures of peripheral blood mononuclear cells of HTLV-2-seropositive individuals have led mainly to the establishment of CD8-expressing transformed T-cell lines. This preferential tropism is, however, not exclusive, since it has been demonstrated that HTLV-2 can infect other mononuclear T-CD4 lymphocytes *in vivo*.

A role for HTLV-2 has been suggested in rare

cases of cutaneous T-cell lymphomas and in some cases of T-CD8 lymphoproliferative disorders. However, whether or not the virus truly has a pathogenic role is unclear [109,110]. A review of the literature relating to the involvement of HTLV-2 in such diseases revealed that there are only five published cases where clear evidence of HTLV-2 infection (by specific serological and/or molecular means) has been demonstrated in CD8 lymphoproliferations. These patients, all originating from the USA, include a case of T-hairy cell leukemia [114], two cases of large granular leukemia [115–117] and two cases of Sézary-like diseases [118]. Furthermore, a critical study of these papers demonstrated that, in none of these cases, was the virus clonally integrated or even detected in the tumor cells. In the so-called T-hairy cell leukemia [114], the virus was oligoclonally integrated into CD8 cells while the clonal tumor cells, which were free of viral infection (negative by Southern blot), were of B-cell type (as in the vast majority of hairy cell leukemias). In one of the two cases of large granular lymphocyte leukemia (LGL), HTLV-2 provirus was detected in the normal CD3+, CD8+ cells, but not in neoplastic large granular lymphocytes of natural killer (NK) phenotype (CD3 and CD 18+), which were free of virus (PCR negative) [117]. In the second case, HTLV-2 was only detected in the DNA of a cell lysate from paraffin-embedded slides of a bone marrow biopsy. In this last patient, who had a clonal proliferation of CD3+, CD8+, CD57+ cells, it was not possible to ascertain the role of HTLV-2 in the pathogenesis of the disease [115,116]. Finally, in the two remaining patients, with MF or Sézary-like syndrome, in whom clonal proliferation was not demonstrated, a search for the presence of HTLV-2 in the tumor cells (by PCR and /or Southern blot) was not performed [118]. Thus, in contrast to HTLV-1, whose etiological role in ATLL is now well established, there is currently neither serological nor molecular evidence that HTLV-2 is etiologically associated with any malignant lympoproliferative disease [112,113,116].

The study of leukemogenic retroviruses requires collaboration between molecular biologists, clinicians and epidemiologists, and long-term prospective studies involving multicenter cohorts of infected individuals, would be necessary to characterize a high-risk biological profile for ATLL, or for that matter for TSP/HAM, among HTLV-1-infected individuals. If this could be accomplished, preventive interventions or preclinical therapies could be envisaged. The development of a vaccine [119] must be pursued through the establishment of acceptable recombinant viral vaccines in proper experimental models, i.e., those in which ATLL and TSP/HAM types of syndromes can be obtained. Finally, the characterization of 'disease susceptibility genes'

is being actively pursued for HTLV-1-associated diseases.

A recent issue of *JAIDS and HR*, **13**, Supplement 1, 1996, provides several articles on the clinical aspects and the physiopathological mechanism of ATLL, giving some new insights into the pathogenicity of HTLV-1-associated diseases.

Acknowledgments

We thank Liliane Lozano and Monique Van Beveren for excellent editorial assistance.

References

1. Poiesz BJ, Ruscetti FW, Gazdar AF, et al. Detection and isolation of type-C retrovirus particles from fresh and cultured lymphocytes of a patient with cutaneous T-cell lymphoma. *Proc. Natl Acad. Sci. USA* 1980, **77**: 7145–7149.
2. Hinuma Y, Nagata K, Hanaoka M, et al. Adult T-cell leukemia: Antigen in an ATL cell line and detection of antibodies to the antigen in human sera. *Proc. Natl Acad. Sci. USA* 1981, **78**: 6476–6480.
3. Yoshida M, Miyoshi I, Hinuma Y. Isolation and characterization of retrovirus from cell lines of human adult T-cell leukemia and its implication in the disease. *Proc. Natl Acad. Sci. USA* 1982, **79**: 2031–2035.
4. Takatsuki K, Uchiayama T, Sagawa K, et al. Adult T-cell leukemia in Japan. In Seno S, Takaku S, Irino S (eds) *Topics in Hematology*. Amsterdam: Excerpta Medica, 1977, p. 73.
5. Yoshida M, Seiki M. Molecular biology of HTLV-I. Biological significance of viral genes in its replication and leukemogenesis. In Gallo RC, Wong-Staal F (eds) *Retrovirus Biology and Human Disease*. New York, Basel: Marcel Dekker, Inc., 1990, pp. 161–186.
6. Cann AJ, Chen SY. Human T-cell leukemia virus types I and II. In Fields BN, Knipe DM, Chanock RM, et al. (eds) *Virology* New York: Raven Press, 1990, pp. 1501–1527.
7. Smith MR, Greene WC. Molecular biology of the type I human T-cell leukemia virus (HTLV-I) and adult T-cell leukemia. *J. Clin. Invest.* 1991, **87**: 761–766.
8. Seiki M, Hattori S, Hirayama Y, et al. Human adult T-cell leukemia virus: Complete nucleotide sequence of the provirus genome integrated in leukemia cell DNA. *Proc. Natl Acad. Sci. USA* 1983, **80**: 3618–3622.
9. Koralnik IJ. Structure of HTLV-I. In *HTLV-I* edited by Hölsberg P and Hafler D. John Wiley and Sons 1996, pp. 65–78.

10. Berneman ZN, Gartenhaus RB, Reitz MS Jr, et al. Expression of alternatively spliced human T-lymphotropic virus type I pX mRNA in infected cell lines and in primary uncultured cells from patients with adult T-cell leukemia/lymphoma and healthy carriers. *Proc. Natl Acad. Sci. USA* 1992, **89**: 3005–3009.

11. Koralnik IJ, Gessain A, Klotman ME, et al. Protein isoforms encoded by the pX region of human T-cell leukemia: Lymphotropic virus type I. *Proc. Natl Acad. Sci. USA* 1992, **89**: 8813–8817.

12. Franchini G, Mulloy JC, Koralnik IJ, et al. The human T-cell leukemia/lymphotropic virus type I p12^{I} protein cooperates with the E5 oncoprotein of bovine papillomavirus in cell transformation and binds the 16 KDa subunit of vacuolar H+ ATPase. *J. Virol.* 1993, **67**: 7701–7704.

12a. Koralnik IJ, Mulloy JC, Andresson T, et al. Mapping of the intermolecular association of human T cell leukaemia/lymphotropic virus type I p121 and the vacuolar H+-ATPase 16 kDa subunit protein. *J. Gen. Virol.* 1995, **76**: 1909–1916.

13. Chen YA, Sankale JL. Other human retroviruses. In Kanki PJ, Kalengayi MR (eds) *AIDS in Africa.* New York: Raven Press, 1994, pp. 67–95.

14. Hjelle B. Human T-cell leukemia/lymphoma viruses. Life cycle, pathogenicity, epidemiology, and diagnosis. *Arch. Pathol. Lab. Med.* 1991, **115**: 440–450.

15. Mueller N. The epidemiology of HTLV-I infection. *Cancer Causes Control* 1991, **2**: 37–52.

16. Tajima K. The T and B-cell malignacy study group and coauthors. The 4th nationwide study of adult T-cell leukemia/lymphoma (ATL) in Japan: Estimates of risk of ATL and its geographical and clinical features. *Int. J. Cancer* 1990, **45**: 237–243.

17. Tajima K, Inoue M, Takezaki T, et al. Ethno-epidemiology of ATLL in Japan with special reference to the Mongoloid dispersal. In Takatsuki K (ed.) *Adult T-Cell Leukemia.* Oxford: Oxford University Press, 1994, pp. 91–112.

18. Blattner WA and Gallo RC. Epidemiology of HTLV-I and HTLV-II infection. In Takatsuki K (ed.) *Adult T-Cell Leukaemia.* Oxford: Oxford University Press, 1994, pp. 45–90.

19. Meeting and Progress Report. Retroviruses and cancer: US–Japan clinico-epidemiological experiences held under the auspices of the US-Japan Bilateral Agreement. *Leukemia* 1994, **8**: 694–704.

20. Kondo T, Kono H, Miyamoto N, et al. Age- and sex-specific cumulative rate and risk of ATL for HTLV-I carriers. *Int. J. Cancer* 1989, **43**: 1061–1064.

21. Kamihira S, Yamada Y, Ikeda S, et al. Risk of adult T-cell leukemia developing in individuals with HTLV-I infection. *Leukemia Lymphoma* 1992, **6**: 437–439.

22. Murphy EL, Hanchard B, Figueroa JP. Modelling the risk of adult T-cell leukemia/lymphoma in persons infected with human T-lymphotropic virus type 1. *Int. J. Cancer* 1989, **43**: 250–253.

23. Kamihira S, Yamada Y, Ikeda S, et al. Risk of adult T-cell leukemia developing in individuals with HTLV-I infection. *Leukemia Lymphoma* 1992, **6**: 437–439.

24. Hino S. Maternal–infant transmission of HTLV-I: Implication for disease. In Blattner WA (ed.) *Human Retrovirology: HTLV.* New York: Raven Press, 1990, pp. 363–374.

25. Katamine S, Moriuchi R, Yamamoto T, et al. HTLV-I proviral DNA in umbilical cord blood of babies born to carrier mothers. *Lancet* 1994, **343**: 1326–1327.

26. Takahashi K, Takezaki T, Oki T, et al. Inhibitory effect of maternal antibody on mother-to-child transmission of human T-lymphotropic virus type I. *Int. J. Cancer* 1991, **49**: 673–677.

27. Williams AE, Fang CT, Slamon DJ et al. Seroprevalence and epidemiological correlates of HTLV-I infection in the US blood donors. *Science* 1988, **240**: 643.

28. Sandler SG, Fang CT, Williams AE. Human T-cell lymphotropic virus type I and II in Transfusion Medicine. *Transf. Med. Rev.* 1991, **5**: 93–107.

29. Gout O, Baulac M, Gessain A, et al. Rapid development of myelopathy after HTLV-I infection acquired by transfusion during cardiac transplantation. *N. Engl. J. Med.* 1990, **322**: 383–388.

30. Williams NP, Tsuda H, Yamaguchi K, et al. Blood transfusion induced opportunistic adult T cell leukemia/lymphoma after Hodgkin's disease. *Leukemia Lymphoma*, 1991, **5**: 435–439.

31. The T- and B-Cell Maligancy Study Group. The third nation-wide study on adult T-cell leukemia/lymphoma (ATL) in Japan: Characteristic patterns of HLA antigen and HTLV-I infection in ATL patients and their relatives. *Int. J. Cancer* 1988, **41**: 505–512.

32. Matutes E, Catovsky D. ATL of Caribbean origin. In Takatsuki K (ed.) *Adult T-Cell Leukemia,* Oxford: Oxford University Press, 1994, pp. 114–138.

33. Gerard Y, Lepere JF, Pradinaud R, et al. Clustering and clinical diversity of adult T-cell leukemia/lymphoma associated with HTLV-I in a remote black population of French Guiana. *Int. J. Cancer* 1995, **60**: 773–776.

34. Matutes E, Schulz T, Andrada Serpa MJ, et al. Report of the Second International Symposium on HTLV in Brazil. *Leukemia* 1994, **8**: 1092–1094.

35. Delaporte E, Klotz F, Peeters M, et al. Non-Hodgkin lymphoma in Gabon and its relation to HTLV-I. *Int. J. Cancer* 1993, **53**: 48–50.

36. Gessain K, Jouannelle A, Escarmant P, et al. HTLV antibodies in patients with non-Hodkin lymphomas in Martinique. *Lancet* 1984, **i**: 1183–1184.

37. Pombo de Oliveira MS, Matutes E, Famadas LC, et al. Adult T-cell leukemia/lymphoma in Brazil and its relation to HTLV-I. *Lancet* 1990, **336**: 987–990.

38. Blank A, Yamaguchi K, Blank M, et al. Six Colombian patients with adult T-cell leukemia/lymphoma. *Leukemia Lymphoma* 1993, **9**: 407–412.

39. Weinberg JB, Spiegel RA, Blazey DL, et al. Human T-cell lymphotropic virus I and adult T-cell leukemia: Report of a cluster in North Carolina. *Am. J Med.* 1988, **85**: 51–58.

40. Ratner L, Griffith RC, Marselle L, et al. A lymphoproliferative disorder caused by human T-lymphotropic virus type I. Demonstration of a continuum between acute and chronic adult T-cell leukemia/lymphoma. *Am. J. Med.* 1987, **83**: 953–958.

41. Takatsuki K, Matsuoka M, Yamaguchi K. ATL and HTLV-I related diseases. In Takatsuki K (ed.) *Adult*

T-Cell Leukemia, Oxford: Oxford University Press, 1994, pp. 1–27.

42. Takatsuki K, Yamaguchi K, Watanabe T, et al. Adult T-cell leukemia and HTLV-I related diseases. In Takatsuki K, Hinuma Y, Yoshida M (eds). *Advances in Adult T-Cell Leukemia and HTLV-I Research*. Tokyo: Japan Scientific Societies Press, Gann Monograph on Cancer Research 1992, Vol. 39, pp. 1–15.

43. Shimoyama BJH and members of the Lymphoma Study Group. Diagnostic criteria and classification of clinical subtypes of adult T-cell leukemia-lymphoma. *Br. J. Haematol.* 1991, **79**: 428–437.

44. Shimoyama M. Treatment of patients with adult T-cell leukemia–lymphoma: An overview. In Takatsuki K, Hinuma Y, Yoshida M (eds). *Advances in Adult T-Cell Leukemia and HTLV-I Research*. Tokyo: Japan Scientific Societies Press, Gann Monograph on Cancer Research 1992, Vol. 39, pp. 43–46.

45. Yamaguchi K, Yoshioka R, Kiyokawa T, et al. Lymphoma type adult T-cell leukemia – a clinicopathologic study of HTLV related T-cell type malignant lymphoma. *Hematol. Oncol.* 1986, **4**: 59–65.

46. Shirono K, Hattori T, Takatsuki K. A new classification of clinical stages of adult T-cell leukemia based on prognosis of the disease. *Leukemia* 1994, **8**: 1834–1837.

47. Levine PH, Cleghorn F, Manns A, et al. Adult T-cell leukemia/lymphoma: A working point-score classification for epidemiological studies. *Int. J. Cancer* 1994, **59**: 491–493.

48. Kamihira S. Hemato-cytological aspects of adult T-cell leukemia. In Takatsuki K, Hinuma Y, Yoshida M (eds). Advances in Adult T-Cell Leukemia and HTLV-I Research. Tokyo: Japan Scientific Societies Press, Gann Monograph on Cancer Research 1992, Vol. 39, pp. 17–32.

49. Shirono K, Hattori T, Hata H, et al. Profiles of expression of activated cell antigens on peripheral blood and lymph node cells from different clinical states of adult T-cell leukemia. *Blood* 1989, **73**: 1664–1671.

50. Uchiyama T, Ishikawa T, Kondo A, et al. Pathophysiology of ATL cells: Cell growth characteristics. In Takatsuki K (ed.) *Adult T-Cell Leukemia*. Oxford: Oxford University Press, 1994, pp. 181–203.

51. Suzushima H, Asou N, Nishimura S, et al. Double-negative (CD4⁻, CD8⁻) T cells from adult T-cell leukemia patients also have poor expression of the T-cell receptor ab/CD3 complex. *Blood* 1993, **81**: 1032–1039.

52. Shimoyama M, Sakurai M, Kamada N. Chromosomal aberrations in adult T-cell leukemia–lymphoma: Summary of a Karyotype Review Committeee Report. In Takatsuki K, Hinuma Y, Yoshida M (eds) *Advances in Adult T-Cell Leukemia and HTLV-I Research*. Tokyo: Japan Scientific Societies Press, Gann Monograph on Cancer Research 1992, Vol. 39, pp. 95–105.

53. Maruyama K, Fukushima T, Kawamura K, et al. Chromosome and gene rearrangements in immortalized human lymphocytes infected with human T-lymphotropic virus type I. *Cancer Res.* 1990, **50**: 56975–57025.

54. Cesarman E, Chadburn A, Inghirami G, et al. Structural and functional analysis of oncogenes and tumor suppressor genes in adult T-cell leukemia/lymphoma shows frequent p53 mutations. *Blood* 1992, **80**: 3205–3216.

55. Sakashita A, Hattori T, Miller C, et al. Mutations of the p53 gene in adult T-cell leukemia. *Blood* 1992, **79**: 477–480.

56. Chadburn A, Athan E, Wieczorek R et al. Detection and characterization of human T-cell lymphotropic virus type I (HTLV-I) associated T-cell neoplasms in an HTLV-I nonendemic region by polymerase chain reaction. *Blood* 1991, **77**: 2419–2430.

57. Wong-Staal F, Hahn B, Manzari V, et al. A survey of human leukemias for sequences of a human retrovirus. *Nature* 1983, **302**: 626–628.

58. Yoshida M, Seiki M, Yamaguchi K, et al. Monoclonal integration of human T-cell leukemia provirus in all primary tumors of adult T-cell leukemia suggests causative role of human T-cell leukemia virus in the disease. *Proc. Natl Acad. Sci. USA* 1984, **81**: 2534–2537.

59. Yamaguchi K, Seiki M, Yoshida M, et al. The detection of human T-cell leukemia virus proviral DNA and its application for classification and diagnosis of T-cell malignancy. *Blood* 1984, **63**: 1235–1240.

60. Tanaka T, Takahashi K, Ideyama S, et al. Demonstration of clonal proliferation of T lymphocytes in early neoplastic disease. Studies with probes for the b-chain of the T-cell receptor and human T-cell lymphotropic virus type I. *J. Am. Acad. Dermatol.* 1989, **21**: 218–223.

61. Clark JW, Gurgo C, Franchini G, et al. Molecular epidemiology of HTLV-I associated non-Hodgkin's lymphomas in Jamaica. *Cancer* 1988, **61**: 1477–1482.

62. Korber B, Okayama A, Donnelly R, et al. Polymerase chain reaction analysis of defective human T-cell leukemia virus type I proviral genomes in leukemic cells of patients with adult T-cell leukemia. *J. Virol.* 1991, **65**: 5471–5476.

63. Furukawa Y, Fujisawa J, Osame M, et al. Frequent clonal proliferation of human T-cell leukemia virus type 1 (HTLV-1)-infected T-cells in HTLV-1-associated myelopathy (HAM-TSP). *Blood* 1992, **80**: 1012–1016.

64. Yamaguchi K, Kiyokawa T, Nakada K, et al. Polyclonal integration of HTLV-I proviral DNA in lymphocytes from HTLV-I seropositive individuals: An intermediate state between the healthy carrier state and smouldering ATL. *Br. J. Haematol.* 1988, **68**: 169–174.

65. Takemoto S, Matsuoka M, Yamaguchi, et al. A novel diagnostic method of adult T-cell leukimia: Monoclonal integration of human T-cell lymphotropic virus type I provirus DNA detected by inverse polymerase chain reaction. *Blood* 1994, **84**: 3080–3085.

66. Wattel E, Vartanian JP, Pannetier C, et al. Clonal expansion of HTLV-I infected cells in asymptomatic and symptomatic carriers without malignancy. *J. Virol.* 1995, **69**: 2863–2868.

67. Shimamoto Y, Suga K, Shibata K, et al. Clinical importance of extraordinary integration patterns of

CHAPTER 14

Pathogenesis of the low-grade B-cell lymphomas

ANDREW D. ZELENETZ AND DAVID BRODEUR

Introduction

The non-Hodgkin's lymphomas (NHLs) comprise a wide range of tumors of the lymphoreticular system which have distinct histological appearances and have been divided by their natural history into three categories: low grade; intermediate grade; and high grade [1]. The low-grade lymphomas (LGLs) are characterized clinically as having a relatively indolent natural history with median survivals of 6–8 years, although there can be substantial variation among the subtypes (see Chapters 40 and 41). Furthermore, despite good clinical responses to therapy, LGLs typically recur and few, if any, patients are cured of their disease.

The Working Formulation (WF) [1] defines three histological subtypes of lymphoma as low grade: small lymphocytic lymphoma (SLL); follicular small cleaved cell lymphoma (FSCL); and follicular mixed small cleaved and large-cell lymphoma (FML). However, as a consequence of the widespread use of cytogenetic, molecular and immunocytochemical analyses, additional pathologically distinct forms of lymphoma have been described [1,2,3]. Several of these entities have natural histories similar to the LGLs included in the WF. Table 14.1 lists the most widely recognized forms of LGL, and some of the distinguishing immunocytochemical and molecular characteristics. This classification is similar to that proposed by the International Lymphoma Study Group [4]. In addition to the entities included in the WF, the LGLs include mantle cell lymphoma (MCL), mucosa-associated lymphoid tissue (MALT) lymphoma, monocytoid B-cell lymphoma (MBCL), cutaneous T-cell lymphoma (CTCL), and enteropathy-associated T-cell lymphoma (EATL). In this chapter, the biology and pathogenesis of the B-cell LGLs will be reviewed. Clinical presentations are included only insofar as they are illustrative of the biology of the tumors. For more in depth discussion as to the clinical course and treatment of these tumors, the reader is referred to Chapters 40, 42, 44 and 48 in this volume. A discussion of the pathogenesis of the T-cell lymphomas can be found in Chapter 17.

Follicular lymphoma

HISTOLOGY AND IMMUNOHISTOCHEMISTRY

Follicular lymphoma (FL) involves the effacement

Table 14.1 Salient characteristics of the low-grade lymphomas*

Pathology	Immunocytochemistry	Molecular lesions
Small lymphocytic (SLL)	sIg+(weak), cIg±, CD5+, CD10−, CD23+, CD43+, CD11a+ [LFA-1]	
Small lymphocytic with plasmacytoid differentiation (SLL-PL)	cIg+, cIg+, CD5−, CD10−, CD23−, CD43±	t(9;14)(p13;q32)
Follicular (FL)	sIg+(strong), cIg−, CD5−, CD10+, CD23±, CD43−	t(14;18)(q32;q21), 90%
small cleaved cell (FSCL) mixed small cleaved and large cell (FML) large-cell lymphoma† (FLCL)		
Mantle cell lymphoma (MCL)	sIg+(moderate), cIg−, CD5+, CD10±, CD23−, CD43+	t(11;14)(q13;q32) >50%
Marginal zone B-cell lymphomas Mucosa-associated lymphoid tissue (MALT) Monocytoid B-cell lymphoma (MBCL)	sIg+, cIg+ (40%), CD5−, CD10− CD23−,CD43±	
Cutaneous T-cell (CTCL) Mycosis fungoides (MF) and Sézary syndrome (SS)	CD4+, CD7−	Variable
Enteropathy-associated T-cell lymphoma (EATL)	CD3+, CD7+, CD4−, CD8−, CD5−, MLA+	TCRβ clonally rearranged

* This table includes several forms of LGL not included in the WF [1] but share similar natural histories. This classification of the LGLs is similar to that proposed by the International Lymphoma Study Group [4]. The B-cell LGLs include SLL, SLL-PL, FL, MCL, MALT lymphoma and MBCL. These express the B-cell antigens CD19, CD20, CD22.
† In the WF [1], FLCL is categorized as an intermediate-grade lymphoma and is included here because of the molecular and immunophenotypic similarity to the other FLs.

of the normal lymph node architecture by irregular nodules composed of neoplastic cells [5]. The clonal cells within the nodules are B-cells that typically express a cell surface immunoglobulin (sIg), most commonly IgM (90%), CD10, CD19, CD20, CD22, and are CD5-negative [6]. FL is the malignant counterpart of the postmitotic centrocyte found in the germinal center (GC) [7–9]. In addition to the clonal cells, the neoplastic nodules are infiltrated by T-cells and the neoplastic B-cells are associated with follicular dendritic cells (FDCs), which appear to be responsible for the maintenance of the follicular architecture [10]. The FDCs in FL are immunopheno-typically similar to FDCs found in normal GCs [11]. The T-cells are polyclonal and are capable of regulating Ig production by the monoclonal B-cells [12]. Interaction of FL cells with FDCs in normal GCs and neoplastic follicles is mediated by the interaction of the β_1 integrin very late antigen-4 (VLA-4) expressed on the neoplastic B-cell and the vascular cell adhesion molecule-1 (VCAM-1) expressed on FDCs [13]. In contrast, intercellular adhesion molecule-1 (ICAM-1), another adhesion molecule expressed on FDCs which is involved in B-cell binding via interaction with lymphocyte function-associated antigen-1 (LFA-1) [14], is variably expressed in neoplastic follicles, although uniformly expressed in normal reactive germinal centers [15]. Subtypes of FL are categorized by the histologic appearance of the clonal B-cell population [1]. In the small cleaved cell variant (FSCL), this population is predominantly composed of small cells about the size of normal lymphocytes, which have angulated irregular nuclei containing condensed chromatin. The proliferative rate of these cells, as determined by expression of the Ki-67 antigen, is very low [16]. In the large-cell variant (follicular large-cell lymphhoma; FLCL), the neoplastic B-cells resemble the large cleaved cell or centroblasts seen in diffuse large-cell lymphomas. The chromatin is not condensed, there are discernible nucleoli and there are few small cleaved cells. The mixed-cell form of FL (FML) is composed of an admixture of the large and small cells with between five and 15 large cells per high-powered field. Despite criteria for distinguishing these subtypes of FL, there is significant interobserver and intraobserver variation [17].

THE t(14;18) CHROMOSOMAL TRANSLOCATION

Cytogenetic analysis has shown that a reciprocal translocation between chromosomes 14 and 18, t(14;18) (q32;q21), is common in FL [18]. This translocation results in the juxtaposition of the immunoglobulin heavy (IgH) chain joining segment (J$_H$) on chromosome 14 to a locus designated *bcl-2* (for *B-cell lymphoma*) on chromosome 18 [19–21] (Figure 14.1). The breakpoints on chromosome 18 cluster into two groups: the major breakpoint region (mbr), which accounts for approximately 65% of the breakpoints, and the minor cluster region (mcr), which accounts for 25% of the breakpoints [19–22]. Most of the remaining breakpoints map to the 30 kb region separating the mbr and mcr, although at least one breakpoint has been described distal to the mcr [23]. The t(14;18) translocation occurs with equal frequency in the three histologic subtypes of FL: FSCL, FML and FLCL. Translocations at the mbr result in the expression of the *bcl-2* gene as a fusion transcript with part of the IgH chain [19,21,24,25]. Cloning and sequencing of the cDNA for the *bcl-2/* IgH fusion transcript has demonstrated an open reading frame capable of encoding a 26 kD protein. As a consequence of the translocation, the intact

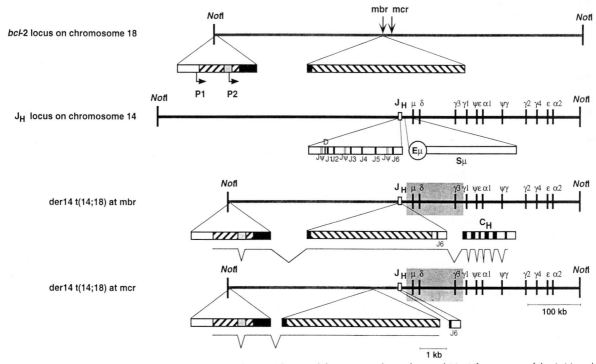

Figure 14.1 Physical and transcription maps of the germline and the expected translocated *Not*1 fragments of the IgH and *bcl-2* loci involved in the t(14;18) chromosomal translocation. The exploded regions of chromosome 18 represent the *bcl-2* gene: 5' untranslated (▨), first intron (▧), coding region (■), and 3' untranslated (◩). The exploded region of chromosome 14 details the structure of the J$_H$ segments. The shaded areas in the der(14) maps represent the typical extent of the interstitial deletion observed in roughly 90% of cases of follicular lymphoma (see text). The thin lines under the exploded regions of the der(14) maps indicated the *bcl-2* transcripts observed in the alternate breakpoint clusters: the major breakpoint region (mbr) and the minor cluster regions (mcr). The mbr is within the 3' noncoding region of the *bcl-2* gene resulting in the generation of a fusion transcript with the IgH locus. The mcr is approximately 30 kb downstream of the third exon and translocations in this cluster generate normal-length *bcl-2* transcripts. Translocations at both the mbr and mcr do not alter the coding region for the Bcl-2 protein. (Reproduced from Zelenetz et al. [30] with permission.)

coding region of the *bcl*-2 gene is markedly overexpressed [25,26].

The molecular anatomy of the der(14) and der(18) chromosomes has been examined in detail [27]. Random 'N' nucleotides are found at the junction between the *bcl*-2 gene and the J_H region on the der(14) chromosome. On the der(18) chromosome the region distal to the *bcl*-2 locus is juxtaposed to a IgH diversity gene element (D) again with interposed 'N' nucleotides. The finding of 'N' sequences at the chromosomal breakpoints, and the deletion of the region between the D element and the J_H segment, is reminiscent of the normal process of D–J_H rearrangement during early B-cell ontogeny. These findings suggest that the t(14;18) translocation occurs as an error of Ig gene rearrangement at the pro-B-cell stage of ontogeny.

Although the t(14;18) translocation appears to occur as an error during D–J_H recombination the molecular events remain uncertain. Analysis of the breakpoints in the mbr revealed that they cluster in three 16 bp regions spanning a 180 bp region [28]. These clusters are characterized by homology to the χ elements involved in procaryotic homologous recombination. Interestingly, similar χ-like elements were found in the D loci, suggesting that the translocation could be mediated by recombination at the χ-like elements. A 45 kD binding protein has been identified which binds to the χ-like elements in the mbr, and homologous sites in the mcr and the IgH locus [29]. Finding these binding sites on both chromosomal partners suggests that χ is involved in the translocation.

In addition to the t(14;18) translocation, a 150–200 kb deletion of the IgH locus on the der(14) chromosome is observed in 90% of cases of FL [30]. This deletion appears to occur subsequent to the t(14;18) translocation and has molecular characteristics suggesting that it is the result of a nonphysiological class switch deletion of the translocated IgH locus. In the majority of cases, these deletions result in a switch to the Cγ1 IgH constant region. However, the precise molecular anatomy of the deletion has not been defined and it has been pointed out that alternative explanations for these deletions exist [31]. The biologic significance of this deletion has not been determined, although its high frequency of occurrence suggests it may have a role in the development of the tumor.

bcl-2

The *bcl*-2 gene is composed of three exons [26]. The product of the *bcl*-2 open reading frame, a 26 kD protein, is encoded by exons 2 and 3, which are separated by a very large 370 kb intron [19,21,25,26].

Exon 1 is untranslated and the 220 bp intron 1 is removed by splicing in only a portion of the transcripts [26]. The gene is predominantly expressed from a GC-rich promoter upstream of exon 1 (P1). A second promoter, which is a classical TATA plus CAAT box, within intron 1 (P2) is also utilized. The 5' untranslated region contains a unique negative regulatory element (NRE), which can decrease the expression of transcripts originating from P1. This element may be critical to the regulation of *bcl*-2 expression during B-cell ontogeny [32]. The message has a long 3' untranslated region and there are several polyadenylation sites. The high levels of *bcl*-2 mRNA in cells bearing a t(14;18) translocation result from increased rates of transcription rather than an alteration in the half-life of the message [26].

The *bcl*-2 gene product prevents programmed cell death (PCD), a term used interchangeably with apoptosis. This was first demonstrated by the ability of *bcl*-2 expression to prolong the survival of an interleukin-3 (IL-3)-dependent pre-B-cell line when deprived of the cytokine [33]. Overexpression of *bcl*-2 has been shown to block cell death induced by a variety of stimuli including: γ- and ultraviolet (UV)-irradiation [34–36], dexamethasone [34,35], chemotherapeutic drugs [37,38], free radicals [39], c-*myc* [40], p53 [41], withdrawal of some cytokines (e.g., IL-3, IL-5) [33,42,43], and *Ced*-9 mutations of *C. elegans* [44]. Not all mediators of PCD are blocked by the overexpression of *bcl*-2; anti-Ig [45], withdrawal of some cytokines (dependent on the particular cell line and cytokine) [42,43], and positive and negative selection of thymocytes [34–46], for example, appear to be regulated by other mechanisms. Intensive efforts eventually led to the localization of the *bcl*-2 gene product to the nuclear envelope, endoplasmic reticulum and the outer mitochondrial membranes; it is, however, absent from the plasma membrane [42,47–49]. In spite of its association with mitochondria, overexpression of *bcl*-2 in cells lacking mitochondrial DNA is still able to inhibit apoptosis, demonstrating that an intact mitochondrial respiratory chain is not necessary for *bcl*-2 activity [50].

The critical role played by *bcl*-2 in the regulation of apoptosis in a variety of systems is beyond the scope of this chapter. The reader is directed to several excellent reviews of this subject [36,51–53].

bcl-2 in normal B-cell development

The regulation of apoptosis is critical during normal B-cell ontogeny. As cells differentiate from pro-B to pre-B to sIg+ B-cells, there is extensive cell loss as a result of PCD. In the pre-pro-B-cells, *bcl*-2 is highly expressed but is downregulated as cells differentiate beyond this stage [54,55]. When sIg is expressed in the mature B-cell the *bcl-2* gene product is again expressed. Downregulation of *bcl-2* expression corresponds to stages of B-cell differentiation in which cells that fail to complete productive heavy and light chain rearrangement or which are self-reactive are eliminated. However, deletion of self-reactive B-cells is not entirely dependent on the downregulation of *bcl-2*, as evidenced by the fact that *bcl-2* transgenic mice with forced expression of a *bcl-2* transgene in lymphoid cells are still able to delete self-reactive B-cells in the bone marrow [56]. The emergence of mature B-cells from the marrow completes the antigen-independent phase of B-cell development.

Upon encountering antigen, B-cells undergo somatic diversification of the antigen receptor by a process of somatic mutation followed by selection. These events occur within the GC [57–59]. In the GC, most cells are destined to be eliminated by apoptosis because they are not selected by presented antigen. Consistent with this, neither the centroblasts, which are the dividing B-cells undergoing somatic mutation found in the dark zone, nor the vast majority of postmitotic centrocytes of the GC, express *bcl-2* as determined by both immunohistochemistry and Western blot analyses [60,61]. Immunohistochemical techniques demonstrate that expression of *bcl-2* in the GC is confined to a small proportion of centrocytes juxtaposed to FDCs in the apical light zone [60,62]. Indeed, expression of *bcl-2* in the majority of cells in a germinal center is strongly suggestive of FL. Interestingly, using *in situ* hybridization with a *bcl-2* antisense probe, messenger RNA can be detected throughout the germinal center, suggesting that control of *bcl-2* expression within the GC is posttranscriptional [62].

Centrocytes are rescued from apoptosis by binding antigen presented by FDCs; this rescue is a complex process and is only in part dependent on the expression of *bcl-2*. Centrocytes purified from GCs will undergo spontaneous apoptosis in culture, which can be blocked by incubation of the cells with monoclonal antibodies (mAbs) reactive with the CD40 cell surface molecule, or by incubation with the natural ligand of CD40, CD40L, normally found on the surface of activated T-cells [61,63]. As a consequence of this activation of CD40, *bcl-2* protein expression is observed; however, expression of the *bcl-2* protein is not detectable at significant levels until approximately 48 hours of culture, suggesting that the survival of centrocytes after CD40 stimulation involves other pathways in addition to the activation of *bcl-2* expression [63]. Cells selected by antigen are able to differentiate into plasma cells or memory B-cells [59]. Indeed, transgenic mice with enforced expression of *bcl-2* in

B-cells have a dramatically expanded memory B-cell compartment, demonstrating an important role for *bcl-2* in the maintenance of B-cell memory [64].

Further evidence of the role of *bcl-2* in the normal immune system has come from the study of *bcl-2* knockout mice. Mice with homozygous deletion of the *bcl-2* proto-oncogene have near control numbers of B- and T-cells at birth [65,66]. However, by 4 weeks of life, B- and T-cells disappear from the blood and bone marrow, and the thymus and spleen undergo involution secondary to apoptosis. These results demonstrate that *bcl-2* is dispensable for lymphocyte development but is necessary for maintenance of a stable immune system. These mice also manifest polycystic kidneys and hypopigmented hair.

Bcl-2 controls cell death by interaction with Bcl-2 homologs

The molecular basis by which Bcl-2 acts has not been fully elucidated. Recent evidence has demonstrated that Bcl-2 is the prototype of a family of related proteins including Bax, Bcl-X$_L$, Mcl-1, Bad, *Caenorhabditis elegans* protein Ced-9 and viral proteins BHRF1 from Epstein–Barr virus (EBV) and LMW5-HL from African Swine Fever virus. These proteins share two homology domains, which have been referred to as BH1 and BH2 [1a,2a]. Bcl-2 controls cell death by heterodimerization. Bax, which can homodimerize or form heterodimers with Bcl-2, will promote apoptosis in response to an apoptotic stimulus when overexpressed. The ability of Bcl-2 to inhibit apoptosis depends on interaction with Bax via the BH1 and BH2 domains [3a]. Korsmeyer and colleagues have proposed a model in which the susceptibility to apoptotic stimuli is regulated by the ratio of Bcl-2 to Bax [4a]. The role of Bax and other Bcl-2 family members in the molecular pathogenesis of human lymphomas remains to be elucidated.

Activation of bcl-2 is not sufficient for lymphomagenesis

Several lines of evidence suggest that activation of *bcl-2* is not sufficient to result in malignant transformation of B-cells. Firstly, recent studies have shown that the t(14;18) translocation can be detected in hyperplastic lymphoid tissue obtained from normal individuals [67,68]. Additional data have been obtained through the study of mice expressing a *bcl-2* minigene construct, which results in enforced expression of *bcl-2* in the B-cell compartment. These animals do not have lymphoma at birth but rather develop marked expansion of circulating memory

B-cells and polyclonal follicular hyperplasia [43,69, 70]. However, these animals do develop aggressive diffuse large-cell lymphomas with a latency period of approximately 18 months, suggesting that this transformation is a multistep process [71]. Molecular analysis of the resulting large-cell lymphomas reveals that about 50% of these tumors have acquired a translocation activating the c-*myc* proto-oncogene. The progeny of crosses between transgenic animals expressing *bcl*-2 and transgenic animals expressing c-*myc*, where both transgenes are under the influence of the immunoglobulin Eμ enhancer, rapidly develop very primitive lymphoid tumors, demonstrating that these molecular events are synergistic in lymphomagenesis [72]. However, it is important to note that the transgenic models do not develop the monoclonal, low-grade FL characteristic of the human disease [69], although the diffuse large-cell lymphomas observed in these animals appear to be akin to the histologically transformed lymphomas which occur in human FL (see section on histologic transformation).

INTERACTION OF FL WITH THE HOST

One of the most intriguing aspects of the natural history of FL is the potential for clinically significant spontaneous regression [73]. Within the involved lymph node, malignant FL cells are found in close proximity to FDCs and polyclonal T-cells [10]. The infiltrating T-cells are predominantly CD4+, although small numbers of CD+8 cells are present. Within an individual patient, the extent of T-cell infiltration is relatively constant in multiple anatomic sites, although among patients the extent of infiltration can vary significantly [10]. The number of infiltrating T-cells correlates with response to therapy with anti-idiotypic monoclonal antibodies [74,75]. These observations suggest that FL cells may be subject to growth regulation by T-cells in a manner similar to nonmalignant centrocytes [76].

FL cells have been shown to proliferate in response to alloreactive CD4+ human T-cell clones [77]. The FL proliferative response required contact with the T-cells and T-cell recognition of alloantigens on the FL cells. The stimulation was enhanced by addition of cytokines IL-2 and IL-4. Isolated FL cells have also been stimulated to proliferate by incubation with IL-4 and stromal cells presenting an anti-CD40 monoclonal antibody [78]. In this system, the proliferating FL cells acquired a blastic morphology with loss of small cleaved cells. That the proliferating cells were derived from the FL clone was established by demonstrating the same t(14;18) breakpoint in the original tumor and proliferating cells.

Thus, FL cells, like normal centrocytes, can be activated via the CD40 receptor. As mentioned above, interaction of CD40L with CD40 activates a *bcl*-2-independent survival pathway in normal centrocytes. However, unlike normal centrocytes, isolated FL cells are resistant to apoptosis [78]; thus, it is unlikely that signaling through CD40 in FL cells is necessary to provide a survival signal. It is more likely that the CD40 pathway provides a proliferative signal to FL cells from infiltrating activated T-cells, possibly in the setting of antigen.

FL CELLS UNDERGO SOMATIC MUTATION

The sIg on lymphoma cells is a tumor-specific antigen which has been exploited therapeutically with anti-idiotypic (anti-Id) mAbs [79]. Significant antitumor responses have been seen when anti-Id mAbs are infused into patients [80–83]. Some patients who had tumor progression following antibody therapy were found to have tumor variants which were idiotype-negative despite persistent expression of sIg [84]. Molecular analysis of these variants revealed that the variable (V) genes expressed were mutated relative to the original tumor specimen. Subsequently it has been demonstrated that the V genes expressed in individual cells of a given FL vary from one to another even in the absence of selection by anti-Id mAbs [85,86]. This microheterogeneity within the tumor is consistent with the process of somatic mutation and is another biological indicator that FL cells are the malignant equivalents of centrocytes.

CLONAL EXPANSION IN FL IS SUBSEQUENT TO ANTIGENIC SELECTION

Since activation of *bcl*-2 alone appears to be insufficient for lymphomagenesis, the development of FL must be a multistep process [76]. By exploiting the microheterogeneity of V gene sequences within FL, it has been demonstrated that clonal expansion occurs subsequent to the initiation of somatic mutation and therefore within the germinal center [87–90]. Analysis of the pattern of mutations which result in an altered protein sequence (replacement [R] mutations) within the complementarity-determining regions (CDRs; the regions of the immunoglobulin which make contact with antigen) and the framework regions (FRs) demonstrates that there is an excess of R mutations in the CDRs and a dearth of these mutations in the FRs. This pattern of mutation is the same as that seen in antigen-driven clonal selection

[91–93]. It suggests that clonal expansion in FL is subsequent to antigenic selection [87–90]. Although the nature of the antigen is unknown, 25% of idiotype proteins isolated from FL react with a panel of known autoantigens [94], thereby raising the possibility that autoantigens may be involved in the pathogenesis of FL. However, IgH V gene usage has been determined in FL and found to be comparable to that of EBV-transformed B-cells [95]. This suggests that the pool of antigens involved in follicular lymphomagenesis is not highly restricted.

HISTOLOGIC TRANSFORMATION

Histologic conversion to an intermediate grade, often diffuse large-cell lymphoma (DLCL), frequently disrupts the indolent clinical course of FL and is generally associated with a poor prognosis [96–98]. The malignant cells in the clone of transformed diffuse lymphoma (tDL) appear to have lost growth modulation by T-cells and can be established as cell lines *in vitro* [99]. The common clonal origin of the FL and tDL has been established by demonstrating that the sIg of the tDL reacts with monoclonal anti-Id antibodies prepared to react against the FL [86]. Further analysis of the pattern of somatic mutation demonstrated that the tDL arose from a single cell, suggesting that additional genetic event(s) were critical to the transformation.

In some cases, the tDL is a very aggressive lymphoid neoplasm which is sIg– and has a t(8;14)(q24;q32) translocation activating the c-*myc* proto-oncogene in addition to the t(14;18) translocation [100,101]. Although this represents an interesting clinical entity [102], the c-*myc* proto-oncogene was found to be rearranged in only 8% of tDL in a series of 38 cases [103]. Interestingly, t(8;14) translocations have been observed in a subset of histologically typical FLs, which lack t(14;18) translocations [104]. The molecular structure of the t(8;14) translocations is distinct from the classical t(8;14) translocation seen in Burkitt's lymphoma. The natural history of these unusual cases appears to be indistinguishable from t(14;18)-positive FL.

p53 mutations have been observed in 30–35% of tDL [105,106]. Immunohistochemical analysis for detection of mutant p53 in pretransformation biopsies of tDL cases with mutant p53 showed rare positive cells [105, 106]. Of note, three of 25 control cases of FL had mutations in p53, one of which subsequently underwent histologic conversion [105]. The presence of p53 mutations in tDL contrasts with *de novo* DLCL, which is rarely associated with mutation of p53 [107]. p53 mutation and c-*myc* translocation are apparently independent transformation pathways for FL as there is no overlap in the cases with these molecular lesions [105]. However, it remains to be demonstrated whether mutant p53 can complement *bcl*-2 in the malignant transformation of lymphocytes, as has been shown for c-*myc* (see page 357). The *bcl*-3 gene is rearranged in a small fraction of tDL (8%) independent of c-*myc* rearrangement [108]. In three tDL cases in which *bcl*-3 was rearranged, the rearrangement could also be detected in the prior FL from the same patient. An additional *bcl*-3 rearrangement was detected in one of 58 cases of FL. In one tDL case, the *bcl*-3 rearrangement was shown to be acquired as an additional molecular lesion during the indolent phase of the disease prior to transformation. In all cases in which the *bcl*-3 gene was rearranged, rearrangement of *bcl*-2 was also detected. Thus, *bcl*-3 rearrangement may not be a transforming event *per se* but rather a progression event during the indolent phase of FL.

It appears that p53 mutation, c-*myc* or *bcl*-3 translocations cannot account for all cases of tDL. Cytogenetic analysis has revealed several recurrent, nonrandom abnormalities in tDL [109–112]. In t(14;18)-positive FL, additional cytogenetic abnormalities have been associated with histologic transformation: del(6q); +7 [or dup(7q)]; +12; and +17 [or i(17q)]. It is likely that there are additional pathways to histologic transformation involving loci within these chromosomal regions.

FL AS A MODEL OF MULTISTEP TRANSFORMATION

From the information presented above it is clear that the pathogenesis of FL involves multiple steps. In this section, the above information is brought together to present a model of follicular lymphomagenesis (see Figure 14.2). Although based on existing data, further work will be necessary to confirm the details of this model, which, as such, should be considered a working hypothesis. The model illustrates the interplay between the development of molecular lesions and normal B-cell ontogeny in the process of tumorigenesis.

The tumor has its origin in the bone marrow, where the t(14;18) translocation occurs at the pro-B-cell stage of development. This event serves to enhance the survival of this particular clone, although the role of the additional interstitial deletion of the der(14) chromosome has yet to be defined. The clone completes productive Ig gene rearrangement, enters the circulation, and eventually migrates to the lymph node. As noted above, cells bearing the t(14;18) translocation can be detected in hyperplastic lymphoid tissue and thus, as reviewed above (page 357)

SOMATIC MUTATION

INTERSTITIAL DELETION

ANTIGENIC SELECTION

PROGRESSION EVENTS
   (*e.g.* p53, c-*myc*, bcl-3, del(6q))

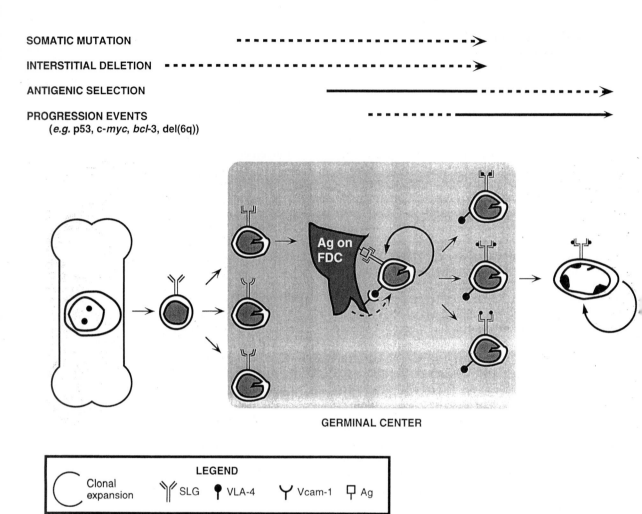

GERMINAL CENTER

LEGEND

Clonal expansion   SLG   VLA-4   Vcam-1   Ag

Figure 14.2 A model for follicular lymphomagenesis and tumor progression. The tumor originates in the bone marrow where the t(14;18) translocation occurs in a pro-B-cell. Potentially multiple virgin B-cells can result if progeny of the t(14;18)-positive pro-B-cell successfully rearrange H and L chains. For simplicity, this is shown as a single successful event. The resultant virgin B-cell migrates to the GC and the V genes undergo somatic mutation. One of the resultant clones is antigenically selected and then is clonally expanded. The dashed arrow emanating from the FDC represents soluble factors (e.g., IL-4) and interaction with surface molecules (e.g., CD40–CD40L) necessary for proliferation. The details of these interactions *in vivo* remain to be elucidated. The progeny then distribute systemically to lymph nodes and bone marrow, and home via integrin/adhesion molecule interaction. Additional somatic mutations can accumulate in these secondary sites and further antigenic selection is possible. Over time, additional genetic events occur, contributing to more aggressive clinical behavior and occasionally to frank transformation. Some of these events can result in antigen-independent growth, since some FLs lose expression of sIg. However, somatic mutations can accumulate and antigenic selection continues up to the time of histologic transformation, after which the mutation rate drops significantly. The existing data make it impossible to determine the timing of the interstitial deletion of the der(14) chromosome, although it is subsequent to the t(14;18) translocation. Refer to the text for additional details.

this event alone is insufficient for lymphomagenesis. Cells from the t(14;18)-positive clone continue to develop on the B-cell pathway and are subject to antigenic selection. Antigenic selection may provide a proliferative signal to the cell, permitting clonal expansion. Subsequently, the clone is distributed throughout the lymphoid system, quite probably via interaction with integrins expressed on FDCs. Additional molecular lesions can accumulate within the FL clone, leading to more aggressive behavior and potentially to histological transformation via several independent pathways.

Mantle cell lymphoma

INTRODUCTION

Definition

MCL does not readily fit into the WF [1], although in the WF it would generally be designated as a diffuse small cleaved cell lymphoma (DSCL). This entity has been referred to in the literature by numerous synonymous designations: centrocytic lymphoma; mantle zone lymphoma; diffuse lymphoma with intermediate differentiation (DLID); DSCL; and lymphomatous polyposis of the gastrointestinal tract [113–119]. Rappaport's original description [120] of diffuse poorly differentiated lymphocytic lymphoma (DPDL) was tainted by the inclusion of both lymphoblastic lymphoma and cases which have more recently been show to be focally follicular. The NCI Classification Project showed a shorter median survival and the possibility of cure in a fraction of patients with DSCL compared with DPDL. DSCL was rarely reported from US institutions but was more frequently seen in the series from Milan [1]. It is now widely recognized that MCL is composed not of small cleaved cells of the germinal center (as implied by the Kiel term 'centrocytic' [117]) but of a malignant derivative of the mantle zone lymphocyte. Aberrant differentiation of these cells is demonstrated by the abnormal presence of CD5 antigen [113]. This nosologic entity should be defined by its cell of origin, rather than the mantle zone pattern of growth, since the latter is present in only a fraction of MCLs and may be demonstrated in small lymphocytic or lymphoplasmacytoid lymphomas as well. Since by histologic, immunophenotypic and cytogenetic criteria, intermediate lymphocytic lymphoma, lymphocytic lymphoma of intermediate differentiation and mantle zone lymphoma all appear to be identical to the centrocytic lymphoma of the Kiel classification, the new term mantle cell lymphoma was proposed to include all of these [119].

Clinical presentation

Typically the middle-aged or elderly patient presents with a systemic malignancy involving lymph nodes, spleen and bone marrow, and occasionally peripheral blood, as well as extranodal disease, such as Waldeyer's ring [114,121,122]. The initial endoscopic presentation of lymphomatous polyposis may be initially confused with familial adenomatous polyposis coli or even inflammatory bowel disease. There are no known toxic, infectious or heritable risk factors.

The median survival of MCL patients of less than 5 years was the shortest among the LGLs [123]; however, unlike the similarly aggressive intermediate-grade lymphomas, a plateau in the survival curve with treatment was not demonstrated [114].

HISTOLOGY AND IMMUNOCHEMISTRY

MCL is typically a diffuse infiltration of monotonous small lymphocytes with irregular nuclei, which, unlike MALT lymphomas, spares the overlying epithelium. The normal mantle zone around adjacent benign germinal centers may be absent, or the tumor may infiltrate the mantle zone of nearby normal germinal centers, giving a nodular pattern of growth [121,124,125]. Large non-cleaved cells are absent and plasmacytoid differentiation and plasma cells are rarely seen. Patients may progress to a blastic form of the disease with a worse prognosis, but transformation to a diffuse large-cell histology is not observed [114,123]. The tumors express mature B-cell differentiation antigens (CD19, CD20 and CD22), sIgM, with or without IgD along with expression of CD5, CD43, and, rarely, CD10 [126]. The surface staining of IgM and IgD is intermediate between the usually dim pattern of SLL/chronic lymphocytic leukemia (CLL) and the bright pattern of FL.

The cell of origin of MCL is believed to be a small CD5+, sIgM+ lymphocyte detectable in fetal circulation. These probably represent virgin B-cells, which form in the bone marrow and go on to form primary germinal centers in the spleen and bone marrow. These correspond in the adult to IgM-positive, alkaline phosphatase-positive cells in the mantle zones of secondary follicles [127,128]. Molecular confirmation that these tumors are derived from virgin B-cells is lacking.

THE t(11;14) CHROMOSOMAL TRANSLOCATION

MCLs have been shown frequently to possess (>50%) of an t(11;14)(q13;q32) translocation [129–135] while the t(14;18)(q32;q21) translocation characteristic of FSCL is not observed. Of the 12 cases of intermediate lymphocytic lymphoma reported by Weisenburger in 1987, three had translocations of the long arm of chromosome 11 to 14q32 IgH, and two others had structural abnormalities of the long arm of chromosome 11 [134]. These findings were confirmed in later studies [130,133]. After the discovery of the recombination of the oncogene c-*myc* with IgH in the t(8;14)(q24;q32) of Burkitt's

Lymphomas arising from cells of the marginal zone

DEFINITION AND CLINICAL PRESENTATION

Mucosa-associated lymphoid tissue (MALT) lymphoma and monocytoid B-cell lymphoma are low-grade neoplastic processes that share morphological and immunohistochemical features, and may represent variants of a single pathologic entity arising from marginal zone cells [169].

Mucosa-associated lymphoid tissue

MALT is a low-grade neoplastic process arising in a specific extranodal epithelial lymphoid compartment typified by Peyer's patches [170–173]. Originally described in the gastrointestinal tract, it is now well recognized in the respiratory tract, salivary glands, ocular adnexa, breast, skin, kidney, prostate, gall bladder, thyroid, thymus and uterine cervix [174, 175]. The unifying feature of these diverse clinical presentations is the ability of the MALT lymphoma cells to home to the epithelium of origin where it gives rise to a localized but low-grade small lymphocytic neoplasm. The extranodal homing of the MALT lymphocyte probably reflects its initial origin in the extranodal germinal center [176,177]. In one review of extranodal lymphomas, 80% of primary low-grade gastric lymphomas, 30% of breast lymphomas and 40% of orbital lymphomas were morphologically consistent with MALT lymphomas [178].

Monocytoid B-cell lymphoma

MBCL is a neoplasm of marginal zone origin closely related to MALT and may be a nodal presentation of the same disease [169,178–182]. This is supported by the observation that involved regional lymph nodes of MALT may have the monocytoid B-cell morphology [183,184]. Concurrent extranodal presentations are common in MBCL, although like the MALT lymphomas the bone marrow is not invariably involved at presentation [180,181,183]. This lymphoma more often occurs in women, and there is a strong association with Sjögren's syndrome and other autoimmune disorders [180,183,185]. In a recently published series of 100 cases [186] of MBCL, 48 had localized and 17 had generalized adenopathy. Twenty-three patients had extranodal disease; 19 of these cases had salivary gland involvement. Twenty-three of 61 cases with bone marrow biopsies had involvement by MBCL.

HISTOLOGY AND IMMUNOCHEMISTRY

MALT-lymphomas and MBCL share similar cytological features. The cells are small sized, the chromatin is densely clumped and the cytoplasm is clear [186]. In the MALT lymphomas, mucosal tissue is diffusely infiltrated by small lymphoid (occasionally with irregular nuclei) or lymphoplasmacytoid cells, which infiltrate the overlying epithelium, as well as the submucosa [187]. The involvement of the epithelium is an important differential diagnostic feature and benign germinal centers may be preserved, giving rise to the impression of 'pseudolymphoma' [188]. Germinal centers may also be densely infiltrated (colonized) by small neoplastic lymphocytes, giving the impression of a follicular lymphoma [189]. There may be an admixture of nodal monocytoid B-cells of marginal zone origin or neoplastic plasma cells in the interfollicular zones. The marginal zone cell lymphomas express sIg: IgM>IgG>IgA [190,191]. CD43 expression is variable, although CD5, CD10 and CD23 expression are absent [191]. Approximately 40% of the tumors express cytoplasmic immunoglobulin (cIg).

CYTOGENETICS AND MOLECULAR GENETICS

No consistent cytogenetic abnormality has been detected in MALT, although the number of tumors examined cytogenetically to date is small [192,193]. A reported t(11;18)(q21;q21.1) translocation in three cases of extranodal lymphoma did not demonstrate rearrangement of the bcl-2 oncogene by Southern blot analysis [194]. Indeed, rearrangement of the bcl-2 gene has been uniformly noted to be absent [189,195].

Because of the variable histologic appearance of the MALT lymphomas, it can at times be difficult to distinguish them from benign reactive processes. One of the tools used to distinguish MALT lymphoma from reactive lymphoid tissue is the presence of IgH gene rearrangement, either by Southern blotting or PCR [196,197]. For example, this may aid in the distinction of lymphoma from myoepithelial sialadenitis [198].

EPIDEMIOLOGY AND RISK FACTORS

MALT lymphoma may present at any adult age [199] and has been reported in a pediatric patient, even in the absence of celiac disease [200]. Patients often have an antecedent history of autoimmune disorder or other chronic inflammation, such as peptic ulcer disease, Hashimoto's thyroiditis or Sjögren's syndrome [201–203].

Unlike the nodal follicular small cleaved lymphoma, extranodal MALT lymphoma frequently presents as a localized, low-grade process, which is effectively managed by surgical excision alone [204], or with the addition of radiotherapy or alkylating agent chemotherapy [205,206]. Relapses tend also to be localized to epithelial tissues and further local control may lead to a long disease-free interval [197].

HISTOLOGIC TRANSFORMATION

High-grade transformation has been described, both in the MALT lymphoma and MBCL [169,175,180, 207–210]. Rearrangement of c-*myc* is probably a component of the transformation, since extranodal large-cell lymphomas (LCLs) are more likely to have c-*myc* rearrangements and less likely to have a t(14;18) translocation than nodal LCLs [211]. Half of the primary gastric LCLs arising in MALT have a c-*myc* rearrangement [212]. However, matched specimens of the low-grade MALT lymphoma and the transformed lymphoma have yet to be examined to determine whether translocation of c-*myc* is present only in the aggressive element.

ANTIGENIC DRIVE AND AUTOIMMUNITY

That antigen may be involved in the proliferative drive of the low-grade MALT lymphomas suggested by the occurrence of subepithelial plasma cell differentiation, blast transformation [173] and colonization of reactive B-cell follicles by tumor cells [173,189]. Serial biopsies in one patient with MALT lymphoma showed a level of somatic mutation in the IgH locus consistent with antigenic selection during a germinal center phase [197,213].

Tumor-derived idiotypes (Id) from three cases of MALT lymphoma have been shown to have autoantibody reactivity to normal tissue components [214]. In case 1, Id reactivity was directed towards FDCs from both the patient and normal lymphoid tissues. In case 2, Id reactivity was seen in postcapillary venules in Peyer's patches and also in the appendix, but not in tonsil or peripheral lymph nodes. In case 3, a broad pattern of reactivity was observed. In addition, proliferation of cultured MALT lymphoma cells can be modulated in some cases by the addition of anti-Id antibodies, supporting the notion that antigen is involved in the pathogenesis of the MALT lymphomas [215]. Finally, MALT B-cells

have been shown to proliferate in the presence of *Helicobacter pylori* [215] (see below). Autoimmunity may be relevant to the generation of gastric MALT lymphoma, and has been demonstrated by the finding of common epitopes in gastric mucosa and *H. pylori*, as well as by the identification of autoantibodies synthesized by the lymphoma cells themselves [214–218].

In the absence of a known etiology, one could postulate that viral infection of epithelial cells provides antigenic stimulation in Hashimoto's disease or Sjögren's syndrome. This may lead to the presentation of autologous epitopes and result in expansion of autoreactive cells. The proliferation at this point may be oligoclonal and an additional molecular lesion may lead to a monoclonal outgrowth. Alternatively, the autoreactive cell may carry a molecular lesion, which gives it a survival or growth advantage as in the case of FL (see page 357). Clonal evolution may lead to the development of cytokine independence and/or T-helper cell independence, and contribute to high-grade transformation and dissemination beyond the initial local area.

HELICOBACTER PYLORI *AND* GASTRIC LYMPHOMA

H. pylori is present in the gastric mucosa of >90% of cases of gastric MALT lymphoma [217] and its incidence correlates well with the prevalence of *H. pylori* in gastric biopsies [219]. MALT is not normally present in the gastric mucosa, but arises as the result of antigenic stimulation, for example, chronic infection with *H. pylori* [220]. In some cases of gastric MALT lymphoma, tumor B-cells proliferate *in vitro* in the presence of *H. pylori*. This effect was observed to be highest in the presence of tumor-infiltrating T-cells. Proliferation was not seen in a case of high-grade gastric MALT lymphoma or in MALT lymphomas arising outside the stomach. There are now many reported series of patients with documented regression of MALT lymphoma after eradication of *H. pylori* infection with antibiotic therapy [218,221,222]. However, long-term follow-up will be required to determine whether the malignant clone has been eradicated in these cases.

CONCLUSIONS

The MALT lymphomas provide an intriguing model of the involvement of antigenic drive in lymphomagenesis. The finding of autoreactive Ids in some cases and reactivity to *H. pylori* in others is strong evidence of this process. The finding that

MALT lymphomas express somatically mutated V genes suggests that these tumors have been selected by their ability to bind antigen with high affinity, although this remains to be proven. Provocatively, some cases appear to regress when the inciting antigen is removed. The applicability of this approach to other potentially antigen-stimulated, low-grade lymphomas will require identification of the relevant antigens, as well as a strategy to eliminate them.

MALT lymphomas cannot arise simply as a response to antigen: since they are clonal proliferations, additional abnormalities must be required. However, the nature of the molecular lesions that contribute to the pathogenesis of these tumors is unknown. Cytogenetics has failed to reveal a consistent chromosomal abnormality. Other approaches will be necessary to identify the genes involved in MALT lymphomagenesis.

Small lymphocytic lymphoma

HISTOLOGY AND IMMUNOHISTOCHEMISTRY

Small lymphocytic lymphoma is closely related to chronic lymphocytic leukemia. Such tumors are typically B-cell neoplasms expressing cell surface IgM and IgD. Both of these tumors express the CD5 antigen observed on T-cell populations and a subfraction of B-cells. One distinguishing characteristic is that SLL often expresses the cell adhesion molecule, LFA-1 (CD11a), which may contribute to the occurrence of SLL as a nodal lymphoma, in contrast to the leukemic picture typical of CLL. A variant of SLL demonstrating plasmacytoid differentiation (SLL-PL) is discussed in the following section as a separate entity. This distinction is made because of the recent association of SLL-PL with a specific chromosomal translocation t(9;14)(p13;q32) and distinct immunohistochemistry.

CYTOGENETICS AND TUMOR PROGRESSION

No consistent cytogenetic abnormality has been described, although several recurrent cytogenetic changes have been observed in a subset of cases. Trisomy 12, the most common abnormality in CLL, and trisomy 18, are seen in more than 10% of cases of SLL but have not been specifically associated with this histology in a large series of cytogenetically characterized NHLs [223]. In this series, trisomy 3

was observed in 30% of cases of SLL, which was significantly more common than the frequency of 7.5% observed in other histologies.

Another recurrent abnormality observed in 26% of cases of SLL is del(6)(q21;q23) [224], which has been observed as a sole karyotypic abnormality in some cases. This abnormality has been significantly associated with SLL in which there are circulating prolymphocytoid cells as well as in prolymphocytic leukemia (PLL). The del(6q) has also been reported as the sole abnormality in a small number of cases of CLL [225–229], in 20% of cases of PLL [230,231], and in approximately 4% of cases of CLL [225–229]. The locus involved in the del(6q) has not yet been identified, although positional cloning has demonstrated loss of heterozygosity of restriction fragment length polymorphisms in this region [232,233].

RICHTER'S TRANSFORMATION

In 1928, Richter described the development of generalized reticular cell sarcoma (large-cell lymphoma in modern terminology) in association with chronic lymphocytic leukemia [234]. Histologic transformation to an aggressive, poor prognosis large-cell lymphoma or leukemia is now well recognized in patients with CLL and SLL. The frequency of transformation or Richter's syndrome (RS) in SL or CLL is lower than the frequency of histologic conversion observed in FL [235]. There are conflicting data regarding the relationship of the origins of the large-cell lymphomas arising in patients with CLL. Some investigations have shown that the transformed lymphoma arose from the same clone of cells as the CLL [236–245], while others have suggested that the large-cell lymphoma arises from a distinct clone [245–252]. In some cases, for example, the low-grade and large-cell lymphomas have distinct Ig gene rearrangements. However, sometimes a careful analysis has revealed a common clonal origin, based on the presence of identical cytogenetic or molecular markers in both low- and high-grade tumors despite discordant Ig rearrangements. Clear discordance among clonal markers has also been observed. For example, in one case of CLL there was a clonal deletion of chromosome 13 involving the RB gene. The transformed lymphoma from the same patient did not have the del(13q) [252], demonstrating that the large-cell lymphoma did not arise from the CLL clone. Thus the data suggest that in most cases RS represents clonal progression from the low-grade tumor, but in some cases a clonally distinct tumor may arise. The explanation for the development of a second neoplastic clone is unknown, although it is possible that a long-lived early B-lineage cell gives rise to both tumors. Such a putative tumor precursor clone could contain genetic lesions, which contribute to clonal survival, but do not result in overt neoplastic transformation. Additional genetic alterations could then lead to the development of the low-grade tumor or RS. Alternatively, the relative immune defect seen in patients with SLL/CLL may predispose to lymphomagenesis. Clearly, further investigations are needed if this phenonmenon is to be understood.

CONCLUSIONS

Little is known about the molecular pathogenesis of SLL. Furthermore, the results presented above suggest that these tumors may arise as a consequence of multiple distinct molecular mechanisms. Further subclassification of these tumors based on correlations between molecular and cytogenetic findings with clinical syndromes, such as the association of del(6q) with SLL/PLL, may clarify this multiplicity.

Small lymphocytic lymphoma with plasmacytoid differentation

HISTOLOGY, IMMUNOHISTOCHEMISTRY AND CLINICAL FEATURES

SLL-PL is distinguished histologically from SLL by the plasmacytoid features of the malignant lymphocytes. Immunochemically, this tumor is of B-cell origin and expresses CD19 and CD20 [178,253]. Both surface and cytoplasmic Ig, usually IgM, are expressed and IgD is typically not expressed. Unlike SLL, the tumor does not express CD5. CD10 and CD23 are also absent while CD43 expression in variable [178]. This tumor has an indolent natural history and unlike the marginal zone cell lymphomas, which can also express cIg, it tends to be disseminated at presentation [253]. Like the other low-grade lymphomas (except MCL), SLL-PL can undergo histological conversion into DLCL.

THE t(9;14) CHROMOSOMAL TRANSLOCATION

In a series of 426 consecutively ascertained and karyotypically abnormal cases of NHL, eight cases were described with a t(9;14)(p13;q32) translocation [253]. Four of them were SLL-PL and in three of these the sole abnormality was a t(9;14). Retrospective review of the two cases of DLCL in this group of eight tumors with t(9;14) revealed an antecedent history of a SLL-PL. Thus, six of the eight cases with this translocation had SLL-PL histology. Although both reciprocal translocation products were present in these tumors, two cases retained only the der(14) chromosome, suggesting that the potential proto-oncogene at 9p13 was translocated to the IgH locus as in the t(14;18) and t(11;14) translocations.

CONCLUSIONS

The designation of SLL-PL as a distinct entity arises from its histological and immunophenotypic differences from SLL/CLL. The possibility that the t(9;14) translocation represents a specific translocation in this lymphoma needs to be further explored. Unfortunately, the proto-oncogene at 9p13 has yet to be identified. Identification of the locus will make possible the preparation of molecular probes, which can be used to determine the incidence of this translocation in a series of SLL-PL by Southern blot hybridization or by fluorescent *in situ* hybridization, and will permit the examination of its role in lymphomagenesis.

Conclusions

The human low-grade B-cell lymphomas represent a challenge to the laboratory and clinical investigator alike. The FLs have demonstrated that cellular homeostasis plays a central role in tumor development. By reducing the rate of cell death, populations of cells accumulate and these expanded clones are at risk for the development of additional genetic lesions. The molecular pathogenesis of MCL has demonstrated that disruption of the cell cycle can contribute to tumorigenesis.

In addition, the LGLs are models of human tumor progression. After an indolent phase, in which treatment may not even be necessary [73], evolution to a more aggressive tumor is common. Often, these changes in behavior are associated with additional cytogenetic abnormalities; sometimes they are accompanied by histologic transformation to higher-grade lymphomas. A further dissection of the molecular events involved in this process of evolution and progression of the neoplastic clone should ultimately provide a greater understanding of the pathogenesis of the low-grade lymphomas.

Despite the significant advances in our understanding of lymphomagenesis that have been made, treatment outcomes have not changed in three decades, and the low-grade tumors remain largely incurable [254]. It is the ultimate goal of studying the molecular pathogenesis of the LGLs to provide more precise diagnoses and more effective therapies. The critical molecular events which have been elucidated may prove to be suitable molecular targets for novel therapeutics.

References

1. The Non-Hodgkin's Lymphoma Pathologic Project. National Cancer Institute sponsored study of classification of non-Hodgkin's lymphomas. Summary and description of a working formulation for clinical usage. *Cancer* 1982, **49**: 2112–2135.

1a. Williams GT, Smith CA. Molecular regulation of apoptosis: Genetic controls on cell death. *Cell* 1993, **74**: 777–779.

2. Warnke RA, Kim H, Fuks Z, et al. The coexistence of nodular and diffuse patterns in nodular and diffuse patterns in nodular non-Hodgkin's lymphomas: Significance and clinicopathologic correlation. *Cancer* 1977, **40**: 1229.

2a. Yang E, Zha J, Jockel J, et al. Bad, a heterodimeric partner for Bcl-x$_L$ and Bcl-2, displaces Bax and promotes cell death. *Cell* 1995, **80**: 285–291.

3. Garvin AJ, Simon R, Young RC, et al. The Rappaport classification of non-Hodgkin's lymphomas: A closer look using other proposed classifications. *Semin. Oncol.* 1980, **7**: 234–243.

3a. Yin XM, Oltvai ZN, Korsmeyer SJ. BH1 and BH2 domains of Bcl-2 are required for inhibition of apoptosis and heterodimerization with Bax. *Nature* 1994, **369**: 321–323.

4. Harris NL, Jaffe ES, Stein H, et al. A revised European–American classification of lymphoid neoplasms: A proposal from the International Lymphoma Study Group. *Blood* 1994, **84**: 1361–1392.

4a. Oltvai ZN, Korsmeyer SJ. Checkpoints of dueling dimers foil death wishes. *Cell* 1994, **79**: 189–192.

5. Nathwani BN, Winberg CD, Diamond LW, et al. Morphologic criteria for the differentiation of follicular lymphoma from florid reactive follicular hyperplasia: a study of 80 cases. *Cancer* 1981, **48**: 1794–1806.

6. Warnke RA, Weiss LM. B-Cell malignant lymphomas: An immunologic perspective. In Berard CW, Dorfman RF, Kaufman N (eds) *Malignant Lymphoma, International Academy of Pathology Monographs.* Baltimore: Williams & Wilkins, 1987, pp. 88–103.

7. Jaffe ES, Shevach EM, Frank MM, et al. Nodular lymphoma – evidence for origin from follicular B lymphocytes. *N. Engl. J. Med.* 1974, **290**: 813–819.

8. Leech JH, Glick AD, Waldron JA, et al. Malignant lymphomas of follicular center cell origin in man. I.

Immunologic studies. *J. Natl. Cancer Inst.* 1975, **54**: 11–21.

9. Glick AD, Leech JH, Waldron JA, et al. Malignant lymphomas of follicular center cell origin in man. II. Ultrastructural and cytochemical studies. *J. Natl. Cancer Inst.* 1975, **54**: 23–36.

10. Dvoretsky P, Wood GS, Levy R, et al. T-Lymphocyte subsets in follicular lymphomas compared to those in non-neoplastic lymph nodes and tonsils. *Human Immunol.* 1982, **13**: 618–625.

11. Petrasch S, Perez-Alvarez C, Schmitz J, et al. Antigenic phenotyping of human follicular dendritic cells isolated from non-malignant and malignant lymphoid tissue. *Eur. J. Immunol.* 1990, **20**: 1013–1018.

12. Braziel RM, Sussman E, Jaffe ES, et al. Induction of immunoglobulin secretion in follicular non-Hodgkin's lymphomas: Role of immunoregulatory T-cells. *Blood* 1985, **66**: 128–134.

13. Freedman AS, Munro JM, Morimoto C, et al. Follicular non-Hodgkin's lymphoma cell adhesion to normal germinal centers and neoplastic follicles involves very late antigen-4 and vascular cell adhesion molecule-1. *Blood* 1992, **79**: 206–212.

14. Koopman G, Parmentier HK, Schuurman HJ, et al. Adhesion of human B-cells to follicular dendritic cells involves both the lymphocyte function-associated antigen 1/intercellular adhesion molecule 1 and very late antigen 4/vascular cell adhesion molecule 1 pathways. *J. Exp. Med.* 1991, **173**: 1279–1304.

15. Ree HJ, Khan AA, Elsakr M, et al. Intercellular adhesion molecule-1 (ICAM-1) staining of reactive and neoplastic follicles. ICAM-1 expression of neoplastic follicle differs from that of reactive germinal center and is independent of follicular dendritic cells. *Cancer* 1993, **71**: 2817–2822.

16. Gerdes J, Dallenbach F, Lennert K, et al. Growth fractions in malignant non-Hodgkin's lymphomas (NHL) as determined *in situ* with the monoclonal antibody Ki-67. *Hematol. Oncol.* 1984, **2**: 365–371.

17. Metter GE, Nathwani BN, Burke JS, et al. Morphological subclassification of follicular lymphoma: Variability of diagnoses among hematopathologists, a collaborative study between the Repository Center and Pathology Panel for Lymphoma Clinical Studies. *J. Clin. Oncol.* 1985, **3**: 25–38.

18. Yunis JJ, Oken NM, Kaplan ME, et al. Distinctive chromosomal abnormalities in histologic subtypes of non-Hodgkin's lymphomas. *N. Engl. J. Med.* 1982, **307**: 1231.

19. Cleary ML, Sklar J. Nucleotide sequence of a t(14;18) chromosomal breakpoint in follicular lymphoma and demonstration of a breakpoint cluster region near a transcriptionally active locus on chromosome 18. *Proc. Natl Acad. Sci. USA* 1985, **82**: 7439–7443.

20. Tsujimoto Y, Gorham J, Cossman J, et al. The t(14;18) chromosome translocations involved in B-cell lymphoma result from mistakes in VDJ joining. *Science* 1985, **229**: 1390–1393.

21. Bakhshi A, Jensen J, Goldman P, et al. Cloning the chromosomal breakpoint of t(14;18) human lymphomas: Clustering around J$_H$ on chromosome 14 and near a transcriptional unit on 18. *Cell* 1985, **41**: 899–906.

22. Cleary ML, Galili N, Sklar J. Detection of a second t(14;18) breakpoint cluster region in follicular lymphomas. *J. Exp. Med.* 1986, **164**: 315–320.

23. Zelenetz AD, Chu G, Galili N, et al. Enhanced detection of the t(14;18) translocation in malignant lymphoma using pulsed-field gel electrophoresis. *Blood* 1991, **78**: 1552–1560.

24. Tsujimoto Y, Cossman J, Jaffe E, et al. Involvement of the *bcl*-2 gene in human follicular lymphomas. *Science* 1985, **228**: 1440–1443.

25. Tsujimoto Y, Croce CM. Analysis of the structure, transcripts, and protein products of bcl-2, the gene involved in human follicular lymphoma. *Proc. Natl Acad. Sci. USA* 1986, **83**: 5214–5218.

26. Seto M, Jaeger U, Hockett R, et al. Alternative promoters and exons, somatic mutation and deregulation of the Bcl-2-Ig fusion gene in lymphoma. *Eur. Mol. Bio. Org. J.* 1988, **7**: 123–131.

27. Bakhshi A, Wright JJ, Graninger W, et al. Mechanism of the t(14;18) chromosomal translocation: Structural analysis of both derivative 14 and 18 reciprocal partners. *Proc. Natl Acad. Sci. USA* 1987, **84**: 2396–2400.

28. Wyatt RT, Rudders RA, Zelenetz AD, et al. BLC2 oncogene translocation is mediated by a χ-like consensus. *J. Exp. Med.* 1992, **175**: 1575–1588.

29. Jaeger U, Purtscher B, Karth GD, et al. Mechanism of the chromosomal translocation t(14;18) in lymphoma: Detection of a 45-Kd breakpoint binding protein. *Blood* 1993, **81**: 1833–1840.

30. Zelenetz AD, Cleary ML, Levy R. A submicroscopic interstitial deletion of chromosome 14 frequently occurs adjacent to the t(14;18) translocation breakpoint in human follicular lymphoma. *Genes Chrom. Can.* 1993, **6**: 140–150.

31. Dyer MJS. Unusual deletions in the immunoglobulin heavy chain locus in follicular B-cell lymphoma with t(14;18)(q32.3;q21.3). *Genes Chrom. Can.* 1993, **8**: 270–272.

32. Young RL, Korsmeyer SJ. A negative regulatory element in the *bcl*-2 5'-untranslated region inhibits expression from an upstream promoter. *Molec. Cell Biol.* 1993, **13**: 3683–3697.

33. Vaux D, Cory S, and Adams J. Bcl-2 gene promotes haemopoietic cell survival and cooperates with c-myc to immortalize pre-B-cells. *Nature* 1988, **335**: 440–442.

34. Sentman CL, Shutter JR, Hockenbery D, et al. bcl-2 inhibits multiple forms of apoptosis but not negative selection in thymocytes. *Cell* 1991, **67**: 879–888.

35. Strasser A, Harris AW, Cory S. *bcl*-2 transgene inhibits T-cell death and perturbs thymic self-censorship. *Cell* 1991, **67**: 889–899.

36. Reed JC. Bcl-2 and the regulation of programmed cell death. *J. Cell Biol.* 1994, **124**: 1–6.

37. Miyashita T, Reed JC. Bcl-2 gene transfer increases relative resistance of S49.1 and WEH17.2 lymphoid cells to cell death and DNA fragmentation induced by glucocorticoids and multiple chemotherapeutic drugs. *Can. Res.* 1992, **52**: 5407–11.

38. Lotem J, Sachs L. Regulation by *bcl*-2, c-*myc*, and p53 of susceptibility to induction of apoptosis by heat shock and cancer chemotherapy compounds in differ-

entiation-competent and -defective myeloid leukemic cells. *Cell Growth Differ.* 1993, **4**: 41–47.

39. Hockenbery DM, Oltvai ZN, Yin X-M, et al. Bcl-2 functions in an antioxidant pathway to prevent apoptosis. *Cell* 1993, **75**: 241–251.

40. Fanidi A, Harrington EA, Evan GI. Cooperative interaction between c-myc and bcl-2 proto-oncogenes. *Nature* 1992, **359**: 554–556.

41. Wang Y, Szekely L, Okan I, et al. Wild-type p53-triggered apoptosis is inhibited by bcl-2 in a v-myc-induced T-cell lymphoma line. *Oncogene* 1993, **8**: 3427–3431.

42. Hockenbery D, Nunez G, Milliman C, et al. Bcl-2 is an inner mitochondrial membrane protein that blocks programmed cell death. *Nature* 1990, **348**: 334–336.

43. Nunez G, London L, Hockenbery D, et al. Deregulated Bcl-2 gene expression selectively prolongs survival of growth factor-deprived cell lines. *J. Immunol. 1990,* **144**: 3602–3610.

44. Vaux DL, Weissman IL, and Kim SK. Prevention of programmed cell death in *Caenorhabditis elegans* by human bcl-2. *Science* 1992, **258**: 1955–1957.

45. Cuende E, Ales-Martinez JE, Ding L, et al. Programmed cell death by bcl-2-dependent and independent mechanisms in B lymphoma cells. *Eur. Mol. Bio. Org. J.* 1993, **12**: 1555–1560.

46. Tao W, Teh S-J, Melhado I, et al. The T-cell receptor repertoire of CD4⁻8⁺ thymocytes is altered by overexpression of the BCL-2 protooncogene in the thymus. *J. Exp. Med.* 1994, **179**: 145–153.

47. Chen-Levy S, Cleary ML. Membrane topology of the Bcl-2 proto-oncogenic protein demonstrated *in vitro*. *J. Biol. Chem.* 1990, **265**: 4929–4933.

48. Monaghan P, Robertson D, Amos AS, et al. Ultrastructural localization of Bcl-2 protein. *J. Histochem. Cytochem.* 1992, **40**: 1819–1825.

49. Krajewski S, Tanaka S, Takayama S, et al. Investigations of the subcellular distribution of the BCL-2 oncoprotein: Residence in the nuclear envelope, endoplasmic reticulum, and outer mitochondrial membrane. *Cancer Res.* 1993, **53**: 4701–4714.

50. Jacobson MD, Burne JF, King MP, et al. Bcl-2 blocks apoptosis in cells lacking mitochondrial DNA. *Nature* 1993, **361**: 365–369.

51. Korsmeyer SJ. Bcl-2 initiates a new category of oncogenes: regulators of cell death. *Blood* 1992, **80**: 879–886.

52. Hockenbery DM. The bcl-2 oncogene and apoptosis. *Semin. Immunol.* 1992, **4**: 413–420.

53. McDonnell TJ, Marin MC, Hsu B, et al. The bcl-2 oncogene: Apoptosis and neoplasia. *Radiat. Res.* 1993, **136**: 307–312.

54. Li Y-S, Hayakawa K, Hardy RR. The regulated expression of B lineage associated genes during B-cell differentiation in bone marrow and fetal liver. *J. Exp. Med.* 1993, **178**: 951–960.

55. Merino R, Ding L, Veis DJ, et al. Developmental regulation of the Bcl-2 protein and susceptibility to cell death in B lymphocytes. *Eur. Mol. Bio. Org. J.* 1994, **13**: 683–691.

56. Nisitani S, Tsubata T, Murakami M, et al. The bcl-2 gene product inhibits clonal deletion of self-reactive

B lymphocytes in the periphery but not in the bone marrow. *J. Exp. Med.* 1993, **178**: 1247–1254.

57. Nieuwenhuis P, Opstelten D. Functional anatomy of germinal centers. *Am. J. Anat.* 1984, **170**: 421–435.

58. MacLennan ICM, Liu YJ, Oldfield J, et al. The evolution of B-cell clones. *Curr. Topics Micro. Immunol.* 1990, **159**: 37–63.

59. MacLennan I. The center of hypermutation. *Nature* 1991, **354**: 352–353.

60. Hockenbery DM, Zutter M, Hickey W, et al. BCL2 protein is topographically restricted in tissues characterized by apoptotic cell death. *Proc. Natl Acad. Sci. USA* 1991, **88**: 6961–6965.

61. Liu Y-J, Mason D, Johnson G, et al. Germinal center cells express bcl-2 protein after activation by signals which prevent their entry into apoptosis. *Eur. J. Immunol.* 1991, **21**: 1905–1910.

62. Chleq-Deschamps CM, LeBrun DP, Huie P, et al. Topological dissociation of BCL-2 messenger RNA and protein expression in human lymphoid tissues. *Blood* 1993, **81**: 293–298.

63. Holder MJ, Wang H, Milner AE, et al. Suppression of apoptosis in normal and neoplastic human B lymphocytes by CD40 ligand is independent of Bc1–2 induction. *Eur. J. Immunol.* 1993, **23**: 2368–2373.

64. Nunez G, Hockenbery D, McDonnell TJ, et al. Bcl-2 maintains B-cell memory. *Nature* 1991, **353**: 71–73.

65. Nakayama K, Nakayama K, Negishi I, et al. Disappearance of the lymphoid system in Bcl-2 homozygous mutant chimeric mice. *Science* 1993, **261**: 1584–1588.

66. Veis DJ, Sorenson CM, Shutter JR, et al. Bcl-2-deficient mice demonstrate fulminant lymphoid apoptosis, polycystic kidneys, and hypopigmented hair. *Cell* 1993, **75**: 229–240.

67. Limpens J, de Jong D, van Krieken JHJM, et al. Bcl-2/J_H rearrangements in benign lymphoid tissues with follicular hyperplasia. *Oncogene* 1991, **6**: 2271–2276.

68. Aster JC, Kobayashi Y, Shiota M, et al. Detection of the t(14;18) at similar frequencies in hyperplastic lymphoid tissues from American and Japanese patients. *Am. J. Path.* 1992, **141**: 291–299.

69. McDonnell TJ, Deane N, Platt FM, et al. Bcl-2 immunoglobulin transgenic mice demonstrate extended B-cell survival and follicular lymphoproliferation. *Cell* 1989, **57**: 79–88.

70. McDonnell TJ, Nunez G, Platt FM, et al. Deregulated Bcl-2-immunoglobulin transgene expands a resting but responsive immunoglobulin M and D-expressing B-cell population. *Molec. Cell Biol.* 1990, **10**: 1901–1907.

71. McDonnell TJ, Korsmeyer SJ. Progression from lymphoid hyperplasia to high-grade malignant lymphoma in mice transgenic for the t(14;18). *Nature* 1991, **349**: 254–256.

72. Strasser A, Haris A, Bath M, et al. Novel primitive lymphoid tumors induced in transgenic mice by cooperation between myc and bcl-2. *Nature* 1990, **348**: 331–333.

73. Horning S, Rosenberg S. The natural history of initially untreated low-grade non-Hodgkin's lymphomas. *N. Engl. J. Med.* 1985, **311**: 1471–1475.

74. Garcia CF, Lowder J, Meeker TC, et al. Differences in host infiltrates among lymphoma patients treated with anti-idiotype antibodies: Correlation with treatment response. *J. Immunol.* 1985, **135**: 4252–4260.

75. Lowder J, Meeker T, Campbell M, et al. Studies on B lymphoid tumors treated with monoclonal anti-idiotype antibodies: Correlation with clinical responses. *Blood* 1987, **69**: 199–210.

76. Zelenetz AD, Campbell MJ, Bahler DW, et al. Follicular lymphoma: A model of lymphoid tumor progression in man. *Ann. Oncol.* 1991, **2**: 115–122.

77. Umetsu DT, Esserman L, Donlon TA, et al. Induction of proliferation of human follicular (B-type) lymphoma cells by cognate interaction with CD4+ T-cell clones. *J. Immunol.* 1990, **144**: 2550–2557.

78. Johnson PWM, Watt SM, Betts DR, et al. Isolated follicular lymphoma cells are resistant to apoptosis and can be grown *in vitro* in the CD40/stromal cell system. *Blood* 1993, **82**: 1848–1857.

79. Hopper JE, Nissonoff A. Individual antigenic specificity of immunoglobulins. *Adv. Immunol.* 1971, **13**: 57–99.

80. Miller RA, Maloney DG, Warnke R, et al. Treatment of B-cell lymphoma with monoclonal anti-idiotype antibody. *N. Engl. J. Med.* 1982, **306**: 517–522.

81. Meeker TC, Lowder J, Maloney DG, et al. A clinical trial of anti-idiotype therapy for B-cell malignancy. *Blood* 1985, **65**: 1349–1363.

82. Brown SL, Miller RA, Horning SJ, et al. Treatment of B-cell lymphoma with anti-idiotype antibodies alone and in combination with alpha interferon. *Blood* 1989, **73**: 651–661.

83. Maloney DG, Brown S, Czerwinski DK, et al. Monoclonal anti-idiotype antibody therapy of B-cell lymphoma: The addition of a short course of chemotherapy does not interfere with the antitumor effect nor prevent the emergence of idiotype-negative variant cells. *Blood* 1992, **80**: 1502–1510.

84. Meeker T, Lowder JN, Cleary ML, et al. Emergence of idiotype variants during therapy of B cell lymphoma with anti-idiotype antibodies. *N. Engl. J. Med.* 1986, **312**: 1685.

85. Levy R, Levy S, Cleary ML, et al. Somatic mutation in human B-cell tumors. *Immunol. Rev.* 1987, **96**: 43.

86. Zelenetz AD, Chen TT, Levy R. Histologic transformation of follicular lymphoma to diffuse lymphoma represents tumor progression by a single malignant B cell. *J. Exp. Med.* 1991, **173**: 197–207.

87. Bahler D, Levy R. Clonal evolution of a follicular lymphoma: Evidence for antigen selection. *Proc. Natl Acad. Sci. USA* 1992, **89**: 6770–6774.

88. Zelenetz A, Chen T, Levy R. Clonal expansion in follicular lymphoma occurs subsequent to antigenic selection. *J. Exp. Med.* 1992, **179**: 1137–1148.

89. Bahler DW, Zelenetz AD, Chen TT, et al. Antigen selection in human lymphomagenesis. *Cancer Res.* 1992, **52**: 5547s–5551s.

90. Zelenetz AD. Bcl-2. In Melchers F, Potter M (eds) *Mechanisms of B-Cell Neoplasia* Basel: Editiones Roche 1993, pp. 359–369.

91. Shlomchik MJ, Marshak-Rothstein A, Wolfowicz CB, et al. The role of clonal selection and somatic

mutation in autoimmunity. *Nature* 1987, **328**: 805–811.

92. Shlomchik MJ, Aucoin AH, Pisetsky DS, et al. Structure and function of anti-DNA autoantibodies derived from a single autoimmune mouse. *Proc. Natl Acad. Sci. USA* 1987, **84**: 9150–9154.

93. Shlomchik M, Mascelli M, Shan H, et al. Anti-DNA antibodies from autoimmune mice arise by clonal expansion and somatic mutation. *J. Exp. Med.* 1990, **171**: 265–296.

94. Dighiero G, Hart S, Lim A, et al. Autoantibody activity of immunoglobulins isolated from B-cell follicular lymphomas. *Blood* 1991, **78**: 581–585.

95. Bahler DW, Campbell MJ, Hart S, et al. Ig V_H gene expression among human follicular lymphomas. *Blood* 1991, **78**: 1561–1568.

96. Hubbard SM, Chabner BA, DeVita VT, et al. Histologic progression in non-Hodgkin's lymphoma. *Blood* 1982, **59**: 258.

97. Acker B, Hoppe RT, Colby TV, et al. Histologic conversion in the non-Hodgkin's lymphomas. *J. Clin. Oncol.* 1983, **1**: 11–16.

98. Ersbøll J, Schultz HB, Perdersen-Bjergaard J, et al. Follicular low-grade non-Hodgkin's lymphoma: Long-term outcome with or without tumor progression. *Eur. J. Haematol.* 1989, **42**: 155–163.

99. Tweeddale ME, Lim B, Jamal N, et al. The presence of clonogenic cell in high-grade malignant lymphoma: A prognostic factor. *Blood* 1987, **69**: 1307–1314.

100. Gauwerky CE, Hoxie J, Nowell PC, et al. Pre-B-cell leukemia with a t(14;18) translocation is preceded by follicular lymphoma. *Oncogene* 1988, **2**: 431.

101. de Jong D, Voetdijk BMH, Beverstock GC, et al. Activation of the c-*myc* oncogene in a precursor-B-cell blast crisis of follicular lymphoma, presenting as composite lymphoma. *N. Engl. J. Med.* 1988, **318**: 1373.

102. de Jong D, Voetdjik B, Ommen G, et al. Translocation t(14;18) as a cause for defective immunoglobulin production. *J. Exp. Med.* 1989, **169**: 613–624.

103. Yano T, Jaffe ES, Longo DL, et al. MYC rearrangements in histologically progressed follicular lymphomas. *Blood* 1992, **80**: 758–67.

104. Ladanyi M, Offit K, Parsa NZ, et al. Follicular lymphoma with t(8;14)(q24;q32): A distinct clinical and molecular subset of t(8;14)-bearing lymphomas. *Blood* 1992, **79**: 2124–2130.

105. Sander CA, Yano T, Clark HM, et al. p53 mutation is associated with progression in follicular lymphomas. *Blood* 1993, **82**: 1994–2004.

106. Lo Coco F, Gaidano G, Louie DC, et al. p53 mutations are associated with histologic transformation of follicular lymphoma. *Blood* 1993, **82**: 2289–2295.

107. Gaidano G, Ballerini P, Grong JZ, et al. p53 mutations in human lymphoid malignancies: Association with Burkitt lymphoma and chronic lymphocytic leukemia. *Proc. Natl Acad. Sci. USA* 1991, **88**: 5413–5417.

108. Yano T, Sander CA, Andrade RE, et al. Molecular analysis of the BCL-3 locus at chromosome 17q22 in B-cell neoplasms. *Blood* 1993, **82**: 1813–1899.

109. Yunis JJ, Frizzera G, Oken MM, et al. Multiple recurrent genomic defects in follicular lymphoma. *N. Engl. J. Med.* 1987, **316**: 79–84.

110. Richardson ME, Quanguang C, Filippa DA, et al. Intermediate- to high-grade histology of lymphomas carrying t(14;18) is associated with additional nonrandom chromosome changes. *Blood* 1987, **70**: 444–447.

111. Armitage JO, Sanger WG, Weisenburger DD, et al. Correlation of secondary cytogenetic abnormalities with histologic appearance in non-Hodgkin's lymphomas bearing t(14;18)(q32;q21). *J. Natl Cancer Inst.* 1988, **80**: 576–580.

112. Levine EG, Juneja S, Arthur D, et al. Sequential karyotypes in non-Hodgkin's lymphoma: Their nature and significance. *Genes Chrom. Cancer* 1990, **1**: 270–280.

113. Close P, Lauder I. Mantle zone lymphoma – is it an entity? *J. Path.* 1990, **160**: 279–281.

114. Lardelli P, Bookman M, Sundeen JJ, et al. Lymphocytic lymphoma of intermediate differentiation: Morphologic and immunophenotypic spectrum and clinical correlations. *Am. J. Surg. Path.* 1990, **14**: 752–763.

115. Triozzi P, Borowitz MJ, and Gockerman JP. Gastrointestinal involvement and multiple lymphomatous polyposis in mantle-zone lymphoma. *J. Clin. Oncol.* 1986, **8**: 804–808.

116. O'Brian DS, Kennedy MJ, Daly PA, et al. Multiple lymphomatous polyposis of the gastrointestinal tract. A clinicopathologically distinctive form of non-Hodgkin's lymphoma of B-cell centrocytic type. *Am. J. Surg. Path.* 1989, **13**: 691–699.

117. Lennert K, Feller AC. In Lennert K (eds) *Histopathology of Non-Hodgkin's Lymphomas*. Berlin: Springer-Verlag, 1992, p. 312.

118. Bennett JM, Catovsky D, Daniel MT, et al. Proposal for the classification of the acute leukemias. *Br. J. Haematol* 1976, **33**: 451–458.

119. Banks PM, Chan J, Cleary ML, et al. Mantle cell lymphoma: A proposal for unification of morphologic, immunologic and molecular data. *Am. J. Surg. Path.* 1992, **16**: 637–640.

120. Rappaport H. Tumors of the hemopoietic system. In *Atlas of Tumor Pathology*, Section 3, Fascicle 8. Washington, DC: Armed Forces Institute of Pathology, 1966.

121. Jaffe ES, Bookman MA, Longo D. Lymphocytic lymphoma of intermediate differentiation – mantle zone lymphoma: A distinct subtype of B-cell lymphoma. *Human Pathol.* 1987, **18**: 877.

122. Pombo de Oliveira MS, Jaffe ES, Catovsky D. Leukaemic phase of mantle zone (intermediate) lymphoma: Its characterisation in 11 cases. *J. Clin. Pathol.* 1989, **42**: 962.

123. Swerdlow SH, Habeshaw JA, Murray LJ, et al. Centrocytic lymphoma: A distinct clinicopathologic and morphologic entity, a multiparameter study of 18 cases at diagnosis and relapse. *Am. J. Path.* 1983, **113**: 181–197.

124. Weisenburger DD, Kim H, and Rappaport H. Mantle-zone lymphoma: A follicular variant of intermediate lymphocytic lymphoma. *Cancer* 1982, **49**: 1429.

125. Katzin W, Linden M, Fishleder A, et al. Immunophenotypic and genotypic characterization of diffuse mixed non-Hodgkin's lymphomas. *Am. J. Path.* 1989, **135**: 615.

126. Cossman J, Neckers LM, Hsu S-M, et al. Low-grade lymphomas: Expression of developmentally regulated B-cell antigens. *Am. J. Path.* 1984, **115**: 117.

127. Perry DA, Bast M, Armitage JO, et al. Diffuse intermediate lymphocytic lymphoma: A clinicopathologic study and comparison with small lymphocytic lymphoma and diffuse small cleaved cell lymphoma. *Cancer* 1990, **66**: 1995–2000.

128. Weisenburger DD, Duggan MJ, Perry DA, et al. Non-Hodgkin's lymphomas of mantle zone origin. *Pathol. Ann.* 1991, **26**: 139–158.

129. Frizzera G, Sakurai M, Notohara K, et al. t(11;14)(q13;32) in B-cell lymphomas (intermediately differentiated lymphocytic and follicular). A report of four cases. *Am. J. Path.* 1991, **95**: 684–691.

130. Leroux D, Le MarcíHadour F, Gressin R, et al. Non-Hodgkin's lymphomas with t(11;14)(q13;q32): A subset of mantle zone/intermediate lymphocytic lymphoma. *Br. J. Haematol* 1991, **77**: 346–353.

131. Medeiros LJ, Van Krieken JH, Jaffe ES, et al. Association of bcl-1 rearrangements with lymphocytic lymphoma of intermediate differentiation. *Blood* 1990, **76**: 2086–2090.

132. Rosenberg CL, Wong E, Petty EM, et al. PRAD1, a candidate BCL1 oncogene: Mapping and expression in centrocytic lymphoma. *Proc. Natl Acad. Sci. USA* 1991, **88**: 9638–9642.

133. Van den Berghe E, De Wolf-Peeters C, Van den Oord J, et al. Translocation (11;14): A cytogenetic anomaly associated with B-cell lymphomas of non-follicle center cell lineage. *J. Path.* 1991, **163**: 13.

134. Weisenburger DD, Sanger WG, Armitage JO, et al. Intermediate lymphocytic lymphoma: Immunophenotypic and cytogenetic findings. *Blood* 1987, **69**: 1617–1621.

135. Williams ME, Swerdlow SH, Meeker TC. Chromosome t(11;14)(q13;q32) breakpoints in centrocytic lymphoma are highly localized at the bcl-1 major translocation cluster. *Leukemia* 1993, **7**: 1437–1440.

136. Tsujimoto Y, Jaffe ES, Cossman J, et al. Clustering of breakpoints on chromosome 11 in human B-cell neoplasms with the t(11;14) chomosome translocation. *Nature* 1985, **315**: 340–343.

137. Rimokh R, Berger F, Cornillet P, et al. Break in the bcl-1 locus is closely associated with intermediate lymphocytic lymphoma subtype. *Genes Chrom. Cancer* 1990, **2**: 223–226.

138. Williams ME, Westermann CD, Swerdlow SH. Genotypic characterization of centrocytic lymphoma: frequent rearrangement of the chromosome 11 bcl-1 locus. *Blood* 1990, **76**: 1387–1391.

139. Athan E, Foitl DR, Knowles DM. BCL-1 rearrangement. Frequency and clinical significance among B-cell chronic lymphocytic leukemias and non-Hodgkin's lymphomas. *Am. J. Path.* 1991, **138**: 591.

140. Williams ME, Swerdlow SH, Rosenberg CL, et al. Characterization of chromosome 11 translocation breakpoints at the bcl-1 and PRAD1 loci in centrocytic lymphoma. *Cancer Res.* 1992, **52**(Suppl.): 5541s–5544s.

141. De Boer CJ, Loyson S, Kluin PM, et al. Multiple breakpoints within the bcl-1 locus in B-cell lymphoma: Rearrangements of the Cyclin D1 gene. *Cancer Res.* 1993, **53**: 4148–4152.

142. Raynaud SD, Bekri S, Leroux D, et al. Expanded range in 11q13 breakpoints with differing patterns of Cyclin D1 expression in B-cell malignancies. *Genes Chrom. Cancer* 1993, **8**: 80–87.

143. Rimokh R, Berger F, Delsol G, et al. Rearrangement and overexpression of the BCL-1/PRAD-1 gene in intermediate lymphocytic lymphomas and in t(11q13)-bearing leukemias. *Blood* 1993, **81**: 3063–3067.

144. Brito-Babapulle V, Pittman S, Melo JV, et al. Cytogenetic studies on prolymphocytic leukemia 1. B-cell prolymphocytic leukemia. *Hematol. Pathol.* 1987, **1**: 27.

145. Raffeld M, Jaffe E. bcl-1, t(11;14), and and mantle cell-derived lymphomas. *Blood* 1991, **78**: 259–263.

146. Tsujimoto Y, Louie E, Bashir MM, et al. The reciprocal partners of both the t(14;18) and the t(11;14) translocations involved in B-cell neoplasms are generated by the same mechanism. *Oncogene* 1988, **2**: 347.

147. Finger LR, Harvey RC, Moore RCA, et al. A common mechanism of chromosomal translocation in T- and B-cell neoplasia. *Science* 1986, **234**: 982–985.

148. Tsujimoto Y, Yunis J, Onorato-Showe L, et al. Molecular cloning of the chromosomal breakpoint of B-cell lymphomas and leukemias with the t(11;14) chromosome translocation. *Science* 1984, **224**: 1403–1406.

149. Withers DA, Harvey RC, Faust JB, et al. Characterization of a candidate bcl-1 gene. *Molec. Cell Biol.* 1991, **11**: 4846–4853.

150. Rosenberg CL, Kim HG, Shows TB, et al. Rearrangement and overexpression of D11S287E, a candidate oncogene on chromosome 11q13 in benign parathyroid tumors. *Oncogene* 1991, **6**: 449–453.

151. Motokura T, Bloom T, Kim HG, et al. A novel cyclin encoded by a bcl-1 linked candidate oncogene. *Nature* 1991, **350**: 512–515.

152. Xiong Y, Connolly T, Futcher B, et al. Human D-type cyclin. *Cell* 1991, **65**: 691–699.

153. Matsushime H, Roussel MF, Ashmun RA, et al. Colony-stimulating factor 1 regulates novel cyclins during the G1 phase of the cell cycle. *Cell* 1991, **65**: 701–713.

154. Tushinski RJ, Oliver IT, Guilbert LJ, et al. Survival of mononuclear phagocytes depends on a lineage-specific growth factor that the differentiated cells selectively destroy. *Cell* 1982, **28**: 71–81.

155. Tushinski RJ, Stanley ER. The regulation of mononuclear phagocyte entry into S phase by the colony stimulating factor CSF-1. *J. Cell Physiol.* 1985, **122**: 221–228.

156. Baldin V, Lukas J, Marcote MJ, et al. Cyclin D1 is a nuclear protein required for cell cycle progression in G1. *Genes Dev.* 1993, **7**: 812–821.

157. Lukas J, Pagano M, Staskova Z, et al. Cyclin D1 protein oscillates and is essential for cell cycle progression in human tumor cell lines. *Oncogene* 1994, **9**: 707–718.

158. Seto M, Yamamoto K, Lida S, et al. Gene rearrangement and overexpression of PRAD1 in

lymphoid malignancy with t(11;14)(q13;q32) translocation. *Oncogene* 1992, **7**: 1401–1406.

159. Rosenberg CL, Motokura T, Kronenberg HM, et al. Coding sequence of the overexpressed transcript of the putative oncogene PRAD1/cyclin D1 in two primary human tumors. *Oncogene* 1993, **8**: 519–521.

160. Lammie GA, Fanti V, Smith R, et al. D11S287, a putative oncogene on chromosome 11q13, is amplified and expressed in squamous cell and mammary carcinomas and linked to bcl-1. *Oncogene* 1991, **6**: 439–444.

161. Schuuring E, Verhoeven E, Mooi W, et al. Identification and cloning of two overexpressed genes, U21B31/PRAD1 and EMS1, within the amplified chromsome 11q13 region in human carcinomas. *Oncogene* 1992, **7**: 355–361.

162. Jiang W, Kahn SM, Zhou P, et al. Overexpression of cyclin D1 in rat fibroblasts causes abnormalities in growth control, cell cycle progression and gene expression. *Oncogene* 1993, **8**: 3447–3457.

163. Quelle DE, Ashmun RA, Shurtleff SA, et al. Overexpression of mouse D-type cyclins accelerates G1 phase in rodent fibroblasts. *Genes Dev.* 1993, **7**: 1559–1571.

164. Hsiao WL, Housey GM, Johnson MD, et al. Cells that overproduce protein kinase C are more susceptible to transformation by an activated H-ras oncogene. *Mol. Cell Biol.* 1989, **9**: 2641–2647.

165. Lovec H, Sewing A, Lucibello FC, et al. Oncogenic activity of cyclin D1 revealed through cooperation with Ha-ras: Link between cell cycle control and malignant transformation. *Oncogene* 1994, **9**: 323–326.

166. Hinds PW, Dowdy SF, Eaton EN, et al. Function of a human cyclin gene as an oncogene. *Proc. Natl Acad. Sci. USA* 1994, **91**: 709–713.

167. Hinds PW, Mittnacht S, Dulic V, et al. Regulation of retinoblastoma protein functions by ectopic expression of human cyclins. *Cell* 1992, **70**: 993–1006.

168. Cobrinik D, Dowdy S, Hinds PW, et al. The retinoblastoma protein and the regulation of cell cycling. *Trends Biochem. Sci.* 1992, **92**: 312–315.

169. Nizze H, Cogliatti SB, von SC, et al. Monocytoid B-cell lymphoma: Morphological variants and relationship to low-grade B-cell lymphoma of the mucosa-associated lymphoid tissue. *Histopathology* 1991, **18**: 403–414.

170. Spencer J, Finn T, Pulford KAF, et al. The human gut contains a novel population of B-lymphocytes which resemble marginal zone cells. *Clin. Exp. Immunol.* 1985, **62**: 607–612.

171. Isaacson P, Wright DH. Malignant lymphoma of mucosa-associated lymphoid tissue: A distinctive type of B-cell lymphoma. *Cancer* 1983, **52**: 1410–1416.

172. Isaacson P, Wright DH. Extranodal malignant lymphoma arising from mucosa-associated lymphoid tissue. *Cancer* 1984, **53**: 2515–2524.

173. Isaacson PG, Spencer J. Malignant lymphoma of mucosa-associated lymphoid tissue. *Histopathology* 1987, **11**: 445–462.

174. Hyjek E, Smith WJ, and Isaacson PG. Primary B-cell lymphoma of salivary glands and its relationship to myoepithelial sialadenitis. *Human Pathol.* 1988, **19**: 766–776.

175. Pelstring RJ, Essell JH, Kurtin PJ, et al. Diversity of organ site involvement among malignant lymphomas of mucosa-associated tissues (MALTomas). *Am. J. Clin. Path.* 1991, **96**: 738–745.

176. Gallatin W, Weissman I, Butcher E. A cell-surface molecule involved in organ-specific homing of lymphocytes. *Nature* 1983, **304**: 30–34.

177. Butcher E. Cellular and molecular mechanisms that direct leukocyte traffic. *Am. J Path.* 1990, **136**: 3–12.

178. Harris NL. Low-grade B-cell lymphoma of mucosa-associated lymphoid tissue and monocytoid B-cell lymphoma. Related entities that are distinct from other low-grade B-cell lymphomas [editorial; comment]. *Arch. Path. Lab. Med.* 1993, **117**: 771–775.

179. Sheibani K, Sohn CC, Burke JS, et al. Monocytoid B-cell lymphoma. A novel B-cell neoplasm. *Am. J. Path.* 1986, **124**: 310–318.

180. Sheibani K, Burke JS, Swartz WG, et al. Monocytoid B-cell lymphoma. Clinicopathologic study of 21 cases of a unique type of low-grade lymphoma. *Cancer* 1988, **62**: 1531–1538.

181. Cogliatti SB, Lennert K, Hansmann ML, et al. Monocytoid B-cell lymphoma: Clinical and prognostic features of 21 patients. *J. Clin. Path.* 1990, **43**: 619–625.

182. Harris NL. Extranodal lymphoid infiltrates and mucosa-associated lymphoid tissue (MALT). A unifying concept [editorial] [see comments]. *Am. J. Surg. Path.* 1991, **15**: 879–884.

183. Ngan BY, Warnke RA, Wilson M, et al. Monocytoid B-cell lymphoma: A study of 36 cases [see comments]. *Human Path.* 1991, **22**: 409–421.

184. Parveen T, Navarro-Roman L, Medeiros J, et al. Low-grade B-cell lymphoma of mucosa associated lymphoid tissue arising out of the kidney. *Arch. Path. Lab. Med. 1993*, **117**: 780–783.

185. Shin SS, Sheibani K, Fishleder A, et al. Monocytoid B-cell lymphoma in patients with Sjogren's syndrome: A clinicopathologic study of 13 patients [see comments]. *Human Path.* 1991, **22**: 422–430.

186. Shin SS, Sheibani K. Monocytoid B-cell lymphoma. *Am. J. Clin. Path.* 1993, **99**: 421–425.

187. Papadaki L, Wotherspoon AC, Isaacson PG. The lymphoepithelial lesion of gastric low-grade B-cell lymphoma of mucosa-associated lymphoid tissue (MALT): An ultrastructural study. *Histopathology* 1992, **21**: 415–421.

188. Faris TD, Saltzstein SL. Gastric lymphoid hyperplasia: A lesion confused with lymphosarcoma. *Cancer* 1964, **17**: 207–212.

189. Isaacson P, Wotherspoon A, Diss T, et al. Follicular colonization in B-cell lymphoma of mucosa-associated lymphoid tissue. *Am. J. Surg. Path.* 1991, **15**: 819–828.

190. Piris MA, Rivas C, Morente M, et al. Monocytoid B-cell lymphoma, a tumor related to the marginal zone. *Histopathology* 1988, **12**: 383–392.

191. Zukerberg L, Medeiros L, Ferry J, et al. Diffuse low-grade B-cell lymphomas: Four clinically distinct subtypes defined by a combination of morphologic and

CHAPTER 15

Pathogenesis of intermediate-grade B-cell lymphomas

RICCARDO DALLA-FAVERA AND GIORGIO CATTORETTI

Introduction

Intermediate-grade lymphomas in the Working Formulation for Clinical Usage encompass an heterogeneous group of tumors including follicular large-cell lymphoma, as well as diffuse large- and diffuse mixed-cell lymphoma. In terms of pathogenesis, however, all types of follicular lymphoma (FL), of both low and intermediate grade, fall into one category and diffuse lymphomas of intermediate grade and perhaps some high-grade large-cell lymphomas into another. The pathogenesis of FL is described in Chapter 14; this chapter will focus on diffuse lymphoma. These tumors will be collectively referred to as diffuse lymphoma with a large-cell component (DLLC) to include the diffuse large- and mixed-cell subtypes.

DLLC represent approximately 50% of B-cell non-Hodgkin's lymphomas (NHL) diagnosed *de novo* [1]. In addition, DLLC can derive from the histologic transformation of FL, so that it is the most important form of NHL in terms of morbidity and mortality. Although this group of NHL is heterogeneous in terms of histology and cell phenotype, all

DLLC represent clonal expansions of mature B-cells, with many phenotypic features of germinal center centroblasts [2]. Given the remarkably complex biological interactions regulating the differentiation and function of mature B-cells in the germinal center (see Chapter 8), it is conceivable that a multitude of complex and poorly understood epigenetic alterations may contribute to the pathogenesis of DLLC. However, in common with other cancer types, there is substantial experimental evidence indicating that DLLC develops as a consequence of the occurrence of specific genetic alterations involving proto-oncogenes and tumor suppressor genes.

Until recently, the only genetic alterations detected in at least some DLLC, those involving the *bcl*-2 and c-*myc* genes, were not specifically associated with DLLC and could be found at higher frequency in other NHL types (see Chapters 14 and 16). More recently, however, some progress has been made with the identification of a novel set of genetic alterations which display a closer association with DLLC and may therefore play a specific role in the pathogenesis of these tumors.

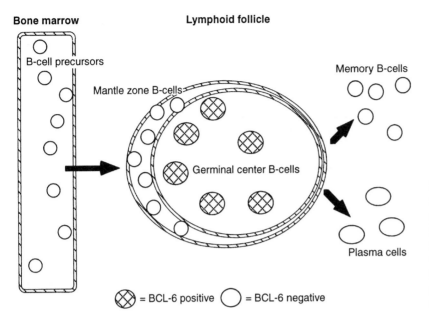

Figure 15.3 Schematic representation of the pattern of the expression of *bcl*-6 during normal B-cell differentiation. B-Cells (centroblasts and centrocytes) within the germinal centers, but not their precursors (virgin B-cells) or progeny (memory B-cells, plasma cells), express *bcl*-6.

the *c-myc* proto-oncogene in Burkitt's lymphoma (Chapter 16). In all cases displaying direct involvement of *bcl*-6, the coding domain is left intact, whereas the 5' regulatory region containing the promoter sequences is either completely removed (when truncation occurs within the first exon or intron) or truncated. As a result, all of the coding exons of the *bcl*-6 gene are linked downstream to heterologous sequences, which, based on cytogenetic analysis, can originate from different chromosomes in different cases.

Analysis of rearranged *bcl*-6 genes and their

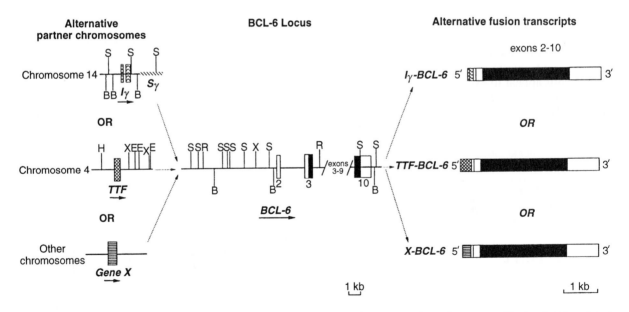

Figure 15.4 Schematic representation of rearranged *bcl*-6 genes in chromosomal translocations affecting 3q27 and their transcriptional products. The left side of the panel shows the alternative partner chromosomes containing promoter regions (IgH, TTF-1, or other not yet identified, called X), which can be found juxtaposed 5' to the *bcl*-6 coding domains (center) in different DLLC carrying 3q27 translocations [14–16]. The right side of the panel shows the respective transcription products of these translocations: noncoding sequences from various chromosome are fused 5' to *bcl*-6 coding sequences.

transcription products in a few DLLC cases indicates that the common functional consequence of these alterations is the juxtaposition of heterologous promoters to the *bcl*-6 coding domain, a mechanism called promoter substitution (Figure 15.4) [14–16]. These recombinations generate chimeric transcripts which initiate from promoters derived from one of the various chromosomal loci that recombine with 3q27 and are spliced to normal *bcl*-6 coding domains, thus permitting expression of a normal *bcl*-6 protein. In a minority of cases carrying *bcl*-6 rearrangements, the breakpoints are located immediately 5' to the promoter region and therefore remove only the putative 5' regulatory sequences. In these cases, it is conceivable that the consequence of the translocation may be the substitution of normal (possibly negative) regulatory sequences with transcriptional enhancers or distantly acting regulatory elements from other chromosomes.

The finding that in some NHL the normal *bcl*-6 promoter is substituted by heterologous regulatory sequences implies that *bcl*-6 expression is deregulated in these tumors. In fact, one common characteristic of the heterologous promoters found linked to *bcl*-6 is that they are active in B-cells, but are not downregulated during B-cell differentiation [14–16]. Thus, one common consequence of these alterations may be to prevent downregulation of *bcl*-6 and, in turn, the differentiation of B-cells into plasma cells. Additional investigations are, however, necessary to establish the oncogenic potential of altered *bcl*-6 genes, as well as to elucidate their specific role in lymphomagenesis.

FREQUENCY OF bcl-6 REARRANGEMENTS IN THE NHL SUBTYPES

When assessed by molecular analysis of tumor DNA, the frequency of *bcl*-6 rearrangements far exceeds that expected from cytogenetic identification of 3q27 aberrations in DLCL (12%) [3], suggesting that BCL-6 rearrangements can occur as a consequence of submicroscopic chromosomal aberrations. Table 15.2 shows that *bcl*-6 rearrangements are detectable in 40% of DLLC, significantly less frequently in FL, and are not observed in other types of NHL or in other lymphoid malignancies, including acute lymphoblastic leukemia (ALL), chronic lymphocytic leukemia (CLL), multiple myeloma and T-cell-derived malignances [13].

Among the heterogeneous lymphomas in the DLLC spectrum, *bcl*-6 rearrangements are significantly more frequent in tumors with a pure diffuse large-cell histology (DLCL) which lack *bcl*-2

Table 15.2 Frequency of *bcl*-6 gene rearrangements in lymphoid tumors

NHL	Histology	% Rearranged
Low grade	SL	0
	SCC-F	11
	MX-F	0
Intermediate grade	MX-D	10
	DLCL	40
	SCC-D	0
High grade	IMB	0
	SNCL	0

NHL, non-Hodgkin's lymphomas; SL, small lymphocytic; SCC-F, follicular small cleaved cell; MX-F, follicular mixed; MX-D, diffuse mixed cell; DLCL, diffuse large cell; SCC-D, diffuse small cleaved cell; IMB, immunoblastic; SNCL, small non-cleaved cell lymphoma. Data from ref. 13.

rearrangements. Considering that DLLC can originate both *de novo* and from the 'transformation' of FL, and that the latter typically carry *bcl*-2 rearrangements, this finding suggests that *bcl*-6 aberrations may be specifically involved in the pathogenesis of *de novo* DLLC (Figure 15.5).

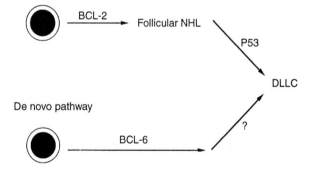

Figure 15.5 Schematic representation of the major pathways leading to DLLC development based on the presence of *bcl*-2, *bcl*-6 and p53 lesions. The scheme does not include other genetic lesions, which are observed at lower frequency and in variable association with *bcl*-2 or *bcl*-6 rearrangements (e.g., *c-myc* alterations) or for which insufficient data are available (NF-κB/Rel). The pathways shown represent common, but not exclusive, combinations of genetic lesions, since rare DLLC cases displaying p53 mutations in the absence of *bcl*-2 rearrangements, or both *bcl*-2 and *bcl*-6 rearrangements, have been described (see text).

demonstrated in Burkitt's lymphoma [8] and 'variant' translocations between the same band on chromosome 8 (q24), and either 2 or 22 were also described [9]. These translocations were present in essentially all Burkitt's lymphomas, from equatorial Africa as well as Europe and the USA, suggesting that they were an essential component of pathogenesis.

HISTOLOGY VERSUS CYTOGENETICS

Pathologists who had worked in Africa soon realized that a fraction of childhood lymphomas occurring in other world regions are histologically indistinguishable from African Burkitt's lymphoma [10–12]. Subsequently, Burkitt's lymphoma was 'defined' as a histological entity at a conference held under the auspices of the World Health Organization [13]. The cellular origins of the lymphoma remained unknown, hence the term 'undifferentiated lymphoma' in the modified Rappaport classification scheme [14], but Lukes and Collins related the cytological appearance of Burkitt's lymphoma to normal cells that they identified in the germinal follicle of lymph nodes – small noncleaved cells – and used this terminology in their classification system [15]. This same terminology was subsequently used in the Working Formulation [16]. Because of variability in the degree of pleomorphism in the cells of some of the tumors felt to fall into these categories, undifferentiated lymphomas in the Rappaport classification scheme and small noncleaved cell lymphomas in the Working Formulation were divided into two categories, Burkitt's lymphoma and non-Burkitt's lymphoma. In the Revised European–American Lymphoma (REAL) classification, the terminology Burkitt and Burkitt-like is preferred [17]. While these categories differ primarily with respect to the degree of cellular pleomorphism, there is no sharp dividing line between them. Burkitt-like lymphomas include cells which are larger than those of Burkitt's lymphoma and also have a higher fraction of cells that contain a single large nucleolus instead of the multiple (typically 2–5) nucleoli of Burkitt's lymphoma. These characteristics are present in B-cell immunoblastic or large-cell (centroblastic) lymphomas, and, not surprisingly, therefore, the Burkitt-like lymphomas also merge, morphologically, with the large-cell lymphomas [18].

While Burkitt's lymphoma is the predominant (but not exclusive) morphological subtype in children, Burkitt-like lymphomas account for a higher proportion of these lymphomas in adults. Some of the latter contain 14;18 translocations [19] as well as 8;14 translocations, while a small fraction (10–20%) of large-cell lymphomas in adults have 8;14 or variant translocations [20]. These fractions may vary, depending upon where the dividing line between large B-cell lymphoma and Burkitt-like lymphoma is drawn. Thus, the histological categories probably do not separate discrete pathobiological entities and, although Burkitt's lymphoma may be relatively homogeneous, Burkitt-like and large-cell lymphomas are clearly not. On the other hand, if the characteristic nonrandom chromosomal translocations were used to define a pathological entity, its histology would extend from small noncleaved cell to large-cell lymphoma. It seems probable that large-cell lymphomas with 8;14 translocations are biologically very similar to Burkitt's lymphomas but have differentiated somewhat further than classical Burkitt's lymphoma. This may relate to the presence of particular molecular abnormalities, but at present, apart from differences in the breakpoint location on chromosome 8, genetic differences have not been described between large-cell and small noncleaved cell lymphomas that contain 8;14 or variant translocations. In addition, immunophenotypic differences are not sufficient to differentiate between these entities (Table 16.1). Since similar or identical histological entities with similar immunophenotypic characteristics may carry quite different genetic lesions, it would appear that the cytogenetic and molecular abnormalities (c-*myc*/immunoglobulin translocations versus *bcl*-2/immunoglobulin translocations) provide definitions of pathobiological entities that (excepting follicular lymphomas) cannot be differentiated by their histological appearances.

In children, no clear biological (immunophenotypic or cytogenetic) or clinical significance has been ascribed to the histological subcategories of small noncleaved cell lymphoma [21], and in the Kiel classification, these are not separated [22]. Interestingly, in O'Conor's original description of the histology of Burkitt's lymphoma in Uganda – a disease which is likely to be much more homogeneous with respect to pathogenesis than small noncleaved cell lymphomas in other countries – he did describe some

Table 16.1 Comparison of immunophenotypic markers between Burkitt's lymphoma and other B-cell lymphomas

	CD5	CD23	CD10
Burkitt's lymphoma	—	—	+
Mantle cell lymphoma	+	—	–/+
MALT lymphoma	—	—	—
Follicular lymphoma	—	–/+	+/–
Large B-cell lymphoma	–/+	–/+	–/+

–/+ indicates that the majority, but not all tumors, are negative for this marker. +/– indicates that most, but not all tumors are positive for this marker.

Table 16.2 Distribution of histological types in malignant lymphoma in East African Children

Histological type*	Number of patients
Stem cell	11
Histiocytic	5
Lymphocytic poorly differentiated	88
Mixed cell	2
Total	106

* Using the Gall and Rappaport classification scheme.

variation in the histological appearance in a series of patients with similar clinical characteristics and gross pathological appearances (Table 16.2) [3]. It seems unlikely, therefore, that in children histological differences connote significant differences in biology.

There is little information that specifically relates to the small noncleaved cell lymphomas which contain 14;18 translocations, although the transformation of follicular lymphomas into small noncleaved cell lymphomas has been described, and such lymphomas may, therefore, be more closely related to large B-cell lymphomas, which contain 14;18 translocations (perhaps they would be diagnosed as such by some pathologists). Rarely, transformed follicular lymphomas with small noncleaved or Burkitt-like morphology have been described in which an 8;14 or variant translocation has been superimposed on a 14;18 translocation, a finding which is consistent with the phenotypic resemblance of Burkitt's lymphoma to a germinal center cell and which may simply represent a relatively uncommon pathway whereby follicular lymphomas may undergo transformation. However, in the absence of more definitive information, this chapter will focus on the small noncleaved cell lymphomas associated with 8;14 or variant translocations, and for simplicity, they will be referred to collectively as Burkitt's lymphoma.

Genesis and significance of the chromosomal translocations associated with Burkitt's lymphoma

The discovery of the nonrandom chromosomal translocations associated with Burkitt's lymphoma provided important insights into pathogenesis, but not until the genes located at the chromosomal breakpoints were identified [23,24]. A common feature of the translocations is involvement of chromosome 8 at band q24 – the location of the c-*myc* oncogene known to be a critical gene in the regulation of cell proliferation. The partner genes to c-*myc* are the immunoglobulin loci on chromosomes 14q32 (heavy chain), 2p11 (kappa), or 22q11 (lambda). In 8;14 translocations, which account for 80% of the translocations associated with Burkitt's lymphoma, c-*myc* is translocated from chromosome 8 to the heavy chain locus on chromosome 14, while in the so-called 'variant' translocations, a part of the light chain constant region is translocated to chromosome 8, distal to the c-*myc* gene. In each case the c-*myc* gene is juxtaposed to an immunoglobulin constant region, whether of heavy or light chain origin.

This observation strongly suggests that the immunoglobulin genes play an important role in pathogenesis – either with respect to the genesis of the translocations or to the functional changes that the translocations bring about, or to both. As discussed elsewhere in this volume, it is probable that the recombinational events that occur early in B-cell ontogeny, the purpose of which is to develop a set of functional but diversely reacting set of immunoglobulin genes, increase the likelihood that a translocation will occur. There is good evidence that the c-*myc* gene is transcriptionally deregulated in Burkitt's lymphoma [25], and it is probable that transcriptional enhancers within the immunoglobulin regions – whether from heavy chain or light chain loci – which have been juxtaposed to c-*myc* by the translocation, cause continuous transcription from c-*myc* (Figure 16.1). Structural changes within the c-*myc* regulatory region (see below) may also be relevant to its deregulation. In 8;14 translocations, this effect is not necessarily mediated through the recognized enhancer situated upstream of the switch-μ region, since the breakpoint, in at least a third of cases, is downstream of the intron in which it resides, such that it is translocated to the reciprocal chromosome 8 and is not in *cis* with the translocated c-*myc* (Figure 16.1). Moreover, the ability of this enhancer to function in Burkitt's lymphoma cell lines is variable [26], suggesting that either other enhancer elements within the immunoglobulin locus, or a different mechanism of transcriptional deregulation altogether may sometimes be operative. Nonetheless, the net consequence of the c-*myc*–immunoglobulin translocation appears to be that the c-*myc* gene is regulated as if it were an immunoglobulin gene, i.e., it is constitutively expressed in these immunoglobulin-synthesizing cells.

While at first sight the transcriptional deregulation of Myc expression might be considered to be sufficient to cause the cell to proliferate indefinitely –

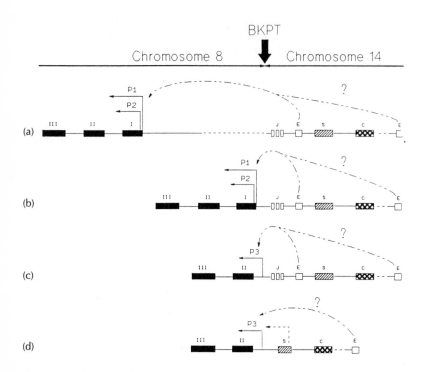

Figure 16.1   Juxtaposition of c-*myc* with Ig sequences. This figure shows the variations in breakpoint locations (BKPT) and the presumptive regulation of c-*myc* (exons I, II and III) by immunoglobulin regulatory elements (E) – the recognized μ enhancer and undefined enhancer elements within the Ig locus. On chromosome 8: (a) far 5' breakpoint; (b) immediate 5' of c-*myc*; (c and d) intron breakpoints. On chromosome 14, (a) (b) and (c) show breakpoints in or close to the J (joining region), and (d) shows a switch-μ breakpoint. In (c) and (d), the major promoters of c-*myc* – P1 and P2 – are deleted by the translocation and transcription is initiated near an intronic promoter, P3. Some transcripts may also initiate from start sites in the juxtaposed switch-μ region(s).

and perhaps, therefore, to be sufficient to induce neoplasia, this is clearly not the case. The regulation of such critical genes as c-*myc* is complex and occurs at a number of levels, each of which may need to be deactivated before aberrant expression can result in neoplasia. For example, beyond the transcriptional controls and the regulation of c-*myc* RNA levels (topics beyond the scope of this discussion), are additional controls at the level of protein–protein interactions. These ensure that the proliferation and differentiation of cells is orderly and occurs in response to appropriate signals. Further, even in the event that all such such regulatory mechanisms are subverted, additional safety mechanisms exist whereby sufficiently deviant cells (in the case in point, expression of Myc in an appropriate context) are diverted to a pathway leading to programmed cell death (apoptosis). Such proliferation and differentiation check points, which ensure that cells meet certain criteria before proceeding through the cell cycle or differentiation sequence, markedly reduce the risk of disordered growth and differentiation, and potentially, therefore, neoplasia. Thus, lymphogenesis entails the selection of a cell clone which has developed a series of mutations that permit it, in spite of its central abnormality (brought about, in the case of Burkitt's lymphoma, by the c-*myc*/immunoglobulin translocation), to overcome the multiple layers of control that would otherwise lead to apoptosis.

THE FUNCTIONS AND REGULATION OF MYC

Myc is known to be a transcription factor, but the biochemical pathways it influences remain to be elucidated. It must activate genes involved in cellular proliferation, since it is known to be induced when cells pass from a nonproliferative state (G_0) to a proliferative state (G_1) [27–29]. It also activates pathways that negatively regulate itself, since there is a well-documented negative feedback loop – an essential element in the regulation of Myc levels [30]. Myc appears to be able to condition cells to undergo proliferation, probably by direct or indirect stimulation of the expression of cyclin D1. Passage through G_1 into S phase, however, requires lifting of the G_1 checkpoint, the primary function of which appears to be to ensure that only cells with intact DNA, and in which there is an appropriate pattern of gene expression (in the context of signals reaching the nucleus from surface receptors), continue into S phase. This process involves phosphorylation of the retinoblastoma protein, Rb, by a cyclin D1/cdk4 complex, with resultant release of the transcription factor, E2F (which is normally bound to Rb). E2F then causes the expression of genes required for DNA synthesis [31]. Simple deregulation of c-*myc* may be insufficient for the cell to pass this checkpoint, as is illustrated by the observation that cells that are artificially induced to express high levels of c-*myc* in the absence of growth factors are diverted into a pathway leading to programmed cell death [32]. It is, therefore, probable that the Burkitt's lymphoma cell has also developed genetic changes that permit passage beyond the G_1 checkpoint. This is discussed further below.

Regulation of Myc transactivation by dimerization

While it is known that Myc can dimerize through its carboxy terminal motifs (basic helix–loop–helix and leucine zipper), as a homodimer it is a very weak transactivator. Another protein, Max, which has strong homology with the carboxy terminal region of Myc, and which is expressed at fairly constant levels in a variety of cell types, is capable of forming heterodimers with Myc, and these Myc:Max hetero-dimers are potent transactivators [33,34]. Max appears to be essential to all Myc functions. Max–Max dimers, in contrast, are transcriptional repressors, and it appears that a stimulus to proliferate, for example, exposure of cells to a growth factor, causes Myc induction to levels vastly in excess of those of Max, such that Myc:Max heterodimers are favored and the target genes of Myc are transactivated. Another protein, or rather, family of proteins capable of forming heterodimers with Max is Mad (there are at least four Mad proteins that are expressed at different points in differentiation). Mad proteins appear to displace Myc from Max in this setting. Mad:Max dimers bind another protein, Sin-3, which is a transcriptional repressor, to form a complex that inhibits the expression of Myc target genes [35].

Myc target genes

While a number of genes that Myc is capable of transactivating have been described (e.g., plasminogen activator, ornithine decarboxylase and a transcript related to α-thymosin), the relevance of these genes to cell proliferation is not clear. Myc, however, has also been shown to bind to, and to increase the transcription of p53, a recognized suppressor of cell growth and an inducer of apoptosis. p53 induces the cyclin/cdk (cyclin-dependent kinase) inhibitor, p21 (Waf-1), which prevents Rb phosphorylation and hence establishes a G_1 block [36]. In at least some cell types p53 also appears to decrease Bcl-2 expression and increase Bax expression (Bax contains a p53 consensus binding sequence in its promoter), thus favoring Bax:Bax dimers and cell death [37]. It has been suggested that p53 induction is an important pathway for Myc-mediated apoptosis, which occurs when Myc continues to be expressed at high level in the absence of growth factor stimulation of the cell. This may be why p53

mutations are rather frequent in Burkitt's lymphoma – this restrictive mechanism is deactivated, permitting the cell to survive in a wider range of environments.

Myc can also downregulate several proteins, including itself [30] and the α-chain of the leucocyte adhesion molecule, LFA-1 [38] – an effect which could be relevant to its role in oncogenesis, since LFA-1 is involved in the recognition of B-cells by T-cells (see below). Myc itself appears to be downregulated by exposure of cells to a number of molecules, including transforming growth factor-β (TGFβ) and interferons [39–41].

A MOUSE MODEL OF LYMPHOMAGENESIS CAUSED BY c-myc DEREGULATION

An important animal model that supports the likelihood that c-*myc* deregulation is an essential, although insufficient element in the pathogenesis of Burkitt's lymphoma is the Eμ-myc mouse [42,43]. Several mouse strains that are transgenic for c-*myc* have been made by transfection of a c-*myc* gene into a fertilized ovum, such that progeny mice contain an extra c-*myc* gene in all their cells. Since the gene is coupled to an immunoglobulin enhancer derived from the μ heavy chain intron (Eμ), the exogenous c-*myc* gene is selectively expressed in lymphoid cells. High levels of Myc protein are expressed early in B-cell differentiation, and result in an expanded, polyclonal precursor population and a deficit of mature B-cells. This strongly suggests that many differentiating cells fail to reach the B-cell pool, presumably because of overexpression of Myc at an inappropriate time and consequent diversion to a programmed cell death pathway. Eμ-myc mice are predisposed to the development of pre-B-cell and B-cell neoplasms, which develop within 100 days in some 30% of mice. Interestingly, the neoplasms are monoclonal, confirming that c-*myc* deregulation is insufficient to cause neoplasia, and suggesting that other mutations are necessary to permit the cell to pass checkpoints in the differentiation sequence that detect aberrant Myc expression and lead to cell death. This conjecture is consistent with the observations that Eμ-myc pre-B-cells do not survive in culture (they die more rapidly than normal pre-B-cells unless supplied with exogenous growth factors) [44], and that massive cell death occurs in B-cells at an intermediate level of differentiation (i.e., between pre-B-cells and mature B-cells) in the bone marrows of Eμ-myc transgenic mice [45].

In an attempt to identify genes that might be mutated or abnormally expressed in the tumor cells, as distinct from the hyperplastic pre-B-cells, mice were infected with Moloney virus, a retrovirus that does not carry an oncogene, but which is capable of inserting into the cell genome, and by virtue of the enhancer sequences present in its long terminal repeat regions, increasing the expression of adjacent genes (either upstream or downstream). $E\mu$-myc mice infected with Moloney virus developed tumors much more rapidly, and by identifying the genes immediately adjacent to the Moloney proviruses (i.e., Moloney genomes inserted into cellular DNA), in the tumors that developed, it was possible to identify several oncogenes (*pim*-1 and *bmi*-1) capable of cooperating with c-*myc* in the induction of tumors [46–48]. Interestingly, these same genes were not overexpressed in lymphomas that developed in $E\mu$-myc mice uninfected with Moloney virus, but this simply demonstrates that there may be multiple pathways to the same functional end result. Similar acceleration of tumor induction, accompanied by a shift to pre-B tumors was observed by crossing $E\mu$-myc mice with mice transgenic for N-ras or Bcl-2, or with knockout mice with p53 homozygously deleted, and infecting $E\mu$-myc mice with retroviruses containing v-*raf* or v-*abl* [44,48]. These results suggest that positive growth signals via aberrant signal transduction (*ras, raf, abl*), or the inhibition of apoptosis (*bcl*-2 or lack of p53) can both cooperate with the deregulated c-*myc* gene in producing B-cell lymphomas, providing support for the model in which aberrant Myc expression must be accompanied by additional genetic changes that deactivate check point executor genes.

THE GENESIS OF c-myc/IMMUNOGLOBULIN TRANSLOCATIONS

As already suggested, the participation of all of three immunoglobulin loci in translocations associated with Burkitt's lymphoma strongly suggests that immunoglobulin gene recombination is in some way involved in the genesis of the chromosomal translocations – and that the translocations occur close to the point in B-cell differentiation when recombination takes place. It has been suggested, in fact, that translocations arise as a consequence of 'mistakes' in recombination. One possible type of mistake would be for the the immunoglobulin gene recombinases (known to include Rag-1 and Rag-2 at least [49]), which recognize specific target sequences in the DNA, to link the immunoglobulin locus to a nonimmunoglobulin gene. This could occur because of the presence of an accessible immunoglobulin recombinase signal sequence, or sequence that resembles a signal sequence on another chromosome.

Presumably, the degree of resemblance would influence the likelihood that such an event would occur. Pseudosignal sequences have been identified throughout the genome, and recombinational errors have been postulated to account for the genesis of the *scl* translocation and the *sil–scl* deletion that occur in T-cell acute lymphoblastic leukemia (ALL), as well as the *bcl*-2 translocation of follicular lymphomas [50,51]. In very few of the breakpoints in Burkitt's lymphomas, however, is the breakpoint associated with physiological signal sequences or convincing pseudosequences.

It is also possible that the altered chromatin pattern in the vicinity of the regions that undergo recombination predisposes to DNA breakage – this could apply to any 'active' chromosomal region, i.e., one in which genes are being transcribed. While ligation could involve immunoglobulin recombinases, it might also be mediated by other enzymes such as the topoisomerases, or the Chi enzyme that may have a role in some 14;18 translocations [52]. In the latter circumstances, there would be no requirement for immunoglobulin-like signal sequences. Whatever the mechanism, only translocations that give rise to a particular functional result would be observed in tumors. While such events are likely to be exceedingly rare, it must be borne in mind that enormous numbers of B-cells are generated on a daily basis – perhaps some 10^{10} mature B-lymphocytes from approximately 10^9 stem cells (extrapolated from mouse experiments [53]). Thus, exquisitely rare events are very likely to be observed in populations over time. In addition, factors that increase the number of B-cells generated or increase the risk of chromosomal breakage will correspondingly increase the probability of a translocation occurring. Osmond has shown, for example, in mice infected with malaria, that significant increases in bone marrow pro-B-cell populations and decreases in mature B-cell populations are readily demonstrable [54]. This finding is entirely consistent with Wedderburn's observations that mice infected with malaria – like mice transgenic for c-*myc* – are more likely to develop lymphoma when simultaneously infected with Moloney leukemia virus [55]. It also provides experimental support for epidemiological evidence suggesting a role for malaria in the pathogenesis of African Burkitt's lymphoma.

Evidence that the translocations in Burkitt's lymphoma occur in precursor B-cells

Additional evidence in support of the likelihood that the c-*myc*/immunoglobulin translocations occur early in B-cell differentiation has been provided by a

Southern blot analysis of the J (joining) region involved in heavy chain recombination. We have shown that, in a significant proportion of Burkitt's lymphomas with an 8;14 translocation (at least half and probably more), the J region on one of the two chromosome 14 alleles is unrearranged [56]. This has several implications. Firstly, since essentially all Burkitt's lymphomas synthesize immunoglobulin, at least one of the immunoglobulin genes must be functionally rearranged. Yet in the majority of Burkitt's lymphomas the breakpoint on chromosome 14 is within an immunoglobulin allele that is not expressed [57,58]. This, coupled to the Southern blot analysis, demonstrates that the translocation usually occurs into an unrearranged immunoglobulin allele – i.e, that the translocation occurred prior to D–J joining, the first element of immunoglobulin gene rearrangement. Since D–J joining usually occurs simultaneously on both alleles of chromosome 14, it is probable that the translocation occurred prior to the initiation of immunoglobulin gene rearrangement, i.e., in a pro-B-cell. The only alternative to this conclusion is that the translocation occurs preferentially into the unrearranged allele of a rare cell that has only rearranged one immunoglobulin gene. Such cells are not observed with any frequency in peripheral blood, so that this possibility does not lessen the likelihood that translocations occur in immature B-cells. Additional indirect evidence for the latter is provided by the observation of rare human lymphoid neoplasms in which an 8;14 translocation is present in an immature B-cell, i.e., one expressing terminal deoxynucleotide transferase (TdT), or with a pre-B-cell phenotype [59–62].

A second finding in the Southern blot analysis described was that a high proportion of the breakpoints on chromosome 14 that were not within switch-μ regions were adjacent to but outside the J region, i.e., the signal sequences at which physiological immunoglobulin gene rearrangements occur were not utilized in the translocation. Thus, the translocations do not appear to be a simple consequence of errors occurring during immunoglobulin gene recombination.

The occurrence of the translocation in a pro-B-cell has several theoretical consequences. It reduces the chances, for example, that the cell will successfully create an antibody molecule – a high proportion of attempts at rearrangement, probably eight out of nine primary attempts, do not result in the production of a functional heavy chain. Since essentially all Burkitt's lymphomas synthesize immunoglobulin, it would appear that a functional immunoglobulin molecule is required for a cell to be fully transformed (rare examples of immunoglobulin-negative Burkitt's lymphoma, if not misdiagnosed, might be explained on the basis of the presence of additional genetic

changes that obviate this requirement). In addition, since several cell divisions are believed to occur during immunoglobulin gene rearrangement [53], one might question why Burkitt's lymphoma is not polyclonal, for progeny cells ought to be able to rearrange their immunoglobulin genes differently – at least at the light chain locus, resulting in both lamda- and kappa-bearing cells.

Requirement for the expression of immunoglobulin

There are several potential explanations for the almost invariable expression of immunoglobulin by Burkitt's lymphoma cells. Firstly, it is probably that the cell bearing a c-*myc*/immunoglobulin translocation will be forced into a programmed cell death pathway unless it is able to make a functioning heavy chain. Evidence from mice in which the μ-membrane exon responsible for permitting insertion of the μ-heavy chain into the cell membrane has been knocked out, suggests that even prior to the selection of cells that have functional surface immunoglobulin molecules (i.e., including both heavy and light chains), failure to express μ-chains, presumably in conjunction with surrogate light chain (polypeptides V pre-B and 14.1), prevents the cell from differentiating beyond an early pre-B-stage [63,64]. This might be considered a differentiation check point, similar in principle to the cell cycle check points in G_1 and G_2, which are concerned with the integrity of the genome. While the check point could, theoretically, be deactivated by one or more mutations, this appears to be a rare event.

In addition to the requirement for a functional antibody, the possibility that antigenic stimulation of the translocation-bearing cell is a necessary component of pathogenesis must also be considered. One piece of evidence that is at least consistent with the latter is the presence of somatic mutations in the hypervariable regions of the heavy chains present in Burkitt's lymphoma cells. These somatic mutations are believed to arise only after a cell has been stimulated by antigen and has undergone activation and passage through a germinal follicle. However, whether a Burkitt's lymphoma cell must actually passage through a germinal center or whether, because of the genetic abnormalities that are present, it continues to differentiate along the B-lymphocyte activation pathway without antigen exposure, can only be surmised at present. This is discussed further below.

The conclusion that the c-*myc*/immunoglobulin translocation occurs in a pro-B-cell is also consistent with the likelihood that the deregulation of the c-*myc* gene is insufficient to cause Burkitt's lymphoma (as is the case in the transgenic mouse model). The lack of expression of both kappa and lambda light chains suggests that additional, rare genetic events (occurring in a single progeny cell) are required.

Location of cells undergoing translocation

The strong evidence that the c-*myc*/immunoglobulin translocations occur in pro-B-cells also suggests that they occur in the bone marrow, since some time before birth, the bone marrow becomes the major site of pluripotential hematopoietic stem cells in humans. Although the bone marrow is not always involved in Burkitt's lymphoma (and is infrequently involved in African Burkitt's lymphoma), since the translocation-bearing cell must undergo further differentiation before it becomes fully transformed, it would be natural to conclude that the cell leaves the bone marrow as it develops beyond a pre-B-cell, as would any other B-cell. While this may well be the case, the possibility that Burkitt's lymphoma cells arise in the Peyer's patches of the ileum cannot be exluded. This location is known to be the major site of production of B-lymphocytes and diversification of the B-cell repertoire in lambs [65], and could be a minor site of lymphopoiesis in children – perhaps increased in some circumstances. This would be entirely consistent with the frequent location of Burkitt's lymphoma in the small intestine. There is no information, at present, that sheds light on this possibility.

STRUCTURAL CHANGES IN c-myc IN BURKITT'S LYMPHOMA

The translocations involving c-*myc* appear always to be associated with structural alterations in the gene, leaving the coding region largely intact. These can be major, i.e., deletion of some or almost all of the regulatory region, or minor, i.e., point mutations in the regulatory region. The extent of the structural alterations is dependent upon the chromosome 8 breakpoint – which varies considerably [66]. In some tumors the breakpoint is outside the gene and its known regulatory region – often as much as several hundred kilobases upstream (for 5'). In other tumors the breakpoint is close to the gene (within, or its 5' flanking region is arbitrarily defined by the HindIII restriction enzyme site approximately two kilobases upstream of the c-*myc* promotors). In the variant translocations the breakpoint is downstream of c-*myc* – ranging from immediately adjacent to the gene to, again, several hundred kilobases downstream [67]. Many of these breakpoints, the exception being those far upstream or downstream of c-*myc*, fall within the transcriptional regulatory region of the

gene, the bulk of which is situated within a region defined by the HindIII site and the beginning of exon II. The first exon of the gene, which includes a number of regulatory elements including the major promotors, P1 and P2, appears to be largely devoted to transcriptional regulation, while additional elements are known to be situated in the first intron [68]. It is clear that the location of the breakpoint on chromosome 8 may be relevant, beyond causing juxtaposition to immunoglobulin enhancers, to the deregulation of the gene. Breakpoints far outside the gene may have little effect, but breakpoints within the regulatory region could have a major impact. In intron breakpoints, for example, the bulk of the regulatory region is separated from the coding region (exons II and III). Even breakpoints 3' of c-*myc* could influence the transcriptional regulation of the gene since enhancer elements situated downstream of the coding region have been recently described [69].

Geographic differences in the chromosomal breakpoint locations

If translocation breakpoints influence the regulation of c-*myc*, e.g., by deleting negative regulatory elements such that the remaining positive elements can act unopposed on the c-*myc* promoters, it might be expected that breakpoint cluster regions could be defined within the overall region within which the chromosome 8 breakpoints are distributed. Indeed, some regions of c-*myc*, for example, the immediate 5' flanking sequences, and the 5' part of the first intron, are relatively frequently the site of a breakpoint, and could be considered to be cluster regions [70,71]. Interestingly, the relative frequency with which different regions of c-*myc* are sites of chromosomal breakpoints varies markedly from one country to another. For example, in an analysis of 120 tumors, we observed that in Burkitt's lymphoma from equatorial Africa (Ghana) 75% of breakpoints are outside the HindIII fragment that encompasses c-*myc* (Figure 16.2a). In contrast, in the United States, only 9% of Burkitt's lymphomas have breakpoints outside the HindIII fragment [70]. If breakpoint locations are divided into three broad groups – far 5' (outside HindIII), immediate 5' (in the 5' flanking region within HindIII) and within the gene itself (actually, downstream of the SmaI site that is just upstream of P1), it is clear that the distribution of these three molecular subtypes of Burkitt's lymphoma is different in the various countries we have examined.

Just as the breakpoint location on chromosome 8 varies, that on chromosome 14 also varies [72]. This could also be relevant to the deregulation of c-*myc*. It is entirely possible, for example, that immunoglobulin enhancer elements vary with respect to the impact

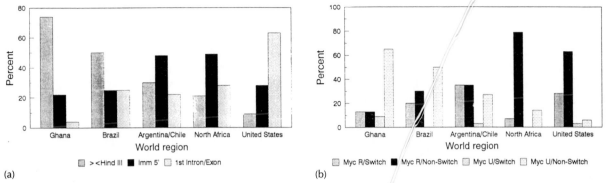

(a)   (b)

Figure 16.2 Geographical differences in breakpoint locations. (a) Proportions of the three major breakpoint regions on chromosome 8 (outside HindIII, immediately upstream of the c-*myc* or within the first intron or exon of c-*myc*) observed in tumors from the world regions shown. Data is based on Southern blot analysis of 120 tumors. (b) Combinations of breakpoints on chromosomes 8 and 14. Chromosome 14 breakpoints are divided into those within and those outside the switch-μ region. Most breakpoints outside the switch-μ region are upstream, close to or within the J (joining) region. Chromosome 8 breakpoints are divided into those with a rearranged (R) c-*myc* gene (i.e., within the HindIII fragment that encompasses c-*myc*) or those outside this fragment (U), most of which will be far upstream of the gene. Data derived from the same tumors shown in (a) except that in three tumors the breakpoint location on chromosome 14 could not be discerned.

they have on c-*myc* transcription according to which c-*myc* regulatory elements are present on the chromosome 8 fragment translocated to chromosome 14. A relationship between the breakpoints on chromosomes 8 and 14 might therefore be expected. While analyses at the sequence level have not been performed, there is a relationship between the breakpoints on each chromosome, since the frequency of various 'combinations' differs (Figure 16.2b) [71]. Breakpoints outside the HindIII fragment on chromosome 8 (and therefore, outside the regulatory region of c-*myc*) that do not result in a rearrangement detectable on standard Southern blot

analysis are generally associated with a breakpoint in the J region of the heavy chain locus, such that the μ intronic enhancer is juxtaposed to c-*myc*. While there is no direct evidence that this has functional significance, the infrequency of breakpoints distant from c-*myc* in combination with switch-μ breakpoints (i.e., in which the μ intronic enhancer is not juxtaposed to c-*myc*) suggests that it does. Other breakpoint combinations appear to vary in frequency in different geographic regions.

The reason for the geographic difference in the distribution of breakpoint locations remains unknown, although it does seem to imply that environmental

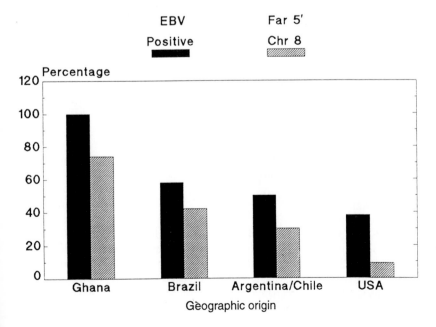

Figure 16.3 Comparison of fraction of EBV-associated tumors and the fraction of tumors with a far 5' breakpoint in Burkitt's lymphomas from the regions shown.

factors influence the breakpoint locations. Perhaps differences in the breakpoint location are determined by the cell type in which the translocation occurs. It is then possible that different proportions of the predominant pro-B-cell population (early, intermediate and late) that undergoes translocation exist in these countries as a consequence of prevailing infectious diseases (e.g., malaria). In this respect, there is some relationship between EBV association and the likelihood of a breakpoint outside HindIII on chromosome 8 (Figure 16.3), although this relationship appears not to hold in North Africa where there are few distant breakpoints but most tumors are EBV-associated.

Mutations in the regulatory region of c-myc

In a high proportion – quite probably all – of the tumors in which a significant proportion of the regulatory region remains coupled to c-*myc*, mutations can be demonstrated in the 3' end of the first exon and within the 5' part of the first intron of the gene [66,70,73]. Several regulatory elements have been demonstrated in these regions, including the myc-inhibitory factor (MIF) binding sites in the first intron [68]. The latter appear to have a negative influence on the major promoters of c-*myc*, P1 and P2, and it appears that mutations in the MIF sites, which are almost invariably present when the chromosome 8 breakpoint is outside the c-*myc*-regulatory region, remove the negative influence of MIF on transcription. Perhaps the combination of MIF mutations and the juxtaposition of the μ-intronic enhancer to c-*myc* are required for c-*myc* deregulation when the chromosome 8 breakpoint is distant from c-*myc*.

Mutations in the coding region of c-myc

A second set of mutations have been identified in the coding region of c-*myc* [74,75]. In Ghanaian tumors almost all of those examined had mutations in the amino-terminal region of the protein, while in American tumors the mutations were scattered throughout the protein (but sparing the dimerization region in the carboxy terminus) [74]. Some clustering of the mutations occurs – particularly in a region containing two phosphorylation sites (threonine 58 and serine 62), and the majority are in the transactivating region of the protein. It is now known that the transactivating properties of c-*myc* can be regulated by the protein p107, a 'pocket protein' that is closely related to the Rb protein and, like the latter, binds and inhibits the function of the transcription factor E2F. In addition to, and analogous to its ability to bind E2F, p107 has been shown to bind to the transactivating region of c-*myc* and to inhibit the ability of

the latter to transactivate other genes (Figure 16.4) [76]. This activity appears to require phosphorylation on threonine 58, which requires prior phosphorylation of serine 62 via a cyclin A/cdk2-dependent mechanism [77]. At least some of the mutations in the c-*myc* transactivating region have been shown to prevent phosphorylation by p107 and thus to deactivate this regulatory mechanism.

The mutations in the protein appear, therefore, to complement transcriptional deregulation by causing functional deregulation. The circumstances, however, in which p107 normally causes inhibition of Myc transactivation are not known. Since cyclin A is expressed during S phase, and is required for cell traversal of S phase, it would appear likely (although experimental evidence has yet to be obtained) that Myc, although expressed throughout the cell cycle, is normally inactivated by cyclin A/cdk2/p107-mediated phosphorylation during S phase. Interestingly, it has recently been shown that E2F is also inactivated by cyclin A/cdk2-mediated phosphorylation during S phase [78]. The significance of these observations remains uncertain, but there can be little doubt that the coding region mutations contribute to functional Myc deregulation.

IMPORTANCE OF p53 MUTATIONS

As discussed already, p53 is a protein that induces G_1 arrest in the presence of DNA damage. Potent inducers of p53 include radiation and chemotherapeutic agents that, by one means or another, induce DNA strand breaks, so creating free DNA ends. However, p53 can also be transactivated by other

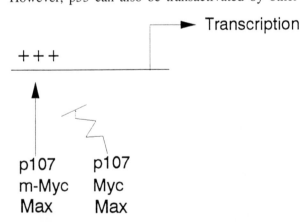

Figure 16.4 Diagrammatic depiction of the influence of mutations in the Myc protein transactivating region on the inhibitory effect of p107 on Myc's ability to transactivate a target gene. m-Myc, Mutated Myc. Myc, normal Myc. The dimerization partner of Myc, Max, is shown forming dimers with both mutated and normal Myc.

genes, including, in certain circumstances, Myc itself [79]. While Myc's ability to induce p53 may depend upon the cellular milieu (and probably only when Myc expression is inappropriate because of the absence of growth factor stimulation), the possibility that Myc could induce expression of a protein capable of inducing cell cycle arrest and apoptosis could well be disadvantageous to the tumor cell. It is perhaps not surprising, therefore, that a rather high fraction of Burkitt's lymphomas (35–50%) contain mutant p53 genes at presentation [80,81]. It seems likely that this primarily relates to further deregulation of cell cycle control mechanisms unrelated to DNA damage.

We have shown that Burkitt's lymphoma cells that contain mutated p53 genes are relatively resistant to chemotherapy and radiation because of their inability to induce p21 (Waf-1) [82,83]. p21, by inhibiting phosphorylation of Rb, causes G_1 arrest, such that cells have an opportunity to repair damaged DNA or, if unable to, or in the presence of conflicting growth signals, to undergo apoptosis. Failure to repair DNA may also be associated with increased genetic instability and hence the accumulation of additional genetic abnormalities that could be relevant to tumor progression and/or chemotherapy responsiveness. Accumulating information suggests that p53 mutations do, in fact, result in resistance to treatment [84,85].

Epstein–Barr virus and Burkitt's lymphoma

EPIDEMIOLOGICAL ASPECTS

EBV DNA is present in all cells of a variable fraction of Burkitt's lymphomas throughout the world – ranging from approximately 95% in equatorial Africa to some 10–20% in Europe and the United States [7]. At first sight this is surprising, for EBV is a ubiquitous virus that infects almost the entire world population. Nasopharyngeal cancer is invariably associated with EBV in all parts of the world – why, therefore, should the fraction of Burkitt's tumors which contain EBV differ in different regions? One possible clue to this is the difference in the age at which EBV infection occurs. In the developing countries EBV seroconversion occurs much earlier (in the first few years of life) than in the industrial nations, where seroconversion takes place throughout the first two or three decades of life [6,7,86]. In contrast, a substantial proportion of individuals in industrial nations (perhaps 50%) are first infected during adolescence or early adulthood (although this varies with socioeconomic status, seroconversion occurring at an earlier age in the less privileged) [6]. Perhaps, as originally suggested by de Thé, early infection with EBV predisposes to the development of EBV-associated Burkitt's lymphoma [87]. This could account for the high incidence of EBV-associated Burkitt's lymphoma in equatorial Africa, and the rarity of EBV-negative cases there. However, EBV-seropositive individuals frequently develop EBV-negative Burkitt's lymphoma [7]. Indeed, EBV is associated with only some 40% acquired immunodeficiency syndrome (AIDS)-associated Burkitt's lymphoma [88,89], yet essentially all human immunodeficiency virus (HIV)-infected patients are EBV-seropositive, and there is good evidence that the body burden of EBV (as measured by EBV-positive cells in the circulation and in peripheral lymph nodes) is higher in such individuals [90].

These data suggest that EBV-associated and EBV-negative Burkitt's lymphoma have different pathogenetic origins, or at least that whether or not EBV has a role in pathogenesis may depend upon environmental and life-style factors. This is borne out by the observation that in Latin American countries the proportion of Burkitt's lymphomas that are EBV-positive is intermediate between equatorial Africa and the USA [7,71]. The intriguing association between chromosome 8 breakpoint locations outside c-*myc* and the likelihood of EBV DNA being present in the tumor cells remains unexplained, although both occur more often in countries with low socioeconomic status [70,91].

The apparent increased risk for EBV-associated Burkitt's lymphoma in populations in which primary EBV infection occurs in early childhood suggests that there are age-related differences in the way EBV is handled. For example, it is possible that EBV replication, or the proliferation of EBV-infected cells is not as effectively contained in children – an argument supported by the infrequency of infectious mononucleosis (a disease that is largely the consequence of a florid nonspecific immune reaction to the presence of EBV-infected cells) in very young children. This could result in the infection of more B-cells, or perhaps a wider range of B-cells (e.g., precursor B-cells) – and thereby a greater likelihood of EBV contributing to pathogenesis. Malaria, which is immunosuppressive, has been shown to be associated with an increased number of circulating EBV-containing cells [92], and it is probable, therefore, that malaria also alters the range and number of B-cells infected by EBV. However, even so, the fraction of B-cells in the body that contain EBV is quite small, suggesting that this virus does make an important contribution to pathogenesis – otherwise the majority of Burkitt's lymphomas would surely be EBV-negative.

Seroepidemiological studies in the West Nile district of Uganda [93] and from a patient who developed Burkitt's lymphoma after Hodgkin's disease [94] indicate that clinical tumor does not develop for many months or even years after primary EBV infection – that this must be the case can also be surmised from the average age of patients with Burkitt's lymphoma in Uganda (approximately 7 years) compared to the age at which EBV infection occurs (100% are infected by the age of 3 years). Burkitt's lymphoma in children less than 2 years of age is almost never observed. Since the doubling time of Burkitt's lymphoma is measured in days, this delay in the clinical appearance of the tumor cannot be accounted for on the basis of the time required for a single cell to develop into a clinically apparent tumor, but presumably relates to the time required for the accumulation of the necessary mutations in a cell clone for it to become neoplastic.

BIOLOGICAL AND MOLECULAR ASPECTS

While it is difficult to reach a conclusion as to whether EBV plays an important pathogenetic role in Burkitt's lymphoma based on epidemiological studies alone, molecular studies provide additional insights and are the most likely eventual source of unequivocal evidence for a pathogenetic role. It is most unlikely that EBV infects tumor cells after lymphomagenesis, since it is not only present in all tumor cells, but is monoclonal, i.e., all cells in the population contain virus with the same number of terminal repeats – i.e., they were all derived from the same EBV-infected cell [95]. However, in order to demonstrate a pathogenetic role for EBV, it will be necessary to demonstrate a molecular pathway through which it can act that is relevant to oncogenesis. Interestingly, although EBV is capable of transforming B-cells *in vitro*, such that they continue to proliferate indefinitely – a capability that has been used in the past to support the likelihood that the virus is of pathogenetic relevance to Burkitt's lymphoma – the program of latent gene products expressed in such cells is quite different from that expressed in Burkitt's lymphoma cells. In transformed B-cells, all six EBV nuclear antigens, EBNAs 1–6, are expressed, along with the latent membrane proteins, LMP-1 and LMP-2, A and B, whereas in Burkitt's lymphoma, only EBNA-1 is expressed [96] (see also Chapter 12). These patterns of latent gene expression are controlled by separate promoters. In the EBNA-1-only pattern, a promoter

immediately upstream of the EBNA-1-coding region, originally believed to be in the BamH1 F fragment (hence generally known as F_p) but now believed to be in the BamH1 Q fragment, is used exclusively, whereas when all latent genes are expressed, one of two promoters (referred to as C_p and W_p because of their locations in the C and W BamH1 restriction fragments of the EBV genome) are used [97]. The full program of latent gene expression almost certainly relates to the need for the virus to cause the cell to enter the cell cycle – i.e., to move from G_0 to G_1 such that the viral genome that entered the cell can be replicated and established in the cell as multiple episomal copies. Several of these genes have been shown to be essential to the transformation of B-lymphocytes. EBNA-1 is a transactivating gene whose only known functions are to regulate the replication of the viral episomes at the time of cell division, and thus ensure that the viral presence is equally maintained in all progeny cells and, in some circumstances to enhance the expression of other viral genes [98]. It is highly probable that all nine latent genes were expressed when EBV first entered a B-cell (or precursor B-cell, since EBV is known to be capable of infecting immature B-cells) destined to become Burkitt's lymphoma, but unlikely that they have a pathogenetic role beyond establishment of EBV infection. They cannot be relevant to the maintenance of the transformed phenotype in Burkitt's lymphoma, since they are not expressed in tumor cells. Whether or not EBNA-1 has a tumorigenic role – presumably by transactivating one or more cellular genes – remains to be seen.

Importance of different EBNA expression programs

One reason for the altered pattern of expression of the EBV latent genes in Burkitt's lymphoma compared to transformed cell lines is clear. All of the latent genes of EBV except for EBNA-1 excite a cytotoxic T-cell response, since they are expressed in the context of HLA class I antigens. This ensures that, in an immunocompetent host, EBV-transformed cells are eliminated by specifically reactive cytotoxic T-cells – hence the self-limited nature of the acute viral infection, including infectious mononucleosis (see Chapter 12). Tumor cells that expressed all latent genes would also be destroyed by T-cells. Of course, the lack of expression of these genes indicates that they cannot be relevant to the proliferative drive of Burkitt's lymphoma cells. The lack of immunogenicity of EBNA-1 was recently shown to be a consequence of the presence of a region of glycine/alanine repeats in this protein [99]. This repeat region appears to inhibit peptide processing, which, coupled to a defect in peptide transporter proteins [100], prevents expression of EBNA-1 epitopes (and those of other proteins into which it is engineered) at the cell surface in the context of human leukocyte antigen (HLA) class I antigens and so EBNA-1 does not excite a T-cell response.

Recently it was shown that small, resting lymphocytes present in the circulation of normal individuals express only EBNA-1 and it is now generally agreed that the viral strategy is to maintain a reservoir of viral genomes in resting B-cells, which, since they express only EBNA-1, do not excite a T-cell cytotoxic response [101,102]. The stability of the number of EBV-containing B-cells in the circulation of individuals treated with acyclovir (which prevents virus replication) indicates that these cells are not being continuously replenished as a result of new infections of B-cells caused by virus release [103] – a possibility considered in earlier years when the virus reservoir was believed to be in epithelial cells in the pharynx. The increase in number of circulating EBV-containing cells, however, in both HIV- and malaria-infected individuals [90,92] suggests that their numbers are regulated, in some way, by T-cells. Indeed, since they are resting cells – the equivalent of either virgin cells or memory cells, both of which appear to survive for only a matter of weeks without exposure to antigen, the intriguing possibility that circulating EBV-infected B-cells are maintained and regulated like memory B-cells must be considered. Normal memory cells probably undergo continual or intermittent replenishment in germinal centers, where antigen is stored in the context of follicular dendritic cells [104]. Antigen exposure would cause activation and expansion of the clone of memory cells. In the case of EBV-infected cells, periodic re-establishment of the full latent gene program could replace this need for antigen, but it would have to take place in a site protected from cytotoxic T-cells capable of destroying cells expressing multiple EBV latent genes (presumably also the germinal center, which contains no CD8 T-cells). Occasional expansion of EBV-infected clones in germinal centers has been documented [105], but whether this is essential to maintenance of the virus reservoir, and whether it entails antigen stimulation, is unknown. Interestingly, EBV possesses at least two means of avoiding apoptosis – its own BHRF-1 gene, which is very much like Bcl-2 in its ability to protect against apoptosis, and the ability to induce cellular Bcl-2 via the viral gene, LMP-1 [106]. This could be of relevance to the follicular center check point whereby only cells stimulated by antigen (i.e., with a sufficiently high-affinity antibody to compete with other cells) are permitted to survive. EBV-activated cells (or EBV-containing cells with low antigen affinity) might be forced into an apoptotic

pathway at this point in the absence of a means to prevent this.

It seems likely, although it has yet to be demonstrated, that the signals provided to normal B-cells within the follicle that result in their becoming either memory cells or plasma cells would apply equally to B-cells harboring EBV that pass through. Perhaps the signal to become resting cells also signals an EBV-promoter switch such that all latent genes except EBNA-1 are no longer expressed. Any cells that persist as activated blasts and express the full latent gene program will, presumably, be destroyed by cytotoxic T-cells on exit from the germinal follicle. Similar events may account for the entry of EBV into the resting B-cell compartment after acute infection.

Presumably resting B-cells can also enter a lytic cycle when passing through epithelial surfaces, e.g., the pharynx (another potential source of loss of EBV-containing B-cells). Recent attempts to demonstrate virus in epithelial cells of the pharynx have not been successful, in line with the notion that the B-cell reservoir is also the source of virus present in saliva [107,108]. This view of the biology of maintenance of the EBV reservoir fits remarkably well with current ideas regarding the phenotype of Burkitt's lymphoma cells (see below).

Mutations in EBNA-1 in Burkitt's lymphoma

The fact that EBV is a harmless parasite with respect to the bulk of the human population is at first sight difficult to reconcile with a potential role in Burkitt's lymphoma. One possibility to account for this, which has been repeatedly considered, is that there are tumorigenic virus strains. The identification of two EBV strains, Types 1 and 2, which are defined on the basis of sequence differences within several EBV genes (EBNAs 2 and 3c, for example) raised the possibility that the oncogenic potential might reside in one of these strains. This has proved not to be the case. Although the majority of EBV-associated Burkitt's lymphomas outside Africa possess Type I EBV, African and HIV-associated Burkitt's lymphomas are equally likely to be associated with Types 1 or 2 EBV [109,110].

In any event, it is not easy to understand how differences in EBV latent genes that are not expressed in the tumor cells could be relevant to viral oncogenesis. The recent demonstration, however, that there is sequence variability in the carboxy terminus of EBNA-1 – specifically, in the DNA binding and dimerization domains – raises the question of an oncogenic virus strain in the context of a gene that *is* expressed in the tumor cells

[111,112]. One of the variant EBNA-1 molecules p-ala is identical to the EBNA-1 present in the cell line B95–8, a marmoset cell line transformed by EBV derived from a patient with infectious mononucleosis; another variant (v-pro) differs at some 15 specific nucleotides from the B95–8 'prototype'. Type 1 and 2 EBV strains (based on EBNA-2 and/or EBNA-3c sequences) may be of either EBNA-1 subtype. We have found that both these EBNA-1 subtypes are present in the peripheral blood lymphocytes of most individuals, but the majority of EBV-positive Burkitt's lymphomas contain yet another variant EBNA-1. The tumor-associated EBNA-1 nearly always differs at a single amino acid residue from both prototype and variant EBNA-1 molecules present in peripheral blood lymphocytes [112a]. This suggests that the tumor-associated mutation provides a selective advantage to the tumor cell by altering the function of EBNA-1 in some way. Since each tumor cell contains multiple EBV genomes, the tumor-associated mutation, which is homozygous, must have been present in the virus that infected the original cell from which the neoplastic clone developed. The mutation does not inhibit the ability of EBNA-1 to influence plasmid replication and thus to regulate the copy number of viral episomes, since mutated EBNA-1 retains its capacity to transactivate ori-P, presumably a *sine qua non* for the continued existence of lymphoblastoid cell lines, which have an absolute requirement for the expression of multiple viral genes.

Additional possible lymphomagenic effects of EBV

EBV may influence the pathogenesis of Burkitt's lymphoma at many points in the pathway and, if it does, its potency as a lymphomagen would be correspondingly increased. It has been proposed, for example, that EBV can expand the population of B-cells that gives rise to Burkitt's lymphoma [113]. If this is so, then presumably such cells would be immature B-cells, since these are the target for the c-*myc*/immunoglobulin translocation. An alternative hypothesis has been proposed – that EBV infects a cell already containing such a translocation and results in full transformation. To date there is no evidence that favors this suggestion [114]. Against it, however, is the observation that EBV-transformed B-cell lines derived from fetal liver have a high risk of developing translocations involving chromosome 14 [115]. Evidence that EBV can induce *Rag* gene expression [116] is also consistent with the possibility that EBV may increase the likelihood that translocations will develop in immature B-cells – perhaps those about to rearrange their immuno-

globulin genes. Recently, we obtained evidence that EBNA-1 could 'collaborate' with the *myc*/immunoglobulin translocation since it is capable of transactivating the c-*myc* gene [7], while the demonstration that mice transgenic for EBNA-1 develop lymphomas [117] strongly supports a role for EBNA-1 in the pathogenetic process.

It would seem that the preponderance of evidence strongly favors a pathogenetic role for EBV in Burkitt's lymphoma, even though the details of the molecular pathways through which it acts remain unknown. EBNA-1, which is not known to play a role in the transformation of B-lymphocytes, has emerged as a possible candidate oncogene. This raises the question why Burkitt's lymphoma is not always associated with EBV. Many answers are possible – perhaps this is a function of the age at which infection by EBV occurs and the prevalence of other potential collaborating factors, such as malaria. But whatever pathogenetic pathways are affected by EBV, similar functional effects could result from mutations in the same pathways. In this case, however, because such changes are likely to arise only in a single cell, as compared to the many virus infected cells, complementation by other genetic lesions is less likely, and EBV-negative Burkitt's lymphoma would be expected to have a much lower incidence than EBV-positive Burkitt's lymphoma – which it does. The possibility that, in EBV-negative Burkitt's lymphoma quite different genetic abnormalities able to complement the c-*myc*/immunoglobulin translocation arise, cannot be excluded.

Cellular origins of Burkitt's lymphoma

The identity of the normal counterpart cell of Burkitt's lymphoma is a topic of some debate. It seems highly probable, for reasons already provided, that the c-*myc*/immunoglobulin chromosomal translocations which constitute an essential, if not sufficient, element in pathogenesis occur in pro-B-cells. Burkitt's lymphoma, however, probably never has a pro-B-cell phenotype and rarely has a pre-B-cell phenotype [60–62], indicating that cells containing a c-*myc*/immunoglobulin translocation must, in order to become neoplastic cells, undergo differentiation at least to the point of expressing surface immunoglobulin consisting of both heavy and light chains. Normal B-cells enter a resting phase shortly after expressing IgM at the cell membrane. Cells which contain a c-*myc*/immunoglobulin translocation, however, cannot enter a resting phase – presumably because of the expression of the deregulated c-*myc* gene. Thus, Burkitt's lymphoma might be considered to be the neoplastic counterpart of a resting B-cell even though Burkitt's lymphoma cells maintain the nuclear chromatin structure of a cell in cycle, and the cytoplasmic apparatus for synthesizing the numerous proteins necessary for cell proliferation. In apparent contradiction to this possibility is the observation that the immunophenotype of Burkitt's lymphoma is similar or identical to that of germinal center cells.

SUPPORT FOR THE 'RESTING CELL' HYPOTHESIS

There are two main arguments, derived from experimental evidence, which support the notion that Burkitt's lymphoma is the neoplastic counterpart of a resting B-cell. The first derives from the lack of expression of the untranslocated c-*myc* gene in Burkitt's lymphoma. The reason for this has long been debated [57]. A favorite hypothesis was that the untranslocated c-*myc* gene is downregulated via a recognized negative feedback loop [30] because of the high expression of c-*myc* from the translocated allele. However, there is also evidence that the chromatin pattern in the nonexpressed allele differs from that in the expressed allele, and that nonexpression is not simply a question of negative feedback regulation [118]. In resting lymphocytes, both c-*myc* genes are made 'inaccessible' by the chromatin structure; the finding that this applies to the untranslocated allele in Burkitt's lymphoma is therefore consistent with the possibility that the normal cell counterpart is a resting cell. The translocation of a c-*myc* allele to an active (immunoglobulin) region on chromosome 14 allows it to escape from the restrictive chromatin pattern on chromosome 8 and permits the gene to be expressed when in the normal cell counterpart it would not be. While the negative feedback loop may well be inactive in Burkitt's lymphoma, this appears to be a common feature of transformed cells [30] and may relate more to the deregulated expression of the c-*myc* gene involved in the translocation than to inhibition of the expression of the normal allele.

The hypothesis that Burkitt's lymphoma cells are the neoplastic counterpart of a resting B-cell is also consistent with the restricted program of EBV latent gene expression (EBNA-1 only) in EBV-associated Burkitt's lymphoma – resting B-cells appear to have a similarly restricted pattern of latent gene expression. This paradigm has the attractive feature that no special mechanism is required to account for the down regulation of the EBV latent gene program

associated with B-cell transformation – it is the same mechanism as that which is normally utilized to create the virus reservoir in resting B-cells. While the details of this mechanism have not been elucidated, it has been demonstrated that the switch in promoter utilization, with alteration of the full EBV latent gene program to an EBNA-1-only phenotype, also occurs when non-B-cells are fused to EBV-transformed lymphoblastoid cells. This at least indicates that the virus uses cellular genes to control its latent gene program [119] and supports the idea that the EBNA-1-only pattern in Burkitt's lymphoma reflects the pattern that would obtain in its normal cell counterpart. The only cell type known, to date, to express EBNA-1 and no other latent genes is a resting B-cell.

Relationship to germinal follicle cells

Although Burkitt's lymphoma is never follicular, transformation of follicular lymphoma into a pre-B-cell leukemia or a Burkitt-like lymphoma, in association with the development of an 8;14 translocation superimposed on the existing 14;18 translocation, has been described [120–127]. In addition, *de novo* small noncleaved cell lymphomas containing both translocations are well known [128]. These observations suggest that 8;14 translocations can occasionally develop in the precursor B-cells of a clone that already contains an 14;18 translocation and which was either subclinical or, in more differentiated progeny, had previously been manifested as a follicular lymphoma. This provides powerful support for the probability that both these translocations arise in presursor B-cells – presumably associated genetic changes determine the degree of differentiation that will occur, and whether the resultant tumor will be a Burkitt-like lymphoma (including L3 ALL) or a precursor B-cell leukemia. The development of either precursor or mature B-cell malignancies in tumors containing both translocations is reminiscent of the mouse Eμ-myc transgenic model in which the lymphomas that arise may have a pre-B- or B-phenotype. In addition, Eμ-myc mice develop lymphomas sooner and at higher frequency when crossed with mouse strains transgenic for *bcl*-2 [48].

Burkitt's lymphoma may also occasionally colonize germinal centers [129]. Pallesen has observed Burkitt's lymphoma in mesenteric lymph nodes draining an ileocecal Burkitt's lymphoma, colonizing the mantle zone of germinal follicles prior to replacing the germinal center [130]. This phenomenon also occurs in the low-grade lymphomas of mucosa-associated lymphoid tissue (MALT) [131] and is quite consistent with the hypothesis that Burkitt's lymphoma is the neoplastic counterpart of a resting B-cell – virgin B-cells and perhaps memory B-cells responding to antigen develop higher-affinity antibodies, which are selected for in germinal follicles. However, it has also been pointed out that the phenotype of Burkitt's lymphoma cells closely resembles that of a subpopulation of large B-cells of the germinal center rather than resting B-cells [132,133] in that both express the B lineage markers CD19 and CD20, as well as a glycolipid antigen, CD77 (originally called BLA), and the common ALL antigen, CD10, and neither express (or express low levels of) B-cell activation markers such as CD23, CD30, CD39 and CD70, or cellular adhesion molecules CD54 (ICAM-1), CD11a/18 (LFA-1) and CD58 (LFA-3) [127–129]. The low level of expression of adhesion molecules as well, sometimes, as HLA molecules by Burkitt's lymphoma cells has been cited as an important element in its ability to escape destruction by cytotoxic T-cells [134,135]. Only EBV-positive tumors are likely, however, to be at significant risk for immune destruction, and a more important means of escaping recognition by T-cells is likely to be the lack of expression, *in vivo*, of immunogenic viral antigens; sensitization of Burkitt's lymphoma cells with EBV peptide epitopes restores recognition and permits lysis by EBV-specific cytotoxic T-cells in spite of low levels of expression of CD11a/18 and CD58. This is probably mediated through ICAM-2, which is expressed at high levels on Burkitt's lymphoma cell lines [136].

Although CD10 is also expressed on precursor cells, such cells also express TdT, and usually CD34, neither of which are present on Burkitt's lymphoma cells, and in concert with CD77 and high levels of expression of surface immunoglobulin, there can be no doubt that Burkitt's lymphoma cells have a mature phenotype. Burkitt's lymphoma cell lines may also secrete immunoglobulin in significant amounts, EBV-negative cell lines secreting considerably more than EBV-positive cell lines [137], and can be induced by treatment with phorbol ester to differentiate into plasmablasts [138] – both consistent with a phenotype of germinal center cells, which may also differentiate in this way if given appropriate signals. At a molecular level, the presence of mutations in the hypervariable region of the heavy immunoglobulin chain in Burkitt's lymphoma cells [139] is also strongly suggestive of a relationship with follicular center cells, since somatic mutations are believed to arise in the germinal center during the process of selection of high-affinity antibodies [140]. More recently, it has been reported that Burkitt's lymphoma expresses the protein Bcl-6, a zinc-finger transcription factor, which is rearranged in a high fraction of large B-cell lymphomas (centroblastic lymphomas) [141,142]. In lymph nodes the expression of this protein has been shown to be confined to germinal center cells. Mutations have been observed in the *bcl*-6 gene in Burkitt's lym-

phoma, as they have in large-cell lymphomas and follicular lymphomas, but, as is the case with mutations in the hypervariable region of the immunoglobulin heavy chain, there are half as many mutations in Burkitt's lymphoma as in follicular lymphomas [143].

Unlike the majority of normal centrocytes, Burkitt's lymphoma cells show little evidence of isotype switching, although occasional Burkitt's lymphomas that express IgG or IgA have been described. Although breakpoints on chromosome 14 do occur within the switch μ region in Burkitt's lymphoma, and occasionally in other switch regions, this does not necessarily imply that they occur at the B-lymphocyte stage at which class switching normally occurs in the germinal center – and most probably to the state of chromatin in the immunoglobulin locus in immature B-cells about to rearrange their immunoglobulin genes, as discussed above.

Finally, the presence of p53 mutations in Burkitt's lymphoma has at least a parallel in follicular lymphomas for, although such mutations are uncommon in primary follicular lymphomas, p53 mutations are quite frequently associated with transformation to a large-cell lymphoma [144].

These observations suggest quite strongly that Burkitt's lymphoma, at least in terms of its predominant phenotype, has progressed beyond the resting, virgin lymphocyte stage to that of a germinal center cell. While follicular dendritic cells, which are required for the formation of germinal follicles, are not present in Burkitt's lymphoma, tingible body macrophages are present. Indeed, the 'starry-sky' appearance that is typical of Burkitt's lymphoma is also typical of germinal centers. Such macrophages can be seen in any rapidly growing tumor, so that their presence cannot be considered to be strong evidence of a germinal center origin. However, they are almost a hallmark of Burkitt's lymphoma, and so may have more significance – they could, for example, be producing growth factors. Their presence also relates to the high rate of apoptosis that is ongoing in Burkitt's lymphoma.

What should be inferred from these observations? Burkitt's lymphoma is clearly not a follicular lymphoma, although cytologically it merges, through Burkitt-like lymphoma, with large B-cell lymphoma (centroblastic lymphoma) – a tumor that is believed to be the neoplastic counterpart of large germinal center cells (centroblasts) – and it may arise in the setting of an underlying follicular lymphoma. Several possible explanations can be considered. Burkitt's lymphoma cells may have differentiated to a stage (at least in some respects – the possibility of discordant differentiation cannot be excluded) that is the equivalent of a follicle center cell but without actually passing through a germinal follicle, and without the need for antigen stimulation. Alternatively, in order for the Burkitt's lymphoma cell to be fully transformed, it must pass through a germinal follicle, i.e., the microenvironment of the follicle is a necessary component of lymphomagenesis. If the latter is the case, then one must ask why. Perhaps antigen stimulation or contact with helper T-cells is required for the potential tumor cell to be fully transformed. The presence of a deregulated c-*myc* gene would not necessarily replace this requirement. As already implied, in the absence of appropriate growth signals, inappropriate expression of c-*myc* would normally lead to cell death, via apoptosis. Indeed, ionomycin-induced apoptosis in Burkitt's lymphoma cells appears to be driven by Myc [144a]. Interestingly, normal germinal center cells (centrocytes), cultured at 37°C *in vitro*, undergo apoptosis unless stimulated by antigen or antigen equivalent (e.g., anti-μ) or CD40 ligand or the equivalent (e.g., an agonal CD40 antibody). In contrast, anti-μ has an inhibitory effect on cell lines derived from Burkitt's lymphoma, and probably induces apoptosis [145]. The significance of this is unclear, although inhibition by anti-μ has been considered to indicate tolerance to antigen in immature B-cells [146]. However, an alternative mechanism whereby Burkitt's lymphoma could escape apoptosis would be to acquire additional genetic lesions. Since the germinal center is the location at which B-cells acquire mutations in the hypervariable region of their immunoglobulin heavy chains, it is entirely possible that cells that pass through a germinal follicle are much more likely to acquire the requisite genetic abnormalities than cells that do not. The specificity of the hypermutational mechanism is unknown, but there is evidence that it can result in mutations even in framework regions of immunoglobulin molecules [147]. It may be the selection process that gives the appearance of specificity. If the hypermutational mechanism is not precise, it could easily explain the presence of mutations in the regulatory and coding regions of translocated c-*myc* in Burkitt's lymphoma, and perhaps even the presence of mutations in other genes – bcl-6 and p53.

While it may appear difficult to reconcile parallels in Burkitt's lymphoma with resting B-cells with the strong evidence that it bears many characteristics of a germinal center cell, it may not be appropriate to assume that the neoplastic clone would correspond in all respects to a specific stage of differentiation. Perhaps the tumor cell has, by selection, utilized those characteristics of adjacent cell stages that are conducive to the neoplastic state. However, what causes the cell to refrain from further differentiation, either into a full memory-cell phenotype or into an immunoblast, is not known. Perhaps it is unable to make contact with CD4 cells, which appear to be

necessary for further differentiation. This could be due to altered expression of adhesion molecules, but it has been observed that Burkitt's lymphoma cells, which express EBNA-1 only, are poor antigen presenting cells due to their failure to process exogenous antigen [148]. In normal B-cells, antigen presentation to CD4 T-cells, in the context of MHC class II molecules, appears to be a prerequisite for progression to a memory cell or plasmacytoid cell [140]. Thus, whether or not there is a cognate antigen to the Burkitt's lymphoma cell immunoglobulin, it may not be able to progress beyond its phenotype as a germinal center cell because of its inability to interact, through a cognate receptor mechanism, with CD4 cells.

Sometimes these constraints may not apply, and the neoplastic cell may be able to progress to the stage of a centroblast or immunoblast, or even beyond. This could account for the presence of 8;14 translocations in large B-cell lymphomas, for the plasmacytoid differentiation observed when Burkitt's lymphoma cells are exposed to phorbol esters [149] and other differentiating agents [150], and for the occasional occurrence, in HIV-positive individuals, of an EBV-positive, 8;14 translocation-bearing tumor with marked plasmacytoid differentiation [151].

Finally, it is important to recognize that Burkitt's lymphoma presents predominantly as a gastrointestinal lymphoma. This would suggest that it is the neoplastic counterpart of lymphocytes, or activated lymphocytes, belonging to the mucosa-associated lymphoid system. Burkitt's lymphoma does differ immunophenotypically from low-grade MALT lymphomas is some respects, e.g., the lack of CD10 expression in the latter (Table 16.1), but this by no means excludes a close relationship. Interestingly, MALT lymphomas, like Burkitt's lymphoma, frequently involve the small bowel, and the lymphoepithelial lesions characteristic of low-grade MALT lymphomas have been described in Burkitt's lymphoma [152]. Moreover, both the tooth buds and lactating breast are infiltrated by mucosal B-cells, and both are sites of preferential involvement by Burkitt's lymphoma (see Chapter 21). Similarly, other characteristic sites for marginal zone lymphomas, i.e., MALT like lymphomas occuring in nonmucosal tissue, are not infrequently involved in Burkitt's lymphoma, e.g., thyroid and salivary glands. MALT lymphomas can also transform into more aggressive lymphomas and, although such transformed tumors are usually diagnosed as centroblastic lymphomas, a higher fraction contain c-*myc*/immunoglobulin translocations than nodal large-cell lymphomas [153,154]. Thus, the possibility that Burkitt's lymphoma is a high-grade MALT lymphoma is worthy of further exploration. Coupled to

114. Lenoir GM, Bornkamm GW. Burkitt's lymphoma, a human cancer model for the study of the multistep development of cancer: Proposal of a new scenario. In Klein G (ed.) *Advances in Viral Oncology*, Vol. 6. New York: Raven Press, 1987.

115. Altiok E, Klein G, Zech L, et al. Epstein–Barr virus-transformed pro-B-cells are prone to illegitimate recombination between the switch region of the mu chain gene and other chromosomes. *Proc. Natl Acad. Sci. USA* 1989, **86**: 6333–6337.

116. Kuhn-Hallek I, Sage DR, Stein L, et al. Expression of recombination activating genes (RAG-1 and RAG-2) in Epstein–Barr virus-bearing B-cells. *Blood* 1995, **85**: 1289–1299.

117. Wilson JB, Levine AJ. The oncogenic potential of Epstein–Barr virus nuclear antigen 1 in transgenic mice. *Curr. Top. Microbiol. Immunol.* 1992, **182**: 375–385.

118. Nishikura K, Murray JM. The mechanism of inactivation of the normal c-myc gene locus in human Burkitt lymphoma cells. *Oncogene* 1988, **2**: 493–498.

119. Contreras-Brodin BA, Anvret M, Imreh S, et al. B-cell phenotype-dependent expression of the Epstein–Barr virus nuclear antigens EBNA2 to EBNA6: Studies with somatic cell hybrids. *J. Gen. Virol.* 1991, **72**: 3025–3033.

120. Pegoraro L, Palumbo A, Erikson J, et al. A 14:18 and an 8:14 chromosome translocation in a cell line derived from an acute B-cell leukemia. *Proc. Natl Acad. Sci. USA* 1984, **81**: 7166–7170.

121. Gauwerky CE, Haluska FG, Tsujimoto Y, et al. Evolution of B-cell malignancy: Pre-B-cell leukemia resulting from MYC activation in a B-cell neoplasm with a rearranged BCL2 gene. *Proc. Natl Acad. Sci. USA* 1988, **85**: 8548–8552.

122. Gauwerky CE, Hoxie J, Nowell PC, et al. Pre-B-cell leukemia with a t(8:14) and a t(14:18) translocation is preceded by follicular lymphoma. *Oncogene* 1988, **2**: 431–435.

123. Gluck WL, Bigner SH, Borowitz MJ, et al. Acute lymphoblastic leukemia of Burkitt's type (L3 ALL) with 8:22 and 14:18 translocations and absent surface immunoglobulins. *Am. J. Clin. Path.* 1986, **85**: 636–640.

124. Aventin A, Mecucci C, Guanyabens C, et al. Variant t(2:18) translocation in a Burkitt conversion of follicular lymphoma. *Br. J. Haematol.* 1990, **74**: 367–369.

125. Lee JT, Innes DJ, Williams ME. Sequential bcl-2 and c-myc oncogene rearrangements associated with the clinical transformation of non-Hodgkin's lymphoma. *J. Clin. Invest.* 1989, **84**: 1454–1459.

126. Mintzer DM, Andreeff M, Filippa DA, et al. Progression of nodular poorly differentiated lymphocytic lymphoma to Burkitt's-like lymphoma. *Blood* 1984, **64**: 415–421.

127. Garvin AJ, Simon RM, Osborne CK, et al. An autopsy study of histologic progression in non-Hodgkin's lymphomas. 192 cases from the National Cancer Institute. *Cancer* 1983, **52**: 393–398.

128. Fifth International Workshop on Chromosomes in Leukemia–Lymphoma. *Blood* 1987, **70**: 1554–1564.

129. Mann RB, Jaffe ES, Braylan RC, et al. Non-endemic Burkitt's lymphoma. *N. Engl. J. Med.* 1976, **295**: 685–691.

130. Palleson G. Burkitt's lymphoma: Diagnostic and taxonomic aspects. In Molander DW (ed.) *Diseases of the Lymphatic System*. New York: Springer Verlag, 1984, pp. 89–102.

131. Isaacson PG, Wotherspoon AC, Disst P. Follicular colonization in B-cell lymphoma of mucosa associated lymphoid tissue. *Am. J. Surg. Path.* 1991, **15**: 819–828.

132. Gregory CD, Turtz T, Edwards CF, et al. Identification of a subset of normal B-cells with a Burkitt's lymphoma (BL)-like phenotype. *J. Immunol.* 1987, **139**: 313–318.

133. Gregory CD, Murray RF, Edwards CF, et al. Down-regulation of cell adhesion molecules LFA-3 and ICAM-1 in Epstein–Barr virus positive Burkitt's lymphoma underlies tumor cell escape from virus-specific T-cell surveillance. *J. Exp. Med.* 1988, **167**: 1811–1824.

134. Billaud M, Rousset F, Calender A, et al. Low expression of lymphocyte function-associated antigen (LFA)-1 and LFA-3 adhesion molecules is a common trait in Burkitt's lymphoma asociated with and not associated with Epstein–Barr virus. *Blood* 1990, **75**: 1827–1833.

135. Masucci MG, Zhang QJ, Gavioli R, et al. Immune escape by Epstein–Barr virus carrying Burkitt's lymphoma: *In vitro* reconstitution of sensitivity to EBV-specific cytotoxic T-cells. *Int. Immunol.* 1992, **11**: 1283–1292.

136. Khanna R, Burrows SR, Suhrbier A, et al. EBV peptide epitope sensitization restores human cytotoxic T-cell recognition of Burkitt's lymphoma cells. Evidence for a critical role for ICAM-2. *J. Immunol.* 1993, **150**: 5154–5162.

137. Benjamin D, Magrath IT, Maguire R, et al. Immunoglobulin secretion by cell lines derived from African and American undifferentiated lymphomas of Burkitt's and non-Burkitt's type. *J. Immunol.* 1982, **129**: 1336–1342.

138. Benjamin D, Magrath IT, Triche T, et al. Induction of plasmacytoid differentiation by phorbol ester in B-cell lymphoma cell lines bearing 8:14 translocations. *Proc. Natl Acad. Sci. USA* 1984, **81**: 3547–3551.

139. Chapman CJ, Mockridge CI, Rowe M, et al. Analysis of VH genes used by neoplastic B-cells in endemic Burkitt's lymphoma shows somatic hypermutation and intraclonal heterogeneity. *Blood* 1995, **85**: 2176–2181.

140. Mclennan ICM. Germinal centers. *Ann. Rev. Immunol.* 1994, **12**: 117–139.

141. Cattoretti G, Chang C-C, Cechova K, et al. Bcl-6 protein is expressed in germinal center B-cells. *Blood* 1995, **86**: 45–53.

142. Onizuku T, Moriyama M, Yamochi T, et al. Bcl-6 gene product, a 92–98 kD nuclear phosphoprotein, is highly expressed in germinal center B-cells and their neoplastic counterpart. *Blood* 1995, **86**: 28–37.

143. Migliazza A, Martinotti S, Chen W, et al. Frequent somatic hypermutation of the 5' non-coding region of the bcl-6 gene in B-cell lymphomas. *Proc. Natl Acad. Sci. USA* 1995, **92**: 2520–2524.

144. Lo Coco F, Gaidano G, Louie CD, et al. p53 mutations are associated with histological transformation in follicular lymphomas. *Blood* 1993, **82**: 2289–2295.

144a. Milner AE, Grand RJA, Waters CM, et al. Apoptosis in Burkitt lymphoma cells is driven by c-*myc*. *Oncogene* 1993, **8**: 3385–3391.

145. Arasi VE, Leiberman R, Sandlund J, et al. Anti-Ig inhibition of Burkitt's lymphoma cell proliferation and concurrent reduction of c-myc and μ heavy chain gene expression. *Cancer Res.* 1989, **49**: 3235–3241.

146. Yao X-R, Scott DW. Expression of protein tyrosine kinases in the Ig complex of anti-μ-sensitive and anti-μ-resistant B-cell lymphomas: Role of the p55^{blk} kinase in signaling growth arrest and apoptosis. *Immunol. Rev.* 1993, **132**: 163–186.

147. Chang B, Casali P. The CDR1 sequences of a major proportion of human germline Ig VH genes are inherently susceptible to amino acid replacement. *Immunol. Today* 1994, **15**: 367–373.

148. de Campos-Lima PO, Torsteinsdottir S, Cuomo L, et al. Antigen processing and presentation by EBV-carrying cell lines: Cell-phenotype dependence and influence of the EBV-encoded LMP1. *Int. J. Cancer* 1993, **53**: 856–862.

149. Benjamin D, Magrath IT, Triche TJ, et al. Induction of plasmacytoid differentiation by phorbol ester in a B-cell lymphoma cell line bearing an 8:14 translocation. *Proc. Natl Acad. Sci. USA* 1984, **8**: 3547–3551.

150. Sandlund JT, Necker LM, Schneller HE, et al. Theophylline induced differentiation provides direct evidence for the deregulation of c-*myc* in Burkitt's lymphoma and suggests participation of immunoglobulin enhancer sequences. *Cancer Res.* 1992, **53**: 127–132.

151. Shad, A, Bhatia B, Magrath IT, et al. Unpublished observation.

152. Isaacson PB, Norton AJ. *Extranodal Lymphomas.* Edinburgh: Churchill Livingstone, 1994.

153. Ladanyi M, Offit K, Jhanwar SC, et al. MYC rearrangement and translocations involving band 8q24 in diffuse large cell lymphomas. *Blood* 1991, **77**: 1057–1063.

154. Raghoebier S, Kramer MHH, Van Krieken JGJM, et al. Essential differences in oncogene involvement between primary nodal and extranodal large cell lymphoma. *Blood* 1991, **78**: 2680–2685.

155. Lewin N, Aman P, Mellstedt, et al. Characterization of EBV-carrying B-cell populations in healthy seropositive individuals with regard to density, release of transforming virus and spontaneous outgrowth. *Int. J. Cancer* 1987, **39**: 472–476.

156. Rowe M, Rowe DT, Gregory CD, et al. Differences in B-cell growth phenotype reflect novel patterns of Epstein–Barr virus latent gene expression in Burkitt's lymphoma cells. *EMBO J.* 1987, **6**: 2743–2751.

157. Osato T, Imai S, Kinoshita T, et al. Epstein Barr virus, Burkitt's lymphoma, and an African tumor promoter. *Adv. Exp. Med. Biol.* 1990, **278**: 147–150.

158. Van Den Bosch C, Griffin BE, Kazembe P, et al. Are plant factors a missing link in the evolution of endemic Burkitt's lymphoma? *Br. J. Cancer* 1993, **68**: 1232–1235.

159. Gunven P, Klein G, Klein E, et al. Surface immunoglobulins on Burkitt's lymphoma biopsy cells from 91 patients. *Int. J. Cancer* 1980, **25**: 711–719.

Table 17.1 Chromosomal rearrangements in T-cell neoplasms

Rearrangement	Disease	Rearranged gene at breakpoint	Activated gene near breakpoint	Encoded protein domain	References
Gene activation					
t(8;14)(q24;q11)	T-ALL	*TCRα* (14q11)	c-*myc* (8q24)	bHLH/ZIP	14,15
t(1;14)(p33;q11)	T-ALL	*TCRδ* (14q11)	*scl/tal-1/tcl*-5 (1p33)	bHLH	8,10,11
t(1;7)(p33;q35)	T-ALL	*TCRβ* (7q35)	*scl/tal-1/tcl*-5 (1p33)	bHLH	22
t(1;3)(p33;p21)	T-ALL	*TCTA (3p21)*	*scl/tal-1/tcl*-5 (1p33)	bHLH	23
t(7;9)(q35;q34)	T-ALL	*TCRβ* (7q35)	*tal*-2 (9q34)	bHLH	12
t(7;19)(q35;p13)	T-ALL	*TCRβ* (7q35)	*lyl*-1 (19p13)	bHLH	7
t(11;14)(p15;q11)	T-ALL	*TCRδ* (14q11)	*rbtn*-1/*ttg*-1 (11p15)	LIM	57,58
t(11;14)(p13;q11)	T-ALL	*TCRα/δ* (14q11)	*rbtn*-2/*ttg*-2 (11p13)	LIM	59,60
t(7;11)(q35;p13)	T-ALL	*TCRβ* (7q35)	*rbtn*-2/*ttg*-2 (11p13)	LIM	62
t(10;14)(q24;q11)	T-ALL	*TCRα* (14q11)	*hox*11 (10q24)	Homeobox	75,211,212
t(7;10)(q35;q24)	T-ALL	*TCRβ* (7q35)	*hox*11 (10q24)	Homeobox	74
t(7;9)(q34;q34)	T-ALL	*TCRβ* (7q34)	*tan*-1 (9q34.3)	Notch	88
t(1;7)(p34;q34)	T-ALL	*TCRβ* (7q34)	*lck* (1p34)	Receptor tyrosine kinase	87
t(14;14)(q11;q32.1)	T-CLL/T-PLL	*TCRα* (14q11)	*tcl*-1 (14q32.1)	Unknown	120,134
inv(14)(q11;q32.1)	T-CLL/T-PLL	*TCRα* (14q11)	*tcl*-1 (14q32.1)	Unknown	120,135
Gene fusion					
Rearrangement	Disease	Fusion gene	Genes involved in fusion	Encoded protein domains	
t(11;19)(q23;p13.3)	T-ALL	*all-1/enl*	*all-1/mll/hrx* (11q23) *enl* (19p13.3)	AT-hook; zinc finger; trithorax; ser–pro rich	100
t(X;11)(q13;q23)	T-ALL	*all-1/afx*	*all-1/mll/hrx* (11q23) *afx* (Xq13)	AT-hook; zinc finger; trithorax; ser–pro rich	213
t(4;16)(q26;p13)	T-lymphoma	*il-2/bcm*	*il-2* (4q26) *bcm* (16p13.1)	Cytokine Unknown	214

T-ALL, T-cell acute lymphoblastic leukemia; T-CLL, T-cell chronic lymphocytic leukemia; T-PLL, T-cell prolymphocytic leukemia; bHLH, basic helix–loop–helix; ZIP, leucine zipper.

this chapter, the clinical designation T-cell acute lymphoblastic leukemia/lymphoma is sometimes used, although it remains unknown whether some genetic abnormalities more often occur in lymphomas rather than leukemias or vice versa.

The cloning of chromosomal breakpoints in T-cell neoplasms has led to the discovery of many new proto-oncogenes associated with these hematologic malignancies. In some cases, proto-oncogenes previously shown to be involved in the pathogenesis of B-cell tumors, such as c-*myc*, have also been shown to be involved in T-cell neoplasia. Similarly, as with B-cell neoplasia, many of the proteins encoded by proto-oncogenes associated with T-cell leukemia/lymphoma have structural features of transcription factors that act in the cell nucleus to regulate the expression of genes. These transcription factor proteins can be classified into three main groups based on their structural domains: basic helix–loop–helix

proteins (bHLH), LIM domain proteins and homeobox proteins (see Table 17.1). The bHLH proteins (c-Myc, Scl/Tal-1, Tal-2, and Lyl-1) form the largest group, whereas only two members of the LIM domain group (Rbtn-1 and Rbtn-2) and a single representative of the homeobox domain group (Hox11) have been implicated to date in precursor T-cell malignancies. Other characterized proto-oncogenes (*lck* and *tan*-1) in precursor T-ALL encode proteins involved in signal transduction. Because fewer consistent chromosomal rearrangements have been associated with mature T-cell neoplasms, only a small number of proto-oncogenes have been implicated in these malignancies. These include the *tcl*-1 gene, involved in the majority of T-cell prolymphocytic leukemias, and the *NFκB*-2/*lyt*-10 transcription factor gene associated with rare cases of cutaneous T-cell lymphoma.

In this chapter, we shall discuss the known

molecular pathogenesis of selected T-cell neoplasms. First, the proto-oncogenes and encoded proteins involved in precursor T-cell leukemia/lymphoma will be described and possible mechanisms of leukemogenesis will be presented. A recurring theme will be the deregulation of the expression of transcription factors, which leads to abnormal cellular proliferation. Next, the possible roles of tumor suppressor genes in the progression of precursor T-cell neoplasms will be briefly discussed. In the second half of the chapter, known genetic defects in mature T-cell neoplasms will be described with emphasis on proto-oncogenes activated in T-cell prolymphocytic leukemia and in some cases of cutaneous T-cell lymphoma. Adult T-cell leukemia/lymphoma (Chapter 13) and T-cell anaplastic large-cell lymphoma (Chapter 18) are discussed elsewhere in this volume.

Precursor T-cell leukemia/lymphoma

GENES ENCODING BASIC HELIX–LOOP–HELIX TRANSCRIPTION FACTOR PROTEINS

The basic domain, helix–loop–helix (bHLH) motif is found in a wide array of transcription factors in organisms ranging from baker's yeast to man (for review, see [2]). This motif was initially identified as a region of sequence homology common to the immunoglobulin enhancer binding protein E2A, the achaete-scute complex of *Drosophila*, the MyoD family of muscle-determination proteins, and the *myc* family of genes [3]. The bHLH motif is defined by the presence of conserved basic residues, a conserved amphipathic α-helix, a nonconserved loop and a second conserved amphipathic α-helix. bHLH proteins such as MyoD and E2A have been shown to form both homodimeric and heterodimeric complexes that bind to DNA [4]. The bHLH complexes recognize and bind to an 'E-box' DNA sequence, which has the general form 5'-CANNTG-3', and can be found in many enhancer regions. Many of these hetero- and homodimeric complexes have been shown to function as transcription activators, leading to the general hypothesis that bHLH genes are transcriptional regulators [4]. bHLH proteins have been grouped into three broad categories: ubiquitously expressed (class A) proteins, such as E2A and Daughterless, tissue-specific (class B) proteins,

such as MyoD, and (class C) proteins, such as c-Myc, which contain a leucine zipper motif in addition to the bHLH motif (bHLH-Zip). Class A proteins may activate transcription as either homodimers or as heterodimeric complexes with the tissue-specific class B proteins [5]. bHLH proteins can often be grouped into subfamilies, based on sequence similarity within the generally nonconserved loop region.

Four genes – c-*myc*, *lyl*-1, *scl/tal*-1 and *tal*-2 – encoding the bHLH domain are involved in chromosomal translocations associated with T-ALL. The c-*myc* gene, first identified as a retroviral oncogene, had previously been shown to be involved in chromosomal translocations in Burkitt's lymphoma, a high-grade B-cell neoplasm [6]. *lyl*-1, *scl/tal*-1 and *tal*-2 were discovered by virtue of their involvement in T-ALL. Two of these genes (*lyl*-1 and *scl/tal*-1) were identified using a similar strategy – a chromosomal breakpoint was cloned using a TCR gene probe, followed by a search for transcription units in the vicinity of the breakpoint. *lyl*-1 was first identified as a transcription unit disrupted by a t(7;19)(q35;p13) involving *TCRβ* [7]. The *scl/tal*-1 gene, originally designated *tcl*-5, was initially cloned through analysis of a t(1;14) translocation present in the DU528 cell line [8–11]. The *tal*-2 gene was cloned by degenerate PCR in a search for *scl/tal*-1-related genes [12].

c-myc

Approximately 2% of T-ALL cases are characterized by the t(8;14)(q24;q11) chromosomal translocation, which juxtaposes segments of the *TCRα* locus at 14q11 to the c-*myc* locus at 8q24. Clinical characterization of pediatric T-ALL cases with the t(8;14)(q24;q11) shows that these cases typically have a high tumor burden, early spread to extramedullary sites and an aggressive clinical course [13]. In T-ALL cases involving c-*myc*, all characterized breakpoints are located downstream of the c-*myc* gene and do not interrupt the coding sequence [14–16]. Molecular studies indicate that the constant (Cα) region of the α-chain of the TCR is juxtaposed distal to the c-*myc* gene on the der(8) chromosome at distances ranging from less than 2 kb to over 40 kb in some cases [14,16]. Thus, t(8;14) translocations involving c-*myc* in T-ALL are similar in orientation to so-called 'variant' translocations involving immunoglobulin light chain loci in Burkitt's lymphoma.

Studies of somatic cell hybrids made from human T-ALL cells containing the t(8;14)(q24;q11) translocation showed that human c-*myc* transcripts were expressed only in hybrids carrying the 8q+ chromosome, but not in hybrids containing the normal chromosome 8 [14]. This finding indicates that translocation of the Cα locus downstream of c-*myc* can result in transcriptional activation of the c-*myc* gene. Sequence analysis of the translocation-associated c-*myc* allele in a T-ALL cell line with a t(8;14)(q24;q11) did not demonstrate any mutations in the coding or regulatory regions of c-*myc* [17]. This finding stands in contrast to c-*myc* mutations commonly found in cases of Burkitt's lymphoma [18], and supports the hypothesis that juxtaposition of the *TCRα* locus to a germline c-*myc* proto-oncogene is sufficient to cause c-*myc* deregulation [17].

The c-Myc protein contains functional domains for transcriptional transactivation, DNA binding, and protein–protein interactions. Important structural elements of c-Myc include a basic amino acid region involved in DNA binding and a helix–loop–helix protein dimerization motif. Unlike other bHLH proteins involved in T-cell ALL, c-Myc also contains a leucine zipper (ZIP) protein dimerization domain. The c-Myc protein is phosphorylated on serine and threonine residues, but not on tyrosine side chains. c-Myc is thought to function in transcriptional regulation through heterodimerization with a protein called Max, which in turn is involved in heterodimerization equilibria with the Mad and Mxi-1 proteins [19,20]. Chromosomal rearrangements that result in deregulated or constitutive c-Myc expression are thought to shift the binding equilibrium toward c-Myc/Max dimers, which activate transcription. Dysregulated transcription of unidentified genes controlled by c-Myc is postulated to lead to uncontrolled cell proliferation and oncogenesis.

scl/tal-1/tcl-5

Within the bHLH family, the gene most frequently involved in T-cell ALL has been designated by three different names: *scl*, *tal*-1 and *tcl*-5. The *scl/tal*-1 gene was first identified at the site of a *TCRδ* breakpoint in the multipotential DU528 cell line, known to contain a t(1;14)(p33;q11) translocation [8,10]. This translocation juxtaposes the *scl/tal*-1 locus to the *TCRδ* locus in a head-to-tail fashion and produces a fusion mRNA that is expressed at high levels in the DU528 cell line. The translocation breakpoint occurs within the 3' untranslated region of the *scl/tal*-1 gene, and preserves the coding sequence. Because the *TCRδ* enhancer is placed in close proximity to the *scl/tal*-1 locus as a result of the translocation, it seems reasonable to presume that unscheduled expression of an *scl/tal–TCRδ* fusion mRNA is caused through the influence of this enhancer. However, the translocation in DU528 proved to be unusual. More commonly, the breakpoints occur within the 5' untranslated region of the gene [11,21]. In addition to the t(1;14) translocations, t(1;7)(p32;q35) [22] and t(1;3)(p34;p21) [23]

translocations have been reported, which involve *scl/tal*-1 and the *TCRβ* and *TCTA* loci respectively (Figure 17.1). All reports of the mapping of *scl/tal*-1 place it between chromosome bands 1p32 and 1p34, but the precise localization of the *scl/tal*-1 locus on chromosome 1p has not been determined.

Much more common than *scl/tal*-1 disruption by chromosomal translocation is disruption of the locus by a site-specific interstitial deletion of chromosome 1, which juxtaposes the *scl/tal*-1 locus with a distinct upstream locus named *sil* (Figure 17.2) [24,25]. Both *sil* and *scl/tal*-1 are transcribed in the same orientation, and a fusion mRNA is formed by *sil* exon 1 splicing to *scl/tal*-1 exon 3 [26]. Because both of these are untranslated exons, the net effect of the rearrangment is to place *scl/tal*-1 under the control of the regulatory elements normally governing *sil* expression. This rearrangement has been attributed to illegitimate V(D)J recombinase activity because it displays all the hallmarks of normal V(D)J recombination, such as site-specificity directed by conserved heptamer sequences, nontemplated 'N' region addition, and variable amounts of exonucleolytic 'nibbling' [24,26]. The frequency of this event ranges from 6% to 26% in a number of childhood T-ALL series whether from the United States [27,28], India [29], Japan [30], China [31] or the Netherlands [32]. However, *sil–scl/tal*-1 juxtaposition has been detected infrequently in adult cases of T-ALL [33]. Interestingly, there seems to be a strong correlation between *scl/tal*-1 rearrangement and committment to the α/β T-cell lineage [34,35]. There is evidence that suggests that this correlation is based on methylation differences within the *scl/tal*-1 locus between α/β and γ/δ T-cells [36]. A map displaying *scl/tal*-1 breakpoints is shown in Figure 17.1.

The Scl/Tal-1 bHLH domain is quite similar to that of Lyl-1 (84% identity of the 58 amino acid motif), although the remainder of these proteins show no obvious homology [25]. Murine Scl is 94% identical to its human homolog protein and maps to a syntenic chromosomal region [37]. Both the murine and human *scl/tal*-1 genes show a complex pattern of alternative splicing in the 5' untranslated region and in the human *scl/tal*-1 gene transcription initiates from at least two distinct promoters in normal tissues [38]. In addition, several malignant T-cell lines and patient samples with an intact *scl/tal*-1 5' regulatory region (i.e., not disrupted by a translocation) have abundant *scl/tal*-1 transcripts which arise from a cryptic promoter within exon 4 [25,39]. Because exon 4 is a coding exon, this transcript cannot produce a full-length Scl/Tal-1 protein, but instead generates a truncated protein lacking the transactivation domain in the amino terminus (see below).

Early studies based on Northern blots and RNase protection assays suggested that *scl/tal*-1 expression

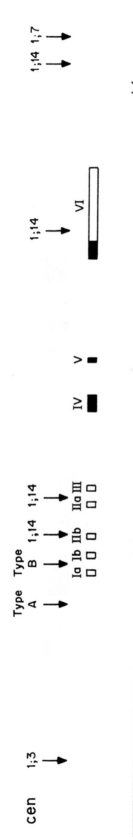

Figure 17.1 *scl/tal*-1 breakpoints and intron/exon structure. Exons are shown as boxes numbered Ia–VI. Protein coding regions are indicated by solid boxes. The sites of t(1;3), t(1;14), and t(1;7) translocations are indicated by arrows. Type A and Type B (also known as tal[d1] and tal[d2]) refer to distinct clusters of *scl/tal*-1 breakpoints, where *scl/tal*-1 is joined to *sil* via an interstitial deletion. Cen, centromere; tel, telomere.

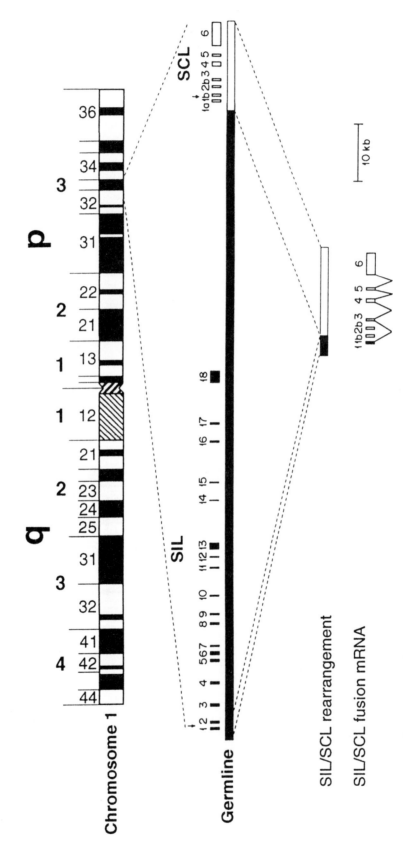

Figure 17.2 Schematic representation of rearrangement between *scl/tal*-1 and *sil* loci. Chromosome 1 banding pattern is as indicated, and the germline *sil* and *scl/tal*-1 genomic structure is indicated. Solid boxes represent *sil* exons; open boxes represent *scl/tal*-1 exons. The arrow represents the points of fusion in the most common form of *sil* and *scl/tal*-1 rearrangement. The two loci are joined as indicated, and a fusion mRNA between *sil* exon 1 and *scl/tal*-1 exon 3 is formed.

SCL protein domains

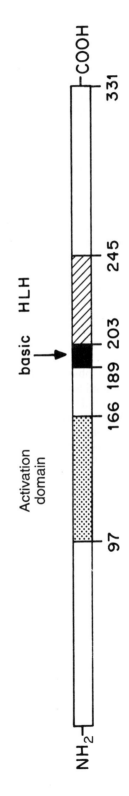

Activation domain

basic HLH

NH₂

97 166 189 203 245 331

COOH

Figure 17.3 Schematic representation of Scl/Tal-1 protein domains (see text).

unscheduled expression of *rbtn*-2 in T-ALL lymphoblasts that have undergone *rbtn*-2 translocations.

Both Rbtn-1 and Rbtn-2 are members of the LIM domain family of proteins. LIM domain proteins contain a cysteine-rich motif that can be regarded as a 'subset' of the zinc-finger motifs (for review, see [62]). The term LIM is an acronym derived from the first three proteins in this family (Lin-11, Isl-1 and Mec-3) to be identified. The LIM domain proteins can be further classified by the presence or absence of a homeodomain (LIM-HD or LIM-only, respectively). Both Rbtn-1 and Rbtn-2 fall into the LIM-only class. The fact that LIM domain proteins complex zinc ions and can potentially form DNA binding structures similar to that of GATA-1 suggests that Rbtn-1 and Rbtn-2 are transcriptional activators. Both Rbtn-1 and Rbtn-2 have recently been shown to possess transcription activation domains near their amino termini [64]. Since transcription activators generally function in multi-subunit complexes, it is of particular interest that both Rbtn-2 and Rbtn-1 have been shown to interact with Scl/Tal-1 *in vivo*, using a yeast two-hybrid assay [65]. Mutational analysis indicated that this interaction was not mediated through the Scl/Tal-1 bHLH domain (see Figure 17.4). Furthermore, a fraction of T-ALL patients have been shown to have rearrangements of both *scl/tal*-1, and *rbtn*-1 or *rbtn*-2 [65]. Much like the bHLH motif discussed above, the LIM domain is conserved throughout evolution, suggesting an important role in growth and/or development [62].

Similar to the *scl/tal*-1 experiments described above, an important clue to the role of *rbtn*-2 in growth and development has come from null mutation experiments. Mice lacking *rbtn*-2 are not viable, and die from lack of yolk-sac erythropoiesis at day 10.5 of embryogenesis [66]. This finding indicates that *rbtn*-2, like *scl/tal*-1, is also essential for normal erythropoiesis. In contrast to the results seen in mice with the *scl/tal*-1 null mutation, in which essentially no monocyte/macrophage colonies were obtained, yolk-sac cultures from the *rbtn*-2 null mutants demonstrated formation of viable monocyte/macrophage colonies.

Unscheduled or dysregulated expression of *rbtn*-1 and *rbtn*-2 has been shown to cause T-cell malignancies in transgenic mice. A *rbtn*-1 transgene, regulated by the *lck* promoter, has been shown to lead to unscheduled expression of *rbtn*-1 in the thymus. The transgenic mice first developed a polyclonal expansion of the T-cell compartment, followed by the appearance of T-cell lymphomas in 4–50% of the animals after a relatively long (9–16 months) latent period [67]. The transgenic line with the highest level of *rbtn*-1 expression developed tumors with the highest frequency, suggesting a

dosage effect of the *rbtn*-1 transgene. The immunophenotype of these tumors (primarily either immature CD4–8+ or CD4+8+) was similar to the immunophenotype of T-ALL patients with *rbtn*-1 translocations [67]. Mice transgenic for a *rbtn*-1 cDNA driven by an insulin promoter did not develop pancreatic tumors or dysplasia, suggesting that the oncogenic effect of *rbtn*-1 was specific to T-lymphocytes [68]. Mice transgenic for an *rbtn*-2 cDNA driven by a CD2 promoter also developed an immature T-cell malignancy. Over 70% of mice expressing the transgene developed a T-cell lymphoblastic lymphoma/leukemia syndrome, with an average latency of approximately 10 months [69]. The incidence of T-cell malignancy varied directly with the level of *rbtn*-2 expression; 96% of mice derived from the transgenic line that expressed the highest level of *rbtn*-2 developed T-cell malignancies, whereas only 30% of animals from a founder that expressed a lower level of *rbtn*-2 developed tumors [69]. The clinical and immunophenotypic features of these tumors was similar to those seen in patients with *rbtn*-2 translocations, with aggressively growing predominantly CD4+8+ tumors present both in the mediastinum and bone marrow.

GENES ENCODING HOMEODOMAIN PROTEINS

hox11

In approximately 4–7% of T-ALLs, the *hox*11 gene at 10q24 is transcriptionally activated by chromosomal rearrangements involving either the *TCRδ* locus at 14q11 or, more rarely, the *TCRβ* locus at 7q34–35 (for review, see [70]). In the t(10;14)(q24;q11) reciprocal translocation, *hox*11 moves from its normal location on the long arm of chromosome 10 to the der(14) chromosome in juxtaposition to a diversity segment of the *TCRδ* gene. In all characterized cases, the chromosomal breakpoint is located at a variable distance upstream of the *hox*11 coding sequence; thus, translocations do not disrupt the coding region of the *hox*11 gene (Figure 17.5). Many of the characterized breakpoints are clustered within a 1 kb region upstream of the *hox*11 transcriptional start site. The most distant characterized breakpoint, associated with the variant t(7;10)(q35;q24), is located about 12 kb upstream of *hox*11. Because most of the breakpoints are clustered close to *hox*11, its molecular rearrangement can be detected reliably by Southern analysis using a *hox*11 probe.

Chromosomal rearrangements involving *hox*11 are thought to result from mistakes in the physiological rearrangement of TCR genes that normally occur

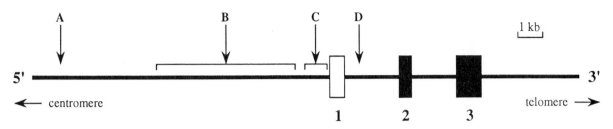

Figure 17.5 Map of the *hox*11 gene on chromosome band 10q24 [71,74]. Noncoding exon 1 is shown as an open box. Coding exons 2 and 3 are represented by filled boxes. A, B, C and D represent chromosomal breakpoint regions located upstream of the coding sequences of the gene. Most characterized breakpoints are located in breakpoint cluster regions B and C.

at an early stage of T-cell differentiation. Specifically, mistakes in V–D–J joining were implicated in six T-cell leukemia cases with the t(10;14)(q24;q11) [71]. *TCRδ* diversity segments were involved in the translocations in all six cases and DNA sequence analysis revealed extra nucleotides inserted at the chromosomal junctions in a similar fashion to those observed in normally rearranged Ig and TCR segments. A heptamer-like recognition sequence, located adjacent to the breakpoint cluster region on chromosome 10, was suggested as a likely target for aberrant recombinations mediated by the V–(D)–J recombinase system. It has also been suggested that S1 hypersensitive sites and potential Z-DNA structures may play a role in some chromosomal rearrangements involving *hox*11 [72,73].

*hox*11, a member of the homeobox gene family, consists of three exons that span a genomic region of approximately 7 kb on 10q24 [74,75]. The gene is transcribed in a centromeric-to-telomeric orientation; the first exon does not contain coding sequence [71]. *Hox11* encodes a predicted 43 kD protein that contains a homeobox domain homologous to that of homeoproteins widely conserved throughout the course of evolution [76]. Most human homeobox genes are organized in clusters on chromosomes 2, 7, 12 and 17. Because *hox*11 is not associated with a known homeobox cluster on chromosome 10, it is sometimes referred to as an 'orphan' homeobox gene.

Homeobox genes were originally discovered through the study of fruit-fly mutations in which one type of body part is replaced by another during the course of development. In *Drosophila* embryonic development, the spatial and temporal expression of homeobox genes determines the basic body plan; homeobox genes are also thought to play a similar master control role in mammalian development. Homeoproteins function as transcription factors that regulate the expression of genes and gene families. The 61 amino acid homeobox domain is a sequence-specific DNA-binding domain with a conserved helix–turn–helix structure. In addition to binding to specific DNA sequences, homeoproteins regulate transcription through transactivation and/or repression domains that flank the homeodomain.

Like other homeoproteins, Hox11 has properties associated with transcription factors and appears to play an important role in development. *In vitro* experiments demonstrate that tagged Hox11 protein localizes to the cell nucleus and that a *hox*11 cDNA construct is capable of transactivating transcription of a reporter gene [77]. Hox11 binds to a specific DNA sequence, GGCGGTAAGTGG, containing a core motif, TAAGTG, consistent with models of homeodomain–DNA interaction [78]. Mice made homozygously deficient in *hox*11 by gene targeting have no spleen but otherwise appear to have a normal phenotype [79]. This surprising result suggests that *hox*11 may be a master gene controlling the development of an entire organ.

The study of the embryonic expression of murine *hox*11 (*tlx*-1) demonstrates a segmentally restricted pattern of expression in structures derived from the anterior branchial arch, the hindbrain and the spleen [80]. No expression of *hox*11 has been detected in murine embryonic and neonatal thymus, indicating that *hox*11 is not normally involved in T-cell development [81]. With the exception of liver, *hox*11 is not transcribed in adult human tissues at a level detectable by Northern analysis. Although *hox*11 is not normally transcribed in human T-cells, abundant transcription of *hox*11 is seen in T-cell leukemias and T-cell lines that contain 10q24 translocations. Thus, the consequence of translocations involving *hox*11, as is the case with *scl/tal*-1 and *rbtn*-1, appears to be constitutive expression in a cell lineage in which the protein is not normally expressed.

Preliminary experimental evidence supports the hypothesis that *hox*11 can function as an oncogene when transcribed inappropriately in some types of cells or tissues. NIH3T3 cells that express *hox*11 grow abnormally in culture and are tumorigenic when injected into athymic nude mice [82]. Transduction of murine bone marrow cells with a *hox*11 expression vector resulted in the immortalization of nonleukemogenic myeloid precursor cells [83]. Transgenic mice in which *hox*11 is expressed in the thymus develop T-cell lymphoblastic leukemia–lymphoma [84]. Taken together, these observations suggest that inappropriate or dysregulated *hox*11 expression may play a role in the initiation and/or progression of leukemia. The precise role of the *hox*11 gene in leukemogenesis remains to be elucidated.

Homeobox genes other than *hox*11 have been implicated in human cancer through the molecular cloning of chromosomal breakpoints. The t(1;19) (q23;p13) translocation in pediatric pre-B-cell acute lymphoblastic leukemia results in the fusion of the *E2A* transcription factor gene on 19p13 with the *pbx*1 homeodomain gene on 1q23 [85]. In the pediatric soft-tissue tumor alveolar rhabdomyosarcoma, the t(2;13)(q35;q14) results in the fusion of the paired-box homeodomain gene *pax*3 on 2q35 with the *fkhr* gene on 13q14 [86]. *Fkhr* is a human homologue of the *Drosophila* fork head homeotic gene. Thus, different homeobox genes seem to be involved in different types of tumors. Furthermore, homeobox genes can play a role in human oncogenesis through the mechanisms of either transcriptional activation or gene fusion, two different consequences of chromosomal rearrangement.

All of the genes discussed above (*c-myc*, *scl/tal-1*, *tal-2*, *lyl-1*, *rbtn-1*, *rbtn-2*, *hox*11), which are thought to be activated by chromosomal translocation, are presumed to produce a wild-type gene product. This presumption is based, in large part, on the appearance of a normal-sized mRNA and/or protein, as well as complete sequence analysis of a handful of cDNAs derived from cell lines or patient samples that harbor the translocations. A detailed search for the presence of point mutations or small (<20 bp) deletions of any of the above genes in the context of T-cell malignancies has not been reported. However, a recent study [18] has demonstrated that point mutations of c-*myc* coding regions occur frequently in Burkitt's lymphoma, a B-cell neoplasm characterized by activation of the c-*myc* gene through a t(8;14). The similarities between Burkitt's lymphoma and the immature T-cell malignancies associated with recurrent translocations (unscheduled activation of a transcription factor associated with juxtaposition to an antigen receptor loci) make one suspect that some of the genes rearranged in T-cell malignancies may also contain point mutations.

GENES ENCODING MISCELLANEOUS PROTEINS

lck

A gene uncommonly activated in T-cell ALL is the *lck* gene, which encodes a receptor tyrosine kinase that is expressed predominantly in lymphoid cells and considered to be involved in TCR signal transduction. The *lck* gene product shows homology to the *src* oncogene and its oncogenic potential has been demonstrated by its activation in murine T-cell lymphomas by retroviral insertion. A rare but recurrent translocation t(1;7)(p34;q34), between the *TCRβ* locus and the untranslated region upstream of *lck*, occurs in human T-cell ALL [87]. The cell lines that contain this translocation overexpress an abundant *lck* mRNA of normal size, suggesting that *lck* has been activated in these patients and that the activation contributes to leukemogenesis.

tan-1

Between 3% and 5% of precursor T-cell leukemias are characterized by a t(7;9)(q34;q34.3) chromosomal rearrangement that results in juxtaposition of the *TCRβ* locus at 7q34–35 with a gene called *tan-1* located on chromosome 9, band q34.3 [88,89]. Leukemias with this nonrandom chromosomal translocation are similar in morphology and immunophenotype to other T-cell lymphoblastic neoplasms. In contrast to most gene rearrangements in precursor T-cell leukemia–lymphoma, however, the translocation breakpoint is located within an intron in the middle of the target gene. Thus, *tan-1* is disrupted by the chromosomal translocation. Studies indicate that the gene product present in malignant cells that carry the t(7;9) is encoded on the der(9) chromosome by the 3' portion of *tan-*1, which is juxtaposed to one of the J segments of the *TCRβ* gene [89]. Because of the difficulty in localizing the band involved in some translocations precisely, it is possible that some cases with t(7;9)(q34;q34) involve *tal-2*, which has been mapped to 9p32–34, rather than *tan-1* [12].

tan-1 is a human homologue of a *Drosophila* gene called *notch*. *notch* belongs to a family of genes that is widely conserved from flies to vertebrates and which encode transmembrane proteins. Studies in *Drosophila* have shown that the Notch protein functions in signal transduction pathways thought to be involved in cell-fate decisions during differentiation and development [90]. The encoded human Tan-1 and *Drosophila* Notch proteins share 46% identity and 62% similarity overall with homologous domains throughout the length of their amino acid sequences. These include epidermal growth factor-like domains, repeated sequences similar to those found in the Lin-12 protein of *C. elegans*, a transmembrane domain and ankyrin-like repeats similar to those that are present in NF-κB subunits (Figure 17.6). *Tan*-1 is transcribed in a telomeric-to-centromeric direction on the long arm of chromosome 9. An 8.2 kb *tan*-1 transcript is found in many tissues, with highest abundance in developing thymus and spleen [88]. The roles of *tan*-1 in the differentiation and/or development of human tissues have yet to be elucidated. However, the expression pattern of the normal *tan*-1 gene and the involvement of a rearranged *tan*-1 gene in precursor T-cell neoplasms suggest that *tan*-1 may play an important role in normal lymphoid development.

Rearrangement of *tan*-1 with the *TCRβ* locus has two important consequences. First, *tan-1* is truncated such that the 5'-portion of the gene is lost. Second, expression of the truncated *tan*-1 gene is placed under the regulatory control of the *TCRβ* locus. Thus, the t(7;9)(q34;q34.3) chromosomal translocation alters both the structure and the expression of *tan*-1. The structural alteration of the encoded Tan-1 protein may shift its cellular location from the plasma membrane to the endoplasmic reticulum and nucleus. Because of its juxtaposition to the *TCRβ* locus, truncated *tan*-1 is presumably constitutively expressed in T-ALL cells. Experimental studies with transduced murine bone marrow cells indicate that truncated forms of *tan*-1 have oncogenic activity in T-cell precursors [89]. The mechanism of oncogenicity is unknown at this time, but one hypothesis, based on structural similarities with NF-κB subunits, is that *tan*-1 may be involved indirectly in the transcriptional control of genes regulated by the nuclear factor NF-κB [89].

all-*1*/mll/hrx

The *all*-1 gene (also known as *mll* or *hrx*) located on 11q23 has recently been cloned by several groups of investigators and has been the subject of intense investigation NF [91–94]. Among genes disrupted by chromosomal translocations, the *all*-1 gene is unique in at least three respects. As opposed to most genes disrupted by chromosomal translocations, where a single type of malignancy is associated with the translocation, this gene is disrupted in an extraordinarily wide range of leukemias and lymphomas [95]. Furthermore, *all*-1 has a large number of 'partner' genes (at least 25) with which it rearranges, including a fascinating event whereby *all*-1 rearranges with a copy of itself to form a partial internal duplication [96]. Lastly, *all*-1 is a target gene for secondary leukemias, induced by topoisomerase II inhibitors; up to 80% of secondary leukemias induced by topoisomerase II inhibitors involve disruption of the *all*-1 locus [97,98]. Although the most common type of leukemias associated with *all*-1 rearrangements are either B-cell precursor ALL or myelomonocytic leukemias, a t(11;19)(q23;p13) translocation has reproducibly been associated with T- ALL [99] as well as with pre-B-ALL and AML. One of the T-ALL cases has been characterized and shown to produce an *all*-1/*enl* fusion mRNA identical to that described previously with pre-B-ALL [100].

TUMOR SUPRESSOR GENES IN PRECURSOR T-CELL NEOPLASMS

The preceding sections have focused on genes activated by chromosomal translocation, similar to the situation seen with classical viral oncogenes. For the last 10 years, it has become apparent that another class of genes, whose deletion or inactivation is associated with malignancy, are often involved in malignant transformation. These genes have been referred to as anti-oncogenes, growth suppressor genes or tumor supresor genes [101]. At least three of these genes, *rb*, p53, and p16, have been implicated in T-cell leukemias and lymphomas.

The first tumor suppressor gene to be identified was the *rb* gene located on the long arm of chromosome 13. The gene is frequently deleted in retinoblastoma, and was one of the first genes to be cloned by a postional cloning approach [102]. As well as its involvement in retinoblastoma, *rb* has been shown to be inactivated in a wide variety of human malignancies, especially lung, breast and prostate cancer, soft tissue sarcomas and osteosar-

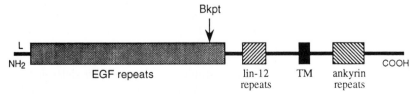

Figure 17.6 Schematic representation of the Tan-1 protein [89]. L, leader sequence; EGF repeats, epidermal growth factor-like repeated motifs; Bkpt, position at which the encoded Tan-1 polypeptide sequence would be disrupted by breakpoints in characterized (7;9)(q34;q34.3) translocations. lin-12 repeats are repeated sequences similar to those found in the *lin*-12 gene of *C. elegans*; TM, transmembrane domain; ankyrin repeats, ankyrin-like repeats.

comas. Additional support for the designation of *rb* as a tumor suppressor gene comes from gene replacement studies, in which exogenous *rb* introduced into a cell line lacking a functional *rb* gene has been shown to result in decreased tumorigenicity of the cell line [103]. In one series, inactivation of *rb* was demonstrated in two of 17 patients with T-ALL [104].

p53 is inactivated by point mutation or deletion in a very wide array of human malignancies; by some estimates, in more than 50% of all human malignancies both copies of p53 have been inactivated. The normal function of p53 is still under intense study, but at least one of its roles appears to be a 'guardian of the genome' [105]. This label has been applied because wild-type p53 acts as a negative regulator of cell growth after induction by a wide array of DNA damage-inducing agents [106]; the arrest takes place during late G_1 of the cell cycle and presumably allows DNA repair to take place prior to cell division or leads to apoptosis [107]. Homozygous mice with a targeted deletion of p53 develop a range of malignancies, the most common of which is a type of T-cell lymphoma [108]. Despite these observations, p53 mutations in newly diagnosed cases of T-ALL appear to be uncommon [109,110], at least in children. However, at relapse, functional inactiva-

tion of both copies of p53 was observed, in one small series, in 50% of samples [111]. Therefore, it would seem that p53 is important to disease progression, as opposed to disease initiation, in patients with T-ALL.

Cyclin-dependent kinase (cdk) inhibitors, a new and expanding class of proteins, are also thought to play a role in T-ALL through alterations in the control of the cell cycle. Cell cycle control is achieved, in .part, through the activation and inactivation of cyclin-dependent protein kinases (Figure 17.7). This process is tightly controlled and depends on the association of cdks with positive regulatory subunits called cyclins, forming cyclin/cdk protein complexes. Active complexes can phosphorylate downstream control proteins, such as Rb, which regulates mammalian cell cycle progression. Rb hyperphosphorylation results in the release of cell cycle block and subsequently in cell division. Inactivation of cdks or cdk/cyclin complexes is achieved through the action of negative regulators called cdk inhibitors (such as p16 and p27) (reviewed in [112, 113]). Thus, mutations in negative regulators of cdks can lead to uncontrolled cellular proliferation.

Homozygous deletions of the p16 gene (also known as *CDKN2*, *MTS*1 or *INK4A*), located at 9p21, occur frequently in association with T-ALL. p16 is a cdk inhibitor, which negatively regulates the cell cycle primarily by its action on Cdk4 or Cdk6. Frequent deletions of the p16 gene in a wide range of malignancies make it a likely candidate for a tumor suppressor gene. The gene was cloned by a variety of strategies; one group cloned the gene using a positional cloning approach in an attempt to discover a gene that predisposes to melanoma [114]. The p16 gene, as well as a closely linked gene with considerable sequence identity (known as p15, *MTS*2 or *INK4B*) were found to be homozygously deleted in almost 50% of a large survey of malignant cell lines [114]. Although there has been considerable debate concerning whether the high frequency of p16 mutations and deletions seen in solid tumor cell lines are an artefact of tissue culture, owing primarily to methodologic difficulties, numerous investigators have confirmed the observation that homozygous deletion of p16 is a frequent event in T-ALL (for review, see [115]). In the largest series, homozygous p16 deletions were detected in up to 80% of T-ALL patients [116,117], making this the most common recurrent genetic lesion in T-ALL. This estimate of 80% may even be an underestimate; because these studies were based on detection of large deletions by Southern blot analysis, point mutations that inactivate p16 would not have been detected. In addition, recent studies have indicated that p16 may be inactivated in certain tumor types by

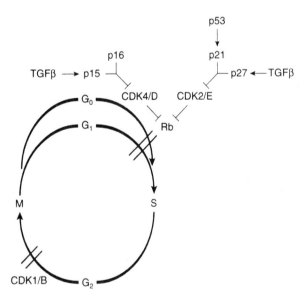

Figure 17.7 Molecular pathways involved in the control of the cell cycle. The double bars represent check points where progression through the cycle may be arrested. Arrows represent activation and blunt-ended bars represent inhibition. p15, p16, p21, p27 are inhibitors of cyclin-dependent kinases (CDKs); p53, tumor suppressor; Rb, retinoblastoma gene product; TGFβ, transforming growth factor β; B, cyclin B; D, cyclin D; E, cyclin E. (Reproduced with permission from [113].)

methylation and consequent silencing of the p16 promoter [118]. Thus, it is possible that virtually all cases of T-ALL produce no functional p16 protein.

In general, deletions of chromosome 9p are relatively large, with the closely linked p15 gene being co-deleted with p16. This raises the question as to whether both p15 and p16 inactivation are required for development of malignancy. While this question has not been definitively answered, a fraction (roughly 20%) of p16 deletions are associated with at least one remaining germline copy of p15 [116], suggesting that p16 rather than p15 deletions may be the critical event. At present, the precise mechanism mediating the contribution of p16 and/or p15 to tumor initiation or progression is unclear. However, functional studies of these proteins and known interactions between cdk/cyclin complexes, p53, and Rb, suggest that the end result of loss of cdk inhibitor activity may be loss of Rb function through hyperphosphorylation. Therefore, a tumor carrying both p15/p16 and p53 mutations, such as T-ALL, would most likely have impaired control of Rb activity, illustrating how the accumulation of mutations can have synergistic or complementary effects that may account for tumor initiation or progression.

Mature T-cell neoplasms

T-cell malignancies of the adult comprise a wide range of disorders of mature T-lymphocytes (post-thymic differentiation), generally referred as peripheral T-cell neoplasms. In the updated Kiel classification, peripheral T-cell neoplasms are subdivided into low- and high-grade forms based on histopathologic criteria [119]. The low-grade forms represent about 5% of the entire spectrum of chronic lymphoproliferative disorders, whereas the high-grade forms comprise 15–20% of the high-grade (intermediate and high-grade in the Working Formulation) lymphoid malignancies. The use of immunophenotypic, cytogenetic and genotypic studies has improved understanding of the nature and classification of these neoplasms, and we can now distinguish several major entities: T-cell chronic lymphocytic leukemia (T-CLL); T-cell prolymphocytic leukemia (T-PLL); large granular lymphocyte (LGL) leukemias; miscellaneous peripheral T-cell lymphomas (PTCL); cutaneous T-cell lymphomas (CTCL); adult T-cell lymphomas (ATCL); and CD30+ anaplastic large-cell lymphomas (ALCL). This section will deal with molecular and genetic aspects of the pathogenesis of some of these entities not covered in other sections, namely T-PLL, LGL leukemias, PTCL and CTCL.

ROLE OF THE tcl-1 GENE IN T-CELL PROLYMPHOCYTIC LEUKEMIA

Rearrangements at the *tcl*-1 locus are observed in 75% of T-cell prolymphocytic leukemia cases [120, 121]. Three different types of rearrangement have been shown to involve the *tcl*-1 locus at 14q32.1 with the *TCR-α/δ* locus at 14q11 (Figure 17.8a–d). These include paracentric inversions of the long arm of chromosome 14, inv(14)(q11;q32.1); simple balanced translocations, t(14;14)(q11;q32.1); and translocations with inverted duplication of the region 14q32–14qter. Translocations between the *tcl*-1 locus and *TCRβ* at 7q35 have been reported much less commonly [122]. In the cases of the 14q paracentric inversion, one breakpoint is in the J region of the *TCRα* locus and the second breakpoint is located centromeric to the *tcl*-1 gene. The portion of chromosome 14 between the two loci inverts, resulting in the juxtaposition of the regulatory regions of the Jα region to the *tcl*-1 locus (Figure 17.8b). In simple balanced translocations, the break in the *tcl*-1 locus occurs telomeric to the gene, and this chromosome is joined to the 14q11 region of the reciprocal chromosome 14; in this case the *TCRα* region is positioned telomeric to the *tcl*-1 locus (Figure 17.8c). Translocations with inverted duplication (observed exclusively in T-CLL arising in patients with ataxia telangectasia) also result in juxtaposition of TCR Jα elements telomeric to the *tcl*-1 locus, but in an orientation similar to that of the paracentric inversions (Figure 17.8d). Chromosomal rearrangements involving the *tcl*-1 locus at 14q32.1 should not be confused with rearrangements involving 14q32.3 sometimes reported in healthy individuals. These rearrangements, such as inv(14) (q11;q32.3) and t(7;14)(q35;q32.3), result from interlocus recombination between *TCRα* or *TCRβ* and the *IgH* locus at 14q32.3 [123–125].

In all three types of chromosomal rearrangement, the *tcl*-1 gene is placed under regulatory control of the TCR locus, whether positioned 5' of the *tcl*-1 gene, as in the case of translocations, or 3' to *tcl*-1, as in the case of inversions. A similar situation exists in Burkitt's lymphoma in which the Ig locus (containing recognized or presumptive enhancer elements) can be located upstream of the c-*myc* oncogene in lymphomas with the t(8;14) chromosomal translocation [6,126] or downstream of c-*myc* in lymphomas with t(8;22) or with t(2;8) chromosomal translocations [127,128]. Similarly, Ig enhancers are found downstream of the *bcl*-2 gene in follicular lymphomas [129,130] and upstream of the *bcl*-2 gene in some cases of B-CLL [131].

The *tcl*-1 gene was identified through positional cloning. The first breakpoints were cloned in 1987–

Table 17.2 Expression of *tcl*-1 mRNA in cell lines

Cell line	Tumor	Translocation	RNA
RS(4;11)	ALL	t (4;11)	–
MV (4;11)	ALL	t (4;11)	–
B1	ALL	t (4;11)	–
ALL380	ALL	t(8;14), t(14;18)	+
ALL-1	ALL	t (9;22)	+
BV173	ALL	t (9;22)	+
RPMI 8866	B-lymphoblastoid	ND	–
GM1500	B-lymphoblastoid	Normal	–
RPMI 8226	Myeloma	Multiple rearrangements	–
U266	Myeloma	Multiple rearrangements	–
P3HR-1	Endemic Burkitt	t (8;14)	+
AKUA	Endemic Burkitt	t (8;14)	+
Daudi	Endemic Burkitt	t (8;14)	+
SKDHL	Sporadic Burkitt	t (8;14)	–
BL 2	Sporadic Burkitt	t (8;22)	–
RS 11846	High-grade B-cell lymphoma	t (14;18), t(8;22)	+
K562	CML	t (9;22)	–
PEER	T-ALL	Multiple rearrangements	–
Jurkat	T-ALL	Multiple rearrangements	–
MOLT-4	T-ALL	t (7;7), 6q–	–
CEM	T-ALL	Multiple rearrangments	–
Sup T1	T-ALL	inv(14) (q11;q32.3)	–
SupT11	T-ALL	t(14;14)(q11;q32.1)	+
HUT 78	T-Sézary syndrome	ND	–

Cell lines with multiple rearrangements do not have translocations or rearrangements at 14q32.1.
ALL, Acute lymphoblastic leukemia; CML, chronic myeloid leukemia; T-ALL, T-cell acute lymphoblasic leukemia; ND, not done.
Adapted from [135].

volving the *tcl*-1 locus, or more rarely t(X;14)(q28; q11) involving the *mtcp*1 locus at Xq28. The activation of the *tcl*-1 gene in a preneoplastic clonal expansion observed in an AT patient has been shown directly, indicating that *tcl*-1 expression in this case represents one of the early steps in leukemogenesis [147].

The early activation of *tcl*-1 in T-cell clonal expansions suggests a role for the encoded protein in the initiation of the neoplastic process. Clonal expansions in AT patients remain preneoplastic for several years and the progression to frank leukemia probably requires the occurrence of secondary genetic events. The functional role(s) of the Tcl-1 protein have not yet been defined, and it is uncertain whether *tcl*-1 belongs to the category of oncogenes that control cell proliferation or to the category of oncogenes that regulate cell survival. Because *tcl*-1 is involved in the initiation of leukemia with a very slow progression, it is reasonable to postulate that the Tcl-1 protein may function in the regulation of programmed cell death, in analogy to the Bcl-2 protein in follicular lymphomas. By extending the life span of the cell, Tcl-1 may allow time for additional genetic mutations to occur, leading to the full development of leukemia.

LARGE GRANULAR LYMPHOCYTE LEUKEMIA

Large granular lymphocytes are a morphologically distinct lymphoid subset comprising 10–15% of peripheral blood mononuclear cells [148]. Two major lineages of LGL have been identified: CD3+ LGL, which probably represent *in vivo* activated cytotoxic T-cells and CD3– LGLs, which are natural killer (NK) cells. Based on clonal cytogenetic abnormalities, TCR gene rearrangement, and clinico-pathological features, it is now recognized that LGL proliferations may be clonally derived from either of their normal counterparts, i.e., CD3+ or CD3– LGL. These disorders correspond to cases previously referred to as Tγ lymphocytosis or Tγ lymphoproliferative disease, CD8+ T-CLL, and T8 lymphocytosis with neutropenia. It has been proposed that these disorders be classified as either T-LGL leukemia, characterized by clonal CD3+ LGL proliferation, or NK-LGL leukemia, characterized by clonal CD3– proliferation [149]. The light microscopic characteristics of LGL cells in both types are similar. The cells are larger than normal lymphocytes, have abundant pale cytoplasm, prominent azurophilic granules, and round or oval nuclei with moderately condensed chromatin and rare nucleoli. Patients with NK-LGL leukemia tend to be younger than those with T-LGL leukemia and have a more aggressive clinical course.

T-LGL CD3+ leukemia cases consistently have TCR gene rearrangements [149], and usually express TCRα/β heterodimers without preferential involvement of a particular TCR variable (V) β-chain family [150]. A fraction of T-LGL leukemia patients (30–50%) have been reported to show serologic evidence of human T-cell leukemia virus (HTLV-1 and HTLV-2) infection and familial retroviral infection has been suggested in some cases [149]. Specific genetic lesions affecting oncogenes and/or tumor suppressor genes have not been reported.

NK-LGL CD3– leukemic cells lack clonal rearrangement of TCR genes [149]. Determination of clonal proliferation in these cases has been performed by cytogenetic analysis [151,152], X-linked gene analysis [153] or Epstein–Barr virus (EBV) DNA analysis with terminal repeat region probes [154]. An interesting finding is that most of the NK-LGL leukemia cases reported to have clonal cytogenetic abnormalities are from Japan. Trisomy 8 and inv(9)(p23;q31) have been observed [152]. EBV has been implicated in the pathogenesis of NK-LGL leukemia, although its association with EBV differs considerably among patient populations, being frequent in Asian patients, but very rare among patients in the Western world [149]. As with T-LGL leukemias, specific genetic lesions affecting oncogenes and/or tumor suppressor genes have not been reported in these forms.

MISCELLANEOUS PERIPHERAL T-CELL LYMPHOMAS

These disorders represent about 15% of the lym-

phomas diagnosed in the Western world and comprise a number of clinical syndromes. There is heterogeneity of T-cell markers and some cases may even lack evidence of T-cell clonality. The majority of patients are adults with generalized disease: the liver, lymph nodes, skin or subcutis, spleen and other viscera may be involved. The clinical course is generally aggressive. Several subtypes of PTCL have been recognized, including T-zone lymphoma, lymphoepithelioid cell lymphoma, angioimmunoblastic T-cell lymphoma, angiocentric lymphoma, intestinal T-cell lymphoma, and anaplastic large-cell lymphoma.

Rearrangement of the TCR genes is present in approximately two-thirds of cases [155, 156]. It has been reported that the γ-locus is more frequently rearranged, and therefore is more useful than the β-locus in the study of PTCL clonality [156]. Rearrangements of the IgH chain gene are also observed in some cases, in particular in angioimmunoblastic T-cell lymphomas, whereas in angiocentric lymphomas rearrangements of the antigen receptor genes are rarely observed. Cytogenetic analysis has shown several types of chromosomal abnormalities in PTCL [157–159]. Trisomy 3 has been observed only in low-grade forms, such as T-zone lymphoma, lymphoepithelioid lymphoma and angioimmunoblastic lymphoma. Trisomy 5 and +X are frequent in angioimmunoblastic lymphomas. Recently, in a combined interphase and metaphase cytogenetic analysis, trisomy 3 and/or +X were found in 32 of 36 patients [159]. In addition, aberrant, unrelated clones were found in about half of these patients, suggesting the occurrence of oligoclonal proliferations in these disorders. Finally, deletions of 6q–, trisomy 7q and monosomy 13 or changes of 13q14 (deletions or translocations) have been found repeatedly in PTCL and, interestingly, they are more frequent in high-grade forms of PTCL, such as pleomorphic medium-to-large cell and immunoblastic lymphoma in the Kiel classification, than in low-grade forms.

CUTANEOUS T-CELL LYMPHOMAS

General description

Primary cutaneous lymphomas (CLs) are among the more frequent types of extranodal non-Hodgkin's lymphomas (NHL) [160]. Based on morphologic, immunophenotypic and, more recently, genotypic criteria, CLs have been classified as either cutaneous T-cell lymphomas (CTCLs) or cutaneous B-cell lymphomas (CBCLs).

CTCLs are the most frequent type of CLs [119]. Their histologic and clinical characteristics have been extensively investigated over the last 10 years [161–165], leading to the definition of a number of pathological entities which, in the Kiel classification, are divided into low-grade and high-grade lymphomas (Table 17.3). Mycosis fungoides (MF) and Sézary syndrome (SS) account for the majority of cases of CTCL. Most of the remaining cases are large-cell lymphomas, including CD30+ large-cell lymphomas, which have an extremely good prognosis whether or not classified as anaplastic [165]. In contrast, primary cutaneous CD30– large-cell lymphomas generally have a poor prognosis. Recent studies have also demonstrated that cutaneous lymphomas, both of B- and T-cell origin, differ from their nodal histological counterparts in immunophenotype, adhesion molecule profile and sometimes with respect to oncogene expression. For example, *bcl*-2 rearrangements are rarely found in cutaneous follicular B-lymphomas [166–168] and the (2;5)(p23; q35) chromosomal translocation is usually absent in cutaneous CD30+ ALCL [169]. These observations indicate that the classification of CTCL should be based on a combination of immunophenotypic, clinical and histologic criteria [170] (Table 17.3).

The vast majority of CTCLs express a helper phenotype (CD4+) [171], but some specific subsets show a suppressor/cytotoxic (CD8+) or γ/δ phenotype

Table 17.3 Classification of cutaneous T-cell lymphoma

Primary CTCL

Low-grade malignant CTCL
Mycosis fungoides
Mycosis fungoides: variants/related disorders
  MF-associated follicular mucinosis
  Pagetoid reticulosis
  Granulomatous slack skin
Sézary syndrome
CD30+ lymphoproliferative disorders*
  Primary cutaneous CD30+ large-cell lymphoma
  Lymphomatoid papulosis
  Borderline cases

High-grade malignant CTCL
CTCL, pleomorphic large cell (CD30–)
CTCL, immunoblastic (CD30–)

Undetermined
CTCL, pleomorphic small/medium cell
CTCL, angiocentric
CD8+ CTCL
Other

* Includes anaplastic, immunoblastic and pleomorphic CD30+ lymphomas.
CTCL, Cutaneous T-cell lymphoma; MF, mycosis fungoides.
From Willemze [170].

(for review, see [172]). CTCLs share the common expression of activation antigens, such as HLA-DR, CD25 and CD71, and the frequent loss of pan-T-cell antigens, such as CD5 and CD7 in MF, and CD2, CD3, CD5 and CD7 in ALCLs and PTLs [173–176]. Furthermore, ALCLs and most PTLs are characterized by CD30/Ki-1 antigen expression [177]. Recently, a new group of subcutaneous lymphomas, owing to proliferation of CD4+, CD8+ or γ/δ post-thymic T-lymphocytes, has been identified [178]. These forms are characterized by a localization to the subcutaneous tissue of the lower extremities and trunk, show an aggressive rapid course and are frequently associated with a hemophagocytic syndrome.

TCR GENE REARRANGEMENT

Although cutaneous T-cell lymphomas, based on morphologic and immunohistochemical criteria, are thought to be clonal expansions of malignant T-lymphocytes, the lack of clonal TCR gene rearrangements by Southern blot analysis has been reported in a variable proportion of cases [179–181]. There are several possible explanations for this:

1. The type of sample analyzed. In some cases of MF, TCR gene rearrangement is detected in peripheral blood cells whereas a germline pattern is observed in skin and the converse may be found in some cases of SS. This finding may result from chromosomal loss or even different degrees of evolution of the neoplastic clone in different sites and emphasizes the importance of testing multiple samples from the same patient.
2. Stage of disease. Early stage MF (stage I–II) may not have a TCR gene rearrangement.
3. Clonal expansion of an early cell frozen at a prearrangement stage of differentiation.
4. The presence of normal or reactive cells in the biopsy specimen. Recently, molecular analysis has been reported for a panel of 38 primary CTCLs including 24 cases of MF at various clinical stages, six cases of small/medium-cell PTL, five cases of medium/large-cell PTL and three cases of ALCL CD30+. All of the cases except one case of ALCL showed clonal rearrangements of TCRβ- and/or γ-chain genes by Southern blot analysis [168]. Interestingly, the negative ALCL case showed an immature phenotypic picture characterized by the absence of the CD3 antigen.

CTCLs with clonal proliferation of γ/δ T-lymphocytes have been reported [182,183]. These cases may explain those CTCL in which TCRβ-chain appears to be in germline configuration, even if the tumor sample analyzed is representative of the malignant cell population.

The presence of more than one clone in a single patient (clonotypic heterogeneity) has been also reported. In particular, Bignon et al. [184] studied skin, lymph node, blood and bone marrow samples of 23 patients with CTCL. Five patients showed more than one clonal rearrangement of the TCR genes at different sites. The most likely explanation for this finding is the evolution of subclones from a single undifferentiated malignant stem cell. Another possible explanation could be the occurrence of contemporary malignant transformation of two or more lymphocytic cells in a micro- or macroenvironment that is prone to the development of lymphoid malignancies.

Ig gene rearrangements have been identified in several of T-cell neoplasias. In particular, Berger et al. [185] detected Ig gene rearrangements in addition to TCR gene rearrangements in the peripheral blood of four of 13 patients with a leukemic phase of CTCL. This phenomenon may result from the non-specificity of the recombinase enzymes responsible for DNA gene rearrangement in T- and B-cells. Another possibility is that the rearrangements are in distinct lymphocyte subsets; for example, the clonal expansion of pathologic T-helper cells could sometimes drive a nonneoplastic B-cell clone that recognizes the TCR idiotype specificity of the malignant T-cell clone.

Clonal TCR gene rearrangements may be detected in some benign cutaneous disorders and do not necessarily indicate malignancy. Lymphomatoid papulosis (LP), for example, is a disease characterized by a dermal proliferation of atypical large cells similar to Reed–Sternberg or cerebriform MF cells with clonal rearrangement of TCR genes [186,187]. Approximately 10–20% of cases of LP may precede or follow a cutaneous T-cell lymphoma, but the remainder have a benign natural history. LP could be a benign neoplasm or a lymphoproliferative process of malignant T-cells with a high incidence of spontaneous resolution.

Finally, the application of PCR technology has significantly improved the sensitivity in detecting a clonal lymphoid population. As discussed above, Southern analysis of lymphoid cutaneous malignancies has a number of limitations, in particular the presence of a large fraction of normal cells in skin biopsies and variable numbers of polyclonal reactive lymphoid cells. Several different strategies have been developed to detect TCR gene rearrangement in CTCL using either RNA [188] or DNA [189]. PCR amplification has been performed on β or γ TCR genes. In particular, the γ gene has been suggested as ideal target because it has a limited V-gene repertoire

and extensive junction diversity. These strategies will allow the diagnosis and staging of CTCL to be made with increased sensitivity and specificity, and therefore at an earlier phase of the disease. This technique could also help in the evaluation of systemic involvement in CTCL and of multiple skin lesions with different clinical appearances.

Chromosomal abnormalities

Cytogenetic analysis has not led to the detection of specific chromosomal abnormalities in CTCL [157–159]. A high frequency of unrelated nonclonal chromosome abnormalities is observed in MF skin samples and peripheral blood lymphocytes in SS, particularly in early stages of the disease. In a recently reported series, about 17% of MF/SS showed this finding, a frequency exceeding that found in malignant lymphoma in general. Clone formation is generally observed in advanced disease. Polyploidy, trisomy 7q, structural aberrations of 6p, and changes of 13q14 were observed in a considerable number of cases of MF and SS [159].

Viral sequences

Involvement of EBV in the pathogenesis of primary CTCL appears to be a rare event. In a recent study, a combined approach based on PCR, RNA *in situ* hybridization and immunohistochemistry was used to detect the presence of EBV in extranodal T-NHL (nasal cavity, gastrointestinal tract lung and skin) [190]. This study indicated that EBV-associated T-NHLs are highly site-restricted: 5/5 nasal, 2/6 pulmonary, 1/12 gastrointestinal and 0/12 cutaneous (6 cases of CD30– and 6 cases CD30+) T-cell lymphomas, supporting the hypothesis that EBV is not involved in the development of primary CTCL.

Recently, the presence of HTLV-1 sequences in peripheral blood mononuclear cells and T-cell lines from SS patients (25 cases), and skin lesions from MF patients (10 cases) has been reported [191]. HTLV-1 *tax/rex* region DNA was detected in 72% of SS-PBMC, 80% of T-cell lines established from SS-PBMC and 30% of skin lesions from MF. HTLV-1 *gag* region sequences were not identified. These data support the presence of a truncated HTLV-1 retrovirus in CTCL. Furthermore, expression of HTLV-1 *tax/rex* RNA was detected in four of eight cases of SS by RNA-PCR, indicating that this viral region is transcribed *in vivo*; in addition, serum antibodies against p27*rex* and p40*tax* were detected in 43% and 29% of SS patients, respectively. Because p27*rex* and p40*tax* have been shown to regulate several genes involved in the proliferation and differentiation of lymphoid cells, one may suggest a role of these viral proteins in neoplastic T-cell activation and/or in the maintenance of the malignant phenotype in a fraction of CTCL.

Oncogene and tumor suppressor gene involvement

The role of known oncogenes and tumor suppressor genes in the pathogenesis of CTCLs is still poorly investigated. A molecular analysis of the putative proto-oncogenes *tal*-1 and *NFκB2/lyt*-10 and the tumor suppressor gene p53 in a panel of 38 primary CTCL has been recently reported [168]. It was found that inactivation of p53 in CTCL is a rare event and that alterations of *tal*-1 and *NFκB2* genes may play a pathogenetic role in a small number of cases.

p53 gene inactivation by point mutation is the most frequent genetic lesion in human cancers, and has been frequently associated with tumor progression (for reviews see [192, 193]). Among lymphoid malignancies, p53 gene mutations have been reported to occur in advanced stages of multiple myeloma and in a minority of malignant NHLs, either highly malignant forms such as Burkitt's lymphoma or transformed follicular lymphomas, or occasionally, in less aggressive tumors, such as B-CLLs (for reviews see [194, 195]). In the study by Neri and coworkers, p53 gene mutations were detected in only one of 38 cases of primary CTCL (a tumoral stage MF) [168]. No p53 mutations were observed in 52 cases of CBCL investigated in the same study, suggesting that p53 inactivation might play a very limited pathogenetic role in CLs. These findings are consistent with the clinical features of these neoplasias. Primary CBCLs as well as the majority of CTCLs are characterized by a low grade of malignancy, indolent clinical course, possible spontaneous resolution of some lesions and good prognosis, particularly those forms expressing CD30 antigen.

Structural alterations of the *tal*-1 gene, a member of the bHLH family of transcription factors [11], have been almost exclusively associated with α/β lineage T-ALLs [34, 35], and it has been proposed, as discussed above, that these are caused by 'illegitimate' V(D)J recombination. The presence of deletions involving the 5' region of the *tal*-1 gene in CTCLs was investigated by a PCR-based approach using two different sets of primers capable of identifying the majority of the reported deletions. In this analysis, rearrangement of the *tal*-1 gene was detected in three of 38 cases of CTCLs, two MFs, and one pleomorphic large-cell lymphoma (PTL) [168]. These patients had an unusually aggressive and rapidly progressive clinical course, with poor response to systemic polychemotherapy. In particular, the PTL patient progressed to immunoblastic lym-

phoma, dying 6 months after diagnosis with massive skin involvement, but without any apparent systemic spread of the disease. These observations extend the spectrum of *tal*-1 gene rearrangements to neoplasms other than T-ALL, and suggest a pathogenetic role for inappropriate *tal*-1 gene expression in a significant proportion of CTCLs.

The *NFκB2/lyt*-10 gene is a member of the *NF-κB/rel* gene family of transcription factors involved in the transcriptional regulation of a large number of cellular and viral genes (for reviews, see [196, 197]). This gene was identified as a putative proto-oncogene (*lyt*-10) involved in a chromosomal translocation t(10;14)(q24;q32) in a case of B-NHL [198] (see description below). In a large analysis of different types of lymphoid malignancies, rearrangement of this gene was found in seven of 400 cases [168, 199] (Neri et al., unpublished results). Interestingly, four of these rearranged cases were primary cutaneous lymphomas, two CBCL and two CTCL. The two CTCL cases were MFs in tumoral stage, but had an atypical, aggressive course and required systemic polychemotherapy: one case had a rapidly fatal course and the other developed peripheral blood involvement 5 years after diagnosis, dying 2 years later with systemic disease. Rearrangements of *NFκB2* were also demonstrated in two of six CTCL analyzed by Takur et al. [200] and in the T-lymphoma cell line, HUT78, derived from a cutaneous lymphoma [200, 201]. These data suggest that *NFκB2/lyt*-10 gene rearrangements may represent a molecular event that preferentially targets CLs among the wide spectrum of lymphoid malignancies.

ROLE OF THE NFκB2/lyt-10 PROTO-ONCOGENE IN CUTANEOUS LYMPHOMAS

In about 10% of low-grade B-cell NHL and, less frequently, in intermediate- and high-grade B-NHL, the chromosome band 10q24 is involved in various aberrations including deletions or translocation with the IgH locus [202]. The involvement of the *hox*11 gene in T-ALL with t(10;14)(q24;q11) and t(7;10) (q35;q24) has been discussed previously in this chapter. However, *hox*11 has not been found to be involved in chromosomal aberrations affecting 10q24 in B-NHL (S. Korsmeyer, personal communication; Neri et al., unpublished results), suggesting the existence of other proto-oncogene loci in this genomic region. To identify other genetic elements involved in chromosomal breakpoints affecting band 10q24, the breakpoint junctions of a t(10;14)(q24; q32) in a case of B-cell lymphoma were cloned and a novel gene identified. This gene was initially named *lyt*-10 (lymphocyte translocation chromosome 10) [198], and then subsequently renamed *NFκB2*, based on its relatedness to the *NF-κB/rel* family [196,197]. Subsequent to the analysis of the first case, similar rearrangements of the *NFκB2/lyt*-10 gene have been found by Southern blot analysis in about 2% of lymphoid malignancies (seven of 400) including various types of B-cell mature neoplasms including myeloma and B-CLL, and both B- and T-cell cutaneous lymphomas ([199] and our own unpublished results).

Molecular characterization of NFκB2/lyt-*10*

The *NFκB2/lyt*-10 gene encodes a member of the NF-κB transcription factor family, found ubiquitously in mammalian cells, which consists of a heterogeneous group of related proteins that can be divided into two main structural classes (for reviews, see [196,197]). The first class is represented by the protein products of the c-*rel/Rel*, p65/RelA and *RelB* genes, which share a conserved N-terminal region of 300 amino acids, called the Rel homology domain. This region is responsible for DNA binding, dimerization, interaction with IκB molecules and nuclear localization. These proteins are further characterized by the presence of distinct transcriptional-activation domains in the C-terminal region. The second class of NF-κB proteins is represented by the p50 (NF-κB1p50) and p52 (NF-κB2p52) subunits, both derived from proteolytic processing of larger precursor proteins (p50/p105 and p52/p100) encoded, respectively, by the *NFκB1* and *NFκB2(lyt*-10*)* genes. These precursor proteins contain an N-terminal Rel homology domain, a polyglycine (poly-G) hinge and a C-terminal ankyrin-like domain. This C-terminal domain contains seven tandem ankyrin repeats and has distinctive functional properties, such as inhibition of the DNA binding activity and sequestering of NF-κB complexes in the cytoplasm. The removal of this domain, probably due to proteolytic processing mediated by the poly-G hinge, gives rise to the active DNA-binding subunits p50 or p52 [203,204]. In unstimulated cells, NF-κB is present in the cytoplasm as an inactive dimeric complex (the most common is the heterodimer constituted by the p50 and p65/RelA subunits) associated with an inhibitory protein, called IκB. Following a variety of stimuli, the complex dissociates from the IκB molecule and moves to the nucleus, where it binds to *cis*-acting DNA consensus sequences (κB sites) found in the promoters/enhancers of inducible genes (for reviews, see [196,197]). The IκB family includes IκB-α (Mad-3/pp40), IkB-γ (a separately expressed C-terminal domain of NF-κBp105 detected in some mouse pre-B-cell lines), IκB-β and the proto-oncogene *bcl*-3. All of these proteins are characterized by the presence of a domain consisting of five to seven ankyrin repeats (for review, see [205]). With the exception of Bcl-3 [206], all of these proteins are able to inhibit DNA binding *in vitro* and to retain NF-κB complexes in the cytoplasm by shielding of the nuclear translocation signal present on the Rel domain of NF-κB proteins.

The *NFκB2* gene is ubiquitously transcribed as a single 3.2 kb mRNA species. In lymphoid cells, there is evidence that *NFκB2* is expressed at low levels in immature B- or T-cells, whereas it is expressed at relatively high levels in mature lymphoid cells. *NFκB2* spans a genomic region of about 8 kb on chromosome 10q24, and contains 24 exons (Figure 17.10) [199]. The first two exons are untranslated and alternatively transcribed, and specific promoter regions containing several functional κB sites have been identified upstream of both exons [207]. At least three main mechanisms are responsible for the regulation of the *NFκB2* gene: (1) induction of gene transcription; (2) processing of the large inactive precursor p100 into the p52 DNA binding subunit; and (3) translocation of p52 from the cytoplasm to the nucleus [203, 204].

Mechanisms of NFκB2/lyt-*10 gene rearrangement*

As mentioned above, the *NFκB2* gene was originally identified as a putative proto-oncogene (*lyt*-10) in a case of B-cell lymphoma where it was found to be involved in a chromosomal translocation t(10;14) (q24;q32) with the *IgH* locus [198]. As a consequence of the translocation, the 5' half of the *NFκB2* gene was juxtaposed to the Cα1 region of the *IgH* locus, generating an *NFκB2*–Cα1 fusion gene which gave rise to a chimeric mRNA *in vivo*. The putative protein encoded by this transcript retained the Rel homology domain and lacked the entire ankyrin domain, which had been replaced by an out-of-frame sequence of the Cα1 region. Because the frequency of 10q24 lesions is about 10% in NHL, it is possible that either some breakpoints are distant from the *NFκB2* locus or that another locus is involved in the majority of breakpoints.

Southern blot analysis [199] and molecular cloning [208] have indicated that rearrangements of *NFκB2* in lymphoid malignancies can occur by two distinct mechanisms: chromosomal translocation with different chromosomal partners (three of eight cases) and, more frequently, interstitial deletions involving the 3' end of the *NFκB2* locus (five of eight cases) (see Figure 17.10). With regard to the translocations, molecular cloning, performed in two

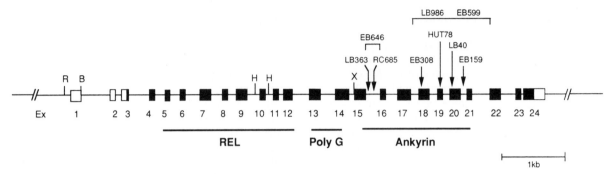

Figure 17.10 Schematic representation of the genomic *NFκB2* locus and breakpoint locations in lymphoid neoplasias. Black boxes indicate translated exons; white boxes indicate untranslated exons. The rel, poly G and ankyrin domains are indicated. Breakpoint locations in cloned cases (LB363, RC685, EB308, HUT78, LB40, EB159) are indicated by arrows; in cases not cloned (EB646, LB986, EB599), the genomic region in which breakpoints occur is indicated by a bracket. Breakpoints in cases rearranged by chromosomal translocation (EB646, LB363, RC685) occur within intron 15 of the *NFκB2* gene (see text).

cases (a B-NHL and a myeloma), indicated the involvement of chromosomes 14q32 and 7q34, respectively. Interestingly, in all of the cases, the breakpoint occurred within intron 15 of the *NFκB2* gene, and nucleotide sequence analysis in two cases showed that the breakpoints occurred close to a pentameric sequence (GGGGT) characteristic of the switch regions of the *IgH* gene [209]. These findings suggest that: (1) band 10q24 in cases involving the *NFκB2* gene may participate in translocations with different chromosomal partners; and (2) rearrangements of *NFκB2* in these cases may result from mistakes in the normal Ig switching mechanisms, which occur in mature B-cells. With regard to the interstitial deletion, fluorescence *in situ* hybridiza-

tion (FISH) analysis of interphase nuclei in two cases (a B-CLL and a CTCL), using unique regions from chromosome band 10q24 (which had rearranged with *NFκB2*) as probes, demonstrated that the distance between the *NFκB2* gene and these unique regions is in the range of a few hundred kilobases, thus indicating that rearrangements of *NFκB2* in these cases may reflect cytogenetically undetectable events. In both of these cases, genomic internal deletions were demonstrated to generate abnormal transcripts that potentially encoded carboxy-terminal truncations of NFκB2. The same molecular mechanism may account for the rearrangement of the *NFκB2/lyt*-10 gene in the T-cell line HUT78 [200,201].

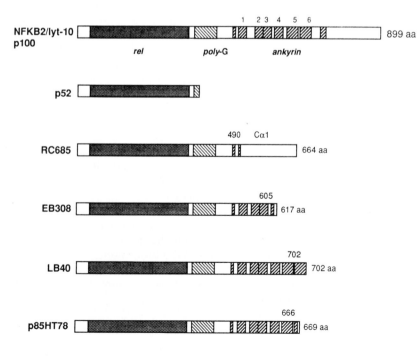

Figure 17.11 Schematic representation of normal and rearranged NFκB2/Lyt-10 proteins. The Rel, poly-G and ankyrin domains are indicated. 1–6, full ankyrin repeats. The tumor-associated truncated NFκB2 proteins, RC685 (57), EB308 (73), LB40 (73), and p85HUT78 (59,60), are aligned under NFκB2/Lyt-10. The number of amino acid residues of the normal NFκB2 protein contained within the predicted truncated proteins is indicated above each scheme. The total polypeptide length of the normal and truncated NFκB2 proteins is shown to the right of each protein.

Deregulation of the NFκB2/lyt-10 gene

Besides the different mechanisms of rearrangement, recombination events involving the C-terminal ankyrin-coding domain of the *NF-κB2* gene can lead to the production of C-terminal truncated proteins which, in some cases (lyt-10/Cα1), are fused with heterologous domains (see scheme in Figure 17.11). Functional analyses of these proteins (lyt-10-Cα1, p85HT78, EB308, LB40) have demonstrated that they localize constitutively in the nucleus, are not subjected to proteolytic processing, and are able to bind to κB sites *in vitro* and *in vivo* [200,201,208, 210]. In particular, functional analysis of the lyt-10/Cα1 and p85HT78 showed that both proteins have retained the ability to mediate transcriptional activation via heterodimerization with p65/RelA but have lost the transrepression activity associated with homodimeric DNA binding. In addition, these two proteins have been found capable of independent transactivation of κB-reporter genes. These findings indicate that tumor-associated NFκB2/lyt-10 proteins may lead to quantitative changes in the composition of NF-κB complexes as well as to qualitative consequences for NF-κB functions. Thus, the overall effect of these alterations could be the constitutive activation of specific subsets of NF-κB-controlled genes, in particular lymphocyte growth genes, which, in turn, may contribute to tumorigenesis. However, attempts to demonstrate *in vitro* transforming ability of constitutively overexpressed *NFκB2/lyt*-10 rearranged genes in lymphoblastoid cells and transgenic animals have failed so far, possibly because of the toxic effect of high levels of active NF-κB2 protein. The use of rearranged *NFκB2* genes under the control of their own regulatory elements in order to avoid overexpression may be a better way to investigate the role of *NFκB2* activation in tumorigenesis.

Synthesis

Many of the proteins encoded by proto-oncogenes involved in T-cell neoplasms have structural features of transcription factors, which act in the cell nucleus to regulate the expression of genes. Those proteins identified to date include members of the basic helix–loop–helix category (c-Myc, Scl/Tal-1, Tal-2 and Lyl-1), the LIM domain group (Rbtn-1 and Rbtn-2), the homeodomain group (Hox11), and the NF-κB/Rel group (NFκB2/Lyt-10). Thus, the abnormal expression of several different types of transcription factors can lead to malignant transformation in T-cells. Studies of the normal functions of the transcription factor proteins indicates that they play important roles in normal cell growth and differentiation. Evidence that some of the different transcription factor proteins may interact with one another (e.g., Scl/Tal-1 with the LIM domain proteins) suggests that some of these proteins may, in fact, help to regulate a common pathway in neoplastic transformation. In addition to transcription factors, at least two of the genes involved in T-cell neoplasms encode proteins (Lck and Tan-1) which normally function in cell signal transduction. The functions of some genes involved in T-cell leukemias (e.g., *all*-1 and *tcl*-1) have not yet been elucidated. Furthermore, it is generally realized that many gene defects in T-cell neoplasms have not yet been identified.

In hematologic malignancy, chromosomal rearrangements are generally believed to be initiating events in the multistep process of neoplastic transformation. Thus, proto-oncogene activation in T-cell malignancies is thought to be a first step down the road toward the malignant phenotype. Tumor suppressor gene loss or inactivation is also believed to play a role in the progression of hematologic malignancies. p53 mutations have been shown to be associated with T-ALL in relapse, but overall the prevalence of p53 mutations in T-cell neoplasms seems to be considerably lower than that found in solid tumors. In contrast, mutation or loss of the p16 gene, which encodes a cyclin-dependent kinase inhibitor, seems to be very common in T-ALL. The identification of oncogene and tumor suppressor gene defects in T-cell neoplasms enables the molecular diagnosis and monitoring of these diseases. More importantly, the identified genes provide potential targets for a new generation of cancer therapies. As in the case of other types of tumors, the study of oncogenes and tumor suppressor genes in T-cell neoplasia has increased our knowledge of normal cell growth and differentiation, and offers hope for better cancer treatment and prevention in the future.

Acknowledgments

PDA acknowledges Ms Elena Greco for artwork and Drs Ilan Kirsch, Richard Baer and Adam Goldfarb for helpful conversations. AN and NSF are grateful to Anna Migliazza, Dino Trecca, Luigia Lombardi, Chih-Chao Chang, Mariano Rocchi, Luca Baldini and Emilio Berti for their contributions to this work. SAS, LV and CMC thank Florencia Bullrich for critical reading of parts of the manuscript. PDA is supported in part by a grant from the American Cancer Society. AN is supported by a grant from

Associazione Italiana Ricerca sul Cancro (AIRC) and by a grant 'Progetto Finalizzato 1993' from the Italian Ministry of Health to Ospedale Maggiore, Milano. CMC is supported by the Falk Medical Research Trust and grants from the National Cancer Institute.

References

1. Boehm T, Rabbitts TH. The human T cell receptor genes are targets for chromosomal abnormalities in T cell tumors. *FASEB J.* 1989, **3**: 2344–2359.
2. Baer R. TAL1, TAL2, and LYL1: A family of basic helix–loop–helix proteins implicated in T cell acute leukemia. *Semin. Cancer Biol.* 1993, **4**: 341–347.
3. Murre C, McCaw PS, Baltimore D. A new DNA binding and dimerization motif in immunoglobulin enhancer binding, daughterless, MyoD, and myc proteins. *Cell* 1989, **56**: 777–783.
4. Weintraub H, Davis R, Tapscott S, et al. The *MyoD* gene family: Nodal point during specification of the muscle cell lineage. *Science* 1991, **251**: 761–766.
5. Murre C, McCaw PS, Vaessin H, et al. Interactions between heterologous helix–loop–helix proteins generate complexes that bind specifically to a common DNA sequence. *Cell* 1989, **58**: 537–544.
6. Dalla Favera R, Bregni M, Erikson J, et al. Assignment of the human c-myc oncogene to the region of chromosome 8 which is translocated in Burkitt lymphoma cells. *Proc. Natl Acad. Sci. USA* 1982, **79**: 7824–7827.
7. Mellentin JD, Smith SD, Cleary ML. *lyl-1*, a novel gene altered by chromosomal translocation in T cell leukemia, codes for a protein with a helix–loop–helix DNA binding motif. *Cell* 1989, **58**: 77–83.
8. Begley CG, Aplan PD, Davey MP, et al. Chromosomal translocation in a human leukemic stem-cell line disrupts the T-cell antigen receptor delta-chain diversity region and results in a previously unreported fusion transcript. *Proc. Natl Acad. Sci. USA* 1989, **86**: 2031–2035.
9. Begley CG, Aplan PD, Denning SM, et al. The gene *SCL* is expressed during early hematopoiesis and encodes a differentiation-related DNA binding motif. *Proc. Natl Acad. Sci. USA* 1989, **86**: 10128–10132.
10. Finger LR, Kagan J, Christopher G, et al. Involvement of the *TCL5* gene on human chromosome 1 in T-cell leukemia and melanoma. *Proc. Natl Acad. Sci. USA* 1989, **86**: 5039–5043.
11. Chen Q, Cheng J-T, Tsai L-H, et al. The *tal-1* gene undergoes chromosome translocation in T-cell acute leukemia and potentially encodes a helix–loop–helix protein. *EMBO J.* 1990, **9**: 415–424.
12. Xia Y, Brown L, Yang CY, et al. *TAL2*, a helix–loop–helix gene activated by the (7;9)(q34;q32) translocation in human T-cell leukemia. *Proc. Natl Acad. Sci. USA* 1991, **88**: 11416–11420.
13. Lange BJ, Raimondi SC, Heerema N, et al. Pediatric leukemia/lymphoma with t(8;14)(q24;q11). *Leukemia* 1992, **6**: 613–618.
14. Erikson J, Finger L, Sun L, et al. Deregulation of *c-myc* by translocation of the α-locus of the T-cell receptor in T-cell leukemias. *Science* 1986, **232**: 884–886.
15. McKeithan TW, Shima E, Le Beau MM, et al. Molecular cloning of the breakpoint junction of a human chromosomal 8;14 translocation involving the T-cell receptor α-chain gene and sequences on the 3' side of *MYC*. *Proc. Natl Acad. Sci. USA* 1986, **83**: 6636–6640.
16. Soudon J, Bernard O, Mathieu-Mahul D, et al. *c-myc* gene expression in a leukemia T-cell line bearing a t(8;14)(q24;q11) translocation. *Leukemia* 1991, **5**: 60–65.
17. Finver SN, Nishikura K, Finger LR, et al. Sequence analysis of the *MYC* oncogene involved in the t(8;14)(q24;q11) chromosome translocation in a human leukemia T-cell line indicates that putative regulatory regions are not altered. *Proc. Natl Acad. Sci. USA* 1988, **85**: 3052–3056.
18. Bhatia K, Huppi K, Spangler G, et al. Point mutations in the c-Myc transactivation domain are common in Burkitt's lymphoma and mouse plasmacytomas. *Nature Genet.* 1993, **5**: 56–61.
19. Amati B, Brooks MW, Levy N, et al. Oncogenic activity of the c-Myc protein requires dimerization with Max. *Cell* 1993, **72**: 233–245.
20. Zervos AS, Gyuris J, Brent R. Mxi1, a protein that specifically interacts with Max to bind Myc–Max recognition sites. *Cell* 1993, **72**: 223–232.
21. Bernard O, Guglielmi P, Jonveaux P, et al. Two distinct mechanisms for the SCL gene activation in the t(1;14) translocation of T-cell leukemias. *Genes Chrom. Cancer* 1990, **1**: 194–208.
22. Fitzgerald TJ, Neale GAM, Raimondi SC, et al. c-tal, a helix–loop–helix protein, is juxtaposed to the T-cell receptor beta chain gene by a reciprocal chromosomal translocation: t(1;7)(p32;q35). *Blood* 1991, **78**: 2686–2695.
23. Aplan PD, Raimondi SC, Kirsch IR. Disruption of the *SCL* gene by a t(1;3) translocation in a patient with T-cell acute lymphoblastic leukemia. *J. Exp. Med.* 1992, **176**: 1303–1310.
24. Brown L, Cheng J-T, Chen Q, et al. Site-specific recombination of the *tal-1* gene is a common occurrence in human T-cell leukemia. *EMBO J.* 1990, **9**: 3343–3351.
25. Aplan PD, Begley CG, Bertness VL, et al. The *SCL* gene is formed from a transcriptionally complex locus. *Mol. Cell. Biol.* 1990, **10**: 6426–6435.
26. Aplan PD, Lombardi DP, Ginsberg AM, et al. Disruption of the human *SCL* locus by 'illegitimate' V(D)J recombinase activity. *Science* 1990, **250**: 1426–1429.
27. Aplan PD, Lombardi DP, Reaman GH, et al. Involvement of the putative hematopoietic transcription factor SCL in T-cell acute lymphoblastic leukemia. *Blood* 1992, **79**: 1327–1333.
28. Bash RO, Crist WM, Shuster JJ, et al. Clinical features and outcome of T-cell acute lymphoblastic leukemia in childhood with respect to alterations at

the *TAL1* locus: A Pediatric Oncology Group study. *Blood* 1993, **81**: 2110–2117.

29. Bhatia K, Spangler G, Advani S, et al. Molecular characterization of *SCL* rearrangements in T-cell ALL from developing countries. *Int. J. Oncol.* 1993, **2**: 725–733.

30. Kikuchi A, Hayashi T, Kobayashi S, et al. Clinical significance of *TAL1* gene alteration in childhood T-cell acute lymphoblastic leukemia and lymphoma. *Leukemia* 1993, **7**: 933–938.

31. Huang W, Kuang S-Q, Huang Q-H, et al. RT/PCR detection of SIL-TAL-1 fusion mRNA in Chinese T-cell acute lymphoblastic leukemia (T-ALL). *Cancer Genet. Cytogenet.* 1995, **81**: 76–82.

32. Janssen JWG, Ludwig W-D, Sterry W, et al. *SIL-TAL1* deletion in T-cell acute lymphoblastic leukemia. *Leukemia* 1993, **7**: 1204–1210.

33. Stock W, Westbrook CA, Sher DA, et al. Low incidence of Tal-1 gene rearrangements in adult acute lymphoblastic leukemia: A Cancer and Leukemia Group B study (8762). *Clin. Cancer Res.* 1995, **1**: 459–463.

34. Macintyre EA, Smit L, Ritz J, et al. Disruption of the *SCL* locus in T-lymphoid malignancies correlates with commitment to the T-cell receptor $\alpha\beta$ lineage. *Blood* 1992, **80**: 1511–1520.

35. Breit TM, Mol EJ, Wolvers-Tettero ILM, et al. Site-specific deletions involving the *tal-1* and *sil* genes are restricted to cells of the T cell receptor α/β lineage: T cell receptor δ gene deletion mechanism affects multiple genes. *J. Exp. Med.* 1993, **177**: 965–977.

36. Breit TM, Wolvers-Tettero ILM, van Dongen JJM. Lineage specific demethylation of *tal-1* gene break-point region determines the frequency of *tal-1* deletions in $\alpha\beta$ lineage T-cells. *Oncogene* 1994, **9**: 1847–1853.

37. Begley CG, Visvader J, Green AR, et al. Molecular cloning and chromosomal localization of the murine homolog of the human helix–loop–helix gene *SCL*. *Proc. Natl Acad. Sci. USA* 1991, **88**: 869–873.

38. Bockamp BO, McLaughlin R, Murrell AM, et al. Lineage-restricted regulation of the murine *SCL/TAL-1* promoter. *Blood* 1995, **86**: 1502–1514.

39. Bernard O, Azogui O, Lecointe N, et al. A third *tal-1* promoter is specifically used in human T cell leukemias. *J. Exp. Med.* 1992, **176**: 919–925.

40. Green AR, Lints T, Visvader J, et al. *SCL* is coexpressed with *GATA-1* in hematopoietic cells but is also expressed in developing brain. *Oncogene* 1992, **7**: 653–660.

41. Mouthon MA, Bernard O, Mitjavila MT, et al. Expression of tal-1 and GATA binding proteins during human hematopoiesis. *Blood* 1993, **81**: 647–655.

42. Hwang L-Y, Siegelman M, Davis L, et al. Expression of the *TAL1* proto-oncogene in cultured endothelial cells and blood vessels of the spleen. *Oncogene* 1993, **8**: 3043–3046.

43. Kallianpur AR, Jordan JE, Brandt SJ. The *SCL/TAL1* gene is expressed in progenitors of both the hematopoietic and vascular systems during embryogenesis. *Blood* 1994, **83**: 1220–1208.

44. Bernard O, Lecointe N, Jonveaux P, et al. Two site-specific deletions and t(1;14) translocation restricted to human T-cell acute leukemias disrupt the 5' part of the tal-1 gene. *Oncogene* 1991, **6**: 1477–1488.

45. Goldfarb AN, Goueli S, Mickelson D, et al. T-cell acute lymphoblastic leukemia – the associated gene *SCL/tal* codes a 42 kd nuclear phosphoprotein. *Blood* 1992, **80**: 2858–2866.

46. Cheng J-T, Hsu H-L, Hwang L-Y, et al. Products of the *TAL1* oncogene: Basic helix–loop–helix proteins phosphorylated at serine residues. *Oncogene* 1993, **8**: 677–683.

47. Hsu H-L, Huang L, Tsan JT, et al. Preferred sequences for DNA recognition by the TAL1 helix–loop–helix proteins. *Mol. Cell. Biol.* 1993, **14**: 1256–1265.

48. Sanchez-Garcia I, Rabbitts TH. Transcriptional activation by TAL-1 and FUS-CHOP proteins expressed in acute malignancies as a result of chromosomal abnormalities. *Proc. Natl Acad. Sci. USA* 1994, **91**: 7869–7873.

49. Shivdasani RA, Mayer EL, Orkin SH. Absence of blood formation in mice lacking the T-cell leukaemia oncoprotein tal-1/SCL. *Nature (Lond.)* 1995, **373**: 432–434.

50. Robb L, Lyons I, Li R, et al. Absence of yolk sac hematopoiesis from mice with a targeted disruption of the *scl* gene. *Proc. Natl Acad. Sci. USA* 1995, **92**: 7075–7079.

51. Leroy-Viard K, Vinit M-A, Lecointe N, et al. Loss of TAL-1 protein activity induces premature apoptosis of Jurkat leukemic T cells upon medium depletion. *EMBO J.* 1995, **14**: 2341–2349.

52. Elwood NJ, Begley CG. Reconstitution of mice with bone marrow cells expressing the *scl* gene is insufficient to cause leukemia. *Cell Growth Diff.* 1995, **6**: 19–25.

53. Robb L, Rasko JEJ, Bath ML, et al. *Scl*, a gene frequently activated in human T cell leukaemia, does not induce lymphomas in transgenic mice. *Oncogene* 1995, **10**: 205–209.

54. Xia Y, Brown L, Tsan JT, et al. The translocation (1;14)(p34;q11) in human T-cell leukemia: Chromosome breakage 25 kilobase pairs downstream of the *TAL1* protooncogene. *Genes Chrom. Cancer* 1992, **4**: 211–216.

55. Kuo SS, Mellentin JD, Copeland NG, et al. Structure, chromosome mapping, and expression of the mouse *Lyl-1* gene. *Oncogene* 1991, **6**: 961–968.

56. Visvader J, Begley CG, Adams JM. Differential expression of the *LYL, SCL*, and *E2A* helix–loop–helix genes within the hemopoietic system. *Oncogene* 1991, **6**: 187–194.

57. Boehm T, Baer R, Lavenir I, et al. The mechanism of chromosomal translocation t(11;14) involving the T-cell receptor Cδ locus on human chromosome 14q11 and a transcribed region of chromosome 11p15. *EMBO J.* 1988, **7**: 385–394.

58. McGuire EA, Hockett RD, Pollock KM, et al. The t(11;14)(p15;q11) in a T-cell acute lymphoblastic leukemia cell line activates multiple transcripts, including Ttg-1, a gene encoding a potential zinc finger protein. *Mol. Cell. Biol.* 1989, **9**: 2124–2132.

59. Boehm T, Foroni L, Kaneko Y, et al. The rhombotin family of cystein-rich LIM-domain oncogenes: Distinct members are involved in T-cell translocations to

human chromosomes 11p15 and 11p13. *Proc. Natl Acad. Sci. USA* 1991, **88**: 4367–4371.

60. Royer-Pokora B, Loos U, Ludwig W-D. *TTG-2*, a new gene encoding a cysteine-rich protein with the LIM motif, is overexpressed in acute T-cell leukemia with the t(11;14)(p13;q11). *Oncogene* 1991, **6**: 1887–1893.

61. Boehm T, Spillanti M-G, Sofroniew MV, et al. Developmentally regulated and tissue-specific expression of mRNAs encoding the two alternative forms of the LIM domain oncogene rhombotin: Evidence for thymus expression. *Oncogene* 1991, **6**: 695–703.

62. Sanchez-Garcia I, Rabbits TH. LIM domain proteins in leukaemia and development. *Semin. Cancer Biol.* 1993, **4**: 349–358.

63. Royer-Pokora B, Rogers M, Zhu T-H, et al. The *TTG-2/RBTN2* T cell oncogene encodes two alternative transcripts from two promoters: The distal promoter is removed by most 11p13 translocations in acute T cell leukemias (T-ALL). *Oncogene* 1995, **10**: 1353–1360.

64. Sanchez-Garcia I, Axelson H, Rabbitts TH. Functional diversity of LIM proteins: Amino-terminal activation domains in the oncogenic proteins RBTN1 and RBTN2. *Oncogene* 1995, **10**: 1301–1306.

65. Wadman I, Li J, Bash RO, et al. Specific in vivo association between the bHLH and LIM proteins implicated in human T cell leukemia. *EMBO J.* 1994, **13**: 4831–4839.

66. Warren AJ, Colledge WH, Carlton MBL, et al. The oncogenic cysteine-rich LIM domain protein Rbtn2 is essential for erythroid development. *Cell* 1994, **78**: 45–57.

67. McGuire EA, Rintoul CE, Sclar GM, et al. Thymic overexpression of *Ttg-1* in transgenic mice results in T-cell acute lymphoblastic leukemia/lymphoma. *Mol. Cell. Biol.* 1992, **12**: 4186–4196.

68. Fisch P, Boehm T, Lavenir I, et al. T-cell acute lymphoblastic lymphoma induced in transgenic mice by the RBTN1 and RBTN2 LIM-domain genes. *Oncogene* 1992, **7**: 2389–2397.

69. Larson RC, Fisch P, Larson TA, et al. T cell tumours of disparate phenotype in mice transgenic for Rbtn-2. *Oncogene* 1994, **9**: 3675–3681.

70. Lichty BD, Ackland-Snow J, Noble L, et al. Dysregulation of *Hox11* by chromosome translocations in T-cell acute lymphoblastic leukemia: A paradigm for homeobox gene involvement in human cancer. *Leuk. Lymphoma* 1995, **16**: 209–215.

71. Kagan J, Joe Y-S, Freireich EJ. Joining of recombination signals on the der 14q- chromosome in T-cell acute leukemia with t(10;14) chromosome translocation. *Cancer Res.* 1994, **54**: 226–230.

72. Boehm T, Mengl-Gaw L, Kees UR, et al. Alternating purine–pyrimidine tracts may promote chromosomal translocations seen in a variety of human lymphoid tumors. *EMBO J.* 1989, **8**: 2621–2631.

73. Lu M, Zhang N, Raimondi S, et al. S1 nuclease hypersensitive sites in an oligopurine/oligopyrimidine DNA from the t(10;14) breakpoint cluster region. *Nucl. Acids Res.* 1992, **20**: 263–266.

74. Kennedy MA, Gonzalez-Sarmiento R, Kees UR, et al. *HOX11*, a homeobox-containing T-cell oncogene on human chromosome 10q24. *Proc. Natl Acad. Sci. USA* 1991, **88**: 8900–8904.

75. Lu M, Gong Z, Shen W, et al. The *tcl-3* proto-oncogene altered by chromosomal translocation in T-cell leukemia codes a homeobox protein. *EMBO J.* 1991, **10**: 2905–2910.

76. Dube ID, Kamel-Reid S, Yuan CC, et al. A novel human homeobox gene lies at the chromosome 10 breakpoint in lymphoid neoplasias with chromosomal translocation t(10;14). *Blood* 1991, **78**: 2996–3003.

77. Dear TN, Sanchez-Garcia I, Rabbitts TH. The *HOX11* gene encodes a DNA-binding nuclear transcription factor belonging to a distinct family of homeobox genes. *Proc. Natl Acad. Sci. USA* 1993, **90**: 4431–4435.

78. Tang S, Breitman ML. The optimal binding sequence of the Hox11 protein contains a predicted recognition core motif. *Nucl. Acids Res.* 1995, **23**: 1928–1935.

79. Roberts CWM, Shutter JR, Korsmeyer SJ. *Hox11* controls the genesis of the spleen. *Nature (Lond.)* 1994, **368**: 747–749.

80. Roberts CWM, Sonder AM, Lumsden A, et al. Developmental expression of *Hox11* and specification of splenic cell fate. *Am. J. Path.* 1995, **146**: 1089–1101.

81. Raju K, Tang S, Dube ID, et al. Characterization and developmental expression of *Tlx-1*, the murine homolog of *HOX11*. *Mech. Develop.* 1993, **44**: 51–64.

82. Sorce L, Li G, Yuan CC, et al. Expression of HOX11, the oncogene deregulated in t(10;14) T-ALL, causes transformation of NIH3T3 cells and facilitates growth of human leukemic cells in immune-deficient mice. *Blood* 1991, **78**: 168a.

83. Hawley RG, Fong AZC, Lu M, et al. The *HOX11* homeobox-containing gene of human leukemia immortalizes murine hematopoietic precursors. *Oncogene* 1994, **9**: 1–12.

84. Hatano M, Roberts CWM, Kawabe T, et al. *Cell* cycle progression, cell death and T cell lymphoma in *HOX11* transgenic mice. *Blood* 1992, **80**: 355a.

85. Nourse J, Mellentin JD, Galili N, et al. Chromosomal translocation t(1;19) results in synthesis of a homeobox fusion mRNA that codes for a potential chimeric transcription factor. *Cell* 1990, **60**: 535–545.

86. Galili N, Davis RJ, Fredericks WJ, et al. Fusion of a fork head domain gene to *PAX3* in the solid tumour alveolar rhabdomyosarcoma. *Nature Genet.* 1993, **5**: 230–235.

87. Tycko B, Smith SD, Sklar J. Chromosomal translocations joining *LCK* and *TCRB* loci in human T cell leukemia. *J. Exp. Med.* 1991, **174**: 867–873.

88. Ellisen LW, Bird J, West DC, et al. *TAN-1*, the human homolog of the Drosophila *Notch* gene, is broken by chromosomal translocations in T lymphoblastic neoplasms. *Cell* 1991, **66**: 649–661.

89. Aster J, Pear W, Hasserjian R, et al. Functional analysis of the *TAN-1* Gene, a human homolog of Drosophila *Notch*. In *Cold Spring Harbor Symposia on Quantitative Biology: The Molecular Genetics of Cancer*. Cold Spring Harbor: The Cold Spring Harbor Laboratory Press, 1994, pp. 125–136.

90. Fortini ME, Artavanis-Tsakonis S. *Notch*: Neurogenesis is only part of the story. *Cell* 1993, **75**: 1245.

91. Cimino G, Moir DT, Canaani O, et al. Cloning of *ALL-1*, the locus involved in leukemias with the t(4;11)(q21;q23), t(9;11)(p22;q23), and t(11;19)(q23;p13) chromosome translocations. *Cancer Res.* 1991, **51**: 6712–6714.

92. Zieman-van der Poel S, McCabe NR, Gill HJ, et al. Identification of a gene, *MLL*, that spans the breakpoint in 11q23 translocations associated with human leukemias. *Proc. Natl Acad. Sci. USA* 1991, **88**: 10735–10739.

93. Gu Y, Nakamura T, Alder H, et al. The t(4;11) chromosome translocation of human acute leukemias fuses the *ALL-1* gene, related to *Drosophila trithorax*, to the *AF-4* gene. *Cell* 1992, **71**: 701–708.

94. Tkachuk DC, Kohler S, Cleary ML. Involvement of a homolog of *Drosophila trithorax* by 11q23 chromosomal translocations in acute leukemias. *Cell* 1992, **71**: 691–700.

95. Thirman MJ, Gill HJ, Burnett RC, et al. Rearrangement of the *MLL* gene in acute lymphoblastic and acute myeloid leukemias with 11q23 chromosomal translocations. *N. Engl. J. Med.* 1993, **329**: 909–914.

96. Schichman SA, Caligiuri MA, Gu Y, et al. *ALL-1* partial duplication in acute leukemia. *Proc. Natl Acad. Sci. USA* 1994, **91**: 6236–6239.

97. Pui C-H, Ribeiro RC, Hancock ML, et al. Acute myeloid leukemia in children treated with epipodophyllotoxins for acute lymphoblastic leukemia. *N. Engl. J. Med.* 1991, **325**: 1682–1687.

98. Gill Super HJ, McCabe NR, Thirman MJ, et al. Rearrangements of the *MLL* gene in therapy-related acute myeloid leukemia in patients previously treated with agents targeting DNA-topoisomerase II. *Blood* 1993, **82**: 3705–3711.

99. Huret JL, Brizard A, Slater R, et al. Cytogenetic heterogeneity in t(11;19) acute leukemia: Clinical, hematological and cytogenetic analyses of 48 patients – Updated published cases and 16 new observations. *Leukemia* 1993, **7**: 152–160.

100. Chervinsky DS, Sait SNJ, Nowak NJ, et al. Complex *MLL* rearrangement in a patient with T-cell acute lymphoblastic leukemia. *Genes Chrom. Cancer* 1995, **14**: 76–84.

101. Sager R. Tumor suppressor genes: The puzzle and the promise. *Science* 1989, **246**: 1406–1412.

102. Friend SH, Bernards R, Rogelj S, et al. A human DNA segment with properties of the gene that predisposes to retinoblastoma and osteosarcoma. *Nature (Lond.)* 1986, **323**: 643–646.

103. Huang HJ, Yee JK, Shew JY, et al. Suppression of the neoplastic phenotype by replacement of the *RB* gene in human cancer cells. *Science* 1988, **242**: 1563–1566.

104. Ahuja HG, Jat PS, Foti A, et al. Abnormalities of the retinoblastoma gene in the pathogenesis of acute leukemia. *Blood* 1991, **78**: 3259–3268.

105. Lane DP. p53, guardian of the genome. *Nature (Lond.)* 1992, **358**: 15–16.

106. Kuerbitz SJ, Plunkett BS, Walsh WV, et al. Wild-type p53 is a cell cycle checkpoint determinant following irradiation. *Proc. Natl Acad. Sci. USA* 1992, **89**: 7491–7495.

107. Lowe SW, Ruley HE, Jacks T, et al. p53-dependent apoptosis modulates the cytotoxicity of anticancer agents. *Cell* 1993, **74**: 957–967.

108. Jacks T, Remington L, Williams BO, et al. Tumor spectrum analysis in p53-mutant mice. *Curr. Biol.* 1994, **4**: 1–7.

109. Felix CA, Nau MM, Takahashi T, et al. Hereditary and acquired p53 gene mutations in childhood acute lymphoblastic leukemia. *J. Clin. Invest.* 1992, **89**: 640–647.

110. Jonveaux P, Berger R. Infrequent mutations in the *p53* gene in primary human T-cell acute lymphoblastic leukemia. *Leukemia* 1991, **5**: 839–840.

111. Yeargin J, Cheng J, Haas M. Role of the p53 tumor suppressor gene in the pathogenesis and in the suppression of acute lymphoblastic T-cell leukemia. *Leukemia* 1992, **6**: 85S–91S.

112. Weinberg RA. The retinoblastoma protein and cell cycle control. *Cell* 1995, **81**: 323–330.

113. Kamb A. Cell-cycle regulators and cancer. *Trends Genet.* 1995, **11**: 136–140.

114. Kamb A, Gruis NA, Weaver-Feldhaus J, et al. A cell cycle regulator potentially involved in genesis of many tumor types. *Science* 1994, **264**: 436–440.

115. Hirama T, Koeffler HP. Role of the cyclin-dependent kinase inhibitors in the development of cancer. *Blood* 1995, **86**: 841–854.

116. Cayuela JM, Hebert J, Sigaux F. Homozygous MTS1 (p16INK4A) deletion in primary tumor cells of 163 leukemic patients. *Blood* 1995, **85**: 854.

117. Takeuchi S, Bartram CR, Seriu T, et al. Analysis of a family of cyclin-dependent kinase inhibitors: *p15/MTS2/INK4B*, *p16/MTS1/INK4A*, and *p18* genes in acute lymphoblastic leukemia of childhood. *Blood* 1995, **86**: 755–760.

118. Herman JG, Merlo A, Mao L, et al. Abnormal DNA methylation frequently inactivates the putative tumor CDKN2/p16 in many types. *Proc. Am. Assoc. Cancer Res.* 1995, **36**: 201.

119. Lennert K, Feller AC. *Histopathology of Non-Hodgkin's Lymphomas (Based on the Updated Kiel Classification)*, 2nd edn. Berlin: Springer-Verlag, 1990.

120. Virgilio L, Isobe M, Narducci MG, et al. Chromosome walking on the *TCL1* locus involved in T-cell neoplasia. *Proc. Natl Acad. Sci. USA* 1993, **90**: 9275–9279.

121. Brito-Babapulle V, Catovsky D. Inversion and tandem duplication involving chromosome 14q11 and 14q32 in T-prolymphocytic leukemia in patients with ataxia-telangectasia. *Cancer Genet. Cytogenet.* 1991, **55**: 1–9.

122. Russo G, Isobe M, Pegoraro L, et al. Molecular analysis of a t(7;14)(q35;q32) chromosome translocation in a T cell leukemia of a patient with ataxia telangiectasia. *Cell* 1988, **53**: 137–144.

123. Aurias A, Couturier J, Dutrillaux A-M, et al. Inversion (14)(q12qter) or (q11.2;q32.3): The most frequently acquired rearrangement in lymphocytes. *Human Genet.* 1985, **71**: 19–21.

124. Hecht F, Hecht BK, Kirsch IR. Fragile sites limited to

lymphocytes: Molecular recombination and malignancy. *Cancer Genet. Cytogenet.* 1987, **26**: 95–104.

125. Welch JP, Lee CLY, Beatty-DeSana JW, et al. Nonrandom occurrence of 7–14 translocations in human lymphocyte cultures. *Nature (Lond.)* 1975, **255**: 241–242.

126. Erikson J, ar-Rushdi A, Driwinga HL, et al. Transcriptional activation of the translocated *c-myc* oncogene in Burkitt lymphoma. *Proc. Natl Acad. Sci. USA* 1983, **80**: 820–824.

127. Croce CM, Thierfelder W, Erikson J, et al. Transcriptional activation of an unrearranged and untranslocated *c-myc* oncogene by translocation of a Cλ locus in Burkitt lymphoma. *Proc. Natl Acad. Sci. USA* 1983, **80**: 6922–6926.

128. Erikson JK, Nishikura K, ar-Rushdi A, et al. Translocation of an immunoglobulin kappa locus to a region 3' of an unrearranged *c-myc* oncogene enhances *c-myc* transcription. *Proc. Natl Acad. Sci. USA* 1983, **80**: 7581–7585.

129. Tsujimoto Y, Cossman J, Jaffe E, et al. Involvement of the *bcl-2* gene in human follicular lymphoma. *Science* 1985, **228**: 1440–1443.

130. Tsujimoto Y, Croce CM. Analysis of the structure, transcripts, and protein products of *bcl-2*, the gene involved in human follicular lymphoma. *Proc. Natl Acad. Sci. USA* 1986, **83**: 5214–5218.

131. Adachi M, Cossman J, Longo D, et al. Variant translocation of the bcl-2 gene to Igλ in chronic lymphocytic leukemia. *Proc. Natl Acad. Sci. USA* 1989, **86**: 2771–2774.

132. Baer R, Heppell A, Taylor AMR, et al. The breakpoint of an inversion of chromosome 14 in a T-cell leukemia: Sequences downstream of the immunoglobulin heavy chain locus are implicated in tumorigenesis. *Proc. Natl Acad. Sci. USA* 1987, **84**: 9069–9073.

133. Mengle-Gaw L, Willard HF, Smith CIE, et al. Human T-cell tumors containing chromosome 14 inversion or translocation with breakpoints proximal to immunoglobulin joining region at 14q32. *EMBO J.* 1987, **6**: 2273–2280.

134. Russo G, Isobe M, Gatti R, et al. Molecular analysis of a t(14;14) translocation in leukemic T-cells of an ataxia telangiectasia patient. *Proc. Natl Acad. Sci. USA* 1989, **86**: 602–606.

135. Virgilio L, Narducci MG, Isobe M, et al. Identification of the *TCL1* gene involved in T-cell malignancies. *Proc. Natl Acad. Sci. USA* 1994, **91**: 12530–12534.

136. Sherrington PD, Fisch P, Taylor AMR, et al. Clonal evolution of malignant and non-malignant T cells carrying t(14;14) and t(X;14) in patients with ataxia telangiectasia. *Oncogene* 1994, **9**: 2377–2381.

137. Stern M-H, Soulier J, Rosenzwajg M, et al. *MTCP-1*: A novel gene on the human chromosome Xq28 translocated to the T cell receptor α/δ locus in mature T cell proliferations. *Oncogene* 1993, **8**: 2475–2483.

138. Fu T-B, Virgilio L, Narducci MG, et al. Characterization and localization of the *TCL-1* oncogene product. *Cancer Res.* 1994, **54**: 6297–6301.

139. Kagan J, Croce CM. Molecular biology of lymphoid malignancies. *Ann. Oncol.* 1991, **2**: 9–21.

140. Solomon E, Borrow J, Goddard AD. Chromosome aberrations and cancer. *Science* 1991, **254**: 1153–1160.

141. Bertness VL, Felix CA, McBride WO, et al. Characterization of the breakpoint of a t(14;14)(q11.2;q32) from the leukemia cells of a patient with T-cell acute lymphoblastic leukemia. *Cancer Genet. Cytogenet.* 1990, **44**: 47–54.

142. Galton DAG, Goldman JM, Wiltshaw E, et al. Prolymphocytic leukemia. *Br. J. Haematol.* 1974, 27: 7–23.

143. Matutes E, Brito-Bapapulle V, Swansbury J, et al. Clinical and laboratory features of 78 cases of T-prolymphocytic cell leukemia. *Blood* 1991, **78**: 3269–3274.

144. Gatti RA, McConville CM, Taylor AMR. Sixth international workshop on ataxia-telangiectasia. *Cancer Res.* 1994, **54**: 6007–6010.

145. Savitsky K, Bar-Shira A, Gilad S, et al. A single ataxia telangiectasia gene with a product similar to PI-3 Kinase. *Science* 1995, **268**: 1749–1753.

146. Kirsch IR. V(D)J recombination and ataxia-telangiectasia: A review. *Int. J. Radiat. Biol.* 1994, **66**: S97–S108.

147. Narducci MG, Virgilio L, Isobe M, et al. *TCL1* oncogene activation in preleukemic T cells from a case of ataxia-telangiectasia. *Blood* 1995, **86**: 2358–2364.

148. Timonen T, Ortaldo JR, Herberman RB. Characteristics of human large granular lymphocytes and relationship to natural killer and K cells. *J. Exp. Med.* 1981, **153**: 569–582.

149. Loughran TP Jr. Clonal diseases of large granular lymphocytes. *Blood* 1993, **82**: 1–14.

150. Davey MP, Starkebaum G, Loughran TP Jr. CD3+ leukemic large granular lymphocytes utilize diverse T-cell receptor Vβ genes. *Blood* 1995, **85**: 146–150.

151. Taniwaki M, Tagawa S, Nishigaki H, et al. Chromosomal abnormalities define clonal proliferation in CD3-large granular lymphocyte leukemia. *Am. J. Hematol.* 1990, **33**: 32–38.

152. Shimodaira S, Ishida F, Kobayashi H, et al. The detection of clonal proliferation in granular lymphocyte-proliferative disorders of natural killer cell lineage. *Br. J. Haematol.* 1994, **90**: 578–584.

153. Tafferi A, Greipp PR, Leibson PJ, et al. Demonstration of clonality, by X-linked DNA analysis, in chronic natural killer cell lymphocytosis and successful therapy with oral cyclophosphamide. *Leukemia* 1992, **6**: 477–480.

154. Kawa-Ha K, Ishihara S, Ninomiya T, et al. CD3-negative lymphoproliferative disease of granular lymphocytes containing Epstein–Barr viral DNA. *J. Clin. Invest.* 1989, **84**: 51–55.

155. Takagi N, Nakamura S, Ueda R, et al. A phenotypic and genotypic study of three node-based, low-grade peripheral T-cell lymphomas: Angioimmunoblastic lymphoma, T-zone lymphoma, and lymphoepithelioid lymphoma. *Cancer* 1992, **69**: 2571–2582.

156. Theodorou I, Raphael M, Bigorgne C, et al. Recombination pattern of the TCR gamma locus in human peripheral T-cell lymphomas. *J. Pathol.* 1994, **174**: 233–242.

157. Schlegelberger B, Himmler A, Godde E, et al.

Cytogenetic findings in peripheral T-cell lymphomas as a basis for distinguishing low-grade and high-grade lymphomas. *Blood* 1994, **83**: 505–511.

158. Schlegelberger B, Himmler A, Bartles H, et al. Recurrent chromosome abnormalities in peripheral T-cell lymphomas. *Cancer Genet. Cytogenet.* 1994, **78**: 15–22.

159. Schlegelberger B, Zhang Y, Weber-Matthiesen K, et al. Detection of aberrant clones in nearly all cases of angioimmunoblastic lymphadenopathy with dysproteinemia-type T-cell lymphoma by combined interphase and metaphase cytogenetics. *Blood* 1994, **84**: 2640–2648.

160. Burg G, Kerl H, Przybilla B, et al. Some statistical data, diagnosis, and staging of cutaneous B-cell lymphomas. *J. Dermatol. Surg. Oncol.* 1984, **10**: 256–277.

161. Burg G, Braun-Falco O. *Cutaneous Lymphomas, Pseudolymphomas and Related Disorders.* Berlin: Springer Verlag, 1983.

162. Su IJ, Wang YC, Chen YC, et al. Cutaneous manifestations of post-thymic T-cell malignancies: Description of five clinicopathologic subtypes. *J. Am. Acad. Dermatol.* 1990, **23**: 653–662.

163. Kerl H, Cerroni L, Burg G. The morphological spectrum of lymphomas of the skin: A proposal for a new classification of cutaneous lymphomas and pseudolymphomas. *Semin. Diagn. Pathol.* 1991, **8**: 55–61.

164. Hastrup N, Hamilton-Dutoit S, Ralfkiaer E, et al. Peripheral T-cell lymphomas: An evaluation of reproducibility of the updated Kiel classification. *Histopathology* 1991, **18**: 99–105.

165. Beljaards RC, Kaudewitz P, Berti E, et al. Primary cutaneous CD30-positive large cell lymphoma: Definition of a new type of cutaneous lymphoma with a favorable prognosis. A multicenter study of 47 patients. *Cancer* 1993, **71**: 2097–2103.

166. Delia D, Borello MG, Berti E, et al. Clonal immunoglobulin gene rearrangements and normal T-cell receptor, bcl-2 and c-myc genes in primary cutaneous lymphomas. *Cancer Res.* 1989, **49**: 4901–4905.

167. Cerroni L, Volkenand M, Rieger E, et al. Bcl-2 protein expression and correlation with the interchromosomal (14;18) translocation in cutaneous lymphomas and pseudolymphomas. *J. Invest. Dermatol.* 1994, **102**: 231–235.

168. Neri A, Fracchiolla NS, Roscetti E, et al. Molecular analysis of cutaneous B- and T-cell lymphomas. *Blood* 1995, **86**: 3160–3172.

169. Bitter MA, Franklin WA, Larson RA. Morphology in Ki-1 (CD30) positive non-Hodgkin's lymphomas is correlated with clinical features and the presence of a unique chromosomal abnormality t(2;5)(p23;q35). *Am. J. Surg. Pathol.* 1990, **14**: 305–316.

170. Willemze R, Beljaards RC, Meijer CJLM, et al. Classification of primary cutaneous lymphomas. Historical overview and perspectives. *Dermatology* 1994, **189**: 8–15.

171. van der Putte SCJ, Toonstra J, van Wicken DF, et al. Aberrant immunophenotypes in mycosis fungoides. *Arch. Dermatol.* 1988, **24**: 373–380.

172. Rest AB, Horn TD. Immunophenotypic analysis of benign and malignant cutaneous lymphoid infiltrates. *Clin. Dermatol.* 1991, **9**: 261–272.

173. Abel EA, Lindae ML, Hoppe RT, et al. Benign and malignant forms or erythroderma: Cutaneous immunophenotypic characteristics. *J. Am. Acad. Dermatol.* 1988, **19**: 1089–1095.

174. Willemze R, De Graaff-Reitsma CB, Cnossen J, et al. Characterization of T-cell subpopulations in skin and peripheral blood of patients with cutaneous T-cell lymphomas and benign inflammatory dermatoses. *J. Invest. Dermatol.* 1983, **80**: 60–66.

175. Vander Valk P, Willemze R, Meijer CJLM. Peripheral T-cell lymphomas: A clinicopathological and immunological study of ten cases. *Histopathology* 1986, **10**: 235–249.

176. Krajewski AS, Myskow MW, Cachia PG, et al. T-cell lymphoma: Morphology, immunophenotype and clinical features. *Histopathology* 1988, **13**: 19–41.

177. Chott A, Kaserer K, Augustin IW, et al. Ki-1 positive large cell lymphoma: A clinicopathologic study of 41 cases. *Am. J. Surg. Pathol.* 1990, **14**: 439–448.

178. Gonzalez CL, Medeiros LJ, Braziel RM, et al. T-cell lymphoma involving subcutaneous tissue. A clinicopathologic entity commonly associated with hemophagocytic syndrome. *Am. J. Surg. Pathol.* 1993, **15**: 17–27.

179. Zelickson BD, Peters MS, Pittelkow MR. Gene rearrangement analysis in lymphoid neoplasia. *Clin. Dermatol.* 1991, **9**: 119–128.

180. Landa NG, Zelickson BD, Peters MS, et al. Lymphoma versus pseudolymphoma of the skin: Gene rearrangement study of 21 cases with clinicopathologic correlation. *J. Am. Acad. Dermatol.* 1993, **29**: 945–953.

181. Terhune MG, Cooper KD. Gene rearrangements and T-cell lymphomas. *Arch. Dermatol.* 1993, 129: 1484–1490.

182. Berti E, Cerri A, Cavicchini S, et al. Primary cutaneous γ/δ T-cell lymphoma presenting as disseminated pagetoid reticulosis. *J. Invest. Dermatol.* 1991, **96**: 718–723.

183. Heald P, Buckley P, Gilliam A, et al. Correlations of unique clinical, immunotypic, and histologic findings in cutaneous gamma/delta T-cell lymphoma. *J. Am. Acad. Dermatol.* 1992, **26**: 865–870.

184. Bignon Y-J, Souteyrand P, Roger H, et al. Clonotypic heterogeneity in cutaneous T-cell lymphomas. *Cancer Res.* 1990, **50**: 6620–6625.

185. Berger CL, Eisenberg A, Soper L, et al. Dual genotype in cutaneous T-cell lymphoma: Immunoglobulin gene rearrangement in clonal T-cell malignancy. *J. Invest. Dermatol.* 1988, **90**: 73–77.

186. Willemze R, Meijer CJ, van Vloten WA, et al. The clinical and histological spectrum of lymphomatoid papulosis. *Br. J. Dermatol.* 1982, **107**: 131–144.

187. Weiss LM, Wood GS, Trela M, et al. Clonal T-cell populations in lymphomatoid papulosis: Evidence of a lymphoproliferative origin for a clinically benign disease. *N. Eng. J. Med.* 1986, **315**: 475–479.

188. Lessin SR, Rook AH, Rovera G. Molecular diagnosis of cutaneous T-cell lymphoma: Polymerase chain reaction amplification of T-cell antigen receptor β-chain gene rearrangements. *J. Invest. Dermatol.* 1991, **96**: 299–302.

189. Bottaro M, Berti E, Biondi A, et al. Heteroduplex analysis of T-cell receptor γ gene rearrangements for

diagnosis and monitoring of cutaneous T-cell lymphomas. *Blood* 1994, **83**: 3271–3278.

190. deBruin PC, Jiwa M, Oudejans JJ, et al. Presence of Epstein–Barr virus in extranodal T-cell lymphomas: Differences in relation to site. *Blood* 1994, **83**: 1612–1618.

191. Ghosh SK, Abrams JT, Terunuma H, et al. Human T-cell leukemia virus type I *tax/rex* DNA and RNA in cutaneous T-cell lymphoma. *Blood* 1994, **84**: 2663–2671.

192. Hollstein M, Sidransky D, Vogelstein B, et al. p53 mutations in human cancers. *Science* 1991, 253: 49–53.

193. Levine AJ, Momand J, Finlay CA. The p53 tumor suppressor gene. *Nature (Lond.)* 1991, **351**: 453–456.

194. Prokocimer M, Rotter V. Structure and function of the p53 in normal cells and their aberrations in cancer cells: Projection on the hematologic cell lineages. *Blood* 1994, **84**: 2391–2411.

195. Imamura J, Miyoshi I, Koeffler HP. p53 in hematologic malignancies. *Blood* 1994, **84**: 2412–2421.

196. Grilli M, Chiu JJ-S, Lenardo MJ. NF-κB and Rel: Participants in a multiform transcriptional regulatory system. *Int. Rev. Cytol.* 1993, **143**: 1–62.

197. Baeuerle PA, Henkel T. Function and activation of NF-κB in the immune system. *Ann. Rev. Immunol.* 1994, **12**: 141–179.

198. Neri A, Chang C-C, Lombardi L, et al. B cell lymphoma-associated chromosomal translocation involves candidate oncogene *lyt-10*, homologous to *NF-κGp50*. *Cell* 1991, **67**: 1075–1087.

199. Fracchiolla NS, Lombardi L, Salina M, et al. Structural alterations of the NF-κB transcription factor *lyt-10* in lymphoid malignancies. *Oncogene* 1993, **8**: 2839–2845.

200. Thakur S, Lin H-C, Tseng W-T, et al. Rearrangement and altered expression of the *NFKB2* gene in human cutaneous T-lymphoma cells. *Oncogene* 1994, **9**: 2335–2344.

201. Zhang J, Chang C-C, Lombardi L, et al. Rearranged *NFKB2* gene in HUT78 T-lymphoma cell line codes for a constitutively nuclear factor lacking transcriptional repressor functions. *Oncogene* 1994, 10: 1931–1937.

202. Offit K, Wong G, Filippa DA, et al. Cytogenetic analysis of 434 consecutively ascertained specimens of non-Hodgkin lymphoma: Clinical correlation. *Blood* 1991, **77**: 1508–1515.

203. Mercurio F, DiDonato JA, Rosette C, et al. p105 and p98 precursor proteins play an active role in NF-κB-mediated signal transduction. *Gene Develop.* 1993, **7**: 705–718.

204. Chang C-C, Zhang J, Lombardi L, et al. Mechanism of expression and role in transcriptional control of the proto-oncogene *NFKB2/LYT-10*. *Oncogene* 1994, **9**: 923–933.

205. Gilmore T, Morin P. The IκB proteins: Members of a multifunctional family. *Trends Genet.* 1993, **9**: 427–433.

206. Zhang Q, DiDonato JA, Karin M, et al. *BCL3* encodes a nuclear protein with can alter the subcellular location of NF-κB proteins. *Mol. Cell. Biol.* 1994, **14**: 3915–3926.

207. Lombardi L, Ciana P, Cappellini C, et al. Structural and functional characterization of the promoter regions of the *NFKB2* gene. *Nucl. Acids Res.* 1995, **23**: 2328–2336.

208. Migliazza A, Lombardi L, Rocchi M, et al. Heterogeneous chromosomal aberrations generate 3' truncations of the *NFKB2/lyt-10* gene in lymphoid malignancies. *Blood* 1994, **84**: 3850–3860.

209. Marcu KB, Lang RB, Stanton LW, et al. A model for the molecular requirements of immunoglobulin heavy chain class switching. *Nature (Lond.)* 1982, **298**: 87–90.

210. Chang C-C, Zhang J, Lombardi L, et al. Rearranged *NFKB2* genes in lymphoid neoplasms code for constitutively active nuclear transactivators. *Mol. Cell. Biol.* 1995, **15**: 5180–5187.

211. Kagan J, Finger LR, Letofsky J, et al. Clustering of breakpoints on chromosome 10 in acute T-cell leukemias with the t(10;14) chromosome translocation. *Proc. Natl Acad. Sci. USA* 1989, **86**: 4161–4165.

212. Hatano M, Roberts CWM, Minden M, et al. Deregulation of a homeobox gene, HOX11, by the t(10;14) in T cell leukemia. *Science* 1991, **253**: 79–82.

213. Corral J, Forster A, Thompson S, et al. Acute leukemias of different lineages have similar *MLL* gene fusions encoding related chimeric proteins resulting from chromosomal translocation. *Proc. Natl Acad. Sci. USA* 1993, **90**: 8538–8542.

214. Laabi Y, Gras MP, Carbonnel F, et al. A new gene, BCM, on chromosome 16 is fused to the interleukin 2 gene by a t(4;16)(q26;p13) translocation in a malignant T cell lymphoma. *EMBO J.* 1992, 11: 3897–3904.

CHAPTER 18

Pathogenesis of Ki-1+ lymphomas

MARSHALL E. KADIN AND MARSHA C. KINNEY

Introduction

In 1981 an antiserum raised by immunization of rabbits with the Hodgkin's disease (HD) cell line L428 was found to stain Hodgkin/Reed–Sternberg (H/RS) cells in tissue sections of HD [1]. In 1982, a monoclonal antibody (Ki-1) raised by immunization of mice with line L428 was found to react with H/RS cells and a subset of large lymphoid cells in the parafollicular area of lymph nodes and tonsils; it was hypothesized that these Ki-1+ cells correspond to the normal counterpart of H/RS cells [2]. Subsequently, Stein and colleagues found that the Ki-1 antibody also reacted with a subset of large-cell lymphomas, which had previously been classified as malignant histiocytosis [3]. These Ki-1+ non-Hodgkin's lymphomas (NHL) were distinguished by anaplastic large cells and a distinctive pattern of lymph node involvement, sparing germinal centers and infiltrating lymph node sinuses, often leading to a mistaken diagnosis of metastatic carcinoma [3]. This lymphoma has become known as Ki-1+ anaplastic large-cell lymphoma (ALCL). In addition to these primary Ki-1+ ALCLs, secondary Ki-1+ ALCLs of similar histology and immunophenotype can arise as a result of progression of low-grade lymphomas (see section entitled Relationship of ALCL to other lymphomas, on page 452). In this chapter we discuss the histology, immunophenotype, cytogenetics and clinicopathologic features of Ki-1+ ALCL in the context of recent developments in the pathogenesis of Ki-1+ ALCL.

Clinical features

Patients with ALCL are generally younger than other patients with NHL with a median age of under 45 years in three recent studies [4–6]. There is a bimodal age distribution with a first peak in the second decade and a second smaller peak after age 60 [7]). The male/female ratio is approximately 1.65:1 [6].

Peripheral lymphadenopathy is present in most patients with relative sparing of the mediastinum (<20%). Extranodal disease is common at presentation (approximately 40%). The most frequent extranodal sites of ALCL are skin, bone, soft tissue, gastrointestinal tract, liver, lung and pleura [4–6,8].

Bone marrow involvement appears to be infrequent, probably <10%, making patients with relapsed ALCL good candidates for autologous bone marrow transplantation. However, a recent study showed that, when immunohistochemistry was performed, subtle bone marrow involvement was detected in 23% of patients with a negative bone marrow biopsy on routine histology, and bone marrow involvement was associated with a significant lower survival [8a].

Most ALCL patients present with advanced Ann Arbor stage III or IV disease [4,6]. Systemic B symptoms occur in about 40% of patients [6,7]. Most published series have reported a disease-free survival (DFS) of about 50% and overall survival (OS) of approximately 70%. The discrepancy between DFS and OS is due to frequent, often delayed, relapses in ALCL [4,6,8]. Greer et al. noted that a few patients with ALCL, particularly those with localized skin lesions, have an indolent course, while others with stage IV disease have a fulminant course [6]. Additionally, patients whose lesions have a relatively monomorphic histology appear to have a worse prognosis [9]. This does not hold true for primary cutaneous large-cell lymphomas in which expression of Ki-1 antigen confers a favorable prognosis regardless of histologic subtype [10].

Bone marrow transplantation has been effective salvage therapy for chemotherapy-resistant Ki-1+ ALCL, achieving complete remissions in about one-half of pediatric [11] and adult patients [4,6]. Because of the expression of the Ki-1 antigen on virtually all ALCL cells and absence of Ki-1 antigen on bone marrow progenitor cells, immunotherapy linking toxins or radionuclides to anti-CD30 antibodies may hold promise for therapy-resistant Ki-1+ ALCL and for eliminating minimal residual disease [12].

Histology

In ALCL, tumor cells commonly infiltrate the paracortical regions and sinuses of lymph nodes (Figure 18.1). Residual primary or secondary follicles are often seen. Occasionally, tumor cells are found at the periphery and even within follicles. There is prominent tumor cell infiltration of the subcapsular sinus and tumor cells may also be found in the medullary or paracortical sinuses. The overall pattern is easily confused with metastatic tumor. Other features are fibrosis, infiltrates of plasma cells or histiocytes, and variable numbers of neutrophils and eosinophils, especially in extranodal sites of lymphoma.

Stein et al. described a cytologic spectrum of large tumor cells with pleomorphic nuclei, clumped heterochromatin, one or more nucleoli, and abundant, often vacuolated cytoplasm, to cells with more regular, rounded vesicular nuclei with basophilic cytoplasm [3]. Agnarsson and Kadin called attention to the variable cytology of Ki-1+ lymphomas, describing in particular Reed–Sternberg (RS)-like cells, cells with convoluted or doughnut-shaped nuclei, and multinucleated cells with a wreath-like arrangement of nuclei (Figure 18.2). Erythrophagocytosis by reactive histiocytes and occasionally by tumor cells [13] appears to be responsible for the frequent diagnosis, prior to its recognition, of ALCL as malignant histiocytosis. Chott et al. emphasized the distinction between pleomorphic RS-like cells and monomorphic large-cells, showing an association with higher-stage disease and poorer prognosis in the monomorphic type [9]. Chan et al. described two major cell types. Type I is a pale cell type and type II is a basophilic, often multinucleated cell [13a].

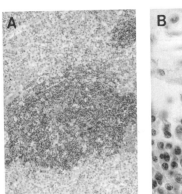 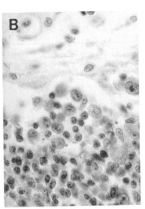 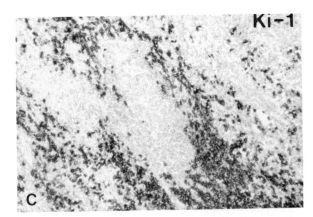

Figure 18.1 Ki-1/CD30+ ALCL. (A) Tumor cells infiltrating the paracortical region of a lymph node, sparing a darkly stained B-cell follicle. (B) Tumor cells in the subcapsular sinus of a lymph node. (C) An immunoperoxidase stain for Ki-1/CD30+ cells surrounding preserved B-cell nodules.

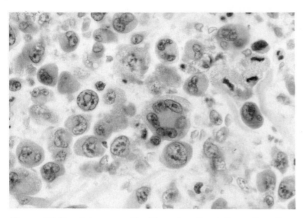

Figure 18.2 A tumor cell with a doughnut-shaped nucleus and a multinucleated cell with a wreath-like arrangement of nuclei in Ki-1/CD30+ ALCL.

Several histologic variants of Ki-1+ ALCL have been recognized (Figure 18.3). A *Hodgkin's-like variant* with RS cells and lacunar-type cells can be easily confused with the syncytial variant of nodular sclerosing HD [13]. A *sarcomatoid variant* with bizarre cells and storiform or myxoid stroma resembles a soft tissue sarcoma [14]. *Histiocyte-rich* [15] and *small-cell predominant variants* [16] may be mistaken for inflammation because of the paucity of large Ki-1+ blasts. We also recognize a clear cell type in which the majority of cells are large Ki-1+ cells. This variant may often have been classified as a peripheral T-cell lymphoma. Although the exact histogenetic relationship among these morphologic variants is not completely understood, early evidence suggests that they have a common pathogenesis in the form of a shared reciprocal translocation, t(2;5)(p23;q35)(see below).

Immunophenotype

Nearly all ALCLs have a phenotype consistent with an origin from an activated T- or B-lymphocyte [3,13]. Thus the tumor cells express lymphocyte activation antigens CD25, CD71 and CD30. Most ALCLs have an aberrant T-cell phenotype consistent with a peripheral T-cell lymphoma. In our experience, CD4 and CD5 are commonly expressed but CD3 is frequently absent [13]. Fewer primary ALCLs have a B-cell phenotype, CD20+, and in paraffin sections may contain cytoplasmic immunoglobulin. In some ALCLs lymphocyte specific antigens are not detected and their lineage is uncertain [17]. Rare cases in which tumor cells express CD30 and histiocyte-associated markers (lysozyme, alpha-

1-anti-chymotrypsin, CD68, CD13) may be derived from the histiocyte/myeloid lineage [18–20].

The differential diagnosis of ALCL from Hodgkin's disease, carcinoma and histiocytic malignancy can be facilitated by immunophenotypic studies (Table 18.1). Expression of EMA, BNH9 and CD45 and usual lack of CD15 distinguishes most ALCLs from HD other than lymphocyte predominance type [13, 21].

The expression of CD30, LCA and the usual absence of cytokeratin distinguishes most cases of ALCL from carcinoma. However, frequent expression of epithelial membrane antigen (EMA) [21] and the often weak or absent expression of leukocyte common antigen (LCA) [22] may lead to difficulty in the distinction between ALCL and anaplastic carcinoma. Moreover, in one study cytokeratins were detected in frozen sections in five of 20 ALCL [23]. Additionally, CD30 expression has been observed in some embryonal [24] and pancreatic [25] carcinomas. These results emphasize the necessity of using a panel of monoclonal antibodies in making the diagnosis of ALCL.

The expression of CD30 and the absence of lysozyme favors a diagnosis of ALCL over true histiocytic neoplasm. However, it is important to note that some ALCL of T-cell lineage can express α-1-antitrypsin and/or α-1-antichymotrypsin which are histiocyte-associated antigens [26], and are often used to support a diagnosis of true histiocytic neoplasm.

Genotype

MOLECULAR ANALYSIS OF ANTIGEN RECEPTOR GENES

In a molecular analysis of DNA from 30 large-cell lymphomas with expression of the CD30 antigen, O'Connor et al. detected clonal rearrangements of T-cell receptor (TCR) genes in 16, of immunoglobulin (Ig) genes in 6, and no rearrangements in 8 cases [17]. Among 16 cases which were genotypically of T-cell lineage, 11 cases lacked the pan-T-cell antigen CD3, which is expressed at the cell surface together with the TCR antigen. This may indicate that these lymphomas have arisen from an early stage of T-cell ontogeny prior to TCR gene rearrangement. Alternatively, CD3 could be lost following transformation, similar to loss of Ig in some transformed B-cells. This possibility would be consistent with the hypothesis that most Ki-1+ ALCL are derived from activated

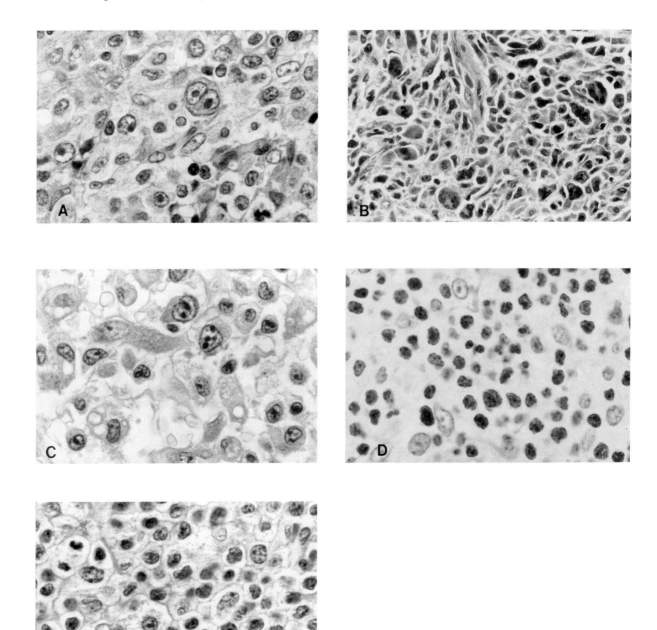

Figure 18.3 Histologic variants of Ki-1/CD30+ ALCL: (A) Hodgkin's-like variant with Reed–Sternberg cell; (B) sarcomatoid variant; (C) histiocyte-rich variant; (D) small-cell variant; (E) clear-cell variant.

T-lymphocytes [3]. Herbst et al. found that 15 of 22 Ki-1+ ALCL had rearrangement of Ig or TCR genes [27]. In seven cases, TCRβ and Ig genes were in germline configuration, although there were at least 20% Ki-1+ cells. Of 13 Ki-1+ ALCL with T-cell phenotype, nine had TCRβ gene rearrangements (two cases had both TCRβ and TCRγ rearrangements) and four cases with at least 50% Ki-1+ cells had a germline pattern with both TCRβ and JH probes. Four Ki-1+ ALCL had a B-cell phenotype.

One of these B-cell ALCLs had rearranged IgH and λ light chain genes; one had rearranged IgH, κ light chain, and TCRβ genes; one had rearrangement of only the TCRγ gene; and one had neither Ig nor TCR gene rearrangements. Two of four cases lacking T- and B-antigens had a TCRβ rearrangement. Because Ki-1+ ALC and HD display rearrangement patterns that are often inadequate for the formation of functionally active antigen receptors, Herbst et al. suggested that they do not represent malignant

Table 18.1 Markers in differential diagnosis of ALCL: antigens detected in paraffin sections

	CD30	CD15	CD45	EMA	BNH.9	Lysozyme	Keratin
ALCL	+	–/+	+/–	+	–/+	—	—
H	+	+	—	—	—	—	—
Carcinoma	—	+/–	—	+	—	—	+
Histiocytosis	—	—	+/–	–/+	—	+	—

+, 75–100%; +/–, 50–75%; –/+, 25–50%; –, 0–25% cases positive for staining of tumor cells.

counterparts of antigen-activated lymphocytes differentiated along a physiological pathway. Instead they cited experimental evidence by Katamine et al. [28] and Gregory et al. [29] that cell lines derived from Epstein–Barr virus (EBV)-immortalized fetal B-cells could have either a complete Ig rearrangement, lack rearrangement, or have a pre-B-cell type rearrangement, i.e., rearranged IgH chain genes and germline Ig light chain genes. They proposed that similar viral transformation of T-cells before and after rearrangement could also occur. These data could provide an experimental basis for the dissociation between genotype and phenotype, which Herbst et al. observed in Ki-1+ ALCL and HD [27].

Pathogenesis

Following the development of the Ki-1 antibody in 1982 and recognition of ALCL in 1985, considerable research has been directed towards understanding the pathogenesis of ALCL and the biology of the Ki-1 (CD30) antigen. The following discussion will summarize these studies and address current questions regarding the function of the CD30 antigen and its ligand (CD30L), the role of the t(2;5)(p23;q35), viruses, the expression of cytokines and structural proteins, and the possible relationship of ALCL to Hodgkin's disease and other lymphomas.

CD30 ANTIGEN

The pattern of CD30 antigen expression is highly restricted in normal tissues. Ki-1/CD30+ cells may be seen in certain inflammatory conditions such as toxoplasmosis and infectious mononucleosis [30]. Less than 0.2% of resting peripheral blood lymphocytes express Ki-1/CD30, and monocytes express Ki-1/CD30 only after extensive manipulation *in vitro* [31].

Ki-1/CD30 antigen has broader reactivity *in vitro*.

Ki-1/CD30 is an activation antigen induced on normal peripheral blood lymphocytes after exposure to mitogens (phytohemagglutinin, staphylococcal protein A), viruses [human T-cell lymphotrophic virus (HTLV)-1 and HTLV-2, EBV] [3] and during mixed lymphocyte cultures [32]. Ki-1/CD30 expression appears relatively late in the process of T-cell activation [33,34]. Ki-1/CD30 is also expressed by many cell lines of lymphoid, promyelocytic and erythroid origin [31,35,36].

Biochemical studies have shown that Ki-1/CD30 antigen exists in several molecular weight forms (57,90,105, and 120 kD) that may be cytoplasmic, membrane-associated or released into the extracellular environment [35,37]. The intracellular Ki-1/57 kD molecule has protein kinase activity whereas the larger membrane-associated form does not [38]. Soluble Ki-1/CD30 can be detected in serum of patients with ALCL and advanced Hodgkin's disease using an ELISA assay [39].

In 1992, Durkop et al. cloned the cDNA encoding the Ki-1/CD30 antigen and reported that the CD30 protein represents a transmembrane receptor, the extracellular domain of which is homologous to the nerve growth factor receptor (NGFR) superfamily. This superfamily includes the low-affinity NGFR; tumor necrosis factor receptors (TNFR)-1 and TNFR-2; T-cell activation antigens OX-40 and CD27; 4-1BB, an inducible T-cell antigen of unknown function; B-cell antigen CD40; Fas, a cell-surface antigen that mediates apoptosis; and SalF19R, an open reading frame (ORF) in Shope sarcoma virus [40]. Like other members of the NGFR superfamily, the intracellular domain of CD30 has no striking sequence homology with other proteins [41]. The intracellular domain is rich in sequences associated with rapid intracellular protein degradation.

Using a chimeric probe consisting of the extracellular domain of CD30 fused to truncated immunoglobulin heavy chains, Smith et al. cloned a protein expressed by the cDNA cognate of the CD30 ligand (CD30L) from the murine T-cell clone 7B9 [42]. The encoded protein is a 239 amino acid type II membrane protein, the C-terminal domain of which shows significant homology to tumor necrosis factor (TNF)α, TNFβ and CD40L. However, CD30L is extensively glycosylated and does not contain the simple pseudo-four-fold sequence repeats that characterize CD40 and TNF receptors. Gruss et al. demonstrated that CD30L is pleiotropic, inducing proliferation of nonmalignant T-cells in the presence of an anti-CD3 co-stimulus and proliferation of the T-cell-like Reed–Sternberg cell line HDLM-2, but inhibiting proliferation through a cytotoxic effect on most CD30+ ALCL cell lines like Karpas 299 [42a]. Thus, expression of CD30 and CD30L could be associated with both autocrine and paracrine modulation of tumor cell growth in HD and Ki-1/ CD30+ ALCL.

The CD30 gene has been localized to chromosome 1p36 [42b]. Interestingly, the gene for TNFR-2 is also localized on chromosome 1 at 1p36.2–p36.3 [43]. An EBV insertion site 1 (EBVS1) is located nearby at 1p35 [44]. 1p36 has been reported to be a target for viral integration [45]. As Fonatsch et al. suggest [42b], expression of CD30 may be a consequence of either genomic instability due to viral integration or control by a viral promoter or activator. The association of EBV, and less frequently, HTLV-1, with ALCL suggests a possible role for viruses in the pathogenesis of this lymphoma whether or not the site of integration is important.

CHROMOSOME ABNORMALITIES ASSOCIATED WITH ALCL

A recurrent translocation, t(2;5)(p23;q35), has been identified in established cell lines [46–48] and fresh tumor cell suspensions [16,46–50] derived from Ki-1/CD30+ ALCL and 'malignant histiocytosis' [46]. Recent cloning of this translocation has shown that it creates a fusion product comprised of promoter sequences from nucleophosmin (NPM), a nucleolar phosphoprotein gene on chromosome 5 at q35, and a previously unidentified protein kinase gene on chromosome 2 at p23, now designated anaplastic lymphoma kinase (ALK) [51]. NPM is highly conserved and appears to be responsible for shuttling ribosomal components between the nucleolus and cytoplasm in late stages of ribosomal assembly [52,53]. Recently, the NPM gene was found to be rearranged in each of five ALCL lines with the t(2;5) but was rearranged in only two of 16 ALCL tumors [53a]. Comparison of the newly identified ALK sequence with known members of the protein tyrosine kinase (*ptk*) gene family [54,55] shows greatest homology to members of the insulin receptor kinase subfamily. This subfamily includes leukocyte tyrosine kinase (*ltk*), tyrosine receptor kinase A (*trka*), the cellular homolog of transforming protein of

avian sarcoma virus (*ros*) and its *Drosophila* homolog Sevenless, the β-chain of the insulin-like growth factor-1 receptor (IGF-1 receptor), and the β-chain of the insulin receptor (IR).

The predicted hybrid protein resulting from the t(2;5) consists of amino-terminal amino acids from NPM linked to the catalytic domain of ALK. ALK is normally expressed by cells in the small intestine, testis and brain, but not by normal lymphoid cells. Unregulated expression of the truncated ALK kinase created by its juxtaposition to the promoter of NPM is likely to contribute to the malignant transformation of the normal counterpart cells of Ki-1/CD30+ ALCL.

Not all ALCL show the t(2;5). In some cases, translocations between 5q35 and chromosome 3 [47] or chromosome 6 [56] have been observed. Sainati et al. demonstrated a novel translocation t(2;13)(23; q34) in a Ki-1/CD30+ ALCL [57]. Ohno et al. found a t(9;14)(p13;q32) in a diffuse ALCL, which expressed Ki-1/CD30 and had an Ig gene rearrangement [58]. In one study, the t(2;5)(p23;q35) was identified in only one of six cases of Ki-1/CD30+ ALCL tested; the remaining cases all showed a 6q– abnormality, common in lymphoid malignancies, as well as other abnormalities [59]. The absence of the t(2;5) may relate to the morphologic heterogeneity of Ki-1/ CD30+ lymphomas. In comparing anaplastic and nonanaplastic CD30+ lymphomas, Bitter et al. [49] found that the t(2;5) was often absent in nonanaplastic lymphomas.

Kinney et al. demonstrated the t(2;5) in each of four Ki-1+ T-cell lymphomas which initially contained a majority of small irregular lymphocytes and a minority of large Ki-1+ blasts [16]. In two of these small-cell variant cases, there was histologic progression to a monomorphic Ki-1/CD30+ ALCL. Gordon et al. found the t(2;5) in three pediatric Ki-1+ peripheral T-cell lymphomas without the typical pathology of ALCL, two large-cell and one mixed large- and small-cell type [60]. The t(2;5) also may not be equally associated with all primary sites of Ki-1/CD30+ ALCL. We have not yet detected the t(2;5) in primary cutaneous Ki-1/CD30+ ALCL [60a]. Two other studies have obtained similar negative results [60b,60c], while a study from France [61d] did detect the t(2;5) by reverse transcriptase polymerase chain reaction and in situ hybridization in a subset of primary cutaneous Ki-1/ CD30+ lymphomas, including lymphomatoid papulosis. These studies were facilitated by the recent cloning of the t(2;5) and the development of reverse transcriptase-polymerase chain reaction (PCR) [61] and polyclonal antibody [61a] methods to detect the translocation or its products.

ONCOGENES IN ALCL

p53, a cell-cycle-dependent nuclear phosphoprotein, is a tumor suppressor gene that plays an important role in the progression of human neoplasms. Loss or alteration of the gene contributes to unregulated growth in neoplasia. Monoallelic loss of portions of the short arm of chromosome 17 in the 17p13.1 region often is associated with mutations of the residual p53 allele. Most of these mutations occur in exons 5–8. Mutant p53 protein has an extended half-life, leading to an increased level of protein which may be detected by immunoprecipitation or by immunostaining. The mutant protein loses the ability to bind to DNA, which is an important characteristic of the normal p53 protein product [62,63]. High levels of p53 expression have been interpreted as abnormal; however, p53 protein can be detected in actively proliferating benign and neoplastic hematopoietic cells [64]. Increased expression of the p53 gene product has been detected in about 75% of primary Ki-1/CD30+ ALCLs [65,66], but the percentage of cases containing p53 gene mutations is relatively low [66], suggesting that expression of elevated p53 gene product may be a result of rapid proliferation in the tumor cell population. Mutations of the p53 gene are more common in relapsed Ki-1/CD30+ ALCL (Ian Magrath, personal communication).

Information regarding other oncogenes is rather limited in ALCL. Myc gene rearrangements were not detected in three ALCLs arising in human immunodeficiency virus (HIV)-positive patients [67], while screening of 70 lymphomas for c-Myb protein revealed it to be present in lymphomas with a high growth fraction, i.e., precursor cell-derived lymphoblastic lymphomas of B- and T-cell type and ALCL (five out of nine cases positive) of T-cell type. The protein was located mainly in the nucleus and in some cases in the cytoplasm as well [68]. The c-*myb* proto-oncogene is the cellular homologue of the transforming gene v-*myb* of the avian myeloblastosis virus and is expressed in hematopoietic tissue, particularly those that are enriched for early stages of hematopoietic differentiation. An increase in c-*myb* expression appears to correlate with cell cycle progression; expression occurs intitially in the nucleus and later, as cells differentiate, in the cytoplasm.

Because of the proximity of the c-*fms* proto-oncogene (which encodes the receptor for the mononuclear phagocyte growth factor, CSF-1) to the q35 breakpoint in the t(2;5), abnormalities of c-*fms* in tumors with the t(2;5) have been sought. However, DNA restriction fragment analysis in a small number of cases showed no involvement of c-*fms* [46,47].

Viruses associated with ALCL

EPSTEIN–BARR VIRUS

EBV is a potent inducer of CD30 expression on lymphoid blasts in vitro [3], suggesting that EBV may play a role in the development of Ki-1/CD30+ lymphomas. Using PCR techniques, EBV genome has been detected in 32–100% of ALCL [69–71]. Lower rates of detection have been reported with Southern blotting [72] and *in situ* hybridization (ISH) [69,70,73]. ISH demonstrated the virus to be in tumor cells [70,71,74–76]. Clonal integration of EBV has been demonstrated in most cases studied by EBV-terminal repeat analysis [67,72,74,77]. Although most ALCLs have a T-cell phenotype, the majority of EBV+ cases have a B- or non-B, non-T-phenotype. This may relate to the fact that many of these cases have been reported in immunocompromised patients with HIV infection [67,77–80] or renal allografts [74], in whom EBV association of ALCL approaches 100%.

EBV gene expression is heterogeneous in ALCL. Latent membrane protein (LMP) has been detected in some cases [70,71,74,80–82], usually not of the T-cell type [70,72]. The highest incidence of LMP expression has been reported in ALCL arising in HIV+ drug users in Italy (nine out of 12 cases) [77]. EBV nuclear antigen-2 (EBNA-2) expression is even less frequent, and has been reported exclusively in B-cell ALCL [71,77]. Three patterns of EBV expression may be seen: LMP–, EBNA-2–, similar to the pattern seen in Burkitt's lymphoma [83]; LMP+, EBNA-2–, described in HD [84] and undifferentiated nasopharyngeal carcinoma [85]; and LMP+, EBNA-2+ characteristic of lymphoblastoid cell lines, atypical lymphoproliferations of B-cell type [83,86], and EBV-induced lymphomas in severe combined immunodefficiency (SCID) mice xenografted with human peripheral blood lymphocytes [87]. The transforming capacity of LMP suggests a role for EBV in the pathogenesis of EBV-associated ALCLs, particularly those of the B-cell or non-B, non-T type. EBV-encoded lytic cycle proteins, BZLF1 and gp 350/250 have not been reported in ALCL [71,82].

HIV

Although most lymphomas occurring in HIV+ patients have been intermediate- to high-grade B-cell lymphomas, other types of lymphoid malignancies have been reported including Hodgkin's disease, T-cell lymphomas, and precursor B- and T-cell malig-

cell shape, long known to be associated with dysplasia and malignancy, may result in the derepression of a mitogenic signal, and thus function in cell activation or malignant transformation [107,108].

The histologic features of Ki-1/CD30+ ALCL, including the cohesiveness of tumor cells and predilection for nodal sinuses and vascular spaces, suggests a role for adhesion molecules in the pathogenesis of this lymphoma, or at least in its cytoarchitecture, but little investigation has been done in this area. The association of EBV and LMP expression in HD and Ki-1/CD30+ ALCL has been discussed. The effector roles of LMP and EBNA on lymphocyte growth *in vitro* have been related to their ability to induce expression of the B-cell activation molecule CD23 and to increase expression of the adhesion molecules LFA-1/CD11a and ICAM-1/CD54. This led Kanavaros et al. [81] to study EBV and expression of adhesion molecules in HD and Ki-1/CD30+ NHL. Among seven ALCLs and 28 nonanaplastic NHL tested, LMP was detected in six CD30+ NHL (one T- and five B-cell). One of the CD30+ cases was an ALCL, B-cell type and the remainder were non-anaplastic NHL. No correlation was found between expression of LMP and detection of CD23, LFA-1/CD11a and ICAM-1/CD54. There were no significant differences in the expression of adhesion molecules in CD30+ versus CD30– cases.

Relationship of ALCL to other lymphomas

Most Ki-1/CD30+ ALCLs arise *de novo* but a minority are 'secondary' resulting from a transformational event in a pre-existing lymphoma. Secondary Ki-1/CD30+ ALCLs can occur in the progression of other T-cell disorders such as angioimmunoblastic lymphadenopathy and angioimmunoproliferative disorder (lymphomatoid granulomatosis) or B-cell disorders, such as follicular lymphoma [109]. Because they follow a prior lymphoma, secondary Ki-1/CD30+ ALCL have a later peak age incidence than primary Ki-1/CD30+ ALCL [7]. They also tend to have a poor prognosis. It is likely, as demonstrated in one case [110], that secondary ALCLs do not possess the t(2;5) associated with primary ALCL. Clearly, considerably more work will be necessary to determine whether this applies in general to secondary ALCL.

There is considerable information regarding the association of Ki-1/CD30+ ALCL with cutaneous T-cell lymphoma (mycosis fungoides) and with HD; special attention will be paid to this.

Cutaneous T-cell lymphoma

Since the skin is the most common extranodal site of ALCL, it may be difficult to distinguish ALCL from tumor-stage mycosis fungoides, which often contains numerous large cells, and from lymphomatoid papulosis and regressing atypical histiocytosis. Primary Ki-1/CD30+ ALCLs usually occur as one to a few large (>2 cm) nodules comprising sheets of large anaplastic, often multinucleated cells, which extend from the upper dermis down into the subcutis. Epidermotropism of malignant cells is uncommon in Ki-1/CD30+ ALCL, in contrast to frequent epidermotropism in mycosis fungoides. In mycosis fungoides, the tumor cells have prominent 'ceribriform' convolutions, generally absent in Ki-1/CD30+ ALCL. In contrast to ALCL, the atypical cells in lymphomatoid papulosis, which are essentially indistinguishable from ALCL cells, occur individually or in small groups surrounded by inflammatory cells. In Ki-1/CD30+ ALCL, except for neutrophils, inflammatory cells are largely confined to the periphery of the lesion. Secondary Ki-1/CD30+ ALCL can occur as a manifestation of tumor progression in both mycosis fungoides and lymphomatoid papulosis [110–112], and a clonal relationship between ALCL and lymphomatoid papulosis has been demonstrated by TCR gene rearrangement studies [112].

There is general agreement that regressing atypical histiocytosis, a term derived from the histiocyte-like morphology of tumor cells in regressing nodules, is not a separate disease but is synonomous with regressing Ki-1/CD30+ ALCL [113].

Hodgkin's disease

Several lines of evidence suggest a histogenetic relationship between CD30+ ALCL and HD. Patients with HD may have coexistent or subsequent Ki-1/CD30+ ALCL [114,115]. Both HD and ALCL have a bimodal age incidence with a first peak in childhood and adolescence, and a second peak after age 50 [7]. In some instances, CD30+ ALCL is difficult to distinguish histologically from the syncytial variant of nodular sclerosis or lymphocyte depletion, reticular type HD. Furthermore, tumor cells in both HD and ALCL are CD30+, CD25+ and express other lymphocyte activation antigens.

Biological similarities also exist. Bullrich et al. recently demonstrated that similar NPM gene rearrangements may identify a certain subtype of ALCL and HD, which may be closely related [53a].

There is considerable evidence to implicate viruses, particularly EBV, in the pathogenesis of some HD and a subset of Ki-1/CD30+ ALCL. Production of IL-6 and IL-9 has been demonstrated in both Ki-1/CD30+ ALCL and HD [95,100a]. Stein et al. [3] have hypothesized that both lymphomas arise from activated B- or T-cells. Viral or host factors, presumably through production of lymphokines, may result in a marked inflammatory response as seen in HD; alternatively, the tumor cell could lose the capacity to produce cytokines or to respond to regulatory factors (e.g., TGFβ), and therefore have a proliferative advantage and an aggressive course as may be seen in Ki-1/CD30+ ALCL.

Despite the similarities in Ki-1/CD30+ ALCL and HD, there are differences in natural history and response to therapy, making it important to distinguish between these two lymphomas. Nodal sites of disease are noncontiguous in more than 50% of patients with ALCL [6] whereas contiguous nodal involvement is characteristic of HD [116]. Inguinal lymph node involvement is common in disseminated ALCL but occurs in only about 5% of HD, especially nodular lymphocyte-predominant Hodgkin's disease (NLPHD). Mediastinal lymphoma is infrequent (<20%) in ALCL [5,6] compared with >60% in HD, particularly the nodular sclerosing type [116]. Extranodal disease is common at presentation in Ki-1/CD30+ ALCL, occurring in 25–65% of patients in different series [4–6,9], compared with <10% (excluding the spleen), in HD [116].

Ki-1/CD30+ ALCL and HD share morphologic similarities. In both disorders the malignant cells are large transformed cells with abundant cytoplasm, large nuclei and prominent nucleoli. Classical Reed–Sternberg cells with bilobed or multiple nuclei and huge inclusion-like nucleoli are a constant feature of HD and are less frequent but do occur in Ki-1/CD30+ ALCL. In Ki-1/CD30+ ALCL, multinucleated cells often have a wreath-like arrangement of nuclei with less prominent nucleoli than in RS cells. Mononuclear tumor cells in ALCL often have markedly convoluted nuclei resulting in the appearance of a doughnut-shaped nucleus.

Sinus infiltration by tumor cells is a characteristic feature of Ki-1/CD30+ ALCL and is rare in HD. Although focal fibrosis is present in Ki-1/CD30+ ALCL, dense bands of collagen fibrosis characteristic of nodular sclerosing HD usually are not present. Eosinophilia, common in HD, is not prominent in most cases of Ki-1/CD30+ ALCL.

Immunophenotyping is useful in distinguishing Ki-1/CD30+ ALCL and HD in borderline cases (Table 18.1). Leu-M1 is seen in 70% of non-lymphocyte-predominant (non-LP) HD but less than 30% in most series of Ki-1/CD30+ ALCL [21,26].

LCA is present on tumor cells in two-thirds of ALCL, especially when frozen tissue is studied, but is present on RS cells in only a minority of HD cases, with the exception of lymphocyte predominance. BNH9, a blood group-related H and Y determinant also expressed on endothelial cells, is present on tumor cells in 24–51% of ALCL but in less than 10% of HD [19,117]. Similarly, EMA is present on tumor cells in most Ki-1/CD30+ ALCL but is rarely detected on RS cells except, once again, in lymphocyte predominance. T-Cell antigens, especially CD2, CD4 and CD5, are present on tumor cells in more than 50% of Ki-1/CD30+ ALCL but less than 25% of HD. In contrast, B-cell antigens, especially L26 (CD20) may be more common in HD with numerous RS cells than in Ki-1/CD30+ ALCL [118,119].

Cytogenetic analysis may be particularly useful in distinguishing ALCL from HD. The t(2,5)(p23;q35) characteristic of T-cell ALCL has not been detected by cytogenetics in HD [120]. A reverse transcriptase PCR designed to detect the t(2;5) did not lead to identification of the fusion product in any of 40 lymph node biopsies of HD (25 nodular sclerosing, 11 mixed cellularity, two lymphocyte depleted, two lymphocyte predominance) suggesting a different molecular pathogenesis for HD and ALCL with the t(2;5) [121]. This does not exclude the possibility that both diseases arise from the same or a closely related precursor cell.

References

1. Stein H, Gerdes J, Kirchner H, et al. Hodgkin and Sternberg–Reed cell antigen(s) detected by an antiserum to a cell line (L428) derived from Hodgkin's disease. *Int. J. Cancer* 1981, **28**: 425–429.
2. Schwab U, Stein H, Gerdes J, et al. Production of a monoclonal antibody specific for Hodgkin and Reed–Sternberg cells of Hodgkin's disease and a subset of normal lymphoid cells. *Nature* 1982, **299**: 65–67.
3. Stein H, Mason DY, Gerdes J, et al. The expression of the Hodgkin's disease associated antigen Ki-1 in reactive and neoplastic lymphoid tissue: Evidence that Reed–Sternberg cells and histiocytic malignancies are derived from activated lymphoid cells. *Blood* 1985, **68**: 848–858.
4. Shulman L, Frisard B, Antin JH, et al. Primary Ki-1 anaplastic large-cell lymphoma in adults: Clinical characteristics and outcome. *J. Clin. Oncol.* 1993, **11**: 937–942.
5. Nakamura S, Takagi N, Kojima M, et al. Clinicopathologic study of large cell anaplastic lymphoma (Ki-1-positive large cell lymphoma) among Japanese. *Cancer* 1991, **69**: 118–129.
6. Greer JP, Kinney MC, Collins RD, et al. Clinical

features of 31 patients with Ki-1 anaplastic large cell lymphoma. *J. Clin. Oncol.* 1991, **9**: 539–547.

7. Lennert K, Feller A. T-Cell lymphomas. In Lennert K, Feller A (eds) *Histopathology of Non-Hodgkin's Lymphomas (Based on the Updated Kiel Classification)*, 2nd edn. Berlin: Springer-Verlag, 1992, pp. 165–221.

8. Kadin M, Anderson J, Chilcote R. Lack of prognostic significance of Ki-1 (CD30) positivity in disseminated pediatric large cell lymphoma. *Blood* 1991, **78**(Suppl. 1): 121a.

8a. Fraga M, Brousset P, Schlaifer D, et al. Bone marrow involvement in anaplastic large cell lymphoma. Immunohistochemical detection of minimal disease and its prognostic significance. *Am. J. Clin. Path.* 1995, **103**: 82–89.

9. Chott A, Kaserer K, Augustin I, et al. Ki-1-positive large-cell lymphoma: A clinicopathologic study of 41 cases. *Am. J. Surg. Path.* 1990, **14**: 439–448.

10. Beljaards RC, Meijer CJLM, Scheffer E, et al. Primary cutaneous CD30-positive large cell lymphoma: Definition of a new type of cutaneous lymphoma with a favorable prognosis. *Cancer* 1993, **71**: 2097–2104.

11. Chakravarti B, Kamani NR, Bayever E, et al. Bone marrow transplantation for childhood Ki-1 lymphoma. *J. Clin. Oncol.* 1990, **8**: 657–660.

12. Pasqualucci L, Wasik MA, Teicher B, et al. Antitumor activity of anti-CD30 immunotoxin (Ber-H2/Saporin) *in vitro* and in SCID mice xenografted with human CD30+ anaplastic large cell lymphoma. *Blood* 1995, **85**: 2139–2146.

13. Agnarsson BA, Kadin ME. Ki-1-positive large-cell lymphoma: A morphologic and immunologic study of 19 cases. *Am. J. Surg. Path.* 1988, **12**: 264–274.

13a. Chan JKC, Ng CS, Hui PK, et al. Anaplastic large-cell Ki-1 lymphoma: Delineation of two morphological types. *Histopathology* 1989, **15**: 11–34.

14. Chan JKC, Buchanan R, Fletcher CDM. Sarcomatoid variant of anaplastic large cell Ki-1 lymphoma. *Am. J. Surg. Path.* 1990, **14**: 383–390.

15. Pileri S, Falini B, Delsol G, et al. Lymphohistiocytic T-cell lymphoma (anaplastic large-cell lymphoma CD30+/Ki-1+ with a high content of reactive histiocytes). *Histopathology* 1990, **16**: 983–988.

16. Kinney MC, Collins RD, Greer JP, et al. A small cell predominant variant of primary Ki-1 (CD30)+ T-cell lymphoma. *Am. J. Surg. Path.* 1993, **17**: 859–868.

17. O' Connor NTJ, Stein H, Gatter KC, et al. Genotypic analysis of large-cell lymphomas which express the Ki-1 antigen. *Histopathology* 1987, **1**: 733–740.

18. Banks PM, Metter J, Allred DC. Anaplastic large cell (Ki-1) lymphoma with histiocytic phenotype simulating carcinoma. *Am. J. Clin. Path.* 1990, **94**: 445–452.

19. Carbone A, Gloghini A, DeRe V, et al. Histopathologic, immunophenotypic, and genotypic analysis of Ki-1 anaplastic large cell lymphomas that express histiocyte-associated antigens. *Cancer* 1990, **66**: 2547–2556.

20. Sakurai S, Nakajima T, Oyama T, et al. Anaplastic large cell lymphoma with histiocytic phenotypes. *Acta Path. Jap.* 1993, **43**: 142–145.

21. Delsol G, Al Saati T, Gatter KC, et al. Coexpression of epithelial membrane antigen (EMA), Ki-1, and interleukin-2 receptor by anaplastic large-cell lymphomas. Diagnostic value in so-called malignant histiocytosis. *Am. J. Path.* 1988, **130**: 59–70.

22. Falini B, Pileri S, Stein H, et al. Variable expression of leucocyte-common (CD45) antigen in CD30 (Ki-1)-positive anaplastic large-cell lymphoma: Implications for the differential diagnosis between lymphoid and non-lymphoid malignancies. *Human Path.* 1990, **21**: 624–629.

23. Gustmann C, Altmannsberger M, Osborn M, et al. Cytokeratin expression and vimentin content in large-cell anaplastic lymphomas and other non-Hodgkin's lymphomas. *Am. J. Path.* 1991, **138**: 1413–1422.

24. Pallesen G, Hamilton-Dutoit SJ. Ki-1 (CD30) antigen is regularly expressed by tumor cells of embryonal carcinoma. *Am. J. Path.* 1988, **133**: 446–450.

25. Schwarting R, Gerdes J, Durkop H, et al. Ber-H2: A new anti-Ki-1 (CD30) monoclonal antibody directed at a formol-resistant epitope. *Blood* 1989, **74**: 1678–1689.

26. Kinney MC, Glick AD, Stein H, et al. Comparison of anaplastic large cell (Ki-1) lymphomas and microvillous lymphomas in their immunologic and ultrastructural features. *Am. J. Surg. Path.* 1990, **14**: 1047–1060.

27. Herbst H, Tippelman G, Anagnostopoulos I, et al. Immunoglobulin and T-cell receptor gene rearrangements in Hodgkin's disease and Ki-1 positive anaplastic large-cell lymphoma: Dissociation between phenotype and genotype. *Leuk. Res.* 1989, **13**: 103–116.

28. Katamine S, Otsu M, Tada K, et al. Epstein–Barr virus transforms precursor B cells even before immunoglobulin gene rearrangements. *Nature* 1984, **309**: 369–372.

29. Gregory C, Kirchgens C, Edwards C. Epstein–Barr virus-transformed human precursor B cell lines: Altered growth phenotype of lines with germline or rearranged but nonexpressed heavy chain genes. *Eur. J. Immunol.* 1987, **17**: 1199–1207.

30. Abbondanzo SL, Sato N, Straus SE, et al. Acute infectious mononucleosis: CD30 (Ki-1) antigen expression and histologic correlations. *Am. J. Clin. Path.* 1990, **93**: 698–702.

31. Andreesen R, Osterholz J, Lohr GW, et al. Human macrophages can express the Hodgkin's cell-associated antigen Ki-1 (CD30). *Am. J. Path.* 1989, **134**: 187–192.

32. Andreeson R, Brugger W, Lohr GW, et al. A Hodgkin cell-specific antigen is expressed on a subset of auto- and alloactivated T (helper) lymphoblasts. *Blood* 1984, **63**: 1299–1302.

33. Chadburn A, Inghirami G, Knowles DM. The kinetics and temporal expression of T-cell activation-associated antigens CD15 (Leu-M1), CD30 (Ki-1), EMA, and CD11c (Leu-M5) by benign activated T cells. *Hematol. Path.* 1992, **6**: 193–202.

34. Ellis RM, Simms PE, Slivnick DJ, et al. CD30 is a signal-transducing molecule that defines a subset of human activated CD45RO+ T cells. *J. Immunol.* 1993, **151**: 2380–2389.

35. Hansen H, Lemke H, Bredfeldt G, et al. The Hodgkin-associated Ki-1 antigen exists in an intracellular and a membrane-bound form. *Biol. Chem. Hoppe-Seyler* 1989, **370**: 409–416.

36. Schaadt M, Burrichter H, Stein H, et al. The cell of origin in Hodgkin's disease. Conclusions from *in vivo* and *in vitro* studies. *Int. Rev. Exp. Path.* 1985, **27**: 185–202.

37. Froese P, Lemke H, Gerdes J, et al. Biochemical characterization and biosynthesis of the Ki-1 antigen in Hodgkin-derived and virus-transformed human B- and T-lymphoid cell lines. *J. Immunol.* 1987, **139**: 2081–2087.

38. Hansen H, Bredfeldt G, Havsteen B, et al. Protein kinase activity of the intracellular but not of the membrane-associated form of the Ki-1 antigen (CD30). *Res. Immunol.* 1990, **141**: 13–31.

39. Josimovic-Alasevic O, Durkop H, Schwarting R. Ki-1 (CD30) antigen is released by Ki-1 positive tumor cells in vitro and in vivo. I. Partial characterization of soluble Ki-1 antigen and detection of the antigen in cell culture supernatants and in serum by an enzyme-linked immunosorbent assay. *Eur. J. Immunol.* 1989, **19**: 157–162.

40. Durkop H, Latza U, Hummel M, et al. Molecular cloning and expression of a new member of the nerve growth factor receptor family that is characteristic of Hodgkin's disease. *Cell* 1992, **68**: 421–427.

41. Rogers S, Wells R, Rechensteiner M. Amino acid sequences common to rapidly degraded proteins. The PEST hypothesis. *Science* 1986, **234**: 364–368.

42. Smith CA, Gruss H-J, Davis T, et al. CD30 antigen, a marker for Hodgkin's lymphoma, is a receptor whose ligand defines an emerging family of cytokines with homology to TNF. *Cell* 1993, **73**: 1349.

42a. Gruss H-J, Boiani N, Williams DE, et al. Pleiotropic effects of the CD30 ligand and CD30-expressing cells and lymphoma cell lines. *Blood* 1994, **83**: 2045–2056.

42b. Fonatsch C, Latza U, Durkop H, et al. Assignment of the human CD30 (Ki-1) gene to 1p36. *Genomics* 1992, **14**: 825–826.

43. Kemper O, Derre J, Cherif D, et al. The gene for the type II (p75) tumor necrosis factor receptor (TNF-RII) is localized on band 1p36.2-p36.3. *Human Genet.* 1991, **87**: 623–624.

44. Lawrence J, Villnave C, Singer R. Sensitive, high-resolution chromatin and chromosome mapping *in situ*: Presence and orientation of two closely integrated copies of EBV in a lymphoma line. *Cell* 1988, **52**: 51–61.

45. Debiec-Rychter M, Zukowski K, Wang C, et al. Chromosomal characterizations of human nasal and nasopharyngeal cells immortalized by human papillomavirus type 16 DNA. *Cytogenetics* 1991, **52**: 51–61.

46. Morgan R, Smith SD, Hecht BK, et al. Lack of involvement of the c-fms and N-myc genes by chromosomal translocation t(2;5)(p23;q35) common to malignancies with features of so-called malignant histiocytosis. *Blood* 1989, **73**: 2155–2164.

47. Rimokh R, Magaud J-P, Berger F, et al. A translocation involving a specific breakpoint on chromosome 5 is characteristic of anaplastic large-cell lymphoma ('Ki-1 lymphoma'). *Br. J. Haematol.* 1989, **71**: 31–36.

48. Fischer P, Nacheva E, Mason DY. A Ki-1 (CD30)-positive human cell line (Karpas 299) established from a high-grade non-Hodgkin's lymphoma, showing a 2;5 translocation and rearrangement of the T-cell receptor β-chain gene. *Blood* 1988, **72**: 234–240.

49. Bitter MA, Franklin WA, Larson RA. Morphology in Ki-1 (CD30)-positive non-Hodgkin's lymphoma is correlated with clinical features and the presence of a unique chromosomal abnormality, t(2;5)(p23;q35). *Am. J. Surg. Path.* 1990, **14**: 305–316.

50. Mason DY, Bastard C, Rimokh R, et al. CD30-positive large cell lymphomas ('Ki-1 lymphoma') are associated with a chromosomal translocation involving 5q35. *Br. J. Haematol.* 1990, **74**: 161–168.

51. Morris SW, Kirstein MN, Valentine MB, et al. Fusion of a kinase gene, ALK, to a nucleolar protein gene, NPM, in non-Hodgkin's lymphoma. *Science* 1994, **263**: 1281–1284.

52. Chan W-Y, Liu Q-R, Borjigin J, et al. Characterization of the cDNA encoding human nucleophosmin and studies of its role in normal and abnormal growth. *Biochemistry* 1989, **28**: 1033–1039.

53. Borer RA, Lehner CF, Eppenberger HM, et al. Major nucleolar proteins shuttle between nucleus and cytoplasm. *Cell* 1989, **56**: 379–390.

53a. Bullrich F, Morris SW, Hummel M, et al. Nucleophosmin (NPM) gene rearrangements in Ki-1-positive lymphomas. *Cancer Res.* 1994, **54**: 2873–2877.

54. Hanks SK, Quinn AM, Hunter T. The protein kinase family: Conserved features and deduced phylogeny of the catalytic domains. *Science* 1988, **241**: 42–52.

55. Taylor SS, Knighton DR, Zheng J, et al. Structural framework for the protein kinase family. *Annu. Rev. Cell Biol.* 1992, **8**: 429–462.

56. Barbey S, Gogusev J, Mouly H, et al. DEL cell line: A 'malignant histiocytosis' CD30+ t(5;6)(q35;p21) cell line. *Int. J. Cancer* 1990, **45**: 546–553.

57. Sainati L, Montaldi A, Stella M, et al. A novel variant translocation t(2;3)(p23;q34) in Ki-1 large-cell anaplastic lymphoma. *Br. J. Haematol.* 1990, **75**: 621–622.

58. Ohno H, Takahisa F, Furukawa T, et al. Molecular analysis of a chromosomal translocation, t(9;14)(p13;q32), in a diffuse large-cell lymphoma cell line expressing the Ki-1 antigen. *Proc. Natl Acad. Sci. USA* 1990, **87**: 628–632.

59. Dekmezian R, Goodacre A, Cabanillas F, et al. The 2;5 translocation: Is it specific for anaplastic (Ki-1) large cell lymphoma? *Lab. Invest.* 1990, **62**: 25A.

60. Gordon BG, Weisenburger DD, Warkentin PI, et al. Peripheral T-cell lymphoma in childhood and adolescence. A clinicopathologic study of 22 patients. *Cancer* 1993, **71**: 257–263.

60a. De Coteau JF, Butmarc JR, Kinney MC, et al. The t(2;5) chromosomal translocation is not a common feature of primary cutaneous CD30+ lymphoproliferative disorders: Comparison with anaplastic large-cell lymphoma of nodal origin. *Blood* 1996, **87**: 3437–3441.

60b. Wood GS, Hardiman DL, Boni R, et al. Lack of the t(2;5) or other mutations resulting in expression of anaplastic lymphoma kinase catalytic domain in CD30+ primary cutaneous lymphoproliferative disorders and Hodgkin's disease. *Blood* 1996, **88**: 1765–1770.

60c. Sarris AH, Luthra R, Papadimitracopoulou V, et al. Amplification of genomic DNA demonstrates the presence of the t(2;5)(p23;q35) in anaplastic large cell lymphoma, but not in other non-Hodgkin's lymphomas, Hodgkin's disease, or lymphomatoid papulosis. *Blood* 1996, **88**: 1771–1779.

60d. Beylot-Barry M, Lamant L, Vergier B, et al. Detection of t(2;5)(p23;q35) translocation by reverse transcriptase polymerase chain reaction and in situ hybridization in CD30-positive cutaneous lymphoma and lymphomatoid papulosis. *Am. J. Pathol.* 1996, **149**: 483–492.

61. Downing JR, Shurtleff SA, Zielenska M. Molecular detection of the t(2;5) translocation of non-Hodgkin's lymphoma by reverse transcriptase-polymerase chain reaction. *Blood* 1995, **85**: 3416–3422.

61a. Shiota M, Takenaga M, Satoh H, et al. Diagnosis of t(2;5)(23;q35)-associated Ki-1 lymphoma with immunohistochemistry. *Blood* 1994, **84**: 3648–3652.

62. Kern SE, Pietenpol JA, Thiagalingam S, et al. Oncogenic forms of p53 inhibit p53-regulated gene expression. *Science* 1992, **256**: 827–830.

63. Vogelstein B, Kinzler KW. p53 function and dysfunction. *Cell* 1992, **70**: 523–526.

64. Danova M, Giordano M, Mazzini G, et al. Expression of p53 protein during the cell cycle measured by flow cytometry in human leukemia. *Leukemia Res.* 1990, **14**: 417–422.

65. Doglioni E, Pelosio P, Mombello A, et al. Immunohistochemical evidence of abnormal expression of the antioncogene-encoded p53 phosphoprotein in Hodgkin's disease and CD30+ anaplastic lymphomas. *Hematol. Path.* 1991, **5**: 67–73.

66. Cesarman E, Inghirami G, Chadburn A, et al. High levels of p53 protein expression do not correlate with p53 gene mutations in anaplastic large cell lymphoma. *Am. J. Path.* 1993, **143**: 845–856.

67. Chadburn A, Cesarman E, Jagirdar J, et al. CD30 (Ki-1) positive anaplastic large cell lymphomas in individuals infected with the human immunodeficiency virus. *Cancer* 1993, **72**: 3078–3090.

68. Bading H, Gerdes J, Schwarting R, et al. Nuclear and cytoplasmic distribution of cellular myb protein in human hematopoietic cells evidenced by monoclonal antibody. *Oncogene* 1988, **3**: 257–265.

69. Ross CW, Schlegelmilch JA, Grogan TM, et al. Detection of Epstein–Barr virus genome in Ki-1 (CD30)-positive, large-cell anaplastic lymphomas using the polymerase chain reaction. *Am. J. Path.* 1992, **141**: 457–465.

70. Kanavaros P, Jiwa NM, De Bruin PC, et al. High incidence of EBV genome in CD30-positive non-Hodgkin's lymphomas. *J. Path.* 1992, **168**: 307–315.

71. Herbst H, Dallenbach F, Hummel M, et al. Epstein–Barr virus DNA and latent gene products in Ki-1 (CD30)-positive anaplastic large cell lymphomas. *Blood* 1991, **78**: 2666–2673.

72. Anagnostopoulos I, Herbst H, Niedobitek G, et al. Demonstration of monoclonal EBV genomes in Hodgkin's disease and Ki-1-positive anaplastic large cell lymphoma by combined Southern blot and in situ hybridization. *Blood* 1989, **74**: 810–816.

73. Brousset P, Rochaix P, Chittal S, et al. High incidence of Epstein–Barr virus detection in Hodgkin's disease and absence of detection in anaplastic large cell lymphoma in children. *Histopathology* 1993, **23**: 181–191.

74. Borisch B, Gatter KC, Tobler A, et al. Epstein–Barr virus-associated anaplastic large cell lymphoma in renal transplant patients. *Am. J. Clin. Path.* 1992, **98**: 312–318.

75. Kumar S, Kumar D, Kingma DW, et al. Epstein–Barr virus-associated T-cell lymphoma in a renal transplant patient. *Am. J. Surg. Path.* 1993, **17**: 1046–1053.

76. Borisch B, Boni J, Burki K, et al. Recurrent cutaneous anaplastic large cell (CD30+) lymphoma associated with Epstein–Barr virus. A case report with 9-year follow-up. *Am. J. Surg. Path.* 1992, **16**: 796–801.

77. Boicchi M, DeRe V, Gloghini A, et al. High incidence of monoclonal EBV episomes in Hodgkin's disease and anaplastic large-cell Ki-1 positive lymphoma in HIV-positive patients. *Int. J. Cancer* 1993, **54**: 53–59.

78. Borisch-Chappuis B, Muller H, Stutte J, et al. Identification of EBV-DNA in lymph nodes from patients with lymphadenopathy and lymphomas associated with AIDS. *Virchows Arch. B Cell Path.* 1990, **58**: 199–205.

79. Carbone A, Gloghini A, Zanette I, et al. Demonstration of Epstein–Barr viral genomes by in situ hybridiation in acquired immune deficiency syndrome-related high-grade and anaplastic large cell CD30+ lymphomas. *Am. J. Clin. Path.* 1993, **99**: 289–297.

80. Hamilton-Dutoit SJ, Rea D, Raphael M, et al. Epstein–Barr virus-latent gene expression and tumor cell phenotype in acquired immundeficiency syndrome-related non-Hodgkin's lymphoma. Correlation of lymphoma phenotype with three distinct patterns of viral latency. *Am. J. Path.* 1993, **143**: 1072–1085.

81. Kanavaros P, Jiwa M, Van Der Valk P, et al. Expression of Epstein–Barr virus latent gene products and related cellular activation and adhesion molecules in Hodgkin's disease and non-Hodgkin's lymphomas arising in patients without pre-existing immunodeficiency. *Human Path.* 1993, **24**: 725–729.

82. Hamilton-Dutoit SJ, Pallesen G. A survey of Epstein–Barr virus gene expression in sporadic non-Hodgkin's lymphomas. Detection of Epstein–Barr virus in a subset of peripheral T-cell lymphomas. *Am. J. Path.* 1992, **140**: 1315–1325.

83. Rowe M, Rowe DT, Gregory CD, et al. Differences in B cell growth phenotype reflect novel patterns of Epstein–Barr virus latent gene expression in Burkitt's lymphoma cells. *EMBO J.* 1987, **6**: 2743–2751.

84. Pallesen G, Hamilton-Dutoit SJ, Rowe M, et al. Expression of Epstein–Barr latent gene products in the tumor cells of Hodgkin's disease. *Lancet* 1991, **337**: 320–322.

85. Fahraeus R, Fu HL, Ernberg I, et al. Expression of

Epstein–Barr virus-encoded proteins in nasopharyngeal carcinoma. *Int. J. Cancer* 1990, **42**: 329–338.

86. Young L, Alfieri C, Hennessy K, et al. Expression of Epstein–Barr virus transformation-associated genes in tissues of patients with EBV lymphoproliferative disease. *N. Engl. J. Med.* 1989, **321**: 1080–1085.

87. Rowe M, Young LS, Crocker J, et al. Epstein–Barr virus (EBV)-associated lymphoproliferative disease in the SCID mouse model: Implications for the pathogenesis of EBV-positive lymphomas in man. *J. Exp. Med.* 1991, **173**: 147–158.

88. Offit K, Ladanyi M, Gangi MD, et al. Ki-1 antigen expression defines a favorable clinical subset of non-B cell non-Hodgkin's lymphoma. *Leukemia-Lymphoma* 1990, **4**: 625–630.

89. Gonzales-Clemente JM, Ribera JM, Campo E, et al. Ki-1+ anaplastic large-cell lymphoma of T-cell origin in an HIV-infected patient. *AIDS* 1991, **5**: 751–755.

90. Pedersen C, Gerstoft J, Lundgren JD, et al. HIV-associated lymphoma: Histopathology and association with Epstein–Barr virus genome related to clinical, immunological, and prognostic features. *Eur. J. Cancer* 1991, **27**: 1416–1423.

91. Anagnostopoulos I, Hummel M, Kaudewitz P, et al. Detection of HTLV-1 proviral sequences in CD30-positive large cell cutaneous T-cell lymphomas. *Am. J. Path.* 1990, **137**: 1317–1322.

92. Tashiro K, Kikuchi M, Takeshita M, et al. Clinicopathological study of Ki-1 positive lymphomas. *Path. Res. Pract.* 1989, **185**: 461–467.

93. Peuchmaur M, Emilie D, Crevon MC, et al. IL-2 mRNA expression in TAC-positive malignant lymphomas. *Am. J. Path.* 1990, **136**: 383–390.

94. Hsu S-M, Waldron JW, Hsu P-L, et al. Cytokines in malignant lymphomas: Review and prospective evaluation. *Human Path.* 1993, **24**: 1040–1057.

95. Merz H, Houssian FA, Orscheschek K, et al. Interleukin-9 expression in human malignant lymphomas: Unique association with Hodgkin's disease and large cell anaplastic lymphoma. *Blood* 1991, **78**: 1311–1317.

96. Kehrl JH, Wakefield LM, Roberts AB, et al. Production of transforming growth factor beta by human T lymphocytes and its potential role in the regulation of T cell growth. *J. Exp. Med.* 1986, **163**: 1037–1050.

97. Newcom SR, Kadin ME, Ansari AA. Production of transforming growth factor-beta activity by Ki-1 positive lymphoma cells and analysis of its role in the regulation of Ki-1 positive lymphoma growth. *Am. J. Path.* 1988, **140**: 709–718.

98. Newcom SR, Tagra KK, Kadin ME. Neutralizing antibodies against transforming growth factor-β potentiate the proliferation of Ki-1 positive lymphoma cells. Further evidence for negative autocrine regulation by transforming growth factor-β. *Am. J. Path.* 1992, **140**: 709–718.

99. Kadin ME, Cavaille-Coll MW, Gertz R. Loss of receptors for transforming growth factor B in human T-cell malignancies. *Proc. Natl Acad. Sci. USA* 1994, **91**: 6002–6006.

100. Agematsu K, Komiyama, A. Ki-1 positive large-cell lymphoma: Multiple lytic bone lesions and interleukin-6. *Leukemia-Lymphoma* 1992, **7**: 309–15.

100a. Merz H, Fliedner A, Orscheschek K, et al. Cytokine

expression in T-cell lymphomas and Hodgkin's disease. Its possible implication in autocrine or paracrine production as a potential basis for neoplastic growth. *Am. J. Path.* 1991, **139**: 1173–1180.

101. Nishihira H, Tanaka Y, Kigasawa H, et al. Ki-1 lymphoma producing G-CSF. *Br. J. Haematol.* 1991, **80**: 556–565.

102. Steinert PM, Roop DR. Molecular and cellular biology of intermediate filaments. *Ann. Rev. Biochem.* 1988, **57**: 593–625.

103. Bilbe G, Delabie J, Bruggen J, et al. Restin: A novel intermediate filament-associated protein highly expressed in Reed–Sternberg cells of Hodgkin's disease. *EMBO J.* 1992, **11**: 2103–2113.

104. Delabie J, Shipman R, Bruggen J, et al. Expression of the novel intermediate filament-associated protein Restin in Hodgkin's disease and anaplastic large-cell lymphoma. *Blood* 1992, **80**: 2891–2896.

105. Kinzler KW, Nilbert MC, Volgelstein B, et al. Identification of a gene located at chromosome 5q1 that is mutated in colorectal carcinomas. *Science* 1991, **251**: 1366–1370.

106. Joslyn G, Carlson M, Thliveris A, et al. Identification of deletion mutations and three new genes at the familial polyposis locus. *Cell* 1991, **66**: 601–613.

107. Bourne HR. Consider the coiled coil [news]. *Nature* 1991, **351**: 188–190.

108. Bourne HR. Suppression with a difference [news]. *Nature* 1991, **353**: 696–698.

109. Hugh J, Poppema S. Ki-1 (CD30) antigen expression on transformed follicular lymphomas. *Lab. Invest.* 1990, **62**: 46A.

110. Davis T, Morton CM, Miller-Cassman R, et al. Hodgkin's disease, lymphomatoid papulosis and mycosis fungoides derived from a common T-cell clone. *N. Engl. J. Med.* 1992, **3216**: 1115–1122.

111. Kaudewitz P, Stein H, Dallenbach F. Primary and secondary cutaneous Ki-1+ (CD30+) anaplastic large-cell lymphomas. Morphologic, immunohistologic, and clinical characteristics. *Cancer* 1989, **135**: 359–367.

112. Volkenandt M, Bertino JR, Shenoy BV, et al. Molecular evidence for a clonal relationship between lymphomatoid papulosis and Ki-1 positive anaplastic large cell lymphoma. *J. Dermatol. Sci.* 1993, **6**: 121–126.

113. Motley RJ, Jasini B, Ford AM, et al. Regressing atypical histiocytosis, a regressing cutaneous phase of Ki-1-positive anaplastic large cell lymphoma. Immunocytochemical, nucleic acid and cytogenetic studies of a new case in view of current opinion. *Cancer* 1992, **70**: 476–483.

114. Pileri S, Mazza P, Zinzani PL, et al. Ki-1 lymphoma and Hodgkin's disease. *Haematol. (Pavia)* 1989, **74**: 333–334.

115. Rosso R, Paulli M, Magrini U, et al. Anaplastic large cell lymphoma, CD30/Ki-1 positive, expressing the CD15/Leu-M1 antigen. Immunohistochemical and morphological relationships to Hodgkin's disease. *Virchows Arch. A. Path. Anat.* 1990, **416**: 229–235.

116. Mauch PM, Kalish LA, Kadin ME, et al. Patterns of presentation of Hodgkin's disease. Implications for etiology and pathogenesis. *Cancer* 1993, **71**: 2062–2071.

Table 19.2 Immunodeficiency Cancer Registry cases: distribution of tumors and immunodeficiencies

Immunodeficiency	Adenocarcinoma	Lymphoma	Hodgkin's disease	Leukemia	Other tumors	Total
Severe combined immunodeficiency	1 (2.4%)	3 (73.8%)	4 (9.5%)	5 (11.9%)	1 (2.4%)	42 (8.4%)
X-linked agammaglobulinemia	3 (14.3%)	7 (33.3%)	3 (14.3%)	7 (33.3%)	1 (4.8%)	21 (4.2%)
Common variable immunodeficiency	20 (16.7%)	55 (45.8%)	8 (6.7%)	8 (6.7%)	29 (24.2%)	120 (24.0%)
IgA deficiency	8 (21.1%)	6 (15.8%)	3 (7.9%)	0 (0%)	21 (55.3%)	38 (7.6%)
Hyper-IgM syndrome	0 (0%)	9 (56.3%)	4 (25.0%)	0 (0%)	3 (18.8%)	16 (3.2%)
Wiskott–Aldrich syndrome	0 (0%)	59 (75.6%)	3 (3.8%)	7 (9.0%)	9 (11.5%)	78 (15.6%)
Ataxia telangiectasia	13 (8.7%)	69 (46.0%)	16 (10.7%)	32 (21.3%)	20 (13.3%)	150 (30.0%)
Other immunodeficiencies	1 (4.0%)	12 (48.0%)	1 (4.0%)	4 (16.0%)	7 (28.0%)	25 (5.0%)
Total immunodeficiency categories	46 (9.2%)	252 (50.4%)	43 (8.6%)	63 (12.6%)	96 (19.2%)	500 (100%)

efficiency of EBV transformation and/or suppresses proliferation of transformed B-cells, thus reducing the likelihood of B-cell lymphoproliferative disease (BLPD) in this particular SCID phenotype. On the other hand, three cases of lymphoma in patients with purine nucleoside phosphorylase (PNP) deficiency (a related enzyme defect with relatively normal B-cell function) are known to the ICR occurring at 4, 6 and 8 years of age. Given the rarity of PNP deficiency, these case reports suggest that lymphoid malignancy occurs with high frequency in children with PNP deficiency, and that such patients should be carefully monitored for this complication and might benefit from correction of the immunodeficiency at the earliest possible opportunity. Most confirmed cases of lymphoproliferative disease in SCID have been reported in X-SCID and Omenn's syndrome. To date no reliable information exists regarding the existence of lymphomas in SCID due to 70 kD zeta-associated protein (ZAP 70) deficiency [18] or RAG-1 or -2 deficiencies [19].

PREDOMINANTLY ANTIBODY DEFICIENCIES

Patients with the disorders classified by the World Health Organization (WHO) as predominantly antibody deficiencies share a propensity toward recurrent and chronic pyogenic infections particularly involving the respiratory tract. ICR tabulation for these disorders indicates that lymphomas are the predominant tumor type, followed by gastrointestinal carcinomas. Extranodal lymphomas are relatively common in patients with common variable immune deficiency or X-linked agammaglobulinemia, and X-linked hypogammaglobulinemia with increased IgM syndrome.

A retrospective North American survey of 96 patients diagnosed with X-linked agammaglobulinemia/hypogammaglobulinemia (XLA) identified only two cases with cancer [20], suggesting a low incidence of cancer compared with certain other immunodeficiency categories. Of the 21 tumors reported to the ICR in patients with X-linked hypogammaglobulinemia, seven (33%) were reported as lymphomas (Table 19.2) involving the gastrointestinal (GI) tract, lymph nodes or multiple sites predominantly (Table 19.3). No central nervous system (CNS) lymphomas were reported. There are two ICR cases of GI carcinomas in XLA. The median age for all tumors is only 1.2 years (similar to that for SCID). Because the majority of XLA cases in the ICR were diagnosed during the 1950s and 1960, it is possible that some XLA cases in the ICR may actually represent boys with SCID, or alternatively with CVID.

Non-Hodgkin's lymphomas are the predominant tumor among cases of CVID in the ICR: 55/120

Table 19.3 Characteristics of non-Hodgkin's lymphomas in the Immunodeficiency Cancer Registry (ICR)*

Immunodeficiency	N	Sex† (M:F)	Median age at diagnosis (years)	Primary tumor sites (%)‡			
				CNS	Gastrointestinal tract	Lymph node	Multiple
Severe combined immunodeficiency	31	23:7	1.6	6.5	3.2	9.7	48.4
X-linked agammaglobulinemia	7	7:0	1.2	0	14.3	14.3	14.3
Common variable immunodeficiency	55	30:23	23.0	1.8	12.7	12.7	25.5
IgA deficiency	6	4:1	9.4	16.7	0	0	0
Hyper-IgM syndrome	9	7:2	7.8	11.1	22.2	22.2	0
Wiskott–Aldrich syndrome	59	59:0	6.2	23.7	6.8	8.5	20.3
Ataxia telangiectasia	69	40:24	8.5	0	8.7	10.1	14.5
Other immunodeficiencies	4	4:0	4.0	0	0	0	0
Total immunodeficiency categories	240	174:57	7.1	7.9	8.8	10.4	21.7

* This table excludes cases of non-Hodgkin's lymphoma in immunodeficiency categories with fewer than two cases reported.
† For 51.3% of ICR cases primary tumor site is other or unknown.
‡ Sex reported where known.

tumor cases (45.8%), followed in decreasing proportion by carcinomas: 20/120 (16.7%) and Hodgkin's disease: 8/120 (6.7%) [7]. Other published reports also stress the high incidence of lymphomas, especially among elderly females [4] and the frequent finding of gastric carcinomas [21,22]. The majority of NHL in CVID appear to be of B-cell origin as judged by immunophenotyping or histopathologic interpretation. However, 14 out of 55 cases were reported to be of T-cell phenotype. In our experience at Minnesota, children with features of CVID have also developed large granular lymphocytosis with neutropenia, a proliferative disorder of natural killer lymphocytes.

IgA deficiency occurs with a higher frequency than most other recognized primary immunodeficiencies (approximately 1:600 in the general population), yet only a handful of tumor cases have been registered with the ICR (35/500 ICR cases), or have appeared in the literature. However, the predominant tumor types recognized in patients with IgA deficiency – adenocarcinomas, including GI carcinomas and NHL – are the same as reported for CVID. There is accumulating evidence that IgA deficiency and CVID can occur in the same kindred, and are associated with an unusually high incidence of shared rare alleles and deletions in the class III region of the MHC complex on chromosome six [23]. They may represent similar abnormalities in Ig class switching during immunoglobulin synthesis. One can argue that most cases of IgA deficiency go undetected, and the incidence of tumors in IgA deficiency is not accurately recognized.

Non-Hodgkin's lymphomas and Hodgkin's disease are recognized complications of X-linked hypogammaglobulinemia with increased IgM (CD40 ligand deficiency). In the recent analysis of archival tissue from the ICR, three out of three cases of Hodgkin's disease were found to be associated with EBV infection as detected by the EBER-1 probe [17].

WELL-CHARACTERIZED IMMUNODEFICIENCIES

Wiskott–Aldrich syndrome

Wiskott–Aldrich syndrome is an X-linked disorder with features of microthrombocytopenia and an associated bleeding diathesis, eczema and susceptibility to bacterial, viral and parasitic infections. While rare cases of nonmalignant tumors of the soft tissues and brain have come to light in Wiskott–Aldrich syndrome patients, lymphoproliferative disorders are overwhelmingly predominant: 59 out of 78 ICR cases (75%). The risk of developing non-Hodgkin's lymphoma in Wiskott–Aldrich syndrome (WAS) approaches 100% by 30 years of age [2]. In a review of tumors in WAS collected at the National Institutes of Health, Cotelingam [24] described an 18% incidence of tumors in 50 patients observed between 1966 and 1982. There were eight cases of non-Hodgkin's lymphoma and one case of Hodgkin's disease. The most common primary site was the brain and median survival after diagnosis in patients who received chemotherapy was less than one year. There were no long-term remissions. In an independent review of tissues from 22 other cases available to the ICR, Dr Glauco Frizzera, in 1987, found 17 out of 22 to represent lymphomas of terminally differentiating B-cells ranging in histology from polymorphic B-cell lymphoma with plasmacytoid features (indistinguishable in appearance from tumors observed in immunosuppressed allograft recipients) to plasmacytic immunocytoma and immunoblastic sarcoma of B-cells (Table 19.4). The median age for development of B-cell tumors was 6.4 years. Nine of 14 cases for which the tumor site was known had involvement of the CNS.

In recent studies of archival ICR tumor material, Ambinder et al. found five out of five lymphomas from WAS patients to stain strongly positive with

Table 19.4 Clinical and pathological features of 22 cases of lymphoproliferative disorders in WAS reviewed by the Immunodeficiency Cancer Registry

ICR histology	ICR No.	Contributors	Reported histology	Age at diagnosis (years)	Survival (years) postdiagnosis	Sites
Pleomorphic immunocytoma (PI)	3001	J. Montgomery	RES hyperplasia	2.3	0	Liver
	3002	R. Buckley E. Green	Myeloid metaplasia	1.7	0	Multiple
	3007	W. Krivit	RCS	6.6	0	Multiple (CNS)
	3012	V. Marinkovick	RCS	3.1	0	Multiple (CNS)
	3036	R. Schwartz Z. Tomkiewicz	Astrocytoma	3.5	0.1	CNS
	3044	C. Huntley	RCS	2.3	0	Multiple
	3045	J. Whisnant	Malignant lymphoma NOS	7.3	Alive	GI
Immunoblastic sarcoma of B-cells	3019	D. McKeell	Histiocytic lymphoma	20.1	0	LN
	3035	M. Tamar	RCS	3.8	0	Multiple (CNS)
	3018	R. Holland K. Heidelberger L. Skendzel	Histiocytic lymphoma	18.8	0.4	CNS
Lymphoplasmacytoid tumor	3003	G. Guin	RCS	1.7	0	Multiple (CNS)
	3031	W. London	Microglioma	8.2	0.9	CNS
	3046	J. Corrigan P. Johnson	Malignant lymphoma Poorly differentiated	3.1	1.6	CNS
Follicular centre cell/polymorphic B-cell lymphoma	3009	J. Miller	Histiocytic lymphoma	6.2	0.1	Multiple (CNS)
PI, polymorphic B-cell lymphoma	3017	M. Schulkind R. Weber	Hodgkin's disease	7.5	1.3	Multiple (CNS)
	3081	A. Filipovich	Polymorphic B-cell lymphoma	8.9	0.2	CNS Pericardium
Hodgkin's disease	3020	P. Periman	Hodgkin's disease	16.9	1.5	LN, spleen, liver
	3050	G. Schechter	Hodgkin's disease	32	Alive	LN, spleen
Immunoblastic sarcoma of T-cells	3027	R. Freeman	Histiocytic lymphoma	17.5	1.1	Skin
	3037	R. Heyn	Histiocytic lymphoma	22.3	3.7	LN
	3043	S. Leiken	Histiocytic lymphoma	2.9	0.5	CNS

RES, Reticuloendothelial system; RCS, reticulum cell sarcoma; NOS, not otherwise specified; GI, gastrointestinal tract; LN, lymph node.

probes for EBER-1 and latent membrane protein-1 (LMP-1) [17]. An important related observation emerged from the analysis of lymphoid tissues from WAS patients that had not yet developed lymphoma, or tissues that were not involved with a histologically identifiable lymphoproliferative process. In tissues from the three patients available for study, numerous scattered EBER-1-positive LMP-1-negative lymphocytes were repeatedly detected. The distribution and frequency of these cells was similar to the pattern observed in patients with acute infectious mononucleosis.

EBV-associated B-cell lymphoproliferative disease has become recognized as a particularly frequent complication following attempts at T-depleted haploidentical bone marrow transplantation in WAS (approximately 50% incidence) [25]; virologic studies of tumor tissues both pre- and posttransplant implicate EBV as an important cofactor in the development of lymphoproliferative disease in WAS patients. Chronic immunoregulatory dysfunction has long been suspected in WAS as reflected by frequent findings of enlarged lymph nodes, splenomegaly and the high incidence of a variety of autoimmune complications.

Ataxia telangiectasia

Ataxia telangiectasia (AT) is an autosomal recessive disorder associated with chromosomal breakage and/or instability. Ataxia due to cerebellar degeneration, oculocutaneous telangiectasia and sinopulmonary infections are common features of this disorder. AT can serve as a model for the association between abnormal chromosomal rearrangement and lymphoid malignancies. Roughly half of reported tumors in AT are non-Hodgkin's lymphomas: 69 out of 150 ICR cases (46%). In addition, 21.3% of ICR cases (32 out of 150) were reported as leukemias. Both B- and T-cell malignancies occur. Following exposure to DNA-damaging agents, such as X-irradiation, AT cells fail to pause and repair damage, but rush on to DNA replication. It appears that one of the functions of the AT gene (localized to 11q22–23) [11] is to activate the normal 'tumor suppressor' gene p53 in response to DNA damage. Among its other roles p53 protein functions as a transcription factor to upregulate expression of a DNA repair gene, GADD45, which triggers the G_1 check point in the cell cycle, allowing damaged DNA to be repaired before the cell enters S phase [26].

In AT, a variable, but limited number of lymphocytes carry productive rearrangements of immunoglobulin and T-cell receptor chains. This finding may explain the variable development of the immune repertoire and the continuous predisposition to acquired cytogenetic changes which can lead to malignant transformation of lymphocytes [27] in this disorder. During normal lymphopoiesis DNA strands must be cut as a prerequisite to productive splicing of templates for immunoglobulin or T-cell receptor (TCR) proteins. In the course of rearrangement, opportunities arise for cut segments to reattach erroneously to mismatched gene sequences from other chromosomes which are simultaneously attempting productive splicing (e.g., 7q34-TCRβ chain sequence may attach to 14q11α-chain gene rather than to a nearby appropriate 7qβ sequence). Since gene rearrangement during lymphopoiesis is relatively error prone, certain 'nonrandom' translocations involving immunoglobulin or TCR genes (cited above) can be found in 1/200–1/500 peripheral blood T-cells in normal individuals [28]. Chromosome analyses comparing AT lymphocytes with normal lymphocytes reveal a 25-fold increase in the incidence of such acquired, 'nonrandom' rearrangements involving the immunoglobulin supergene family in AT [28].

Study of translocations observed in B- and T-cell malignancies from AT patients suggests that two mechanisms are commonly associated with malignant transformation: (1) translocations between members of the pair of number 14 chromosomes followed by clonal deletion of one of the two translocation partners; and (2) translocations of 14q32, the joining regions of Ig heavy genes (and less often 2p12 and 22q11, immunoglobulin light chain regions) with 8q24 (c-*myc*). The latter cytogenetic changes in AT lymphoid malignancies bear remarkable similarities to rearrangements observed in lymphoid tumors from normal individuals [29]. Thus, the AT defect appears to magnify a common mechanism of lymphomagenesis.

IMMUNODEFICIENCIES ASSOCIATED WITH OTHER DISEASES

The hyper-IgE syndrome first described in 1966 as Job's syndrome is characterized clinically by desquamating eczematoid skin rash, staphylococcal abscesses and draining otitis media [30]. Markedly elevated IgE levels are usually detected, while other laboratory abnormalities including eosinophilia, neutrophil chemotactic defects and alterations in T-cell subsets or function are variable. Several cases of lymphoma have been reported in hyper-IgE syndrome – both in the literature [31], and to the ICR. Owing to inconsistencies in the use of strict criteria for the diagnosis of hyper-IgE syndrome, the inheritance pattern remains unclear, and it has been difficult to estimate the risk of lymphoma. However, a recent study of serum cytokines in six patients with well-documented hyper-IgE syndrome has revealed a profound deficiency of circulating alpha interferon, a negative regulatory signal for terminal B-cell activation, proliferation and IgE synthesis in six of six patients studied [32]. This observation leads us to speculate that in hyper-IgE syndrome T-cell immunoregulatory abnormalities may underlie the overproduction of IgE and also contribute to the risk of lymphomas.

X-Linked lymphoproliferative syndrome, first published as Duncan's syndrome [33], has been postulated to represent an unusual susceptibility to overwhelming EBV infection. This disorder carries a high risk of B-cell lymphoma in the boys who survive infectious mononucleosis. Histopathologically, lymphomas in XLP are variable, but some tumors bear considerable resemblance to posttransplant EBV-related BLPD, and the GI tract is a frequent primary site [34]. In addition to susceptibility to EBV infection, XLP patients demonstrate variable susceptibility to other opportunistic infections and display an attenuated ability to form a variety of specific antibodies [35].

PHAGOCYTIC DEFECTS

Chediak–Higashi syndrome (CHS) is the only genetically determined immunodeficiency classified as a primary phagocytic defect which has historically been associated with a significant risk of 'cancer'. This rare autosomal recessive disease is characterized by partial albinism, frequent pyogenic infections and abnormal granules in both polymorphonuclear cells and lymphoid cells. In addition to neutrophil dysfunction, CHS patients have been reported to have variable dysfunction of natural killer and T-cells in the laboratory. The majority of CHS patients eventually develop a systemic complication termed the 'accelerated phase' which is universally fatal (unless successful marrow transplantation can be performed). This process is manifested with fevers, heptosplenomegaly and lymphadenopathy, pancytopenia, coagulopathy, widespread lymphohistiocytic organ infiltrates, and has been frequently diagnosed as malignancy. Based on a review of pathologic descriptions from the literature and multiple immunologic and virologic analyses of tissues from seven patients with CHS in the accelerated phase seen at our institution (four of these cases are reviewed in [36]), we favor the possibility that this disorder is a reactive lymphohistiocytic proliferation consistent with hemophagocytic lymphohistiocytosis (HLH) [37], typically following exposure to EBV (see description of HLH below).

Although historical data in CHS are probably unreliable for estimating cancer risk, we cannot discount the possibility that CHS patients may have an increased risk of true lymphomas compared to the general population. Cases characteristic of Hodgkin's disease [38] and T-cell lymphoma [39] have been published in CHS patients.

HEMOPHAGOCYTIC LYMPHOHISTIOCYTOSIS

HLH is the term adopted by the Histiocyte Society [37] to describe a life-threatening hemodestructive syndrome which occurs in several disorders, including both a congenital disease with autosomal recessive inheritance called familial hemophagocytic lymphohistiocytosis (FHL) [40] and an acquired form termed viral- or infection-associated hemophagocytic syndrome (VAHS or IAHS) [41]. Clinical presentation of HLH usually includes prolonged fever, failure to thrive, irritability and hepatosplenomegaly. Associated laboratory features include pancytopenia, hypertriglyceridemia and hypofibrinogenemia. The characteristic histopathologic finding is diffuse infiltration, primarily of the liver, spleen, bone marrow, lymph nodes and brain, by activated non-Langerhan histiocytes actively phagocytizing blood cells. Foci of lymphoid proliferation also occur. It is currently believed that HLH represents an exaggerated immune response which escapes from normal regulatory control mechanisms [42]. The immune dysregulation may be primary, as in the inherited form of FHL, XLP syndrome, or CHS, or it may be secondary, as in VAHS/IAHS. HLH can also occur as a secondary complication of lymphoma when tumor-derived factors (cytokines) may suppress normal host immune responses or release factors which stimulate hemophagocytosis [43].

Indeed, persistent T-cell activation and overproduction of cytokines have been proposed as major factors in the pathophysiology of HLH. Patients with active HLH have many markers of T-cell activation, including increased class II expression by T-cells, marked elevation of serum soluble interleukin-2 (IL-2) receptors [44], and increased levels of soluble CD8 [45]. Inflammatory cytokines such as serum interferon-γ, interleukin-6 (IL-6) and tumor necrosis factor are also elevated in the sera of patients, and increased levels correlate with disease activity [46].

The most consistent immunologic abnormality described in HLH has been impaired natural killer (NK) function [47]. Interestingly, reversible loss of NK function has also been reported in patients with CHS [48] and in boys with X-linked lymphoproliferations [49].

The biological basis of increased susceptibility to lymphoproliferative disorders in patients with immunodeficiencies

At least three major biological factors, occurring alone or in conjunction with one another, contribute to the high incidence of non-Hodgkin's lymphoma or BLPD in immunodeficient hosts. These are: (1) the ubiquity of the Epstein–Barr virus; (2) host defects in immunoregulation resulting in imbalanced cytokine production; and (3) genetic defects resulting in imprecise and/or ineffective rearrangement of immunoglobulin and T-cell receptor genes during lymphopoiesis (as described above for ataxia telangiectasia).

EBV infection is a major cofactor in many, but not all, B-cell lymphoproliferative processes. Immunodeficient hosts can acquire EBV through primary infection, through transfer with organs or tissues at transplant, or from blood transfusions.

EBV can also be reactivated during immunosuppressive therapy. During primary infection, EBV immortalizes B-lymphocytes *in vivo*, resulting in polyclonal activation and proliferation. BCRF-1, one of the EBV genes, has been found to inhibit the production of tumor necrosis factor and interferon gamma by host T-lymphocytes – lymphokines, which normally synergize to kill virus-infected cells. In this way, BCRF-1, which bears marked sequence homology to cellular interleukin-10, may protect the EBV-infected cells from destruction.

In the normal host, EBV-driven lymphoproliferation is thought to be primarily controlled by EBV-specific autologous cytotoxic T-cells [which are major histocompatibility complex (MHC) restricted], with a lesser role being played by humoral responses, antibody-dependent cellular cytotoxicity, NK cell activity, and possibly endogenous interferons. This complex of EBV-specific immunologic control is delicately balanced to maintain the EBV in latency following primary infection. In the immunodeficient host, suppressor and cytotoxic functions (both antigen-specific and MHC-restricted, as well as nonspecific) are often defective, and the production of regulatory cytokines which maintain the conditions favoring viral latency may become unbalanced, permitting virus production and infection of additional clones of B-cells. However, the role of virus replication and infection of additional cells in this process is not known – latently infected B-cells capable of proliferation may be more than sufficient

to account for the consequences of impairment of EBV-specific immunity.

It is hypothesized that B-cells which are already EBV-transformed may have a growth advantage in the setting of polyclonal lymphocyte proliferation. The high mitotic index of EBV-transformed cells increases the probability of mutations involving proto-oncogenes or tumor suppressor genes giving rise to populations of B-cells which will no longer be susceptible to ambient regulatory stimuli. Some of these resistant clones may carry cytogenetic rearrangements.

While EBV has been found in virtually all tumor samples of posttransplant BLPD (both solid organ and bone marrow), the association between EBV and primary immunodeficiencies is not universal. In a retrospective analysis of paraffin sections bequested to the ICR, 16 'lymphomas' were evaluated for the presence of the EBV genome using probes for EBER by *in situ* hybridization and LMP-1 with immunoperoxidase staining. The histopathology of each specimen was also independently determined using current criteria for classification of lymphoid tumors. All specimens consistent with NHL had either diffuse large-cell or immunoblastic histologies. NHL in SCID (2/2) and WAS (5/5) were both EBER-1 and LMP-1 positive. On the other hand, two out of two NHL in AT patients and one case of immunoproliferative small intestine disease in a patient with combined immunodeficiency were EBER-1 negative. In a similar review of lymphoproliferative lesions in patients with CVID from the National Institutes of Health (NIH), EBV was identified in one of two NHL by *in situ* hybridization [50]. Interestingly, all five cases of 'lymphoma' reclassified as Hodgkin's disease from the ICR were found to contain EBER-1-positive and LMP-1-positive Reed–Sternberg cells (two AT patients and three patients with X-linked hyper-IgM syndrome). The EBER-1-positive HD cases had either nodular sclerosis or mixed cellularity histology [17].

While these findings emphasize the importance of EBV as a cofactor in lymphoproliferative disorders connected with immunodeficiencies, it is clear that other factors, possibly other microbes, and/or significant endogenous immunoregulatory dysfunction are at play in the pathogenesis of 'lymphomas' in the context of immunodeficiency.

The second circumstance favoring the development of lymphoproliferative disorders in immunodeficient hosts is defective immunoregulation following B- and T-cell activation. Although their number, subset distribution and functional repertoire may not be normal, virtually all immunodeficient patients (with the exception of certain forms of SCID) possess B- and/or T-cells capable of activation. Indeed, owing to circumstances peculiar to the immunodeficient settings, stimulation of some subsets of lymphocytes may be unusually intense and/or prolonged. The majority of patients with primary immunodeficiencies (as listed in Table 19.1) have defects in formation of specific protective antibodies such that they are unable to eliminate respiratory and gastrointestinal pathogens promptly and are therefore prone to chronic antigenic stimulation. T-Cells which are chronically stimulated produce a variable array of lymphokines that favor lymphocyte multiplication. Some of these lymphokines can promote the recruitment of cytotoxic T-cells, and others favor B-cell proliferation.

At the same time, relative or selective deficiencies in the production of downregulating lymphokines are found in many immunodeficient settings. It appears likely that the T-cell subset similar to the murine T_{H1} population, which produces interferons and IL-2, is quantitatively or qualitatively reduced in many primary immunodeficiency states. On the other hand, increased levels of cytokines which are believed to be critical to normal terminal B-cell differentiation such as IL-4 and IL-10 (characteristic of T_{H2} type cells) have been documented in patients with primary and secondary immunodeficiencies who have developed EBV-associated BLPD [51].

In summary, there is developing information pertinent to the mechanisms whereby the abnormalities present in various primary immunodeficiencies contribute to the observed increased incidence of lymphoproliferative disorders in these syndromes. Two important categories of abnormalities in this respect are the defects that impair DNA repair and thus hinder successful Ig and TCR gene rearrangements, and the functional imbalances in cytokine production by activated subsets of T-helper cells and/or other immune cells, that promote terminal B-cell proliferation and/or inhibit the development of cytotoxic effector cells.

References

1. Filipovich AH, Heinitz KJ, Robison L, et al. The Immunodeficiency Cancer Registry. A research resource. *Am. J. Ped. Hem. Oncol.* 1987, **9**: 183–184.
2. Perry GS III, Spector BD, Schuman LM, et al. The Wiskott–Aldrich syndrome in the United States and Canada (1892–1979). *J. Pediat.* 1980, **97**: 72–78.
3. Morrell D, Cromatie E, Swift M. Mortality and cancer incidence in 263 patients with ataxia-telangiectasia. *J. Natl Cancer Inst.* 1986, **77**: 89–92.
4. Cunningham-Rundles C, Siegal FP, Cunningham-Rundles S, et al. Incidence of cancer in 98 patients with common varied immunodeficiency. *J. Clin. Immunol.* 1987, **7**: 294–299.
5. Scientific Group on Immunodeficiency. Primary immunodeficiency diseases. Report of a WHO sponsored meeting. *Immunodeficiency Rev.* 1989, **1**: 173–205.
6. Gatti RA, Good RA. Occurrence of malignancy in immunodeficiency diseases. A literature review. *Cancer* 1971, **28**: 89–98.
7. Noguchi M, Yi H, Rosenblatt HM, et al. Interleukin-2 receptor gamma chain mutation results in X-linked severe combined immunodeficiency in humans. *Cell* 1993, **73**: 147–157.
8. Tsukada S, Saffran DC, Rawlings DJ, et al. Deficient expression of a B-cell cytoplasmic tyrosine kinase in human X-linked agammaglobulinemia. *Cell* 1993, **72**: 279–290.
9. Callard RE, Armitage RJ, Fanslow WC, et al. *Immunol. Today* 1993, **14**: 559–564.
10. Derry JMJ, Ochs HD, Francke U. Isolation of a novel gene mutated in Wiskott–Aldrich syndrome. *Cell* 1994, **78**: 635–644.
11. Gatti RA, Berkel I, Boder E, et al. Localization of an ataxia-telangiectasia gene to chromosome 11q22–23. *Nature* 1988, **336**: 577–580.
12. Driscoll DA, Budarf ML, Emanuel BS. A genetic etiology for DiGeorge syndrome: Consistent deletions and microdeletions of 22q11. *Am. J. Human Genet.* 1992, **50**: 924–933.
13. Kersey JH, Spector BD, Good RA. In Klein G, Weinhouse S, Haddow A (eds) *Advances in Cancer Research*. New York: Academic Press, 1973, pp. 211–230.
14. Filipovich AH, Shapiro RS. Tumors in patients with common variable immunodeficiency. *J. Immunol. Immunopharmacol.* 1991, **XI**: 43–46.
15. Filipovich AH, Stoker V, Robison L, et al. Lymphomas in severe combined immunodeficiency syndrome (SCID): Report of the Immunodeficiency-Cancer Registry (ICR). *Blood* 1984, **64**: 155a.
16. Kersey HJ, Filipovich AH, Spector BD, et al. Lymphoma after thymus transplantation. *N. Engl. J. Med.* 1980, **302**: 301–302.
17. Ambinder RF, Mann RB, Barletta JM, et al. Association of Epstein–Barr virus (EBV) with Hodgkin's disease (HD) in patients with primary immunodeficiency and frequent detection of EBV in lymphoid tissue without neoplastic involvement in Wiskott–Aldrich syndrome (WAS): A survey of EBV in archival tissues from the Immunodeficiency Cancer Registry (ICR). *Blood* 1992, **80**: 118a.
18. Chan AC, Kadlecek TA, Elder ME, et al. ZAP-70 deficiency in an autosomal recessive form of severe combined immunodeficiency. *Science* 1994, **264**: 1599–1601.
19. Schwarz K, Hansen-Hagge TE, Bartram CR. Recombinase deficiency in mouse and man. *Immunodeficiency* 1993, **4**: 249–250.
20. Lederman HM, Winkelstein JA. X-linked agammaglobulinemia: an analysis of 96 patients. *Medicine* 1985, **64**: 145–156.
21. Hermans PE, Diax-Buxo JA, Stobo JD. Idiopathic late onset immunoglobulin deficiency. Clinical observations in 50 patients. *Am. J. Med.* 1976, **61**: 221–237.

22. Kinlen LJ, Webster AD, Bird A, et al. Prospective study of cancer in patients with hypogammaglobulinemia. *Lancet* 1985, **1**: 263–266.
23. Schaffer FM, Palermos J, Zhu ZB, et al. Individuals with IgA deficiency and common variable immunodeficiency share polymorphisms of major histocompatibility complex class III genes. *Proc. Natl Acad. Sci.* 1989, **86**: 8015–8019.
24. Cotelingam JD, Witebsky FG, Hsu SM, et al. Malignant lymphoma in patients with the Wiskott–Aldrich syndrome. *Cancer Invest.* 1985, **3**: 515–522.
25. Fischer A, Friedrich W, Fasth A. Reduction of graft failure by a monoclonal antibody (anti-LFA-1 CD11a) after HLA nonidentical bone marrow transplantation in children with immunodeficiencies, osteopetrosis, and Fanconi's anemia: a European Group for Immunodeficiency/European Group for Bone Marrow Transplantation report. *Blood* 1991, **77**: 249–256.
26. Prokocimer M, Rotter V. Structure and function of p53 in normal cells and their aberrations in cancer cells. *Blood* 1994, **84**: 2391–2411.
27. Hecht F, McCaw BK. Chromosome instability syndromes. In Mulvivill JJ (ed.) *Genetics of Human Cancer*. New York: Raven Press, 1977, pp. 105–123.
28. Hecht F, Hecht BKM. Chromosome changes connect immunodeficiency and cancer in ataxia-telangiectasia. *Am. J. Ped. Hem. Oncol.* 1987, **9**: 185–189.
29. Finger LR, Harvey RD, Moore RC, et al. A common mechanism of chromosomal translocation in T- and B-cell neoplasia. *Science* 1986, **234**: 982–985.
30. Davis SD, Schaller J, Wedgwood RJ. Job's syndrome, recurrent, 'cold', staphylococcal abcesses. *Lancet* 1966, **1**: 1013–1015.
31. Bale JF Jr, Wilson JF, Hill HR. Fatal histiocytic lymphoma of the brain associated with hyperimmunoglobulinemia-E and recurrent infections. *Cancer* 1977, **39**: 2386–2390.
32. Kamat D, Mathur A, Shapiro RS, et al. Deficiency of circulating alpha interferon (IFNα) in hyper immunoglobulin syndrome (HIES). *Ped. Res.* 1992, **31**: 151A.
33. Purtilo DT, Cassel C, Yang JPS, et al. X-linked recessive progressive combined variable immunodeficiency (Duncan's disease). *Lancet* 1975, **1**: 935–940.
34. Harrington DS, Weisenburger DD, Purtilo DT. Malignant lymphoma in the X-linked lymphoproliferative syndrome. *Cancer* 1987, **59**: 1419–1429.
35. Purtilo DT, Grierson HL. Methods of detection of new families with X-linked lymphoproliferative disease. *Cancer Genet. Cytogenet.* 1991, **51**: 143–153.
36. Rubin CM, Burke BA, McKenna RW, et al. The accelerated phase of Chediak–Higashi syndrome. An expression of the virus-associated hemophagocytic syndrome? *Cancer* 1985, **56**: 524–530.
37. Henter JI, Elinder G, Soder O, et al. Hypercytokinemia in familial hemophagocytic lymphohistiocytosis. *Blood* 1991, **78**: 2918–2922.
38. Tan C, Eteubanas E, Lieberman P, et al. Chediak–Higashi syndrome in a child with Hodgkin's disease. *Am. J. Dis. Child.* 1971, **121**: 135–139.
39. Argyle JC, Kjeldsberg CR, Marty J, et al. T-cell lymphoma and the Chediak–Higashi syndrome. *Blood* 1982, **60**: 672–676.
40. Farquhar JW, Claireaux AF. Familial haemophagocytic reticulosis. *Arch. Dis. Child.* 1952, **27**: 519–525.
41. Risdall RJ, McKenna RW, Nesbit ME, et al. Virus-associated hemophagocytic syndrome: A benign histiologic proliferation distinct from malignant histiocytosis. *Cancer* 1979, **44**: 993–1002.
42. Stark B, Cohen IJ, Pecht M, et al. Immunologic dysregulation in a patient with familial hemophagocytic lymphohistiocytosis. *Cancer* 1987, **60**: 2629–2636.
43. Jaffe ES, Costa J, Fauci AS, et al. Malignant lymphoma and erythrogocytosis simulating malignant histiocytosis. *Am. J. Med.* 1983, **75**: 741–749.
44. Komp DM, McNamara J, Buckley P. Elevated soluble interleukin-2 receptor in childhood hemophagocytic histiocytic syndromes. *Blood* 1989, **73**: 2128–2132.
45. Henter JI, Elinder G, Soder O, et al. Hypercytokinemia in familial hemophagocytic lymphohistiocytosis. *Blood* 1991, **78**: 2918–2922.
46. Holtman H, Janka GE, Weidner E, et al. Impaired natural killer cell function in familial hemophagocytic lymphohistiocytosis. *Immunology* 1982, **162**: 364–371.
47. Perez N, Virelizier JL, Arenazan-Seisdedos F, et al. Impaired natural killer activity in lymphohistiocytosis syndrome. *J. Pediatr.* 1984, **104**: 569–573.
48. Ladisch S, Poplack DG, Holiman B, et al. Immunodeficiency in familial erythrophagocytic lymphohistiocytosis. *Lancet* 1976, **1**: 581–583.
49. Harada S, Bechtold T, Seeley TD, et al. Cell-mediated immunity to Epstein–Barr virus (EBV) and natural killer (NK)-cell activity in the X-linked lymphoproliferative syndrome. *Int. J. Cancer* 1982, **30**: 739–744.
50. Sander CA, Medeiros LJ, Weiss LM, et al. Lymphoproliferative lesions in patients with common variable immunodeficiency syndrome. *Am. J. Surg. Pathol.* 1992, 16: 1170–1182.
51. Mathur A, Kamat DM, Filipovich AH, et al. Immunoregulatory abnormalities in patients with Epstein–Barr virus-associated B-cell lymphoproliferative disorders. *Transplantation* 1994, **57**: 1042–1045.

CHAPTER 20

Pathology and pathogenesis of non-Hodgkin's lymphomas associated with HIV infection

DANIEL M. KNOWLES

Introduction

Approximately one year after the initial cases of acquired immune deficiency syndrome (AIDS) were described, Doll and List reported a young immunocompromised homosexual man with Burkitt's lymphoma [1]. A few months later, Ziegler and colleagues reported four cases of advanced stage Burkitt's-like lymphoma in immunocompromised homosexual men [2,3]. Subsequently, a large, multi-institutional study of homosexual men who developed malignant lymphoma [4], several large clinical series of AIDS-associated lymphoma reported from the endemic areas of Los Angeles [5,6], Houston [7] and New York City [8,9], as well as numerous other reports of smaller numbers of cases of AIDS-associated lymphoma [10–12], led to widespread recognition of this new aspect of the AIDS epidemic. These reports encouraged the Centers for Disease Control and Preventon (CDC) to expand its criteria for the diagnosis of AIDS in 1987 to include human immunodeficiency virus (HIV)-seropositive individuals who develop intermediate or high-grade non-Hodgkin's lymphoma (NHL) of B-cell or indeterminate phenotype, even in the absence of opportunistic infections and Kaposi's sarcoma [13]. AIDS-associated NHLs displaying clinical, morphologic and immunologic characteristics similar to the cases initially described in the United States have been observed with increasing frequency worldwide [14–19].

Non-Hodgkin's lymphoma is now widely recognized as the second most common neoplasm occur-

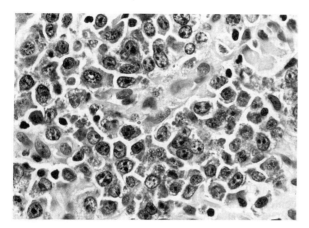

Figure 20.2   An AIDS-associated large-cell, immunoblastic, plasmacytoid lymphoma. The neoplastic cells are larger and show more variabilty in size and shape than those comprising small, noncleaved cell lymphoma and large-cell lymphoma. The nuclei are sometimes eccentrically placed and are surrounded by abundant amphophilic cytoplasm containing a paranuclear *hof* that imparts a plasmacytoid appearance to the malignant cells (H & E, × 630).

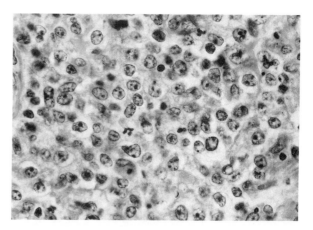

Figure 20.3   An AIDS-associated large, noncleaved cell lymphoma. The neoplastic cells contain moderately abundant cytoplasm and generally round regular nuclei containing a single nucleolus lying adjacent to the nuclear membrane (H & E, × 630). (Reproduced with permission from Knowles and Chadburn [20].)

Immunophenotypic and immunogenotypic characteristics

The vast majority of AIDS-associated NHLs express monotypic surface immunoglobulin and/or B-cell-associated antigens CD19, CD20 and CD22 and lack T-cell-associated antigens, consistent with derivation from the B-cell lineage [4–6,9,18,37–39]. Most AIDS-associated SNCC lymphomas express monotypic surface immunoglobulin, usually IgMκ; approximately 75% express CD10, and only about 10% express CD21, the C3d/Epstein–Barr virus receptor. In contrast, approximately 50% of LC and IBP lymphomas express monotypic surface immunoglobulin of variable isotype, approximately 30% express CD10, and about 67% express CD21 [9,39]. These findings suggest that most AIDS-associated B-cell NHLs exhibit immunophenotypes similar to those expressed by morphologically comparable B-cell NHLs unassociated with HIV infection occurring in the general population [9,39].

AIDS-associated NHLs displaying B-cell immunophenotypes consistently exhibit clonal immunoglobulin heavy chain and light chain gene rearrangements, and lack clonal T-cell receptor beta-chain gene rearrangements – molecular confirmation of their B-cell derivation [9,37,39–41]. On Southern

blot analysis one or two high-intensity, rearranged bands of immunoglobulin heavy chain gene origin are usually observed, and one or more faint, rearranged bands may also be present [37] (Figure 20.4). The high-intensity bands represent the malignant clonal B-cell population, which often carries a rearranged c-*myc* gene (discussed below). The faint, rearranged bands may represent additional minor B-cell clones. Such clones have been identified in approximately 20% of hyperplastic lymph nodes obtained from HIV-infected individuals who have the persistent generalized lymphadenopathy (PGL) syndrome [37]. These clones lack evidence of malignant transformation, such as c-*myc* gene rearrangements. They may persist in some lymph nodes that become replaced by malignant lymphoma, thus accounting for the additional faint, rearranged bands observed in these cases.

Sites of disease

One of the major characteristics of patients with AIDS-associated NHL is the presence of widely disseminated disease, including a high frequency of extranodal involvement, at initial presentation. Approximately two-thirds of patients have stage III or IV disease and another 20% have stage IE disease initially [9,15,19]. However, even those patients who have stage IE disease usually have large, bulky tumor masses. Thus, very few patients present with localized lymph node-based disease [4,6,9,27]. The

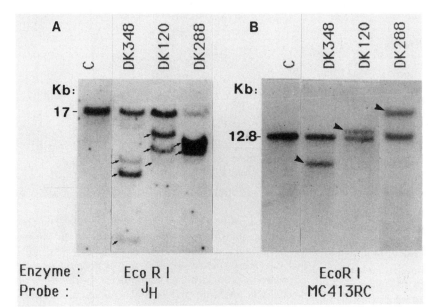

Figure 20.4 Southern blot hybridization analysis of AIDS-associated non-Hodgkin's lymphomas for rearrangements of the immunoglobulin heavy chain gene and the c-*myc* gene. Aliquots of DNA extracted from the indicated cases and from normal human placenta (C, control) were digested with EcoRI and hybridized to an immunoglobulin heavy chain joining region (JH) probe (panel A, left) and to probe MC413RC, representative of the third exon of the c-*myc* gene (panel B, right). Arrows indicate rearranged bands. The control lane (C) shows the germline configuration. All three AIDS-associated NHLs examined here exhibit clonal immunoglobulin heavy chain gene and c-*myc* gene rearrangement. All AIDS-associated NHLs exhibiting a B-cell immunophenotype display clonal immunoglobulin heavy chain gene rearrangements, indicative of a clonal B-cell derivation. Some of the neoplasms display more than two rearranged bands, often of varying intensity, in addition to the germline band. These bands may represent minor B-cell clones that are present in addition to the dominant malignant B-cell lymphoma. (Reproduced with permission from Knowles and Dalla-Favera [41a].)

most frequently involved extranodal sites are the CNS, the gastrointestinal tract and the bone marrow [4,6,9,15,18,27,42,43]. Patients with non-AIDS-associated intermediate- and high-grade NHLs may present with extranodal disease as well. However, the extranodal sites of lymphomatous involvement in AIDS-associated NHL are relatively distinct. This is primarily because of the greatly increased incidence of primary CNS lymphoma [4,38,43–45] but also because certain extranodal locations that are uncommonly observed as primary sites of NHL in non-HIV-infected individuals, such as the rectum, anus and heart, among others, are frequent sites of origin of AIDS-associated NHL [4,38,43, 46–49].

CENTRAL NERVOUS SYSTEM

The CNS is the most common extranodal site of involvement by AIDS-associated NHL [32,43]. Approximately 20–40% of patients who have AIDS-associated NHL, especially those who have bone marrow infiltration, have CNS involvement at presentation [4,6,7,9,27]; two-thirds of the patients have CNS involvement at autopsy [50]. The majority of patients who have systemic malignant lymphoma with secondary CNS involvement have leptomenin-

geal infiltration and lack solid parenchymal masses [50] (Figure 20.5). Neoplastic cells may be present in cerebrospinal fluid (CSF) samples obtained from these individuals [32,38,51].

In addition to the high frequency of secondary CNS involvement, as many as 20% of all AIDS-associated NHLs present as intracranial parenchymal lesions limited to the CNS, that is, are primary CNS lymphomas [4,21,27,50,52] (Figure 20.6). In fact, AIDS is now the most common risk factor for the development of primary CNS lymphoma. In a recent review of 1286 adults with AIDS, primary CNS lymphoma was found in eight patients at presentation and subsequently developed in 25 additional patients [53]. In contrast, spontaneous primary CNS lymphoma occurs uncommonly, primarily in elderly individuals, and constitutes less than 1.5% of all primary brain tumors [54].

AIDS-associated primary CNS lymphomas are intracranial parenchymal tumors. The lesions are often quite large, sometimes over 3 cm [55,56]. They most commonly occur in the cerebrum, but they also frequently occur in the basal ganglia, cerebellum and brainstem [45,56–59]. They are characterized by multifocality, indistinct borders, and a granular surface grossly [45]. They are nearly always found to be multicentric upon microscopic examination at autopsy [45,50,59] (Figure 20.6). The neoplastic

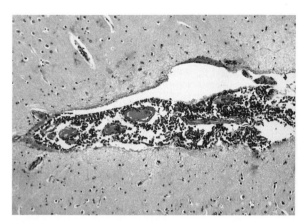

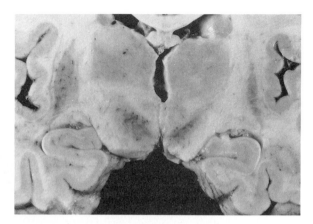

Figure 20.5 Secondary CNS involvement by a NHL. An HIV-positive heterosexual woman presented with massive bone marrow replacement and peripheral blood involvement by B-cell acute lymphoblastic leukemia or Burkitt's lymphoma in leukemic phase, accompanied by meningeal signs. Malignant lymphoid cells were identified in a cerebrospinal fluid sample. Examination at autopsy revealed extensive leptomeningeal infiltration by neoplastic lymphoid cells without solid parenchymal masses, consistent with secondary CNS involvement (H & E, × 100). (Reproduced with permission from Knowles and Chadburn [20].)

Figure 20.6 An AIDS-associated primary CNS NHL. The infiltrative nature of the lymphoma is manifested on the left by the uniform enlargement of the thalamus and subthalamic area whereas its tendency to be multifocal is illustrated by more localized tumor foci in the dorsolateral thalamus (arrowhead) and contralateral temporal white matter (arrow) (figure courtesy of Dr James Powers, University of Rochester). (Reproduced with permission from Knowles and Chadburn [20].)

cells are characteristically distributed along vascular channels as perivascular cellular cuffs [45,56,59]. Frank meningeal involvement, including the presence of diagnostic malignant cells in the CSF, is only observed in 15–25% of cases [44,45]. The great majority of AIDS-associated primary CNS lymphomas display IBP and LC morphology [9,18,44, 45,50,52,56,59]; most AIDS-associated SNCC lymphomas observed in the CNS represent secondary involvement.

GASTROINTESTINAL TRACT

The gastrointestinal tract appears to be the second most common extranodal site of involvement by AIDS-associated NHL. Approximately 30% of patients have gastrointestinal tract involvement at presentation [9,38], and the majority of patients have gastrointestinal tract and liver involvement at autopsy [50]. The gastrointestinal tract is also a common primary site of origin of AIDS-associated NHL [9,38]. The most frequent sites of origin within the gastrointestinal tract are the stomach and the small intestine [38], but any region from the oropharynx to the rectum and anus, including the liver [60,61], may serve as a primary site of NHL. Some patients have extensive lymphomatous involvement of the entire gastrointestinal tract [38].

A newly recognized frequent manifestation of AIDS is the occurrence of malignant lymphoma in the rectum and anus of homosexual men [38,46–48]. Primary anorectal lymphoma occurs infrequently in the general population. Malignant lymphomas of all histologic types comprise less than 1% of all malignant tumors of the rectum [46,62] and rectal lymphomas represent only approximately 5% of all gastrointestinal tract lymphomas [62–64]. Primary anorectal lymphomas occurring in the general population affect men and women equally, usually occur in the sixth and seventh decades, generally develop high up in the rectum and often exhibit low-grade histology [47,51]. In contrast, AIDS-associated primary anorectal lymphomas usually occur in young homosexual men, median age approximately 35 years, who practice passive anal intercourse with multiple anonymous sexual partners. The lymphomas usually occur in the lower rectum and anal canal, and exhibit SNCC, IBP and LC morphologies. Although most patients initially present with stage IE disease, nearly all of them develop disseminated lymphoma and the median survival is only approximately 7 months [46–48]. The development of anorectal lymphoma in homosexual men in association with AIDS at a specific site of sexual activity is intriguing but the significance is unknown. Anal intercourse has been shown to be a risk factor for the development of anal carcinoma, however [65,66], and by analogy, anal intercourse may play a con-

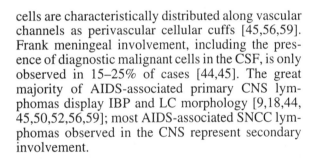

tributory role in the development of anorectal lymphoma as well.

OTHER EXTRANODAL SITES

AIDS-associated NHLs have been reported to arise and/or present in virtually every anatomic site, including the orbit [9,67,68], oral cavity [4,9,18,27], mandible [9,67,69], skin [9,67], salivary glands [9,70], heart [43,49,71], lungs [9,18,43,67], muscles [18], bones [4,18,27], kidneys [4,15,43], testis [9,18] and the adrenal glands [9,43]. Neoplastic cells may even be present in the peripheral blood [9,20] (Figure 20.7). Involvement of these extranodal sites is often a manifestation of widely disseminated disease. However, in many instances, the malignant lymphoma appears to have actually arisen in the particular extranodal site. For example, Constantino and colleagues [71] reported a malignant lymphoma originating in the heart of a 34-year-old IVDA; we have observed two similar cases. Kaplan and associates [72] reported a Burkitt's lymphoma originating in the common bile duct and Levecq and colleagues [73] reported a high-grade B-cell lymphoma arising in an ileostomy stoma in a 73-year-old heterosexual man who had contracted AIDS via transfusion. Regardless of the causative factors, it is clear that AIDS-associated NHLs may arise and/or present in virtually any extranodal site, no matter how isolated or obscure. Therefore, malignant lymphoma should always be considered when a member of an AIDS-risk group presents with a tumor mass, regardless of the site or mode of presentation. Moreover, the atypical presentation of a diffuse aggressive NHL involving an unusual extranodal

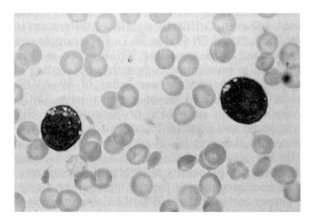

Figure 20.7 Peripheral blood involvement by AIDS-associated small, noncleaved cell lymphoma (Wright stain, × 1000). (Reproduced with permission from Knowles and Dalla-Favera [41a].)

site should always raise a suspicion for HIV infection.

BODY CAVITIES

We recently identified a distinct subset of AIDS-associated NHLs possessing distinct immunophenotypic and molecular genetic characteristics that preferentially arise in and/or involve the body cavities [74]. Almost 20 such cases have now been described in the literature [74–77]. The lymphomas exhibit exclusive or dominant involvement of the pleural, pericardial and/or peritoneal cavities. A lymphomatous effusion, sometimes massive, is the most common presentation. This may or may not be accompanied by a body cavity-based tumor mass. However, sometimes, an obvious tumor mass is lacking even at autopsy. The tumor remains confined to one or more body cavities throughout the clinical course in approximately two-thirds of patients [74–77], although the tumor may spread to visceral or distant sites. The median survival is similar to that of other AIDS-associated NHLs [9], i.e., about 6 months [74–77].

Nearly all the body cavity-based lymphomas reported thus far have been classified as IBP lymphoma; occasional cases have been classified as LC and rare cases as SNCC lymphoma [74–77]. In our experience, these lymphomas usually display marked cellular pleomorphism. They are composed of large round or ovoid to polygonal tumor cells possessing abundant acidophilic to amphophilic cytoplasm, and large, round and regular to highly irregular and even hyperconvoluted nuclei containing one or more nucleoli. A variable proportion of the cells contain an eccentrically placed nucleus accompanied by a paranuclear *hof*, suggesting plasmacytoid differentiation. Pleomorphic binucleate and multinucleate lymphoma cells containing multiple prominent nucleoli reminiscent of Reed–Sternberg cells may be present. Mitotic figures, many of which are atypical, are usually numerous [20,39,74,75] (Figures 20.8 and 20.9).

The neoplastic cells comprising the majority of body cavity-based lymphomas express an indeterminate immunophenotype. They express leukocyte common antigen, but lack surface and cytoplasmic immunoglobulin and B-cell, T-cell and myelomonocytic lineage-restricted antigens. They express various antigens associated with activation, however, including HLA-DR, CD23, CD38, CD71, BL-2, BL-3 and Ki-24. Less than 25% of cases express immunoglobulin or B-cell lineage-specific antigens [74–77]. Thus, the tumor cells are devoid of cell surface antigens associated with the early and middle stages of B-cell differentiation and express antigens

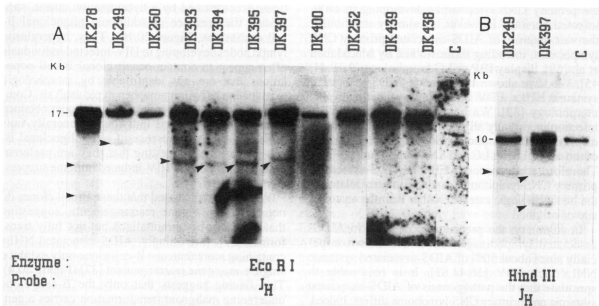

Figure 20.10 Immunoglobulin gene rearrangement analysis of histopathologically benign and immunophenotypically polyclonal lymph nodes obtained from patients who have persistent generalized lymphadenopathy syndrome. The DNA extracted from the indicated cases and from normal human placenta (C, control) were digested with EcoRI or HindIII, and hybridized to an immunoglobulin heavy chain joining region (JH) probe. Arrows indicate rearranged bands. The control lane (C) shows the germline configuration. Many of these hyperplastic lymph nodes display one or more rearranged bands, often of low intensity, indicating the presence of one or more small clonal B-cell expansions. The rearranged bands are sometimes accompanied by a hybridization smear, suggesting the presence of additional oligoclonal B-cell populations. These results suggest that the hyperplastic lymph nodes of HIV-infected persons often contain occult clonal B-cell populations that are not identifiable by morphologic examination or by immunophenotypic analysis. (Reproduced from Pelicci et al. [37] with permission from the Rockefeller University Press by copyright.)

activated c-*myc* gene into EBV-infected lymphoblasts obtained from HIV-infected patients leads to their malignant conversion [106]. Lastly, chromosomal abnormalities frequently occur in the hyperplastic lymph nodes of HIV-infected persons who later develop NHL [107].

Nevertheless, AIDS-associated NHL is preceded by hyperplastic lymphadenopathy in only approximately one-third of individuals [4,9] and only about 5–10% of patients who have PGL actually develop malignant lymphoma [102,108]. It has been reported that patients who previously have PGL significantly more frequently have NHL restricted to lymph nodes [18]. Nevertheless, a high proportion of these malignant lymphomas apparently develop in extranodal sites [9]. Finally, once again, only 50% or less of AIDS-associated systemic NHLs contain clonal EBV [16,41,82]. Therefore, the precise relationship between EBV infection, PGL and the development of NHL in AIDS remains incompletely understood.

ROLE OF PROTO-ONCOGENES

We have shown that approximately 80% of AIDS-associated systemic NHLs exhibit activating alterations involving the c-*myc* proto-oncogene [37,41,82] (Figure 20.4). However, c-*myc* gene alterations are not distributed randomly among different categories of AIDS-associated NHL. Instead, in our experience, all AIDS-associated NHLs displaying SNCC (Burkitt's and non-Burkitt's) morphology and the lymphoma cell lines derived from them, but only about one-third of those displaying LC and IBP morphology, exhibit c-*myc* gene rearrangements (Table 20.3) [82,87]. In contrast, c-*myc* gene rearrangement occurs infrequently among LC and IBP lymphomas occurring in the general population unassociated with AIDS [109], except perhaps in the gastrointestinal tract [110].

Given the high proportion of AIDS-associated NHLs that display c-*myc* gene alterations and the preferential association of this genetic lesion with a specific histopathologic category, it is likely that

Table 20.3 Genetic lesions in AIDS-associated non-Hodgkin's lymphomas

| Genetic lesion | Total | Histopathology | | |
		SNCC	LC	IBP
EBV	42%	31%	25%	100%
bcl-1	0	0	0	0
bcl-2	0	0	0	0
bcl-6	14%	0	25%	19%
c-myc	79%	100%	50%	25%
ras	15%	19%	0	20%
p53	37%	63%	0	0
Rb	0	0	0	0

SNCC, small noncleaved cell; LC, large cell; IBP, immunoblastic, plasmacytoid.

c-myc gene rearrangement contributes to the pathogenesis of AIDS-associated NHL. Several lines of evidence support this conclusion. These include the fact that transgenic mice carrying Ig-*myc* chimeric constructs develop an increased incidence of B-cell lymphoma [111] and that transfection of activated *c-myc* genes into EBV-immortalized lymphoblasts isolated from AIDS patients leads to their malignant transformation [106]. The mechanism by which rearrangement of the *c-myc* proto-oncogene contributes to the pathogenesis of AIDS-associated NHLs may be analogous to the mechanism operational in non-AIDS-associated Burkitt's lymphomas, namely by disrupting the normal control of c-*myc* gene expression. Theoretically, it is possible that one or more biological alterations occurring in AIDS favors the occurrence of chromosomal translocations involving the *c-myc* oncogene. Alternatively, cells in which these translocations have occurred may acquire specific biologic properties that render them especially well suited to expand and progress toward malignancy in the context of immune deficiency. One such alteration may be the downregulation of the integrin recepton leukocyte function-associated antigen 1 (LFA-1) which has been shown to be controlled by c-*myc* in B-cells [112]. Burkitt's lymphoma cells have been shown to lack LFA-1, which is involved in immunorecognition by T-cells and are unable to elicit either autologous or allogeneic T-cell responses *in vitro* [113,114]. Obviously, the effects of such alterations would be markedly amplified in the context of the severe immune deficiency associated with AIDS.

It is now known that several differences exist between endemic (African) and sporadic (Western) Burkitt's lymphoma (Table 20.4). More than 90% of cases of endemic Burkitt's lymphoma are associated with EBV infection and these malignant cells express

Table 20.4 Differences between endemic and sporadic Burkitt's lymphoma

Characteristics	Endemic	Sporadic
EBV associated	+	—
Fc receptor	+	—
C3d (EBV) receptor	+	—
IgM secretion	—	+
c-myc gene breakpoints	Outside *c-myc*	Close to or within *c-myc*
IgH gene breakpoints	Rarely Sμ	More often Sμ

Reproduced with permission from Knowles and Dalla-Favera [41a].

Fc and EBV receptors but do not secrete IgM. In contrast, only a small proportion of sporadic Burkitt's lymphoma is associated with EBV infection and these malignant cells usually lack Fc and EBV receptors and secrete IgM [115]. In addition, we have shown that the translocations involving chromosome 8 may lead to deregulation of the c-*myc* gene via different molecular mechanisms which differ according to the geographical origin of the tumor [109,116–118]. The c-*myc* gene is activated by point mutations or small rearrangements occurring within regulatory regions spanning its first exon–first intron border in t(8;14) associated with endemic (African) Burkitt's lymphoma and the variant translocations t(2;8), t(8;22) associated with both endemic and sporadic (Western) Burkitt's lymphoma. In contrast, the c-*myc* gene is activated by truncations occurring within its first exon, first intron or 5' flanking sequences in t(8;14) associated with sporadic Burkitt's lymphoma [109,116–118]. The pattern of chromosome 14 involvement in t(8;14) is also heterogeneous. c-*myc* recombines preferentially with the joining region of the immunoglobulin heavy chain gene in all Burkitt's lymphomas; the less common immunoglobulin gene switch region breakpoints are more often associated with a rearranged c-*myc* gene and with sporadic Burkitt's lymphoma than with endemic Burkitt's lymphoma (see Chapter 16) [109,116–118]. Thus, the pathogenesis of endemic and sporadic Burkitt's lymphoma differs, perhaps as a consequence of differences in the state of differentiation of the target cells in which the translocational events occur [118].

We have shown that virtually all AIDS-associated SNCC lymphomas exhibit c-*myc* gene rearrangements but that the majority lack EBV DNA sequences and proteins, and also lack Fc and C3d (EBV) receptors [9,37,39,41,82] – characteristics similar to those of sporadic Burkitt's lymphoma [115]. Moreover, we have also shown that the molecular mechanisms leading to c-*myc* gene activation in AIDS-associated NHLs are similar to those in sporadic Burkitt's lymphoma [41,82,109,119]. Therefore, the bulk of the immunologic and molecular genetic evidence suggests that the majority of AIDS-associated NHLs more closely resemble sporadic than endemic Burkitt's lymphoma (Table 20.4).

The *bcl*-2 oncogene is associated with t(14;18) and occurs preferentially in low- and intermediate-grade lymphomas of follicular center cell derivation [120,121]. The putative oncogene *bcl*-1 is associated with t(11;14) and occurs in about 5% of NHLs and lymphoid leukemias (LL) [122], most commonly low-grade mantle cell (centrocytic) lymphomas [123]. We have demonstrated, and others have also found, that AIDS-associated NHLs consistently lack rearrangements of the *bcl*-2 oncogene as well as rearrangements of the putative oncogene *bcl*-1 (Table 20.3) [41,74,122], indicating that AIDS-associated NHLs are not derived from follicular center or mantle zone B-cells, and are not related to follicular center cell and mantle cell lymphomas.

In the process of cloning the chromosomal junctions of translocations involving band 3q27 [124], we identified a candidate oncogene, *bcl*-6, which is structurally altered as a consequence of the translocations [125]. The *bcl*-6 gene codes for a zinc-finger protein sharing homologies with several transcription factors [125,126]. Rearrangements of the *bcl*-6 gene result in translocations within its 5' noncoding regulatory sequences, which presumably leads to deregulated protein expression [125]. We have shown that rearrangements of the *bcl*-6 gene occur in approximately 45% of diffuse large-cell lymphoma but not in follicular lymphoma, SNCC (Burkitt's and Burkitt's-like) lymphoma, acute lymphoblastic leukemia, chronic lymphocytic leukemia or multiple myeloma [127]. Thus, *bcl*-6 gene rearrangements are specifically associated with diffuse large-cell lymphoma. Recently, we demonstrated that this is true among AIDS-associated NHLs as well. We found that 25% and 19% of AIDS-associated LC and IBP lymphomas, respectively, but not SNCC lymphomas, exhibit *bcl*-6 gene rearrangements (Table 20.3) [128]. This is irrespective of the presence or absence of EBV. However, *bcl*-6 gene rearrangements were not detected in any cases containing c-*myc* gene rearrangements or p53 mutations. These findings further support the notion that distinct molecular pathways exist in AIDS lymphomagenesis.

Activation of the *ras* proto-oncogene family by single nucleotide substitutions at codons 12,13 and 61 has been associated with a large number of human malignancies [129]. We recently demonstrated that mutations involving codons 12 or 13 of the N-*ras* gene are detectable in approximately 18% of precursor B-cell acute lymphoblastic leu-

kemias and mutations involving codon 61 of the N-*ras* gene are detectable in approximately 32% of cases of multiple myeloma/plasmacytoma [130, 131]. We were unable to detect mutations involving the H-, K- and N-*ras* genes in any of 143 non-HIV-associated NHLs or LLs. In contrast, we found point mutations involving *ras* genes in four of 27 (15%) AIDS-associated NHLs, one IBP and three SNCC lymphomas (Table 20.3) [82]. The N-*ras* gene was involved in three cases (two A→T transversions at codon 61 and one G→A transition at codon 12) and the K-*ras* gene was involved in one case (G→A transition at codon 12). Thus, *ras* gene mutations represent a potentially distinctive feature of AIDS-associated NHLs compared to non-HIV-associated NHLs of comparable morphology. Although the evidence is still quite preliminary, such differences in the patterns of proto-oncogene alteration suggest that distinct pathogenetic mechanisms may be operational in AIDS-associated lymphomagenesis.

ROLE OF TUMOR SUPPRESSOR GENES

Tumor suppressor genes such as the p53 and retinoblastoma (Rb) genes are believed to play a significant role in the development and progression of human neoplasia when their disruption or loss relieves cells from normal negative regulatory signals [132]. The p53 gene, mapping to the short arm of chromosome 17 (band 17p13), encodes a nuclear phosphoprotein that is believed to play an essential role in cell cycle control [132]. Inactivation of the p53 gene in human tumors is usually the result of point mutations occurring in the coding sequence of exons 5 through 9 in one allele, with or without loss of the corresponding allele [133,134]. p53 mutation and/or monoallelic loss of a variable portion of the short arm of chromosome 17 occurs relatively frequently in many human malignancies [135,136]. Using a single strand conformational polymorphism assay in conjunction with direct DNA sequencing, we demonstrated that p53 gene mutations are also preferentially associated with certain clinicopathologic categories of lymphoid malignancy [137,138]. These are Burkitt's lymphoma and leukemia, B-cell chronic lymphocytic leukemia, the clinically aggressive stage of large-cell transformation of B-cell chronic lymphocytic leukemia referred to as Richter's syndrome [137] and adult T-cell lymphoma/leukemia [138]. Mutations involving the p53 gene loci occur infrequently among NHLs and LLs belonging to other clinicopathologic categories [137]. Thus, p53 gene mutations appear to be highly relevant to the development and/or progression of specific categories of lymphoid neoplasia, analogous to their role in solid tumors and the role of dominantly acting oncogenes in lymphoid neoplasia.

We demonstrated that p53 gene mutations occur in approximately 37% of AIDS-associated systemic NHLs [82]. However, the mutations are not randomly distributed among different histologic categories. We found that approximately 60% of SNCC lymphomas exhibit mutations of p53 gene exons 5 through 9, while LC and IBP lymphomas consistently lack p53 gene mutations (statistical significance $P<0.05$) (Table 20.3). A single base pair substitution leading to a missense or occasionally to a nonsense mutation occurs in 75% of abnormal p53 genes. Gross rearrangements occur in the remaining 25% of cases [82]. Transitions at CpG dinucleotides, the most frequent type of mutation in many human tumors [133,134], represent a high proportion of the mutational events. In some cases, p53 gene mutations are accompanied by loss of the other allele. Therefore, p53 gene inactivation in AIDS-associated NHLs occurs by molecular mechanisms similar to those described in other human tumors [134] and the mutational spectrum is similar to that described in NHLs arising in immunocompetent persons [137].

The pathogenetic relevance of p53 gene inactivation in AIDS-associated lymphomagenesis is underscored by the highly specific clustering of p53 gene mutations in AIDS-associated NHLs belonging to the SNCC category and the lymphoma cell lines derived from them [87]. Furthermore, the frequency of p53 gene inactivation in AIDS-associated SNCC lymphoma is twice that of non-AIDS-associated SNCC lymphoma [82]. The SNCC lymphomas also consistently exhibit c-*myc* gene rearrangement [82]. The very frequent simultaneous occurrence of p53 tumor suppressor gene inactivation and c-*myc* proto-oncogene deregulation in the same tumor *in vivo* [82] and lymphoma cell line *in vitro* [87] suggests that cells carrying an activated c-*myc* oncogene may be under pressure to subsequently delete a p53-dependent pathway. This hypothesis is supported by preliminary observations suggesting that the c-*myc* protein may be involved in regulation of p53 gene expression [139].

The Rb gene, located on chromosome 13q14 [140], encodes phosphorylated proteins of 110 to 114 kD normally present in all human tissues that are believed to inhibit cell growth [141]. Mutational inactivation of the Rb gene has been documented in a large variety of malignant tumors, suggesting that functional loss of the Rb gene is involved in the initiation and/or progression of many human malignancies [142]. Point mutations, encountered in 80% of lesions, represent the most frequent mechanism of Rb tumor suppressor gene inactivation; gross rearrangements or large intragenic deletions occur much less commonly [143]. We found that a small but significant proportion of diffuse aggressive NHLs occurring sporadically in the general population unassociated with HIV infection lack detectable Rb protein, indicating acquired Rb gene mutations/deletions [144]. These findings suggest that Rb gene mutations/deletions may play an important role in the development and/or progression of a subset of lymphoid neoplasms, analogous to their role in certain solid tumors. We failed, however, to find any evidence of Rb gene inactivation among 27 AIDS-associated NHLs (Table 20.3) [82] and three AIDS-associated NHL cell lines [87] using a variety of technical approaches. These results suggest that Rb gene mutations/deletions occur very infrequently, if at all, in AIDS-associated NHLs, and therefore do not play an important role in their development or progression.

Other hematopoietic neoplasms

In addition to diffuse aggressive NHL, a variety of other hematopoietic neoplasms have been reported in persons who have AIDS, are HIV-seropositive, or are at increased risk for developing AIDS. These include B-cell acute lymphoblastic leukemia [20, 145–151], plasmacytoma and multiple myeloma [11,152–158], low-grade B-cell NHLs and lymphocytic leukemias [4–6,27,159–161], Hodgkin's disease [8,9,15,20,162–174], precursor T-cell lymphoblastic lymphoma [175–177], cutaneous T-cell lymphoma [178–180], peripheral T-cell lymphoma [181–184], human T-cell lymphoma/leukemia virus-1 (HTLV-1)-associated adult T-cell lymphoma/leukemia [185,186], CD30 (Ki-1) positive anaplastic large-cell lymphoma [18,19,187,188], angiocentric immunoproliferative lesions [189–191], suppressor T-cell chronic lymphocytic leukemia, T8 lymphocytosis, T-gamma lymphoproliferative disease [9, 11,192–194], and acute myeloid leukemia [20,195–197]. However, these neoplasms occur only sporadically in AIDS risk group individuals and there is no definitive epidemiologic evidence to suggest that the incidence of these neoplasms has increased in parallel with the AIDS epidemic. Since the relationship of these hematologic neoplasms to HIV infection and AIDS is generally unclear, these neoplasms are not recognized as meeting the criteria for the diagnosis of AIDS in HIV-infected individuals by the CDC at the present time.

A notable exception should be made for B-cell acute lymphoblastic leukemia, approximately a dozen or more cases of which have been reported, pri-

virtually 100% of CNS and body cavity-based lymphomas contain EBV but apparently lack c-*myc* gene rearrangement. In the case of SNCC lymphoma, 100% exhibit c-*myc* gene rearrangements, two-thirds contain p53 mutations, one-third contain EBV, and none exhibit *bcl*-6 gene rearrangements. In contrast, in the case of IBP lymphoma, 100% contain EBV, 25% display c-*myc* gene rearrangements, 20% display *bcl*-6 gene rearrangements, and none contain p53 gene mutations. These findings suggest that the etiology of NHL in the setting of HIV infection is diverse and that more than one pathogenetic mechanism is operational in their development and progression. In addition to B-cell NHL, other hematopoietic neoplasms, including Hodgkin's disease and various malignancies of B-cell, T-cell and myeloid cell derivation, have been described in HIV-infected individuals. Growing epidemiologic evidence suggests that the incidence of Hodgkin's disease may be increased in HIV-infected persons. However, the significance of the occurrence of other hematopoietic neoplasms in HIV-seropositive persons is unclear since these neoplasms have not increased in parallel with the AIDS epidemic. The incidence of B-cell NHL is, however, increasing as HIV-infected individuals live longer. It has been estimated that AIDS-associated NHLs will account for 50% of all new cases of B-cell NHL diagnosed in the United States by the year 2000. Thus, it is imperative that AIDS lymphomagenesis remain an active area of clinical and scientific investigation.

References

1. Doll DC, List AF. Burkitt's lymphoma in a homosexual. *Lancet* 1982, **i**: 1026–1027.
2. Centers for Disease Control. Diffuse, undifferentiated non-Hodgkin's lymphoma among homosexual males – United States. *Morbid. Mortal. Week. Rep.* 1982, **31**: 277–279.
3. Ziegler JL, Miner RC, Rosenbaum E, et al. Outbreak of Burkitt's like-lymphoma in homosexual men. *Lancet* 1982, **ii**: 631–633.
4. Ziegler JL, Beckstead JA, Volberding PA, et al. Non-Hodgkin's lymphoma in 90 homosexual men: Relation to generalized lymphadenopathy and the acquired immunodeficiency syndrome (AIDS). *N. Eng. J. Med.* 1984, **311**: 565–570.
5. Levine AM, Meyer PR, Begandy MK, et al. Development of B-cell lymphoma in homosexual men. *Ann. Intern. Med.* 1984, **100**: 7–13.
6. Levine AM, Gill PS, Meyer PR, et al. Retrovirus and malignant lymphomas in homosexual men. *JAMA* 1985, **254**: 1921–1925.
7. Kalter SP, Riggs SA, Cabanillas F, et al. Aggressive non-Hodgkin's lymphomas in immunocompromised homosexual males. *Blood* 1985, **55**: 655–659.
8. Ioachim HL, Cooper MC, Hellman GC: Lymphomas in men at high risk for acquired immunodeficiency syndrome (AIDS). *Cancer* 1985, **56**: 2831–2842.
9. Knowles, DM, Chamulak GA, Subar M, et al. Lymphoid neoplasia associated with the acquired immunodeficiency syndrome (AIDS): The New York University Medical Center Experience with 105 patients (1981–1986). *Ann. Intern. Med.* 1988, **108**: 744–753.
10. Snider WD, Simpson DM, Aronyk KE, et al. Primary lymphoma of the nervous system associated with acquired immune-deficiency syndrome. *N. Eng. J. Med.* 1983, **308**: 45.
11. Kaplan MH, Susin M, Pahwa SG, et al. Neoplastic complications of HTLV-III infection. Lymphomas and solid tumors. *Am. J. Med.* 1987, **82**: 389–396.
12. Ahmed T, Wormser GP, Stahl RE, et al. Malignant lymphomas in a population at risk for acquired immune deficiency syndrome. *Cancer* 1987, **60**: 719–723.
13. Centers for Disease Control. Revision of the CDC surveillance case definition for acquired immunodeficiency syndrome. *Morbid. Mortal. Week. Rep.* 1987, **36** (suppl.): 1S–15S.
14. Payan MJ, Gambarelli D, Routy JP, et al. Primary lymphoma of the brain associated with AIDS. *Acta Neuropathol. (Berl.)* 1984, **64**: 78–80.
15. Monfardini S, Tirelli U, Vaccher E, et al. Malignant lymphomas in patients with or at risk for AIDS: A report of 50 cases observed in Italy. *J. Natl Cancer Inst.* 1988, **80**: 855–860.
16. Hamilton-Dutoit SJ, Pallesen G, et al. Identification of EBV-DNA in tumour cells of AIDS-related lymphomas by in-situ hybridization. *Lancet* 1989, **i**: 554–555.
17. Hamilton-Dutoit SJ, Pallesen G, Franzmann MB, et al. AIDS-related lymphoma: Histopathology, immunophenotype, and association with EBV as demonstrated by in situ nucleic acid hybridization. *Am. J. Pathol.* 1991, **138**: 149–163.
18. Raphael J, Gentihomme O, Tulliez M, et al. Histopathologic features of high grade non-Hodgkin's lymphomas in acquired immunodeficiency syndrome. *Arch. Pathol. Lab. Med.* 1991, **115**: 15–20.
19. Carbone A, Tirelli U, Vaccher E, et al. A clinicopathologic study of lymphoid neoplasias associated with human immunodeficiency virus infection in Italy. *Cancer* 1991, **68**: 842–852.
20. Knowles DM, Chadburn A. Lymphadenopathy and the lymphoid neoplasms associated with the acquired immune deficiency syndrome (AIDS). In Knowles DM (ed.) *Neoplastic Hematopathology.* Baltimore: Williams and Wilkins, 1992, pp. 773–836.
21. Beral V, Peterman T, Berkelman R, Jaffe H. AIDS-associated non-Hodgkin's lymphoma. *Lancet* 1991, **337**: 805–809.
22. Levine AM. Non-Hodgkin's lymphomas and other malignancies in the acquired immunodeficiency syndrome. *Semin. Oncol.* 1987, **14** (Suppl. 3): 34–39.
23. Harnly ME, Swan SH, Holly EA, et al. Temporal trends in the incidence of non-Hodgkin's lymphoma

and selected malignancies in a population with a high incidence of acquired immunodeficiency syndrome. *Am. J. Epidemiol.* 1988, **128**: 261–267.

24. Pluda JM, Yarchoan R, Jaffe E, et al. Development of non-Hodgkin lymphoma in a cohort of patients with severe human immunodeficiency virus (HIV) infection on long-term antiretroviral therapy. *Ann. Intern. Med.* 1990, **113**: 276–282.

25. Moore RD, Kessler H, Richman DD, et al. Non-Hodgkin's lymphoma in patients with advanced HIV infection treated with zidovudine. *JAMA* 1991, **265**: 2208–2211.

26. Gail MH, Pluda JM, Rabkin CS, et al. Projection of the incidence of non-Hodgkin's lymphoma related to acquired immunodeficiency syndrome. *J. Natl Cancer Inst.* 1991, **83**: 695–701.

27. Lowenthal DA, Straus DJ, Campbell SW, et al. AIDS-related lymphoid neoplasia: The Memorial Hospital experience. *Cancer* 1988, **61**: 2325–2337.

28. Khojasteh A, Reynolds RD, Khojasteh CA. Malignant lymphoreticular lesions in patients with immune disorders resembling acquired immunodeficiency syndrome (AIDS): Review of 80 cases. *South. Med. J.* 1986, **79**: 1070–1074.

29. De Jarlais DC, Marmor M, Thomas P, et al. Kaposi's sarcoma among four different AIDS risk groups. *N. Engl. J. Med.* 1984, **310**: 1119.

30. Beral V, Peterman TA, Berkelman RC, et al. Kaposi's sarcoma among persons with AIDS: A sexually transmitted disease? *Lancet* 1990, **335**: 123–128.

31. Knowles DM, Chadburn A. The neoplasms associated with AIDS. In Joshi W (ed.) *Pathology of AIDS and other Manifestations of HIV Infection.* New York: Igaku-Shoin, 1990, pp. 83–120.

32. Levine AM. Acquired immunodeficiency syndrome-related lymphoma. *Blood* 1992, **80**: 8–20.

33. Ragni MV, Lewis JH, Bontempo FA, et al. Lymphoma presenting as a traumatic hematoma in an HTLV-III antibody positive hemophiliac. *N. Engl J. Med.* 1985, **313**: 640.

34. Rechavi G, Ben-Bassat I, Berkowicz M, et al. Molecular analysis of Burkitt's leukemia in two hemophilic brothers with AIDS. *Blood* 1987, **70**: 1713–1717.

35. The Non-Hodgkin's Lymphoma Classification Project: National Cancer Institute sponsored study of classification of non-Hodgkin's lymphomas: Summary and description of a working formulation for clinical usage. *Cancer* 1982, **49**: 2112–2135.

36. Rappaport H. Tumors of the hematopoietic system. *Atlas of Tumor Pathology*, Sect. 3, Fasc. 8. Washington, DC: Armed Forces Institute of Pathology, 1966.

37. Pelicci PG, Knowles DM, Arlin Z, et al. Multiple monoclonal B-cell expansions and c-myc oncogene rearrangements in AIDS-related lymphoproliferative disorders: Implications for lymphomagenesis. *J. Exp. Med.* 1986, **164**: 2049–2060.

38. Levine AM, Gill PS. AIDS-related malignant lymphoma: Clinical presentation and treatment approaches. *Oncology* 1987, **1**: 41–46.

39. Knowles DM, Chamulak GA, Subar M, et al. Clinico-pathologic, immunophenotypic, and molecular genetic analysis of AIDS-associated lymphoid neoplasia: Clinical and biologic implications. *Path. Annual* 1988, **23**: 33–67.

40. Groopman J, Sullivan JL, Mulder C, et al. Pathogenesis of B-cell lymphoma in a patient with AIDS. *Blood* 1986, **67**: 612–615.

41. Subar M, Neri A, Inghirami G, et al. Frequent c-myc oncogene activation and infrequent presence of Epstein–Barr virus genome in AIDS-associated lymphoma. *Blood* 1988, **72**: 667–671.

41a. Knowles DM, Dalla-Favera R. AIDS-associated malignant lymphoma. In Broder S, Merrigan TC, Bolognesi D (eds) *Textbook of AIDS Medicine.* Baltimore: Williams and Wilkins, 1994, pp. 431–463.

42. Kaplan LD, Abrams DI, Feigal E, et al. AIDS-associated non-Hodgkin's lymphoma in San Francisco. *JAMA* 1989, **261**: 719–724.

43. Levine AM. Reactive and neoplastic lymphoproliferative disorders and other miscellaneous cancers associated with HIV infection. In De Vita VT Jr, Hellman S, Rosenberg SA (eds) *AIDS: Etiology, Diagnosis, Treatment and Prevention*, 2nd edn. Philadelphia, PA: Lippincott, 1989, p. 263.

44. Gill PS, Levine AM, Meyer PR, et al. Primary central nervous system lymphoma in homosexual men: Clinical, immunologic, and pathologic features. *Am. J. Med.* 1985, **78**: 742–748.

45. So YT, Beckstead JH, Davis RL. Primary central nervous system lymphoma in acquired immune deficiency syndrome: A clinical and pathological study. *Ann. Neurol.* 1986, **20**: 566–572.

46. Burkes RL, Meyer PR, Gill PS, et al. Rectal lymphoma in homosexual men. *Arch. Intern. Med.* 1986, **146**: 913–915.

47. Ioachim HL, Weinstein MA, Robbins RD, et al. Primary anorectal lymphoma: A new manifestation of the acquired immune deficiency syndrome (AIDS). *Cancer* 1987, **60**: 1449–1453.

48. Lee MH, Waxman M, Gillooley JF. Primary malignant lymphoma of the anorectum in homosexual men. *Dis. Col. Rect.* 1986, **29**: 413–416.

49. Gill PS, Chandraratna AN, Meyer PR, et al. Malignant lymphoma: Cardiac involvement at initial presentation. *J. Clin. Oncol.* 1987, **5**: 216–224.

50. Loureiro C, Gill PS, Meyer PR, et al. Autopsy findings in AIDS-related lymphoma. *Cancer* 1988, **62**: 735–739.

51. Subar M, Chadburn A, Knowles DM. Gastrointestinal neoplasms in the acquired immunodeficiency syndrome. In Kotler DP (ed.) *Gastrointestinal and Nutritional Manifestations of the Acquired Immunodeficiency Syndrome.* New York: Raven Press, 1991, pp. 93–117.

52. Formenti SC, Gill PS, Lean E, et al. Primary central nervous system lymphoma in AIDS: Results of radiation therapy. *Cancer* 1989, **63**: 1101–1107.

53. Levy RM, Janssen RS, Bush TJ, et al. Neuroepidemiology of acquired immunodeficiency syndrome, In Rosenblum ML, Levy RM, Bredesen DE (eds) *AIDS and the Nervous System.* New York: Raven Press, 1988, pp. 13–27.

54. Henry JM, Heffner RR Jr, Dillard SH, et al. Primary malignant lymphomas of the central nervous system.

Cancer 1974, **34**: 1293–1302.

55. Gill PS, Graham RA, Boswell W, et al. A comparison of imaging, clinical and pathologic aspects of space occupying lesions within the brain in patients with acquired immunodeficiency syndrome. *Am. J. Physiol. Imaging* 1986, **1**: 134–141.

56. Goldstein JD, Dickson DW, Moser FG, et al. Primary central nervous system lymphoma in acquired immunodeficiency syndrome: A clinical and pathologic study with results of treatment with radiation. *Cancer* 1991, **67**: 2756–2765.

57. Baumgartner JE, Rachlin JR, Beckstead JH, et al. Primary central nervous system lymphomas: Natural history and response to radiation therapy in 55 patients with acquired immunodeficiency syndrome. *J. Neurosurg.* 1990, **73**: 206–211.

58. Ciricillo SF, Rosenblum ML. Use of CT and MR imaging to distinguish intracranial lesions and to define the need for biopsy in AIDS patients. *J. Neurosurg.* 1990, **73**: 720–724.

59. MacMahon EME, Glass JD, Hayward SD, et al. Epstein Barr virus in AIDS-related primary central nervous system lymphoma. *Lancet* 1991, **338**: 969–973.

60. Reichart CM, O'Leary TJ, Levens DL, et al. Autopsy pathology in the acquired immune deficiency syndrome. *Am. J. Pathol.* 1983, **112**: 357–382.

61. Caccamo D, Pervez NK, Marchevsky A. Primary lymphoma of the liver in the acquired immunodeficiency syndrome. *Arch. Pathol. Lab. Med.* 1986, **110**: 553–555.

62. Van den Heule B, Taylor CR, Terry R, et al. Presentation of malignant lymphoma in the rectum. *Cancer* 1982, **49**: 2602–2607.

63. Loehr WJ, Mujahed Z, Zahn FD, et al. Primary lymphoma of the gastrointestinal tract: A review of 100 cases. *Ann. Surg.* 1969, **170**: 232–238.

64. Dragosics B, Bauer P, Radaszkiewicz T. Primary gastrointestinal non-Hodgkin's lymphomas: A retrospective clinicopathologic study of 150 cases. *Cancer* 1985, **55**: 1060–1073.

65. Daling JR, Weiss NS, Klopfenstein LL, et al. Correlates of homosexual behavior and the incidence of anal cancer. *JAMA* 1982, **247**: 1988–1990.

66. Peters RK, Mack TM. Patterns of anal cancinoma by gender and marital status in Los Angeles County. *Br. J. Cancer* 1983, **48**: 629–636.

67. DiCarlo EF, Anderson JB, Metroka CE, et al. Malignant lymphomas and the acquired immunodeficiency syndrome. *Arch. Pathol. Lab. Med.* 1986, **110**: 1012–1016.

68. Brooks HL, Downing J, McClure JA, et al. Orbital Burkitt's lymphoma in a homosexual man with acquired immune deficiency. *Arch. Ophthalmol.* 1984, **102**: 1533–1537.

69. Whang-Peng J, Lec EC, Sieverts H, et al. Burkitt's lymphoma in AIDS: Cytogenetic study. *Blood* 1984, **63**: 818–822.

70. Ioachim HL, Ryan JR, Blaugrund SM. Salivary gland lymph nodes: The site of lymphadenopathies and lymphomas associated with human immunodeficiency virus infection. *Arch. Pathol. Lab. Med.* 1988, **112**: 1224–1228.

71. Constantino A, West TE, Gupta M, et al. Primary cardiac lymphoma in a patient with acquired immune deficiency syndrome. *Cancer* 1987, **60**: 2801–2805.

72. Kaplan LD, Kahn J, Jacobson M, et al. Primary bile duct lymphoma in the acquired immunodeficiency syndrome (AIDS). *Ann. Intern. Med.* 1989, **110**: 161–162.

73. Levecq H, Hautefeuille M, Hoang C, et al. Primary stomal lymphoma: An unsual complication of ileostomy in a patient with transfusion-related acquired immune deficiency syndrome. *Cancer* 1990, **65**: 1028–1032.

74. Knowles DM, Inghirami G, Ubriaco A, et al. Molecular genetic analysis of three AIDS-associated neoplasms of uncertain lineage demonstrates their B-cell derivation and the possible pathogenetic role of the Epstein–Barr virus. *Blood* 1989, **73**: 792–799.

75. Walts AE, Shintaku IP, Said JW. Diagnosis of malignant lymphoma in effusions from patients with AIDS by gene rearrangement. *Am. J. Clin. Pathol.* 1990, **94**: 170–175.

76. Feiner HD, Rizk CC, Finfer MD. Frequent 'null cell' status of lymphomas in the pleura in HIV positive patients. *Lab. Invest. (Abst.)* 1989, **60**: 28A.

77. Karcher DS, Dawkins F, Garrett CT, et al. Body cavity-based non-Hodgkin's lymphoma (NHL) in HIV-infected patients: B-cell lymphoma with unusual clinical, immunophenotypic, and genotypic features. *Lab. Invest. (Abst.)* 1992, **66**: 80A.

78. Stein H, Gerdes J, Lemke H, et al. Evidence of Sternberg cells being derived from activated lymphocytes. In Neth L, Gallo R, Greaves M, Janka G (eds) *Haematology and Blood Transfusion*, Vol. 29. *Modern Trends in Human Leukemia VI*. Berlin: Springer-Verlag, 1985, pp. 441–444.

79. Thorley-Lawson DA, Nadler LM, Bhan AK, et al. BLAST-2 (EBVCs), an early cell surface marker of human B cell activation, is superinduced by Epstein–Barr virus. *J. Immunol.* 1985, **134**: 3007–3012.

80. Rothman R, Tourani JM, Andrieu JM. AIDS associated non-Hodgkin's lymphoma. *Lancet* 1991, **338**: 884–885.

81. Levine AM, Sullivan-Halley J, Pike MC, et al. HIV-related lymphoma: Prognostic factors predictive of survival. *Cancer* 1991, **68**: 2466–2472.

82. Ballerini P, Gaidano G, Gong JZ, et al. Multiple genetic lesions in AIDS-related non-Hodgkin lymphoma. *Blood* 1993, **81**: 166–176.

83. Montagnier L, Gruest J, Chamaret S, et al. Adaptation of lymphadenopathy associated virus (LAV) to replication in EBV-transformed B lymphoblastoid cell lines. *Science* 1984, **225**: 63–66.

84. Saxinger WC, Levine PH, Dean AG, et al. Evidence for exposure to HTLV-III in Uganda before 1973. *Science* 1985, **227**: 1036–1038.

85. Laurence J, Astrin SM. Human immunodeficiency virus induction of malignant transformation in human B lymphocytes. *Proc. Natl Acad. Sci. USA* 1991, **88**: 7635–7639.

86. Ganser A, Carlo-Stella C, Bartram CR, et al. Establishment of two Epstein–Barr virus negative Burkitt cell lines from a patient with AIDS and B-cell lymphoma. *Blood* 1988, **72**: 1255–1260.

87. Gaidano G, Parsa NZ, Tassi V, et al. In vitro

establishment of AIDS-related lymphoma cell lines: Phenotypic characterization, oncogene and tumor suppressor gene lesions, and heterogeneity in Epstein–Barr virus infection. *Leukemia* 1993, **7**: 1621–1629.

88. Shibata D, Brynes RK, Nathwani B, et al. Human immunodeficiency viral DNA is readily found in lymph node biopsies from seropositive individuals. *Am. J. Pathol.* 1989, **135**: 697–702.

89. Louie S, Daoust PR, Schwartz RS.: Immunodeficiency and the pathogenesis of non-Hodgkin's lymphoma. *Semin. Oncol.* 1980, **7**: 267–284.

90. Penn I. Lymphomas complicating organ transplantation. *Transplant. Proc.* 1983, **15**(Suppl.): 2790–2797.

91. de Thé G, Geser A, Day NE, et al. Epidemiological evidence for casual relationship between Epstein–Barr virus and Burkitt's lymphoma from Ugandan prospective study. *Nature* 1978, **274**: 756–761.

92. Klein G, Klein E. Evolution of tumors and the impact of molecular oncology. *Nature* 1985, **315**: 190–195.

93. Hanto DW, Frizzera G, Purtillo DT, et al. Clinical spectrum of lymphoproliferative disorders in renal transplant recipients and evidence for the role of Epstein–Barr virus. *Cancer Res.* 1981, **41**: 4253–4261.

94. Shearer WT, Ritz J, Finegold M, et al. Epstein–Barr virus associated B-cell proliferations of diverse clonal origins after bone marrow transplantation in a 12 year old patient with severe combined immunodeficiency. *N. Engl. J. Med.* 1985, **312**: 1152–1159.

95. Cleary ML, Sklar J. Lymphoproliferative disorders in cardiac recipients are multiclonal lymphomas. *Lancet* 1989, **ii**: 489–493.

96. Birx DL, Redfield RR, Tosato G. Defective regulation of Epstein–Barr virus infection in patients with acquired immunodeficiency syndrome (AIDS) or AIDS-related disorders. *N. Engl. J. Med.* 1986, **14**: 874–879.

97. Barriga F, Whang-Peng J, Lee E, et al. Development of a second clonally discrete Burkitt's lymphoma in a human immunodeficiency virus-positive homosexual patient. *Blood* 1988, **72**: 792–795.

98. Petersen JM, Tubbs RR, Savage RA, et al. Small non-cleaved Burkitt-like lymphoma with chromosome t(8,14) translocation and Epstein–Barr virus nuclear associated antigen in a homosexual man with acquired immune deficiency syndrome. *Am. J. Med.* 1985, **78**: 141–148.

99. Neri A, Barriga F, Knowles DM, et al. Epstein–Barr virus infection precedes clonal expansion in Burkitt's and AIDS-associated lymphoma. *Blood* 1991, **77**: 1092–1095.

100. Wang D, Liebowitz D, Kieff E. An EBV membrane protein expressed in immortalized lymphocytes transforms established rodent cells. *Cell* 1985, **43**: 831–840.

101. Seligmann M, Chess L, Fahey JL, et al. AIDS – An immunologic re-evaluation. *N. Engl. J. Med.* 1984, **311**: 1286–1292.

102. Metroka CE, Cunningham-Rundles S, Pollack MS, et at. Generalized lymphadenopathy in homosexual men. *Ann. Intern. Med.* 1983, **99**: 585–591.

103. Mathur-Wagh U, Enlow RW, Spigland I, et al. Longitudinal study of persistent generalised lymphadenopathy in homosexual men: Relation to acquired immunodeficiency syndrome. *Lancet* 1984, **i**: 1033–1038.

104. Chaganti RSK, Jhanwar SC, Koziner B et al. Specific translocations characterize Burkitt's-like lymphoma of homosexual men with the acquired immunodeficiency syndrome. *Blood* 1983, **61**: 1265–1268.

105. Shibata D, Weiss LM, Nathwani BN, et al. Epstein–Barr virus in benign lymph node biopsies from individuals infected with the human immunodeficiency virus is associated with concurrent or subsequent development of non-Hodgkin's lymphoma. *Blood* 1991, **77**: 1527–1533.

106. Lombardi L, Newcomb EW, Dalia-Favera R. Pathogenesis of Burkitt lymphoma: Expression of an activated c-myc oncogene causes the tumorigenic conversion of EBV-infected human B lymphoblasts. *Cell* 1987, **49**: 161–170.

107. Alonso ML, Richardson ME, Metroka CE, et al. Chromosome abnormalities in AIDS-associated lymphadenopathy. *Blood* 1987, **69**: 855–858.

108. Mathur-Wagh U, Mildvan D, Senie RT. Follow-up at 4½ years on homosexual men with generalized lymphadenopathy. *N. Engl. J. Med.* 1985, **313**: 1542–1543.

109. Dalla-Favera R. Chromosomal translocations involving the c-myc oncogene and their role in the pathogenesis of B-cell neoplasia. In Brugge J, Curran T, Harlow E, McCormick F (eds) *Origins of Human Cancer. A Comprehensive Review.* Cold Spring Harbor, NY: Cold Spring Harbor Laboratory Press, 1991, p. 543.

110. Van Krieken JHJM, Raffeld M, Raghoebier S, et al. Molecular genetics of gastrointestinal non-Hodgkin's lymphomas: Unusual prevalence and pattern of c-myc rearrangements in aggressive lymphomas. *Blood* 1990, **76**: 797–800.

111. Adams JM, Harris AW, Pinkert CA, et al. The c-myc oncogene driven by immunoglobulin enhancers induces lymphoid malignancy in transgenic mice. *Nature* 1985, **318**: 533–538.

112. Inghirami G, Grignani F, Sternas L, et al. Down-regulation of LFA-1 adhesion receptors by c-myc oncogene in human B lymphoblastoid cells. *Science* 1990, **250**: 682–686.

113. Clayberger C, Wright A, Medeiros LJ, et al. Absence of cell surface LFA-1 as a mechanism of escape from immunosurveillance. *Lancet* 1987, **2**: 533–536.

114. Inghirami G, Wieczorek R, Zhu BY, et al. Differential expression of LFA-1 molecules in non-Hodgkin's lymphoma and lymphoid leukemia. *Blood* 1988, **72**: 1431–1434.

115. Magrath IT. Burkitt's lymphoma as a human tumor model: New concepts in etiology and pathogenesis. In Pochedly C (ed.) *Pediatric Hematology/Oncology Reviews.* New York: Praeger, 1985, pp. 1–51.

116. Pelicci PG, Knowles DM, MaGrath I, et al. Chromosomal breakpoints and structural alterations of the c-myc locus differ in endemic and sporadic forms of Burkitt lymphoma. *Proc. Natl Acad. Sci. USA* 1986, **83**: 2984–2988.

117. Neri A, Barriga F, Knowles DM, et al. Different regions of the immunoglobulin heavy-chain locus are involved in chromosomal translocations in distinct pathogenetic forms of Burkitt lymphoma. *Proc. Natl Acad. Sci. USA* 1988, **85**: 2748–2752.

118. Shiramizu B, Barriga F, Neequaye J, et al. Patterns of chromosomal breakpoint locations in Burkitt's lymphoma: Relevance to geography and Epstein–Barr virus association. *Blood* 1991, **77**: 1516–1526.

119. Lanfrancone L, Pelicci PG, Dalla-Favera R: Structure and expression of translocated c-myc oncogenes: Specific differences in endemic, sporadic and AIDS-associated forms of Burkitt lymphomas. *Curr. Topics Microbiol. Immunol.* 1986, **132**: 257–265.

120. Tsujimoto Y, Cossman J, Jaffe E, et al. Involvement of the bcl-2 gene in human follicular lymphoma. *Science* 1985, **228**: 1440–1443.

121. Weiss LM, Warnke RA, Sklar J, et al. Molecular analysis of the t(14,18) chromosomal translocation in malignant lymphomas. *N. Engl. J. Med.* 1987, **317**: 1185–1189.

122. Athan E, Foitl DR, Knowles DM. bcl-1 gene rearrangement: Frequency and clinical significance among B cell chronic lymphocytic leukemias and non-Hodgkin's lymphomas. *Am. J. Pathol.* 1991, **138**: 591–597.

123. Raffeld M, Jaffe ES. bcl-1, t(11,14), and mantle cell-derived lymphomas. *Blood* 1991, **78**: 259–263.

124. Ye BH, Rao PH, Chaganti RSK, et al. Cloning of BCL-6, the locus involved in chromosome translocations affecting band 3q27 in B-cell lymphoma. *Cancer Res.* 1993, **53**: 2732.

125. Ye BH, Lista F, Lo Coco F, et al. Alterations of a zinc-finger encoding gene, BCL-6, in diffuse large cell-lymphoma. *Science* 1993, **262**: 747.

126. Kerckaert J-P, Deweindt C, Tilly H, et al. LAZ3, a novel zinc-finger encoding gene, is disrupted by recurring chromosome 3q27 translocations in human lymphoma. *Nature Genet.* 1993, **5**: 66.

127. Lo Coco F, Ye BH, Lista F, et al. Rearrangements of the BCL6 gene in diffuse large-cell non-Hodgkin's lymphoma. *Blood* 1994, **83**: 1757–1759.

128. Gaidano G, Lo Coco F, Ye BH, et al. Rearrangements of the BCL-6 gene in AIDS-associated non-Hodgkin lymphoma: Association with diffuse large-cell subtype. *Blood* 1994, **84**: 397–402.

129. Bos JL. Ras oncogenes in human cancer: A review. *Cancer Res.* 1989, **49**: 4682–4689.

130. Neri A, Knowles DM, McCormick F, et al. Analysis of ras oncogene mutations in human lymphoid malignancies. *Proc. Natl Acad. Sci. USA* 1988, **85**: 9268–9272.

131. Neri A, Baldini L, Ferrero D, et al. Frequency and type of ras oncogenes in lymphoid malignancies. In *Molecular Diagnostics of Human Cancer. Cancer Cells*, Vol. 7. Cold Spring Harbor, NY: Cold Spring Harbor Laboratory, 1989, pp. 101–105.

132. Gaidano G, Dalla-Favera R. Proto-oncogenes and tumor suppressor genes. In Knowles DM (ed.) *Neoplastic Hematopathology*. Baltimore: Williams & Wilkins, 1992, pp. 245–262.

133. Hollstein M, Sidransky D, Vogelstein B, Harris CC. p53 mutations in human cancers. *Science* 1991, **253**: 49–53.

134. Levine AJ, Momand J, Finlay CA. The p53 tumor suppressor gene. *Nature*, 1991, **351**: 453–456.

135. Baker SJ, Fearon ER, Nigro JM, et al. Chromosome 17 deletion and p53 gene mutations in colorectal carcinomas. *Science* 1989, **244**: 217–221.

136. Nigro JM, Baker SJ, Preisinger AC, et al. Mutations in the p53 gene occur in diverse human tumour types. *Nature* 1989, **342**: 705–708.

137. Gaidano G, Ballerini P, Gong JZ, et al. p53 mutations in human lymphoid malignancies: Association with Burkitt's lymphoma and chronic lymphocytic leukemia. *Proc. Natl Acad. Sci. USA* 1991, **88**: 5413–5417.

138. Cesarman E, Chadburn A, Inghirami G, et al. Structural and functional analysis of oncogenes and tumor suppressor genes in adult T cell leukemia/lymphoma (ATLL) reveals frequent p53 mutations. *Blood*, 1992, **80**: 3205–3216.

139. Ronen D, Rotter V, Reisman D. Expression from the murine p53 promoter is mediated by factor binding to a downstream helix-loop-helix recognition motif. *Proc. Natl Acad. Sci. USA* 1991, **88**: 4128–4132.

140. Dryja TP, Rapaport JM, Joyce JM, et al. Molecular detection of deletions involving band q14 of chromosome 13 in retinoblastoma. *Proc. Natl Acad. Sci. USA* 1986, **83**: 7391–7394.

141. Ludlow JW, Shon J, Pipas JM, et al. The retinoblastoma susceptibility gene product undergoes cell cycle-dependent dephosphorylation and binding to and release from SV40 large T. *Cell* 1990, **60**: 387–396.

142. Goodrich DW, Lee WH. The molecular genetics of retinoblastoma. *Cancer Surveys* 1990, **9**: 529–554.

143. Yandell DW, Campbell TA, Dayton SH, et al. Oncogenic point mutations in the human retinoblastoma gene: Their application to genetic counseling. *N. Engl. J. Med.* 1989, **321**: 1689–1695.

144. Haber MM, Inghirami G, Dalla-Favera R, et al. Retinoblastoma (Rb) gene product expression in B cell non-Hodgkin's lymphomas (NHLs) and lymphoid leukemias (LLs). *Lab. Invest.* 1991, **64**: 73A.

145. Berman M, Minowada J, Lewy JM, et al. Burkitt cell acute lymphoblastic leukemia with partial expression of T-cell markers and subclonal chromosome abnormalities in a man with acquired immunodeficiency syndrome. *Cancer Genet. Cytogenet.* 1985, **16**: 341–347.

146. Gill PS, Meyer PR, Paviova Z, et al. B cell acute lymphocytic leukemia in adults. Clinical, morphologic, and immunologic findings. *J. Clin. Oncol.* 1986, **4**: 737–743.

147. Ernberg I, Bjorkholm M, Zech L, et al. An EBV genome carrying pre-B cell leukemia in a homosexual man with characteristic karyotype and impaired EBV-specific immunity. *J. Clin. Oncol.* 1986, **4**: 1481–1488.

148. Rossi G, Gorla R, Cadeo GP, et al. Acute lymphoblastic leukemia of B cell origin in an anti-HIV positive intravenous drug abuser. *Br. J. Haematol.* 1988, **68**: 140–141.

149. Flanagan P, Chowdhury V, Costello C. HIV-associated

B cell ALL. *Br. J. Haematol.* 1988, **69**: 287.

150. Milpied N, Bourhis JH, Garand R, et al. B cell ALL in an anti-HIV positive patient: Achievement of a complete response with aggressive chemotherapy. *Br. J. Haematol.* 1988, **70**: 501–502.

151. Bernheim A, Berger R. Cytogenetic studies of Burkitt lymphoma–leukemia in patients with acquired immunodeficiency syndrome. *Cancer Genet. Cytogenet.* 1988, **32**: 67–74.

152. Israel AM, Koziner B, Strauss DJ. Plasmacytoma and the acquired immunodeficiency syndrome. *Ann. Intern. Med.* 1983, **99**: 635–636.

153. Vandermolen LA, Fehir KM, Rice L. Multiple myeloma in a homosexual man with chronic lymphadenopathy. *Arch. Intern. Med.* 1985, **145**: 745–746.

154. Gold JWM, Weikel CS, Godbold J, et al. Unexplained persistent lymphadenopathy in homosexual men and the acquired immune deficiency syndrome. *Medicine* 1985, **64**: 203–213.

155. Thomas MAB, Ibeis LS, Wells JV, et al. IgA kappa multiple myeloma and lymphadenopathy syndrome associated with AIDS virus infection. *Aust. NZ J. Med.* 1986, **16**: 402–404.

156. Karnad AB, Martin AW, Koh HK, et al. Nonsecretory multiple myeloma in a 26 year old man with acquired immunodeficiency syndrome, presenting with multiple extramedullary plasmacytomas and osteolytic bone disease. *Am. J. Hematol. 1989,* **32**: 305–310.

157. Voelkerding KV, Sandhaus LM, Kim HC, et al. Plasma cell malignancy in the acquired immune deficiency syndrome. *Am. J. Clin. Pathol. 1989,* **92**: 222–228.

158. Gold JE, Schwam L, Castella A, et al. Malignant plasma cell tumors in HIV-infected patients. *Cancer* 1990, **66**: 363–368.

159. Sewell HF, Walker F, Bennett B, et al. Chronic lymphocytic leukaemia contemporaneous with HIV infection. *Br. Med. J.* 1987, **294**: 938–939.

160. Turner RR, Brynes RK, Nathwani BN, et al. Low grade B-cell lymphomas and leukemias in homosexual men. *Lab. Invest.* 1988, **58**: 96A.

161. Ioachim HL, Dorsett B, Cronin W, et al. Acquired immunodeficiency syndrome associated lymphomas: Clinical, pathological, immunologic and viral characteristics of 111 cases. *Hum. Pathol.* 1991, **22**: 659–673.

162. Robert NJ, Schneiderman H. Hodgkin's disease and the acquired immunodeficiency syndrome. *Ann. Intern. Med.* 1984, **101**: 142–143.

163. Schoeppel JL, Hoppe RT, Dorfman RF, et al. Hodgkin's disease in homosexual men with generalized lymphadenopathy. *Ann. Intern. Med.* 1985, **102**: 68–70.

164. Scheib RG, Siegel RS. Atypical Hodgkin's disease and the acquired immunodeficiency syndrome. *Ann. Intern. Med.* 1985, **102**: 554.

165. Baer DM, Anderson ET, Wilkinson LS. Acquired immune deficiency syndrome in homosexual men with Hodgkin's disease. *Am. J. Med.* 1986, **80**: 738–740.

166. Unger PD, Strauchen JA. Hodgkin's disease in AIDS complex patients: Report of four cases and tissue immunologic marker studies. *Cancer* 1986, **58**: 821–825.

167. Prior E, Goldberg AF, Conjalka MS, et al. Hodgkin's disease in homosexual men: An AIDS-related phenomenon? *Am. J. Med.* 1986, **81**: 1085–1088.

168. Temple JJ, Andes WA. AIDS and Hodgkin's disease. *Lancet* 1986, **2**: 454–455.

169. Cid JA, Cid JL, Sanudo EF, et al. AIDS and Hodgkin's disease. *Lancet* 1986, **ii**: 1104–1105.

170. Alfonso PG, Sanudo EF, Carretero JM, et al. Hodgkin's disease in HIV-infected patients. *Biomed. Pharmacother.* 1988, **42**: 321–325.

171. Serrano M, Bellas C, Campo E, et al. Hodgkin's disease in patients with antibodies to human immunodeficiency virus: A study of 22 patients. *Cancer* 1990, **65**: 2248–2254.

172. Ree HJ, Strauchen JA, Khan M, et al. HIV-associated Hodgkin's disease: Clinicopathologic studies of 24 cases. Preponderance of mixed cellularity type characterized by the occurrence of fibro-histiocytoid stromal cells. *Cancer* 1991, **67**: 1614–1621.

173. Ames ED, Conjalka MS, Goldberg AF, et al. Hodgkin's disease and AIDS. Twenty-three new cases and a review of the literature. *Hematol. Oncol. Clin. North Am.* 1991, **5**: 343–356.

174. Gold JE, Altarac D, Ree HJ, et al. HIV-associated Hodgkin Disease: A clinical study of 18 cases and review of the literature. *Am. J. Hematol.* 1991, **36**: 93–99.

175. Ciobanu N, Andreeff M, Safai B, et al. Lymphoblastic neoplasia in a homosexual patient with Kaposi's sarcoma. *Ann. Intern. Med.* 1983, **98**: 151–155.

176. Presant CA, Gala K, Wiseman C, et al. Human immunodeficiency virus-associated T-cell lymphoblastic lymphoma in AIDS. *Cancer* 1987, **60**: 1459–1461.

177. Ruff P, Bagg A, Papadopoulos K. Precursor T-cell lymphoma associated with HIV-1 infection: First reported case. *Cancer* 1989, **64**: 39–42.

178. Goldstein J, Becker N, DelRowe J, et al. Cutaneous T cell lymphoma in a patient infected with human immunodeficiency virus type 1: Use of radiation therapy. *Cancer* 1990, **66**: 1130–1132.

179. Crane GA, Variakojis D, Rosen ST, et al. Cutaneous T cell lymphoma in patients with human immunodeficiency virus infection. *Arch. Dermatol.* 1991, **127**: 989–994.

180. Parker SC, Fenton DA, McGibbon DH. Homme rouge and the acquired immunodeficiency syndrome. *N. Eng. J. Med.* 1990, **321**: 906–907.

181. Howard MR, McVerry BA. T-cell lymphoma in a haemophiliac positive for antibody to HIV. *Br. J. Haematol.* 1987, **67**: 115.

182. Nasr SA, Byrnes RK, Garrison CP, et al. Peripheral T-cell lymphoma in a patient with acquired immune deficiency syndrome. *Cancer* 1988, **61**: 947–951.

183. Sternlieb J, Mintzer D, Kwa D, et al. Peripheral T cell lymphoma in a patient with the acquired immunodeficiency syndrome. *Am. J. Med.* 1988, **85**: 445.

184. Herndier BG, Shiramizu BT, Jewett NE, et al. Acquired immunodeficiency syndrome-associated T-

cell lymphoma: Evidence for human immunodeficiency virus type 1-associated T-cell transformation. *Blood* 1992, **79**: 1768–1774.

185. Kobayashi M, Yoshimoto S, Fujishita S, et al. HTLV-1 positive T-cell lymphoma-leukemia in an AIDS patient. *Lancet* 1984, **i**: 1361–1362.

186. Shibata D, Brynes R, Rabinowitz A, et al. HTLV-1 associated adult T cell leukemia lymphoma in a patient infected with HIV-1. *Ann. Intern. Med.* 1989, **111**: 871–875.

187. Gonzalez-Clemente JM, Ribera JM, Campo E, et al. Ki-1 positive anaplastic large cell lymphoma of T cell origin in an HIV infected patient. *AIDS* 1991, **5**: 751–755.

188. Ghadburn A, Cesarman E, Jagidar J, et al. CD30 (Ki-1) positive anaplastic large cell lymphomas in HIV infected individuals. *Cancer* 1993, **72**: 3078–3090.

189. Montillo P, Dronda F, Moreno S, et al. Lymphomatoid granulomatosis and the acquired immunodeficiency syndrome. *Ann. Intern. Med.* 1987, **106**: 166–167.

190. Anders KH, Latta H, Chang BS, et al. Lymphomatoid granulomatosis and malignant lymphomas of the central nervous system in the acquired immunodeficiency syndrome. *Hum. Pathol.* 1989, **20**: 326–334.

191. Gold JE, Ghali V, Brown JC, et al. Angiocentric immunoproliferative lesions, T cell non-Hodgkin's lymphoma and the acquired immune deficiency syndrome: A case report and review of the literature. *Cancer* 1990, **66**: 2407–2413.

192. Harper ME, Kaplan MH, Marselle LM, et al. Concomitant infection with HTLV-1 and HTLV-III in a patient with T8 lymphoproliferative disease. *N. Eng. J. Med.* 1986, **315**: 1073–1078.

193. Guillon JM, Fouret P, Mayaud C, et al. Extensive T8-positive lymphocytic visceral infiltration in a homosexual man. *Am. J. Med.* 1987, **82**: 655–661.

194. Ghali V, Castella A, Louis-Charles A, Agranovsky E, Croxson ST: Expansion of large granular lymphocytes (natural killer cells) with limited antigen expression (CD2+, CD3−, CD4−, CD8−, CD16+, NKH-1−) in an HIV-positive homosexual male. *Cancer* 1990, **65**: 2243–2247.

195. Napoli VM, Stein SF, Spira TJ, Raskin D. Myelodysplasia progressing to acute myeloblastic leukemia in an HTLV-III virus-positive homosexual man with AIDS-related complex. *Am. J. Clin. Pathol.* 1986, **86**: 788–791.

196. Darne C, Solal-Celigny P, Herrera A, et al. Acute myelofibrosis and infection with the lymphadenopathy-associated virus/human T-lymphotropic virus type III. *Ann. Intern. Med.* 1986, **104**: 130–131.

197. Willumsen L, Ellegaard J, Pedersen B. HIV infection in acute myeloblastic leukemia. *Am. J. Clin. Pathol.* 1987, **88**: 536–537.

198. Bennett JM, Catovsky D, Daniel M-T, et al. Proposals for the classification of acute leukemias. French–American–British (FAB) co-operative group. *Br. J. Haematol.* 1976, **33**: 451–458.

199. Minerbrook M, Schulman P, Budman DR, et al.

200. Magrath IT, Jain V, Jaffe ES. Small noncleaved cell lymphoma. In Knowles DM (ed.) *Neoplastic Hematopathology.* Baltimore: Williams & Wilkins, 1992, pp. 749–772.

201. Hewell PA, Alexanian R. Multiple myeloma in young persons. *Ann. Intern. Med.* 1976, **84**: 441–443.

202. Salahuddin SZ, Albashi DV, Hunter EA, et al. HTLV-III infection of EBV-genome-positive B-lymphoid cells with or without detectable T4 antigens. *Int. J. Cancer* 1987, **39**: 198–202.

203. Horning SJ, Rosenberg SA. The natural history of initially untreated low grade non-Hodgkin's lymphomas. *N. Engl. J. Med.* 19?? **311**: 1471–1984.

204. Audouin J, Diebold, J, Pallesen G. Frequent expression of Epstein–Barr virus latent membrane protein-1 in tumour cells of Hodgkin's disease HIV-positive patients. *J. Pathol.* 1992, **167**: 381–384.

205. Biggar RJ, Horm J, Goedert JJ, Melbye M. Cancer in a group at risk of acquired immunodeficiency syndrome (AIDS) through 1984. *Am. J. Epidemiol.* 1987, **126**: 578–586.

206. Bernstein L, Levin D, Mench H, Ross RK. AIDS-related secular trends in cancer in Los Angeles county men: A comparison by marital status. *Cancer Res.* 1989, **49**: 466–470.

207. Roithmann S, Tourani JM, Andrieu JM. Hodgkin's disease in HIV-infected intravenous drug abusers. *N. Engl. J. Med.* 1990, **323**: 275–276.

208. Tirelli U, Vaccher E, Rezza G, et al. Hodgkin disease and infection with the human immunodeficiency virus (HIV) in Italy. *Ann. Intern. Med.* 1988, **108**: 309–310.

209. Hessol NA, Katz MH, Liu JY, et al. Increased incidence of Hodgkin disease in homosexual men with HIV infection. *Ann. Intern. Med.* 1992, **117**: 309–311.

210. Stevenson M, Volsky B, Hedenskog M, et al. Immortalization of human T lymphocytes after transfection of Epstein–Barr virus DNA. *Science* 1986, **233**: 980–984.

211. Jones JF, Shurin S, Abramowsky C, et al. T-cell lymphoma containing Epstein–Barr viral DNA in patients with chronic Epstein–Barr virus infections. *N. Engl. J. Med.* 1988, **318**: 733–741.

212. Harabuchi Y, Yamanaka N, Kataura A, et al. Epstein–Barr virus in nasal T-cell lymphomas in patients with lethal midline granuloma. *Lancet* 1990, **335**: 128–130.

213. Schneider DR, Picker LJ. Myelodysplasia in the acquired immune deficiency syndrome. *Am. J. Clin. Pathol.* 1985, **84**: 144–152.

214. Spector BD, Perry GS III, Kersey JH. Genetically determined immunodeficiency disease and malignancy: Report from the immunodeficiency-cancer registry. *Clin. Immunol. Immunopathol.* 1978, **11**: 12–29.

199. (cont.) Burkitt's leukemia: A re-evaluation. *Cancer* 1982, **49**: 1444–1448.

CHAPTER 21

Lymphomas of mucosa-associated lymphoid tissue

DENNIS H. WRIGHT

Introduction

The concept of mucosal lymphomas was proposed a little over a decade ago in a paper noting the close morphologic similarities between the small intestinal lesions in a patient with Mediterranean lymphoma and the stomach lesions in a patient with low-grade gastric lymphoma [1]. In a subsequent paper, Isaacson and Wright [2] noted the clinical, histopathologic and immunohistochemical features in common between stomach, salivary gland, lung and thyroid lymphomas and proposed that this was due to their common origin from mucosa-associated lymphoid tissue (MALT). It is, in retrospect, remarkable that before that time non-Hodgkin's lymphomas were categorized on the basis of their cytology and growth pattern, irrespective of their site of origin. Thus, the

study of 1175 cases of non-Hodgkin's lymphomas, that formed the basis of the Working Formulation, published in 1982 [3], included nodal and extranodal lymphomas but made no distinction between these in terms of histology or survival analysis. Isaacson and Wright based their proposal, that many lymphomas at extranodal sites exhibit morphologic and behavioral characteristics in keeping with an origin from the mucosal immune system, on earlier studies using the adoptive transfer of lymphoid cells in syngeneic mice that had established the existence of this system [4–6]. In these experiments, labeled lymphocytes, derived from mesenteric lymph nodes, showed preferential homing to the gut. Those derived from bronchial lymph nodes showed a propensity to localize in the lungs, whereas the majority of peripheral lymph node cells returned to their sites of origin [4]. It was shown that the estrous cycle influenced the migration of mesenteric lymph node cells to the lower genital tract [5], and that these cells home to the mammary glands in late pregnancy and lactation [6]. These selective homing patterns are mediated, at least in part, by adhesion molecules expressed on venules [7].

Isaacson and Wright [1,2] originally considered lymphomas of MALT to be follicle center cell derived, i.e., that they were derived from the follicle centers within MALT. This interpretation was, in part, based on the observation of light chain restriction within germinal centers in the tumors. This apparent monoclonality of germinal centers was subsequently shown to be due to follicular colonization by tumor cells, a characteristic of MALT lymphomas not appreciated at the time, and the error was compounded by the use of frozen section immunohistochemistry with its poorer morphological definition. In a study of primary B-cell gastric lymphoma, Isaacson et al. [8] noted that all gastric MALT lymphomas contained germinal centers and, while these often appeared reactive, immunohistochemistry identified their neoplastic nature, i.e., light chain restriction. In this publication they noted the constant presence of characteristic perifollicular centrocyte-like cells that were phenotypically different from follicle center cells. In a study of ten primary gastric lymphomas, using novel monoclonal antibodies reactive in paraffin-embedded tissues, Myhre and Isaacson [9] reassessed the histogenesis of this tumor. They concluded that primary gastric lymphoma is a tumor of centrocyte-like (CCL) cells occasionally showing plasmacytic differentiation and that the follicles, within the tumor, are reactive but that selective invasion of these reactive follicles by neoplastic CCL cells leads to the appearance of malignancy. They noted that CCL cells bear close morphologic and immunophenotypic similarities to splenic marginal zone cells. In a review of lymphomas of MALT, Isaacson and Spencer [10] noted that CCL cells have the same immunophenotype as marginal zone B-cells that are found within the dome area of Peyer's patches and that selectively infiltrate the dome epithelium [11]. They concluded that, given the cytological appearance and situation in relation to follicles and dome epithelium, these cells are almost certainly the benign equivalent of the neoplastic CCL cells. This hypothesis is consistent with the marginal zone distribution of CCL cells in MALT lymphomas and their propensity to invade mucosal epithelium.

A large proportion of lymphomas presenting at extranodal sites are high grade and show none of the features of low-grade MALT lymphomas. Reactive germinal centers are overgrown and obliterated, the lymphoma is composed of blast cells rather than CCL cells, and plasma cell differentiation does not occur. Such tumors are often indistinguishable from high-grade, nodal, B-cell lymphomas. However, in low-grade lymphomas of MALT, blastic transformation may be seen and low-grade and high-grade lymphomas may coexist. Isaacson and Chan [12] studied a series of gastric lymphomas and noted that the chance of finding a low-grade MALT lymphoma associated with a high-grade lymphoma was related to the number of surgical blocks taken from the specimen. They further established that the immunoglobulin phenotype was common between the low- and high-grade lymphoma. It would, thus, appear that the natural history of MALT lymphomas, in common with that of other low-grade B-cell lymphomas, is for transformation to high-grade lymphoma to occur after a variable period of time.

The concept that many extranodal lymphomas are derived from MALT goes some way to explain not only their histological characteristics but also their clinical behavior. Many of these tumors remain localized to their site or organ of origin, and do not show the wide dissemination characteristic of most low-grade B-cell lymphomas. This could be related to the propensity of MALT lymphocytes to home back to their site of stimulation or to undergo terminal differentiation. The observation that MALT lymphomas derived from one mucosal site may metastasize to other mucosal sites reflects the concept of a common mucosal defense system whereby MALT lymphocytes stimulated at one mucosal surface home also to other mucosal sites [4,5].

In their original publication, Isaacson and Wright [2] described MALT lymphomas in recognized sites of the mucosal immune system, such as the gastrointestinal tract, bronchus and salivary gland. Their categorization of thyroid lymphomas as MALT lymphomas could be rationalized on the grounds that embryologically the thyroid gland is foregut derived. In recent years, lymphomas with MALT characteristics have been described in nonmucosal sites, such as the skin and the kidney. These lymphomas show the histological, immunohistochemical and biological features of MALT lymphomas, namely that they are composed of monocytoid or CLL cells that have a marginal zone distribution and show follicular colonization and plasma cell differentiation. They often arise in pre-existing inflammatory infiltrates and usually contain reactive germinal centers, features that have led to their categorization, in the past, as pseudolymphomas. They may remain localized for long periods of time and have a good prognosis. The tumor cells express surface immunoglobulin (usually IgM) and a substantial number synthesize cytoplasmic immunoglobulin. They express the B-cell antigens, CD19, 20, 22 and 79a, but they are negative for CD5, CD10 and CD23. The International Lymphoma Study Group has proposed that such lymphomas should be categorized as marginal zone B-cell lymphomas, thus avoiding the use of the term 'MALT lymphoma' for tumors arising at nonmucosal sites [13].

Pathology

LOW-GRADE

The cell of origin of low-grade MALT lymphomas is thought to be a marginal zone lymphocyte [13]. Most characteristically these cells have oval, sometimes indented nuclei, with a moderate amount of clear cytoplasm (centrocyte-like cells, monocytoid cells) [9] (Figures 21.1 and 21.2). In some lymphomas of MALT, particularly in the lung, the cells have more rounded nuclei and may closely resemble small lymphocytes [14–16]. In low-grade lymphomas of MALT the CCL cells invade epithelial structures, forming so-called lymphoepithelial lesions. These vary according to the organ involved. In the stomach, lymphoepithelial lesions are formed by small groups of CCL cells invading and destroying gastric glands [9,10] (Figure 21.3). Infiltration by single cells does not constitute a lymphoepithelial lesion. Similar, although usually less well defined, lesions can be seen in the bronchial epithelium in lymphomas of MALT of the lung [14–16]. In the thyroid gland the CCL cells fill out thyroid follicles, giving a very characteristic appearance [17,18]

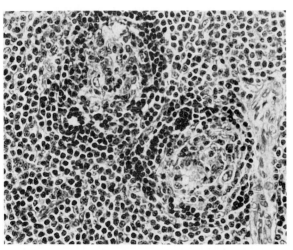

Figure 21.2 A high-power view of the lymphoma shown in Figure 21.1. Two reactive germinal centers are surrounded by a dark mantle zone. Marginal zone cells (centrocyte-like cells) surround these reactive follicles.

(Figures 21.4 and 21.5). This must, however, be distinguished from the invasion of follicles by T-lymphocytes and macrophages, frequently seen in Hashimoto's disease. In salivary tissue, CCL cells infiltrate and surround epimyoepithelial islands with an intensity that is not seen in Sjögren's syndrome [19,20] (Figure 21.6). They may also form lymphoepithelial lesions with duct epithelium, similar to those seen in the stomach.

Approximately 30% of low-grade lymphomas of MALT show plasmacytic differentiation. The plasma cell infiltrates are always sharply demarcated from the CCL cells, a finding in keeping with the concept that these cells have been part of the MALT

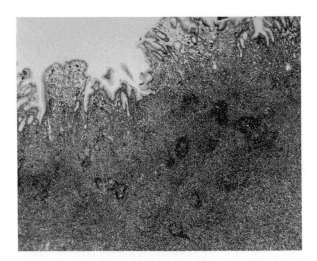

Figure 21.1 A low-power view of a low-grade MALT lymphoma of the stomach. Isolated germinal centers with dark mantle zones can be seen. These are surrounded by and partly infiltrated by sheets of paler-staining marginal zone cells.

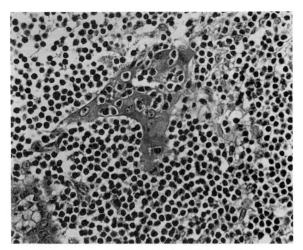

Figure 21.3 A low-grade gastric MALT lymphoma. A distorted gastric gland infiltrated by marginal zone cells forms a typical lymphoepithelial lesion.

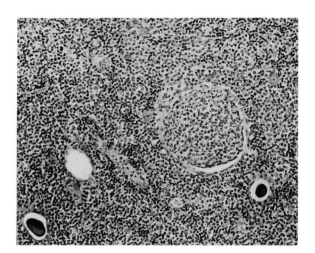

Figure 21.4 A low-grade MALT lymphoma of thyroid showing filling out of a thyroid acinus by marginal zone cells.

circulation and have returned to the mucosal surface as differentiated cells. If these cells had differentiated locally from the CCL cells, one would expect to see intermediate forms with less sharp separation between the two cell types. The plasma cells never show mucosal invasion to form lymphoepithelial lesions. They frequently show immunoglobulin inclusions and occasionally immunoglobulin crystals, which may be extruded into the extracellular tissue. Undoubtedly, some cases of plasmacytoma reported at mucosal sites, in the past, have been MALT lymphomas exhibiting extreme plasmacytic differentiation. Occurring at mucosal sites, often on the background of an inflammatory process, MALT-lymphomas frequently contain reactive plasma cells.

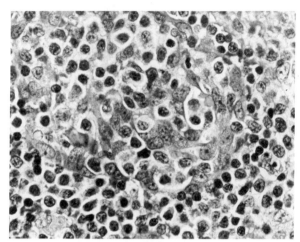

Figure 21.6 A low-grade MALT lymphoma of salivary gland showing a myoepithelial island. Darkly staining, oval-shaped epithelial and myoepithelial cells are seen to be interspersed with marginal zone cells, which have abundant clear cytoplasm.

It is important, therefore, that plasma cell differentiation in the tumor is confirmed by immunoglobulin staining.

A further characteristic feature of low-grade MALT lymphomas is the propensity to invade and replace pre-existing reactive germinal centers (follicular colonization) [20–22] (Figure 21.7). This often gives the tumors a nodular appearance and may lead to the erroneous diagnosis of follicle center cell lymphoma. The cells that replace the germinal centers may appear as CCL cells, or show blastic or plasmacytic differentiation.

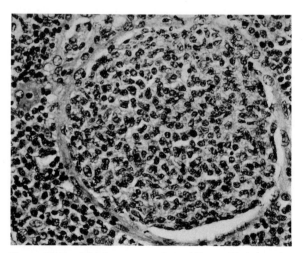

Figure 21.5 A higher power view of Figure 21.4 showing the characteristic morphology of the marginal zone cells within the thyroid acinus.

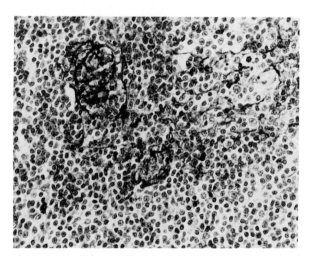

Figure 21.7 A low-grade gastric MALT lymphoma stained with an antibody to CD21 to show follicular dendritic cells. The dendritic network of a reactive germinal center is expanded and dispersed by infiltrating marginal zone cells.

HIGH-GRADE

Blast cells, highlighted by Giemsa staining, are seen in low-grade lymphomas of MALT. They occur singly or in small aggregates amongst the CCL cells, never amongst the plasma cells. Sometimes they are seen within mucosal lymphatics. Large aggregates of blast cells indicate progression to high-grade lymphoma [12,20]. The majority of high-grade lymphomas of MALT consist of sheets of blast cells resembling centroblasts or immunoblasts. Varying degrees of pleomorphism may be encountered. The identification of low-grade areas, within such tumors, establishes their identify as MALT lymphomas. Lymphoepithelial lesions cannot usually be identified in high-grade MALT lymphomas using routine histology. However, immunohistochemistry may identify extensive epithelial invasion in the thyroid and at other sites where the invaded epithelium is protected from erosion [23].

Diagnosis of lymphomas of MALT in endoscopic biopsies

The increasing use of diagnostic endoscopic biopsies presents pathologists with the problem of identifying lymphomas of MALT in small tissue samples and differentiating them, in the case of low-grade MALT lymphomas, from inflammatory lesions and, in the case of high-grade lymphomas, from other neo-

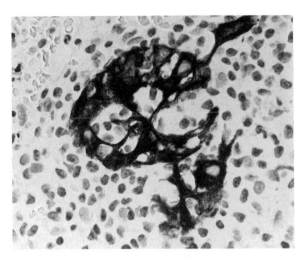

Figure 21.9   The section illustrated in Figure 21.8 shows clusters of tumor cells within a disrupted gastric gland forming a typic lymphoepithelial lesion.

plasms. The diagnostic features of low-grade MALT lymphomas in endoscopic biopsies are the presence of a dense, monomorphous infiltrate of centrocyte-like cells, lymphoepithelial lesions and, in a proportion of cases, plasma cell differentiation. The specificity of lymphoepithelial lesions has been questioned by some authors. Zuckerberg et al. [24] in a comparison of 25 low-grade gastric MALT lymphomas and 58 benign inflammatory infiltrates found that prominent lymphoepithelial lesions were not observed in benign inflammatory infiltrates. The identification of lymphoepithelial lesions is important in the distinction between mantle cell lymphomas of the gastrointestinal tract (lymphomatous polyposis) and low-grade lymphomas of MALT. Immunohistochemical stains for cytokeratins or epithelial membrane antigen provide a valuable means of highlighting and identifying lymphoepithelial lesions [20] (Figures 21.8 and 21.9). The presence of Dutcher bodies (immunoglobulin inclusions protruding into the nucleus) was also a feature of MALT lymphomas not seen in inflammatory lesions [24]. Where a biopsy remains inconclusive, further biopsies may be requested or other techniques used to substantiate a diagnosis of lymphoma. These include the use of immunohistochemistry to determine light chain restriction [25]. The success of this technique will depend upon the quality of the biopsy and the technical skills of the laboratory. It is easier to identify immunoglobulin in plasma cells than in centrocyte-like cells; however, plasmacytic differentiation is observed in only one-third of low-grade MALT lymphomas. Monoclonality may be established using molecular biological techniques [26–28]. In particular, PCR may be applied to small, endoscopic biopsies. It is important, however, that

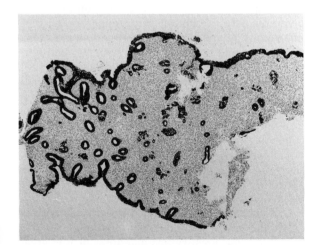

Figure 21.8   An endoscopic biopsy of a gastric MALT lymphoma stained to show low molecular weight cytokeratin with the antibody CAM 5.2. The regular structure of many of the gastric glands has been disrupted by infiltrating tumor cells forming typical lymphoepithelial lesions.

such studies are interpreted in association with the histology and not used as the primary means of diagnosing MALT lymphomas.

Stomach

The stomach, an organ that lacks organized lymphoid tissue in its physiological state, is the most common site of MALT lymphomas. *Helicobacter pylori* infection induces lymphoid proliferations in the stomach that may closely resemble low-grade MALT lymphoma [20,29] and it is thought that MALT lymphomas develop from these lesions [30–32]. Patients with gastric MALT lymphomas most frequently present with dyspepsia. The tumor has a peak incidence in the sixth and seventh decades, but may be seen in the third decade of life. In most reported series of gastric MALT lymphomas, the sex incidence varies from unity to 1.4:1 [33,34]. Grossly, the tumors most frequently occur in the antrum and appear as areas of mucosal flattening or fine mammilation in which one or more shallow ulcers are seen. It has been shown that some tumors are multifocal in their distribution in the stomach [35], which means that gastrectomy alone, even when resection margins are clear of tumor, cannot be accepted as a curative procedure.

The association between *Helicobacter pylori* gastritis and gastric MALT lymphomas has been shown in individual patients and by epidemiological studies [31,32]. *H. pylori* infection is also associated with gastric adenocarcinoma [36,37], which probably accounts for the reports of synchronous gastric adenocarcinoma and MALT lymphoma [38,39]. Cells of three low-grade gastric MALT lymphomas were shown to exhibit T-cell-dependent proliferation and increased tumor-specific immunoglobulin synthesis in response to stimulation with specific strains of *H. pylori* [40]. Cells from two high-grade gastric MALT lymphomas, a low-grade MALT lymphoma of salivary gland, a low-grade MALT lymphoma of thyroid and a nodal lymphocytic lymphoma showed no response. In a companion study [41], six patients with low-grade gastric MALT lymphoma and *H. pylori* infection were treated with antibiotics, resulting in eradication of *H. pylori*. In five of these patients, repeated biopsies showed no evidence of lymphoma. These studies suggest that low-grade gastric MALT lymphomas, at least for some stage of their evolution, are driven by *H. pylori* antigens and that eradication of this organism can lead to tumor regression.

Gastric MALT lymphomas may show distant spread to other mucosal sites, such as the small intestine, but spread to bone marrow and peripheral lymph nodes, such as is seen in most low-grade B-cell lymphomas, is distinctly uncommon. Spread to local lymph nodes occurs in less than half the cases. Within the lymph nodes, the tumor cells may show a marginal zone distribution around reactive follicles or they may colonize the follicles, giving the appearances of a follicular lymphoma. However, in contrast to follicle center cell lymphomas which show high levels of Bcl-2 expression and relatively low proliferation fractions, colonized follicles show low Bcl-2 expression and high proliferation fractions [20].

Prognosis is related to stage and grade. In two large, retrospective series [33,34], treated with surgery and chemotherapy and/or radiotherapy, the 5-year survival was in the region of 90% and the 10-year survival between 60% and 70%. Low-grade lymphomas had significantly better survival probabilities than high-grade lymphomas. These figures contrast with a 20% survival at 6 years of nodal immunocytomas, the category into which many low-grade MALT lymphomas were placed (and which includes tumors carrying a poor prognosis) before their recognition as a distinct entity [42].

Intestine

Lymphomas of the small and large intestine are more heterogeneous than gastric lymphomas which are predominantly of MALT type. They include enteropathy-associated T-cell lymphoma (see below), Burkitt-like lymphomas of the ileocaecal region that occur predominantly in children and young adults, lymphomatous polyposis (mantle cell lymphoma), plasmacytomas and occasional follicle center cell lymphomas, as well as tumors of MALT derivation [20]. MALT lymphomas are more common in the small, than in the large, intestine. They occur typically in elderly patients and may form annular ulcerating lesions or polypoid masses. Presentation is most commonly with abdominal pain, weight loss, obstruction or bleeding. These tumors may be low grade and show the same histological features as low-grade MALT lymphomas of the stomach. High-grade lymphomas have the morphology of nodal high-grade B-cell lymphomas and are often categorized as centroblastic or immunoblastic. Multiple blocks may, however, identify residual areas of low-grade MALT lymphoma. Other clues to the MALT origin are the low expression of Bcl-2 protein, association with lymphomas at other MALT sites, such as the stomach, and their tendency to remain localized (stage IE and IIE). The prognosis of MALT lymphomas of the intestine, as judged from limited reports, appears to be less favorable than that of gastric MALT lymphomas [43,44]. Immunoproliferative small intestinal disease (IPSID) is a form of MALT lymphoma affecting the upper small intestine, in which the neoplastic plasma cells secrete α heavy chain without light chains. The disease occurs almost exclusively in the Middle East. It is the subject of Chapter 22 and is not dealt with further in this chapter.

Waldeyer's ring

Waldeyer's ring is the second most common site of extranodal lymphomas after the gastrointestinal tract. Lymphoid tissue in the oropharynx is situated at the interface between the gut-associated and systemic lymphoid tissues, making it a potential site for MALT lymphomas. The organization of lymphoid tissue in Waldeyer's ring has similarities to the organization of MALT, including the absence of sinuses, the introduction of antigen through cryptal epithelium and the presence of a marginal zone-related subpopulation of B-cells. Chan et al. [45] were the first to suggest that some lymphomas of Waldeyer's ring may be of MALT derivation. More recently, Paulsen and Lennert [46] reviewed 329 cases of low-grade, non-Hodgkin's lymphoma of Waldeyer's ring and identified 12 of these as MALT lymphomas. These cases were identifed by their centrocyte-like morphology and perifollicular growth pattern and, in some cases, by follicular colonization and plasmacytic differentation. In all cases, the centrocyte-like cells invaded the reticulated epithelium of the crypts and the respiratory epithelium, although the authors did not consider that they formed typical lymphoepithelial lesions. This latter point is debatable, since the epithelium of the tonsillar crypts is normally heavily infiltrated by lymphocytes, making it difficult to know what criteria should be used to identify a lymphoepithelial lesion at this site. Further support for the concept that some non-Hodgkin's lymphomas of Waldeyer's ring are of MALT origin, is the observation that synchronous and metachronous involvement of Waldeyer's ring is recorded in patients with gastrointestinal lymphomas, despite the lack of direct lymphatic communication between these sites [47,48]. In addition, a significant population of patients with Waldeyer's ring lymphomas relapse in the gastrointestinal tract [49–51], an association not seen in patients with lymphomas at other sites in the head and neck [50]. Two-thirds of B-cell non-Hodgkin's lymphomas arising in Waldeyer's ring are high

grade and may not, therefore, be recognized morphologically as MALT lymphomas [52].

It is of interest that only 3.6% of the low-grade, non-Hodgkin's lymphomas of Waldeyer's ring, reported by Paulsen and Lennert [46], were categorized as being MALT lymphomas. This contrasts with almost 100% of low-grade B-cell non-Hodgkin's lymphomas of the stomach being of MALT derivation. This probably reflects the fact that most MALT lymphomas arise in aquired reactive lymphoid tissue, associated with infections or autoimmune disease. It may be that, in these circumstances, antigen drive combined perhaps with defective T-cell control are prerequisites for the emergence of neoplastic B-cells.

Liver and biliary tract

Primary non-Hodgkin's lymphomas of the liver are uncommon and only two have been reported that have the morphology of MALT lymphomas [20]. One of these was found in a liver removed from a patient with chronic, active hepatitis prior to transplantation. The other was in a patient with no associated liver disease. The histology showed reactive lymphoid follicles in the portal tracts surrounded by centrocyte-like cells that formed lymphoepithelial lesions with bile ducts.

Two cases of primary MALT lymphoma of the gall bladder have been reported in the literature [53,54]. Both were incidental findings, one in a patient undergoing cholecystectomy for cholelithiasis and the other in a patient undergoing colectomy for carcinoma of the colon. In both cases, the lymphoma contained reactive lymphoid follicles surrounded by centrocyte-like cells that formed lymphoeipthelial lesions with the gall bladder epithelium. Both also showed monotypic plasma cell differentiation.

Salivary glands

Organized lymphoid tissues are not seen in normal salivary glands, although they are part of the mucosal immune system and transport secretory IgA. Lymphoid tissue accumulates around salivary gland ducts in the condition designated as myoepithelial sialadenitis (MESA), which may be associated with Sjögren's syndrome [55]. The organization of the lymphoid tissue and its relationship to duct epithelium is similar to that seen in MALT in the gastrointestinal tract. The risk of lymphoma in patients with Sjögren's syndrome and MESA is over 40 times greater than that of the general population [20].

The distinction between MESA and low-grade MALT lymphoma of salivary gland may be difficult and the slow progression of these cases led to the use of the term 'benign lymphoepithelial lesion of salivary gland' before MALT lymphomas at this site were recognized [56–58]. Immunohistochemistry and molecular biological techniques have been used to establish the monoclonal nature of these proliferations [59,60]. Histologically, ducts may show dilatation, as a result of obstruction, but frequently undergo a proliferative change to form epimyoepithelial islands. These islands become infiltrated by, and surrounded by, centrocyte-like or monocytoid cells (Figure 21.6). The clear cytoplasm of these cells gives a characteristic pale halo around the epimyoepithelial islands. Reactive lymphoid follicles are seen within the lesion and these may undergo follicular colonization. Plasma cell differentiation may also occur.

Metastasis to lymph nodes may give rise to the characteristic marginal zone distribution in centrocyte-like cells, giving the appearance of so-called monocytoid B-cell lymphomas. Spread to lymph nodes is often accompanied by an intense proliferation of epithelioid cells in which individual or clusters of centrocyte-like cells are surrounded by epithelioid cells [61]. Low-grade MALT lymphomas of salivary glands may show progression to high-grade lymphomas [20]. In general, MALT lymphomas of the salivary gland show a slow progression with periods as long as 29 years recorded between the appearance of salivary gland enlargement and the diagnosis of lymphoma [55]. An association with MALT lymphomas at other sites has been recorded [55].

Respiratory system

The bronchial tree is considered to be part of the mucosal immune system [4], although the presence of bronchus-associated lymphoid tissue (BALT) has been disputed. However, although organized lymphoid tissue is not found in normal lungs, it is seen in response to some infections. In follicular broncheolitis, a condition associated with Sjögren's syndrome and other autoimmune disease, lymphoid follicles showed the same relationship to overlying bronchial epithelium as is seen in MALT of the gastrointestinal tract [62]. MALT lymphomas of the lung may arise in the setting of such acquired lymphoid tissue, as at other sites.

Low-grade MALT lymphomas of the lung show the characteristic features seen at other sites [63–66]. Reactive germinal centres are surrounded and eventually colonized by centrocyte-like cells. These cells infiltrate bronchiolar and bronchial epithelium forming lymphoepithelial lesions and plasmacytic differentiation may occur. At the periphery of the tumor, lymphoid cells show interstitial infiltration along alveolar walls giving the appearance of lymphocytic interstitial pneumonia. This may cause problems of differential diagnosis in small biopsies, necessitating the use of immunohistochemistry or molecular biology to establish the monoclonality of the infiltrate. High-grade MALT lymphomas of the lung are much rarer than low-grade tumors. They can be recognized as MALT lymphomas by the finding of residual areas of low-grade tumor or by their propensity to infiltrate bronchial epithelium in the manner of MALT lymphomas [23].

Low-grade MALT lymphomas are very indolent in their clinical evolution and are not infrequently detected as a result of a routine chest X-ray, rather than as a consequence of the investigation of symptoms. They may be associated with MALT lymphomas at other sites. Most patients are stage IE at presentation and survival, following resection alone, or resection and radiotherapy or chemotherapy, appears to be excellent [14,64,65,67].

Kaplan et al. [68] noted three primary non-Hodgkin's lymphomas of the trachea recorded in the literature and added a fourth case of their own. This case showed the features of a low-grade lymphoma of MALT forming lymphoepithelial lesions with the tracheal epithelium and submucosal plasmacytic differentiation. The patient was disease free, 12 months following surgical excision and local radiation.

Thyroid

Malignant lymphoma of the thyroid arises in the setting of Hashimoto's disease or lymphocytic thyroiditis [17,18]. The relative risk of patients with Hashimoto's disease developing lymphoma of the thyroid is 67 [69]. Lymphoid tissue in Hashimoto's disease, or lymphocytic thyroiditis, recapitulates many of the features of MALT seen in the gastrointestinal tract and the majority of lymphomas, at this site, are believed to be MALT lymphomas. Although the thyroid would not usually be regarded as a mucosal site, it is derived from the fore-gut and low-grade lymphomas of the thyroid show all the characteristic features of MALT lymphomas.

Lymphoepithelial lesions in low-grade thyroid MALT lymphomas are formed by tumor cells infiltrating and filling out thyroid acini (Figures 21.4 and 21.5). The majority of thyroid lymphomas are high grade and these also show infiltration of thyroid epithelium to form lymphoepithelial lesions [23]. This feature is not identifiable with routine stains but is highlighted by immunohistochemistry for cyto-keratins or epithelial membrane antigen. Follicular colonization has been well described in thyroid MALT lymphomas [22]. Plasma cell differentiaton is common in these tumors and may be so marked that the tumors are miscategorized as plasmacyto-mas. Immunohistochemistry, or molecular biologi-cal techniques, can be used to establish the clonality of MALT lymphomas of the thyroid and to separate them from Hashimoto's disease in borderline cases. In contrast to most other MALT lymphomas that usually synthesize IgM heavy chain, MALT lym-phomas of the thyroid most frequently synthesize IgG heavy chain [20].

Lymphoma of the thyroid occurs predominantly in late middle and old age and shows a marked female preponderance. The prognosis appears to be much worse if the tumor shows capsular invasion. MALT lymphomas of the thyroid are associated with MALT lymphomas at other sites, the associa-tion between thyroid and gastrointestinal lymphomas having been recognized for many years [70].

Thymus

Three cases of low-grade MALT lymphoma have been described in the thymus [71,72]. All had thymic enlargement as a result of a multicystic thymic mass. One patient had a preceding 25-year history of Sjögren's syndrome. The lymphomas displayed the typical histological features of low-grade MALT lymphoma forming lymphoepithelial lesions with the epithelium of Hassall's corpuscles. Two patients had lymph node involvement but are alive, 3 and 2 years following thymectomy, having received chemo-therapy or radiotherapy. One patient, without lymph node involvement, is well, 6 years following thymec-tomy without further treatment.

Breast

Primary breast lymphomas fall into two clinico-pathological groups [73,74]. The first presents wtih bilateral, diffuse disease during pregnancy or lacta-tion, is rapidly progressive and histologically cor-responds to Burkitt's lymphoma (see below). The second occurs predominantly in older women who present with solitary breast lumps, clinically simulat-ing breast carcinoma. Hugh et al. [73] concluded that the majority of the second group were MALT lymphomas, based on the evidence of their histologi-cal appearance, including the formation of lym-phoepithelial lesions with breast ducts, the possible chronic inflammatory precursor lesion and the pat-tern of recurrence with the frequent involvement of other MALT sites. In contrast, Bobrow et al. [74], in a study of eight B-cell lymphomas of breast, iden-tified one as a follicle center cell lymphoma but concluded that the remaining seven high-grade lymphomas, although lacking t(14;18), showed no features of lymphomas of MALT. It would be surprising if lymphomas arising in a recognized site of MALT [6] were not lymphomas of MALT.

Urogenital tract

The lower female genital tract is recognized as part of the mucosal immune system, influenced by estrogen [5]. MALT lymphomas have rarely been recognized at this site with one MALT lymphoma recorded in the cervix [54] and possibly two in the fallopian tube [20,75]. Most ovarian lymphomas are of high grade and include Burkitt's lymphoma (see below). It is, as yet, uncertain whether any of these tumors are of MALT type.

Low-grade MALT lymphomas have been des-cribed in the prostate gland [20,54]. The majority of lymphomas of the male genital tract occur in the testis and are high grade. The relationship of these tumors to either the mucosal or the systemic immune system is, as yet, uncertain.

Primary lymphomas of the kidney are rare. Two low-grade MALT lymphomas have been described at this site [54,76]. These show the typical morpho-logical features of low-grade MALT lymphomas, including the formation of lymphoepithelial lesions with the renal tubules. One of these patients had Sjögren's syndrome and simultaneous malignant lymphoma of the parotid gland. MALT lymphomas have been described in the urinary bladder where they mimic and are often misdiagnosed on biopsy specimens as chronic cystitis [77–79]. They arise on a background of follicular cystitis and cystitis cystica. The centrocyte-like cells form lymphoepithel-ial lesions with the epithelium in areas of cystitis cystica. Plasmacytic differentiation beneath the uro-thelium is common. These lymphomas may follow an indolent course. Their increased frequency in women is probably due to the greater incidence of cystitis in females.

Ocular adnexae

The great majority of lymphomas of the orbit are low grade and of the B-cell phenotype. Approximately, one-third arise in the conjunctiva [80], one-third in the lacrimal gland and one-third elsewhere in the orbit [20]. Isaacson and Norton [20] argue that the majority of these cases are low-grade MALT lymphomas. The lymphomas in the conjunctiva and lacrimal gland show lymphoepithelial lesions, and may surround or colonize follicles. The tumor cells have the morphology of small lymphocytes, CCL cells or monocytoid cells. They are CD20 and CD22-positive and negative for CD10. Although some CD5-positive tumors have been reported, a finding that would suggest lymphocytic or mantle cell lymphoma, it is not clear to what extent the CD5 positivity is due to infiltrating T-lymphocytes. Fifteen to 20% of patients with stage IE ocular disease go on to develop disease elsewhere, after periods as long as 22 years, with involvement of other MALT sites, such as the lung and salivary glands [81].

Skin

It is now recognized that an uncommon group of low-grade B-cell lymphomas of skin, often categorized as lymphoplasmacytic lymphomas or immunocytomas, have features of marginal zone or MALT lymphomas [20,54]. They most often present as single or multiple violatious nodules or plaques. They may be associated with lymphomas at other MALT sites, but most frequently appear to be confined to the skin and to recur at this site. Histologically, they show all the characteristics of MALT lymphomas with a marginal zone distribution around reactive follicles, follicular colonization and plasmacytic differentiation. They may form lymphoepithelial lesions, either in hair follicles or in sweat gland ducts. The frequent presence of reactive germinal centres may lead to misdiagnosis as a reactive or inflammatory lesion, although immunohistochemistry or molecular biological techniques will usually establish the monoclonality of the infiltrate [82]. It is probable that these lymphomas arise in a setting of an inflammatory lesion, such as Lyme disease [20]. Transformation to high-grade B-cell lymphoma may be seen in a minority of cases.

Monocytoid B-cell lymphomas

Monocytoid B-cell lymphoma was described as a novel B-cell neoplasm in 1986 [83]. Many of the cases described in this and subsequent publications [84–88] had evidence of autoimmune disease, particularly Sjögren's syndrome [88]. In several of the cases, the lymphomas involved the salivary gland or mucosal sites and were indistinguishable from MALT lymphomas. Studies from the Kiel Lymphoma Registry, of 21 cases of monocytoid B-cell lymphoma, showed that seven of them had concomitant or subsequent lymphomas of MALT [89]. Further studies, by the same group, of the draining lymph nodes from 58 gastric MALT lymphomas found the pattern of monocytoid B-cell lymphoma in 10 of them [90]. Monocytoid B-cell lymphomas have the same cytomorphology and immunophenotype as MALT lymphomas and share with them the characteristics of marginal zone distribution, follicular colonization and plasma cell differentiation [61]. It, thus, appears that monocytoid B-cell lymphomas and MALT lymphomas are closely related entities with monocytoid B-cell lymphoma frequently representing spread of a MALT lymphoma to lymph nodes [13].

Burkitt's lymphoma

It has been proposed that endemic Burkitt's lymphoma is derived from cells of MALT [91]. The argument in favor of this hypothesis is that Burkitt's lymphoma involves many MALT sites and tends not to involve peripheral lymph nodes, spleen or bone marrow. The massive, diffuse, bilateral breast tumors that occur in females who develop Burkitt's lymphoma, during pregnancy or lactation can be seen as a recapitulation of the migration of mucosal B-blasts to the breasts at this time [92]. Derivation from mucosal lymphocytes may also account for the age-dependent localization of Burkitt's lymphoma to the jaw [93], in which all four quadrants of the maxilla and mandible are frequently involved. The toothbud is essentially a downgrowth of mucosal epithelium into the jaw which, at the time of active tooth development, contains substantial amounts of lymphoid tissue (unpublished personal observation). This lymphoid tissue is no longer apparent by the mid-teens, which would account for why jaw tumors are most frequent in the youngest children with Burkitt's lymphoma and least frequent in the oldest. The molecular biology of Burkitt's lymphoma, in particular c-*myc* dysregulation, would explain why the behavior of this tumor is so different from that of other MALT lymphomas, and why, for example, the tumor cells do not show differentiation towards plasma cells. It is of interest that Burkitt's lymphoma does appear to show the characteristic epithelial infiltration, seen in other MALT lymphomas, with the formation of lymphoepithelial lesions [20].

T-Cell lymphomas of mucosa-associated lymphoid tissue

T-cells constitute part of the mucosal immune system in which they function both as regulators of immunoglobulin production and as effector cells in cell-mediated immunity. Phenotypically distinct subpopulations of T-cells are found in the Peyer's patches, submucosa and within the epithelium (intraepithelial lymphocytes). The function of intraepithelial lymphocytes is uncertain. Their numbers and the proportion expressing $\gamma\delta$ T-cell receptors is increased in celiac disease. The association of these cells with villus atrophy and their responsiveness to

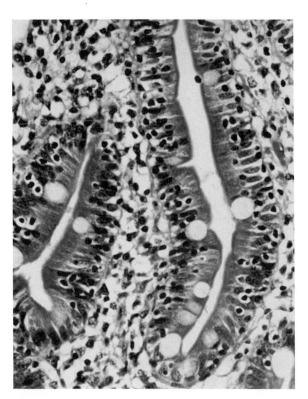

Figure 21.11 A higher-power view of Figure 21.10 showing intraepithelial lymphocytes.

gluten withdrawal and rechallenge, suggests that they play a central role in mediating mucosal damage in this disease. Patients with celiac disease have an increased prevalence of malignant lymphomas, predominantly of the small intestine, that appear to arise from intraepithelial T-lymphocytes.

Fairley and Mackie [94] first reported the association of sprue and malignant lymphoma attributing the malabsorption to lymphatic obstruction. Gough et al. [95], however, reported three patients with lymphoma and steatorrhea, and reviewed 29 other patients reported in the literature in whom malabsorption frequently predated the diagnosis of lymphoma, in some instances by as much as 20–25 years. They proposed that the lymphomas were a complication of idiopathic steatorrhea, rather than the cause. Subsequent studies have generally supported this concept [96–98].

Isaacson and Wright [99] reported 18 patients with small intestinal lymphoma with villus atrophy and intraepithelial lymphocytosis in the adjacent, uninvolved bowel (Figures 21.10 and 21.11). Five of these patients had an established diagnosis of adult onset celiac disease before the diagnosis of lymphoma. They proposed that these tumors were of a single, histogenetic type and, based on the morphology and distribution of the tumor cells and the limited immunohistochemical markers available at

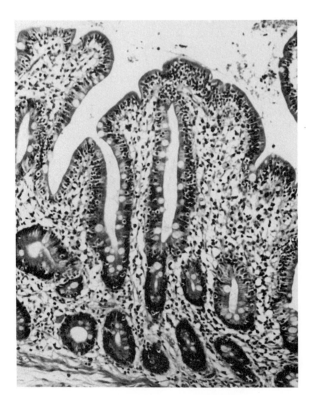

Figure 21.10 Enteropathic bowel adjacent to an enteropathy-associated T-cell lymphoma showing villus atrophy, crypt hyperplasia and marked intraepithelial lymphocytosis.

the time, designated the tumors as malignant histiocytosis of the intestine. Subsequent studies, using molecular biological techniques to identify clonal rearrangements of the T-cell receptor genes and improved immunohistochemistry, showed the tumor cells to be of the T-cell lineage [100]. The tumor cells also expressed the activation marker CD30 and a novel integrin $\beta 7$ subunit expressed on intraepithelial T-cells and recognized by the antibody HML1 (CD103) [101]. The tumor is now generally designated as enteropathy-associated T-cell lymphoma (EATCL) [102].

Most patients with EATCL present in the fifth to the seventh decades of life with acute intestinal obstruction or perforation, preceded by weight loss and abdominal pain. Patients with established celiac disease often become unresponsive to a gluten-free diet with recrudescence of features of severe malabsorption. Pyrexia, finger clubbing and icthyotic skin rashes may occur. Signs and symptoms of an abdominal catastrophy usually lead to laparotomy with resection of diseased bowel. The resected bowel is often edematous and proximally dilated, and shows one or more circumferential ulcers on the mucosal surface. Gross features of a neoplastic process, in the form of tumor masses, may not be apparent. Mesenteric lymph node enlargement is usual, but this may be due either to reactive hyperplasia or lymphoma. Ulcers are most frequently located in the upper small intestine but may be found throughout the bowel, including, rarely, the stomach and colon. The prognosis of EATCL is extremely poor, with an average survival of less than 6 months from diagnosis [103], although occasional long-term survivors have been reported [104]. This poor prognosis is, in part, related to the clinical state in which patients often present, following a major abdominal catastrophy on top of malnutrition due to preceding malabsorption.

Histologically, EATCL are high-grade lymphomas showing varying degrees of pleomorphism (Figure 21.12). The tumor cells are usually accompanied by a large number of inflammatory cells, associated with the intestinal ulceration. In some instances, these can obscure small collections of tumor cells giving the appearance of an inflammatory ulcer. It has been suggested that most, if not all, cases of ulcerative enteritis associated with celiac disease are, in fact, cryptic lymphomas [105]. In such cases, the tumor cells may be highlighted with immunohistochemistry using antibodies to CD30. Phenotypically, most EATCL express CD3 and CD8 in keeping with an origin from intraepithelial lymphocytes [104]. Their possible origin from intraepithelial lymphocytes is further supported by the observation that the tumor cells themselves frequently show epitheliotropism (Figures 21.13–21.15), a fea-

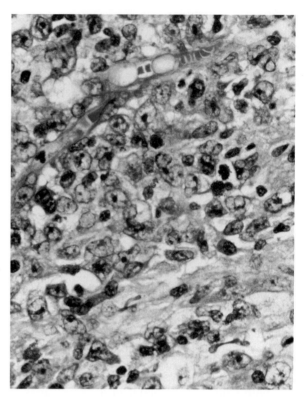

Figure 21.12 An enteropathy-associated T-cell lymphoma. Large blastic cells with vesicular nuclei and prominent, often central nucleoli, are admixed with histiocytes and small lymphocytes.

ture that may be highlighted by CD30 staining.

Not all authors have accepted the view that EATCL is a complication of celiac disease. Hourihane and Weir [106] postulated that the enteropathy

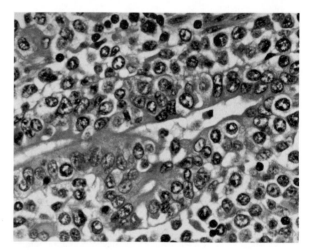

Figure 21.13 A high-power view of an enteropathy-associated T-cell lymphoma showing infiltration of glandular epithelium by blastic tumor cells.

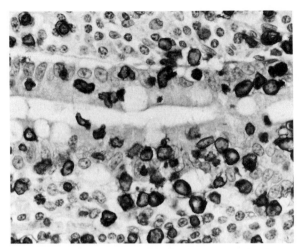

Figure 21.14 The same case as that illustrated in Figure 21.13 stained for CD3. CD3-positive small lymphocytes and tumor cells can be seen infiltrating glandular epithelium.

associated with the lymphoma was a prelymphomatous infiltrate analagous to mycosis fungoides. They suggested that the high-grade lymphoma resulted from transformation of this low-grade enteropathic infiltrate. O'Farrelly et al. [102] compared 76 patients with uncomplicated celiac disease and 16 patients with EATCL. They found differences in these two groups, with respect to antibody levels to α-gliadin, response to gluten withdrawal, HLA groups and sex ratio, and suggested that there are two forms of enteropathy, one benign and sensitive to wheat protein and the other analagous to mycosis fungoides. In contrast to the findings of O'Farrelly et al. [102], others have observed similar expression of HLA serotypes in celiac disease and EATCL with a high proportion of cases in both groups expressing HLA DR3.

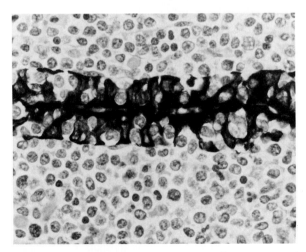

Figure 21.15 The same case as illustrated in Figure 21.13 stained for low molecular weight cytokeratin. This stain highlights the epitheliotropism of the tumor cells.

HLA polymorphisms can be detected at the DNA level using polymerase chain reaction amplification, followed by oligonucleotide probing or DNA sequencing. Susceptibility to celiac disease is associated with an HLA DQ heterodimer encoded by DQA1*0501 and DQB1*0201 genes in *cis* or *trans* configuration [107]. In a recent study of 47 patients with EATCL and 91 patients with uncomplicated celiac disease, genotype frequencies were compared with 151 unrelated control individuals [108]. Ninety-one per cent of the celiac disease patients were of the DQA1*0501, DQB1*0201 genotype, compared with 93% of the EATCL patients and 23% of the controls. DRB1*03 frequencies were also elevated in both patient groups, compared with controls. These results suggest that EATCL arises in individuals with the DQA1*0501, DQB1*0201 celiac disease predisposing genotype. However, the frequencies of DRB1*03, 04 heterozygotes was significantly increased in the EATCL group, compared with uncomplicated celiac disease patients and controls. Conversely, there was a significant decrease in DRB1*07 frequencies in the EATCL patients, compared with the uncomplicated celiac disease patients. In addition, none of the 38 DQA1*0501, DQB1*0201 EATCL patients were homozygous for DQB1*0201, compared with 53% of the DQA1*0501, DQB1*0201 celiac disease patients and 38% of the DQA1*0501, DQB1*0201 controls. These findings suggest that additional HLA-DR/DQ-associated alleles acting independently or in association with DQA1*0501, DQB1*0201 may represent risk factors for EATCL. Age of onset data in a group of celiac disease patients suggested that DQB1*0201 homozygosity may predispose to early age of onset, which may account for the absence of this genotype in EATCL, which is predominantly associated with adult onset celiac disease.

Alfsen et al. [109] studied a single case of EATCL and identified a clonal T-cell receptor gene rearrangement in the enteropathic bowel, distant to the tumor. Unfortunately, the authors were unable to undertake clonality studies on the main tumor mass. They suggested that the high-grade lymphoma had arisen as a result of transformation of the low-grade neoplasm present in the enteropathic bowel, supporting the analogy with mycosis fungoides proposed by Hourihane and Weir. The difficulty in obtaining fresh tissue from patients with EATCL made it hard to enlarge this study. However, the detection of T-cell receptor gene rearrangements is now possible using the polymerase chain reaction on sections of routinely processed, paraffin-embedded tissues. Primers for T-cell receptor β and γ genes, used in combinations that allow detection of approximately 90% of T-cell receptor gene rearrangements, were used to study 14 cases of EATCL [104]. Clonal T-cell rearrangements were identified in 13 of the 14 tumors and in the enteropathic bowel in 11 cases. In ten of these cases, the amplified DNA was the same size in the enteropathic bowel as in the tumor, and in two cases nucleotide sequencing showed identity between the amplified band from the enteropathic bowel and that from the tumor.

These findings could be the result of intramucosal spread of tumor cells into the enteropathic bowel. They might be taken as support for the mycosis fungoides hypothesis or that clonal T-cell populations emerge from the intraepithelial lesions of celiac disease and subsequently transform into high-grade tumors. Evidence against intramucosal cell spread was the inability to identify tumor cells by morphology or immunohistochemistry, and the fact that the blocks of enteropathic bowel were often taken at a distance from the tumor with intervening blocks negative for clonal gene rearrangements. Evidence against the mycosis fungoides hypothesis, i.e., that the enteropathy is the result of a low-grade lymphoma, was the failure to indentify clonal T-cells in all blocks of enteropathic bowel. The data best fit the hypothesis that clonal evolution occurs within the reactive intraepithelial T-cells of celiac disease. One patient in this series was diagnosed as having celiac disease in childhood and treated with a gluten-free diet until the age of 12 when he resumed a normal diet. At the age of 47, he presented with abdominal pain, weight loss and melena and an EATCL was resected. He was given postoperative chemotherapy and restarted on a gluten-free diet. Nine years later he re-presented with small bowel obstruction and a lymphomatous stricture was resected. The patient was given a further course of chemotherapy, and he is alive and well 16 years after his first resection. Identical clonal T-cell receptor β gene rearrangements were found in both resected tumors. The adjacent enteropathic bowel did not show the same rearrangement of the β gene but both showed identical rearrangements of the γ gene. It seems improbable that the recurrence, 9 years after the first resection, was caused by regrowth of high-grade tumor cells, which exhibit a high proliferation index, and more likely that the recurrence evolved from a low-grade clone in the residual enteropathic bowel.

One of the reasons why some authors have been reluctant to accept EATCL as a complication of celiac disease is the fact that few patients with EATCL give a clear-cut history of celiac disease since childhood, and most present with adult-onset celiac disease or have no proven history of gluten-sensitive enteropathy. The reason for this apparent paradox may lie in the fact that there are many patients with subclinical, latent or undiagnosed celiac disease in the community [110]. These individuals consume a normal diet, whereas patients diagnosed as having celiac disease will be managed by gluten withdrawal. There is some evidence that adherence to a gluten-free diet protects patients with celiac disease from malignancy and returns them to a normal life expectancy [111]. Patients with latent celiac disease, taking a normal diet, may, therefore, be the population at greatest risk of developing EATCL. Gluten may provide the antigen drive that allows, or causes, the neoplastic progression in intraepithelial lymphocytes in susceptible individuals and may have the same relationship to EATCL as has been proposed for *Helicobacter pylori* in relationship to gastric MALT lymphoma.

References

1. Isaacson P, Wright DH. Malignant lymphoma of mucosa-associated lymphoid tissue. A distinctive type of B-cell lymphoma. *Cancer* 1983, **52**: 1410–1416.
2. Isaacson P, Wright DH. Extranodal malignant lymphoma arising from mucosa-associated lymphoid tissue. *Cancer* 1984, **53**: 2515–2524.
3. National Cancer Institute sponsored study of classifications of non-Hodgkin's lymphomas. Summary and description of a Working Formulation for clinical usage. *Cancer* 1982, **49**: 2112–2135.
4. McDermott MR, Bienenstock J. Evidence for a common mucosal immunologic system. 1. Migration of B-immunoblasts into intestinal, respiratory and genital tissues. *J. Immunol.* 1979, **122**: 1892–1898.
5. McDermott MR, Clark DA, Bienenstock J. Evidence for a common mucosal immunologic system. 2. Influence of the estrus cycle on B-immunoblast migration into genital and intestinal tissues. *J. Immunol.* 1980, **124**: 2536–2539.
6. Roux ME, McWilliams M, Phillips-Quagliata JM, et al. Origin of IgA-secreting plasma cells in the mammary gland. *J. Exp. Med.* 1977, **146**: 1311–1321.
7. Butcher EC. Cellular and molecular mechanisms that direct leucocyte traffic. *Am. J. Pathol.* 1990, **136**: 3–11.
8. Isaacson PG, Spencer J, Finn T. Primary B-cell gastric lymphoma. *Hum. Pathol.* 1986, **17**: 72–82.
9. Myhre MJ, Isaacson PG. Primary B-cell gastric lymphoma – A reassessment of its histogenesis. *J. Pathol.* 1987, **152**: 1–11.
10. Isaacson PG, Spencer J. Malignant lymphoma of mucosa-associated lymphoid tissue. *Histopathology* 1987, **11**: 445–462.
11. Spencer J, Finn T, Isaacson PG. Gut-associated lymphoid tissue: A morphological and immunocytochemical study of the human appendix. *Gut* 1985, **26**: 672–679.
12. Chan JKC, Ng CS, Isaacson PG. Relationship between high-grade lymphoma and low-grade B-cell mucosa-

associated lymphoid tissue lymphoma [MALToma] of the stomach. *Am. J. Pathol.* 1990, **136**: 1153–1164.

13. Harris NL, Jaffe ES, Stein H, et al. A revised European–American classification of lymphoid neoplasms: A proposal from the International Lymphoma Study Group. *Blood* 1994, **84**: 1361–1392.

14. Herbert A, Wright DH, Isaacson PG, et al. Primary malignant lymphoma of the lung: Histopathologic and immunologic evaluation of nine cases. *Hum. Pathol.* 1984, **15**: 415–422.

15. Addis BJ, Hyjek E, Isaacson PG. Primary pulmonary lymphoma: A reappraisal of its histogenesis and its relationship to pseudolymphoma and lymphoid interstitial pneumonia. *Histopathology* 1988, **13**: 1–17.

16. Li G, Hansmann ML, Zwingers T, et al. Primary lymphomas of the lung: Morphological, immunohistochemical and clinical features. *Histopathology* 1990, **16**: 519–531.

17. Anscombe AM, Wright DH. Primary malignant lymphoma of the thyroid – A tumour of mucosa-associated lymphoid tissue: Review of 76 cases. *Histopathology* 1985, **9**: 81–97.

18. Hyjek E, Isaacson PG. Primary B-cell lymphoma of the thyroid and its relationship to Hashimoto's thyroiditis. *Hum. Pathol.* 1988, **19**: 1315–1326.

19. Hyjek E, Smith WJ, Isaacson PG. Primary B-cell lymphoma of salivary glands and its relationship to myoepithelial sialadenitis. *Hum. Pathol.* 1988, **19**: 766–776.

20. Isaacson PG, Norton AJ. *Extranodal Lymphomas.* Edinburgh: Churchill Livingstone 1994.

21. Isaacson PG, Wotherspoon AC, Diss T, et al. Follicular colonisation in B-cell lymphoma of MALT. *Am. J. Surg. Pathol.* 1991, **15**: 819–828.

22. Isaacson PG, Androulakis-Papachristou A, Diss T, et al. Follicular colonisation of thyroid lymphoma. *Am. J. Pathol.* 1992, **41**: 43–52.

23. Bateman AC, Wright DH. Epitheliotropism in high-grade lymphomas of mucosa-associated lymphoid tissue. *Histopathology* 1993, **23**: 409–415.

24. Zuckerberg LR, Ferry JA, Southern JF, et al. Lymphoid infiltrates of the stomach. Evaluation of histologic criteria for the diagnosis of low-grade gastric lymphoma on endoscopic biopsy specimens. *Am. J. Surg. Pathol.* 1990, **14**: 1087–1099.

25. Spencer J, Diss TC, Isaacson PG. Primary B-cell gastric lymphoma. A genotypic analysis. *Am. J. Pathol.* 1989, **135**: 557–564.

26. Diss TC, Peng H, Wotherspoon AC, et al. Detection of monoclonality in low-grade B-cell lymphomas using the polymerase chain reaction is dependent on primer selection and lymphoma type. *J. Pathol.* 1993, **169**: 291–295.

27. Osborne BM, Pugh WC. Practicality of molecular studies to evaluate small lymphocytic proliferations in endoscopic gastric biopsies. *Am. J. Surg. Pathol.* 1992, **16**: 838–844.

28. Sukpanichnant S, Vnencak-Jones CL, McCurley TL. Determination of B-cell clonality in paraffin-embedded endoscopic biopsy specimens of abnormal lymphocytic infiltrates and gastrointestinal lymphoma by polymerase chain reaction. *Am. J. Clin. Pathol.* 1994, **102**: 299–305.

29. Genta RM, Hamner HW, Graham DY. Gastric lymphoid follicles in *Helicobacter pylori* infection: Frequency, distribution and response to triple therapy. *Hum. Pathol.* 1993, **24**: 577–583.

30. Wotherspoon AC, Ortiz-Hidalgo C, Falzon MR, et al. *Helicobacter pylori*-associated gastritis and primary B-cell gastric lymphoma. *Lancet* 1991, **338**: 1175–1176.

31. Doglioni C, Wotherspoon AC, Moschini A, et al. High incidence of primary gastric lymphoma in north eastern Italy. *Lancet* 1992, **339**: 834–835.

32. Parsonnet J, Hansen S, Rodriguez L, et al. *Helicobacter pylori* infection and gastric lymphoma. *N. Engl. J. Med.* 1994, **330**: 1267–1271.

33. Cogliatti SB, Schmid U, Schumacher U, et al. Primary B-cell gastric lymphoma: A clinico-pathological study of 145 patients. *Gastroenterology* 1991, **101**: 1159–1170.

34. Radaszkiewicz T, Dragosics B, Bauer P. Gastrointestinal malignant lymphomas of the mucosa-associated lymphoid tissue: Factors relevant to prognosis. *Gastroenterology* 1992, **102**: 1628–1638.

35. Wotherspoon AC, Doglioni C, Isaacson PG. Low-grade gastric B-cell lymphoma of mucosa-associated lymphoid tissue (MALT). A multi-focal disease. *Histopathology* 1992, **20**: 29–34.

36. Nomura A, Stemmermann GN, Chyou P-H, et al. *Helicobacter pylori* infection and gastric carcinoma among Japanese Americans in Hawaii. *N. Engl. J. Med.* 1991, **325**: 1132–1136.

37. Parsonnet J, Friedman GD, Vandersteen DP, et al. *Helicobacter pylori* infection and the risk of gastric carcinoma. *N. Engl. J. Med.* 1991, **325**: 1127–1131.

38. Shani A, Schutt AJ, Weilend LH. Primary gastric malignant lymphoma, followed by gastric adenocarcinoma: Report of 4 cases and review of the literature. *Cancer* 1978, **42**: 2039–2044.

39. Baron BW, Bitter MA, Baron JM, et al. Gastric adenocarcinoma after gastric lymphoma. *Cancer* 1987, **60**: 1876–1882.

40. Hussell T, Isaacson PG, Crabtree JE, et al. The response of cells from low-grade B-cell gastric lymphomas of mucosa-associated lymphoid tissue to *Helicobacter pylori*. *Lancet* 1993, **342**: 571–574.

41. Wotherspoon AC, Doglioni C, Diss TC, et al. Regression of primary low-grade B-cell gastric lymphoma of mucosa-associated lymphoid tissue type after eradication of *Helicobacter pylori*. *Lancet* 1993, **342**: 575–577.

42. Lennert K, Feller AC. *Non-Hodgkin's Lymphomas*, 2nd edn (based upon the updated Kiel Classification). Berlin: Springer Verlag, 1990.

43. Shepherd NA, Hall PA, Coates PJ, et al. Primary malignant lymphoma of the colon and rectum. A histopathological and immunohistochemical study of 45 cases with clinico-pathological correlations. *Histopathology* 1988, **12**: 235–252.

44. Domizio P, Owen RA, Shephard NA, et al. Primary lymphoma of the small intestine: A clinico-pathological study of 119 cases. *Am. J. Surg. Pathol.* 1993, **17**: 429–432.

45. Chan JKC, Ng CS, Lo STH. Immunohistological characterisation of malignant lymphomas of the

Waldeyer's ring, other than the nasopharynx. *Histopathology* 1987, **11**: 885–899.

46. Paulsen J, Lennert K. Low-grade B-cell lymphoma of MALT type in Waldeyer's ring. *Histopathology* 1993, **24**: 1–11.
47. Rudders RA, Ross ME, DeLellis RA. Primary extranodal lymphoma, response to treatment and factors influencing prognosis. *Cancer* 1978, **42**: 406–416.
48. Ree HJ, Rege VB, Kinsley RE, et al. Malignant lymphoma of Waldeyer's ring, following gastrointestinal lymphoma. *Cancer* 1980, **46**: 1528–1535.
49. Saul SH, Kapadia SB. Primary lymphoma of Waldeyer's ring. Clinico-pathologic study of 68 cases. *Cancer* 1985, **56**: 157–166.
50. Jacobs C, Weiss L, Hoppe RT. The management of extranodal head and neck lymphomas. *Arch. Oto. Laryng. Head Neck Surg.* 1986, **112**: 654–658.
51. Shirato H, Tsuji H, Arimoto T, et al. Early stage head and neck non-Hodgkin's lymphoma: The effect of tumor burden on prognosis. *Cancer* 1986, **58**: 2312–2319.
52. Menarguez J, Mollejo M, Carrion R, et al. Waldeyer ring lymphomas. A clinico-pathological study of 119 cases. *Histopathology* 1994, **24**: 13–22.
53. Mosnier JF, Brousse N, Sevestre C, et al. Primary low-grade B-cell lymphoma of the mucosa-associated lymphoid tissue arising in the gall bladder. *Histopathology* 1992, **20**: 273–275.
54. Pelstring RJ, Essell JH, Kurtin PJ, et al. Diversity of organ site involvement among malignant lymphomas of mucosa-associated tissues. *Am. J. Clin. Pathol.* 1991, **96**: 738–745.
55. Schmid U, Helbron D, Lennert K. Development of malignant lymphoma in myoepithelial sialadenitis (Sjögren's syndrome). *Virchows Arch. A (Pathol. Anat.)* 1982, **395**: 11–43.
56. Azzopardi JG, Evans DJ. Malignant lymphoma of parotid associated with Mikulicz disease (benign lymphoepithelial lesion). *J. Clin. Pathol.* 1971, **24**: 744–752.
57. Anderson LG, Talal N. The spectrum of benign to malignant lymphoproliferation in Sjögren's syndrome. *Clin. Exp. Immunol.* 1971, **10**: 199–221.
58. Gleeson MJ, Cawson RA, Bennett MH. Benign lymphoepithelial lesion: A less than benign disease. *Clin. Oto. Laryngol.* 1986, **11**: 47–51.
59. Zulman J, Jaffe R, Talal N. Evidence that the malignant lymphoma of Sjögren's syndrome is a monoclonal B-cell neoplasm. *N. Engl. J. Med.* 1978, **299**: 1215–1220.
60. Fishleder A, Tubbs R, Hesse B, et al. Uniform detection of immunoglobulin gene rearrangement in benign lymphoepithelial lesions. *N. Engl. J. Med.* 1987, **316**: 1118–1121.
61. Ortiz-Hidalgo C, Wright DH. The morphological spectrum of monocytoid B-cell lymphoma and its relationship to lymphomas of mucosa-associated lymphoid tissue. *Histopathology* 1992, **21**: 555–561.
62. Yousem SA, Colby TV, Carrington CB. Follicular bronchitis/bronchiolitis. *Hum. Pathol.* 1985, **16**: 700–706.
63. Herbert A, Wright DH, Isaacson PG, et al. Primary malignant lymphoma of the lung: Histopathologic and immunologic evaluation of nine cases. *Hum. Pathol.* 1984, **15**: 415–422.
64. Addis BJ, Hyjek E, Isaacson PG. Primary pulmonary lymphoma: A reappraisal of its histogenesis and its relationship to pseudolymphoma and lymphoid interstitial pneumonia. *Histopathology* 1988, **13**: 1–17.
65. Li G, Hansmann ML, Zwingers T, et al. Primary lymphomas of the lung. Morphological, immunohistochemical and clinical features. *Histopathology* 1990, **16**: 519–531.
66. Chetty R, Close PM, Timme AH, et al. Primary biphasic lymphoplasmacytic lymphoma of the lung. A mucosa-associated lymphoid tissue lymphoma with compartmentalization of plasma cells in the lung and lymph nodes. *Cancer* 1992, **69**: 1124–1129.
67. Koss NM, Hochholzer L, Nichols PW, et al. Primary non-Hodgkin's lymphoma and pseudolymphoma of lung: A study of 161 patients. *Hum. Pathol.* 1983, **14**: 1024–1038.
68. Kaplan MA, Pettit CL, Zukerberg LR, et al. Primary lymphoma of the trachea with morphologic and immunophenotypic characteristics of low-grade B-cell lymphoma of mucosa-associated lymphoid tissue. *Am. J. Surg. Pathol.* 1992, **16**: 71–75.
69. Holm L-E, Blomgren H, Löwhagen T. *Cancer* risks in patients with chronic lymphocytic thyroiditis. *N. Engl. J. Med.* 1985, **312**: 601–604.
70. Brewer DB, Orr JW. Struma reticulosa: A consideration of the undifferentiated tumours of the thyroid. *J. Pathol. Bact.* 1953, **65**: 193–208.
71. Isaacson PG, Chan JKC, Tang C, et al. Low-grade B-cell lymphoma of mucosa-associated lymphoid tissue arising in the thymus. A thymic lymphoma mimicking myoepithelial sialadenitis. *Am. J. Surg. Pathol.* 1990, **14**: 342–351.
72. Takagi N, Nakamura S, Yamamoto K, et al. Malignant lymphoma of mucosa-associated lymphoid tissue arising in the thymus of a patient with Sjögren's syndrome. A morphologic, phenotypic and genotypic study. *Cancer* 1992, **69**: 1347–1355.
73. Hugh JC, Jackson FI, Hanson J, et al. Primary breast lymphoma. An immunohistologic study of 20 new cases. *Cancer* 1990, **66**: 2602–2611.
74. Bobrow LG, Richards MA, Happerfield LC, et al. Breast lymphomas: A clinico-pathologic review. *Hum. Pathol.* 1993, **24**: 274–278.
75. Ferry JA, Young RH. Malignant lymphoma, pseudolymphoma and hematopoietic disorders of the female genital tract. *Pathol. Ann.* 1991, **26**: 227–263.
76. Parveen T, Navarro-Roman L, Medeiros J, et al. Low-grade B-cell lymphoma of mucosa-associated lymphoid tissue arising in the kidney. *Arch. Pathol. Lab. Med.* 1993, **117**: 780–783.
77. Abraham NZ Jr, Maher TJ, Hutchinson RE. Extranodal monocytoid B-cell lymphoma of the urinary bladder. *Mod. Pathol.* 1993, **6**: 145–149.
78. Pawade J, Banerjee SS, Harris M, et al. Lymphomas of mucosa-associated lymphoid tissue arising in the urinary bladder. *Histopathology* 1993, **23**: 147–151.
79. Kuhara H, Tamura Z, Suchi IT, et al. Primary malignant lymphoma of the bladder. A case report. *Acta. Pathol. Jap.* 1990, **40**: 764–769.

80. Wotherspoon AC, Diss TC, Pan LX, et al. Low-grade B-cell lymphoma of the conjunctiva: A mucosa-associated lymphoid tissue (MALT) type lymphoma. *Histopathology* 1993, **23**: 417–424.

81. Medeiros LJ, Harris NL. Immunohistologic analysis of small lymphocytic infiltrates of the orbit and conjunctiva. *Hum. Pathol.* 1990, **21**: 1126–1131.

82. LeBoit PE, McNutt S, Reed JA, et al. Primary cutaneous immunocytoma. A B-cell lymphoma that can easily be mistaken for cutaneous lymphoid hyperplasia. *Am. J. Surg. Pathol.* 1994, **18**: 969–978.

83. Shibani K, Sohn CC, Burke JS, et al. Monocytoid B-cell lymphoma. A novel B-cell neoplasm. *Am. J. Pathol.* 1986, **124**: 310–318.

84. Shibani K, Burke JS, Schwartz WG, et al. Monocytoid B-cell lymphoma. Clinico-pathological study of 21 cases of a unique type of low-grade lymphoma. *Cancer* 1988, **62**: 1531–1538.

85. Ng CS, Chan JKC. Monocytoid B-cell lymphoma. *Hum. Pathol.* 1987, **18**: 1069–1071.

86. Piris MA, Rivas C, Morente M, et al. Monocytoid B-cell lymphoma. A tumour related to the marginal zone. *Histopathology* 1988, **12**: 383–392.

87. Ngan B-Y, Warnke RA, Wilson M, et al. Monocytoid B-cell lymphoma; a study of 36 cases. *Hum. Pathol.* 1991, **22**: 409–421.

88. Shin SS, Shibani K, Fishleder A, et al. Monocytoid B-cell lymphoma in patients with Sjögren's syndrome; a clinico-pathologic study of 13 patients. *Hum. Pathol.* 1991, **22**: 422–430.

89. Cogliatti SB, Lennert K, Hansmann M-L, et al. Monocytoid B-cell lymphoma; clinical and prognostic features of 21 patients. *J. Clin. Pathol.* 1990, **43**: 619–625.

90. Nizze H, Cogliatti SB, VonSchilling C, et al. Monocytoid B-cell lymphoma; morphological variants and relationship to low-grade B-cell lymphoma of the mucosa-associated lymphoid tissue. *Histopathology* 1991, **18**: 403–414.

91. Wright DH. In Lenoir G, O'Conor G, Olweny CLM (eds) *Burkitt's Lymphoma: A Human Cancer Model.* IARC Scientific Publications Number 60: Histogenesis of Burkitt's lymphoma; a B-cell tumour of mucosa-associated lymphoid tissue. Lyon: International Agency for Research on Cancer, 1985, pp. 37–45.

92. Shepherd JJ, Wright DH. Burkitt's tumour presenting as bilateral swellings of the breast in women of child bearing age. *Br. J. Surg.* 1967, **54**: 776–780.

93. Burkitt D. Burkitt's lymphoma: General features and facial tumours. In Burkitt DP, Wright DH (eds) *Burkitt's Lymphoma.* Edinburgh: E&S Livingstone, 1970, pp. 6–15.

94. Fairley NH, Mackie FP. The clinical and biochemical syndrome in lymphadenoma and allied diseases involving the mesenteric lymph glands. *Br. Med. J.* 1937, **1**: 375–380.

95. Gough KR, Read AE, Naish JM. Intestinal reticulosis as a complication of idiopathic steatorrhea. *Gut* 1962, **3**: 232–239.

96. Harris OD, Cooke WT, Thompson H, et al. Malignancy in adult celiac disease and idiopathic steatorrhea. *Am. J. Med.* 1967, **42**: 899–912.

97. Swinson CM, Slavin G, Coles EC, et al. Coeliac disease and malignancy. *Lancet* 1983, **1**: 111–115.

98. Thompson H. Necropsy studies on adult onset coeliac disease. *J. Clin. Path.* 1974, **27**: 710–721.

99. Isaacson PG, Wright DH. Intestinal lymphoma associated with malabsorption. *Lancet* 1978, **1**: 67–70.

100. Isaacson PG, Spencer J, Connolly CE, et al. Malignant histiocytosis of the intestine; a T-cell lymphoma. *Lancet* 1985, **2**: 688–690.

101. Stein H, Dienemann D, Sperling M. Identification of a T-cell lymphoma category derived from intestinal mucosa-associated T-cells. *Lancet* 1988, **2**: 1053–1054.

102. O'Farrelly C, Feighery C, O'Brian DS, et al. Humoral response to wheat protein in patients with coeliac disease and enteropathy-associated T-cell lymphoma. *Br. Med. J.* 1986, **293**: 908–910.

103. Mead GM, Whitehouse JM, Thompson J, et al. Clinical features and management of malignant histiocytosis of the intestine. *Cancer* 1987, **60**: 2791–2796.

104. Murray H, Cuevas EC, Jones DB, et al. A study of the immunohistochemistry and T-cell clonality of enteropathy-associated T-cell lymphomas. *Am. J. Pathol.* 1995, **146**: 509–519.

105. Isaacson PG, Wright DH. Malignant histiocytosis of the intestine; its relationship to malabsorption and ulcerative jejunitis. *Hum. Pathol.* 1988, **9**: 661–677.

106. Hourihane DO'B, Weir DG. Malignant celiac syndrome. *Gastroenterology* 1970, **29**: 130–139.

107. Sollid MN, Thorsby E. HLA susceptibility genes in celiac disease: Genetic mapping and role in pathogenesis. *Gastroenterology* 1993, **105**: 910–922.

108. Howell WM, Leung ST, Jones, DB, et al. HLA-DRB, DQA and DQB polymorphism in coeliac disease and enteropathy-associated T-cell lymphoma: Common features and additional risk factors for malignancy. *Human. Immunol.* 1995, **43**: 29–37.

109. Alfsen GC, Beiske K, Bell H, et al. Low-grade intestinal lymphoma of intraepithelial T-lymphocytes with concomitant enteropathy-associated T-cell lymphoma; case report suggesting a possible histogenetic relationship. *Hum. Pathol.* 1989, **20**: 909–913.

110. Catassi C, Rätsch I-M, Fabiani E, et al. Coeliac disease in the year 2000; exploring the iceberg. *Lancet* 1994, **343**: 200–203.

111. Holmes GKT, Prior P, Lane MR, et al. Malignancy in coeliac disease, effect of a gluten-free diet. *Gut* 1989, **30**: 333–338.

Pathological findings

The disease can be divided into two major phases, the first phase of which is further subdivided. Phase 1a is a reactive lymphoplasmacytic infiltration (IPSID) of the intestinal mucosa of the upper gastrointestinal tract causing wide separation of the crypts of Lieberkühn and obliteration of the villous architecture without significant impairment of the surface epithelium. This infiltrate can also be found in the mesenteric lymph nodes. The lymphoplasmacytic infiltration is detectable only on intestinal biopsy, since on macroscopic (endoscopic) examination the gut appears normal. This phase is probably reversible by antibiotic therapy. In phase 1b the infiltrate is composed of abnormal lymphoplasmacytic cells. Macroscopically there is a diffuse thickening of mucosal folds which is sometimes associated with a nodular mucosal pattern. This is probably a transitional phase and is not reversible. Phase 2 is a lymphoma with diffuse infiltration of the gut: the disease extends from the gut epithelium to the mesenteric and retroperitoneal lymph nodes. Extra-abdominal involvement is rare. Of special interest is the finding that the spleen is frequently small and fibrotic, as described in celiac disease.

Histologically, the malignant phase is characterized by an abnormal plasmacytoid, centroblastic and/or centrocytic infiltrate and the presence of large immunoblasts, sometimes resembling Reed–Sternberg cells, that can predominate in the infiltrate. It has been suggested that these large immunoblasts result from dedifferentiation of the monoclonal plasma cells [18–21], but they could also arise from immature precursors of the plasma cells situated in Peyer's patches [19–21].

The detailed histopathological description of this entity has been reported by Rappaport et al. [22], Nassar et al. [23] and has been extensively reviewed by Haghighi and Wolf [14].

These observations have led to the following hypothesis concerning the evolution of the disease. In underprivileged populations, repeated gastrointestinal tract infections in a host with an appropriate genetic background may result in a local lymphoplasmacytic response. The abnormal gut is the portal of entrance for additional 'noxious' agents and antigens that further stimulate the lymphatic tissue. Spontaneous or environmentally induced mutations in the proliferating pool result in chromosomal translocations, oncogene rearrangement and activation that can result in a malignant transformation. Although cytogenetic abnormalities have been reported in a number of cases, a specific consistent abnormality has not been described [24]. It is probable that the predominant stage of differentiation of cells in the proliferating pools at the time of the transforming event will influence the cytological pattern and hence the heterogeneity; lymphoplasmacytic, centrocytic (small cleaved cell), centroblastic (large cleaved or noncleaved cell), mixed or immunoblastic lymphoma will result. Histological evolution has been proven [14], although whether dedifferentiation of the infiltrating cells or clonal evolution in a proliferating pool is the cause remains to be determined.

Clinical features and diagnosis

The age distribution and clinical manifestations of primary intestinal lymphoma with malabsorption do not vary in different geographical regions [4–14]. Abdominal pain, chronic severe intermittent diarrhea and weight loss in young adults of both sexes are the main features in all series. The diarrhea is mainly a result of steatorrhea, and a protein-losing enteropathy has been reported [14]. Peripheral edema, tetany and clubbing have been observed in about 50% of patients. Peripheral lymphadenopathy and hepatosplenomegaly are very rare and in their presence intestinal lymphoma is an unlikely diagnosis [8].

At presentation, abdominal masses occur in 30–50 per cent of the patients. This finding is a late manifestation of the disease and its frequency will depend in part on the quality of the medical services in the region and on the time taken to diagnose the disease. The clinical course is frequently indolent with spontaneous remissions. Some patients have been diagnosed 1–4 years after the onset of symptoms.

Unfortunately, routine laboratory tests are not diagnostic. The abnormalities result from malabsorption as evident by steatorrhea and hypoproteinemia; less frequently hypocalcemia, hypomagnesemia and hypokalemia are seen. The cholesterol levels are frequently very low; hypochromic anemia is usually present and elevated alkaline phosphatase, often of intestinal origin, is a common finding [8]. The presence of α-heavy chain in the serum, urine, saliva and intestinal fluids is diagnostic, but not essential to the diagnosis, since it has been detected in the serum in only 25–60% of patients with primary intestinal lymphoma in developing countries. Therefore, the question of whether this protein abnormality is an integral part of the clinical syndrome of intestinal lymphoma with malabsorption remains unresolved.

Haghighi and Wolf [14] and Doe et al. [18] have developed an immunoselection method in which immunoelectrophoresis is performed in a gel containing a specially developed anti-Fab α-antiserum, which provides a very sensitive screening method for detecting α-heavy-chain disease (αHCD). This method, however, has not been applied to systematic screening of intestinal lymphoma patients, and therefore present estimates of the prevalence of α-heavy chain in the serum of patients with this clinical entity may be underestimated.

X-Rays of the gastrointestinal tract can be helpful, although the pattern is not specific. Barium studies in IPSID patients frequently show a malabsorption pattern which is more prominent in the upper small intestine. A coarse pseudopolypoid mucosal pattern, strictures and segmentation, and pressure by extrinsic masses, are observed in patients with intestinal lymphoma [4,8].

Immunoglobulin abnormalities in αHCD

Immunochemical studies indicate that the αHCD proteins have intact carboxy-terminal regions, and that their alterations involve the deletion of most of the V and all of the CH1 domains [25]. The precise boundaries of the deletions differ from case to case. The normal sequence usually resumes at the beginning of the hinge region of CH2 domain. These deletions are sometimes internal and some αHCD proteins contain a short part of the normal 5' V region amino terminus [25,26]. In all 17 αHCD proteins characterized in which there was an internal V region deletion, the residues corresponding to the V-D-J junctions were missing [27–29]. In a few cases, a portion of J_H sequence remained, indicating the occurrence of a complicated rearrangement process, such as two noncontiguous deletions [28–30]. In several cases the deleted V regions included or were replaced by short abnormal sequences without homology to any known sequence [30–33]. Sometimes the amino acid sequence of secreted αHCD proteins begins at the amino-terminal end with the CH2 domain [25], everything 5' of this has been deleted. It is most likely that the amino-terminal sequences encoded by inserted nonimmunoglobulin residues were cleaved intracellularly before secretion. The deletion of V_H sequences usually does not prevent the cleavage of the signal peptide that is required for protein secretion.

The abnormal proteins may confer a selective advantage; they may function as defective cell receptors leading to continuous signal transduction. Surface immunoglobulins serve as B-cell receptors

and binding of a specific antigen results in signal transduction mediated by the immunoglobulin (Ig)-associated Iga and Igb molecules, leading to the activation of a cascade of kinases. In many respects this phenomenon is analogous to the activation of cell surface growth factor receptors by their specific ligand. Molecular events that alter the structure of growth factor receptors such as the epidermal growth factor receptor (EGFR), the macrophage colony-stimulating factor receptor (M-CSFR) and the fibroblast growth factor receptor (FGFR) convert them into activated oncogenes. In the EGFR, for example, the truncation of the extracellular domain results in the abrogation of the inherent inhibitory effect of the intracellular catalytic domain. In normal receptors the binding of EGF releases the kinase activity and the signal transduction cascade is initiated. The kinase activity of the truncated receptor, known as the erb-B oncogene, is constitutively switched on, irrespective of the presence of the ligand (Figure 22.1a). One can speculate that the mutant α-heavy-chain proteins act in a similar fashion, leading to continuous lymphocyte stimulation resulting in malignant transformation (Figure 22.1b). Another possible selective advantage for B-cells producing Ig molecules with deleted V regions could be the escape from the network control mediated by anti-idiotypic antibodies.

Molecular abnormalities of Ig genes in αHCD

The large deletions in the variable region sequences of Ig genes in αHCD resemble the large deletions demonstrated in mutant severe combined immunodeficiency (SCID) mice. The latter have been shown to result from a basic defect in the V-D-J recombinase activity [34]. The deletions could occur during the V-D-J rearrangement in the early pre-B-cells, during secondary V_H to V_H-D-J_H rearrangement, but, alternatively, they could be independent of physiological gene rearrangements [35,36]. The deletions usually involve the genomic sequences including the CH1 exon and include, in most cases, some switch region sequences. The molecular mechanisms resulting in CH1 deletions might represent faulty isotype switch processes owing to illegitimate recognition of cryptic switch signal sequences. It is of interest that all αHCD proteins characterized so far belong to the α1 subclass [25]. The α1 constant region gene is located 5' to the α2 gene. It might be speculated that aberrant isotype switch processes more often involve the more proximal gene segment. This is consistent with

EGF receptor

erbB oncogene

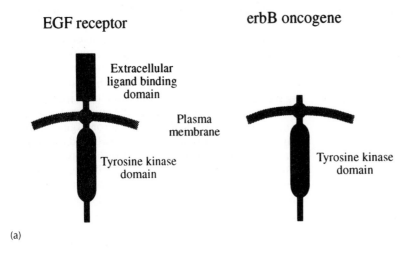

(a)

Surface Ig

Surface alpha
heavy chain

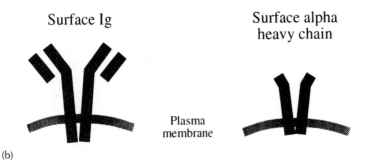

(b)

Figure 22.1 (a) The structure of the EGF receptor and of its truncated version, the erb B oncogene. (b) The structure of normal surface immunoglobulin receptor Ig and of the truncated α-heavy chain.

the strong underrepresentation of most 3'-located genes in other heavy chain diseases. For example, $\gamma2$ and $\gamma4$ are underrepresented in γHCD. The switch sequences of the most upstream-located genes such as Mμ, $\gamma3$, $\gamma1$ and $\alpha1$ might be more susceptible to abnormal deletions than are switch regions of the downstream-located constant region gene segments. An alternative explanation for this finding is that there is selective pressure for the emergence of cells expressing these Ig classes.

In a case of nonsecretory αHCD, a deletion of the polyadenylation signal 3' to the CH3 exon has been demonstrated [37]. Owing to this deletion, only a membrane-bound version of the αHCD protein is produced. Analysis of several cases of αHCD mRNA revealed that in addition to deletion of V and CH1 sequences, insertions of in-frame sequences of unknown origin were found between the leader peptide and the normal CH2 and CH3 coding sequences [38]. These inserts are of variable length (42–105 base pairs) and differ from each other. Such non-Ig sequences probably account for the unusual N termini reported in several αHCD proteins. At the DNA level, the insertions are hundreds of base pairs long and usually show no homology with any known human sequences. The inserted sequences differed from the GC-rich 'N' sequences introduced normally at V-D-J junctions by the terminal deoxynucleotide transferase enzyme [38]. In one rearranged gene, the inserted DNA contained two short sequences that were homologous to a leader-V_H intron and to a satellite I DNA [39], but were not related to known transposable genetic elements introduced in some rearranged murine immunoglobulin genes [40,41]. The inserted sequences did not hybridize with normal human genomic DNA.

Two hypotheses have been suggested for the origin of these inserted sequences [38]. Firstly, they could be of nonhuman origin, possibly derived from the genomes of infectious agents. Epidemiologic findings and the response of the early phase to antibiotic therapy support the involvement of an infectious agent, although it is difficult to imagine why the postulated agent would undergo recombination with the α-heavy-chain locus. Further, the absence of similarities between the inserted sequences in several αHCD cDNAs and the genomic sequences of known infectious agents does not support this option. An alternative possibility is that the inserted sequences represent highly rearranged sequences derived from the Ig gene locus. In one case of αHCD, the characterization of the inserted sequences, indeed, suggested the latter possibility [39].

αHCD cells do not usually secrete light chains. In a few αHCD cases, L-chain determinants were detected in αHCD cells but not in the serum or urine. Despite this, monoclonal rearrangements of light chain genes do occur. It is of interest that in all ten cases of αHCD studied so far, rearrangements of the kappa light chain genes were found, whereas the lambda genes were in the germline configuration [38]. A truncated kappa mRNA was demonstrated in some of these cases [38–42]. In one case of non-secretory αHCD the mRNA size was comparable to that found in the murine MPC11 myeloma, in which a truncated kappa chain devoid of a V domain has been described [42]. These findings may indicate the occurrence of similar genomic alterations in both heavy and light chain loci in αHCD.

The high prevalence of α-heavy-chain proteins in primary intestinal lymphoma in developing countries suggests that there is a selective advantage favoring the proliferation of cells producing α-heavy chain during the evolution of the disease. It is possible that the heavy chain protein confers a selective advantage upon these cells but does not cause malignant transformation. The observation that all α-heavy-chain proteins described so far have been α1 and not α2 proteins [20] suggests that an external selective pressure may operate on IgA1-producing cells. Figure 22.2 illustrates the main difference between IgA1 and IgA2 protein. The hinge domain of IgA1 is 13 amino acids longer than

that of IgA2. Many bacteria have been shown to possess active IgA1 proteases [43]. The cleavage sites for these enzymes are clustered in the short segment of the IgA1 hinge domain. Enteric growth of the IgA1 protease-producing bacteria could suppress the proliferation of IgA1-producing cells and so that only cells that synthesize the aberrant α1-heavy chain proteins would be resistant to the proteolytic activity, because of the deletions involving the hinge or neighboring sequences. Antibiotic treatment would be expected to eliminate this selective pressure and could thus explain the reversibility of this process.

Several features of IPSID are highly reminiscent of the MALT lymphomas [44,45] described in Chapter 21. Both these disorders have an increased incidence in developing countries and both respond to antibiotic treatment in early stages, but not during advanced stages of the disease. The demonstration of a role for *Helicobacter pylori* in MALT lymphomas supports the possibility that an infectious agent may be involved in IPSID.

References

1. Fairley NH, Mackie FP. Clinical and biochemical syndrome in lymphadenoma and allied diseases involving mesenteric lymph glands. *Br. Med. J.* 1937, **1**: 375–380.
2. Gray GM, Rosenberg SA, Cooper AD, et al. Lymphomas

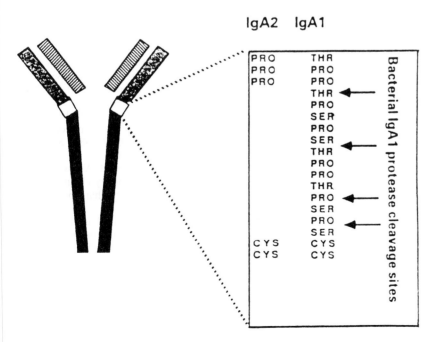

IgA2 IgA1

IgA2	IgA1
PRO	THR
PRO	PRO
PRO	PRO
	THR ←
	PRO
	SER
	PRO
	SER
	THR ←
	PRO
	PRO
	THR
	PRO ←
	SER
	PRO ←
	SER
CYS	CYS
CYS	CYS

Bacterial IgA1 protease cleavage sites

Figure 22.2 Comparison of the hinge region sequences in normal IgA2 and IgA1 α-heavy chains. IgA1 has a 13 amino acid sequence that is the target sequence for several bacterial IgA1 proteases.

PART 4

Presentation, staging and follow-up studies

CHAPTER 23

The non-Hodgkin's lymphomas: presenting features

JACOB D. BITRAN AND JOHN E. ULTMANN

Introduction

In this chapter we will review the presenting symptoms and signs of patients with non-Hodgkin's lymphomas (NHL). The symptoms patients note and the signs they manifest are varied, and will be influenced by the anatomic sites of lymphatic tissue involvement, the type of clonal lymphocytic proliferation (B-cell versus T-cell versus null cell), the architectural appearance of the lymph node (follicular versus diffuse), and the etiologic agents or immunologic diseases associated with or that terminate in NHL.

Symptoms and signs based on anatomic sites of involvement

The presenting symptoms and signs in two of every three patients with NHL are painless lymph node enlargement. The presence of any enlarged lymph node (1 cm or greater in size) *per se* should not make the clinician unduly suspicious of a malignant lymphoma. In both children and adults, palpable inguinal lymph nodes 0.5 cm–2 cm in size may be found during a routine physical examination; these nodes are palpable as a consequence of repeated inflammatory stimuli. In children, enlarged lymph nodes in the cervical or axillary regions may also be present, owing to past infections [1]. Lymph node enlargement is a manifestation of antigenic stimulation or lymph nodal infiltration. The antigenic stimulus may be infectious or inflammatory (Table 23.1) and the infiltrate within the node may be malignant or caused by an inflammatory response. Thus, it is important to take a careful history that includes a review of recent travel to regions where certain types of infections may be endemic (Q fever, Rocky Mountain spotted fever, tularemia), a careful questioning of any occupational or recreational infectious exposure (anthrax, brucellosis) or recent exposure to drugs (Dilantin®). Important factors that help in assessing the significance of enlarged lymph nodes are: age, the region of lymphadenopathy, the physical characteristics of the enlarged lymph nodes, and obviously the clinical setting [2]. In adults, enlarged lymph nodes (greater than 1 cm) in regions other than the inguinal region constitute a pathologic finding which requires a diagnostic work-up, unless there is a known underlying cause (Table 23.1). The physical characteristics of enlarged lymph nodes are helpful in defining the possible etiology. With infections, involved lymph nodes are asymmetrically enlarged, tender, matted together and the overlying skin may be erythematous. Nodes involved by metastatic carcinoma are usually hard and fixed to the underlying tissues. Enlarged nodes involved by lymphomas tend to be firm, nontender and usually

Table 23.1   Etiologies of lymphadenopathy

Infectious

Viral
Adenovirus, cytomegalovirus, Epstein–Barr virus, hepatitis virus, human immunodeficiency virus (HIV), lymphogranuloma venereum, rubella, rubeola, trachoma
Rickettsial
Q Fever, Rocky Mountain spotted fever
Protozoan
Amebiasis, cat scratch disease, toxoplasmosis
Bacterial
Anthrax, brucellosis, chancroid, diphtheria, leprosy, listeriosis, *Mycobacterium* tuberculosis, atypical *Mycobacterium*, plague, rat bite fever, tularemia
Fungal
Blastomycosis, coccidiomycosis, histoplasmosis, ring worm, sporotrichosis
Spirochetal
Leptospirosis, syphilis

Immunologic

Carbamazepine, Dilantin, graft-versus-host disease, hemolytic anemia, rheumatoid arthritis, serum sickness, systemic lupus erythematosus

Neoplastic

Acute leukemias, chronic lymphatic leukemia, chronic myelogenous leukemia, myelosclerosis, Hodgkin's disease, non-Hodgkin's lymphomas, metastatic carcinomas or sarcomas

Other

Addison's disease, amyloidosis, chronic granulomatous disease, necrotizing lymphadenitis, dermatopathic lymphadenitis, follicular hyperplasia, Gaucher's disease, mucocutaneous lymph node syndrome, multifocal Langerhans cell (eosinophilic) granulomatosis, necrotizing lymphadenitis, Neiman–Pick disease, sarcoid, silicone, sinus histiocytosis, thyrotoxicosis, vaccinia

matted. In adults, we suggest a biopsy be performed on newly enlarged lymph node (greater than 1 cm) if an underlying etiology cannot be established within 4 weeks. In some patients a repeat biopsy may be warranted if the first biopsy fails to yield a clear diagnosis. In children, we suggest a biopsy be performed on newly enlarged lymph nodes greater than 2 cm if an etiology cannot be established within 4 weeks. Multiple asymmetric sites of involvement should arouse particular concern.

As previously stated, patients with NHL present with symptoms of painless lymph nodal enlargement. The most commonly involved site is the neck then, in descending frequency, inguinal or axillary regions. Sometimes patients complain of multiple sites of enlarged lymph nodes. They may describe occasional regression or even spontaneous disappearance, an occurrence that should not necessarily allay suspicion since spontaneous regression is observed in as many as 20% of patients with low-grade lymphomas [3]. The presence of epitrochlear, femoral or supraclavicular adenopathy always requires a biopsy. Patients with enlargement of lymphoid tissue in Waldeyer's ring have a high likelihood of NHL and a biopsy should be undertaken without delay. After a complete history and physical examination, blood counts, serum chemistries, prothrombin time, partial thromboplastin time and chest X-ray are performed. If a diagnosis cannot be established a suitably placed lymph node should be biopsied. At the time of biopsy, a portion of the lymph node should be reserved for culture and separate portions (placed in saline or tissue culture medium) for immunophenotyping by flow cytometry and cytogenetic analysis. If possible, an additional piece of the lymph node is frozen such that molecular studies can be conducted if indicated. It is important to coordinate the biopsy procedure and tissue triage with the pathologist who, ideally, should be on hand at the time of the procedure to supervise the division and distribution of the tissue. The surgeon should preferentially biopsy enlarged cervical lymph nodes; in the absence of enlarged cervical lymph nodes, enlarged axillary lymph nodes may be biopsied. Inguinal lymph nodes should be avoided unless there is no other nodal region bearing enlarged lymph nodes.

Patients with NHL may also present with symptoms referable to thorax, abdomen or an extranodal site of involvement. In approximately 20% of patients with NHL, the presenting symptoms are caused by mediastinal adenopathy and may include cough, chest discomfort, or occasionally a superior vena caval syndrome (common in T-cell, rarely in B-cell lymphoma). Many patients with mediastinal adenopathy are asymptomatic and the only evidence of a mediastinal mass is an abnormal chest X-ray.

NHL frequently involves the retroperitoneal, mesenteric and pelvic lymph nodes. Retroperitoneal adenopathy usually causes no symptoms unless the nodal involvement is extensive. Massive retroperitoneal adenopathy can lead to chronic abdominal pain, abdominal fullness and early satiety. Mesenteric masses and pelvic masses may lead to visceral obstruction or perforation. Involvement of the gastrointestinal tract occurs in 16% of patients with NHL (most frequently in malignant lymphoma, diffuse, large cleaved or noncleaved cells, and mucosa-associated lymphoid tissue (MALT) lymphomas) and can lead to abdominal pain or visceral obstruction. In patients with α-heavy-chain disease, or with diffuse involvement of the gastrointestinal tract by lymphoma, patients present with severe malabsorption, weight loss, diarrhea, and steatorrhea. In the Middle East, α-heavy-chain disease often mimics familial Mediterranean fever (FMF) and must be considered in the differential diagnosis of FMF.

Retroperitoneal adenopathy when massive can also cause obstructive uropathy. Patients will complain of polyuria and nocturia (owing to impaired renal concentrating ability), malaise, anorexia, lassitude and headache long before they notice a decreasing urinary output. The abrupt development of hypertension frequently accompanies either acute or subacute ureteric obstruction. Renal tubular acidosis, hyperkalemia and renal salt wasting are early biochemical signs of ureteric obstruction. Pelvic masses may also lead to obstructive uropathy as a result of bladder involvement. Rarely, NHL involves one or both kidneys; when it does flank pain or fullness may be present. Despite extensive involvement of one or both kidneys, symptoms of acute renal failure rarely develop.

NHL can occur primarily in the central nervous system (CNS). In the brain, the presenting symptoms are those of any other space-occupying lesion in this location: headache, nausea, vomiting and focal neurologic deficits. Primary lymphomas of the brain are typically diffuse large cell, cleaved and noncleaved, and much more frequently occur in patients following organ transplantation or in patients with AIDS. NHL can occur in the globe of the eye or in retro-orbital tissues (particularly MALT lymphomas). Ocular lymphomas cause visual disturbances and visual loss; retro-orbital lymphomas cause unilateral proptosis, diplopia and extraocular muscle palsy.

Other symptoms of NHL are dependent on the extranodal sites of involvement. Lymphoma of the testes causes symptoms of a testicular mass; ovarian lymphomatous involvement that of a pelvic mass; lymphoma of the thyroid causes thyroid enlargement and/or a thyroid mass and, rarely, leads to symptoms of hypothyroidism. Lymphoma of the breast leads to symptoms and signs indistinguishable from breast cancer or can cause generalized breast enlargement. Skin involvement by a T-cell lymphoma causes purple colored nodules; mycosis fungoides causes erythematous plaques. Bone involvement causes pain, especially associated with weight bearing. Lytic bone disease is typically found on X-ray and is indistinguishable from any other lesion destroying bone. NHL (particularly MALT lymphomas) of the salivary glands leads to masses or may be associated with the Mikulicz's syndrome (painless parotid and lacrimal gland swelling). Bone marrow involvement can produce anemia, thrombocytopenia or neutropenia; the presenting complaints are fatigue, malaise, easy bruisability and sometimes fever consequent upon infection.

Systemic symptoms such as fever, night sweats and weight loss occur in 20–30% of patients with NHL. Rarely, patients may also complain of pruritus or alcohol intolerance. Systemic symptoms, which more commonly occur with intermediate- or high-grade lymphomas and with advanced stage correlates with a worse prognosis. While most patients with systemic symptoms also have complaints of lymphadenopathy, occasionally a patient's sole complaints may be those of systemic symptoms, and thus NHL must also be considered in patients with fever of unknown origin or unexplained weight loss.

INVESTIGATION OF THE PATIENT WITH EXTRANODAL DISEASE

In patients without adenopathy, the establishment of a diagnosis may entail a broader range of investigations including initial blood counts, serum chemistries, coagulation studies, chest X-ray and possibly other imaging studies. Abnormal masses must be biopsied, and the tissue obtained handled as described for a lymph node biopsy. Sometimes the diagnosis can be established by bone marrow examination (aspiration and biopsy are recommended), or by examination of serous effusions. There are instances when an extranodal site is the only site to biopsy. Extranodal NHL almost always has a diffuse architecture and seldom has a follicular pattern. If a diagnosis of NHL has been made on an extranodal site, it is sometimes advisable to biopsy a lymph node, if one is available, to obtain a more accurate picture of the nodal architecture.

Once a definitive diagnosis of NHL is made, staging studies should be undertaken, followed by appropriate therapeutic decisions.

Presenting symptoms and signs according to the subtypes of the Working Formulation

In the 'Working Formulation' [4] NHL is divided into three categories that correlate with clinical course, low-grade malignant lymphoma, intermediate-grade malignant lymphoma and high-grade malignant lymphoma. A fourth miscellaneous category consists of composite lymphoma, mycosis fungoides, true histiocytic lymphoma, extramedullary plasmacytoma and unclassified malignant lymphomas (see Chapter 3).

LOW-GRADE LYMPHOMAS

Low-grade malignant lymphomas include small lymphocytic lymphoma; follicular, small cleaved cell lymphoma; and follicular mixed, small cleaved and large cleaved cells (up to 30%) lymphoma. 'Mantle zone' lymphoma, not originally included in the Working Formulation, also appropriately belongs in this category [5]. Low-grade lymphomas are, for the most part, derived from B-lymphocytes. Patients with these types of malignant lymphoma usually present with a complaint of enlarged lymph nodes in either the cervical or inguinal regions, that have increased (sometimes with intermittent regression) in size over a period of months. The physical findings confirm the presence of generalized peripheral lymphadenopathy characterized by discrete rubbery lymph nodes. Epitrochlear involvement is frequent. A careful ear, nose and throat examination may disclose involvement of Waldeyer's ring in 16–33% of patients with low-grade lymphomas. When NHL involves Waldeyer's ring there is frequently gastrointestinal (GI) involvement with lymphoma. In patients with low-grade lymphomas, the spleen is often palpable and the liver may be enlarged. A careful examination of the skin is warranted to detect the purple–red papules characteristic of lymphomatous involvement. While a minority of patients (10%) may have truly limited stage (stage I or II) low-grade malignant lymphoma, the majority have stage III or IV disease, which is easily documented by physical examination or further staging (see Chapter 24).

INTERMEDIATE-GRADE LYMPHOMAS

The intermediate-grade lymphomas include follicular, large cleaved cell lymphoma; diffuse small cleaved cell lymphoma; diffuse, mixed small- and large-cell lymphoma (less than 30%); and diffuse, large-cell lymphoma (comprising large cleaved cells, or large noncleaved cells, with or without sclerosis). Because of its similar clinical presentation and response to combination chemotherapy, we have also included diffuse, large-cell, immunoblastic lymphoma in the intermediate-grade lymphomas. From a clinical standpoint, the intermediate-grade lymphomas (large cell, follicular or diffuse; large cell, immunoblastic; and diffuse mixed) can be thought of as a single group. Immunologically, 85% of them are composed of transformed B-lymphocytes and 15% of transformed T-lymphocytes. The presenting complaint is usually lymphadenopathy, usually in cervical or inguinal regions. However, the lymph nodes do not increase or decrease in size, as may occur with low-grade lymphomas. Rather, lymph node growth is progressive and often accompanied by 'B' symptoms. The presenting symptoms in up to 33% of patients with intermediate-grade malignant lymphoma are referrable to extranodal sites of involvement and include abdominal pain, intermittent nausea or vomiting (GI involvement), unilateral or bilateral painless testicular enlargement (testis), or headache, memory impairment, dementia or hemiparesis (CNS). The physical findings confirm the presence of enlarged lymph nodes in one or multiple sites. Frequently, the lymph nodes are matted together and appear to the examiner as a single large nodal mass. Abdominal masses exceeding 6 cm frequently occur in patients with diffused mixed or diffuse, large-cell lymphomas.

Patients with diffuse large-cell, large cleaved or noncleaved cell lymphomas have two distinctive presentations that deserve special attention. Patients with the sclerosing form of large-cell lymphoma involving the mediastinum generally present with symptoms of cough, dyspnea, chest pain and superior vena cava (SVC) syndrome. The physical findings show thoracic and neck vein distension, facial edema, conjunctival sufflation and occasionally arm edema [6]. Peripheral adenopathy may or may not be present. Another distinctive presentation is that associated with the anaplastic subtype of diffuse large-cell lymphoma which occurs predominantly in children and adolescents. The presenting symptoms are usually a cutaneous nodule or nodules, with or without peripheral lymphadenopathy. Immunophenotyping reveals expression of the CD30 antigen (Ki-1 antigen or Hodgkin's-associated antigen) and there is often a t(2;5)(p23;q35) chromosomal translocation [7].

HIGH-GRADE LYMPHOMAS

The high-grade malignant lymphomas include lymphoblastic lymphoma, convoluted and nonconvoluted, and small noncleaved, Burkitt's and non-Burkitt's lymphomas. Lymphoblastic lymphoma is a disease that predominantly affects adolescent males, less often females. The presenting symptoms frequently include shortness of breath or dyspnea on exertion, which results from a mediastinal mass and associated pleural effusions or pericardial effusions which are present in some 70% of patients. The physical findings may include a SVC syndrome and/or dullness to percussion at the lung bases. Symptoms referable to the abdomen are rare. Lymphoblastic lymphoma is usually of T-cell origin and in a leukemic phase is indistinguishable from acute lymphoblastic leukemia. Small noncleaved lymphoma of Burkitt's type is the most common childhood tumor in Africa. Typically, children present with a large rapidly growing mass in the head and neck region, particularly in the jaws or orbit. In contrast, American patients with Burkitt's lymphoma, which is also predominantly a childhood

lymphoma, nearly always present with abdominal symptoms caused by intra-abdominal masses and/or ascites. Occasionally patients may have intussusception or symptoms of acute appendicitis. CNS involvement occurs in 10% of patients with Burkitt's lymphoma at the time of presentation. Patients with high-grade lymphomas may also present with disease in the pharynx, or at other extranodal sites.

NONTUMORAL PRESENTATIONS

Rarely, patients with NHL of any histological subtype may present with symptoms that are unrelated to lymphadenopathy or abdominal masses. These may include fatigue (anemia), petechiae (thrombocytopenia), alterations in mental state (hypercalcemia or dementia) or an ascending polyneuropathy (Guillain–Barré). Such symptoms are paraneoplastic manifestations of NHL. Of the varied paraneoplastic

Table 23.2   Paraneoplastic syndromes associated with non-Hodgkin's lymphomas

Syndrome	Mechanism	Associated especially with
Hematologic		
Hemolytic anemia		
Autoimmune	Coombs' positive (IgG)	'B-Cell' lymphomas
Hypersplenism	Splenic sequestration	
Thrombocytopenia		
Autoimmune	Antiplatelet antibody	'B-Cell' lymphomas
Hypersplenism	Splenic sequestration	
Evan's syndrome (autoimmune anemia and thrombocytopenia)		
Leukocytosis	Unregulated production of GM-CSF, G-CSF, M-CSF, IL-1, IL-3	'B-Cell' lymphomas
Pancytopenia	Marrow infiltration	
Thrombocytosis	Unregulated production of IL-6, IL-11	
Metabolic		
Hypercalcemia	IL-1B	'T-Cell' lymphomas, HTLV-1
Gout	Hyperuricemia	
Lactic acidosis	Accelerated anaerobic metabolism	Large-cell lymphomas
	Impaired hepatic clearance	
Fever	Unregulated production of TNF	
Neurologic		
Angioendotheliosis (multiple infarcts or dementia)	Fibroblast growth factor, IL-1B, transforming factor-B	
Progressive multifocal leukoencephalopathy	? virus, antibody	
Guillain–Barré	? virus, antibody	
Dermatologic		
Leser–Trélat (sudden seborrheic keratosis)		

syndromes (listed in Table 23.2), a few deserve special consideration. The occurrence of hemolytic anemia, either autoimmune or as a result of hypersplenism, is heralded by symptoms of fatigue, malaise, breathlessness and jaundice. Autoimmune hemolytic anemia can antedate the occurrence of NHL, so that NHL must always be considered as a possible underlying cause. Symptoms of malaise, fatigue, easy bruisability and fever, coupled with the physical findings of pallor, petechiae and ecchymosis, must prompt consideration of pancytopenia and marrow infiltration by NHL. Patients with human T-cell leukemia virus HTLV-1 T-cell lymphoma typically present with malaise, lethargy, nausea, weakness, polyuria and polydipsia, which are the consequences of hypercalcemia. The physical findings are those of diffuse adenopathy, skin nodules, plaques, papules and/or erythroderma. Cranial nerve involvement may be found on physical examination. The symptoms of hypercalcemia, which are caused by interleukin-1B, tend to dominate all other symptoms.

Occasionally, patients with non-Hodgkin's lymphoma may present with neurologic symptoms. Symptoms of headache and nausea, coupled with physical findings of cranial nerve palsy are usually associated with meningeal involvement. Meningeal involvement is relatively common in patients with intermediate-, high-grade, and HTLV-1-associated non-Hodgkin's lymphoma. An epidural mass can complicate any of the NHLs and, rarely, patients may present with such findings. Thus, the symptom of back pain, which worsens with a Valsalva maneuver or coughing, and extremity weakness is indicative of spinal canal encroachment until proven otherwise.

Paraneoplastic neurologic disorders tend to focus the attention away from any complaints of peripheral adenopathy. One potentially misleading presentation is that caused by angioendotheliosis. Angioendotheliosis is a proliferative disorder of endothelial cells provoked by angiogenic peptides produced by lymphoma cells [8]. A family member usually notes the abrupt onset of dementia or a patient may complain of the abrupt onset of weakness. The alert clinician may suspect an underlying lymphoma in the presence of lymphadenopathy. Computed tomography and magnetic resonance imaging merely show the occurrence of multiple strokes. The importance of this paraneoplastic disorder is that it responds to primary therapy for the lymphoma and has a relatively good prognosis. Progressive multifocal leukoencephalopathy and Guillain–Barré syndrome can occasionally complicate the course of NHL. However, patients with NHL rarely present with symptoms of either disorder.

Complaints of skin eruptions can be presenting symptoms of cutaneous T-cell lymphomas. The physical findings reveal reddish purple nodules, plaques or erythroderma and generalized lymphadenopathy. While metabolic disorders such as gout, lactic acidosis or hypoglycemia can complicate the course of malignant lymphoma, rarely do patients present with such symptoms.

Diseases associated with an increased risk of NHL

Certain diseases predispose patients to NHL (Table 23.3). There is compelling evidence that viral transformation of lymphocytes, in some circumstances, can predispose to the development of NHL (Table 23.3). Epstein–Barr virus is associated with Burkitt's

Table 23.3   Diseases associated with an increased risk of NHL

Viruses

   Epstein–Barr virus (EBV)
   Human T-cell leukemia/lymphoma virus (HTLV-1)
   Human immunodeficiency virus (HIV)

Immunodeficiency disease

   Ataxia telangiectasia syndrome
   Wiskott–Aldrich syndrome
   Common variable immunodeficiency syndrome
   Klinefelter's syndrome
   Acquired hypogammaglobulinemia
   Bloom's syndrome
   Iatrogenic (organ transplantation)

Autoimmune disorders

   Rheumatoid arthritis
   Adult Still's disease
   Felty's syndrome
   Systemic lupus erythematosus
   Mixed connective tissue disease
   Sjögren's syndrome
   Nontropical sprue
   Hashimoto's thyroiditis
   Cryoglobulinemia

Drugs or chemical exposure

   Cyclosporine
   Diphenylhydantoin
   Carbamazepine
   Dioxin (Agent Orange)?
   Chemotherapy

Radiation exposure

lymphoma and, as previously discussed, HTLV-1 with adult T-cell lymphoma. Human immunodeficiency virus (HIV) is the cause of the acquired immunodeficiency syndrome (AIDS), and AIDS patients are at increased risk of NHL. AIDS-related NHL are usually of intermediate or high grade and of 'B-cell' origin. The challenge to the clinician, in this patient population, is when to suspect NHL. Many patients with HIV will have fever, weight loss and peripheral adenopathy simply on the basis of HIV and, as such, a lymph node biopsy is not indicated in every HIV or AIDS patient. Moreover, many patients with an AIDS-related lymphoma frequently do not present with peripheral lymphadenopathy. Certain symptoms and signs in HIV-infected patients, for example, the abrupt onset of fever and weight loss, may indicate the development of NHL. Adenopathy from HIV almost *never* involves the mediastinum or retroperitoneum; thus, adenopathy in these locations is NHL until proven otherwise [9]. Altered mental states or seizures in an AIDS patient may be a manifestation of toxoplasmosis, cryptococcosis or NHL of the brain. The sudden onset of hepatic or splenic enlargement may indicate NHL within liver or spleen. AIDS-related lymphoma should always be considered in the differential diagnosis of fever, altered mental status, lymphadenopathy or pancytopenia in this patient population, and the physician must have a relatively low threshold for the performance of a biopsy.

Immunodeficiency disease syndromes such as ataxia telangiectasia, common variable immunodeficiency, Wiskott–Aldrich syndrome and Bloom's syndrome are frequently complicated by the occurrence of a high-grade NHL. Similarly, patients with rheumatoid arthritis, Felty's syndrome, systemic lupus erythematosus, Sjögren's syndrome and nontropical sprue are at risk for diffuse, large-cell lymphoma of B-cell origin [10]. In both these disease settings, the presenting symptoms and signs are identical to those of *de novo* NHL.

Drug and chemical exposure have been linked to NHL. Diphenylhydantoin and carbamazepine can cause lymph node enlargement and lymph node hyperplasia, which is sometimes difficult to distinguish from NHL [11]. Exposure to dioxin (Agent Orange) has been linked with an increased risk of follicular lymphoma. Prior radiation therapy or chemotherapy for Hodgkin's disease also increases the risk for NHL.

Immunosuppression following organ transplantation, particularly when induced by cyclosporin or OKT3, increases the risk of NHL. Patients who have undergone organ transplantation are at increased risk for primary CNS lymphomas [12–14]. The symptoms they develop are related to a space-occupying lesion in the CNS: headache, nausea and vomiting and focal neurologic deficits (in contrast to AIDS CNS lymphoma, which usually causes dementia and seizures) [14]. Patients on long-term cyclosporin are at risk for immunosuppression-associated lymphoproliferative disease (we prefer this term because the proliferation is often polyclonal rather than monoclonal, usually manifested as diffuse lymphadenopathy) [12]. While this form of lymphoproliferative disease has the histologic appearance of a high-grade or intermediate-grade malignant lymphoma, it is not always a true lymphoma and may sometimes regress upon withdrawal of cyclosporin or OKT3 [13]. The presenting complaints are those of diffuse lymphadenopathy and the physical findings confirm this.

Lymphoid and histiocytic disorders that may either mimic NHL or terminate in NHL

There are a variety of disorders that may mimic NHL (Table 23.4). In many of the diseases listed in Table 23.4, symptoms such as fever, malaise and weight loss are identical to the 'B' symptoms that accompany NHL. Additionally, lymphadenopathy, mediastinal masses or hepatosplenomegaly mimic the physical findings of NHL. Angioimmunoblastic lymphadenopathy with dysproteinemia (AILD) is a lymphoproliferative disorder characterized by proliferation of immunoblasts bearing the CD4 receptor in association with vascular proliferation. Patients with AILD present with symptoms indistinguishable from NHL, and diagnosis must be established by a lymph node biopsy. AILD is not a malignant neoplasm, but can evolve into a large-cell immunoblastic lymphoma. One third of immunoblastic lymphomas developing in AILD are of T-cell phenotype. Lymphoid granulomatosis (LG), polymorphic reticulosis (PMR) and midline malignant reticulosis (MMR) are overlapping diseases of unknown etiology, and are currently grouped together as angiocentric immunoproliferative lesions (AIL). They involve the upper respiratory tract, (nasopharynx, oropharynx, sinuses and trachea) and lungs [15]. Patients with nasal involvement complain of nasal discharge, midline ulcers or hemoptysis. Patients with pulmonary involvement have symptoms of dyspnea, cough, fever and occasionally hemoptysis. Histologically, there is an infiltrate of atypical large lymphocytes, plasma cells, eosinophils and histiocytes encircling and invading blood vessels. The

Table 23.4   Atypical lymphoid disorders and histiocytic disorders that mimic NHL

Disease	Symptoms and signs	Pathologic characteristics	Terminates in NHL
Angioimmunoblastic lymphadenopathy with dysproteinemia (AILD)	Fever, malaise, weight loss, generalized adenopathy, hepatosplenomegaly, plasmacytosis, Coombs'-positive hemolytic anemia	Effacement of nodal architecture by vascular proliferation, immunoblasts, plasma cells, mature lymphocytes, occasional necrosis. Immunoblasts are CD4+	Yes – Large-cell immunoblastic lymphoma
Angiocentric immunoproliferative lesion	Nasal discharge, midline ulcer, hemoptysis. Dyspnea, fever, cough, occasionally hemoptysis. Papulovesicular eruption on skin, rarely has mononeuritis multiplex	Atypical large lymphocytes, plasma cells, eosinophils and histiocytes invading blood vessels	Yes – Large-cell immunoblastic lymphoma T-cell phenotype
Lymphomatoid papulosis	Skin lesions – red–brown papules, occasionally central necrosis, resolve in 3–4 weeks and cause atrophic scars	Patchy parakeratosis, acanthosis exocytosis of mononuclear cells. Lymphohistiocytic infiltration of dermis, bizarre cells resembling Reed–Sternberg cells (Ki-1 positive)	Yes – Cutaneous T-cell lymphoma
Histiocytic necrotizing lymphadenopathy (Kikuchi's disease)	Disease of women, asymptomatic cervical lymphadenopathy	Atypical mature histiocytes effacing nodes, erythrophagocytosis	No – Self-limited disease
Sinus histiocytosis with massive lymphadenopathy (Rosai–Dorfman)	Fever, bilateral cervical lymphadenopathy, hypergammaglobulinemia	Sinus histiocytosis, lymphoerythrophagocytosis by histiocytes	No – Protracted benign course
Angiofollicular lymph nodal hyperplasia (Castleman's disease)	Fever, sweats, weight loss, fatigue, asymptomatic mediastinal mass, hypergammaglobulinemia	Follicular hyperplasia, collagen or hyaline material about capillaries	No/Infrequently
Malignant histiocytosis	Fever, wasting, lymphadenopathy, abdominal pain, pancytopenia, DIC. Painful lymphadenopathy. Especially axillary and supraclavicular nodes. Maculopapular lesions	Effacement of the nodal architecture by large neoplastic cells with immunoblastic features; CD30 and other markers include CD21+, CD4+ and T-9+	No
Familial erythrophagocytic lymphohistiocytosis	Disease of infants, adenopathy, fever, hepatosplenomegaly, pancytopenia	Histiocytes with hematopoietic elements, erythrophagocytosis	No
Histiocytic syndromes Solitary and multifocal eosinophilic granuloma	Pain in bone, multiple bone. Cough, SOB in 20%. Ages 20–40	Histiocytes with eosinophilic granulocytes	No
Hand–Schuller–Christian	SOB, bone pain, polyuria, polydipsia, exophthalmos (bone defects, diabetes, insipidus, exophthalmos). Age: childhood, occasionally middle age	Histiocytes and eosinophils	No
Letterer–Siwe	Age: newborn to 3 years. Anorexia, irritability, failure to thrive, scaly seborrhea, adenopathy, hepatosplenomegaly	Histiocytes and eosinophils	No

DIC, disseminated intravascular coagulation; SOB, shortness of breath.

lymphocyte population bears the CD15 and CD30 (Hodgkin's-associated) antigen. AIL terminates in a large-cell immunoblastic lymphoma of T-cells in 50% of patients unless appropriate treatment is administered.

Lymphomatoid papulosis is a skin disease characterized by the occurrence of red–brown papules occurring in crops and resolving into atrophic scars in 3–4 weeks. It occurs in patients aged 8–60 years of age and sometimes terminates in a cutaneous T-cell lymphoma. Kikuchi's disease, Castleman's disease and sinus histiocytosis with massive lymphadenopathy all produce symptoms that mimic NHL, but none of these diseases, with the possible exception of the systemic form of Castleman's disease, terminates in NHL. Malignant histiocytosis, familial erythrophagocytic lymphohistiocytosis, and the histiocytic syndromes all cause symptoms and signs that mimic NHL, but these diseases do not terminate in NHL. NHL may, however, be associated with a hemophagocytic syndrome which often presents as fever, jaundice, disseminated intravascular coagulation and pancytopenia. These NHLs are of T-cell origin, may be associated with EBV, and are more common in SE Asia [16–18]. Thus, NHL must be considered as an underlying cause for a hemophagocytic syndrome, particularly in SE Asia.

References

1. Zuelzer WW, Kaplan J. The child with lymphadenopathy. *Semin. Hematol.* 1975, **12**: 323–334.
2. Peterson, BA, Fizzera, G (eds). Benign lymphoproliferative disorders. *Semin. Oncol.* 1993, **20**: 553–661.
3. Portlock CS, Rosenberg SA. No initial therapy for Stage III and IV non-Hodgkin's lymphomas of favorable histologic types. *Ann. Intern. Med.* 1979, **90**: 10–13.
4. National Cancer Institute sponsored study of classification of non-Hodgkin's lymphomas: Summary and description of a working formulation for clinical usage. The Non-Hodgkin's Lymphoma Pathologic Classification Project. *Cancer* 1982, **49**: 2112–2135.
5. Weisenburger DD, Nathwani BN, Diamond LW, et al. Malignant lymphoma, intermediate lymphocytic type: A clinico-pathologic study of 42 cases. *Cancer* 1981, **48**: 1415–1425.
6. Lazzarino M, Orlandi E, Pauli M, et al. Primary mediastinal B-cell lymphoma with sclerosis: An aggressive tumor with distinctive clinical and pathologic features. *Clin. Oncol.* 1993, **11**: 2306–2313.
7. LeBeau MM, Bitter MA, Larson RA, et al. The t(2;5) (p23;q35): A recurring chromosomal abnormality in Ki-1 positive non-Hodgkin's lymphoma. *Leukemia* 1989, **3**: 866–871.
8. Petito CK, Gottlieb GJ, Dougherty JH, et al. Neoplastic angioendotheliosis: Ultrastructural study and review of the literature. *Ann. Neurol.* 1978, **3**: 393–399.
9. Kalter SP, Riggs SA, Cabanillas F, et al. Aggressive non-Hodgkin's lymphoma in immunocompromised homosexual males. *Blood* 1985, **66**: 655–659.
10. Gridley G, Klippel JH, Hoover RN, et al. Incidence of cancer among men with the Felty's syndrome. *Ann. Intern. Med.* 1994, **120**: 35–39.
11. Segal GH, Clough ND, Tubbs RR. Autoimmune and iatrogenic causes of lymphadenopathy. *Semin. Oncol.* 1993, **20**: 611–626.
12. Swinnen LJ, Constanzo-Nordin MR, Fisher SG, et al. Increased incidence of lympho-proliferative disorder after immunosuppression with monoclonal antibody OKT3 in cardiac transplant recipients. *N. Engl. J. Med.* 1990, **323**: 1723–1728.
13. Starzl TE, Porter KA, Iwatsuki S, et al. Reversibility of lymphomas and lympho-proliferative lesions developing under cyclosporine-steroid therapy. *Lancet* 1984, **1**: 583–587.
14. Fine HA, Mayer RJ. Primary central nervous system lymphoma. *Ann. Intern. Med.* 1993, **119**: 1093–1104.
15. Thompson GP, Utz JP, Rosenow EC III, et al. Pulmonary lymphoproliferative disorders. *Mayo Clin. Proc.* 1993; **68**: 804–817.
16. Jaffe ES, Costa J, Fauci AS, et al. Malignant lymphoma and erythrophagocytosis simulating malignant histiocytosis. *Am. J. Med.* 1983, **75**: 741–749.
17. Falini B, Pileri S, De Solas I, et al. Peripheral T-cell lymphomas associated with hemophagocytic syndrome. *Blood* 1990, **75**: 434–444.
18. Wong KF, Chan JKC. Reactive hemophagocytic syndrome – A clinicopathological study of 40 patients in an oriental population. *Am. J. Med.* 1992, **93**: 177–180.

CHAPTER 24

Staging systems and staging investigations

LENA SPECHT

Definition and purpose of staging

Staging is the process of defining the extent of a malignant disease within a given patient. A valid staging classification for the non-Hodgkin's lymphomas (NHLs) is of paramount importance for the following reasons:

1. The stage of the disease should provide important prognostic information, aiding the clinician in predicting, with some accuracy, the outcome of the disease for a patient or a group of patients, thus defining risk groups.
2. The results of the staging investigations should assist the clinician in selecting and planning the most appropriate therapeutic program for the individual patient. Depending on the estimated prognosis decisions are made as to how aggressive or conservative treatment should be for a particular patient. Moreover, the investigations should provide information regarding the imminence of potential complications, which may necessitate prompt action. Involvement of certain sites may require specially designed treatment. If local treatment, i.e., radiotherapy or surgery, is contemplated, precise anatomic delineation of the disease is needed for planning radiotherapy, or determining feasibility and extent of surgical procedures.
3. The staging classification should assist in the evaluation of treatment results. In the context of clinical trials the stage of the disease may be used beforehand to define eligibility and stratification criteria, and afterwards in the statistical analysis to allow adjustments for more valid comparisons.
4. The staging classification should provide a widely accepted descriptive system facilitating the exchange of information among different institutions and, ultimately, assisting in the comparison of groups of cases, particularly with regard to the results of different therapeutic programs.

Staging systems

THE CURRENT STANDARD STAGING SYSTEM

The tumor node metastasis (TNM) classification employed for other malignancies is not a workable staging system for the NHLs, because the site of origin of the disease is often unclear, and there is no way to differentiate among T, N and M [1,2]. An

Table 24.2 Stage distribution of 1014 cases of NHLs, separated into histologic subtypes, from the Non-Hodgkin's Pathologic Classification Project [12]

Histologic subtype	Stage (%)			
	I	II	III	IV
Low grade				
Small lymphocytic	3	8	8	81
Follicular, small cleaved cell	8	10	16	66
Follicular, mixed cell	15	12	28	46
Intermediate grade				
Follicular, large cell	15	12	15	58
Diffuse, small cleaved cell	9	19	12	60
Diffuse, mixed cell	19	26	13	42
Diffuse, large cell	16	30	10	44
High grade				
Immunoblastic	23	29	16	33
Lymphoblastic	7	20	2	72
Small, noncleaved cell	13	21	9	57

cannot be realistically expected that a single system will be satisfactory as a staging classification for all the different subgroups of the NHLs, some of which are not even yet completely defined.

PROPOSED NEWER STAGING SYSTEMS

The need for better staging systems for the NHLs has been widely recognized and has led to the proposal of a number of alternative staging classifications for some of the subgroups of the NHLs. For intermediate- and high-grade NHLs in adults combinations of prognostic factors defining risk groups or 'stages' have been proposed both for early (see Table 24.3) and for advanced disease (see Table 24.4). The prognostic factors employed in these proposals do not differ greatly. Most of them are tumor-related, based on measures of tumor mass and tumor dissemination ultimately reflecting the total tumor burden, or based on biological factors (LDH, β_2-microglobulin) in turn reflecting the total tumor burden and possibly also the growth characteristics of the tumor. In some of the proposals other factors are included which are not tumor-related, but which must rather be defined as patient features determining tolerance to treatment (e.g., age, performance status) [21,27,34,44,59,64]. Although both types of prognostic factors, tumor-related and patient-related, are clearly important for prognosis, it would seem advisable to keep them clearly separate. Staging means defining the extent of the disease within the patient. Neither age nor performance status contributes to this objective. Moreover, if one decides to rely on the staging classification for selecting patients for more intensive treatment, one would want to use

Table 24.3 Proposed staging systems for early intermediate- and high-grade NHLs

Princess Margaret Hospital [54]

Risk factors	Disease bulk (defined in the study), extensive stage IIA or stage I–IIB, age
Group 1	Age < 60 years and no other risk factors
Group 2	Patients not in groups 1 or 3
Group 3	Age ≥ 70 years and large bulk irrespective of stage; age 60–69 years and extensive stage, and medium or large bulk; age < 60 years and extensive stage, and large bulk

Dana–Farber [42]

Risk factors	Two discontiguous sites of involvement, ≥ 2 sites of involvement, disease ≥ 10 cm
Minimal disease	No risk factors
Extended disease	One or more risk factors

Stanford [38]

Risk factors	Mass ≥ 10 cm, > 2 sites of involvement
Favorable	No risk factors
Unfavorable	One or both risk factors

MD Anderson [56]

Risk factors	Extensive disease (criteria outlined in the study), high LDH
Low risk	No risk factors
Intermediate risk	One risk factor
High risk	Both risk factors

Table 24.4 Proposed staging systems for advanced intermediate- and high-grade NHLs

Dana–Farber [48,49]

Risk factors	Performance status (PS) $\geq$ 2 (ECOG), maximum mass size $\geq$ 10 cm, $\geq$ 2 extranodal sites
Low risk	No risk factors
Moderate risk	PS < 2 and 1 other risk factor
Poor risk	PS < 2 and 2 other risk factors, or PS $\geq$ 2 regardless of other risk factors

MD Anderson clinical system [36,58]

Risk factors	Tumor burden (definition outlined in the study), LDH
Stage A	Low tumor burden and normal LDH
Stage B	Low tumor burden and high LDH, or intermediate tumor burden and low LDH
Stage C	Intermediate tumor burden and high LDH, or high tumor burden and low LDH
Stage D	High tumor burden and high LDH

MD Anderson serological system [55]

Risk factors	β_2-Microglobulin $\geq$ 3.0 mg/l, LDH $\geq$ 250 U/l
Low risk	No risk factors
Intermediate risk	One risk factor
High risk	Both risk factors

MD Anderson 'tumor score' system [45]

Risk factors	Score of 1 for each variable: Ann Arbor stage III–IV, B symptoms, LDH $\geq$ 250 U/l, β_2-microglobulin $\geq$ 3.0 mg/l, bulky site (defined in the study) (1 score for each site)
Low risk	Tumor score 0–2
High risk	Tumor score $\geq$ 3

Memorial Sloan–Kettering [26]

Risk factors	Level of site involvement (LSI), LDH
Stage I	Any LSI and low LDH
Stage II	LSI group I–II (peripheral and/or extranodal sites) and medium LDH
Stage III	LSI group I–II and high LDH, or LSI group III–IV (retroperitoneal or bulky mediastinal disease) and medium LDH
Stage IV	LSI group III–IV and high LDH

Vancouver [34]

Risk factors	B symptoms, > 1 extranodal site, > 2 nodal sites, age > 60 years

Patients divided into 5 groups according to number of risk factors present (0–4)

Groupe d'Études des Lymphomes Agressif [23]

Risk factors	High LDH, Ann Arbor stage III–IV, $\geq$ 2 extranodal sites, tumor mass $\geq$ 10 cm
Low risk	No risk factors
Intermediate risk	Normal LDH and 1–2 other risk factors, or high LDH and no other risk factors
Poor risk	Normal LDH and 3 other risk factors, or high LDH and at least 1 other risk factor

Non-Hodgkin's Pathologic Classification Project [51]

Risk factors	Nonlocalized disease, tumor mass $\geq$ 10 cm, mediastinal involvement, $\geq$ 2 extranodal sites, LDH > 225, age $\geq$ 65 years
Group A	Localized disease (1–2 contiguous nodal sites or 1 extranodal site with or without 1 contiguous nodal site)
Group B	Nonlocalized disease and no other risk factors
Group C	Nonlocalized disease, with one or more other risk factors

National Cancer Institute [63]

Risk factors	Nonlocalized disease, any mass > 10 cm, LDH > 500, $\geq$ 3 extranodal sites, B symptoms, performance status $\leq$ 70 (Karnofsky)
Stage I	Localized nodal or extranodal disease (Ann Arbor stage I or IE)
Stage II	Nonlocalized disease and no other risk factors
Stage III	Nonlocalized disease plus any other risk factors

International Index [47]

Risk factors	Ann Arbor stage III–IV, > 1 extranodal site, high LDH, age > 60 years, performance status $\geq$ 2 (ECOG)
Low risk	0–1 risk factors
Low intermediate risk	2 risk factors
High intermediate risk	3 risk factors
High risk	4–5 risk factors

Age-adjusted International Index [47]

Risk factors	Ann Arbor stage III–IV, high LDH, performance status $\geq$ 2 (ECOG)
Low risk	0 risk factors
Low intermediate risk	1 risk factor
High intermediate risk	2 risk factors
High risk	3 risk factors

Table 24.7 Staging systems for specific histologic subtypes of childhood NHLs

Uganda Cancer Institute [85], for Burkitt's lymphoma (endemic)

Stage A	Single extra-abdominal tumor
Stage AR	Completely resected intra-abdominal tumor without extra-abdominal tumor
Stage B	Multiple extra-abdominal tumors
Stage C	Intra-abdominal tumor with or without a single jaw tumor
Stage D	Intra-abdominal tumor with extra-abdominal sites other than a single jaw tumor

Proposed NCI [62], for small noncleaved cell/undifferentiated lymphomas (sporadic)

Stage I	Single extra-abdominal tumor
Stage IR	Resected (>90%) intra-abdominal tumor
Stage II	Multiple extra-abdominal sites excluding bone marrow and CNS
Stage IIIA	Unresected intra-abdominal tumor; epidural tumor not otherwise in stage IV
Stage IIIB	Intra- and extra-abdominal tumor except bone marrow
Stage IVA	Bone marrow involvement without abdominal or CNS tumor
Stage IVB	Bone marrow and abdominal tumor without CNS disease
Stage IVC	CNS disease (malignant CSF pleiocytosis/cranial nerve palsies)

Proposed NCI [62], for lymphoblastic lymphoma

Stage I	Single extrathoracic tumor
Stage II	Multiple extrathoracic tumors excluding bone marrow and CNS
Stage IIIA	Single mediastinal (thymic) tumor
Stage IIIB	Mediastinal tumor with pleural effusion
	Mediastinal tumor with extrathoracic tumor excluding bone marrow and CNS
Stage IVA	CNS disease (malignant CSF pleiocytosis/cranial nerve palsies) without bone marrow involvement
Stage IVB	Bone marrow and intrathoracic tumor (without CNS or extrathoracic tumor)
Stage IVC	Bone marrow and extrathoracic tumor (without CNS)
Stage IVD	Bone marrow and CNS disease
(Stages IV B, C, and D are probably better diagnosed as acute lymphoblastic leukemia)	

securing an adequate surgical biopsy, which must be reviewed by an experienced hematopathologist. If necessary, fresh biopsy material must be obtained by a repeat biopsy.

The staging procedures should establish the extent of the disease as accurately as strictly necessary for the rational planning of treatment, estimation of prognosis and evaluation of response. What pro-

Table 24.8 Required staging procedures for all patients with NHLs

1. History, including the duration and growth rate of lymph node enlargement, and the presence or absence of B symptoms and symptoms suggesting extralymphatic involvement

2. Physical examination, including evaluation of all lymph node regions, recording site and size of all abnormal lymph nodes, inspection of Waldeyer's ring, evaluation of the presence or absence of hepatosplenomegaly, inspection of the skin and detection of palpable masses

3. Laboratory studies:
   a. Complete blood count
   b. Serum lactate dehydrogenase (LDH) and β_2-microglobulin levels
   c. Evaluation of renal function (serum creatinine, uric acid, electrolytes)
   d. Evaluation of liver function (liver enzymes, bilirubin and serum alkaline phosphatase)

4. Radiologic studies:
   a. Standard posteroanterior and lateral chest radiographs
   b. Abdominopelvic CT scan

5. Bilateral posterior iliac crest bone marrow biopsies and peripheral blood smear

cedures are in fact necessary depends on the typical distribution of the disease, which in turn is dependent on the histology and the initial localization of the disease. However, a number of staging procedures are required for all patients with NHLs, regardless of histology and initial presentation. These procedures are listed in Table 24.8. Under certain circumstances supplementary or alternative staging procedures may be indicated (listed in Table 24.9).

A careful history is important. The date that a mass was first observed and its subsequent growth rate should be ascertained. The presence and duration of the different B symptoms of the Ann Arbor classification should be noted. Symptoms suggesting extralymphatic involvement (e.g., bone pain, gastrointestinal complaints, neurologic symptoms, cardiopulmonary symptoms) should be enquired into, and if confirmed should lead to further investigations in order to establish whether they are due to lymphoma.

The physical examination should include a careful evaluation of all lymph node regions, including the preauricular, occipital, epitrochlear, femoral and popliteal nodes, which are more often involved in the NHLs than in Hodgkin's disease. If there is uncertainty about involvement of lymph nodes in a peripheral region, ultrasonography may be helpful [92]. The site and size of abnormal lymph nodes should be recorded, preferably on a schematic drawing of the body of the kind shown in Figure 24.1. A schematic drawing often gives a better description of initial involvement for later comparison than a laborious verbal description. Waldeyer's ring should be inspected either by indirect laryngoscopy or by direct fiberoptic examination; the latter is preferable for viewing the nasopharynx. Examination of Waldeyer's ring is particularly important in patients with involvement of high neck nodes or the gastrointestinal (GI) tract. Hepatosplenomegaly should be noted, although the correlation with

Table 24.9 Supplementary or alternative staging procedures indicated under certain circumstances

For evaluation of peripheral nodal regions:
  Ultrasound
For evaluation of the chest:
  CT scan
  Gallium scintigraphy
For evaluation of the abdomen:
  Lymphangiography
  Ultrasound
  (Percutaneous liver biopsy)
  (Laparotomy)
For evaluation of the bone marrow:
  Magnetic resonance imaging (MRI)

tumor involvement is not very strong [14,16,93–95]. Inspection of the skin and biopsy of suspicious lesions should be performed. Palpable masses, e.g., in salivary glands, thyroid, breast, abdomen, testicles or bones should be detected.

Laboratory studies should include a complete blood count. The blood count does not correlate very well with bone marrow involvement [96,97], but it provides baseline pretreatment values. LDH and β_2-microglobulin are important because they are indirect measures of the total tumor burden and hence of great prognostic value. Serum creatinine, uric acid and electrolytes are important for identifying patients at risk for the development of tumor lysis syndrome. Impaired renal function may also suggest ureteral obstruction from retroperitoneal tumor, which may necessitate hemodialysis or temporary urinary diversion before treatment of the lymphoma is initiated. Liver function tests, particularly for alkaline phosphatase, may be abnormal but correlate poorly with hepatic involvement [93,98,99].

Standard posteroanterior and lateral chest radiographs remain the mainstay of evaluating intrathoracic disease and should be performed in all patients with NHL [100]. Mediastinal and/or hilar adenopathy will be detected in 18–25% of patients [16,101,102]. Pleural effusion is found in 8–10%, usually associated with mediastinal adenopathy [101–103]. However, pleural effusion requires pathologic verification, as it quite often consists of a transudate without malignant cells. Parenchymal lung involvement is seen in 3–6% [101,103]. Linear tomography of the chest may provide additional information, but it will rarely change the patient's stage and is seldom indicated [104,105].

Computed tomography (CT) of the thorax delineates more precisely the anatomic extent of lymphadenopathy in the mediastinum and involvement of the chest wall or pericardium than conventional chest radiographs or tomography [100,106]. However, histologic proof confirming the CT results is generally lacking. Chest CT is not required for routine staging purposes but may be indicated in certain circumstances. If intrathoracic disease is present and radiotherapy is to be part of the treatment, CT is needed for the optimal design of treatment portals. In patients with localized disease outside the thorax, who might be candidates for radiotherapy as the only treatment modality, chest CT may detect otherwise invisible lymphadenopathy and thereby change the treatment strategy. CT is useful whenever findings on conventional chest radiographs require clarification, and may be useful for monitoring response to treatment of mediastinal, pericardial or chest wall disease. Otherwise, chest CT is not generally necessary [106].

Gallium-67 scintigraphy is not recommended as part of the routine staging because of its variable sensitivity, ranging in different studies from 18% to 92% [107–111]. However, the sensitivity may be improved by higher doses of gallium and more advanced technology, and is much better in intermediate- and high-grade NHLs, being invariably higher in small noncleaved cell lymphomas, than in low-grade lymphomas [107–109,111–113]. Because of the normal uptake in the liver and the relatively slow excretion through the intestine, abdominal and pelvic images may be difficult to interpret [110,111]. Gallium-67 scintigraphy is better suited for imaging of the mediastinum, but conventional chest radiographs and CT scans are quite sensitive for detecting mediastinal lymphadenopathy, and gallium scintigraphy rarely provides important new information [100,109,111]. Gallium scintigraphy may be useful for measuring response to therapy [111,114–116] and should be considered in the initial staging of patients with intermediate- and high-grade NHLs with bulky disease in order to obtain a baseline value for later comparison, because the evaluation of response to treatment in these cases may frequently be complicated by a residual mass of unknown significance. A high number of false positives, at least in the abdomen, has been reported in surgically restaged patients but this may be related to misinterpretation of bowel uptake – a problem which may be lessened by adminstering laxatives and rescanning after 24–48 hours (if due to bowel, the pattern will normally alter) [117].

Abdominopelvic CT scan is now the standard test for evaluation of the abdomen in patients with NHLs. In series of patients staged with laparotomy the frequencies of involvement have been 50–60% for para-aortic nodes, 50–60% for mesenteric nodes (most commonly seen in the follicular subtypes), 30–50% for the spleen (most commonly in the follicular subtypes), 15–30% for the liver, 5–20% for the GI tract (more often in children than in adults), and less than 5% for the urinary tract [16,94,100,118,119]. CT scanning is able to detect involvement of lymph nodes provided they are enlarged, which is often the case in NHLs. Involvement of the liver and spleen is frequently diffuse with tumor deposits often less than 1 cm in size, and such lesions are usually not detectable with CT scan (or any other currently available imaging technique). Organ size is an unreliable predictor of involvement. Overall, the accuracy of abdominopelvic CT scan compared with laparotomy for detecting intra-abdominal disease is over 80%, a figure which is not surpassed by any other noninvasive technique [100,120–122].

Lymphangiography has an overall accuracy of 90% compared with laparotomy for detecting involve-ment of para-aortic and iliac lymph nodes [100,123, 124]. However, only retroperitoneal lymph nodes up to the level of the renal vessels can be visualized by lymphangiography. Because upper abdominal lymph nodes, particularly the mesenteric nodes, and other abdominal structures are frequently involved in the NHLs, abdominal CT scan is the preferred test [125–128]. In about 10% of patients with normal abdominal CT scans lymphangiography will prove abnormal [125] – for example, in cases where retroperitoneal lymph nodes are not enlarged but the nodal architecture is abnormal. The lymphangiogram is also a predictor, although a somewhat imprecise one, of intra-abdominal disease outside the directly visualized areas [16,102,124]. Less than 25% of patients with negative lymphangiograms will have disease in the spleen or mesenteric nodes and virtually none will have disease in the liver. Conversely, 50–80% of patients with positive lymphangiograms will have disease in the spleen or mesenteric nodes, and 20–50% will have liver involvement. Lymphangiography should therefore be considered in a patient with a normal abdominal CT scan if a positive lymphangiography would change treatment strategy.

With an adequate abdominal ultrasound examination, abdominal disease can be detected with about the same accuracy as a CT scan [100]. However, technical difficulties such as the presence of gas or bone often preclude examination of all abdominal and pelvic structures. The quality of ultrasound examination is, moreover, highly dependent on the ultrasonographer. The images generated by ultrasound are generally difficult for clinicians to interpret and they cannot easily be used in the planning of radiation fields. Ultrasound may, however, be very useful in patients, typically children, with little retroperitoneal fat, where CT scans cannot delineate lymph nodes properly. Ultrasound may also be extremely helpful in situations where the abdominal CT scan is difficult to interpret because segments of the bowel do not fill with contrast and may be mistaken for lymphoma. The role of magnetic resonance imaging (MRI) in evaluating intra-abdominal disease in the NHLs is still unclear [129,130]. Radionuclide liver/spleen scans have not generally proved useful [100,105].

Invasive procedures in the abdomen are rarely indicated. Percutaneous or peritoneoscopy-directed liver biopsy has been reported to detect liver involvement in up to 42% of patients with NHLs, particularly in follicular subtypes [15]. However, most of the patients also had bone marrow involvement or were already in stage III, so that treatment would not, in the large majority, have been changed by the liver biopsy result. Staging laparotomy with splenectomy has been performed on large numbers of patients, and the information thus gathered has provided us with invaluable data on the intra-abdominal distribution of the NHLs [14–16,94,99,102,131]. Today, however, staging laparotomy for NHLs is rarely performed. With the treatment strategies presently used in most centres the large majority of patients will receive chemotherapy, and only patients with localized, low-grade NHLs are candidates for radiotherapy alone. As there is no evidence that outcome for the latter patients is adversely affected by minimal initial treatment, even if occult, asymptomatic intra-abdominal disease is present, there seems to be no indication for laparotomies in these patients. However, laparotomies are still performed for diagnostic (and sometimes therapeutic) purposes in gastrointestinal NHLs.

Bone marrow involvement is very common in the NHLs. In the large amount of patient material made available for the original Non-Hodgkin's Lymphoma Pathologic Classification Project bone marrow involvement was observed in 30–71% of low-grade, 10–34% of intermediate-grade, and 12–50% of high-grade NHLs [12]. Hence, bone marrow examination is mandatory in the staging of all patients with NHLs. Marrow biopsy is necessary since marrow aspiration is inferior in identifying marrow involvement [97,132]. Bilateral posterior iliac crest biopsy is recommended, because marrow involvement is usually focal, and performing more than one biopsy may increase the detection of involvement by up to 30% [14,97,102,133]. Examination of a peripheral blood smear, usually performed in conjunction with the examination of the bone marrow biopsy, may reveal lymphoma cells in about 10% of patients, usually in the low-grade NHLs [134]. Newer techniques such as flow cytometry, Southern blot analysis, and polymerase chain reaction are far more sensitive than conventional morphologic assessment, and can detect lymphoma cells in blood and bone marrow in a much larger proportion of patients [135–142]. However, whether the results of these highly sensitive analyses should, in future, influence staging and treatment of patients with NHLs is as yet unknown. Hence these techniques should still be regarded primarily as research tools [137,143].

MRI seems to be very sensitive for the detection of bone marrow involvement [144–146]. In patients, where marrow involvement is suspected in spite of negative random biopsies, and where a positive marrow would change treatment strategy, an MRI may be used to identify focal areas of involvement. However, the specificity of MRI for detection of marrow involvement is questionable [145], and suspicious areas should be biopsied for histological confirmation.

PROCEDURES INDICATED IN PATIENTS WITH SPECIFIC SYMPTOMS

In addition to the staging procedures required in all patients to establish the extent of disease, additional procedures may be indicated in the individual patient if certain specific symptoms are present. The more commonly performed additional procedures are listed in Table 24.10. These procedures are not routinely recommended because the yield of positive results is too low in asymptomatic patients.

Neurologic symptoms should always prompt careful examination. General CNS dysfunction or cranial nerve abnormalities may be caused by leptomeningeal involvement or less commonly by intraparenchymal lesions [147–154]. Contrast-enhanced CT or MRI scanning and lumbar puncture with examination of the cerebrospinal fluid (CSF) should be carried out. MRI may sometimes show lesions not visible on CT scan. If these tests are negative in spite of continued symptoms, additional lumbar punctures must be carried out. Immunohistochemical stains may demonstrate a monoclonal population of cells in the CSF even if they appear cytologically benign. Elevated tumor markers (LDH and β_2-microglobulin) in the CSF may provide circumstantial evidence for lymphomatous invasion of the CNS [153,155].

Symptoms of spinal cord dysfunction, most often caused by compression from epidural lesions [148, 149,153], should also be promptly evaluated. Myelography (or CT scan) after intrathecal contrast injection, or, the more frequently performed MRI of the spinal cord, should establish the diagnosis [100,156]. Epidural lesions frequently coexist with leptomeningeal involvement and examination of the CSF should also be carried out [152,153].

Visual symptoms may be caused by ocular involvement (vitreous, retina or choroid), by involvement of extraocular orbital structures, or by leptomeningeal or parenchymal brain involvement. Examinations should include a careful ophthalmologic evaluation, including ophthalmoscopy and slit-lamp examination, CT or MRI scans of the orbits and brain, and a lumbar puncture with examination of the CSF [100,155,156].

A patient with bone pain and swelling should undergo a bone scan. A bone scan should also be considered in patients with an elevated alkaline phosphatase. Radionuclide bone scans are highly sensitive – more sensitive than conventional radiographs – as an indicator of bone involvement [100,157,158]. However, bone scans are not as specific as conventional radiographs, and areas positive on the bone scan should be confirmed by

Table 24.10 Procedures indicated in patients with specific symptoms

Neurologic symptoms
    General CNS dysfunction or cranial nerve abnormalities
        CT or MRI of brain
        Lumbar puncture with examination of cerebrospinal fluid
    Spinal cord dysfunction
        Myelography or MRI of spinal cord
        Lumbar puncture with examination of cerebrospinal fluid
    Visual symptoms
        Ophthalmologic evaluation, including slit-lamp examination
        CT or MRI of orbits and brain
        Lumbar puncture with examination of cerebrospinal fluid
Bone pain or swelling
    Bone scan, positive areas confirmed by plain radiographs (and biopsy, if needed)
Gastrointestinal complaints
    Barium studies of the gastrointestinal tract
Cardiac symptoms
    Echocardiogram

plain radiographs or, if more complicated bone structures such as the facial bones are shown to be positive, by CT scans (and biopsied if need be). Bone involvement is found in less than 10% of patients without specific symptoms [16] and a bone scan is not recommended as a routine staging procedure [100].

Patients with GI complaints should undergo barium studies of the GI tract. The abdominal CT scan is not very sensitive for detection of intrinsic bowel involvement and the routine staging procedures cannot be relied upon to rule out GI involvement. Although GI involvement is a fairly common extranodal manifestation of NHLs [61], virtually all patients with GI involvement have signs or symptoms leading to further investigations, and routine barium studies on all patients are therefore not warranted [100,101, 159,160].

Finally, patients with cardiac symptoms should be evaluated with an echocardiogram to detect cardiac and pericardial involvement.

PROCEDURES INDICATED FOR PATIENTS WITH SPECIFIC HISTOLOGIC SUBTYPES AND/OR DISEASE LOCALIZATIONS

The NHLs can involve virtually any organ or tissue. However, different subgroups of NHLs have differing patterns of spread and involvement of nodal or extranodal areas. These differences reflect the biological characteristics of the tumor cells. In general, low-grade lymphomas are composed of B-lymphocytes that readily circulate and home to B-cell-dependent portions of the lymphoid system. The low-grade NHLs are therefore nearly always disseminated at the time of diagnosis (see Table 24.2). The growth pattern of the low-grade lymphoma cells is nondestructive, however, and they rarely invade privileged sites such as the CNS. Conversely, intermediate- and high-grade NHLs are composed of malignant cells that are less likely to circulate and, hence, these NHLs are somewhat more likely to remain localized (see Table 24.2). However, the growth pattern of the intermediate- and high-grade lymphoma cells is highly destructive, and consequently they have a marked propensity to invade extranodal structures, including privileged sites such as the CNS.

Within the broad histologic subtypes of the Working Formulation, subgroups are now being identified based on clinical, histopathologic, immunologic and cytogenetic studies. These subgroups often have characteristic patterns of anatomic distribution and spread [161–178]. Recent research into homing receptor molecules on the surface of lymphoma cells is beginning to shed light on the mechanisms responsible for the specific disease patterns of different NHLs [76,179–187]. Such receptors recognize molecules on the surface of normal cells in various anatomic localizations (e.g., high endothelial cells) causing exit from the vascular compartments or localization within tissues. In the future we may become capable of more precisely characterizing different NHLs in a more logical and rational way on the basis of the expression of receptor molecules of this kind. This may conceivably lead to the ability to predict the pattern of dissemination in different subgroups of NHLs with greater accuracy than is presently possible, and thus enable us to design optimal staging strategies in individual patients. For the time being, the routine staging procedures and procedures prompted by specific symptoms suffice for the majority of patients with NHL. Additional studies are recommended for patients with specific histologic subtypes and/or specific disease locations (listed in Table 24.11). The following recommendations are based on our present knowledge of patterns of involvement that have a direct bearing on prognosis and the treatment strategy.

Patients with lymphoblastic lymphoma or small noncleaved cell lymphoma have a high potential for the development of leptomeningeal disease, in some series in excess of 25%, and lumbar puncture with examination of the cerebrospinal fluid is mandatory in all such patients [32,87,88,148,150–153, 188,189]. Patients with intermediate- and other high-grade NHLs with stage IV disease (particularly, bone marrow involvement) or with involvement of the testes, paranasal sinuses, or epidural space also have an increased risk (in the order of 20%) of developing leptomeningeal disease, and a lumbar puncture as part of the staging procedures is recommended [150–152,154,188,190–195]. Patients with testicular NHLs should also be examined carefully for involvement of Waldeyer's ring and skin, since the risk of involvement of either is about 10% [191].

Primary brain NHLs are usually parenchymal lesions, which are multifocal in roughly half of immunocompetent patients and in nearly all AIDS patients [155,156]. Patients should therefore be evaluated with contrast-enhanced CT or MRI of the brain and orbits, preferably before corticosteroids are instituted, since corticosteroids can cause contrast-enhancing lesions to shrink or disappear. At least 1/3 of patients have positive CSF, and examination of the CSF should be part of the staging procedures for all such patients, except in cases where a lumbar puncture would be considered unsafe [155,192]. The eye, being a direct extension of the CNS, is reported to be involved in 20% of patients with primary brain NHLs at diagnosis, if carefully examined [192]. Typically, the vitreous, retina or choroid are involved. The initial evaluation of patients with primary brain NHLs should therefore include a careful ophthalmologic evaluation including slit-lamp examination. Patients presenting with NHLs of the ocular structures (as opposed to the extraocular orbital structures) should be investigated in the same way as patients with primary brain NHLs. Patients presenting with primary CNS NHLs will virtually never have systemic lymphoma at the time of diagnosis, hence routine staging procedures would be expected to be negative and should not delay treatment [155,156].

Patients with NHLs involving the nasal cavity, nasopharynx, paranasal sinuses or extraocular orbital structures should be examined with CT or MRI of the relevant area to define the anatomic extent of the disease, including possible invasion of bony structures. This is important for the planning of radiation portals and for follow-up.

Patients with involvement of Waldeyer's ring have an increased risk of involvement of the GI tract, either at presentation or at relapse. In most series the

Table 24.11 Procedures indicated for patients with specific histologic subtypes and/or specific disease localizations

Lymphoblastic lymphoma (all)
Small noncleaved cell lymphoma (all)
Intermediate- or high-grade lymphoma and stage IV disease (particularly bone marrow involvement) or involvement of testis, paranasal sinus or epidural space
    Lumbar puncture with examination of cerebrospinal fluid
Brain, ocular structures
    CT or MRI of brain and orbits
    Lumbar puncture with examination of cerebrospinal fluid
    Ophthalmologic evaluation, including slit-lamp examination
Nasal cavity, nasopharynx, paranasal sinuses, orbit
    CT or MRI of the head and neck
Waldeyer's ring, thyroid
    Barium studies of the GI tract
Breast
    Bilateral mammogram
Stomach (nonlaparotomized patients)
    Endoscopic ultrasound
Bone
    Bone scan

lymphoma: An analysis of 105 cases. *Cancer* 1982, **49**: 586–595.

153. Recht LD. Neurologic complications of systemic lymphoma. *Neurol. Clin.* 1991, **9**: 1001–1015.

154. Young RC, Howser DM, Anderson T, et al. Central nervous system complications of non-Hodgkin's lymphoma. The potential role for prophylactic therapy. *Am. J. Med.* 1979, **66**: 435–443.

155. DeAngelis LM. Primary central nervous system lymphoma. *Princip. Pract. Oncol. Updates* 1992, **6**: 1–13.

156. Hochberg FH, Miller DC. Primary central nervous system lymphoma. *J. Neurosurg.* 1988, **68**: 835–853.

157. Anderson KC, Kaplan WD, Leonard RCF, et al. Role of 99mTc methylene diphosphonate bone imaging in the management of lymphoma. *Cancer Treat. Rep.* 1985, **69**: 1347–1351.

158. Schechter JP, Jones SE, Woolfenden JM, et al. Bone scanning in lymphoma. *Cancer* 1976, **38**: 1142–1148.

159. Brooks JJ, Enterline HT. Primary gastric lymphomas. A clinicopathologic study of 58 cases with long-term follow-up and literature review. *Cancer* 1983, **51**: 701–711.

160. Taal BG, Burgers JMV, van Heerde P, et al. The clinical spectrum and treatment of primary non-Hodgkin's lymphoma of the stomach. *Ann. Oncol.* 1993, **4**: 839–846.

161. Isaacson PG. Pathology of malignant lymphomas. *Curr. Opin. Oncol.* 1992, **4**: 811–820.

162. Sundeen JT, Longo DL, Jaffe ES. CD5 expression in B-cell small lymphocytic malignancies. Correlations with clinical presentation and sites of disease. *Am. J. Surg. Pathol.* 1992, **16**: 130–137.

163. Harris NL. Extranodal lymphoid infiltrates and mucosa-associated lymphoid tissue (MALT). A unifying concept. *Am. J. Surg. Pathol.* 1991, **15**: 879–884.

164. Isaacson PG, Spencer J. Malignant lymphoma of mucosa-associated lymphoid tissue. *Histopathology* 1987, **11**: 445–462.

165. Pelstring RJ, Essell JH, Kurtin PJ, et al. Diversity of organ site involvement among malignant lymphomas of mucosa-associated tissues. *Am. J. Clin. Path.* 1991, **96**: 738–745.

166. Bookman MA, Lardelli P, Jaffe ES, et al. Lymphocytic lymphoma of intermediate differentiation: Morphologic, immunophenotypic, and prognostic factors. *J. Natl Cancer Inst.* 1990, **82**: 742–748.

167. Jaffe ES, Bookman MA, Longo DL. Lymphocytic lymphoma of intermediate differentiation – mantle zone lymphoma: A distinct subtype of B-cell lymphoma. *Hum. Pathol.* 1987, **18**: 877–880.

168. Raffeld M, Jaffe ES. bcl-1, t(11;14), and mantle cell-derived lymphomas. *Blood* 1991, **78**: 259–263.

169. Weisenburger DD, Sanger WG, Armitage JO, et al. Intermediate lymphocytic lymphoma: Immunophenotypic and cytogenetic findings. *Blood* 1987, **69**: 1617–1621.

170. Banerjee SS, Heald J, Harris M. Twelve cases of Ki-1 positive anaplastic large cell lymphoma of skin. *J. Clin. Pathol.* 1991, **44**: 119–125.

171. Bitter MA, Franklin WA, Larson RA, et al. Morphology in Ki-1(CD30)-positive non-Hodgkin's lymphoma is correlated with clinical features and the presence of a unique chromosomal abnormality, t(2;5)(p23;q35). *Am. J. Surg. Pathol.* 1990, **14**: 305–316.

172. Greer JP, Kinney MC, Dollins RD, et al. Clinical features of 31 patients with Ki-1 anaplastic large-cell lymphoma. *J. Clin. Oncol.* 1991, **9**: 539–547.

173. Kadin ME. Ki-1-positive anaplastic large-cell lymphoma: A clinicopathologic entity? *J. Clin. Oncol.* 1991, **9**: 533–536.

174. Penny RJ, Blaustein JC, Longtine JA, et al. Ki-1-positive large cell lymphomas, a heterogenous group of neoplasms. Morphologic, immunophenotypic, genotypic, and clinical features of 24 cases. *Cancer* 1991, **68**: 362–373.

175. Shulman LN, Frisard B, Antin JH, et al. Primary Ki-1 anaplastic large-cell lymphoma in adults: Clinical characteristics and therapeutic outcome. *J. Clin. Oncol.* 1993, **11**: 937–942.

176. Jaffe ES. Pathologic and clinical spectrum of post-thymic T-cell malignancies. *Cancer Invest.* 1984, **2**: 413–426.

177. Takagi N, Nakamura S, Ueda R, et al. A phenotypic and genotypic study of three node-based, low-grade peripheral T-cell lymphomas: Angioimmunoblastic lymphoma, T-zone lymphoma, and lymphoepithelioid lymphoma. *Cancer* 1992, **69**: 2571–2582.

178. Jaffe ES, Cossman J, Blattner WA, et al. The pathologic spectrum of adult T-cell leukemia/lymphoma in the United States. *Am. J. Surg. Pathol.* 1984, **8**: 263–275.

179. Bashir R, Coakham H, Hochberg F. Expression of LFA-1/ICAM-1 in CNS lymphomas: Possible mechanism for lymphoma homing into the brain. *J. Neuro-Oncol.* 1992, **12**: 103–110.

180. Freedman AS, Munro JM, Morimoto C, et al. Follicular non-Hodgkin's lymphoma cell adhesion to normal germinal centers and neoplastic follicles involves very late antigen-4 and vascular cell adhesion molecule-1. *Blood* 1992, **79**: 206–212.

181. Horst E, Meijer CJLM, Radaszkiewicz T, et al. Adhesion molecules in the prognosis of diffuse large-cell lymphoma: Expression of a lymphocyte homing receptor (CD44), LFA-1 (CD11a/18), and ICAM-1 (CD54). *Leukemia* 1990, **4**: 595–599.

182. Jalkanen S, Joensuu H, Söderström K-O. Lymphocyte homing and clinical behavior of non-Hodgkin's lymphoma. *J. Clin. Invest.* 1991, **87**: 1835–1840.

183. Kern WF, Spier CM, Hanneman EH, et al. Neural cell adhesion molecule-positive peripheral T-cell lymphoma: A rare variant with a propensity for unusual sites of involvement. *Blood* 1992, **79**: 2432–2437.

184. Möller P, Eichelmann A, Koretz K, et al. Adhesion molecules VLA-1 to VLA-6 define discrete stages of peripheral B lymphocyte development and characterize different types of B-cell neoplasia. *Leukemia* 1992, **6**: 256–264.

185. Möller P, Eichelmann A, Mechtersheimer G, et al. Expression of β1-integrins, H-CAM (CD44) and LECAM-1 in primary gastro-intestinal B-cell lymphomas as compared to the adhesion receptor profile of the gut-associated lymphoid system, tonsil and

peripheral lymph node. *Int. J. Cancer* 1991, **49**: 846–855.

186. Pinto A, Carbone A, Gloghini A, et al. Differential expression of cell adhesion molecules in B-zone small lymphocytic lymphoma and other well-differentiated lymphocytic disorders. *Cancer* 1993, **72**: 894–904.

187. Steeter PR, Berg EL, Rouse BTN, et al. A tissue-specific endothelial cell molecule involved in lymphocyte homing. *Nature* 1988, **331**: 41–46.

188. Ersbøll J, Schultz HB, Thomsen BLR, et al. Meningeal involvement in non-Hodgkin's lymphoma: Symptoms, incidence, risk factors and treatment. *Scand. J. Haematol.* 1985, **35**: 487–496.

189. Magrath IT, Sariban E. Clinical features of Burkitt's lymphoma in the USA. In Lenoir GM, O'Conor GT, Olweny CLM (eds). *Burkitt's lymphoma: A human cancer model. IARC Scientific Publications*, No. 60. Lyon: International Agency for Research on Cancer, 1985, pp. 119–127.

190. Crellin AM, Vaughan Hudson B, Bennett MH, et al. Non-Hodgkin's lymphoma of the testis. *Radiother. Oncol.* 1993, **27**: 99–106.

191. Doll DC, Weiss RB. Malignant lymphoma of the testis. *Am. J. Med.* 1986, **81**: 515–524.

192. DeAngelis LM, Yahalom J, Heinemann M-H, et al. Primary CNS lymphoma: Combined treatment with chemotherapy and radiotherapy. *Neurology* 1990, **40**: 80–86.

193. Brugère J, Schlienger M, Gérard-Marchant R, et al. Non-Hodgkin's malignant lymphomata of upper digestive and respiratory tract: Natural history and results of radiotherapy. *Br. J. Cancer* 1975, **31**(Suppl. 2): 435–440.

194. Gospodarowicz MK, Sutcliffe SB, Brown TC, et al. Patterns of disease in localized extranodal lymphomas. *J. Clin. Oncol.* 1987, **5**: 875–880.

195. Jacobs C, Hoppe RT. Non-Hodgkin's lymphomas of head and neck extranodal sites. *Int. J. Radiat. Oncol. Biol. Phys.* 1985, **11**: 357–364.

196. Saul SH, Kapadia SB. Primary lymphoma of Waldeyer's ring. Clinicopathologic study of 68 cases. *Cancer* 1985, **56**: 157–166.

197. Mc Dermott EWM, Cassidy N, Heffernan SJ. Perforation through undiagnosed small bowel involvement in primary thyroid lymphoma during chemotherapy. *Cancer* 1992, **69**: 572–573.

198. Tupchong L, Hughes F, Harmer CL. Primary lymphoma of the thyroid: Clinical features, prognostic factors, and results of treatment. *Int. J. Radiat. Oncol. Biol. Phys.* 1986, **12**: 1813–1821.

199. Giardini R, Piccolo C, Rilke F. Primary non-Hodgkin's lymphomas of the female breast. *Cancer* 1992, **69**: 725–735.

200. Musshoff K. Klinische stadieneinteilung der Nicht-Hodgkin-lymphome. *Strahlentherapie* 1977, **153**: 218–221.

201. Azab MB, Henry-Amar M, Rougier P, et al. Prognostic factors in primary gastrointestinal non-Hodgkin's lymphoma. A multivariate analysis, report of 106 cases, and review of the literature. *Cancer* 1989, **64**: 1208–1217.

202. Weingrad DN, Decosse JJ, Sherlock P, et al. Primary gastrointestinal lymphoma: A 30-year review. *Cancer* 1982, **49**: 1258–1265.

203. Gospodarowicz MK, Bush RS, Brown TC, et al. Curability of gastrointestinal lymphoma with combined surgery and radiation. *Int. J. Radiat. Oncol. Biol. Phys.* 1983, **9**: 3–9.

204. Hockey MS, Powell J, Crocker J, et al. Primary gastric lymphoma. *Br. J. Surg.* 1987, **74**: 483–487.

205. Lim FE, Hartman AS, Tan EGC, et al. Factors in the prognosis of gastric lymphoma. *Cancer* 1977, **39**: 1715–1720.

206. Blackledge G, Bush H, Dodge OG, et al. A study of gastro-intestinal lymphoma. *Clin. Oncol.* 1979, **5**: 209–219.

207. Maor MH, Velasquez WS, Fuller LM, et al. Stomach conservation in stages IE and IIE gastric non-Hodgkin's lymphoma. *J. Clin. Oncol.* 1990, **8**: 266–271.

208. Rossi A, Lister TA. Primary gastric non-Hodgkin's lymphoma: A therapeutic challenge. *Eur. J. Cancer* 1993, **29A**: 1924–1926.

209. Tio TL, den Hartog Jager FCA, Tytgat GNJ. Endoscopic ultrasonography in detection and staging of gastric non-Hodgkin lymphoma. *Scand. J. Gastroenterol.* 1986, **21** (Suppl. 123): 52–58.

210. Ostrowski ML, Unni KK, Banks PM, et al. Malignant lymphoma of bone. *Cancer* 1986, **58**: 2646–2655.

proteins. Thus, one set of studies indicates that human CD4+ T-cells (but not CD8+ T-cells) synthesize and secrete their own transferrin [3]. Secreted transferrin might be useful in scavenging for iron in extravascular environments where transferrin concentrations would be decreased. Alternatively, secreted transferrin might also act as a trophic factor for other cells (such as B-cells) once bound to ferric iron.

Unlike T-cells, B-cells appear to express low but detectable levels of surface transferrin receptors in a resting state, as assessed by flow cytometric techniques [4,5]. Moreover, the level of TfR expression begins to rise quickly as a result of increased transcriptional activity that occurs within 2–4 hours after any one of three distinct activation protocols is employed; i.e., anti-μ, anti-δ or LPS [4,5]. These protocols all represent strong T-cell-independent stimuli, and it probably should not be assumed that any perturbation of a resting B-cell is sufficient to trigger this type of response. Indeed, when human B-cells from peripheral blood are stimulated with staphylococcal protein A, the induction of TfR expression seems to be dependent upon the presence of a T-cell-derived B-cell growth factor [6].

Circulating monocytes do not express transferrin receptors. However, they do begin to express TfRs during the activation and maturation sequence that leads to macrophage formation [7]. At this point, a very interesting difference emerges between these cells and lymphocytes. It appears that macrophages do not respond to an iron load by downregulating their TfRs; in fact, macrophages upregulate their TfR expression in the presence of excess iron [8]. It has been proposed that this is relevant to the role of the macrophage as a storage site for iron [9]. A paradox is created, however, since ferritin levels also rise at the same time that increased iron-responsive-element binding protein (IRE-BP) activity is detected. It is not yet clear how macrophages manage to overcome the inverse regulatory relationship that otherwise exists between the TfR and ferritin in most cell types, but the difference in gene regulation and/or cell physiology must be related to the fact that macrophages store iron.

Resting natural killer (NK) cells, like T-cells and unlike B-cells, do not appear to express TfRs. When NK cells are activated, TfR expression can be detected at fairly high levels and peak expression occurs just prior to the peaks of thymidine incorporation and HLA-DR expression [10]. These results resemble those seen with T-cells and, in themselves, do not suggest that the TfR plays any unique or unusual role insofar as the metabolic requirements of the NK cell itself is concerned. A controversial issue that has attracted some attention, however, is whether NK cells might somehow utilize the transferrin

receptor complex expressed on target cells as a binding ligand for attachment. The controversy may dissipate as we learn more about how NK cell receptors interact with class I HLA molecules on target cells [10a] and how that interaction might be effected by transferrin receptors, which can be in close proximity to class I HLA molecules [10b].

In summary, iron homeostasis is managed in different ways by the major cellular participants in the immune response. This suggests rather clearly that differential management of iron-dependent metabolic functions plays an integral part in producing the distinctive physiology of each cell type.

Aspects of iron physiology that pertain to neoplastic lymphoid cells

Although there is no comprehensive review of the alterations in iron metabolism that occur in malignant lymphoid cells, there is a steadily growing group of relevant and interesting observations, and we shall begin with those that pertain to TfR expression.

The first point is that TfR expression level tends to be correlated with lymphoma grade and growth rate [11–16]. Thus, in one early study it was found that high-grade non-Hodgkin's lymphomas (NHL) contained an average of 22.5% OKT-9+ lymphocytes while low-grade lesions contained an average of 2.5% [11]. In a second early study it was found that TfR expression level was correlated with both the rate of spontaneous DNA synthesis and with grade [12] and a third early study further confirmed the relationship with grade [13]. A fairly extensive subsequent study was generally confirmatory but it was also noted that: (1) low-grade follicular lymphomas expressed more TfRs than other low-grade lymphomas; (2) diffuse small cleaved cell tumors had lower levels of TfR expression than other intermediate-grade tumors; and (3) diffuse immunoblastic lymphomas expressed lower levels of TfRs than other types of high-grade lymphomas [14]. Both chronic and acute forms of lymphoid leukemias tend to have lower-level TfR expression unless they are of T-cell origin [15,16].

The next point is that T-cell neoplasms tend to have higher levels of TfR expression than B-cell neoplasms [15–18]. Thus, it was noted in early work that T-cell lymphoblastoid cell lines express almost twice as many TfRs as B-cell lines (about 60 000 versus 30 000, respectively) [17]. Subsequent studies then showed that in T-cell acute lymphoblastic leukemia (ALL) most of the cells express high numbers of TfRs at presentation while, in contrast, in precursor B-cell ALL a smaller proportion of cells express lower numbers of TfRs [15,16]. The fact that T-cell neoplasms often have higher growth rates than B-cell neoplasms may account for such differences in many cases. In some diseases, however, additional factors are clearly relevant. Thus, in T-cell leukemias arising from human T-cell lymphotropic virus-1 (HTLV-1) infection, TfRs are expressed at very high levels at the cell surface, and it appears that this results from defective receptor phosphorylation and internalization [18].

Although any alteration in the behavior of the TfR would be considered significant in relation to iron metabolism in malignant cells, other types of changes have also been observed. Thus, it has been noted that certain T-cell lines are able to synthesize and secrete transferrin [TF; molecular weight (MW) = 80 kD] [19] and this may serve as an autocrine feedback loop once the TF molecules acquire iron from the external environment. Although similar behavior has been observed with normal T-cells (see above), transferrin production no doubt occurs under the control of the normal activation program in these cells. In addition, it has been observed that some lymphoid cell lines are clearly capable of acquiring iron from iron salts in the total absence of TF *in vitro* [20]. Such a capacity could, theoretically, provide a growth advantage to tumor cells under conditions of limited iron availability but it remains to be shown that such behavior has real relevance *in vivo*.

A final area of concern in relation to iron metabolism in malignant cells is that of serum ferritin. It now appears that lymphoid cells can and do express receptors for ferritin [21]. It has also been shown by *in vitro* studies that, once bound, ferritin can inhibit normal lymphocyte activation [21]. It is not clear at this time, however, whether serum ferritin inhibits or promotes the growth of neoplastic lymphoid cells.

Gallium scintigraphy for detection of malignant lymphomas

In 1969 Edwards and Hayes [22] reported on studies of ^{67}Ga citrate localization in patients with Hodgkin's disease. Their initial interest was to exploit the bone-localizing characteristics of gallium [23]. Much to their surprise, Edwards and Hayes discovered that ^{67}Ga localized not only in bone but also in tumor tissue.

In the first 10 years following this discovery, ^{67}Ga imaging was attempted in almost all malignant tumors in which detection and staging was important and otherwise difficult. The results of this survey were then reported in a number of comprehensive reviews [24–28]. Many mechanisms have been proposed to explain how ^{67}Ga localizes in tumors. Although not all investigators agree, there is some consensus that gallium acts as an analog of ferric ion.

GALLIUM AS AN IRON ANALOG

In the early 1970s it was first demonstrated (and subsequently confirmed) that ^{67}Ga in serum was bound tightly to the iron-transport protein, TF [29,30]. It was also shown that TF, owing to its iron binding ability, stimulated ^{67}Ga incorporation into cultured tumor cells [31,32]. A wide variety of other iron binding molecules – desferrioxamine [33,34], lactoferrin (LF)[35] and ferritin [36,37] – bound ^{67}Ga with high affinity. This led to the hypothesis that ^{67}Ga was handled as an iron analog [38]. However, animal [39] and human [40] studies showed great disparity in the biodistribution of ^{59}Fe and ^{67}Ga. Iron localized in hematopoietic tissues and red blood cells (RBCs) but not in most tumor tissue. In contrast, ^{67}Ga had a very high affinity for tumor tissue but low affinity for RBCs or marrow. In addition, ^{67}Ga remained in liver, spleen and other tissue much longer than ^{59}Fe. Hoffer [38] originally suggested that this pronounced difference was related to the unique oxidation–reduction properties of each. For iron to be absorbed in the gastrointestinal (GI) tract, and eventually incorporated into hemoglobin and cytochrome enzymes in the mitochondria, iron must cycle between its two physiologically stable states Fe^{2+} and Fe^{3+} [41–43]. In contrast, Ga^{3+} is the only stable state for gallium under physiological conditions [44], such that gallium is unable to participate in metabolic pathways in which reduction is necessary.

More recent evidence [45–49] suggests that the aqueous solubility of the two metals is as important as the redox properties in determining their biodistributions. In a physiological environment and at trace levels, gallium exists primarily (98%) as gallate, ($Ga(OH)_4$; MW=125 D) and is soluble, whereas iron is not. Therefore, iron, not ^{67}Ga, requires a chelate of some type, e.g., TF, for *in vivo* transport. Gallium binding to TF is very sensitive to physiochemical parameters, particularly bicarbonate and TF concentrations and pH [45,47,50]. The conditions in normal blood are optimal for ^{67}Ga:TF complex formation, but if concentrations of bicarbonate or TF are reduced at the tumor site or *in vitro*, hydroxyl ions can effectively compete with TF for the radionuclide, leading to more gallate formation [45]. Therefore, ^{67}Ga can shift between TF and the gallate depending upon the TF concentration. In patients with normal TF concentration and iron saturation in the blood, the gallate concentration is only 1% of the total injected activity [51]. However, if the concentration of unsaturated TF were to be lowered from 40 to 5 μM by an increase in TF saturation, this would increase gallate concentration to 7% and increase the amount of activity that would pass out in the urine.

TRANSFERRIN RECEPTORS AS ^{67}Ga TRANSPORTERS

Larson and coworkers [52] were the first to extend the iron analog concept to specifically include TfRs. They proposed, based on careful studies, both *in vivo* [53,54] and *in vitro* [52,53], that 'a tumor-associated TfR is the functional unit responsible for the affinity of gallium for certain neoplasms.' Autoradiographic and cell organelle isolation studies demonstrated that ^{67}Ga was incorporated into the lysosomes of viable tumor cells [55–60]. With the normal concentration of Fe*TF in the blood, the TfR are saturated with Fe*TF and cells must upregulate the number of TfR to increase iron uptake [42]. TfRs are mainly regulated to meet the iron requirements of DNA synthesis, specifically, those of ribonucleotide reductase [43]. This is a nonheme iron enzyme, which catalyzes the first rate-limiting step in DNA synthesis, conversion of ribonucleotides to deoxyribonucleotides. In rapidly proliferating tumor cells with a high level of DNA synthesis, upregulation of the surface TfR would also lead to increased ^{67}Ga uptake. An increased number of TfRs has been detected in a variety of tumor cells [52,61,62].

While TfRs appeared to be important to the localization of ^{67}Ga in neoplastic cells, recent experiments with animals that congenitally lack TF show that good tumor ^{67}Ga uptake still occurs [63], a result that is not easily explained. This finding coincides with emerging evidence that cells in certain circumstances can acquire iron, and possibly ^{67}Ga, independently of TF [64–66]. This alternate iron transport system is not affected by cellular growth rate, induction of DNA synthesis, cell division or depletion of cellular iron [64,65]. Moreover, this system has an affinity for iron chelates which is a few orders of magnitude lower than iron for TF. Since ^{67}Ga can easily form gallate *in vivo*, which is

similar in size to these iron chelates, the radionuclide could be taken up by this system in the absence of TF. Indeed, Chitambar and Zivkovic [66] showed ^{67}Ga uptake in cultured TfR-positive cells in the absence of TF, but this uptake constituted only about 10% of TF-stimulated uptake in the same period of time. Hoffer and coworkers [67], using a nude mouse tumor model demonstrated that an anti-TfR monoclonal antibody reduced the percentage uptake of the injected dose per gram of ^{67}Ga in the tumors to 25% of control values. Thus, when the effective TF concentration is reduced or absent, this alternate system, although slower, may be responsible for all the ^{67}Ga accumulation. However, in normal circumstances the TF-dependent system appears to be mainly responsible for ^{67}Ga uptake.

The importance of ^{67}Ga scintigraphy as a diagnostic tool lies both on its ability to identify tumor masses and to differentiate viable tumor from nonviable tumor and/or nontumor tissues. There are some data that suggest that cell viability and DNA synthesis influence ^{67}Ga uptake. Iosilevsky et al. [68] showed that both ^{67}Ga and deoxyglucose uptake in a tumor model had a parallel decline after chemotherapy and radiotherapy, and that the inhibition of tumor ATP production caused a similar decline in ^{67}Ga incorporation [69]. More recently, the response to radiotherapy was monitored in a tumor model using metabolic tracers for glucose metabolism, DNA, RNA and protein synthesis. The uptake of these tracers was compared to [67]Ga [70]. While ^{67}Ga uptake did not reflect the early response to radiation treatment, diminished ^{67}Ga uptake closely followed the diminution in glucose metabolism, except for an increase in ^{67}Ga uptake 1 day after irradiation, probably caused by TF saturation. The DNA synthesis indicator and ^{67}Ga, but not the indicator of glucose metabolism, were able to differentiate between viable and nonviable tumor. [67]Ga and Fe uptake in synchronized mouse tumor cells both peak at the G_2 phase of the cell cycle, i.e., immediately preceding mitosis [71]. Nonradioactive gallium interferes with DNA synthesis by the specific inhibition of ribonucleotide reductase [72,73] and not DNA polymerases as has been proposed [74]. The TF-dependent ^{67}Ga transport system is thus intimately connected with cell division.

While data from model systems may provide useful insight into the uptake mechanism, there is evidence from patient studies that also supports the importance of TfR and cell proliferation in ^{67}Ga localization. Gallium nitrate shows its greatest effect as a therapeutic agent in large-cell lymphomas [43], which frequently express large numbers of TfR. In a study of 29 patients with NHL, all cases identified as 'low grade' were TfR negative, while 'high-grade' lymphomas had up to 28% TfR-positive cells and 'intermediate grade' had 10–15% positive cells [75]. In an immunohistochemical study of tumor tissues from patients with hepatocellular carcinomas (in which ^{67}Ga uptake is particularly high) 33 out of 34 samples were TfR-positive and more intensely stained than surrounding liver parenchyma [76]. Studies in patients with NHL or Hodgkin's lymphoma [77], lung cancer (squamous cell and adenocarcinomas) [78] and thyroid tumors (adenocarcinomas, anaplastic carcinomas and malignant lymphomas) [79] have demonstrated correlations between TfR expression and ^{67}Ga uptake [77,78]. In the thyroid tumors, the S/G$_2$M fraction of cells, measured in DNA content histograms, and proliferative indices of the tumor tissues were significantly greater in patients with positive ^{67}Ga scans than in patients with ^{67}Ga-negative scans.

Finally, TF plays a pivotal role in delivering ^{67}Ga to normal tissues. When the available ^{67}Ga binding sites were reduced in a variety of animals, either by iron injections, because of congenital lack of TF, or by irradiation or chemotherapy, the normal tissue (liver, spleen, bone marrow) uptake of ^{67}Ga was depressed, whole-body excretion was enhanced and activity in bone was unaffected or increased [63, 80–84]. These data closely parallel results from patient studies. Chen et al. [85] showed that the small intestine was the major contributor (60%) to ^{67}Ga excretion into the GI tract and bile made a 20% contribution. Increasing the TF saturation, thus reducing the unsaturated iron binding capacity, substantially reduced ^{67}Ga in the GI tract. Excess iron is also excreted via the small intestine [42].

After almost two decades of research, the evidence strongly suggests that iron and ^{67}Ga follow similar but not identical pathways. The divergence of pathways is the result of the distinct chemistry of these two metals. In particular, iron cycles between two oxidation states *in vivo* and ^{67}Ga cannot, while ^{67}Ga can form a soluble species at neutral pH. The tumor localization mechanisms for ^{67}Ga may be complex and are certainly influenced by a variety of factors. However, data from many laboratory investigations and data from clinical patient studies continue to support Larson's original concept that TfRs are rate limiting in ^{67}Ga uptake. Thus, ^{67}Ga imaging is best thought of as an *in vivo* detector of TfR status and, because of this, as an indicator of active tumor cell proliferation.

CURRENT ROLE OF GALLIUM SCINTIGRAPHY IN NHL

Gallium scintigraphy has been used in patients with NHL for more than two decades. A number of literature reports document highly variable results using this test to detect, stage and/or evaluate treatment response in such patients. In general, however, the current technique of gallium scintigraphy using 'high-dose' gallium citrate administrations (10 mCi doses in adults) and tomographic imaging technology or single photon emission computed tomography (SPECT) has been shown to have a high sensitivity for detecting viable tumor sites in NHL patients.

After an early enthusiastic reception as a lymphoma-imaging test [86,87], gallium citrate scanning for NHL fell into disrepute in the early 1980s following the publication of a paper by Longo et al. [88]. Unfortunately, the gallium scintigraphy technique in this study employed 'low-dose' (1–3 mCi) gallium citrate administrations, and low-sensitivity instruments and scanning techniques. Further, clinical examination, plain and tomographic X-ray studies (not CT) and laparotomy were considered to be the 'gold standards' against which ^{67}Ga scintigraphy was judged. These investigators found, not surprisingly, that the sensitivity of gallium scintigraphy (52%) was poor and that the test failed to have a significant impact on the staging of disease. When this paper appeared in the medical literature, perhaps because it originated from the National Institutes of Health (NIH), it had a widespread negative impact on the use of ^{67}Ga scintigraphy in NHL patient management [89].

Data that demonstrated good to excellent sensitivity for detecting sites of NHL using the newer techniques of 'high-dose' gallium, and more modern scintigraphy techniques and instrumentation, were soon to appear [90–92]. New papers described better than 85% sensitivity for detecting sites of disease: in the Anderson–Kaplan study, 92% sensitivity and nearly 100% specificity were reported in NHL. Equally important, these authors re-emphasized the role of gallium as a functional study, able to discriminate inactive tumor tissue or scar tissue from viable tumor, and thus a valuable tool for the assessment of therapy results. However, the enthusiastic message of these early 1980s studies was diminished, perhaps, in the oncology world by a 1985 paper [93], minimizing the utility of gallium scintigraphy. This appeared in a review of the management of NHL published by the American Cancer Society in its widely disseminated journal, *CA*.

The addition of tomographic techniques to gallium scintigraphy began in the decade of the 1970s with the Anger tomoscanner but the advent of the more widely produced computerized tomographic gamma cameras (SPECT) in the 1980s provided increased sensitivity in the instrumentation to enhance the better results already demonstrated with the higher gallium doses given for tumor scintigraphy [94,95]. These two factors, higher gallium doses and new SPECT cameras with increased sensitivity, moved gallium tumor scintigraphy into the modern era.

A number of recent papers demonstrate the utility of ^{67}Ga scintigraphy in detecting NHL sites involving the gastrointestinal tract [96], pulmonary hila [97] and in determining recurrence after treatment [98–102]. These modern data all show that ^{67}Ga scintigraphy is helpful in staging lymphoma patients. Used after patients are treated, ^{67}Ga scintigraphy appears to be both a sensitive and specific test for restaging patients, and may even be a useful predictor of clinical outcome.

As a practical matter, because the physical half-life of ^{67}Ga is approximately 3 days, other required nuclear medicine studies, such as ^{99m}Tc-methylene disphosphonate (MDP) bone scintigraphy, should be performed prior to ^{67}Ga imaging to avoid complications in the bone scintigraphic technique caused by ^{67}Ga photon scatter into the ^{99m}Tc windows. Also, because ^{67}Ga is excreted in part via the GI tract, the requirement for repeated images following mild catharsis of patients should be anticipated for accurate interpretation of ^{67}Ga uptake in the abdominal/pelvic region.

Bone scintigraphy

Bone scintigraphy with ^{99m}Tc-MDP is the best and least expensive method for performing a skeletal survey to detect bone involvement by NHL. Approximately 1–20% of patients will have bone involvement. Bone scintigraphy is also readily repeated at appropriate intervals to assess the effect of therapeutic regimens, especially in the first few years following diagnosis. Bone abnormalities detected by scintigraphy should be further evaluated with a radiograph because, although scintigraphy is a very sensitive procedure, it does not provide specificity in determining the cause of altered radionuclide uptake. Not all abnormal sites in the scintigram will necessarily be caused by lymphoma; degenerative disease, trauma, benign bone lesions, etc., can all give false-positive indications of skeletal lymphoma. Comparison of directed radiographs and ^{67}Ga citrate scintigrams can often be helpful in determining the exact etiology of abnormal sites on the bone scintigram.

Patterns of more diffuse increased uptake in the long bones, and particularly increased uptake in the region of the metaphyses, can indicate marrow involvement.

Sites of previous marrow biopsy will frequently show increased radionuclide activity for variable periods after the biopsy procedures and should not be misinterpreted. Those patients receiving treatment regimens that include steroids are at increased risk for avascular necrosis, which will be apparent in a bone scintigram; but the pattern of altered bone uptake will change with evolution of the bone necrosis. Finally, areas of bone included in radiation therapy ports can show increased or decreased uptake of skeletal-seeking radiopharmaceuticals – both ^{99m}Tc-MDP and ^{67}Ga – so that knowledge of the skeletal areas that received external beam irradiation is essential for accurate interpretation of subsequent bone scintigrams [103].

Positron emission tomography

A potentially exciting area of imaging research is the use of positron emission tomography (PET) with short-lived radiopharmaceuticals for physiological imaging of tumors, including lymphomas. The advantage of PET derives from the nature of positron tomography, which allows for more precise quantification of radioactivity in small lesions. In addition to positron-emitting isotopes of gallium, there are a number of metabolic-cycle radiopharmaceuticals, such as fluorine-18 2-fluorodeoxyglucose (^{18}F-FDG) which show potential as agents to permit improved imaging of lymphomas [104].

Recent papers have shown that, in patients with untreated lymphomas (both Hodgkin's and various grades of NHL) of the head and neck, the degree to which their tumors accumulated ^{18}F-FDG was correlated with prognosis [105]. PET equipment has generally been restricted to academic research hospitals until recently because of the large associated costs and the short half-life of ^{18}F, requiring close proximity of a supplier. However, new evidence suggests that ^{18}F-FDG uptake, even if imaged on less expensive but properly collimated planar or SPECT gamma cameras, can be used to stage and evaluate treatment responses in lymphoma patients [106].

Other nuclear medicine tests applicable to NHL patients

99mTc-Sestamibi [hexakis(2-methoxyisobutylisoni-trile] is a relatively new myocardial perfusion agent which has also been used for imaging various tumors. This cationic, lipophilic compound accumulates passively in cells, driven by negative membrane potentials generated across plasma and mitochondrial membranes [107–109]. Mechanisms of efflux from cells for this compound are not yet fully understood, but one route appears to involve P-glycoprotein, an energy-dependent multidrug resistance membrane protein for which 99mTc-Sestamibi is a substrate [110].

In vitro, studies have demonstrated increased 99mTc-Sestamibi uptake in carcinoma cells compared to nontransformed cell lines [111]. This is probably the result of the higher negative mitochondrial membrane potentials maintained by malignant cells [112–114]. *In vivo*, 99mTc-Sestamibi has also been used to image both primary and metastatic tumors [115–118]. Visualization of tumors of the lung [115,119], breast [119,120], thyroid [119,121], kidneys [119], bone [116,117] and Burkitt's lymphoma [119] have been reported.

Several case reports of 99mTc-Sestamibi tumor visualization in patients with NHL have appeared in the literature to date. These include a primary cardiac lymphoma [122] and a primary thyroid lymphoma [123], both of which resolved scintigraphically and clinically after therapy. Lastly, in a report by Aktolun et al. [119], Sestamibi was successful in imaging NHL in lymph nodes in one of two patients.

Given its ideal imaging characteristics, dosimetry, ease of preparation and the ability to image soon after injection, 99mTc-Sestamibi will hopefully become a useful agent in the detection and monitoring of NHL. However, further studies are needed to define its sensitivity and specificity in these malignancies.

Evaluation of myocardial function during and after chemotherapy

Anthracyclines are among the most widely used drugs in the treatment of human solid tumors, leukemias and some lymphomas. The main toxicities that limit the therapeutic use of anthracyclines are myelosuppression and cardiotoxicity, the latter being a function mainly of the cumulative dose of anthracycline received. Patients with tumors that may still be responsive to anthracyclines often cannot be safely given more of these drugs because the patients have reached a cumulative dose above which they are more likely to incur a high risk of cardiotoxicity [124]. In patients who are long-term survivors of chemotherapy regimens that included anthracyclines, there is concern that anthracycline-induced cardiotoxicity, even if subclinical, may ultimately lead to a reduction in life span following successful treatment. It is clear that the ability to predict and prevent anthracycline-induced myocardial toxicity will enhance an oncologist's ability to use these drugs effectively in treating patients with NHL.

The routine use of multiple-gated cardiac blood pool (MUGA) scintigraphy to evaluate a patient's left (and right) ventricular ejection fractions is an effective way to monitor cardiac toxicity from chemotherapy and/or radiotherapy. This test records quantitative images of the cardiac blood pool during the cardiac cycle by synchronizing the recording of scintillation data with the electrocardiogram (ECG). Use of the ECG as a signal occurring at a fixed time in relation to the mechanical activity of the heart to trigger or 'gate' the recording of the scintillation counts permits the repetitive sampling of each specific phase of the cardiac cycle from each of many cycles until a statistically significant scintillation count density is recorded. These data are then analyzed to produce a quantitative evaluation of both global and regional ventricular function. This is determined by measuring the changes in either the activity or the volume of the ventricular chamber from systole to diastole [125].

Technetium-99m-labeled autologous red blood cells are most often used as the intravascular radionuclide carrier for this test. An aliquot of the patient's own erythrocytes is prelabeled with tin from a stannous pyrophosphate bone scan pharmaceutical. After a 15–20 minute incubation, the proper dose of 99mTc-pertechnetate is added, which then binds to a component of the erythrocyte. This method produces an excellent intravascular radionuclide signal which does not 'leak' significantly into the interstitial space for several hours. The unbound portion of the 99mTc dose clears rapidly from the body via renal excretion, thus providing a good image of the intravascular blood pool. Because 99mTc has a physical half-life of only 6 hours, the radiation dosimetry is within an acceptable range, permitting repeated studies over the lifetime of a patient without discernible harm.

For an oncology patient about to begin chemotherapy, it is important to obtain a baseline MUGA study followed by serial studies in the intervals between treatments. Figure 25.1 gives a suggested schema for proper use of the radionuclide angiogram. Although a significant fraction of patients who receive high total doses of the anthracyclines will develop cardiac toxicity, the degree of toxicity encountered by individual patients is somewhat idiosyncratic. Thus, each patient should probably be monitored. Alexander et al. [126] first used serial radionuclide ventriculography to measure cardiac performance in patients undergoing doxorubicin treatment. Because no patients had signs of significant toxicity until a cumulative dosage of 350 mg/m² body surface area was reached, serial repeat MUGA studies were suggested once this total dose was reached. Subsequently, significant decreases in the measured left ventricular ejection fraction

(LVEF) were found to be a sensitive indication of impending congestive heart failure (CHF) produced by cardiotoxicity. Mild cardiotoxicity occurred when the LVEF decreased by 10% (10 ejection fraction units) but there were no clinical signs of CHF. Moderate cardiotoxicity, still without clinically evident CHF, was defined as a decline of at least 15% (15 ejection fraction units) to a final level of 45% or less. This degree of LVEF dysfunction was predictive of subsequent clinical CHF if doxorubicin was continued. Severe cardiotoxicity was observed with signs of CHF whenever the LVEF was less than 30%. These absolute values must, of course, be transposed for the normal LVEF range as determined by the technique used in one's own reference nuclear cardiology laboratory [127].

Subsequent reports showed that for patients with pre-existing cardiovascular disease leading to a decreased baseline LVEF (i.e., prechemotherapy), there was no significant increase in doxorubicin cardiotoxicity with doses under 350 mg/m². Thus, the same criteria with respect to reductions in LVEF as used in patients with normal LVEF baseline values can be applied (i.e., an absolute decrease of 10% or fall below 30%) [128]. An attempt to further increase the sensitivity of this test by adding an exercise-induced stress to the work of the left ventricle did not become widely accepted, probably because of the resultant decrease in the specificity of the test [127,129], even though the sensitivity was improved.

Finally, patients with pre-existing myocarditis of varying etiologies (mediastinal radiation therapy [130–132], infectious diseases [133], etc.) may be more sensitive to chemotherapy-induced myocarditis and probably should be monitored with extra caution.

Imaging of lymphoma using radiolabeled antibodies

Numerous trials of unconjugated monoclonal antibody (mAb) for the therapy of lymphoma have been carried out since the initial successful report of Miller et al. [134]. More recently, the use of radiolabeled antibodies for imaging and therapy of lymphomas and leukemias has shown promise [135–147].

TARGET ANTIGENS

Many tumor-associated antigens have been identified using mAbs [148]. As a result of new know-

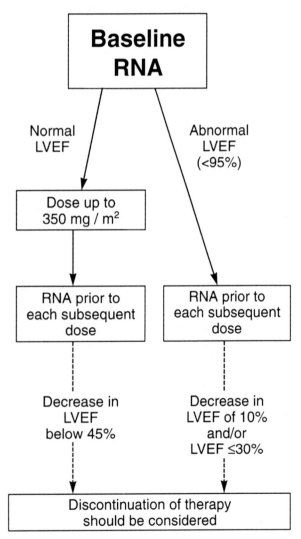

Figure 25.1   Suggested schema for the use of radionuclide angiograms to follow chemotherapy patients who receive adriamycin.

ledge of the biochemical and molecular character of these antigens, they can be crudely classified according to their functional–structural relationships [148]. Among their functions are signaling and membrane transport, cell–cell communications, and cell–matrix interactions. The function of many of these antigens, however, such as those in which the binding sites are on carbohydrate side chains, is not completely clear. Many tumor antigens are frequently found during the early stages of differentiation and may not be expressed, or are expressed only at low levels in normal adult tissues. Tumor targeting, therefore, depends on the preferential expression of the antigen in a tumor compared to its expression in normal tissues.

Most markers of malignant B- and T-cell lymphomas are also present on normal lymphocytes and many are expressed during different stages of development. An international classification categorizing these 'cluster determinants' has been adopted in order to facilitate communication [149]. These antigens are usually complex structures and the functions of many of them have not been fully elucidated. Clinical trials in B-cell malignancies have targeted B-cell antigens, including idiotypes, CD20, CD37, CD21 and HLA-DR [150–153]. In T-cell malignancies, T-cell antigens such as CD5 and CD25 have been targeted [154–156]. Hodgkin's-associated antigens, such as ferritin and CD30, have also been targeted [157–159]. The most tumor-specific antigens are either antigen receptor idiotypes, or mutated or otherwise structurally altered proteins that are present as a consequence of genetic changes in the tumor cells. The need to develop anti-idiotypic reagents on a patient-by-patient basis has made them impractical either as imaging agents or therapeutic reagents, and the targeting of truly tumor-specific molecules, e.g., fusion proteins, suffers from the fact that they may not be expressed on the cell surface. Such approaches are in their infancy. Recently, it has been recognized that certain lymphomas have cross-reacting idiotypes and it is possible that the need to develop unique reagents may partly be overcome by developing panels of anti-idiotypic mAbs [160].

Most lymphoma-associated antigens selected for targeting in clinical trials are cell surface structures that are not shed; therefore, the formation of circulating complexes and consequent blocking of mAb binding to tumor cells has not been widely studied [136,150]. Circulating carcinoembryonic antigen (CEA) and TAG-72 (a mucin-like glycoprotein) in GI tumors are examples in which targeting was observed in spite of elevated serum levels of the circulating antigen [161,162]. Clinical trials using unlabeled antibody in patients with adult T-cell leukemia/lymphoma (ATLL) have shown that cir-

culating interleukin-2 receptor (IL-2R) levels must be considered in designing dosing strategies, but they do not necessarily preclude successful targeting, since many of the patients responded to therapy in spite of circulating IL-2R [163]. In contrast, Parker et al. [146] reported a high level of circulating idiotype in serum that significantly impeded tumor targeting of B-cell lymphoma. Therefore, it appears that circulating antigen may have an effect on antibody biodistribution, but that this effect is variable depending on the particular tumor and host. It is possible that, at the levels of antibody used in most studies, circulating antigen may not impede binding to tumor.

Antigenic modulation is the process by which antigens on the cell surface undergo redistribution in the presence of antibody [137,164,165]. As a result, there is disappearance of the antigen from the cell surface. In the case of antigens such as CD5, this occurs very quickly, resulting in internalization of the antigen–antibody complex [137, 164]. While some antigens modulate quickly, others show very low or undetectable modulation. This has significant implications for imaging and therapy, since an internalized antibody undergoes metabolism, and the fate of the radiolabel is then largely dependent on the properties of the radionuclide rather than the antibody [166–168]. In the case of repeated dosing, it is important to understand the timing of modulation, since binding of the radiolabeled mAb depends on the presence of the antigen on the cell surface.

RADIOLABELING

The major criteria for selecting a radionuclide for labeling antibodies used for imaging are: (1) acceptable physical properties; (2) the required labeling procedure should preserve the immunoreactivity of the antibody; and (3) the radionuclide should be firmly bound chemically to the antibody.

The physical properties that are desirable for use for imaging include: (1) γ-ray energy near the optimal range for existing instrumentation (140 keV); (2) a lack of particulate emission (α or β); and (3) a half-life adequate to trace the process of interest. Other desirable characteristics are: (1) ease and stability of labeling; and (2) advantageous result from metabolism such that the radionuclide remains in the tumor and yet clears from normal tissues. A variety of methods have been used to radiolabel antibodies for tumor imaging [169–171]. Two general methods include direct labeling with iodine [169] and ^{99m}Tc [172], and indirect labeling methods using chelating agents that bind radiometals such as ^{111}In or ^{99m}Tc [173,174].

Most iodinated antibodies used in clinical trials have been labeled using the Chloramine T [175] and iodogen methods [176], although other methods, such as the Bolton–Hunter reagent, which conjugates a preiodinated molecule, have also been used [169]. Because of problems frequently encountered with dehalogenation and release of radionuclide from the tumor site, other iodination methods, which are thought to produce a more stable chemical bond, are being considered [177–180].

[131]I has been the most frequently used radionuclide for imaging and therapy because of its ready availability, the existence of well-established and simple labeling procedures (Chloramine T and Iodogen) and low cost. However, [131]I γ-emission energy (364 keV) is not ideally suited to current instrumentation, since it requires high-energy collimators and is inefficiently detected by the γ-camera, resulting in poorer count rates and lower resolution than with other isotopes. In addition, ^{131}I has β-emissions that cannot be imaged but produce a significant, undesirable, radiation dose to patients.

[123]I is another isotope of iodine with a γ-emission (159 keV) that is very close to the ideal range. Its half-life, although short (13.3 hours), may be adequate for imaging when the chosen antibody localizes early (<48 hours) to tumor, or when used with fragments of antibody. Potential disadvantages are that ^{123}I is produced in a cyclotron, is more expensive than ^{131}I and must be used shortly after production.

As an alternative to radioiodination, the conjugation of chelates to antibodies and labeling with radiometals has potential advantages [174]. Most methods involve conjugating a modified diethylene-triamine penta-acetic acid (DTPA) molecule (bifunctional chelate) to the lysine residues within antibodies and the incorporation of ^{111}In or other radiolabels. In the initial methods, either DTPA mixed anhydride [181] or cyclic anhydride–DTPA [182] were used and, although successful in clinical trials, many of the first-generation chelates were somewhat unstable and imaging was consequently hampered by high accumulation of free tracer in the normal liver and bone marrow. In addition, these chelates showed unstable binding of ^{90}Y, an isotope useful in treatment. In an attempt to decrease the accumulation of tracer in the liver, several newer chelates have been synthesized and appear promising in preclinical evaluation [173,174].

[111]In is a cyclotron-produced radiometal that has been used extensively for radiolabeling cells and antibodies. Its γ-ray emissions, although somewhat higher than the ideal, are superior to those of ^{131}I and can be detected efficiently by existing instrumentation. The high abundance of its emissions and its 67.4-hour physical half-life are well-suited for diagnostic imaging with currently available antibodies.

^{99m}Tc has an ideal energy emission (140 keV) for imaging, and is commercially available from a ^{99m}Mo generator. Nevertheless, its short half-life (6 hours) is a significant disadvantage for labeling intact immunoglobulins (Igs), since most antibody–tumor systems require >24 hours for optimal targeting with intact IgG. Nevertheless, its use with fragments appears promising. The direct methods for labeling with ^{99m}Tc have demonstrated improved stability in imaging of nonhematologic solid tumors [183] but await evaluation in lymphoma.

One of the main goals of radiolabeled mAb imaging studies is to determine the kinetics and to optimize the delivery of antibody to tumor so that therapeutic trials may be undertaken. For this reason, investigators have pursued the concept of a 'matched pair' of radionuclides, where one radionuclide with good characteristics for imaging would be utilized for diagnostic and pharmacokinetic analysis, and a second radionuclide with similar chemistry would then be substituted for therapeutic purposes. Although not a 'matched pair' in this sense, some success has been achieved by using ^{131}I at low doses in diagnostic studies (or ^{123}I could be used) and the same isotope at high doses for therapy [139]. Other matched pairs are ^{111}In and ^{90}Y [184], and ^{99m}Tc and ^{186}Re or ^{188}Re [185].

The number of reported studies in lymphomas in which only imaging with radiolabeled antibodies was attempted is very limited. Most imaging studies have been performed as a component of therapeutic trials, which required imaging for dosimetry purposes. Even so, very few trials with very small patient numbers have been conducted, and most have been phase I studies in which only feasibility and toxicity have been explored (Table 25.1).

B-CELL LYMPHOMAS

MB-1

Two groups have reported their experience with ^{131}I-labeled MB-1 as part of radioimmunotherapy trials of B-cell lymphoma [139,186–188]. MB-1 is a murine IgG1 mAb directed against CD37. This antigen is present on virtually all human B-cells and 90% of human B-cell lymphomas, and in low concentrations in other hematopoietic elements including granulocytes and T-cells [151]. In a dose-escalation trial, Press et al. reported that 10 mg/kg of mAb resulted in optimum targeting, defined as that resulting in the best tumor-to-normal-tissue dosimetry [139]. Of the six patients studied, the tumor could be

Table 25.1 Imaging of leukemias and lymphomas with monoclonal antibodies

mAb	Disease	Antigen	Number of patients	Isotope	Dose (mg)	Dose (mCi)	Reference
MB-1	B-cell lymphoma	CD37	10	^{131}I	0.5/m^2–10/m^2	5–10 DX 232–608 RX	139
MB-1	B-cell lymphoma	CD37	12	^{131}I	40–200	3–7 DX 25–161 RX	188
LYM-1	B-cell lymphoma	Anti-HLA-DR	1	^{131}I	5–6	5 DX 20–63 RX	191
LYM-1	B-cell lymphoma and CLL	Anti-HLA-DR	5	^{131}I	1–8	2.3–11 DX 17–60 Q 2–6 wks RX 37–324 RX	140
LYM-1	B-cell lymphoma	Anti-HLA-DR	18	^{123}I ^{131}I	0.05–0.5	2–6 DX 30–60 Q 2–6 wks RX	190
B1	B-cell lymphoma	Anti-HLA-DR	5	^{67}Cu	5–20 pre-dose 3–31	0.06–3.5 DX and RX	192
B1	B-cell lymphoma	CD20	6	^{131}I	0, 135, 685 pre-dose 15	34–66 RX	193
OKB7	B-cell lymphoma	CD21	18	^{131}I	0.1, 0.5, 1, 5, 15, 40	2 DX	197
LL2	B-cell lymphoma	Undefined	16	^{131}I	0.2–3.9	<10 DX 18.0–58.2 RX	147
Anti-Id	B-cell lymphoma	Anti-Id (IgMk)	1	^{111}In	50–600	0.5 and 2 (^{111}In) DX 10 (^{90}Y) RX	146
T101	CTCL Sézary (1)	CD5	6	^{131}I	10 or 8–16	5–13 DX 98–145 RX	142
T101	CLL	CD5	4	^{131}I	10	5 DX 25–50 RX	210
T101	CTCL	CD5	11	^{111}In	1, 10, 50	5 DX	136

CLL, Chronic lymphocytic leukemia; CTCL, cutaneous T-cell lymphoma; DX, diagnostic study; RX, therapeutic study.

localized with MB-1 in four. Similar imaging results could be obtained with lower antibody mass in 11 of 12 patients [188].

Lym-1

Imaging and biodistribution studies using iodinated Lym-1 prior to radioimmunotherapy have been performed by DeNardo et al. [140,189–192]. Lym-1 is a murine IgG2a that reacts with polymorphic variants of HLA-DR, which are expressed in 40% of B-cell chronic lymphocytic leukemia (CLL), a large number of B-cell malignancies and a small subset of normal B-lymphocytes [152]. In most imaging studies, ^{123}I or ^{131}I has been used as a prelude to therapeutic administrations [140,189–192]. While imaging results appeared quite successful for targeting known sites of disease, the exact sensitivity for tumor detection was not reported. Biodistribution studies have demonstrated a dose–response curve with more favorable localization with doses of 5–50 mg than with lower doses.

CD20

Kaminski et al. have reported their experience with B1 mAb [193]. B1 is an IgG2a that recognizes CD20, an antigen that is present on both normal B-cells as well as on various B-cell malignancies [194]. Previous immunotherapy studies with another anti-CD20 mAb have been reported [195]. Dose-escalation studies have been performed [193] but enhancement of tumor localization with increasing antibody doses was variable. In a separate trial 25 of 26 patients receiving ^{131}I B1 also had localized tumor [196].

OKB7

Scheinberg et al. evaluated the use of ^{131}I OKB7 murine mAb in patients with non-Hodgkin's B-cell lymphoma [197,198]. OKB7 is an IgG2b reactive with CD21 (Epstein–Barr virus receptor, CR2) [199]. This antigen is restricted to a subset of peripheral blood B-lymphocyte, lymph node and spleen follicular B-cells, and it is also present on most NHL and CLLs. In an imaging trial with ^{131}I OKB7, localization was seen in seven out of 13

8. Testa U, Petrini M, Quarnata MT, et al. Iron up-modulates the expression of transferrin receptors during monocyte–macrophage maturation. *J. Biol. Chem.* 1989, **264**: 13181-13187.

9. Testa U, Petrini M, Quaranta MT, Pelosi E, Kuhn L, Peschle C. Differential regulation of iron-responsive element-binding protein in activated lymphocytes versus monocytes–macrophages. In Albertini A, Lenfant CL, Mannucci PM, et al. (eds) *Biotechnology of Plasma Proteins*. Current Studies in Hematology and Blood Transfusion, 58th edn. Basel: Karger, 1991, pp. 158–163.

10. London L, Perussia B, Trinchieri G. Induction of proliferation *in vitro* of resting human natural killer cells: Expression of surface activation antigens. *J. Immunol.* 1985, **134**: 718–727.

10a. Yokoyama WM. Natural killer cell receptors specific for major histocompatibility complex class I molecules. *Proc. Natl Acad. Sci. USA* 1995, **92**: 3081–3085.

10b. Matyus L, Bene L, Heiligen H, et al. Distinct association of transferrin receptor with HLA class I molecules on HUT-102B and JY cells. *Immunol. Lett.* 1995, **44**: 203–208.

11. Habeshaw, JA, Lister TA, Stansfield AG, et al. Correlation of transferrin receptor expression with histological class and outcome in non-Hodgkin lymphoma. *Lancet* 1983, March 5: 498–501.

12. Kvaly S, Langholm R, Kaalhus O, et al. Transferrin receptor and B-lymphoblast antigen – their relationship to DNA synthesis, histology and survival in B-cell lymphomas. *Int. J. Cancer* 1984, **33**: 173–177.

13. Oudemans P, Brutel-de-la-Riviere G, Hart G, et al. Determination of transferrin receptors on frozen sections of malignant B-cell lymphomas by immunofluorescence with a monoclonal antibody. *Cancer* 1986, **58**: 1252–1259.

14. Medeiros L, Picker L, Horning S, et al. Transferrin receptor expression by non-Hodgkin's lymphomas. Correlation with morphologic grade and survival. *Cancer* 1988, **61**: 1844–1851.

15. Esserman L, Takahashi S, Rojas V. An epitope of the transferrin receptor is exposed on the cell surface of high-grade but not low-grade human lymphomas. *Blood* 1989, **74**: 718–729.

16. Petrini M, Pelosi-Testa E, Sposi N, et al. Constitutive expression and abnormal glycosylation of transferin receptor in acute T-cell leukemia. *Cancer Res.* 1989, **49**: 6989–6996.

17. Larrick J, Cresswell P: Transferrin receptors on human B and T lymphoblastoid cell lines. *Biochim. Biophys. Acta.* 1979, **583**: 483–490.

18. Vidal C, Matsushita S, Colamonici O, et al. Human T lymphotropic virus I infection deregulates surface expression of the transferrin receptor. *J. Immunol.* 1988, **141**: 984–988.

19. Kitada S, Hays E: Transferrin-like activity produced by murine malignant T-lymphoma cell lines. *Cancer Res.* 1985, **82**: 3537–3540.

20. Seligman PA, Kovar J, Schleicher RB, Gelfand EW. Transferrin-independent iron uptake supports B lymphocyte growth. *Blood* 1991, **78**: 1526–1531.

21. Fargion S, Fracanzani AL, Cislaghi V, et al. Characteristics of the membrane receptor for human H-ferritin. Albertini A, Lenfant CL, Mannucci PM, et al. (eds) In *Biotechnology of Plasma Proteins*. Current Studies in Hematology and Blood Transfusion, 58th edn. Basel: Karger, 1991, pp. 164–170.

22. Edwards CL, Hayes RL. Tumor scanning with gallium citrate. *J. Nucl. Med.* 1969, **10**: 103–105.

23. Dudley HC, Maddox GE. Deposition of radio gallium (Ga-67) in skeletal tissues. *J. Pharmacol. Exp. Ther.* 1949, **96**: 224–227.

24. Hoffer PB, Bekerman C, Henkin ER (eds). *Gallium-67 Imaging, Part 3, Neoplastic Diseases*. New York, John Wiley & Sons, 1978.

25. Freeman LM, Blaufox MD. Gallium-67 citrate. *Semin. Nucl. Med.* 1978, **3**: 181–270.

26. Halpern S, Hagan P. Gallium-67 citrate imaging in neoplastic and inflammatory disease. In Freeman LM, Weissman HS (eds): *Nuclear Medicine Annual*. New York: Raven Press, 1980, pp. 219–265.

27. Hoffer PB. Status of gallium-67 in tumor detection. *J. Nucl. Med.* 1980, **21**: 394–398.

28. Bekerman C, Hoffer PB, Bitran JD. The role of gallium-67 in the clinical evaluation of cancer. *Semin. Nucl. Med.* 1984, **14**: 296–323.

29. Gunasekera SW, King LJ, Lavender PJ. The behavior of tracer gallium-67 towards serum proteins. *Clin. Chim. Acta.* 1972, **39**: 401–406.

30. Vallabhajosula SR, Harwig JF, Siemsen JK, et al. Radiogallium localization in tumors: Blood binding, transport and the role of transferrin. *J. Nucl. Med.* 1980, **21**: 650–656.

31. Harris AW, Sephton RG. Transferrin promotion of ^{67}Ga and ^{59}Fe uptake by cultured mouse myeloma cells. *Cancer Res.* 1977, **37**: 3634–3638.

32. Sephton RG, Harris AW. Gallium-67 citrate uptake by cultured tumor cells, stimulated by serum transferrin. *J. Natl Cancer Inst.* 1975, **54**: 1263–1266.

33. Larson SM, Rasey JS, Grunbaum Z, et al. Pharmacologic enhancement of ^{67}Ga tumors to blood ratios for EMT-6 sarcoma. *Radiology* 1979, **130**: 241–243.

34. Hoffer PB, Samuel A, Bushberg JT, et al. Effect of desferoxamine on tissue and tumor retention of Ga-67: Concise communication. *J. Nucl. Med.* 1979, **20**: 248–251.

35. Hoffer PB, Huberty J, Khayam-Bashi H. The association of Ga-67 and lactoferrin. *J. Nucl. Med.* 1977, **18**: 713–717.

36. Clausen J, Edeling C-J, Fogh J. [67]Ga Binding to human serum proteins and tumor components. *Cancer Res.* 1974, **34**: 1931–1937.

37. Hegge FN, Mahler DJ, Larson SM. The incorporation of Ga-67 into the ferritin fraction of rabbit hepatocytes *in vivo*. *J. Nucl. Med.* 1977, **18**: 937–939.

38. Hoffer PB. Gallium: Mechanisms. *J. Nucl. Med.* 1980, **21**: 282–284.

39. Sephton RG, Hodgson GS, De Abrew S, et al. Ga-67 and Fe-59 distributions in mice. *J. Nucl. Med.* 1978, **19**: 930–935.

40. Logan KJ, Ng PK, Turner CJ, et al. Comparative pharmacokinetics of ^{67}Ga and ^{59}Fe in humans. *Int. J. Nucl. Med. Biol.* 1981, **8**: 271–276.

41. Aisen P, Listowsky I. Iron transport and storage proteins. *Ann. Rev.* 1980, **49**: 357–393.

42. Crichton RR, Ward RJ. Iron metabolism – new perspectives in view. *Biochemistry* 1992, **31**: 11255–11264.

43. Taetle R. The role of transferrin receptors in hemopoetic cells growth. *Exp. Hematol.* 1990, **18**: 360–365.

44. Cotton FA, Wilkinson G. *Advanced Inorganic Chemistry*, 5th edn. New York: Interscience, 1988, pp. 215–230.

45. Harris WR, Pecoraro VL. Thermodynamic binding constants for gallium transferrin. *Biochemistry* 1983, **22**: 292–299.

46. Weiner RE, Schreiber GJ, Hoffer PB, et al. Compounds which mediate Ga-67 transfer from lactoferrin to ferritin. *J. Nucl. Med.* 1985, **26**: 908–916.

47. Weiner RE. The role of phosphate-containing compounds on the transfer of ^{67}Ga and ^{111}In from transferrin to ferritin. *J. Nucl. Med.* 1989, **30**: 70–79.

48. Baes CF Jr, Mesmer RE. *The Hydrolysis of Cations*. New York: Wiley-Interscience, 1976, pp. 318–319.

49. Neilands JB. Microbial envelope proteins related to iron. *Annu. Rev. Microbiol.* 1982, **36**: 285–309.

50. Tsan MF, Scheffel U, Tzen KY. Factors affecting the binding of Gallium-67 in serum. *Int. J. Nucl. Med. Biol.* 1980, **7**: 270–273.

51. Weiner RE, Spencer RP, Dambro TJ, et al. ^{67}Ga distribution in a man with both a decrease in transferrin and hepatic ^{67}Ga concentration. *J. Nucl. Med.* 1992, **33**: 1701–1703.

52. Larson SM, Rasey JS, Allen DR, et al: Common pathway for tumor cell uptake of gallium-67 and iron-59 via a transferrin receptor. *J. Natl Cancer Inst.* 1980, **64**: 41–53.

53. Larson SM, Rasey JS, Nelson NJ, et al. The kinetics of uptake and macromolecular binding of ^{67}Ga and ^{59}Fe by the EMT-6 sarcoma-like tumor of Balb/c mice. In *Radiopharmaceuticals II: Proceedings of the 2nd International Symposium on Radiopharmaceuticals*. New York: Society of Nuclear Medicine 1979, pp. 277–308.

54. Larson SM, Rasey JS, Allen DR, et al. A transferrin-mediated uptake of gallium-67 by EMT-6 sarcoma. II. Studies *in vivo* (BALB/c mice) (concise communication). *J. Nucl. Med.* 1979, **20**: 843–846.

55. Hayes RL, Nelson B, Swartzendruber DC, et al. Gallium-67 localization in rat and mouse tumors. *Science* 1970, **167**: 289–290.

56. Thesingh CW, Driessen OMJ, Daems WTh, et al. Accumulation and localization of gallium-67 in various types of primary lung carcinoma. *J. Nucl. Med.* 1978, **19**: 28–30.

57. Swartzendruber DC, Nelson B, Hayes RL. Gallium-67 localization in lysomomal-like granules of leukemic and nonleukemic murine tissues. *J. Natl Cancer Inst.* 1971, **46**: 941–952.

58. Brown DH, Byrd BL, Carlton JE, et al. A quantitative study of the subcellular localization of ^{67}Ga. *Cancer Res.* 1976, **36**: 956–963.

59. Berry JP, Escaig F, Poupon MF, et al. Localization of gallium in tumor cells. Electron microscopy, electron probe microanalysis and analytical ion microscopy. *Int. J. Nucl. Med. Biol.* 1983, **10**: 199–204.

60. Manfredi OL, Weiss LR. Gallium-67 citrate in human tumors. *New York State J. Med.* 1978, **78**: 884–887.

61. DeAbrew S. Assays for transferrin and transferrin receptors in tumor and other mouse tissues. *Int. J. Nucl. Med Biol.* 1981, **8**: 217–221.

62. Enns CA, Shindelman JE, Tonik SE, et al. Radioimunochemical measurement of the transferrin receptor in human trophoblast and reticulocyte membranes with a specific antireceptor antibody. *Proc. Natl Acad. Sci.* 1981, **78**: 4222–4225.

63. Sohn M-E, Jones BJ, Whiting JH, et al. Distribution of gallium-67 in normal and hypotransferinemic tumor-bearing mice. *J. Nucl. Med.* 1993, **34**: 2135–2143.

64. Basset P, Quesneau Y, Zwiller J. Iron-induced L1210 cell growth: Evidence of a transferrin-independent iron transport. *Cancer Res.* 1986, **46**: 1644–1647.

65. Kaplan J, Jordan I, Sturrock A. Regulation of the transferrin-independent iron transport system in cultured cells. *J. Biol. Chem.*. 1991, **266**: 2997–3004.

66. Chitambar CR, Zivkovic Z. Uptake of gallium-67 by human leukemic cells: Demonstration of transferrin receptor-dependent and transferrin-independent mechanisms. *Cancer Res.* 1987, **47**: 3929–3934.

67. Chan SM, Hoffer PB, Maric N, et al. Inhibition of gallium-67 uptake in melanoma by an anti-human transferrin receptor monoclonal antibody. *J. Nucl. Med.* 1987, **28**: 1303–1307.

68. Iosilevsky G, Front D, Betman L, et al. Uptake of gallium-67 citrate and (2 H-3) deoxyglucose in the tumor model following chemotherapy and radiotherapy. *J. Nucl. Med.* 1985, **26**: 278–282.

69. Higashi T, Kobayashi M, Wakao H, et al. The relationship between Ga-67 accumulation and ATP metabolism in tumor cells *in vitro*. *Eur. J. Nucl. Med.* 1989, **15**: 152–156.

70. Kubota K, Ishiwata K, Kubota R, et al. Tracer feasibility for monitoring tumor radiotherapy: A quadruple tracer study with fluorine-18-fluorodeoxyglucose or fluorine-18-fluorodeoxyuridine, L-[methyl-^{14}C]methionine, [6-^{3}H]thymidine, and gallium-67. *J. Nucl. Med.* 1991, **32**: 2118–2123.

71. Higashi T, Wakao H, Yamaguchi M, et al. The relationship between Ga-67 accumulation and cell cycle in malignant tumor cells *in vitro*. *Eur. J. Nucl. Med.* 1988, **14**: 155–158.

72. Chitambar CR, Matthaeus WG, Antholine WE, et al. Inhibition of leukemic HL60 cell growth by transferrin-gallium: Effects on ribonucleotide reductase and demonstration of drug synergy with hydroxyurea. *Blood* 1988, **72**: 1930–1936.

73. Hedley DW, Tripp EH, Slowiaczek P, et al. Effect of gallium on DNA synthesis by human T-cell lymphoblasts. *Cancer Res.* 1988, **48**: 3014–3018.

74. Waalkes TF, Sanders K, Smith RG, et al. DNA polymerases of Walker 256 carcinoma. *Cancer Res.* 1974, **34**: 385–391.

75. Gupta AD, Shah VI. Correlation of transferrin receptor expression with histologic grade and imunophenotype in chronic lymphocytic leukemia and non-

Hodgkin's lymphoma. *Hemat. Pathol.* 1990, **4**: 37–41.

76. Sciot R, Paterson AC, Van Eyken P, et al. Transferrin receptor expression in human hepatocellular carcinoma: An immunohistochemical study of 34 cases. *Histopathology* 1988, **12**: 53–63.

77. Feremans W, Bujan W, Neve P, et al. CD71 phenotype and the value of gallium imaging in lymphomas. *Am. J. Hematol.* 1991, **36**: 215–216.

78. Tsuchiya Y, Nakao A, Komatsu T, et al. Relationship between gallium 67 citrate scanning and transferrin receptor expression in lung diseases. *Chest* 1992, **102**: 530–534.

79. Higashi T, Watanabe Y, Yamaguchi M, et al. The relationships between the Ga-67 uptake and nuclear DNA feulgen content in thyroid tumors: Concise communication. *J. Nucl. Med.* 1982, **23**: 988–992.

80. Bradley WP, Alderson PO, Eckelman WC, et al. Decreased tumor uptake of Gallium-67 in animals after whole-body irradiation. *J. Nucl. Med.* 1978, **19**: 204–209.

81. Chilton HM, Witcofshi RL, Watson NE, et al. Alteration of gallium-67 distribution in tumor-bearing mice following treatment with methotrexate: Concise communication. *J. Nucl. Med.* 1981, **22**: 1064–1068.

82. Scheffel U, Wagner HN Jr, Klein JL. Gallium-67 uptake by hepatoma: Studies in cell cultures, perfused livers, and intact rats. *J. Nucl. Med.* 1985, **26**: 1438–1444.

83. Sephton RG, Martin JJ. Modification of distribution of gallium-67 in man by administration of iron. *Brit. J. Radiol.* 1980, **53**: 572–575.

84. Hayes RL, Rafter JJ, Byrd BL, et al. Studies of the *in vivo* entry of Ga-67 into normal and malignant tissue. *J. Nucl. Med.* 1981, **22**: 325–332.

85. Chen DC, Scheffel U, Camargo EE, et al. The source of gallium-67 in gastrointestinal contents: Concise communication. *J. Nucl. Med.* 1980, **21**: 1146–1150.

86. Greenlaw RH, Weinstein MB, Brill AB, et al. ^{67}Ga-citrate imaging in untreated malignant lymphoma: Preliminary report of (the) cooperative group. *J. Nucl. Med.* 1974, **15**: 404–407.

87. Johnston GS, Mae FG, Benua RS, et al. Gallium-67 citrate imaging in Hodgkin's disease: Final report of (The) cooperative group. *J. Nucl. Med.* 1977, **18**: 692–698.

88. Longo DL, Schilsky RL, Bleu L, et al. Gallium-67 scanning: Limited usefulness in staging patient with non-Hodgkin's lymphoma. *Am. J. Med.* 1980, **68**: 695–700.

89. McLaughlin AF, Magee MA, Greenough R, et al. Current role of gallium scanning in the management of lymphoma. *Eur J. Nucl. Med.* 1990, **16**: 755–771.

90. McLaughlin AF, Chu J, Howman-Giles R. Whole body gallium scanning in malignant lymphoma – its role in 1980. *Austral. N. Zealand J. Med.* 1981, **11**: 438.

91. Kaplan WD, Anderson KC, Leonard RCF. High dose gallium imaging in the evaluation of lymphoma. *J. Nucl. Med.* 1983, **24**: 50.

92. Anderson KC, Leonard RCF, Cavellos GP. High dose gallium imaging in lymphoma. *Am. J. Med.* 1983, **75**: 327–331.

93. Ultman JE, Jacobs RH. The non-Hodgkin's lymphomas. *CA* 1985, **35**: 66–87.

94. Tumeh SS, Rosenthal DS, Kaplan WD, et al. Lymphoma-evaluation with GA-67 SPECT. *Radiology* 1987, **164**: 111–114.

95. Front D, Israel O, Sapir EE, et al. Ga-67 SPECT before and after treatment of lymphoma. *Radiology* 1990, **175**: 515–519.

96. Kataoka M, Kawamura M, Tsuda T, et al. The role of gallium-67 imaging in non-Hodgkin's lymphoma of the gastrointestinal tract. *Eur. J. Nucl. Med.* 1990, **17**: 142–147.

97. Chammpion PE, Groshar D, Hoper HR, et al. Does gallium uptake in the pulmonary hila predict involvement by non-Hodgkin's lymphoma? *Nucl. Med. Commun.* 1992, **13**: 730–737.

98. Kaplan WD, Jackelson MS, Herman TS, et al. Gallium-67 imaging: A predictor of residual tumor viability and clinical outcome in patients with diffuse large-cell lymphoma. *J. Clin. Oncol.* 1990, **8**: 1966–1970.

99. Israel O, Front D, Epelbaum R, et al. Residual mass and negative gallium scintigraphy in treated lymphoma. *J. Nucl. Med.* 1990, **31**: 365–368.

100. Kaplan WD. Residual mass and negative gallium scintigraphy in treated lymphoma – When is the gallium scan really negative? *J. Nucl. Med.* 1990, **31**: 369–371 (editorial).

101. Front D, Ben-Haim S, Israel O, et al. Lymphoma: predictive value of Ga-67 scintigraphy after treatment. *Radiology* 1992, **182**: 359–363.

102. Front D, Bar-Shalom R, Epelbaum R. Early detection of lymphoma recurrence with gallium-67 scintigraphy. *J. Nucl. Med.* 1993, **34**: 2101–2104.

103. King MA, Weber DA, Casarett GW, et al. A study of irradiated bone. Part II: changes in Tc-99m pyrophosphate bone imaging. *J. Nucl. Med.* 1980, **21**: 22–30.

104. Paul R. Comparison of fluorine-18–2-fluorodeoxy-glucose and gallium-67 citrate imaging for detection of lymphoma. *J. Nucl. Med.* 1987, **28**: 288–292.

105. Okada J, Yoshikawa K, Imazeki K, et al. The use of FDG-PET in the detection and management of malignant lymphoma: Correlation of uptake with prognosis. *J. Nucl. Med.* 1991, **32**: 686–691.

106. Hoekstra OS, Ossenkoppele GJ, Golding R, et al. Early treatment response in malignant lymphoma, as determined by plain fluorine-18-fluorodeoxyglucose scintigraphy. *J. Nucl. Med.* 1993, **34**: 1706–1710.

107. Chiu ML, Kronauge JF, Piwnica-Worms D. Effect of mitochondrial and plasma membrane potentials on accumulation of hexakis (2-methoxyisobutylisonitrile) technetium (I) in cultured mouse fibroblasts. *J. Nucl. Med.* 1990, **31**: 1646–1653.

108. Piwnica-Worms D, Kronauge JF, Chiu ML. Uptake and retention of hexakis [2-methoxy isonitrile] technetium [I] in cultured chick myocardial cells: Mitochondrial and plasma membrane potential dependence. *Circulation* 1990, **82**: 1826–1838.

109. Piwnica-Worms D, Kronauge JF, Chiu ML. Enhance-

ment by tetra-phenylborate of technetium-99m-MIBI uptake kinetics and accumulation in cultured chick myocardial cells. *J. Nucl. Med.* 1991, **32**: 1992–1999.

110. Piwnica-Worms D, Chiu ML, Budding M, et al. Functional imaging of multi-drug resistant P-glyco-protein with an organotechnetium complex. *Cancer Res.* 1993, **53**: 977–984.

111. Delmon-Moigen LI, Piwnica-Worms D, Van der Abbeele AD, et al. Uptake of the cation hexakis (2-methoxy-isobutyl-isonitrile)-technetium-99m by human carcinoma cell lines *in vitro. Cancer Res.* 1990, **50**: 2198–2202.

112. Summerhayes IC, Lampidis TJ, Bernal SD, et al. Unusual retention of rhodamine 123 by muscle and carcinoma cells. *Proc. Natl Acad. Sci. USA* 1982, **79**: 5292–5296.

113. Davis S, Weiss MJ, Wong JR, et al. Mitochondrial and plasma membrane potentials cause unusual ac-cumulation and retention of rhodamine 123 by human breast adenocarcinoma-derived MCF-7 cells. *J. Biol. Chem.* 1985, **260**: 13844–13850.

114. Chen LB. Mitochondrial membrane potential in living cells. *Ann. Rev. Cell Biol.* 1988, **4**: 155–181.

115. Hassan IM, Sahweil A, Constantinides C, et al. Uptake and kinetics of Tc-99m hexakis 2-methoxy isobutyl isonitrile in benign and malignant lesions in the lungs. *Clin. Nucl. Med.* 1989, **14** : 333–340.

116. Caner B, Kitapci M, Aras T, et al. Increased accumula-tion of hexakis (2-methoxyisobutyliso-nitrile) tech-netium (I) in osteosarcoma and its metastatic lymph nodes. *J. Nucl. Med.* 1991, **32**: 1977–1978.

117. Caner B, Kitapci M, Erbengi G, et al. Increased accumulation of Tc-99m MIBI in undifferentiated mesenchymal tumor and its metastatic lung lesions. *Clin. Nucl. Med.* 1992, **17**: 144–145.

118. Caner B, Kitapci M, Unlu M, et al. Technetium-99m-MIBI uptake in benign and malignant bone lesions. a comparative study with technetium-99m-MDP. *J. Nucl. Med.* 1992, **33**: 319–324.

119. Aktolun C, Bayhan H, Kir M. Clinical experience with Tc-99m MIBI imaging in patients with malig-nant tumors. Preliminary results and comparison with T1-201. *Clin. Nucl. Med.* 1992, **17**: 171–176.

120. Campeau RJ, Kronemer KA, Sutherland CM. Con-cordant uptake of Tc-99m sestamibi and T1-201 in unsuspected breast tumor. *Clin. Nucl. Med.* 1992, **17**: 936–937.

121. O'Driscoll CM, Baker F, Casey MJ, et al. Localization of recurrent medullary thyroid carcinoma with tech-netium-99m-methoxyisobutylnitrile scintigraphy: A case report. *J. Nucl. Med.* 1991, **32**: 2281–2283.

122. Medolago G, Virotta G, Piti A, et al. Abnormal uptake of technetium-99m hexakis-2-methoxyisobu-tylisonitrile in a primary cardiac lymphoma. *Eur. J. Nucl. Med.* 1992, **19**: 222–225.

123. Scott AM, Kostakoglu L, O'Brien JP, et al. Com-parison of technetium-99m-MIBI and thallium-201-chloride uptake in primary thyroid lymphoma. *J. Nucl. Med.* 1992, **33**: 1396–1398.

124. Chabner BA, Myers CE. Anti-tumor antibiotics. In DeVita VT, Hellman S, Rosenberg SA (eds) *Cancer – Principles and Practice of Oncology*, 4th edn. Phila-delphia: J.B. Lippincott, 1993, pp. 376–381.

125. Strauss HW, Pitt B. Gated blood pool imaging. In Strauss HW, Pitt B (eds) *Cardiovascular Nuclear Medicine*. St. Louis: C.V. Mosby, 1979, pp. 126–139.

126. Alexander J, Dainiak N, Berger HJ, et al. Serial assessment of doxorubicin cardiotoxicity with quan-titative radionuclide angiocardiography. *N. Engl. J. Med.* 1979, **300**: 278–283.

127. Gottdiener JS, Mathisen DJ, Borer JS, et al. Doxoru-bicin cardiotoxicity: Assessment of late left ventricu-lar dysfunction by radionuclide cineangiography. *Ann. Intern. Med.* 1981, **94**: 430–435.

128. Choi BW, Berger HJ, Schwartz PE, et al. Serial radionuclide assessment of doxorubicin cardiotoxicity in cancer patients with abnormal baseline resting left ventricular performance. *Am. Heart J.* 1983, **106**: 638–643.

129. McKillop JH, Bristow MR, Goris ML, et al. Sensitivity and specificity of radionuclide ejection fractions in doxorubicin cardiotoxicity. *Am. Heart J.* 1983, **106**: 1048–1056.

130. Burns RJ, Bar-Shlomo BZ, Druck MN, et al. Detec-tion of radiation cardiomyopathy by gated radio-nuclide angiography. *Am. J. Med.* 1983, **74**: 297–302.

131. Von Hoff DD, Layard M, Basa P. Risk factors for doxorubicin induced congestive heart disease. *Ann. Intern. Med.* 1979, **91**: 701–717.

132. Billingham ME, Bristow MR, Glatstein E, et al. Adriamycin cardiotoxicity: Endomyocardial biopsy evidence of enhancement by irradiation. *Am. J. Surg. Pathol.* 1977, **1**: 17–23.

133. Das SK, Brady TJ, Thrall JH, et al. Cardiac function in patients with prior myocarditis. *J. Nucl. Med.* 1980, **21**: 689–693.

134. Miller RA, Maloney DG, Warnke R, et al. Treatment of B-cell lymphoma with monoclonal anti-idiotype antibody. *N. Engl. J. Med.* 1982, **306**: 517–519.

135. Bunn PA, Carrasquillo JA, Keenan AM, et al. Successful imaging of malignant non-Hodgkin's lymphoma using radiolabeled monoclonal antibody. *Lancet* 1984, **ii** :1219–1221.

136. Carrasquillo JA, Bunn PA, Keenan AM, et al. Radioimmuno-detection of cutaneous T-cell lym-phoma with In-111 T101 monoclonal antibody. *N. Engl. J. Med.* 1986, **315**: 673–680.

137. Shawler DL, Miceli MC, Wormsley SB, et al. Induction of *in vivo* and *in vitro* antigenic modulation by the anti-human T-cell monoclonal antibody T101. *Cancer Res.* 1984, **44**: 5921–5927.

138. Carrasquillo JA, Mulshine IL, Bunn PA, et al. Tumor imaging of indium-111 T101 monoclonal antibody is superior to iodine-131 T101 in cutaneous T-cell lymphoma. *J. Nucl. Med.* 1987, **28**: 281–287.

139. Press OW, Eary JF, Badger CC, et al. Treatment of refractory non-Hodgkin's lymphoma with radiolabeled MB-1 (Anti-CD37) antibody. *J. Clin. Oncol.* 1988, **7**: 1027–1038.

140. DeNardo S, DeNardo C, O'Grady L, et al. Pilot studies of radio-immunotherapy of B-cell lymphoma and leukemia using I-131 Lym-l monoclonal antibody. *Antibody Immunoconj. Radiopharm.* 1988, **1**: 17–33.

141. Zimmer AM, Kaplan EH, Kazikiewiez JM, et al.

Pharmacokinetics of I-131 T101 monoclonal antibodies in patients with chronic lymphocytic leukemia. *Antibody Immunoconj. Radiopharm.* 1988, **1**: 291–302.

142. Rosen S, Zimmer A, Goldman-Leikin R, et al. Radioimmuno-detection and radioimmunotherapy of cutaneous T-cell lymphomas using an I-131-labeled monoclonal antibody: An Illinois Cancer Council study. *J. Clin. Oncol.* 1987, **5**: 562–573.

143. Carde P, Manil L, da Costa L, et al. Hodgkin's disease immunoscintigraphy: Use of the anti Reed–Sternberg cells HRS-I monoclonal antibody in 9 patients. *Proc. Am. Soc. Clin. Oncol.* 1988, **7**: 227.

144. Vriesendorp HM, Herpst JM, Leichner PK, et al. Polyclonal yttrium-90 labeled antiferritin for refractory Hodgkin's disease. *Int. J. Radial. Oncol.* 1989, **17**: 815–821.

145. Lenhard R, Order S, Spunberg J, et al. Isotopic immunoglobulin: A new systemic therapy for advanced Hodgkin's Disease. *J. Clin. Oncol.* 1985, **3**: 1296–1300.

146. Parker BA, Vassos AB, Halpern SE, et al. Radioimmuno-therapy of human B-cell lymphoma with Y-90 conjugated anti-idiotype monoclonal antibody. *Cancer Res.* 1990, **50**: 1022s–1028s.

147. Goldenberg DM, Horowitz JA, Sharkey RM, et al. Targeting, dosimetry, and radioimmunotherapy of B-cell lymphomas with iodine-131-labeled LL2 monoclonal antibody. *J. Clin. Oncol.* 1991, **9**: 548–564.

148. Herlyn L, Menrad A, Koprowski H. Structure, function, and clinical significance of human tumor antigens. *J. Natl Cancer Inst.* 1990, **82**: 1183–1188.

149. Knapp W, Dorken B, Rieber P, et al. (eds). *Leukocyte Typing IV*. Oxford: Oxford University Press, 1989.

150. Nadler LM, Stashenko P, Hardy R, et al. Serotherapy of a patient with a monoclonal antibody directed against a human lymphoma-associated antigen. *Cancer Res.* 1980, **40**: 3147–3154.

151. Link M, Bindl L, Meeker T, et al. A unique antigen on mature B cells defined by a monoclonal antibody. *J. Immunol.* 1986, **137**: 3013–3018.

152. Epstein AL, Marder RJ, Winter JN, et al. Two new monoclonal antibodies, Lym-l and Lym-2, reactive with human-B-lymphocytes and derived tumors, with immunodiagnostic and immunotherapeutic potential. *Cancer Res.* 1987, **47**: 830–840.

153. Pawlak-Byczkowska EJ, Hansen HJ, Dion AS, et al. Two new monoclonal antibodies, EPB-1 and EPB-2, reactive with human lymphoma. *Cancer Res.* 1989, **49**: 4568–4577.

154. Royston I, Majda JA, Baird SM, et al. Human T-cell antigens defined by monoclonal antibodies: The 65,000 dalton antigen off T-cells (T65) is also found on chronic lymphocytic leukemia cells bearing surface immunoglobulin. *J. Immunol.* 1980, **57**: 553–564.

155. Robb RJ, Greene WC, Rusk CM. Low and high affinity cellular receptors for interleukin 2, implications for the level of Tac antigen. *J. Exp. Med.* 1984, **160**: 1126–1146.

156. Ledbetter JA, Frankel AE, Herzenberg LA, et al. Human Leu T-cell differentiation antigen: Quantitative expression on normal lymphoid cells and cell lines. In Hammerling GJ, Hammerling U, Kearney JG (eds) *Research Monographs in Immunology*, Vol. 3, *Monoclonal Antibody and T-Cell Hybridoma*. New York: Elsevier/North-Holland Biomedical Press, 1981, pp. 16–22.

157. Pfreudshuh M, Mommertz E, Meissner M, et al. Hodgkin and Reed–Sternberg cell associated monoclonal antibodies HRS-I and HRS-2 react with activated cells of lymphoid and monocytoid origin. *Cancer Res.* 1988, **8**: 217–224.

158. Josimovic-Alasevic O, Durkop H, Schwarting R, et al. Ki-1(CD30) antigen is released by Ki-1-positive tumor cells *in vitro* and *in vivo*. I. Partial characterization of soluble Ki-1 antigen and detection of the antigen in cell culture supernatants and in serum by an enzyme-linked immunosorbent assay. *Eur. J. Immunol.* 1989, **19**: 157–162.

159. Order SE, Porter M, Hellman S. Hodgkin's disease: Evidence for a tumor-associated antigen. *N. Engl. J. Med.* 1971, **285**: 471–474.

160. Rudders RA, Levin A, Jespersen D, et al. Crossreacting human lymphoma idiotypes. *Blood* 1992, **80**: 1039–1044.

161. Carrasquillo JC. Radioimmunoscintigraphy with polyclonal or monoclonal antibodies. In Zalutsky M (ed.) *Antibodies in Radiodiagnosis and Therapy*. Boca Raton, FL: CRC Press, 1989, p. 169.

162. Carrasquillo JA, Sugarbaker P, Colcher D, et al. Radioimmunoscintigraphy of colon cancer with I-131 B72.3 monoclonal antibody. *J. Nucl. Med.* 1988, **29**: 1022–1030.

163. Waldmann TA, Goldman CK, Bongiovanni KF, et al. Therapy of patients with human T-cell lymphotrophic virus-I-induced adult T-cell leukemia with anti-Tac, a monoclonal antibody to the receptor for interleukin 2. *Blood* 1988, **72**: 1805–1816.

164. Schroff RW, Farrell MM, Klein RA, et al. T65 antigen modulation in a phase 1 monoclonal antibody trial with chronic lymphocytic leukemia patients. *J. Immunol.* 1988, **133**: 1641–1648.

165. Wang BS, Kelley KA, Lumanglas AL, et al. Internalization and shedding of Lym-1 monoclonal antibody following interaction with surface antigens of a cultured human B-cell lymphoma. *Cell Immunol.* 1989, **123**: 283–293.

166. Naruki Y, Carrasquillo JA, Reynolds JC, et al. Differential cellular metabolism of In-111, Y-90 and I-125 radiolabeled T101, anti-CD5, monoclonal antibody. *Nucl. Med. Biol.* 1990, **17**: 201–207.

167. Press OW, Farr AG, Borroz I, et al. Endocytosis and degradation of monoclonal antibodies targeting human B-cell malignancies. *Cancer Res.* 1989, **49**: 4906–4912.

168. Press OW, Hansen JA, Farr A, et al. Endocytosis and degradation of murine anti-human CD3 monoclonal antibodies by normal and malignant T-lymphocytes. *Cancer Res.* 1989, **48**: 2249–2257.

169. Eary JF, Krohn KA, Kishore R, et al. Radiochemistry of halogenated antibodies. In Zalutsky M (ed.) *Antibodies in Radiodiagnosis and Therapy*. Boca Raton, FL: CRC Press, 1989, pp. 84–102.

170. Srivastava SC, Mease RC. Progress in research on ligands, nuclides and techniques for labeling monoclonal antibodies. *Nucl. Med. Biol.* 1991, **18**: 589–603.

171. Eckelman WC, Paik CH. Labeling antibodies with metals using bifunctional chelates. In Zalutsky M (ed.) *Antibodies in Radiodiagnosis and Therapy.* Boca Raton, FL: CRC Press, 1989, pp. 103–128.

172. Rhodes BA, Zamora PA, Newell KD, et al. Tc-99m labeling of murine monoclonal antibody fragments. *J. Nucl. Med.* 1986, **27**: 685–693.

173. Meares CF, Moi MK, Diril H, et al. Macrocyclic chelates of radiometals for diagnosis and therapy. *Br. J. Cancer* 1990, **62** (Suppl.): 21–26.

174. Gansow OA. Newer approaches to the radiolabeling of monoclonal antibodies by use of metal chelates. *Nucl. Med. Biol.* 1991, **18**: 369–381.

175. McCnonahey PH, Dixon FJ. A method of trace iodination of proteins for immunologic studies. *Int. Arch. Allergy Appl. Immunol.* 1966, **29**: 185–189.

176. Fraker PJ, Speck JC. Protein and cell membrane iodination with a sparingly soluble chloramide, 1,3,4,6-tetrachloro-3a,6a-diphenylglycouril. *Biochem. Biophys. Res. Commun.* 1978, **80**: 849–857.

177. Wilbur DS, Hadley SW, Hylarides MD, et al. Development of a stable radioiodinating reagent to label monoclonal antibodies for radiotherapy of cancer. *J. Nucl. Med.* 1989, **30**: 216–226.

178. Garg PK, Slade SK, Harrison CL, et al. Labeling proteins using aryl iodide acylation agents: Influence of meta vs para substitution on *in vivo* stability. *Nucl. Med. Biol.* 1989, **16**: 669–673.

179. Pittman RC, Carew TE, Glass CK, et al. A radioiodinated, intracellularly trapped ligand for determining the sites of plasma protein degradation *in vivo*. *Biochem. J.* 1983, **212**: 791–800.

180. Ali SA, Warren SD, Richter KY, et al. Improving the tumor retention of radioiodinated antibody: Aryl carbohydrate adducts. *Cancer Res.* (Suppl.) 1990, **50**: 783s–788s.

181. Krejcarek GE, Tucker Kl. Covalent attachment of chelating groups to macromolecules. *Biochem. Biophys. Res. Commun.* 1977, **77**: 581–585.

182. Hnatowich DJ, Childs RL, Lanteigne D, et al. The preparation of DTPA-coupled antibodies radiolabeled with metallic radionuclides: An improved method. *J. Immunol. Meth.* 1983, **65**: 147–157.

183. Schwarz A, Steinstrabber A. A novel approach to Tc-99m labeled monoclonal antibodies. *J. Nucl. Med.* 1987, **28**: 721 (Abstract).

184. Carrasquillo JA, Kramer B, Fleisher T, et al. In-111 versus Y-90 T101 biodistribution in patients with hematopoietic malignancies. *J. Nucl. Med.* 1991, **32**: 970 (Abstract).

185. Eary JF, Durack L, Williams D, et al. Considerations for imaging Re-188 and Re-186 isotopes. *Clin. Nucl. Med.* 1990, **15**: 911–916.

186. Bernstein ID, Eary JF, Badger CC, et al. High dose radiolabeled antibody therapy of lymphoma. *J. Natl Cancer Inst.* 1989, **82**: 47–50.

187. Eary JF, Press OW, Badger CC, et al. Imaging and treatment of B-cell lymphoma. *J. Nucl. Med.* 1990, **31**: 1257–1268.

188. Kaminski MS, Fig L, Zasadny KR, et al. Imaging, dosimetry and radioimmunotherapy with iodine-131 labeled Anti-CD37 antibody in B-cell lymphoma. *J. Clin. Oncol.* 1992, **10**: 1696–1711.

189. DeNardo S, DeNardo G, O'Grady L, et al. Treatment of B-cell malignancies with I-131 Lym-l monoclonal antibodies. *Int. J. Cancer* 1988, **3**: 96–101.

190. DeNardo GL, DeNardo SL, Meares CF, et al. Pharmacokinetics of copper-67 conjugated Lym-1, a potential therapeutic radioimmunoconjugate, in mice and in patients with lymphoma. *Antibody Immunoconj. Radiopharm.* 1991, **4**: 777–785.

191. DeNardo SJ, DeNardo GL, O'Grady LF, et al. Treatment of a patient with B-cell lymphoma by I-131 LYM-1 monoclonal antibodies. *Int. J. Biol. Markers* 1987, **2**: 49–53.

192. DeNardo GL, DeNardo SJ, O'Grady LF, et al. Fractionated radioimmunotherapy of B-cell malignancies with 131-I-Lym-1. *Cancer Res.* 1990, **50** (Suppl.): 1014s–1016s.

193. Kaminski MS, Zasadny KR, Francis IR, et al. Radioimmunotherapy of B-cell lymphoma with 131-I-Anti-B1 (Anti-CD20) antibody. *N. Engl. J. Med.* 1993, **329**: 459–465.

194. Nadler LM, Ritz J, Hardy R, et al. A unique cell surface antigen identifying lymphoid malignancies of B-cell origin. *J. Clin. Invest.* 1981, **67**: 134–140.

195. Press O, Appelbaum F, Ledbetter J, et al. Monoclonal antibody 1F5 (anti-CD-20) serotherapy of human B-cell lymphomas. *Blood* 1987, **69**: 584–591.

196. Press OW, Eary JF, Appelbaum FR, et al. Radiolabeled-antibody therapy of B-cell lymphoma with autologous bone marrow support. *N. Engl. J. Med.* 1993, **329**: 1219–1224.

197. Scheinberg DA, Straus DJ, Yeh SD, et al. A phase I toxicity, pharmacology, and dosimetry trial of monoclonal antibody OKB7 in patients with non-Hodgkin's lymphoma: Effects of tumor burden and antigen expression. *J. Clin. Oncol.* 1990, **8**: 792–803.

198. Czuczman MS, Straus DJ, Divgi CR, et al. Phase I dose escalation trial of 131-I-labeled monoclonal antibody OKB7 in patients with non-Hodgkin's lymphoma. *J. Clin. Oncol.* 1993, **11**: 2021–2029.

199. Knowles DM II, Tolidijian B, Marboe CC, et al. Distribution of antigens defined by OKB monoclonal antibodies on benign and malignant lymphoid cells and on non-lymphoid tissues. *Blood* 1984, **63**: 886–896.

200. Baum RP, Niesen A, Hertel A, et al. Initial clinical results with Tc-99m labeled monoclonal antibody fragment LL2 for radioimmuno-detection of B-cell lymphomas. *Antibody Immunoconj. Radiopharm.* 1992, **5**: 334 (Abstract).

201. Blend MJ, Seevers RH, Kozloff M, et al. Radioimmunodetection in patients with non-Hodgkin's lymphoma using monoclonal antibody IMMU-LL2. *Antibody Immunoconj. and Radiopharm.* 1992, **5**: 333 (Abstract).

202. Meeker TC, Lowder J, Maloney DG, et al. A clinical trial of anti-idiotype therapy for B-cell malignancy. *Blood* 1985, **65**: 1349–1363.

203. Meeker T, Lowder J, Cleary ML, et al. Emergence of idiotype variants during treatment of B-cell lymphoma with anti-idiotype antibodies. *N. Engl. J. Med.* 1985, **312**: 1658–1665.

203a. Larsen SM, Carrasquillo JA, Reynolds JC, Hellstrom I, Hellstrom KE, Mulshine JL, Mattis LE. Therapeutic applications of radiolabelled antibodies: Current situation and prospects. *Nucl. Med. Biol., Int. J. Radiat. Appl. Instrum. Part B*, 1986, **13**: No. 2, 207–213.

204. Dillman RO, Beuaregard JC, Shawler DL, et al. Continuous infusion of T101 monoclonal antibody in chronic lymphocytic leukemia and cutaneous T-cell lymphoma. *J. Biol. Resp. Mod.* 1986, **5**: 394–410.

205. Jones PL, Brown BA, Sands H. Uptake and metabolism of 111-In-labeled monoclonal antibody B6.2 by the rat liver. *Cancer Res.* 1990, **50** (Suppl.): 852s–856s.

206. Miller RA, Maloney D, Warnke R, et al. Considerations for treatment with hybridoma antibodies. In Mitchell MS, Oettgen HFF (eds) *Hybridomas in Cancer Diagnosis and Treatment*. New York: Raven Press, 1982, pp. 133–147.

207. Dillman RO, Sobol RE, Collins H, et al. T101 monoclonal antibody therapy in chronic lymphocytic leukemia. In Mitchell MS, Oettgen HFF (eds) *Hybridomas in Cancer Diagnosis and Treatment*. New York:, Raven Press, 1982, pp. 151–171.

208. Bunn PA Jr, Edelson R, Ford SS, et al. Patterns of cell proliferation and cell migration in the Sezary syndrome. *Blood* 1981, **57**: 452–463.

209. Miller RA, Coleman CN, Fawcett HD, et al. Sezary syndrome: A model for migration of T lymphocytes to skin. *N. Engl. J. Med.* 1980, **303**: 89–92.

210. Zimmer AM, Rosen ST, Spies SM, et al. Radioimmunotherapy of patients with cutaneous T-cell lymphoma using an iodine-131-labeled monoclonal antibody: Analysis of retreatment following plasmapheresis. *J. Nucl. Med.* 1988, **29**: 174–180.

211. Rosen ST, Zimmer AM, Goldman-Leikin R, et al. Progress in the treatment of cutaneous T-cell lymphomas with radiolabeled monoclonal antibodies. *Nucl. Med. Biol.* 1989, **16**: 667–668.

212. Carrasquillo JA, Foon KA, Mulshine JM, et al.

Radioimmunoscintigraphy of chronic lymphocytic leukemia (CLL) with monoclonal antibodies. *J. Nucl. Med.* 1987, **28**: 602–603 (Abstract).

213. Weinstein JN, Parker RJ, Keenan AM, et al. Monoclonal antibodies in the lymphatics: Toward the diagnosis and therapy of tumor metastases. *Science* 1982, **218**: 1334–1337.

214. Keenan AM, Weinstein JN, Mulshine IL, et al. Immunolymphoscintigraphy in patients with lymphoma after subcutaneous injection of indium labeled T101 monoclonal antibody. *J. Nucl. Med.* 1987, **28**: 4246.

215. Keenan AM, Weinstein JN, Carrasquillo JA, et al. Immunolymphoscintigraphy and the dose dependence of indium labeled T101 monoclonal antibody in patients with cutaneous T-cell lymphoma. *Cancer Res.* 1987, **47**: 6093–6099.

216. Order S, Bloomer W, Jones A, et al. Radionuclide immunoglobulin lymphangiography. A case report. *Cancer* 1975, **35**: 1487–1492.

217. Mulshine JL, Carrasquillo JA, Weinstein JM, et al. Direct intralymphatic injection of radiolabeled In-111 T101 in patients with cutaneous T-cell lymphoma. *Cancer Res.* 1991, **51**: 688–695.

218. Dillman RO, Beauregard JC, Halpern SE, et al. Toxicities and side effects associated with intravenous infusions of murine monoclonal antibodies. *J. Biol. Response Modifiers* 1986, **5**: 73–84.

219. Reynolds JC, Del Vecchio S, Sakahara H, et al. Antimurine antibody response to mouse monoclonal antibodies: Clinical findings and implications. *Nucl. Med. Biol.* 1989, **16**: 121–125.

220. Dillman RO. Human antimouse and antiglobulin responses to monoclonal antibodies. *Antibody Immunoconj. Radiopharm.* 1990, **3**: 1–15.

221. Winter G, Milstein C. Man-made antibodies. *Nature* 1991, **349**: 293–299.

CHAPTER 26

Other imaging techniques in non-Hodgkin's lymphomas

JEAN-NOËL BRUNETON, PIERRE-YVES MARCY, BERNARD PADOVANI
AND MICHEL-YVES MOUROU

Introduction

The frequent involvement of a broad range of extranodal sites in the non-Hodgkin's lymphomas necessitates a correspondingly broad range of imaging studies, if the extent of disease at the time of diagnosis and the response to treatment are to be accurately assessed [1,2]. The purposes of pretreatment imaging are two-fold:

1. To determine whether disease is localized or widespread, and to estimate tumor bulk. This information has important implications for therapy and prognosis, and is essential for meaningful evaluation of the results of clinical trials.
2. To provide a baseline against which treatment response (or lack of response) can be measured. This information is essential to the overall management of the patient, including the choice of salvage therapy, should there be disease progression or recurrence at some point.

While the mainstay of imaging studies in the 1980s was computed tomographic (CT) scanning of the chest and abdomen [3–5], regardless of the age of the patient and histological subtype of the lymphoma, in the 1990s much more account is taken of the type of lymphoma in determining the anatomical regions to be imaged, while technological progress has permitted more accurate determination of the extent of disease. For example, in children, T-cell lymphoblastic lymphomas predominantly involve the chest, and abdominal spread is usually absent or of minor degree, while B-cell tumors nearly always involve the abdomen [6,7]. In adults, primary stomach lymphomas of the mucosa-associated lymphoid tissue (MALT) type tend to remain localized to the stomach, draining lymph nodes or other mucosal sites, but uncommonly spread to more distant sites. Thus, histological information determines, to a considerable extent, the focus of imaging studies. Examples of newer techniques that permit more detailed examination of particular anatomic regions are endosonographic imaging of the stomach and the use of magnetic resonance imaging (MRI) to detect bone marrow involvement, and lesions in the central nervous system that would not be visible by computed tomography (CT) scanning. MRI, which is taking on an increasingly important role in the evaluation of the patient with non-Hodgkin's lymphoma, also has the potential to provide unique information about the nature of residual masses. While these newer techniques on occasion provide invaluable assistance to the clinician, they are expensive and, particularly in the case of repeated surveillance studies posttherapy, have considerably increased the cost of management [8]. Cost effectiveness has, therefore, become an issue of considerable concern.

In this chapter we shall discuss the value of ultrasound (US), CT, MRI, and other imaging techniques for the staging and follow-up of patients with non-Hodgkin's lymphoma (NHL). We shall also address the issue of the evaluation of residual masses, and pay particular attention to the problems that arise in evaluating patients with immunodeficiency-associated lymphomas, particularly human immunodeficiency virus (HIV)-associated lymphomas.

Ultrasonography

NODAL EXAMINATION

Exploration of the abdominal and pelvic regions by ultrasound is often hampered by abdominal gas. The definition of nodal involvement is, thus, based solely on size (diameter over 1.5 cm) but NHL in these regions is frequently bulky [3]. In our experience, detection of superficial adenopathies is improved by the use of high-frequency transducers providing better quantitative analysis and treatment monitoring; subclinical superficial nodal recurrences have also been successfully visualized [9,10]. US is more accurate than CT or MR, which should be reserved for exploration of the deep regions of the trunk [11,12]. Lymphomatous adenopathies tend to be confluent and strongly hypoechoic, sometimes with posterior reinforcement (cyst-like) (Figures 26.1 and 26.2) [13]. Central hypervascularity may be revealed by color Doppler. US is particularly useful for the examination of the abdomen in children (the major site for B-cell lymphomas). Although the combined use of US and CT optimizes results, in many regions of the world, the combined use of US and lymphography can compensate for the absence of an expensive CT unit.

EXTRANODAL EXAMINATION

US can permit visualization of abnormalities in the spleen, liver and kidney [14], organs which are involved in nearly 20% of all NHL patients [15]. Morphologic findings range from a normal appearance, despite subclinical involvement, to homogeneous hypertrophy, hypoechoic multinodular disease, or a solitary tumor mass (which may be a primary lymphoma) [3,14,16,17]. The diagnostic

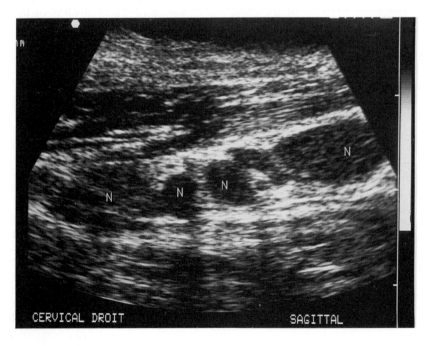

Figure 26.1 Cervical sonogram revealing numerous small hypoechoic nodular masses (N) corresponding to lymphadenopathy caused by NHL.

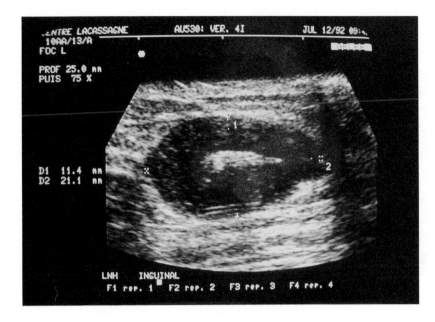

Figure 26.2 Inguinal sonogram visualizing a strongly hypoechoic node with a central echoic hilum (corresponding to vascular structures demonstrated by color Doppler).

value of US is exemplified by its high degree of both sensitivity and specificity – figures of 89% and 95% have been reported by Weiss [17] in a study in which hepatic US was performed in concert with histological examination.

Certain superficial disease sites are excellent indications for US: the thyroid [18], the ocular region [19] and the testis [20]. The appearance under US may even be highly suggestive of the diagnosis, as in testicular lymphoma, where hypoechoic striations may be visualized radiating out from the hypoechoic mediastinum testis (owing to infiltration of the intratesticular lymphatics).

GASTRIC ENDOSONOGRAPHY

Gastric endosonography is a particularly valuable technique because, although gastric lymphoma accounts for less than 5% of all gastrointestinal tract tumors [21], it is the main gastrointestinal site of NHL [3]. Primary gastric NHL is relatively rare compared to the frequency of subclinical secondary gastric involvement, as demonstrated by gastroscopic studies with systematic multiple biopsies of all nongastrointestinal lymphomas, in which Seitz, for example, was able to demonstrate gastric involvement in 21% of cases [22]. Primary B-cell gastric lymphoma is often of MALT origin [23], and complete excision is possible in 63% of cases [21]. The prognosis for patients in all stages is 44% at 10 years [21] but can be as high as 85% at 5 years for stage I disease [24]. The accuracy of endoscopy has improved over recent years; the method currently has a sensitivity of

98% for the diagnosis of malignancy and 64% for definitive diagnosis [25].

Endosonography can readily detect involvement of the second and third layers of the gastric wall, and the presence of mucosal ulcerations [26]. Irregular, hypoechoic thickening of the submucosa with complete destruction of the layers of the stomach wall is a typical finding [27] (Figure 26.3). In addition to this infiltrative form of gastric lymphoma, Palazzo [28] has described two other US patterns: superficial involvement, sometimes with a polypoid or nodular form, and a tumoral mass, which cannot be distinguished from adenocarcinoma using US. The classification of Schüder et al. [27], derived from the TNM classification for gastric cancer, describes the extent of both tumor infiltration (ES T_L 1: confined to the submucosa; ES T_L 2: confined to the muscularis propria or the subserosa; ES T_L 3: through the entire gastric wall; ES T_L 4: involvement of neighboring structures) and the extent of nodal involvement (N_L 0: lymph nodes not involved; N_L 1: nodal involvement). The diagnostic accuracy of endosonography varies from 80% to 95%, depending on the location of the tumor, while the sensitivity for the detection of nodal involvement is between 44% and 100%. Inflammatory nodes are responsible for numerous false-positive errors [26–28]. The major limitation of endosonography is underestimation of the degree of superficial tumoral spread, which occurs in 37.5% of all low-grade lymphomas [28]. Endosonography is, of course, also useful for posttreatment surveillance [26] (Figure 26.4).

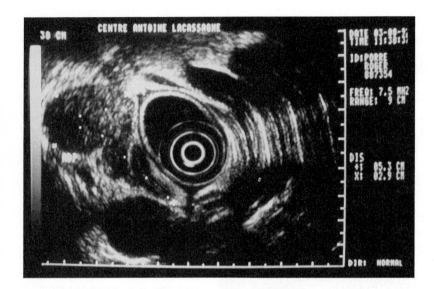

Figure 26.3 Gastric endosonogram showing nodular NHL infiltration of the submucosa.

US-GUIDED BIOPSY

Aspiration biopsy of superficial nodal regions may be performed under US guidance to improve the technical adequacy of samples and to reduce the risk of injury to vascular structures [13]. Cavanna [29] has proposed systematic aspiration biopsy of the spleen for the staging of NHL and did not observe any complications in his series. US-guided aspiration biopsy may also be indicated for the investigation of an anterior mediastinal mass, especially when the tumor is in contact with the chest wall. Easy localization of the internal mammary vessels prior to biopsy avoids vascular injury and Andersson et al. [30] observed only one false-negative error in a series of 28 aspiration biopsies performed on anterior mediastinal masses.

MEDIASTINUM

Wernecke et al. [31] proposed the utilization of US for imaging of the mediastinum as part of the treatment monitoring of lymphomas. He found that alterations in both the size of the mass and the degree of echogenicity were helpful in evaluating disease regression or recurrence. Response to therapy was revealed by a reduction in node diameter and a progressive increase in echogenicity until such time as the node could no longer be visualized, owing to the absence of delimitation from the peripheral connective tissue. While laterosternal US does not provide any information on nodes in the hilar regions, subcarinal nodes or posterior mediastinal nodes, US may be more accurate than CT in certain

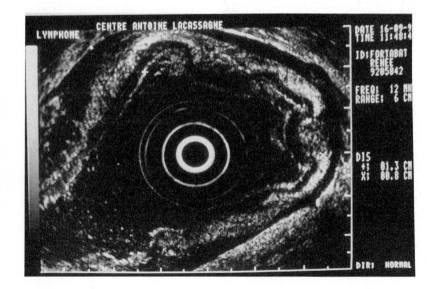

Figure 26.4 Esophageal endosonogram depicting nodal infiltration by NHL.

cases, for example, in permitting better detection of residual masses [31]. In addition, although US is highly dependent on operator skill [32], it can advantageously complement standard plain films in regions of the world where CT scanners are uncommon because of their cost.

Computed tomography

Computed tomography, which is now widely available, at least in industrial nations, has several advantages over US. The technique is reproducible (which is important for monitoring), the short imaging time improves patient tolerance, and the results are not operator-dependent, and are accessible to radiologists and clinicians who did not perform the study. Drawbacks of the method include the associated irradiation, the use of iodinated contrast agents (oral and intravenous), and especially the absence of multiplane images (even though current technological modifications permit three-dimensional reconstructions); in addition, the current high cost of CT scanners still limits their availability and precludes or drastically restricts their installation in a number of countries [33].

NODAL EXAMINATION

CT is currently the 'gold standard' for thoracic and abdominal imaging of lymphomas. The indications listed in the literature for thoracic CT for NHL vary, whereas chest CT is of undisputed value for pretherapy staging of Hodgkin's disease (HD) [34]. Some authors favor systematic thoraco-abdominal CT as part of pretherapy NHL staging [20,35], whereas others [2,36] consider chest radiology sufficient because thoracic NHL generally presents as stage III disease from the outset, with both cervical and abdominal lymphadenopathy and standard chest radiographs often normal. Further, CT of the chest rarely leads to modification of staging or treatment because pulmonary involvement is unlikely. Nevertheless, CT is unquestionably indicated when an abnormality consistent with neoplasia (particularly lymphadenopathy) is seen on the chest radiograph, since this is associated with an increased risk of pulmonary disease. This applies even more so when the patient would otherwise have stage 1 disease. CT is also more valuable than standard plain films for posttherapy follow-up [37] (Figure 26.5).

CT has replaced lymphography for exploration of the abdomen [38] but CT, like abdominal US, relies solely on volumetric data, i.e., the presence of enlarged nodes or abnormal masses. Lymph nodes are considered to be pathologically enlarged when intraperitoneal or retroperitoneal nodes have a transverse diameter of over 1 cm, when there are multiple nodes, or over 1.5 cm for a solitary mass. Diffuse disease corresponds to intraperitoneal and/or retroperitoneal lymphomatous masses that appear as a conglomerate of soft tissue masses with a bulky

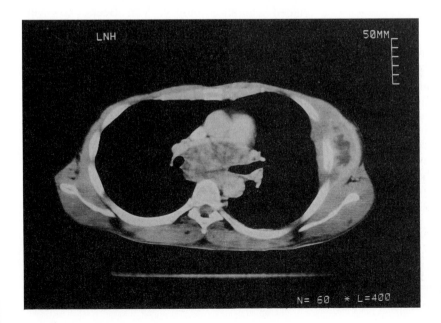

Figure 26.5   Surveillance of a patient with NHL: posterior mediastinal recurrence with involvement of the left chest wall.

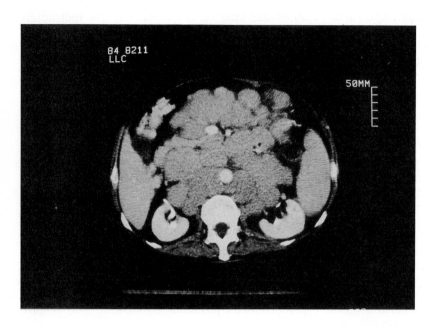

Figure 26.6   Abdominal CT showing involvement of multiple intraperitoneal and retroperitoneal nodes with no signs of vascular thrombosis.

appearance (Figure 26.6). Such masses, in the presence of bowel that has been well filled by oral contrast, do not normally present diagnostic difficulties. When bowel loops are not filled with contrast, however, it may sometimes be difficult to discern whether a given image represents unopacified bowel or a lymphomatous mass. In addition, since CT is limited to providing volumetric data, it is not possible to determine whether small lesions are benign or malignant. CT cannot provide information, as lymphography can, on architectural (i.e., intranodal) abnormalities of lymph nodes, chronic granulomatous involvement or lymphoid hyperplasia.

VISCERAL LOCALIZATIONS

Despite long experience of CT, recent advances with the technique have been reported in the literature, either in connection with a more detailed description of visceral localizations, based on large series, or the development of new techniques. Matsumoto [39] described the differences, as visualized by CT, between NHL and squamous cell carcinoma of the maxillary sinus. NHL tends to present as a bulky tumor without any aggressive bone destruction, as opposed to carcinoma, which is locally invasive.

Similarly, morphologic differences have been demonstrated in the lung, especially during transformation from low- to high-grade lymphoma [40]. Lewis described the most common features encountered in his series of pulmonary lymphomas as, in decreasing order of frequency, peribronchial thick-

ening, multiple nodules and pleural effusion [41]. Other less suggestive appearances have also been reported, including stretched and irregularly narrowed bronchi [42] and an unusual appearance of the 'angiogram sign' (intact vascular network within consolidated lung of low attenuation on CT), which is usually seen in bronchiolo-alveolar lobar cancers [43] (Figure 26.7).

A number of series have reported conflicting results with respect to the value of CT. In pancreatic lymphoma, for example, Prayer reports pancreatic involvement to be manifested usually as a mass associated with lymphadenopathy [44]. Such an appearance, he suggests, should prompt a CT-guided aspiration biopsy. Van Beers, however, considers lymphoma a likely diagnosis only in the presence of extrapancreatic spread towards neighboring organs and considers there to be no specific sign for differential diagnosis from cancer [45] (Figure 26.8). Since the diagnosis must be established histologically, debates regarding the likelihood of a given abnormality being caused by lymphoma rather than carcinoma could be considered somewhat academic.

The increased number of reports on CT evaluation of renal NHL has helped to define the CT findings that occur when there is renal lymphoma. We now know that multiple renal masses or perirenal masses should prompt a search for NHL even in the absence of lymphadenopathy [46], and that CT is more accurate than US for the imaging of renal lymphoma in both adults and children [47].

Dynamic CT (which helps the analysis of hemodynamics within a tumor) allows better evaluation of the features of lymphoma in the stomach [48].

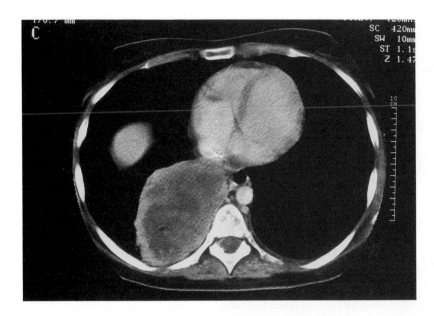

Figure 26.7 Nonspecific density in the right lower lobe: CT-guided percutaneous biopsy correctly diagnosed this pulmonary site of NHL.

Localized or diffuse thickening of the gastric wall secondary to thickening of the submucosal layer is accurately demonstrated by fast scanning; moderate enhancement is noted after iodinated contrast agent injection, and depiction of contrast-filled vessels in the submucosal layer is particularly suggestive of NHL [48].

CT-GUIDED ASPIRATION BIOPSY

CT-guided aspiration biopsy has become a routine diagnostic procedure, especially for chest lesions.

Sensitivity for the diagnosis of thoracic NHL is 73–81% [49,50] when only one aspiration biopsy is performed. In one study, the performance of several aspiration biopsies increased the sensitivity to 95% [49]. This is particularly important to keep in mind when biopsy is performed for the detection of recurrence. Intermediate-grade lymphomas and low-grade follicular NHL present several diagnostic problems including the occasional presence of extensive sclerosis, which may make it difficult to obtain a tissue sample with adequate cellularity for histologic diagnosis [49] (Figure 26.9).

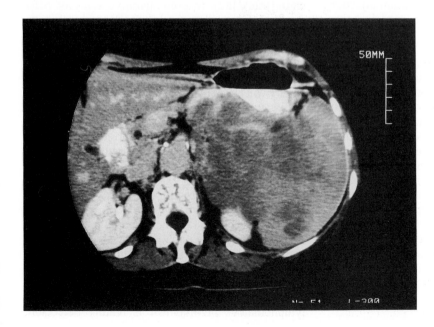

Figure 26.8 Bulky NHL lesion infiltrating the body and tail of the pancreas; note the disease spread towards the posterior gastric wall and especially towards the spleen.

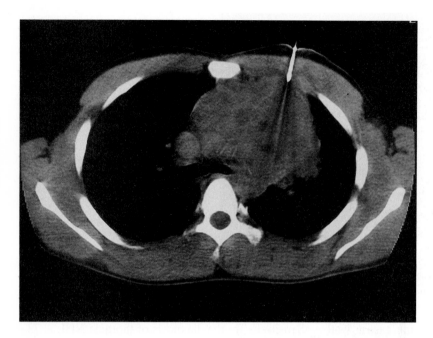

Figure 26.9 CT-guided biopsy of an NHL lesion in the anterior mediastinum.

Magnetic resonance imaging

MRI will undoubtedly compete increasingly with CT for NHL imaging in the future. The advantages of MRI include multiplane exploration (coronal scans are especially useful for exploration of the chest, providing satisfactory analysis of the aortopulmonary window and the subcarinal region, while sagittal scans are indicated for adequate examination of the subclavicular region), the absence of an obligatory need for contrast medium injection (although contrast medium can be used in some circumstances), and a potential for tissue characterization, permitting the diagnosis of fibrosis. The drawbacks include motion-related artefacts, the classic contraindications of MRI (especially synchronous pacemaker and cerebral aneurysm clips), a high cost compared to CT, a current availability that is generally inferior to CT, a longer imaging time than for CT scans and, in an overall manner, poorer patient tolerance. In children, in particular, spatial resolution is not always satisfactory and the imaging time is still too long. Our recent analysis of the value of MRI for the imaging of lymphomas included characterization of the appearance of lymphomatous tissue, NHL staging by MRI, correlation with bone marrow aspiration/biopsy, description of appearances of lymphoma in organs and viscera, the role of MRI in follow-up, and future applications in connection with clinical trials and studies on animal models.

CURRENT APPLICATIONS OF MRI

With a 1.5 Tesla MRI unit, lymphomatous nodal tissue appears less opaque (hypointense) than fat and discretely hypointense relative to muscle in T_1-weighted sequences, but isointense to fat and hyperintense to muscle in T_2-weighted sequences (Figures 26.10 and 26.11). These appearances are the same regardless of the grade of NHL [50].

The first studies of the value of MRI for disease staging were focused on the abdomen [51] and the entire trunk [52]. In a comparative study of MRI, standard plain films and lymphography for the detection of disease sites [52], MRI proved better than standard radiographs in 21% of cases, concurred with lymphography in 97% of cases and demonstrated bone marrow involvement in 19% of cases (which, of course, lymphography could not), a finding which modified the staging of HD or NHL in 15% of cases [52].

Bone marrow, MRI and cytologic studies have been performed by a number of teams [53–55], and all pelvic sites suspected, on the basis of MRI, to be positive were biopsied. MRI appears useful, regardless of the histologic type of NHL (Figure 26.12). Bone marrow involvement is the rule in low-grade malignancies, reflecting the systematic nature of the disease. In high-grade malignancies, however, bone marrow involvement is an indicator of poor prognosis and reflects dissemination of disease. On T_1-weighted sequences, yellow (fatty) marrow presents a more or less homogeneous signal such that lymphomatous involvement is readily detectable.

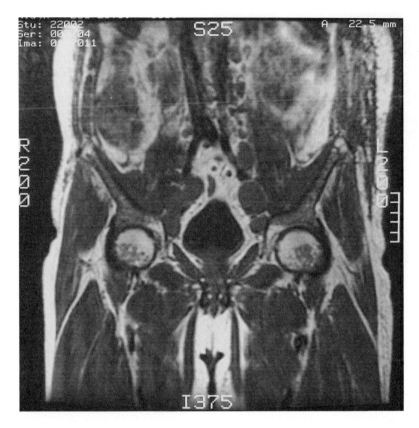

Figure 26.10   MRI (T_1-weighted sequence): nodal pelvic masses with the same signal intensity as muscle but less than that of fat.

Thus, examination of the pelvis can be improved by accurate prebiopsy localization of probable sites of involvement by MRI, which eliminates the numerous false-negative results obtained when bone marrow aspiration biopsies are performed blind. Bone regions containing hematopoietic red marrow, however, present diagnostic difficulties and this problem is therefore greater in younger age groups, since the amount of red marrow decreases progressively with age. Fat suppression sequences (STIR) or chemical

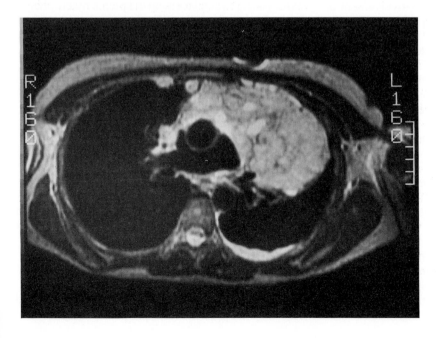

Figure 26.11   MRI (T_2-weighted sequence): NHL in the left anterior mediastinum with a signal intensity higher than that of fat or muscle; note the associated small left pleural effusion.

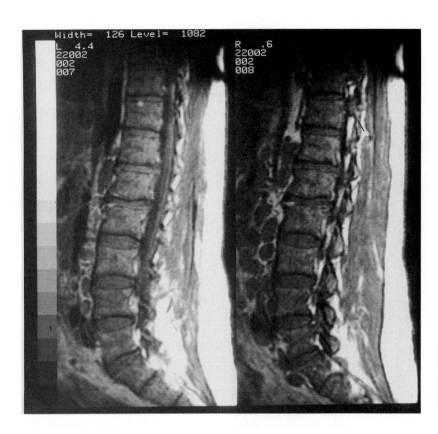

Figure 26.12   MRI of the spine (T_1-weighted sequence): diffuse bone marrow disease associated with retroperitoneal node involvement.

shift imaging have been used, and appear to improve the performances of MRI, since bone appears black and tumoral areas exhibit a high-intensity signal on images obtained with these techniques [56]. MRI is effective for the detection of marrow involvement in high-grade lymphomas but is not as good for low-grade lymphomas, where medullary involvement is moderate. This is not a major problem, though, since most patients with low-grade lymphomas have bone marrow involvement. The detection of areas of signal attenuation, however, is not synonymous with tumor infiltration, since decreased signal intensity of bone marrow has a number of possible causes, including tumoral infiltration, myelofibrosis, or recolonization by hematopoietic cells, i.e., areas of active hematopoiesis [57]. This can pose difficulties with interpretation in patients who are anemic, particularly after bleeding, since regions of red marrow may extend and the signal pattern may be altered. To surmount the problem of varying amounts of red and yellow marrow in different age groups, a reference map showing the topographic distribution of the red marrow as a function of age has been advocated [58], but diagnostic dilemmas unrelated to this require histologic adjudication.

Primary hepatic NHL has no specific MRI features [59] but a homogeneous high-intensity signal may be observed on T_2-weighted sequences, some-times with lobulation of the mass, which is frequently solitary. Utilization of superparamagnetic iron oxide improves the imaging of splenic lymphoma, which has a significantly higher signal than the normal or benign spleen. This situation reflects reduced phagocytosis of the superparamagnetic iron oxide owing to displacement of splenic macrophages by the lymphoma cells and/or immunologic suppression of macrophage activity [60]. However, necrotic or fibrotic tumor, posttherapy, will also fail to have the appearance of normal splenic tissue.

Thanks to the possibility of multiplane scans and the method's excellent contrast resolution, MRI is the only technique at this time that can accurately demonstrate the various components of spinal lymphoma [61].

MRI is superior to CT for the identification of lymphoma at a number of additional localizations, in particular in the central nervous system, a topic discussed in the section on immunodeficient subjects. Posttreatment follow-up by MRI is analyzed in the section on residual masses.

NEWER MRI TECHNIQUES

Numerous MRI reports have published clinical applications of new techniques, frequently studied first in animal treatment models. Multiplane MRI scans improve the design of fields for radiotherapy and appear better than CT for the imaging of thoracic involvement, regardless of the type of lymphoma. Carlsen has reported changes in a CT simulation-based initial treatment plan following MRI in 20% of cases [62]. Coronal scans optimize beam centering by allowing image superimposition on a simulator using a substrascope (MRI simulation) [63]. Analysis of the spleen by the Isis technique allows ^{31}P-nuclear magnetic resonance (NMR) spectroscopy, which utilizes signals from the three phosphates of ATP, phosphomonesters (PME), phosphodiesters (PDE) and inorganic phosphate (Pi). Kaiser has suggested that lymphomatous involvement is revealed by an increase in the PM +Pi/beta ATP quotient and an increase in PDE/beta ATP quotient, corresponding to an increase in metabolism of the phospholipid membrane by augmentation of cell turnover. However, this study was carried out in only 15 patients and further confirmatory studies will be necessary [64]. Spectroscopy with ^{31}P-NMR may improve treatment monitoring because an increase in the PDE/beta ATP quotient indicates tumor response to chemotherapy [65]. MRI can also distinguish the various grades of NHL, as an inhomogeneous tumor appearance corresponds to a high-grade malignancy [66]. The inhomogeneity index described by Rehn et al. [66] is an expression of the degree of homogeneity on T_1- and T_2-weighted sequences using gadolinium injection, which improves the detection of high-grade lymphomas. Despite the small number of patients studied, this imaging method seems to be valuable in the follow-up of low-grade lymphomas (for the detection of transformation to a high-grade lesion) [67].

Various contrast agents for MRI have been tested in animals and used in clinical studies. Opacification of the gastrointestinal tract using superparamagnetic particles improves the ability to interpret abdominal MRI studies and permits the differentiation of lymphadenopathy or other lymphomatous masses from the normal digestive tract [68]. The most interesting studies to date concern the identification of lymphoma in lymph nodes and the bone marrow. Following intravenous injection of superparamagnetic iron oxide in the rat, normal nodes exhibit a reduction in signal intensity whereas no modification is observed in tumoral nodes [69,70]. In the rabbit, injection of superparamagnetic iron oxide causes a decrease in the signal intensity of the red and the yellow marrow, especially on echo gradient studies. This feature should improve MRI detection of small areas of bone marrow infiltration [71]. It is likely that MRI, currently indicated to assess bone marrow involvement and CNS disease, will have an increasing role to play in the future – perhaps particularly with respect to identifying the nature of the abnormal image.

Other imaging techniques

Lymphography has been progressively abandoned for staging and follow-up of NHL in favor of CT [72–74]. CT is not only less invasive but it also provides comparable results, with a maximum of 9% discordant results, to lymphography [72,74]. North et al. [74] compared CT and lymphography in 164 cases of NHL; lymphography was abnormal while CT was normal in only two patients, whereas lymphography was normal but CT revealed nodal abnormalities in 12 patients. While lymphography can demonstrate minimal modifications in nodes during staging and especially follow-up, this technique has become obsolete now that chemotherapy is administered routinely, and the rate of false-negative errors with CT, owing to small lesions, has decreased as a consequence of the success of modern treatment protocols.

Gastrointestinal lesions are currently evaluated primarily by endoscopy; barium studies no longer play the same role as they did 15 years ago and are now indicated solely for examination of the small intestine [75]. CT and US can usefully complement endoscopic data, in particular by demonstrating the typical appearance of the wall of the digestive tract that is often associated with lymphomatous infiltration [76].

Residual masses

A persistent residual mass is noted in 20–40% of patients after treatment; this raises the problem of their nosology and the most appropriate management [41]. As mentioned previously, mediastinal US using parasternal and substernal approaches can sometimes help differentiate fibrosis from recurrent disease in this anatomical location, but this requires considerable operator experience [31,32]. CT can accurately determine the volume of the residual mass, and define targets for surveillance or for aspiration biopsy (Figure 26.13). Depending on the context, mere surveillance by CT or aspiration biopsy were the only alternatives before the introduction of MRI [77,78]. However, size assessment alone is insufficient to confirm complete absence of viable tumor, since masses that have regressed in size may still contain tumoral cells refractory to

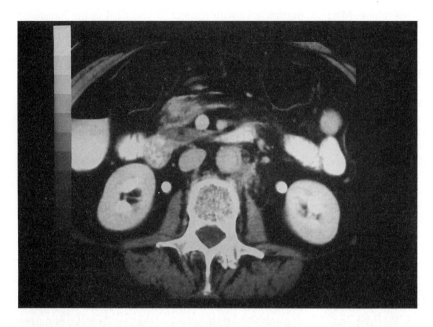

Figure 26.13 Abdominal CT showing a residual mass in the left latero-aortic region that remained stable over 1 year on follow-up scans.

chemotherapy [79]. Several studies have compared modifications in the MRI signal with changes in tumor size [50,79,80]. Although no linear relationship exists between size regression and a decrease in tumor signal intensity on T_2-weighted sequences, an association of these two findings is highly suggestive of residual fibrous scarring. Persistence of a high-intensity signal on T_2-weighted sequences remains a controversial finding. In its early stages, fibrosis consists mainly of fibroblasts and endothelial cells, and is often edematous and rich in mobile protons. This may explain the high-intensity signal observed on T_2-weighted sequences. In addition to inflammatory or necrotic reorganization, fat deposits can also increase the signal intensity on T_2-weighted sequences, making a fat suppression sequence indispensable [80]. These factors necessitate cautious interpretation of follow-up MRI scans, which should preferably be obtained at least 6 months after the start of therapy, if CT has not demonstrated any recurrence in the meantime. Fibrosis will be more mature and less likely to give a high-intensity signal on T_2-weighted sequences. Lymphomas in which there is a fibrotic element, which may be extensive, may also lead to interpretation difficulties. Lymph nodes that are predominantly composed of fibrous tissue and contain little tumor show minimal reduction in size and T_2-weighted signal immediately following treatment [50].

The value of percutaneous biopsy performed under US or CT guidance was mentioned earlier, with emphasis placed on the value of multiple biopsies to improve the accuracy of cytologic diagnosis [49]. The limitations of fine-needle aspiration include false-negative errors related to inadequate tissue samples, sometimes resulting from the presence of fibrosis. In such cases, and when transformation from a low-grade to a higher-grade malignancy is suspected, use of a core biopsy needle or surgical biopsy is indicated.

NHL and immunodeficiency

NHL is more frequent in transplant recipients than in the general population, in particular following the administration of high doses of cyclosporin. Acquired immunodeficiency syndrome (AIDS) patients also have a markedly higher incidence of high-grade lymphoma. In such patients, NHL is more common than HD, and particularly aggressive forms of NHL predominate, namely Burkitt's lymphoma, and large-cell immunoblastic lymphoma. Extranodal manifestations are the rule, and there is a predilection for the central nervous system and digestive tract. These lymphomas, in the context of HIV infection, have a poor prognosis and tend to recur early [81].

Cerebral lymphoma is considerably more common in AIDS patients (more than 14 times) than in the general population [81] and accounts for 25% of all cases of NHL in AIDS [82]. The main diagnostic problem is the differentiation from cerebral abscesses and toxoplasmosis. MRI features suggestive of a lymphomatous process include lesions over 2 cm [83], a periventricular location in the white matter, a solitary lesion, and a weak mass effect (owing to the infiltrative character of the lesion) [84]. On unenhanced CT, a high-density lesion may suggest the diagnosis because toxoplasmosis and other abscesses are hypodense in such studies. Subependymal enhancement has been observed for 38% of NHL following administration of an iodinated contrast agent [85], whereas this phenomenon is rarely seen with toxoplasmosis. The absence of enhancement after iodinated medium injection nearly rules out a diagnosis of lymphoma. Hemorrhage, which is well detected by MRI, suggests toxoplasmosis because NHL is rarely hemorrhagic except in patients with a history of corticosteroid therapy or irradiation [83]. Jensen and Brant-Zawadzju [86] emphasized the value of T_2-weighted sequences, which can demonstrate small non-enhancing lesions. Gadolinium injection may produce homogeneous enhancement suggestive of lymphoma but, occasionally, a ring-enhancing lesion, typical of toxoplasmosis, proves to be lymphoma, although the wall of lymphomatous lesions is thick, while it is thin in case of toxoplasmosis [85]. Finally, irregular and sinuous contrast uptake is strongly suggestive of lymphoma. Evaluation of response to antitoxoplasmosis therapy requires a repeat examination 10 days after treatment; this interval is sufficient for the detection of progression in a lymphomatous lesion and such a finding should prompt stereotactic biopsy (Figures 26.14 and 26.15) [83,87].

CT appears well suited for exploration of the abdomen and often reveals visceral involvement, particularly in the liver, spleen, kidneys or omentum [88]. The demonstration of deep abdominal lymphadenopathy should suggest not only the possibility of NHL, but also of Kaposi's sarcoma or a mycobacterial infection [89]. Nodes smaller than 15 mm

(a)

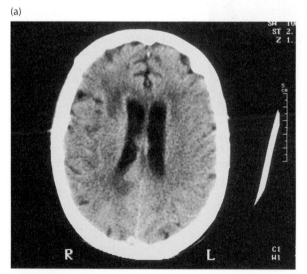

(c)

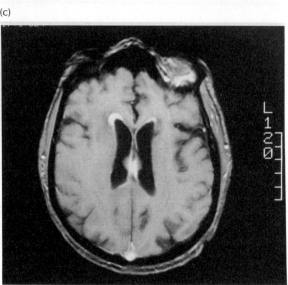

(b)

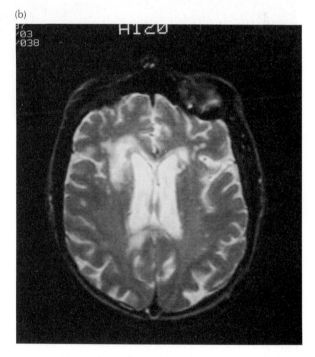

Figure 26.14   Primary NHL in an AIDS patient: hypodense periventricular masses (a). The lesions are better visualized on the T_2-weighted sequence (b) and on the T_1-sequence after intravenous gadolinium injection (c).

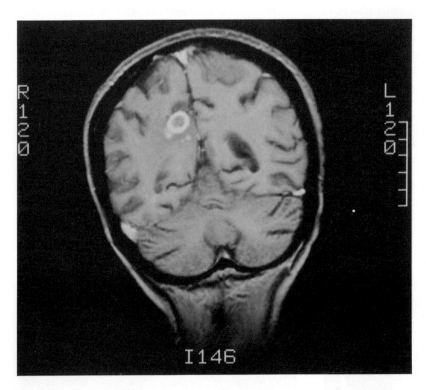

Figure 26.15 MRI after intravenous gadolinium injection (T_1-weighted sequence): annular enhancement of a small lesion (15 mm) corresponding to primary NHL in an AIDS patient.

merely reflect nonspecific reactive hyperplasia in the context of AIDS and do not require biopsy.

Diagnostic evaluation of the chest is much more difficult owing to the nonspecificity of CT signs and the frequent association of several intercurrent pathologies. For example, Kaposi's sarcoma affects up to 20% of AIDS patients and is often contemporary with a *Pneumocystis carinii* infection [90]. Thoracic lymphadenopathy in the context of AIDS may be indicative of Kaposi's sarcoma, NHL, or a mycobacterial infection. Associated pulmonary abnormalities, pleural effusion or hilar lymphadenopathy should prompt a search for cutaneous involvement with Kaposi's sarcoma [90,91]. Not all thoracic 'tumors' in AIDS patients are lymphoma or Kaposi's sarcoma. Eagar et al. reported two patients with chest masses and hilar adenopathies with pleural effusion due to *Pneunocystis carinii* infection [92]. Thus, a definitive diagnosis may need to be established by surgical biopsy in immunodeficient patients if an infectious etiology cannot be established by bronchiolo-alveolar lavage and/or endobronchial biopsy (69% to 91% versus 17% to 60%) [93]. The definitive diagnosis of chest masses in immunodeficient patients is, thus, dependent upon on a constellation of clinical, radiologic, bacteriologic and histologic findings. In particularly difficult cases, only alterations in the appearance of lesions after antiinfectious or lymphoma-specific treatment leads to the establishment of a diagnosis.

Acknowledgment

The authors wish to thank Nancy Rameau for translation of the manuscript.

References

1. Castellino RA. The non-Hodgkin lymphomas: Practical concepts for the diagnostic radiologist. *Radiology* 1991, **178**: 315–321.
2. Frija J, D'Agay MF, Brice P, et al. Imagerie des lymphomes. *Rev. Immunol. Med.* 1993, **5**: 457–468.
3. Bruneton JN, Schneider M. *Radiology of Lymphomas*. Berlin: Springer Verlag, 1986.
4. Jing BS. Diagnostic imaging of abdominal and pelvic lymph nodes in lymphoma. *Radiol. Clin. North Am.* 1990, **28**: 801–831.
5. Shirkhoda A, Ros PR, Farah J, et al. Lymphoma of the solid abdominal viscera. *Radiol. Clin. North Am.* 1990, **28**: 785–799.
6. Cohen MD, Siddiqui A, Weetman R, et al. Hodgkin disease and non-Hodgkin lymphomas in children: Utilization of radiological modalities. *Radiology* 1986, **158**: 499–505.
7. White L, Siegel SE, Quah TC. Non-Hodgkin's lymphomas in children. I. Patterns of disease and classification. *Crit. Rev. Oncol. Hematol.* 1992, **13**: 55–71.

8. Kagan AR, Steckel RJ. Post-treatment surveillance studies for lymphoma patients. *Invest. Radiol.* 1992, **27**: 543–545.

9. Bruneton JN. *Ultrasonography of the Neck.* Berlin: Springer Verlag, 1987.

10. Bruneton JN, Normand F, Balu-Maestro C, et al. Lymphomatous superficial lymph nodes: US detection. *Radiology* 1987, **165**: 233–235.

11. Sakai F, Sone S, Kiyono K, et al. Computed tomography of neck lymph nodes involved with malignant lymphoma: Comparison with ultrasound. *Radiat. Med.* 1991, **9**: 203–208.

12. Andreula CF, Farchi G, Pavone V, et al. I. Linfonodi del collo. Diagnosi mediante risonanza magnetica con tecniche a eco di gradiente. *Radiol. Med. (Torino)* 1991, **81**: 417–421.

13. Bruneton JN, Padovani B, Marcy PY. Echographie des ganglions superficiels. *J. Radiol.* 1994, **75**: 373–381.

14. Goerg C, Schwerk WB. Ultrasound of extranodal abdominal lymphoma. A review. *Clin. Radiol.* 1991, **44**: 92–97.

15. Freeman C, Berg JW, Cutler SJ. Occurrence and prognosis of extranodal lymphoma. *Cancer* 1972, **29**: 252–260.

16. Soyer P, Van Beers B, Teillet-Thiebaud F, et al. Hodgkin's and non-Hodgkin's hepatic lymphoma: Sonographic findings. *Abdom. Imag.* 1993, **18**: 339–343.

17. Weiss A, Weiss H, Gruhn K. Organmanifestationen maligner Lymphome. Ergebnisse einer jahrigen sonographischen Verlaufsbeobachtung von 550 patienten. *Ultraschall. Med.* 1989, **10**: 284–289.

18. Kasagi K, Hatabu H, Tokuda Y, et al. Lymphoproliferative disorders of the thyroid gland: radiological appearances. *Br. J. Radiol.* 1991, **64**: 569–575.

19. Peterson K, Gordon KB, Heinemann MH, et al. The clinical spectrum of ocular lymphoma. *Cancer* 1993, **72**: 843–849.

20. Tweed CS, Peck RJ. A sonographic appearance of testicular lymphoma. *Clin. Radiol.* 1991, **43**: 341–342.

21. Morton JE, Leyland MJ, Vaughan Hudson G, et al. Primary gastrointestinal non-Hodgkin's lymphoma: A review of 175 British National Lymphoma Investigation cases. *Br. J. Cancer* 1993, **67**: 776–782.

22. Seitz JF, Giovannini M, Monges G, et al. Intérêt de la fibroscopie digestive haute dans le bilan d'extension initial des lymphomes malins non hodgkiniens extra-digestifs. Résultats chez 101 patients. *Gastroenterol. Clin. Biol.* 1990, **14**: 961–965.

23. Seifert E, Schulte F, Weismuller J, et al. Endoscopic and bioptic diagnosis of malignant non-Hodgkin's lymphoma of the stomach. *Endoscopy* 1993, **25**: 497–501.

24. Jaser N, Sivula A, Franssila K. Primary gastric non-Hodgkin's lymphoma in Finland, 1972–1977. Clinical presentation and results of treatment. *Scand. J. Gastroenterol.* 1990, **25**: 1052–1059.

25. Schwartz RJ, Conners JM, Schmidt N. Diagnosis and management of stage IE and stage IIE gastric lymphomas. *Am. J. Surg.* 1993, **165**: 561–565.

26. Caletti G, Ferrari A, Brocchie E, et al. Accuracy of endoscopic ultrasonography in the diagnosis and staging of gastric cancer and lymphoma. *Surgery* 1993, **113**: 14–27.

27. Schuder G, Hilderbrandt V, Kreifler-Haag D, et al. Role of endosonography in the surgical management of non-Hodgkin's lymphoma of the stomach. *Endoscopy* 1993, **25**: 509–512.

28. Palazzo L, Roseau G, Ruskone-Fourmestraux A, et al. Endoscopic ultrasonography in the local staging of primary gastric lymphoma. *Endoscopy* 1993, **25**: 502–508.

29. Cavanna L, Civardi G, Fornari F, et al. Ultrasonically guided percutaneous splenic tissue core biopsy in patients with malignant lymphomas. *Cancer* 1992, **69**: 2932–2936.

30. Andersson T, Lindgren PG, Elvin A. Ultrasound guided tumor biopsy in the anterior mediastinum. An alternative to thoracotomy and mediastinoscopy. *Acta Radiol.* 1992, **33**: 423–426.

31. Wernecke K, Vassalo P, Hoffman G, et al. Value of sonography in monitoring the therapeutic response of mediastinal lymphoma: comparison with chest radiography and CT. *Am. J. Roentgenol.* 1991, **156**: 265–272.

32. Marglin SI, Laing FL, Castellino RA. Current status of mediastinal sonography in the post-treatment evaluation of patients with lymphoma. *Am. J. Roentgenol.* 1991, **157**: 469–470.

33. Fishman EK, Kuhlman JE, Jones RJ. CT of lymphoma: Spectrum of disease. *Radiographics* 1991, **11**: 647–669.

34. North LB, Libshitz HI, Lorigan JG. Thoracic lymphoma. *Radiol. Clin. North Am.* 1990, **28**: 745–762.

35. Khoury MB, Godwin JD, Halvorsen R, et al. Role of chest CT in non-Hodgkin lymphoma. *Radiology* 1986, **158**: 659–662.

36. Zagoria RJ, Muss HB, Wolfman NT, et al. Computed tomography versus chest radiography: Impact on management of patients with lymphoma. *Cancer Invest.* 1990, **8**: 357–364.

37. Antinori A, Ammassari A, Murri R, et al. Primary central nervous system lymphoma and brain biopsy in AIDS. *Lancet* 1993, **341**: 1411–1412.

38. Jing BS. Diagnostic imaging of abdominal and pelvic lymph nodes in lymphoma. *Radiol. Clin. North Am.* 1990, **28**: 801–831.

39. Matsumoto S, Shibuya H, Tajera S, et al. Comparison of CT findings in non-Hodgkin lymphoma and squamous cell carcinoma of the maxillary sinus. *Acta Radiol.* 1992, **33**: 523–527.

40. Cordier JF, Chailleux E, Lauque D, et al. Primary pulmonary lymphomas. A clinical study of 70 cases in nonimmunocompromised patients. *Chest* 1993, **103**: 201–208.

41. Lewis ER, Caskey CI, Fishman EK. Lymphoma of the lung: CT findings in 31 patients. *Am. J. Roentgenol.* 1991, **156**: 711–714.

42. Bosanko CMM, Korobkin M, Fantone JC, et al. Lobar primary pulmonary lymphoma: CT findings. *J. Comput. Assist. Tomogr.* 1991, **15**: 679–682.

43. Vincent JM, Ng YY, Norton AJ, et al. CT 'angiogram sign' in primary pulmonary lymphoma. *J. Comput. Assist. Tomogr.* 1992, **16**: 829–831.

44. Prayer L, Schrawitzki H, Mallek R, et al. CT in

pancreatic involvement of non-Hodgkin lymphoma. *Acta Radiol.* 1992, **33**: 123–127.

45. Van Beers B, Lalonde L, Soyer P, et al. Dynamic CT in pancreatic lymphoma. *J. Comput. Assist. Tomogr.* 1993, **17**: 94–97.

46. Cohan RH, Dunnick NR, Leder RA, et al. Computed tomography of renal lymphoma. *J. Comput. Assist. Tomogr.* 1990, **14**: 933–938.

47. Weinberger E, Rosenbaum DM, Pendergrass TW. Renal involvement in children with lymphoma: Comparison of CT with sonography. *Am. J. Roentgenol.* 1990, **155**: 347–349.

48. Minami M, Kawauchi N, Itai Y, et al. Gastric tumors: Radiologic–pathologic correlation and accuracy of T staging with dynamic CT. *Radiology* 1992, **185**: 173–178.

49. Wittich GR, Nowels KW, Korn RL, et al. Coaxial transthoracic fine-needle biopsy in patients with a history of malignant lymphoma. *Radiology* 1992, **183**: 175–178.

50. Negendank WG, Al Katib AM, Karenes C, et al. Lymphomas: MRI contrast characteristics with clinical–pathologic correlations. *Radiology* 1990, **177**: 209–216.

51. Skillings JR, Bramwell V, Nicholson RL, et al. A prospective study of MRI in lymphoma staging. *Cancer* 1991, **67**: 1838–1843.

52. Tesoro-Tess JD, Balzarini L, Ceglia E, et al. MRI in the initial staging of Hodgkin's disease and non-Hodgkin lymphoma. *Eur. J. Radiol.* 1991, **12**: 81–90.

53. Assoun J, Poey C, Attal M, et al. Envahissement médullaire au cours des lymphomes. Corrélation biopsie ostéo-médullaire et IRM. *Rev. Immunol. Med.* 1993, **5**: 15–21.

54. Guckel F, Semmler W, Dohner H, et al. Kernspintomographische darstellung von knochenmarkinfiltrationen bei malignen Lymphomen. *Rofo. Fortschr. Geb. Rontgenstr. Nucklearmed.* 1989, **150**: 26–31.

55. Shields AF, Porter BA, Churchley S, et al. The detection of bone marrow involvement by lymphoma using MRI. *J. Clin. Oncol.* 1987, **5**: 225–230.

56. Rosen BR, Fleming DM, Kushner DL, et al. Hematologic bone marrow disorders: quantitative chemical shift MR imaging. *Radiology* 1988, **169**: 799–804.

57. Smith SR, Williams CE, Davier JM, et al. Bone marrow disorders: Characterization with quantitative MR imaging. *Radiology* 1989, **172**: 805–810.

58. Weinreb JC. MR imaging of bone marrow: A map could help. *Radiology* 1990, **177**: 23–24.

59. Soyer P, Van Beers B, Grandin C, et al. Primary lymphoma of the liver. MR findings. *Eur. J. Radiol.* 1993, **16**: 209–212.

60. Weissleder R, Elizondo G, Stark DD, et al. The diagnosis of splenic lymphoma by MR imaging: Value of superparamagnetic iron oxide. *Am. J. Roentgenol.* 1989, **152**: 175–180.

61. Li MH, Holtas S, Larsson EM. MR imaging of spinal lymphoma. *Acta Radiol.* 1992, **33**: 338–342.

62. Carlsen SE, Bergin CJ, Hoppe RT. MR imaging to detect chest wall and pleural involvement in patients with lymphoma: Effect on radiation therapy planning. *Am. J. Roentgenol.* 1993, **160**: 1191–1195.

63. Flentje M, Zierhut D, Schraube P, et al. Integration of coronal MRI into radiation treatment planning of mediastinal tumors. *Strahlenther. Onkol.* 1993, **169**: 351–357.

64. Kaiser WA, Kombost T, Traber F, et al. Erste Ergebnisse der in-vivo-31 P-NMR-Spektroskopie der Milz bei Patienten mit Splenomegalie. *Rofo. Fortschr. Geb. Rontgenstr. Neuren. Bildgeb. Verfahr.* 1993, **159**: 180–186.

65. Smith SR, Martin PA, Davies JM, et al. The assessment of treatment response in non-Hodgkin's lymphoma by image guided 31P MR spectroscopy. *Br. J. Cancer* 1990, **61**: 485–490.

66. Rehn SM, Nyman RS, Glimelius BLG, et al. Non-Hodgkin lymphoma: Predicting prognostic grade with MR imaging. *Radiology* 1990, **176**: 249–253.

67. Rehn S, Sperber GO, Nyman R et al. Quantification of inhomogeneities in malignancy grading of non-Hodgkin lymphoma with MR imaging. *Acta Radiol.* 1993, **34**: 3–9.

68. Lonnemark M, Hemmingsson A, Bach-Gansmo T, et al. Superparamagnetic particles as oral contrast medium in MR imaging of malignant lymphoma. *Acta Radiol* 1991, **32**: 232–238.

69. Hamm B, Taupitz M, Hussmann P, et al. MR lymphography with iron oxide particles: Dose–response studies and pulse sequence optimization in rabbits. *Am. J. Roentgenol.* 1992, **158**: 183–190.

70. Weissleder R, Elizondo G, Wittenberg J, et al. Ultrasmall superparamagnetic iron oxide: An intravenous contrast agent for assessing lymph nodes with MR imaging. *Radiology* 1990, **175**: 494–498.

71. Seneterre E, Weissleder R, Jaramillo D, et al. Bone marrow: ultrasmall superparamagnetic iron oxide for MR imaging. *Radiology* 1991, **179**: 529–533.

72. Kok T, Jurgens PJ, Van Minden SH, et al. Unterschiedliche Beurteilung der Stadieneinteilung des Hodgkin- und non-Hodgkin-lymphomes (NHL) mit Computertomographie und Lymphographie durch verschiedene untersucher. *Aktuelle Radiol.* 1993, **3**: 238–241.

73. Moskovic E, Fernando I, Blake P, et al. Lymphography. Current role in oncology. *Br. J. Radiol.* 1991, **64**: 421–427.

74. North LB, Wallace S, Lindell MM Jr, et al. Lymphography for staging lymphomas: Is it still a useful procedure? *Am. J. Roentgenol.* 1993, **161**: 867–869.

75. Iida M, Suekane H, Tada S, et al. Double-contrast radiographic features in primary small intestinal lymphoma of the 'Western' type: Correlation with pathologic findings. *Clin. Radiol.* 1991, **44**: 322–326.

76. Smith C, Kubicka RA, Thomas CR Jr. Non-Hodgkin lymphoma of the gastrointestinal tract. *Radiographics* 1992, **12**: 887–899.

77. Uematsu M, Kondo M, Tsutsui T, et al. Residual masses on follow-up CT in patients with mediastinal non-Hodgkin's lymphoma. *Clin. Radiol.* 1989, **40**: 244–247.

78. Whelan JS, Reznek RH, Daniell SJ, et al. CT and US guided core biopsy in the management of non-Hodgkin's lymphoma. *Br. J. Cancer* 1991, **63**: 460–462.

79. Rahmouni A, Tempany C, Jones R, et al. Lymphoma: Monitoring tumor size and signal intensity with MR imaging. *Radiology* 1993, **188**: 445–451.

80. Lee JKT, Glazer HS. Controversy in the MR imaging appearance of fibrosis. *Radiology* 1990, **177**: 21–22.

81. Ioachim HL, Dorsett B, Cronin W, et al. AIDS-associated lymphomas: Clinical, pathologic, immunologic, and viral characteristics of 111 cases. *Hum. Pathol.* 1991, **22**: 659–673.

82. Kaplan LD. IDS associated lymphoma. *Baillière's Clin. Haematol.* 1990, **3**: 139–151.

83. Cordoliani YS, Derosier C, Pharaboz C, et al. Primary cerebral lymphoma in patients with AIDS: MR findings in 17 cases. *Am. J. Roentgenol.* 1992, **159**: 841–847.

84. Ciricillo SF, Rosenblum ML. Use of CT and MR imaging to distinguish intracranial lesions and to define the need of biopsy in AIDS patients. *J. Neurosurg.* 1990, **73**: 720–724.

85. Dina TS. Primary central nervous system lymphoma versus toxoplasmosis in AIDS. *Radiology* 1991, **179**: 823–828.

86. Jensen MC, Brant-Zawadzju M. MR imaging of the brain in patients with AIDS: Value of routine use of IV gadopentetate dimeglumine. *Am. J. Roentgenol.* 1993, **160**: 153–157.

87. Levy RM, Russell E, Yungbluth M, et al. The efficacy of image-guided stereotactic brain biopsy in neurologically symptomatic acquired immunodeficiency syndrome patients. *Neurosurgery* 1992, **30**: 186–189.

88. Townsend RR. CT of AIDS-related lymphoma. *Am. J. Roentgenol.* 1991, **156**: 969–974.

89. Herts BR, Megibow AJ, Birnbaum BA, et al. High-attenuation lymphadenopathy in AIDS patients: Significance of findings at CT. *Radiology* 1992, **185**: 777–781.

90. Heitzman ER. Pulmonary neoplastic and lymphoproliferative disease in AIDS: A review. *Radiology* 1990, **177**: 347–351.

91. Dodd GD III, Ledesma-Medina J, Baron RL, et al. Posttransplant lymphoproliferative disorder: Intrathoracic manifestations. *Radiology* 1992, **184**: 65–69.

92. Eagar GM, Friedland JA, Sagel SS. Tumefactive Pneumocystis carinii infection in AIDS: report of three cases. *Am. J. Roentgenol.* 1993, **160**: 1197–1198.

93. Janzen DL, Padley SPG, Adler BD, et al. Acute pulmonary complications in immunocompromised non-AIDS patients: Comparison of diagnostic accuracy of CT and chest radiography. *Clin. Radiol.* 1993, **47**: 159–165.

PART 5

General principles of management

CHAPTER 27

Complications in the management of non-Hodgkin's lymphomas

AZIZA T. SHAD

Introduction

With the continuing rise in the incidence of cancer [including non-Hodgkin's lymphomas (NHL)] and the current trend of treating malignancies more aggressively, an increasing number of patients are at risk for complications arising from either the disease itself or as unwanted side-effects of treatment. Thus, the successful management of the NHL, as for all other cancers, not only involves the administration of specific therapy, but the treatment of the multiple complications, which may arise either acutely, i.e., before or during therapy, or later, i.e., months or years after the completion of treatment. It is imperative that all physicians who care for patients with cancer are familiar with such complications, since timely and appropriate medical care is essential if they are to be treated effectively, while modifications of treatment regimens in order to avoid them may sometimes be justifiable.

Complications frequently encountered during cancer management can be divided into three broad categories, each of which can be further subdivided into various subcategories as shown in Tables 27.1–27.3. These categories are given below.

TUMOR-RELATED COMPLICATIONS

These include:

1. Complications that arise as a result of the physical encroachment of tumor masses on vital structures or from the large bulk of tumor at diagnosis, e.g., airway obstruction, superior and inferior vena caval obstruction, pleural and pericardial effusions, cardiac tamponade or arrythmias, raised intracranial pressure, spinal cord compression and pulmonary embolism.
2. Metabolic complications including the tumor lysis syndrome, hypercalcemia, hypo/hyperglycemia and SIADH.
3. Complications related to lymphomatous involvement of the gastrointestinal tract, such as intestinal obstruction, hemorrhage and fistulae.
4. Complications such as cardiac arrest – associated with the administration of anesthetics in patients with large mediastinal masses.
5. Cytokine-mediated complications, such as cancer cachexia and fever.

this disease had symptoms of SVC obstruction at diagnosis.

SVCS is rare in the pediatric population. The most common cause today is vascular thrombosis secondary to cardiovascular surgery for congenital heart disease, or, more importantly, catheterization for venous access [9]. However, malignant tumors, particularly NHL, continue to head the list as the most common cause of SVC obstruction in children. The next most common cause is histoplasmosis, which may be seen in patients from areas where this infection is endemic [10]. An extensive review of the literature by Issa et al. [11] in 1983 revealed 150 reported cases of SVCS in childhood. Of these, only 24 (16%) were neoplastic in origin, 16 of them resulting from NHL and one from Hodgkin's lymphoma (HL). In another study, Pokorny and Sherman [12] described 109 children with mediastinal masses, including 24 with lymphoma. SVCS occurred in 3 (20%) of 15 children with NHL and in none of 9 with HL. An interesting, recent study of patients from the Chaim Sheba Medical Center in Israel demonstrated that the main cause of SVCS in their pediatric population was NHL [13]. Over a period of 11 years, 9 of 11 patients (11 months–12 years) who presented with SVCS had NHL and 2 had HL. In another review, of the 121 children with mediastinal masses who presented to the Royal Children's Hospital, Melbourne, the most common cause found was NHL (36 cases) [14]. These studies reiterate the fact that NHL is still the most frequent neoplastic cause of SVC obstruction in children.

The anatomy of the SVC, with its thin wall and close apposition to the vertebral column, make it particularly vulnerable to compression or invasion by malignancies arising in the mediastinum. It is surrounded by lymph nodes that drain the right and lower left sides of the chest, and the thymus in the anterior, superior mediastinum. Thus, involvement of the thymus or adjacent lymph nodes by tumor can cause compression of the SVC. Prolonged compression and/or invasion frequently results in intraluminal thrombosis (which may be exacerbated by the low-pressure flow within the SVC) and complete occlusion of the vein, although lymphomas, being less invasive and more rapidly growing than carcinomas, more often cause compression without thrombosis [15]. The trachea and right main stem bronchus, although relatively rigid when compared to the SVC, can also be easily compressed by tumor in children. The small intraluminal diameter of the trachea in children compared to adults can only accomodate minimal edema; thus symptoms of respiratory obstruction often occur rapidly. The degree and rapidity of obstruction that occurs secondary to compression, clotting and edema determines the severity of the symptoms and

signs. Collateral vessels enlarge in compensation but fail to relieve the obstruction adequately in most instances.

Both adults and children with SVC obstruction can present with a wide range of clinical symptoms, which commonly include cough, hoarseness, chest pain, dyspnea and orthopnea. Respiratory distress and hoarseness were the prominent symptoms in all 11 children with T-cell lymphoma who presented to the Chaim Sheba Medical Center, Israel [13]. Armstrong et al. [3] found that dyspnea, often associated with swelling of the trunk or extremities, was the most common presenting symptom in both bronchogenic carcinomas and lymphomas. Other less common but more sinister symptoms suggesting cerebral edema are those of dizziness, headache, anxiety, epistaxis, distorted vision, altered mental status and syncope, the latter often aggravated by bending [1,4,15–17]. Signs of SVCS include swelling, plethora and cyanosis of the face, neck and arms with prominence of collateral veins, diaphoresis, wheezing and stridor. There may be associated pleural or pericardial effusions. The presence of a pleural effusion may indicate simultaneous obstruction of the thoracic duct, although direct involvement of the pleura is also likely. The presence of laryngeal and/or cerebral edema has often been stated to indicate a poor prognosis in patients with SVC obstruction [4,5], but these complications are rare and have not been clearly shown to be an immediate consequence of SVC obstruction – they may be more likely caused by direct compression of airways, or invasion of the brain by tumor [18]. An unusual finding, not reported in children but sometimes seen in adults in association with SVCS, is spinal cord compression [19]. This again probably relates most often to direct compression by tumor rather than venous congestion or infarction. In adults, the onset of SVCS caused by malignant tumor is often insidious (depending on the histology), with symptoms developing over a period of a few weeks, in contrast to children and adolescents in whom they may rapidly progress in a few days.

In a patient who presents with clinical evidence of SVC obstruction, an efficient radiological work-up can help in establishing the diagnosis, guide attempts at pathologic confirmation, and aid in management decisions [20]. Routine studies of demonstrable ability include chest X-rays, ultrasound, computed tomography (CT) and magnetic resonance imaging (MRI) scans, venography and nuclear flow studies.

A chest X-ray can usually be obtained expeditiously and almost always demonstrates a right-sided mediastinal mass or mediastinal widening. Armstrong et al. [3] found a superior mediastinal mass in 59% of all patients with an SVCS, with a right-sided hilar mass in an additional 19%. Pleural and pericardial effusions, hilar adenopathy and evidence of tracheal compression may also be seen on chest X-ray. A CT scan of the chest has the advantage of providing more accurate information on the location of the obstruction and is useful for guiding subsequent attempts at biopsy via mediastinoscopy, bronchoscopy or percutaneous fine-needle aspiration. A peripheral venogram may be helpful in determining the patency of the venous system as well as the establishment and efficiency of collateral circulation [21,22] but this is a more invasive procedure which requires the use of iodinated contrast material. It is also associated with an increased risk of bleeding or thrombus formation, and therefore has largely been replaced by radionuclide flow studies. Gallium single photo emission CT (SPECT) may be of value in selected cases [23]. MRI of the mediastinum has several advantages over a CT, including the ability to image in several different planes and to visualize blood flow directly without the use of iodinated contrast material [24,25]. However, it has some disadvantages such as the length of time needed for scanning (which may not be ideal in a patient with SVCS and respiratory distress) and high cost.

A histological diagnosis of malignancy is essential prior to initiation of antineoplastic therapy. However, it is wise to avoid biopsy of a large mediastinal mass if possible, because of its relative inaccessibility and the potential for complications [26]. Children with SVCS or SMS tolerate invasive diagnostic procedures poorly. Patients with large mediastinal masses are at increased risk for developing complications during the induction of anesthesia [1,27] (primarily because of airway obstruction) or during the surgical procedure itself. Difficulty in intubation, acute cardiac arrest as well as increased bleeding from engorged mediastinal veins have been described [18,28]. If tracheal intubation is performed (either as an emergency procedure for respiratory arrest or electively for diagnostic purposes), it may be difficult to extubate the patient until significant reduction in the size of the mediastinal mass has been achieved. In consequence, some authors have recommended therapy with corticosteroids (which may induce only minimum shrinkage) or mediastinal radiotherapy before performing a biopsy [18]. This course should only be undertaken when there is no alternative to mediastinal biopsy and the latter is considered to be too risky to undertake.

Clearly, because of the risks associated with anesthesia, the least invasive procedure likely to establish a diagnosis of lymphoma should be chosen in patients with a mediastinal mass. A simple blood count may show evidence of leukemia or a fine-needle aspiration or biopsy of an enlarged peripheral lymph node under local anesthesia may provide the diagnosis. Detailed characterization of cells from a pleural effusion (including immunophenotyping), if present, should be performed and the bone marrow should always be examined for involvement prior to a surgical procedure. If the tumor is confined to the mediastinum, however, then biopsy via a mediastinoscope or parasternal mediastinotomy is warranted, if deemed safe. Mediastinoscopy provides better access to paratracheal masses than mediastinotomy, which is the procedure of choice for anterior mediastinal tumors [15]. It has been reported to be a safe and effective technique for establishing a histological diagnosis in SVCS when less invasive techniques have been unsuccessful [29]. A major concern is the risk of bleeding with mediastinoscopy in the presence of SVCS, but data from several published series suggest that this is an uncommon problem [30,31]. An alternative method to establish the diagnosis in patients with advanced SVCS is ultrasound-guided transthoracic needle aspiration biopsy. In two recent reports [32,33], the diagnostic yield, using this method in 41 patients with advanced SVCS, was between 83% and 100%. None of the patients were reported to have had any complications.

Clearly, in patients with lymphoma causing SVC obstruction, it is appropriate to institute treatment expeditiously. It is worth pointing out, however, that the presence of SVC obstruction itself does not appear to be life threatening. It is the accompanying tracheal compression and respiratory embarrassment that prompts emergency management [34,35]. Ligation of the SVC in dogs is not fatal, and symptoms abate in one week [18]. Fatalities caused by venous obstruction *per se*, have not been indisputably demonstrated in the literature and patients have survived for as long as 28 years with unrelieved SVC obstruction [18]. Indeed, autopsy evidence in a series of almost 2000 cases with malignant SVC obstruction treated by radiotherapy and the observation of spontaneous resolution in 44 patients not treated with radiotherapy [35] strongly suggest that in SVC sydrome overall, resolution of symptoms is probably most often the result of the development of a collateral circulation rather than relief of the SVC obstruction itself. These large series, however, contain few patients with lymphomas (only three were included in the latter series) and caution is required in applying the lessons learned from SVC obstruction caused by carcinomas to SVC obstruction caused by lymphomas because of the difference in growth rate of these tumors.

Nevertheless, these observations do suggest that emergency treatment is not indicated simply because of the presence of SVC obstruction, and that an uncomplicated SVC syndrome does not represent sufficient grounds for immediate irradiation without the establishment of a pathological diagnosis.

Chemotherapy can bring about rapid resolution of SVC obstruction caused by NHL and is emerging as the treatment of choice in this situation. This is already the case in aggressive, high-grade lymphomas, where a considerable reduction of tumor bulk can be achieved with a single cycle of chemotherapy, and is particularly relevant in children where the most common NHL causing SVC obstruction is lymphoblastic lymphoma, in which overall survival is not improved by the addition of mediastinal radiation to chemotherapy [16]. In fact, in younger patients, radiation may cause additional problems, such as tracheal edema, resulting in postirradiation respiratory embarrassment, and may significantly increase the risk of late pulmonary or cardiac toxicity. Radiotherapy should thus be reserved for tumors that are less likely to respond quickly to chemotherapy.

When radiotherapy is utilized, the field usually includes all gross tumor plus a tumor-free margin. The mediastinal, hilar and supraclavicular lymph nodes are also usually irradiated, but this will depend upon plans for subsequent chemotherapy [17]. Although the total radiation dose and rate of administration are dependent on the type of tumor, the patient's condition and the degree of local disease extension, relatively low-dose therapy is preferable, when radiation is being used purely as emergency therapy, e.g., to a total of 1200 cGy, to avoid local complications such as esophagitis, including recall esophagitis with subsequent chemotherapy. Irradiation of a large volume of bone marrow may also significantly impair the ability to deliver subsequent chemotherapy effffectively. Anthracyclines, usually an important component of NHL treatment, enhance radiation damage, so that the risk of added toxicity, especially esophagitis, pericarditis and myocardial damage, is significantly increased if mediastinal irradiation is used. Tumors such as lymphoblastic lymphoma, which are extremely radioresponsive, can undergo rapid dissolution with doses as little as 200 cGy. Almost 75% of patients with SVCS syndrome who receive radiation experience symptomatic relief within 3–4 days after initiation of treatment, while 90% are symptom free by the end of the first week [26]. In the 10% of patients whose symptoms do not improve within the first week of therapy, one should either reconsider the diagnosis, or suspect thrombosis and consider treatment with anticoagulants.

Rarely, a patient may need other emergency measures, such as a decompressive SVC bypass. It is recommended that an SVC bypass be considered early in the occasional patient who presents with profound cerebral or laryngeal edema, extensive thrombosis of the SVC, or severe hypertension and in whom a tissue diagnosis requires a mediastinal exploration [34].

Neurological emergencies

Involvement of the central nervous system (CNS) by malignant lymphoma has been well described [35–40], its overall incidence ranging between 5% and 11% some time during the course of NHL [35,40]. The most frequent type of neurological involvement reported is meningeal infiltration, followed by spinal cord compression [40–42], although some series report the opposite [43]. CNS involvement can either be a presenting feature or occur at relapse (in isolation or accompanied by systemic disease). Prior to the advent of CNS prophylaxis, cerebral and meningeal disease frequently occurred in patients who had achieved clinical remission, as is shown by Levitt et al. [35] in their series of 30 patients, 12 of whom relapsed within 9 months of the initiation of therapy. Risk factors for the development of CNS involvement include a histological diagnosis of high-grade lymphoma (82% of patients described by Young et al. had diffuse histology as compared to 3% with nodular lymphoma [40]), advanced disease at presentation and associated bone marrow involvement.

Lymphomatous infiltration or compression of nervous tissue by a mass can occur in any part of the nervous system including the leptomeninges, cranial nerves, brain, spinal cord and peripheral nerves, resulting in neurological emergencies, such as paraplegia, cranial nerve or nerve plexus palsies, meningeal infiltration and intracerebral tumor. Lymphomatous masses arising from extradural locations (e.g., skull, orbit, nasopharynx, paraspinal) may also impinge upon adjacent nervous tissue. Radicular and spinal cord compression are the most common severe neurological complications seen in NHL [39].

The signs and symptoms of nervous system involvement can therefore be extremely diverse, and include relatively nonspecific, although potentially serious symptoms, such as headache, backache or seizures. The single most common presenting sign seen in patients with lymphomatous leptomeningitis is cranial nerve palsies, particularly involving the facial, oculomotor or abducens nerves [35,40]. Sometimes, more definite features of raised intracranial pressure, such as papilledema, bradycardia and vomiting are present, and localizing signs, such as motor weakness and sensory changes, may also be observed. Occasionally, patients may present with signs and symptoms indicative of a localized radiculopathy only, as reported by Levitt et al. [35]. In their series of 24 patients who had CNS involvement at presentation, five had features confined only to involvement of the lumbosacral (3) or brachial plexus (2). All five patients had negative myelograms, positive cerebrospinal fluid (CSF) cytologies, and lymphomatous infiltration of root and plexus documented at post mortem.

Meningeal involvement

Examination of the CSF is essential in establishing a diagnosis of lymphomatous meningitis (a positive yield can be obtained in almost 97% of all cases) and a lumbar puncture should always be performed at the commencement of treatment, except in the presence of an intracranial lesion, which may have the potential to induce herniation of intracranial structures through the tentorium cerebelli or foramen magnum. Primary diffuse infiltration of the cerebral parenchyma can be difficult to diagnose and often presents with generalized neurological deterioration and seizures, although there may also be localizing signs. The possibility that these symptoms and signs could be the result of intracranial hemorrhage or thrombosis, particularly in a patient who deteriorates neurologically while undergoing therapy (especially if thrombocytopenic, on heparin therapy or with a coagulation disorder), should be considered, for management of such a patient will be quite different.

Lymphomatous leptomeningitis usually responds well to intrathecal chemotherapy (usually via lumbar puncture or Ommaya reservoir) with methotrexate or cytarabine, and/or high-dose systemic administration of these drugs. Cranial irradiation may also be used in some circumstances, traditionally in the case of primary intracerebral lymphomas (although some investigators are eliminating radiation even in this situation) and high-dose corticosteroids are given in the presence of raised intracranial pressure.

Spinal cord compression

Spinal cord compression is a rare presentation of NHL, occurring in about 0.1–10.2% of patients as reported in different series [36,38,39,44]. It is most commonly caused by extradural disease, either owing to an isolated deposit within the spinal canal or by extension from an adjacent nodal mass or bone involvement. Less commonly, it may arise subdurally or within the spinal cord, when the disease may behave like a primary cerebral lymphoma, recurring within the CNS. The most frequent site of extradural compression appears to be the lower thoracic spine (T7–T12) followed by the lumbar and cervical spines and sacrum [36–39,45].

Extradural presentations of lymphoma have been described in all age groups, including childhood, but tend to cluster in the fifth to sixth decades [36,37,45].

In spite of the rarity of its occurrence, malignant lymphoma is still one of the most common causes of spinal cord compression. This complication has been reported as a late manifestation of NHL but is more often a presenting feature [36,38,45,46]. Patients may have rapidly or more slowly progressive symptoms, depending upon the growth rate of the lymphoma. Back pain is one of the most common symptoms and may precede the onset of myelopathy by a few days to a few months [36,38,39,45]. Any patient with proven or suspected cancer and unexplained back pain should be considered to have spinal cord compression and evaluated without delay (Table 27.4). Other presenting symptoms include paresthesias and/or weakness of the lower extremities, with complete paralysis and bladder dysfunction occurring in the most severe cases. On physical examination, the most common findings include a discrete sensory level, hyperreflexia and paraparesis or paraplegia [38]. Aggressive, rapidly growing lymphomas can result in painless paraplegia within hours; hence it is imperative that suspected paraspinal disease be evaluated and treated immediately in

Table 27.4 Evaluation and management of back pain in a patient with suspected or proven malignancy

Obtain complete history followed by a detailed neurological examination.

1. Evidence of rapidly progressive, severe neurological deficit indicative of cord or conus involvement:
   a. Immediate institution of high-dose steroids (dexamethasone)
   b. Emergency X-ray of the spine, MRI and/or metrizamide myelogram
   c. If evidence of spinal cord compression: treat with surgery, radiotherapy or chemotherapy as appropriate*

2. Stable neurological examination with mild deficits indicative of cauda involvement:
   a. Immediate institution of steroids (dexamethasone)
   b. X-ray of the spine, MRI and/or metrizamide myelogram within 24 hours
   c. Treat with chemotherapy or radiotherapy as appropriate

3. Normal neurological examination with no evidence of neurological deficits:
   a. X-ray of the spine, bone scan, CT scan/MRI within 48–96 hours
   b. Treat with chemotherapy once diagnosis has been obtained

Any patient with cancer and back pain should be considered to have spinal cord compression until proven otherwise.

* The therapeutic modality used will depend upon factors such as type of lymphoma, clinical situation (primary versus relapse), etc.

order to avoid irreversible neurological damage. Occasionally, infarction of the cord may occur, owing to compression of the spinal arteries, and such patients are unlikely to recover full function.

Plain films of the spine are usually unremarkable, especially in the case of primary spinal epidural lymphoma, and lack of bony involvement on plain film or CT scan can provide an important clue to diagnosis; thus extradural compression of the cord in the presence of normal radiographs should immediately arouse suspicion of a lymphoma [47]. Occasionally, lytic bony lesions and paraspinal lymphomatous masses may be detected on plain films. MRI, with gadolinium diethylenetriamine penta-acetic acid (DTPA), is the method of choice, today, for accurate determination of the level of the spinal cord block and has virtually replaced contrast myelography. Not only is MRI an excellent study for the demonstration of epidural disease, associated intra-parenchymal spread of tumor and small lesions compressing nerve roots in the cauda equina region, but it is also noninvasive, safer and takes less time to complete (which is of crucial importance in a patient with spinal cord compression) [48]. However, metrizamide myelography followed by spinal CT is still used in centers where MRI facilities are not available. In the absence of other sites of tumor, a laminectomy may be required to establish a histological diagnosis.

Current treatment of spinal cord compression consists of a combination of steroids and chemotherapy/radiotherapy to the spine (Table 27.4). A decision to utilize decompressive surgery should be made after taking into consideration factors such as the degree of paresis, histology of the lymphoma and whether the spinal cord compression is a manifestation of initial presentation or relapse. If the history is suggestive of rapidly progressive spinal cord dysfunction, high-dose steroids (dexamethasone) should be given immediately to try to reduce local edema and lessen the degree of compression, besides exerting a lympholytic effect. A laminectomy may be indicated in patients who present with spinal cord compression secondary to recurrence, particularly when it presents in a previous irradiated region [49]. Chemotherapy should be thought of as a primary therapeutic option for the treatment of spinal cord compression [37,44] and is probably more effective than radiotherapy in highly chemosensitive tumors such as Burkitt's lymphoma (which is also relatively radioresistant), lymphoblastic lymphoma and intermediate-grade lymphomas. The avoidance of radiation, where possible, has the advantage of not adding to myelosuppression because of irradiation of vertebral bone-marrow, or increasing the risk of severe esophagitis, and cardiac or pulmonary toxicity, when compres-

sion is in the thoracic spine. This is not a minor consideration in tumors where chemotherapy provides the only real chance of a cure.

Pleural and pericardial effusions

Pleural involvement

NHL that presents with mediastinal involvement is usually associated with malignant pleural or pericardial effusions that may be clinically silent and only detectable on a chest X-ray or CT scan, or large enough to cause significant respiratory distress. Leukemias and lymphomas account for approximately 13% of malignant pleural effusions, while 16% of patients with lymphoma are said develop a pleural effusion in the course of their disease [50]. Thoracocentesis is indicated for confirmation of diagnosis, relief from respiratory distress or occasionally for elimination of a potential reservoir for drugs such as methotrexate, which are used early on in the treatment of high-grade lymphoma [48]. Pleural effusions provide an excellent source of malignant cells for cytological and immunophenotypic diagnosis [51].

The most effective therapy for a malignant effusion is treatment of the underlying lymphoma. In a newly diagnosed patient with respiratory distress, it may be sufficient to remove fluid just once, since the initiation of specific therapy should prevent reaccumulation. However, an existing pleural effusion can be exacerbated by the hydration necessary for prevention of tumor lysis in patients with extensive disease, or prior to the institution of chemotherapy, especially with agents such as cyclophosphamide and methotrexate. Thus, repeated therapeutic thoracocentesis or an indwelling chest tube may sometimes become necessary for symptomatic relief while awaiting response to chemotherapy. Because rapid response to therapy is the rule, pleurodesis with a sclerosing agent [52–54] after complete drainage of the pleural fluid is only indicated for palliation of tumors refractory to chemotherapy. Of all the sclerosing agents, tetracycline seems to be the most effective and is thought to have the fewest side-effects [55]. If tetracycline fails, surgical pleurectomy may become necessary in patients with refractory disease.

Pericardial involvement

Pericardial effusion can occur either through hematogenous spread or as a result of direct extension from adjacent lymph nodes. Although less common than pleural effusions, it is a far more serious complication of lymphoma because of the risk of life-threatening cardiac tamponade (the inability of the left ventricle to mantain output, usually because of extrinsic pressure or rarely because of an intrinsic mass). Thus, suspicion of a malignant pericardial effusion mandates rapid evaluation and, depending on the duration and severity of symptoms, urgent treatment. In those cases where gradual accumulation of fluid occurs within the pericardial sac, symptoms of cough and dyspnea develop slowly, and tamponade is less likely. However, the rapid accumulation of even a few hundred milliliters can cause tamponade, and result in symptoms resembling heart failure, namely, the sudden onset of cough, chest pain, dyspnea, orthopnea and non-specific abdominal pain [26,48].

M-mode or two-dimensional echocardiography, which demonstrates two echoes, one from the cardiac muscle and the other from the pericardium, is probably the most useful test for determining the presence and severity of both a pericardial effusion and cardiac tamponade [26,48]. It should be performed whenever a pericardial effusion is suspected because of the symptoms described above, or in the presence of a pericardial rub, characteristic low-voltage QRS complexes with ST segment elevation and T-wave flattening or inversion on an electrocardiogram, or because of suggestive radiological findings of cardiomegaly with the typical 'waterbag shadow'. When there are signs of cardiac tamponade, such as pulsus paradoxus, hypotension and elevated venous pressure, pericardiocentesis should be performed without delay. This procedure both relieves tamponade and provides fluid for diagnostic cytology. As with pleural effusions caused by lymphoma, pericardial fluid usually stops accumulating after the initiation of chemotherapy. Radiotherapy should be avoided, if possible, because of the potential for cardiac damage, particularly if an anthracycline is included in the planned drug regimen. Continuous drainage of the pericardium with a catheter or surgical construction of a pericardial window may be necessary while awaiting a response to chemotherapy, if reaccumulation of fluid is rapid after pericardiocentesis or for palliation in patients with refractory lymphomas. In the latter circumstance, the instillation of tetracycline into the pericardial sac has successfully prevented the accumulation of pericardial fluid without causing constrictive pericarditis, as seen in 15 of 22 and 30 of 33 patients described by Shepherd and Davis et al. [53,54].

Pulmonary embolism secondary to a large intra-abdominal mass

The association of cancer and a hypercoagulable state, often leading to pulmonary embolism, is well known [56–60]. Almost all cancer patients, including those with lymphoma, are at increased risk of developing thromboembolism some time during the course of their disease, with a reported clinical incidence somewhere between 1% and 11% [57,60]. Abnormal results on routine coagulation studies suggesting hypercoagulability, namely, elevated levels of fibrin degradation products, thrombocytosis and hyperfibrinogenemia, have been described in up to 90% of these patients [57,58]. Besides hypercoagulability, several other important mechanisms, such as stasis, recent surgery with its associated immobility, paraplegia and chemotherapy also contribute to the pathogenesis of thromboembolic disease in cancer patients, particularly those with abdominal lymphomas [56,59].

By direct compression or distortion of the inferior vena cava (IVC), large abdominal lymphomas may cause venous obstruction and secondary stasis. As a result, the patient may present with a significant, intraluminal thrombus which sometimes causes distal edema (particularly if multiple venous channels are obstructed) or may be silent. The possibility of a thrombus in the IVC and its associated risk of pulmonary embolism should be kept in mind whenever a patient presents with a large intra-abdominal mass, and evaluation of venous flow, either by Doppler ultrasound or B-mode ultrasonography and duplex scanning is often indicated [57,60]. The latter technique is preferred because of its high sensitivity and concomitant imaging of the surrounding soft tissues. Tumor masses in close proximity to, or compressing, major veins are easily identified [60]. CT scans with contrast and MRI scans are also useful in the diagnosis of venous thrombosis [60].

Once a clot has been suspected or identified in the IVC prior to therapy, immediate measures should be undertaken to prevent a possible episode of pulmonary embolism. This necessitates intervention at the start of chemotherapy, either in the form of anticoagulation, or physical containment of the thrombus (placement of a filter). The period of highest risk for an embolus is immediately after the initiation of chemotherapy, when there is rapid and significant reduction in the size of the abdominal tumor [56–60]. Anticoagulation, especially with heparin, can be hazardous because of the risk of gastrointestinal bleeding from involvement of bowel, coupled with thrombocytopenia secondary to bone marrow involvement, chemotherapy or heparin itself. In addition, anticoagulation by oral drugs, such as warfarin, is difficult to control when potentially hepatotoxic chemotherapeutic agents (e.g., methotrexate) are to be administered.

Recently, the introduction of low molecular weight heparin (LMWH) for the treatment of thromboembolism has led to a greater than 50% reduction in bleeding episodes and mortality, compared to treatment with standard heparin [56–60], and LMWH may be appropriate for some patients, particularly in the absence of gastrointestinal disease. An alternative to heparin treatment is the emergency placement of an intraluminal device in the IVC below the renal veins, e.g., a Hunter–Session balloon or Greenfield filter (umbrella). Although only nonrandomized studies addressing this method have been published, preliminary results suggest that the placement of a percutaneous Greenfield filter in the IVC is preferred over anticoagulation therapy in high-risk patients, e.g., cancer patients at high risk for bleeding following chemotherapy [61–63]. Some authors even suggest that filter placement should be used as a primary means of preventing pulmonary embolus in patients with cancer and thromboembolic disease [61–63]. In the event of a suspected episode of pulmonary embolism, an attempt should be made to establish the diagnosis, either by utilization of lung scanning, and, if the patient is stable, pulmonary angiography. However, in an unstable patient, this may be difficult to achieve, in which case, an alternative approach employed, could be to look for coincident deep vein thrombosis in the lower extremities. In either event, antifibrinolytic therapy should be initiated immediately, with close monitoring for complications, primarily bleeding. In the event of an hemorrhage, treatment should be stopped, and red cell transfusions, along with fresh-frozen plasma or cryoprecipitate to replenish the fibrinogen, initiated immediately. Additional platelet transfusions may also be required in a thrombocytopenic patient. Usual recommendations for anticoagulation therapy are to continue with LMWH or oral anticoagulants (if feasible) for at least 3–6 months after an acute episode [64]. However, each patient needs to be evaluated individually and it is possible that, in the face of ongoing, intensive treatment, patients may need to stop anticoagulant therapy during the period of severe thrombocytopenia immediately following a cycle of chemotherapy, in order to avoid hemorrhagic complications.

Obstructive uropathy

A frequently encountered complication of large intra-abdominal and pelvic lymphomas is obstruction of the ureters and urinary bladder, resulting in acute or subacute urinary retention. Renal ultrasound is the simplest test to document obstructive uropathy, and the size of the kidney, extent of hydronephrosis and the amount of residual renal cortex are extremely helpful in determining the potential for restoration of renal function, which is usually very high in this situation [26,48]. A CT scan may be required to determine the actual site of obstruction, which is often not well defined on renal ultrasound.

Once diagnosed, an effort should be made to relieve the obstruction as soon as possible. Ureteric obstruction can best be managed by hemodialysis (to normalize serum electrolyte, uric acid, urea and creatinine levels) followed by appropriate chemotherapy. Placement of ureteral stents or nephrostomy tubes is not normally recommended because of the risk of perforation or leakage, thus increasing the risk of infection and delaying chemotherapy [65]. However, in circumstances where hemodialysis is not available, e.g., developing countries, this may be a reasonable course of action. Peritoneal dialysis, even in the presence of abdominal lymphoma, has also been used with success.

Pharyngeal obstruction

A complication seen sometimes with high-grade lymphomas is pharyngeal obstruction secondary to a large neck mass, resulting in difficulty in swallowing. Usually, the mass is large enough to cause some airway compromise at the same time. Chemotherapy for the underlying lymphoma is the indicated treatment.

METABOLIC COMPLICATIONS

Hyperuricemia and the tumor lysis syndrome

Hyperuricemia is a well-recognized occurrence at presentation in patients with extensive hematopoietic neoplasms, particularly NHL [22]. Along with other metabolic complications, it occurs predominantly in the B-cell lymphomas (small noncleaved cell and large B-cell) and to a lesser extent, in lymphoblastic lymphomas, all of which have a high growth fraction [66–68]. Rapid turnover of these tumor cells, rich in nucleic acids, especially DNA, leads to an increase in the solute burden on the kidneys, resulting in renal complications that include oliguric acute renal failure prior to treatment, an exacerbation after the initiation of chemotherapy and, sometimes, sudden death [69–72] (Table 27.5). Both hyperuricemia and hyperuricosuria – from two to five times the normal rate – can occur [73,74]. Uric acid nephropathy, leading ultimately to renal failure correlates directly with the tumor burden [69–71,75–77] and, therefore, tends to be associated with a worse prognosis. Tumor lysis syndrome, which is a combination of hyperuricemia, hyperkalemia and hyperphosphatemia with hypocalcemia, occurring shortly after the initiation of chemotherapy, does not occur in patients who present with a low tumor burden or in whom all tumor has been resected at diagnosis.

Table 27.5 Characteristics of renal failure associated with tumor lysis syndrome

	Type of nephropathy		
	Uric acid	Phosphate	Xanthine
Hyperkalemia	++	+	+/−
Uricosemia	++	+	+
Hyperphosphatemia	+	++	+
Predisposing factors	Aciduria	Alkaluria	Allopurinol
Time of onset	Before and after starting therapy	Within 48 hours after starting therapy	After starting allopurinol
Prevention	Hydration, alkalinization, allopurinol	Hydration	Hydration

+, Increase in potassium, urate and phosphate levels in plasma; ++, marked increase in potassium, urate and phosphate levels in plasma; +/−, mild to no increase in potassium, urate and phosphate levels in plasma.

Whereas it is important to initiate specific therapy as soon as possible, starting chemotherapy in the presence of hyperuricemia and an impaired urinary output without corrective measures is likely to result in the death of the patient, probably from hyperkalemia, because potassium released from tumor cells cannot be excreted efficiently in the absence of an adequate urine flow. Therefore, the biochemical abnormalities must be corrected before the initiation of specific therapy (although this by no means guarantees that a tumor lysis syndrome will not occur). This period of biochemical correction should not normally exceed 24–48 hours. Reduction of serum uric acid to normal levels can usually be accomplished within this time by alkaline diuresis and allopurinol administration, unless there is additional renal compromise owing to ureteric obstruction, or rarely, massive involvement of the kidneys by tumor. In a review of 37 patients with advanced-stage Burkitt's lymphoma who were treated with induction chemotherapy, renal failure was present at the outset in eight of the patients, two of whom required dialysis for uric acid nephropathy before chemotherapy could be instituted [76]. When hemodialysis is instituted, chemotherapy is normally commenced after the completion of a period of hemodialysis, when biochemical parameters are close to normal. Since further dialysis is unlikely to be required for at least a few hours, the possibility of removing drugs (e.g., cyclophosphamide) by dialysis is, in this way, minimized. There is little comparative information on cyclophosphamide elimination via normal kidneys versus hemodialysis.

In Europe, some protocols, e.g., the COP regimen in the French Pediatric Oncology Society (SFOP) protocol LMB81, call for the use of a 'pre-phase', that is, low-dose chemotherapy given a week before initiation of the major induction regimen, to lessen the risk of tumor lysis [78,79]. Uricase, an enzyme that directly degrades uric acid and rapidly reduces uricosemia, is also available in some European countries.

It is advisable to manage patients at highest risk for developing tumor lysis syndrome initially in a critical care unit because of the intensive monitoring required. Vigorous hydration with 0.5 N saline (or equivalent sodium content) in the region of 4500–5500 ml/m^2 of body surface area every 24 hours, liberal use of diuretics where necessary (e.g., intravenous furosemide, 2–3 mg every 2–3 hours) and allopurinol (initially 10 mg/kg/day in three divided doses) should be commenced immediately in this group of patients in order to maintain a high urine flow (as much as 250–350 ml/m^2/hour or even more in patients at highest risk) for the first few days after the initiation of chemotherapy. This is to ensure that the high solute load created by tumor lysis (primarily composed of phosphates and oxypurines) is accommodated without the onset of hyperkalemia or acute renal failure. Because of relatively poor solubility of phosphates in alkaline urine and the risk of intratubular deposition, it is preferable to maintain the urine pH at about 7 and not to administer bicarbonate during chemotherapy.

Both allopurinol and its metabolite oxypurinol are strong inhibitors of the enzyme xanthine oxidase, and markedly reduce the conversion of xanthine and hypoxanthine to uric acid. This results in the excretion of purines in three forms that are independently soluble in urine [69]. Alkalinization of the urine to a pH of approximately 7 increases the solubility of acid and xanthine. At this pH, uric acid is 10–12 times more soluble [80], and xanthine more than twice as soluble, than at pH 5. The solubility of hypoxanthine differs little at either pH. High-dose allopurinol ensures that a significant proportion of purine metabolites is excreted as xanthine and hypoxanthine, but if urate production is totally inhibited, there is an increased risk of xanthine nephropathy [81]. The objective of allopurinol therapy is, therefore, to increase the total amount of oxypurine that can be excreted in a given volume of urine rather than to inhibit uric acid formation completely.

Under physiological conditions, the solubility product for total calcium and phosphate is 4.6×10^{-6} mol/l [69,82]. When this product is exceeded (as mentioned above), calcium phosphate salts may be precipitated in the renal parenchyma and other soft tissues. Hyperphosphatemia, which may give rise to hypocalcemia and renal failure, occurs within 48 hours of the onset of chemotherapy, is maximal on the 2nd and 3rd days, and may last for up to 7 days [83]. For this reason, hypocalcemia should not be treated unless symptomatic (presenting with tetany or cardiac arrythmias), and intravenous calcium chloride should be given with great caution, if at all. Rarely, hemodialysis may be required for symptomatic hypocalcemia.

The acute tumor lysis syndrome was originally recognized because of sudden death occurring as a direct consequence of hyperkalemia, which may occur within hours of starting therapy. Thus, potassium supplements should be avoided shortly before and during the first few days of therapy, except in exceptional circumstances. Ideally, the patient should be mildly hypokalemic prior to the start of chemotherapy. Hyperkalemia is most unlikely to occur in the presence of a high urine output and, in fact, urine flow is the key to the management of the tumor lysis syndrome. As long as a high urine flow can be maintained, other interventions are unlikely to be needed. If this is not the case, rapid progression of biochemical abnormalities will occur, necessitating emergency hemodialysis.

One problem that can considerably complicate the management of the tumor lysis syndrome is a tendency for fluids to collect in a third space, including serous effusions (ascites, and sometimes pleural effusions), or even limb edema from venous and/or lymphatic obstruction. In such patients, vigorous hydration is complicated by weight gain and an inappropriately low urine flow. This situation can usually be managed by the judicious use of diuretics and careful monitoring of the central venous pressure or pulmonary wedge venous pressure. How-

ever, if an acceptable urine output cannot be maintained, hemodialysis should be instituted.

Hypercalcemia of malignancy

Hypercalcemia is defined as a serum calcium level greater than 2.6 mmol/l (10.5 mg/dl). Levels above 3.0 mmol/l (12.0 mg/dl) may cause transitional disturbances in virtually every organ system, while those above 5.0 mmol/l (20.0 mg/dl) can be fatal [48]. Hypercalcemia is the most common life-threatening metabolic disorder associated with cancer, usually occurring in about 10–20% of patients with advanced malignancy [83a]. It is, however, an uncommon complication of malignant lymphoma, and is generally encountered only in HTLV-1-associated adult T-cell lymphomas and some childhood NHLs such as Burkitt's lymphoma (rarely), and lymphoblastic lymphoma widely metastatic to bone [83b,83c].

Malignant hypercalcemia can be caused by two primary pathophysiologic mechanisms. The first is a result of excessive bone resorption, usually associated with bony metastases. Normal calcium homeostasis is mantained when there is a balance between bone resorption and bone deposition. Bone resorption is stimulated by parathyroid hormone (PTH), prostaglandin E2, polypeptide growth factors, osteoclast activating factor (OAF) and osteoclasts [84]. Hypercalcemia of malignancy is mediated by these same bone-resorbing factors, which can be produced or stimulated by the tumor itself [85]. The second mechanism leading to hypercalcemia is the syndrome of humoral hypercalcemia of malignancy, which occurs secondary to the ectopic production of PTH-like factor by malignant tumors, including lymphomas [86–89]. Although this syndrome is characterized by end-organ manifestations of PTH-like effects, actual production of PTH has rarely been documented. However, related peptides have recently been identified [89]. OAF has been found in association with hypercalcemia in patients with multiple myeloma and Burkitt's lymphoma [90,91].

Hypercalcemia most often occurs in patients with large tumor burdens and may be precipitated by dehydration or immobilization. Once the plasma calcium level rises, homeostatic mechanisms are activated to normalize the serum calcium level. If these mechanisms cannot keep up with the rapidly rising serum calcium, the hypercalcemia itself begins to cause renal dysfunction, with a decrease in the glomerular filtration rate and concentrating ability of the kidneys, resulting in dehydration and consequent worsening of the hypercalcemia. Anorexia and vomiting, a direct effect of hypercalcemia, cause further volume depletion. As a result, there is decrease in the urinary output and, unless aggressively treated, a hypercalcemic crisis can ensue rapidly [92].

There is little correlation between serum calcium levels and the severity of signs and symptoms of hypercalcemia. However, a relationship has been noted between clinical manifestations and the rate of rise of the calcium level [83a], the presence of other metabolic abnormalities and the extent of the patient's underlying debility from cancer [26]. Effects of hypercalcemia can be seen on the gastrointestinal (GI), renal, cardiovascular, neurologic and skeletal systems (Table 27.6). GI symptoms include nausea, vomiting, constipation and abdominal pain, while CNS symptoms are initially vague, being manifested as weakness, somnolence and lethargy, a symptom complex that can be mistaken for intracerebral involvement by lymphoma. Polyuria, precipitation of calcium phosphate in the renal tubules and stones can occur [83a]. Hypercalcemia of any degree can cause some increase in myocardial contractility and irritability, but serum calcium levels over 4.0 mmol/l (16 mg%) can result in fatal cardiac arrhythmias [83a,83d]. Bony symptoms, in the form of bone pain, fractures and skeletal deformities, are often found in the presence of hypercalcemia [85].

Treatment of hypercalcemia secondary to lymphoma must include both, specific therapy for the hypercalcemia in addition to treatment for the underlying lymphoma (Table 27.6). Acute hypercal-

Table 27.6 Clinical presentation and treatment of hypercalcemia of malignancy

Signs and symptoms

Gastrointestinal
  Anorexia, nausea, vomiting, constipation, abdominal pain and ileus

Cardiovascular
  Bradycardia, arrythmias, bundle branch block

Renal
  Polyuria, nocturia, dehydration, calcium phosphate stones

Central nervous system
  Lethargy, apathy, depression, psychoses, stupor and coma

Musculoskeletal
  Hypotonia, bone pain, fractures

Treatment

Vigorous hydration with saline diuresis
Thyrocalcitonin
Mithramycin
Biphosphonates
Gallium nitrate
Corticosteroids

cemia needs to be treated aggressively in an effort to prevent its deleterious consequences. A serum calcium level of more than 3.5 mmol/l (14 mg%) should be considered a medical emergency and treated in an intensive care unit with close cardiac monitoring. In patients with a serum calcium level less than 3.5 mmol/l (14 mg%), saline repletion with standard furosemide (1 mg/kg) diuresis usually provides adequate control while definitive treatment for the lymphoma is being initiated. With higher serum calcium levels, a more vigorous forced diuresis is recommended for adults, using volumes of normal saline up to 3 times the maintenance requirement with furosemide (2–3 mg/kg) every 2 hours, with the goal of achieving a urine output of at least 500 ml/hour [93]. Urine output, electrolytes and magnesium should be closely monitored during therapy as almost half the patients with hypercalcemia are hypokalemic at presentation, and require potassium and magnesium replacement during saline diuresis.

There are a number of pharmacological agents available for the treatment of hypercalcemia that does not respond to the above measures. In an acute crisis, agents such as thyrocalcitonin [3–8 units/kg intravenously (i.v.)] can be administered in conjunction with the saline diuresis. The calcitonin acts within 1–2 hours to reduce serum calcium by inhibiting bone resorption. However, almost 25% of patients may not respond and resistance has been noted with repeated administration [83d,94]. Mithramycin, an antineoplastic antibiotic (25 μg/kg i.v.), is also recommended for use in an emergency situation and is usually effective within 12–35 hours [88,95]. Long-term use of Mithramycin is not feasible because of hepatotoxicity [95]. Recently, a number of biphosphonates (e.g., etidronate, 7.5 mg/kg i.v.) and gallium nitrate have been approved for the treatment of hypercalcemia of malignancy [96–99], and found to be effective in restoring normal calcium levels in anywhere from 47% to 85% of patients. Rarely, hemodialysis may be necessary in unresponsive cases.

Chronic hypercalcemia may be treated with oral phosphates, weekly doses of Mithramycin or, in the case of lymphomas, corticosteroids. The latter are believed to work by decreasing the intestinal absorption and renal excretion of calcium. These measures provide only temporary amelioration, however, and control of the underlying lymphoma is clearly the treatment of choice.

Syndrome of inappropriate antidiuretic hormone secretion

Syndrome of inappropriate antidiuretic hormone secretion (SIADH) is a paraneoplastic syndrome characterized by dilutional hyponatremia in the face

severity of neutropenia in patients receiving chemotherapy for a variety of cancers, and after BMT [137,138] (see Chapter 29). In contrast, results of a recent NCI protocol for the treatment of small noncleaved cell (SNCC) and large-cell lymphoma in children and adults, which utilized GM-CSF, did not demonstrate any significant decrease in the duration of neutropenia or documented infections, but did demonstate an increase in the duration of thrombocytopenia [139], suggesting that it should not be assumed that CSFs will always be of value. Further, treatment with colony-stimulating factors is not without side-effects, and fever, rashes, myalgias, bone pain, capillary leak syndromes in adult patients and severe atypical neuropathy (discussed below) have been seen with the administration of these factors in conjunction with chemotherapy [140,141]; G-CSF appears to be less toxic than GM-CSF. Guidelines for the administration of CSFs have been proposed.

The frequency of fever and neutropenia in some studies has been sufficiently high as to suggest the use of prophylactic antibiotics [141]. This, however, is a controversial area. Numerous studies have been conducted to evaluate the value of both nonabsorbable antibiotics (e.g., gentamycin, vancomycin, polymyxin and colistin) and absorbable oral antibiotics (e.g., trimethoprim-sulphamethoxazole, erythromycin and quinolones) in preventing either the acquisition or the decrease in the number of potentially pathogenic, colonizing organisms in a neutropenic host [141]. In recent years, most investigators have utilized the flouroquinolones (norfloxacin and ciprofloxacin) for prophylaxis, since these agents can be taken orally, are well absorbed and give high systemic drug levels [142,143]. Although these studies have clearly demonstrated a reduction in Gram-negative infections, no significant reduction in Gram-positive infections or infection-related mortality rates has been observed. In addition, reports of organisms resistant to the quinolones are increasing in frequency, leading to concern that overuse of these drugs will negate their benefit [144,145]. Contrary to these reports, Gilbert et al. recently described their experience with the prophylactic use of a combination of oral ciprofloxacin and rifampin in patients undergoing autologous BMT (ABMT) for breast cancer [146]. A total of 99 women received this combination of antibiotics after receiving high-dose chemotherapy followed by bone marrow rescue. The incidence of fever was reduced from 98% to 57%, documented infections from 42% to 13%, and bacteremia from 18% to 0% (*P*<0.001) in patients who received ABMT and stem cell support; while documented infections were reduced from 74% to 17% (*P*<0.001), and bacteremia from 29% to 7% in patients who received bone marrow purged with

chemotherapy and monoclonal antibodies. There was a very low incidence of Gram-positive infections (unlike other studies), and no episodes of breakthrough bacteremia or sepsis were reported. These results support further investigation of the use of prophylactic antibiotic regimens in high-risk patient populations.

A significant decrease in the incidence of herpetic gingivostomatitis, pneumocystis pneumonia, CMV infection and candidial infections has been demonstrated with the prophylactic use of antiviral, antiparasitic and antifungal agents (namely, acyclovir, trimethoprim-sulphamethoxazole, gancyclovir and fluconazole) in neutropenic patients [147–149], and in particularly intensive, chemotherapy protocols or following BMT.

Anemia and thrombocytopenia

Chemotherapy-related temporary aplasia of the bone marrow is the most common cause of anemia in a patient with NHL. This anemia is further exaggerated by ongoing, external blood losses that occur either in association with thrombocytopenia (epistaxis or occult gastrointestinal tract bleeding) or secondary to repeated sampling for diagnostic tests. An additional component of the anemia of most cancer patients is the 'anemia of chronic disease', which is characterized by defective iron reutilization and diminished serum concentrations of erythropoietin (Epo) [150]. Treatment of chemotherapy-associated anemia is usually with packed red cell transfusions, not only for symptomatic patients, but also for those who have a borderline hemoglobin (close to 8 g/dl) and have just received an intensive cycle of chemotherapy. Irradiated blood products are preferred to minimize the risk of transfusion-associated graft-versus-host disease. However, blood transfusions are costly and inconvenient, besides being associated with the risk of transmitting infections, making it imperative to look for other alternatives to increase the hemoglobin level.

One such alternative to blood transfusion that is currently being investigated is the use of the hematopoetic growth factor Epo [151,152]. To date, several hundred anemic cancer patients have been entered in clinical trials and treated with Epo. Preliminary results look promising, and appear to indicate that Epo can alleviate anemia and dramatically reduce transfusion requirements in patients on chemotherapy.

Chemotherapy-associated bone marrow ablation is also the most common cause of thrombocytopenia in a cancer patient. Severe thrombocytopenia (a count less than $10\,000/\text{mm}^3$) puts a patient at high risk for hemorrhage and must be treated with prophylactic platelet transfusions. These transfusions are not without risk also, and problems with refractoriness, transfusion reactions, alloimmunization and hepatitis constantly have to be dealt with in patients who are undergoing chemotherapy. Alternatives to platelet transfusions that are currently being explored include the use of hematopoietic growth factors such as IL-3, IL-6 and IL-11 [152a]. The recently discovered thrombopoietin is likely to prove valuable in hastening recovery from chemotherapy induced thrombocytopenia.

ABDOMINAL EMERGENCIES

Typhlitis/neutropenic enterocolitis

Typhlitis is being increasingly recognized as a serious complication of aggressive chemotherapy for hematological and solid tumors. Typhlitis, from the Greek word *typhlon* meaning cecum, is a necrotizing inflammation of the cecum, sometimes extending into the ileum and ascending colon. Bacterial invasion of the mucosa is responsible for the inflammation, which can rapidly progress to infarction and perforation. *Clostridium septicum* is the bacterial organism most commonly implicated, followed by *Pseudomonas aeruginosa* [153]. Other terms used for typhlitis include neutropenic enterocolitis, necrotizing enterocolitis and ileocecal syndrome.

Typhlitis occurs specifically in immunodeficient patients, usually in the setting of severe neutropenia. Initially described as a complication of leukemia [154,155], it has subsequently been associated with lymphoma [156], aplastic anemia [157], immunosuppression following renal transplantation [158], the use of aggressive chemotherapy in patients with solid tumors [159,160] and in association with AIDS [161]. The pathogenesis of typhlitis is multifactorial. Implicating factors (besides those just mentioned) include intramural hemorrhage and massive bacterial invasion [153–155,160]. However, severe neutropenia and the microbiologic environment of the colon are the two most essential predisposing conditions necessary for the development of typhlitis. The cecum seems to be most vulnerable site compared to other parts of the large intestine because of its unique properties, namely, decreased vascular perfusion, decreased lymphatic drainage and greater distensibility and wall tension [155]. Direct cytotoxicity to the cecal mucosa from aggressive chemotherapy, utilizing drugs such as doxorubicin, Ara-C, methotrexate and taxol, etc., results in breaks in the cecal mucosa, which then serves as a portal of entry for bacteria [155,159,160].

Typhlitis is defined clinically as fever with abdominal pain, usually in the right lower quadrant, in the setting of grade 4 neutropenia (absolute neutrophil count <500/mm^3). It has, however, been seen to present in the absence of fever [39]. Other accompanying findings include nausea and vomiting, abdominal distension, diarrhea, rebound tenderness and occult blood in the stool [159]. The diagnosis is usually confirmed byultrasound [162] or CT scan [163]. Ultrasound findings of the characteristic 'target or halo' sign of a solid mass with an echogenic center (collapsed mucosa and intestinal contents) and hypoechoic periphery (thickened bowel wall) in the setting of abdominal pain in a neutropenic patient is diagnostic of typhlitis (Figure 27.1). CT findings in typhlitis usually include symmetric bowel wall thickening, pericecal inflammation and, if perforation has occurred, a pericecal soft tissue mass (Figure 27.2).

The management of neutropenic enterocolitis is controversial, especially with regard to the necessity and timing of surgical intervention [154,164]. However, in recent years, initial conservative management has become more acceptable [159]. Mortality is high, in the range of 50% to almost 100% with either surgical intervention or conservative treatment. If diagnosed early, a majority of patients can be managed medically with broad-spectrum antibiotics coupled with anaerobic coverage (clindamycin, metronidazole, imipenem) to cover for Gram-negative pathogens and gastrointestinal anaerobes. Surgery is indicated in the face of clinical deterioration in spite of intensive medical management. The details of the role of surgery in typhlitis is discussed elsewhere in Chapter 31.

Patients who do not fit the description of typhlitis, but have signs and symptoms of enterocolitis, may have antibiotic-related pseudomembranous or clostridial enterocolitis (discussed earlier).

NEUROLOGICAL COMPLICATIONS FOLLOWING CHEMOTHERAPY

Neurological complications in the form of transient seizures, encephalopathy and ascending myelopathy have been described in patients following the systemic or intrathecal administration of chemotherapeutic agents, such as methotrexate, cytosine arabinoside (ara-C), cisplatin and ifosfamide, all of which are extremely effective drugs for the treatment of high-grade lymphoma [48,165–167]. Methotrexate and ara-C continue to remain the two most commonly implicated drugs. However, these complications are uncommon, being seen in less than 3% of the patients receiving these agents [166,167].

In most instances, seizures occur as a result of the direct effect of the drug on the CNS. They can be seen, either following the use of systemic, high-dose chemotherapy (in particular, methotrexate, ara-C or

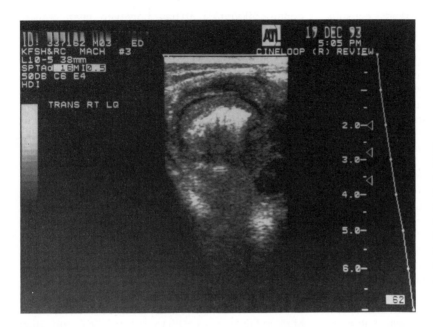

Figure 27.1 Ultrasound of the right lower abdominal quadrant demonstraing the 'halo sign' of a solid mass with an echogenic center (collapsed mucosa and intestinal contents), and hypoechoic periphery (thickened bowel wall). This is characteristic of typhlitis in a neutropenic patient. (Courtesy of Dr Alan Gray, Department of Radiology, King Faisal Special Hospital and Research Center, Saudia Arabia.)

ifosfamide) with or without associated intrathecal therapy, or following chemotherapy in patients who have received a prior insult such as cranial irradiation in the past [48,165]. Focal or generalized seizures can also occur as a result of metabolic abnormalities, such as SIADH or other electrolyte disturbances, after the administration of drugs, such as vincristine, cyclophosphamide and cisplatin. Most chemotherapy-related seizures are usually transient in nature, may be associated with temporary abnormalities on CT or MRI scans, and, once controlled, seldom require antiseizure medication for more than a few months.

Much more serious neurological complications are those of acute encephalopathy following the use of high-dose methotrexate and/or ara-C, and myelopathy following the intrathecal administration of the same drugs, either together or separately [165–167]. Myelopathy is the most frequently cited, serious neurological complication of intrathecal ara-C and methotrexate therapy. Prolonged drug clearance as a result of leptomeningeal tumor, the presence of preservatives in these chemotherapeutic agents (e.g., benzyl alcohol), total cumulative intrathecal dose and other causes of reduced CSF flow have also been implicated as being contributory [165,167,168]. Pat-

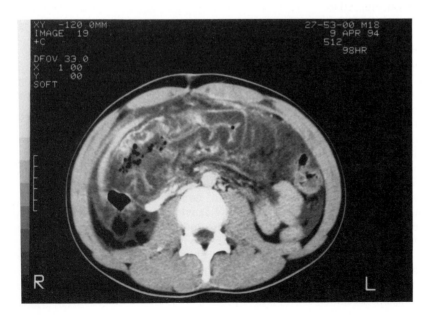

Figure 27.2 CT scan of the abdomen in a patient with neutropenic enterocolitis demonstrating massive edema and thickening of the bowel wall. (Courtesy of Dr Nilo Avila, Department of Diagnostic Radiology, Clinical Center, NIH, Bethesda, MD.)

ients with this syndrome characteristically present within a few days to a week after the administration of chemotherapy with symptoms of radicular or back pain, weakness of the extremities, numbness, paresthesias or sphincter dysfunction, which can rapidly progress, in some cases to paraplegia or quadraplegia. If there is associated encephalopathy, cranial nerve palsies, ataxia, visual impairment, seizures and coma may also ensue. A CT scan of the brain may initially be normal, but the more sensitive MRI may still show swelling of the thoracic or lumbar spinal cord, or the presence of other transient abnormalities, such as 'venous infarcts'. CSF examination is usually significant for an elevation of the total protein, with a marked elevation in the level of the myelin basic protein content, which is barely detectable in the CSF of normal subjects. Rising levels of this protein are found to correlate with disease progression [169]. In most cases, the patient's neurological symptoms improve after the initial event and there is a corresponding fall in the myelin basic protein. However, there are several reports of fatal outcomes and irreversible neurological damage [165–168].

Subacute or acute myeloencephalopathy is a rare, serious neurological side-effect, the mechanism of which is poorly understood. Thus it is difficult to make recommendations for its prevention. However, it has been suggested that an interval of 48–72 hours between successive doses of intrathecal therapy [165], along with serial determination of CSF myelin basic protein, in patients at risk for developing treatment-related neurotoxicity [167] may help lower the chances of developing this complication.

Another set of neurological complications seen in patients receiving vincristine include peripheral neuropathy and cranial nerve palsies. The neuropathy is usually confined to the hands and feet (glove and stocking distribution), but may be more extensive at times. Severe vincristine neuropathy may also be manifested as palatal palsy and ptosis. A complete neurological examination should be performed on every patient prior to administration of each dose of vincristine.

METABOLIC COMPLICATIONS

Treatment of the underlying lymphoma can result in certain metabolic complications, such as SIADH and hyperglycemia. Both these complications are drug related and easily correctable. The most common cause of SIADH in oncology is the administration of chemotherapeutic agents, such as vincristine, cyclophosphamide or morphine [170,171]. SIADH usually coincides with severe vincristine neurotoxicity,

suggesting a direct effect on the supraoptic nuclei, while cyclophosphamide reduces free water clearance. This effect of cyclophosphamide is especially difficult to manage, in the face of the aggressive hydration needed to prevent hemorrhagic cystitis. The presentation and management of SIADH is the same as that caused by the lymphoma itself, and has already been discussed in detail previously.

Hyperglycemia is another troublesome, treatment-related complication that is frequently encountered in practice. It usually occurs as a result of the administration of steroids (either for the treatment of lymphoma or prevention of emesis), alone, or in conjunction with dextrose-containing intravenous fluids and other chemotherapeutic agents, such as asparaginase. The hyperglycemia can usually be controlled by a reduction in the dose of the steroid; rarely insulin may be required where a dose reduction is not possible or is ineffective.

CARDIAC COMPLICATIONS

Most treatment protocols for NHL today incorporate anthracyclines, such as doxorubicin and daunorubicin. Clinical use of these agents can be associated with both an acute and a chronic cardiomyopathy that is often debilitating and not infrequently fatal. It is hypothesized that one of the mechanisms of cardiac toxicity involves anthracycline activation by the cardiac mitochondria, causing the anthracyclines to release free radicals, which are cardiotoxic [171a]. Factors that can increase the risk of cardiomyopathy in patients receiving anthracyclines include mediastinal radiation therapy, uncontrolled hypertension, administration of individual doses of anthracyclines more than 50 mg/m^2 every 3–4 weeks and the coadministation of other chemotherapeutic agents, such as cyclophosphamide in high doses [171b].

Acutely, patients may present with arrhythmias and conduction abnormalities, which can range in severity from benign supraventricular tacycardia to complete heart block. Another manifestation of acute toxicity, sometimes seen within a short interval of anthracycline administration, is the 'myocarditis–pericarditis syndrome', which, in its most severe form, is characterized by the onset of florid, congestive heart failure and pericarditis. Patients who develop this syndrome present with an acute and steep decline in their left ventricular function [documented by radionuclide cineangiography (MUGA)], which is transient in most cases. Near complete recovery is usually seen, although in the rare case, death may ensue rapidly [171b].

The chronic cardiomyopathy associated with anthracyclines is related to their cumulative dose. Although there is considerable, individual variation, almost 50% of patients have been found to develop clear-cut functional impairment, confirmed by endomyocardial biopsy, by the time they receive 500 mg/m^2 of an anthracycline [171b].

Since anthracycline-induced cardiomyopathy is a direct consequence of reduced myocardial contractility, it is important to measure the change in contractility at periodic intervals, while the patient is on therapy. Although no method by itself is 100% accurate, the commonly used tests include echocardiography (usually used to measure the shortening fraction) and MUGA (used to measure ejection fraction). Commonly used guidelines for stopping anthracyclines include an ejection fraction of less than 45%, a shortening fraction of 30% or less, or a drop of greater than 15% in the ejection fraction from pretreatment values. There is usually synchrony in the results obtained by echocardiography and MUGA scans, but falsely low ejection fractions (10–20% less than pretreatment values), with normal myocardial contractility on echocardiogram, have been seen with several NHL patients after administration of a cumulative dose less than 250 mg/m^2 resulting in early discontinuation of anthracyclines (personal communication, I.T. Magrath). This poses a dilemma, as anthracyclines are very effective in the treatment of lymphoblastic and large-cell lymphomas, and premature discontinuation may not be in the best interest of the patient.

Table 27.9 Emetogenic potential of selected chemotherapeutic agents and time course of the nausea and vomiting

	Onset (hours)	Duration (hours)
I. Very high emetogenic potential (> 90%)		
Cisplatin	1–4	12–96
Cyclophosphamide	6–8	8–24
Cytarabine	1–3	3–8
Dacarbazine	1–2	2–4
II. High emetogenic potential (60–90%)		
Carboplatin	2–6	1–48
Carmustine	2–6	4–6
Dactinomycin	2–5	4–24
Daunorubicin	1–3	4–24
Doxorubicin	1–3	4–24
III. Moderate emetogenic potential (30–60%)		
Ifosfamide	2–3	12–72
Etoposide	2–3	8–12
Epirubicin	1–3	4–24
Asparaginase	2–4	8–24
IV. Low emetogenic potential (0–30%)		
Methotrexate	—	—
6-Mercaptopurine	—	—
Vincristine	—	—

NAUSEA AND VOMITING

Nausea and vomiting are two of the most distressing side-effects of cancer chemotherapy encountered today, and when severe and prolonged, can result in pronounced physiological debilitation and psychological distress.

Numerous chemotherapeutic agents used in the treatment of lymphomas can cause nausea and vomiting. A list of the emetogenic potential of various chemotherapeutic agents is presented in Table 27.9.

Various antiemetic regimens have been evaluated over the years. In randomized, comparative clinical trials, high and repeated doses of corticosteroids have been consistently shown to be effective and well tolerated [172,173]. In patients undergoing moderately emetogenic chemotherapy, dexamethasone and methylprednisolone have been found to be superior to the phenothiazines [174]. However, the with the advent of the serotonin (5-hydroxytryptamine [5HT-3]) antagonists, which are highly effective antiemetic agents, the management of this difficult problem has become simpler. Recent studies comparing the antiemetic combination of a serotonin antagonist (granisetron) and dexamethasone with that of granisetron or dexamethasone administered alone, have demonstrated the superiority of the combination regimen in prevention of chemotherapy-induced emesis. Table 27.10 outlines some of the commonly used antiemetic agents/regimens.

MUCOSITIS

Oropharyngeal mucositis is a major complication of intensive chemotherapy regimens, radiation to the head and neck area, and BMT [139,175,176]. Not only can it be severe enough to cause debilitating pain and interfere with swallowing, speech and nutrition, it can also be a site of bleeding (especially in the severely thrombocytopenic patient), or portal of entry for systemic infection.

Normally, the oral mucosa is regenerated every 7–14 days. Both chemotherapy and radiation therapy can interfere with cellular mitosis and reduce the ability of the oral mucosa to regenerate. Oral complications can begin as early as 3 days following the administration of chemotherapy or radiation, and typically include dryness (xerostomia), generalized mucosal erythema with associated pain and dysphagia (mucositis), gingival bleeding, and discrete oral ulcerations (stomatitis).

Stomatitis occurs with a variety of chemotherapeutic agents including daunorubicin, doxorubicin, bleomycin, dactinomycin, 5-flourouracil, methotrexate and melphalan. Oral problems due to radiotherapy are the result of local tissue changes from

Table 27.10 Commonly prescribed antiemetic agents

Drug	Dose	Type of nausea controlled
Agents with weak antiemetic activity		
Dexamethasone (Decadron)	Oral: 10–20 mg every 4–8 hours IV: 8–20 mg every 4–8 hours	Best used in combination with other antiemetic agents, e.g., ondansetron and metoclopramide
Dronabinol (Marinol)	Oral: 5 mg/m^2 every 2–4 hours for 4–6 doses	Significant adverse effects, very expensive, erratic absorption
Agents with moderate antiemetic activity		
Metoclopramide (Reglan)	Oral: 20 mg every 4 hours IV: 1–3 mg/kg every 2–3 hours for 2–6 doses	Effective with moderate dose cisplatin and non-cisplatin combination chemotherapy. Extrapyramidal side-effects common
Prochlorperazine (Compazine)	Oral: 10–20 mg every 4 hours IV: 10–30 mg every 4–6 hours	Sedation and extrapyramidal reactions with higher doses
Agents with strong antiemetic activity		
Ondansetron (Zofran)	Oral: adults – 8 mg, 1/2 hour prior to chemotherapy, then 4 and 8 hours after chemotherapy on day 1.4 mg t.i.d. for the next 2 days Children (4–11 years) – 4 mg with same dosing schedule IV: 0.15 mg/kg infusion prior to and 4 and 8 hours after chemotherapy	Most effective against cisplatin and dose-intensive, combination chemotherapy regimens
Adjunctive agents		
Diphenhydramine (Benadryl)	Oral: 25–50 mg IV: 25–50 mg	Used with metoclopramide and prochlorperazine to prevent extra pyramidal side-effects
Lorazepam (Ativan)	Oral: 1–2 mg IV: 1–2 mg	Used as an anxiolytic and for prevention of extrapyramidal side-effects

direct radiation to the head and neck, and the severity of mucositis depends on the type of ionizing radiation, the volume of irradiated tissue, the dose per day and the cumulative dose.

To assess the severity of the mucositis, both in terms of pain and the ability of the patient to maintain adequate nutritional intake, a mucositis grading system can be helpful. A commonly used grading system is that of the NCI, demonstrated in Table 27.11 [177].

Table 27.11 National Cancer Institute grading system for oral mucositis

Grade 0	No mucositis
Grade 1	Painless ulcers, erythema or mild soreness
Grade 2	Painful erythema, edema or ulcers, can eat
Grade 3	Painful erythema, edema or ulcers, cannot eat
Grade 4	Patient requires parenteral or enteral support

A standardized approach for the prevention and treatment of chemotherapy and radiation-induced mucositis is essential. Effective prevention of mucositis requires a comprehensive oral examination of the patient (preferably prior to, or soon after commencement of chemotherapy), to identify problems, such as poor oral hygiene, peridontal disease, dental caries, orthodontic appliances, ill-fitting prostheses and any other potential source of infection. Other prophylactic measures usually employed at the onset of chemotherapy, include chlorhexidine (Peridex), saline and sodium bicarbonate rinses, and, at some centers, oral acyclovir and nystatin/fluconazole for herpetic or fungal infections.

Regimens frequently used (with varying degrees of success) for the treatment of mucositis and its associated pain include (either alone or in combination) a local anesthetic, such as lidocaine or dyclone, Maalox or Mylanta, diphenhydramine, nystatin or sucralfate. Other less commonly used agents include allopurinol, topical capsaicin, vitamin E mouthwash, prostaglandins and antibiotics. Prolonged administration of oral and parenteral narcotics is required in cases of severe mucositis. A recombinant human transforming frowth factor-β (rhTGF-β) oral rinse and gultamine are currently under evaluation for safety and efficacy in the prevention of mucositis experienced by patients enrolled on dose-intensive treatment protocols. TGF-beta is a multifunctional cytokine with the ability to reversibly inhibit cell growth in nonmesenchymal tissues, by lengthening or arresting cells in the G_0/G_1 phase of the cell cycle. The mechanism of action of glutamine is unknown.

DERMATOLOGICAL TOXICITY

Chemotherapeutic agents can produce both local and systemic dermatological toxicities. Local toxicity occurs in the tissues surrounding the site of drug administration, and is usually manifested by phlebitis, pain, erythema, discoloration of veins, and tissue necrosis secondary to extravasation of a drug, all of which can cause serious morbidity.

The most common systemic toxicity is alopecia, followed by erythematous rashes, pruritis, dermatitis and hyperpigmentation. These are all transient toxicities, usually associated with minimal physical morbidity. Table 27.12 lists the commonly implicated drugs and the toxicities associated with them.

UNUSUAL DRUG TOXICITIES

Besides the known toxicities associated with chemo-

therapeutic agents, there are some reports of rare and unusual side effects of frequently used drugs, such as vincristine, cytarabine, methotrexate, taxol and doxorubicin. These toxicities have been observed when the drug is used either alone, or in combination with another chemotherapeutic agent or colony-stimulating factor.

An unusual dose-limiting, dermatological toxicity known as plantar–palmar erythrodysesthesia was recently observed by Uziely et al. in two complementary phase 1 studies utilizing liposomal doxorubicin [178]. Patients who received three or more courses of 60 mg/m^2 liposomal doxorubicin every 3 weeks developed a temporary, painful desquamating dermatitis primarily affecting the palms of the hands and soles of the feet. The incidence of this toxicity (also called hand–foot syndrome) decreased dramatically on increasing the interval between doses, suggesting a relationship between the syndrome and the cumulative effect of doxorubicin. Weintraub et al. recently reported several cases of severe atypical neuropathy in association with a high cumulative dose of vincristine and colony-stimulating factors, on NCI protocol 89-C-41 (for the treatment of high-grade NHL) [141]. This syndrome was characterized by the acute onset of excruciating pain, unrelieved by narcotics, in the lower extremities and usually accompanied by profound weakness that lasted from weeks to months. It appeared that the colony-stimulating factors decreased the threshold for vincristine toxicity. Table 27.13 lists some of these unusual drug toxicities.

Table 27.12   Dermatological toxicities of chemotherapeutic agents

Drug	Alopecia	Extravasation	Effect on veins*	Dermatitis	Hyperpigmentation†	Nails‡
Cyclophosphamide	+	—	—	—	—	+
Doxorubicin	+	+	+	+	+	+
Daunorubicin	+	+	+	+	+	—
Dactinomycin	+	+	—	+	+	—
Etoposide	+	Rare	—	—	—	—
5-Fluorouracil	+	Rare	+	+	+	+
Toxol	+	—	+	—	—	—
Vincristine	+	+	+	—	—	
Bleomycin	Rare	—	—	+	+	+
Ifosfamide	Rare	—	—	—	—	—
Methotrexate	Rare	—	—	+	+	—
Cisplatin	—	Rare	—	—	—	—
Cytarabine	—	—	—	+	—	

+, Frequently associated with; —, not associated with.
* Effect on veins includes erythema, urticaria, phlebitis and discoloration.
† Pattern of distribution of hyperpigmentation varies with different drugs.
‡ Nail changes range from pigmentation and brittleness to slowed growth and loss.

Table 27.13   Unusual toxicities of selected chemotherapeutic agents

Drugs	Toxicity	References
Cytarabine	Pericarditis	179
Doxorubicin	Palmar–plantar erythrodysesthesia	178
Methotrexate	Severe cutaneous necrosis	180
Vincristine	Visual hallucinations	181
Vincristine + CSFs	Severe atypical neuropathy	141
Taxol + doxorubicin	Typhlitis	160

CSFs, Colony-stimulating factors.

COMPLICATIONS RELATED TO CYTOKINE ADMINISTRATION

Hematopoetic growth factors have made a significant impact on the prevention of infections associated with chemotherapy-induced neutropenia, shortening of the duration of neutropenia following high-dose chemotherapy and stem cell transplantation, and reducing the degree of chemotherapy-associated anemia. However, they are not free of toxicity, a factor that needs to be considered prior to prescribing them routinely in patients undergoing chemotherapy.

The three recombinant hematopoetic factors available for commercial use in the USA today are G-CSF, GM-CSF and Epo. Other factors currently being studied in controlled trials include the interleukins (IL-3, IL-6, IL-1 and IL-11), PIXY321 (GM-CSF/IL-3 fusion protein) and stem cell factor. Most toxicities are common to all these factors and are usually dependent on their receptor sites and cascade effects of secondary cytokine release [152a]. Frequently encountered toxicities include transient bone pain, fever, rash and myalgias, the incidence of these being lowest with G-CSF. Pleural and pericardial effusions have been reported in patients who received GM-CSF [182,183], as have problems with prolonged thrombocytopenia during chemotherapy [139]. Doses of greater than 30 μg/kg of GM-CSF have been implicated in the etiology of the pulmonary capillary leak syndrome, which is characterized by signs and symptoms similiar to the adult respiratory distress syndrome. Occasionally anaphylactic reactions have been documented with the initial dose of GM-CSF. Frequently encountered laboratory abnormalities associated with the use of G-CSF and GM-CSF include mild to moderate elevations of LDH and liver enzymes, abnormal clotting times and hypoalbuminemia. The elevation of LDH in patients with NHL and several other cancers can be misleading, as it is frequently a good marker of tumor progression. However, the elevation that occurs with the concomitant administration of colony-stimulat-ing factors is only transient, and a normal LDH level is observed upon stopping the factor. No specific side-effects of Epo have been described.

CENTRAL LINE-RELATED COMPLICATIONS

Indwelling, temporary central venous catheters and long-term silastic venous catheters, such as Hickmans and Broviac catheters, have become ubiquitous with the treatment of cancer today. However, these devices are not without their problems. Frequently encountered complications include, infection, thrombosis and SVCS. Only the first two complications will be discussed briefly in this section as SVCS has been discussed in detail previously.

Although Gram-positive bacterial infections (particularly *Staph. epidermis*) are the most common causes of catheter-related infections, other organisms such as resistant corynebacteria (CDC-JK), *Bacillus* species, atypical mycobacteria, Gram-negative organisms (especially *Acinetobacter* species) and fungi, can occasionally be the offending agents [125].

The majority of catheter-related bacteremias, especially those associated with coagulase-negative staphylococci, can usually be treated with appropriate antibiotics (e.g., vancomycin), and do not necessitate catheter removal from patients. It is recommended, however, that the antibiotic infusions be rotated amongst the different ports in a multi-lumen catheter for complete eradication of the organism [125]. However, in the face of bacteremia lasting more than 48 hours, the catheter should be removed. *Bacillus* species and *Candida albicans* are more difficult to eradicate with antibiotics alone, and when they are isolated, the catheter should be removed promptly. Other infections that necessitate line removal include exit site infections with Gram-negative bacteria (e.g., *Pseudomonas aeruginosa*), mycobacteria (e.g., *Mycobacterium cheloneii*), and fungi (*Aspergillus*), and tunnel infections.

Thrombosis of the central veins is a recognized

complication of central venous catheters [184]. Fibrin sheath formation around indwelling silastic catheters is frequently seen in patients who undergo venography to rule out occlusion. The incidence of clinical thrombosis associated with catheters is reported to be anywhere from 4% to 12% [185] and urokinase is routinely recommended to lyse the occluding thrombus [186]. Deep venous thrombosis of the arm has also been reported in patients with central indwelling catheters [187]. As the risk of pulmonary embolism is high in this situation, anti-coagulants should be instituted as soon as the diagnosis is established (with the help of venography and CT scan with contrast media) in order to minimize clot propagation, allow collateral channels to remain open and reduce the risk of pulmonary embolism. Good results have been reported when thrombolytic agents are given together with anti-coagulants in the early stages [188]. Another frequently encountered complication in immunosuppressed patients in intensive care units is that of septic venous thrombosis (the simultaneous occurrence of central venous catheter infection, central venous thrombosis and ongoing bacteremia after removal of the catheter). Therapy for this serious complication includes a prolonged course of intravenous antibiotics and full-dose heparinization after prompt removal of the catheter [184].

Late complications of therapy

In recent years, the improved treatment of NHL has resulted in an increase in the number of patients who achieve long-term survival. Consequently, late complications of treatment have become a much more important consideration. Clearly, now that long-term survival of a high proportion of the patients is achievable, efforts to increase survival rates even further by means of more aggressive therapy must be weighed not only against the additional risk of immediate toxicity, but also against the risk of long-term complications which may decrease the quality of subsequent survival. On the other hand, reductions in therapy for 'good-risk' patients in order to minimize toxicity may also decrease survival rates – an equally unacceptable situation. Nonetheless, it is particularly important in good-risk patients to examine treatment protocols critically for components that add little to therapy but may significantly increase toxicity. One area of current controversy in this regard is the use of combined chemotherapy and radiotherapy – a combination that has a particular propensity to give rise to late complications.

The development of late complications represents a particularly serious problem in children, since growth and development are often affected, and there is a potentially greater loss to society in terms of man-years of useful life. Although the toxicities of radiation and chemotherapy are sometimes additive, as seen in second malignancies, late complications often differ markedly, since radiation causes toxicity in the radiation field, such as pulmonary fibrosis, constrictive pericarditis, intellectual dysfunction and endarteritis of a variety of tissues, leading, for example, to chronic renal and bowel disease, hypothyroidism and the impairment of growth of bone and soft tissues. Chemotherapy, on the other hand, may affect any organ or tissue, although late effects are often associated with a specific drug, such as busulfan, which can cause pulmonary fibrosis, and high-dose methotrexate, which may cause leukoencephalopathy. A detailed discussion on each of the late effects, including second malignancies can be found in Chapter 36.

References

1. Halpern S, Chatten J, Meadows AT, et al. Anterior mediastinal masses: Anaesthesia hazards and other problems. *J. Pediatr.* 1983, **102**: 407–410.
2. Loeffler JS, Leopold KA, Recht A, et al. Emergency pre biopsy radiation for mediastinal masses: Impact on subsequent pathological diagnosis and outcome. *J. Clin. Oncol.* 1986, **4**: 716–719.
3. Armstrong BA, Perez CA, Simpson JR, et al. Role of radiation management in SVC syndrome. *Int. J. Radiat. Oncol. Biol. Phys.* 1987, **13**: 531–535.
4. Lochridge SK, Knibbe WP, Doty DB. Obstruction of the SVC. *Surgery* 1979, **85**: 14–20.
5. Parish JM, Marschke RF, Dines DE, et al. Etiological considerations in SVC syndrome. *Mayo Clin. Proc.* 1981, **56**: 407–410.
6. Perez CA, Presant CA, Van Amburg A. Management of SVC syndrome. *Semin. Oncol.* 1978, **5**: 123–127.
7. Shimm DS, Logue GL, Rigsby LC. Evaluating the SVC syndrome. *J. Am. Med. Assoc.* 1981, **245**: 951–955.
8. Lazzarino M, Orlandi E, Paulli M, et al. Primary mediastinal B-cell lymphoma with sclerosis: An aggressive tumor with distinct clinical and pathological features. *J. Clin. Oncol.* 1993, **11**: 2306–2310.
9. Janin Y, Becker J, Wise L, et al. SVC syndrome in childhood and adolescence. A review of the literature and report of 3 cases. *J. Pediatr. Surg.* 1982, **17**: 290–295.
10. Pate JW, Hammon J. SVC syndrome and NHL. *Ann. Surg.* 1985, **161**: 778–785.
11. Issa PY, Brihi ER, Janin Y. SVC syndrome in childhood. Report of 10 cases and review of the literature. *Pediatrics* 1983, **71**: 337–342.

12. Pokorny WJ, Sherman JO. Mediastinal masses in infants and children. *J. Thorac. Cardiovasc. Surg.* 1974, **68**: 869–875.

13. Yellin A, Mandel M, Rechavi G, et al. Superior vena cava syndrome associated with lymphoma. *Am. J. Dis. Child.* 1992, **146**: 1060–1063.

14. Simpson I, Campbell PE. Mediastinal masses in childhood: A review from a pathologist's point of view. *Prog. Pediatr. Surg.* 1991, **27**: 92–102.

15. Nieto AF, Doty DB. SVC obstruction: Clinical syndrome, etiology and treatment. *Curr. Prob. Cancer* 1986, **10**: 441–484.

16. O'Brien RT, Matlak ME, Condon VR, et al. SVC syndrome in children. *West J. Med.* 1981, **135**: 143–147.

17. Levitt SH, Jones TK, Kilpatrick SJ. Treatment of malignant SVC obstruction: A randomized study. *Cancer* 1969, **24**: 447–451.

18. Ahmann FR. A reassessment of the clinical implications of SVC syndrome. *J. Clin. Oncol.* 1984, **2**: 961–969.

19. Carabell SC, Goodman RL. Superior vena cava syndrome. In DeVita VT Jr, Hellman S, Rosenberg (eds) *Principles and Practice of Oncology*, 2nd edn. New York: Lippincott, 1985, pp. 1855–1860.

20. Abner A. Approach to the patient who presents with SVC obstruction. *Chest* 1993, **103**: 394S–397S.

21. Stanford W, Doty DB. The role of venography and surgery in the management of patients with SVC obstruction. *Ann. Thorac. Surg.* 1986, **41**: 158–162.

22. Stanford W, Jolles H, Ell, S, et al. SVC obstruction: A venographic classification. *Am. J. Roentgenol.* 1987, **148**: 259–265.

23. Swayne LC, Kaplan IL. Gallium SPECT detection of neoplastic intravascular obstruction of the SVC. *Clin. Nucl. Med.* 1989, **14**: 823–827.

24. Khimji T, Zeiss J. MRI vs CT and US in the evaluation of a patient presenting with SVC syndrome. *Clin. Imaging* 1992, **16**: 269–272.

25. Webb WR, Sostman HD. MR Imaging of thoracic disease. *Radiology* 1992, **182**: 621–624.

26. Markman M. Common complications and emergencies associated with cancer and its therapy. *Cleveland Clin. J. Med.* 1994, **61**: 105–114.

27. Neumann GG, Weingarten AE, Abramowitz RM, et al. The anaesthetic management of the patient with an anterior mediastinal mass. *Anaesthesiology* 1984, **60**: 144–147.

28. Northrip DR, Bohman BK, Tsueda K. Total airway obstruction and SVC syndrome in a child with an anterior mediastinal tumor. *Anaesth. Analg.* 1986, **65**: 1079–1082.

29. Jahangiri M, Taggart DP, Goldstraw P. Role of mediastinoscopy in SVC obstruction. *Cancer* 1993, **71**: 3006–3010.

30. Yellin A, Rosen A, Reichert N, et al. SVC syndrome: The myths, the facts. *Am. Rev. Respir. Dis.* 1990, **141**: 1114–1120.

31. Chen RC, Bongard F, Klein SR. A contemporary perspective on SVC syndrome. *Am. J. Surg.* 1990, **160**: 207–211.

32. Chen CH, Kuo ML, Shih JF, et al. US guided needle aspiration biopsy in the diagnosis of advanced SVC syndrome. *Chinese Med. J.* 1992, **50**: 119–122.

33. Ko JC, Yang PC, Yuan A, et al. SVC syndrome: Rapid histological diagnosis by US guided trans-thoracic needle aspiration biopsy. *Am. J. Resp. Crit. Care Med.* 1994, **149**: 783–787.

34. Baker GL, Barnes HJ. SVC syndrome: Etiology, diagnosis and treatment. *Am. J. Crit. Care* 1992, **1**: 54–59.

35. Levitt LJ, Dawson DM, Rosenthal DS, et al. CNS involvement in the NHL's. *Cancer* 1980, **45**: 545–550.

36. Perry JR, Dheodhare SS, Bilbao JM, et al. The significance of spinal cord compression as the initial manifestation of lymphoma. *Neurosurgery* 1993, **32**: 157–161.

37. Eeles RA, O'Brien P, Horwich A, et al. NHL presenting with extradural spinal cord compression: Functional outcome and survival. *Br. J. Cancer* 1991, **63**: 126–129.

38. Lyons MK, O'Neill BP, Marsh WR, et al. Primary spinal epidural NHL: Report of 8 patients and review of the literature. *Neurosurgery* 1992, **30**: 675–678.

39. Correale J, Monteverde DA, Bueri JA, et al. Peripheral nervous system and spinal cord involvement in lymphoma. *Acta Neurol. Scand.* 1991, **83**: 45–51.

40. Young RC, Hauser DM, Anderson T. CNS complications in NHL: The role for prophylactic therapy. *Am. J. Med.* 1979, **66**: 435–443.

41. Lewis DW, Packer RJ, Raney B, et al. Incidence, presentation and outcome of spinal cord disease in children with systemic cancer. *Pediatrics* 1986, **78**: 438–443.

42. Nowacki P, Dolinska D, Stankiewicz S, et al. Neurological complications in high-grade NHL's: Clinico-neuropathological correlations. *Neurol. Neurochir. Pol.* 1992, **26**: 334–342.

43. Aysun S, Topcu M, Gunay M, et al. Neurological features as initial presentations of childhood malignancies. *Pediatr. Neurol.* 1994, **10**: 40–43.

44. Oviatt DL, Kirshner HS, Stein RS, et al. Successful chemotherapeutic treatment of epidural compression in NHL. *Cancer* 1982, **49**: 2446–2449.

45. Laing RJ, Jakubowski J, Kunkler R, et al. Primary spinal presentation of NHL: A reappraisal of management and prognosis. *Spine* 1992, **17**: 117–120.

46. Haddad P, Thaell JF, Kiely JM, et al. Lymphoma of the spinal extradural space. *Cancer* 1976, **37**: 1485–1488.

47. Botterell EH, Fitzgerald GW, et al. *Cancer Med. Assoc. J.* 1959, **80**: 791–795.

48. Lange B, D'Angio G, et al. Oncologic emergencies. In Pizzo P, Poplack D (eds) *Principles and Practice of Pediatric Oncology* 2nd edn. Philadephia: JB Lippincott, 1993, pp. 951–972.

49. Friedman M, Kim TH, Panahon AM, et al. Spinal cord compression in malignant lymphoma. *Cancer* 1976, **37**: 1485–1488.

50. Mckenna RJ, Khalil M, Ener MS, et al. Pleural and pericardial effusions in cancer patients. *Curr. Prob. Cancer* 1985, **9**: 1–4.

51. Salyer WR, Eggleston JC, Erozan YS, et al. Efficacy

of pleural needle biopsy and pleural fluid cytopathology in the diagnosis of malignant neoplasms involving the pleura. *Chest* 1975, **67**: 536–539.

52. Spain RC, Whittlesey D. Respiratory emergencies in patients with cancer. *Semin. Oncol.* 1989, **16**: 471–489.

53. Shepherd FA, Ginsberg JS, Evans WK, et al. Tetracycline sclerosis in the management of malignant pericardial effusion. *J. Clin. Oncol.* 1985, **13**: 1678–1682.

54. Davis S, Rambotti P, Grignani F. Intra-pericardial tetracycline sclerosis in the treatment of malignant pericardial effusion. *J. Clin. Oncol.* 1984, **2**: 631–636.

55. Bayly TC, Kisner DL, Sybert A, et al. Tetracycline and quinacrine in the control of malignant pleural effusions: A randomized trial. *Cancer* 1978, **41**: 1188–1192.

56. Donati MB. Cancer and thrombosis. *Hemostasis* 1994, **24**: 128–131.

57. Dhami MS, Bona RD. Using anti-coagulants safely: Guidelines for therapeutic and prophylactic regimens. *Post Graduate Med.* 1991, **93**: 121–122.

58. Sarasin FP, Eckman MH. Management and prevention of thrombo-embolic events in 86 patients with cancer related hypercoagulable states. *J. Gen. Intern. Med.* 1993, **8**: 476–486.

59. Rickles FR, Levine M, Edwards RL, et al. Hemostatic alterations in cancer patients. *Cancer Metastasis Rev.* 1992, **11**: 237–248.

60. Naschitz JE, Yeshurun D, Lev LM. Thromboembolism in cancer. Changing trends. *Cancer* 1993, **71**: 1384–1390.

61. Rosen MP, Porter DH, Kim D. Reassessment of venacaval filter use in patients with cancer. *J. Vascular Interven. Radiol.* 1994, **5**: 501–506.

62. Magnant JG, Walsh DB, Juravsky R, et al. Current use of IVC filters. *J. Vascular Surg.* 1992, **16**: 701–716.

63. Greenfield LJ, Michna BA. 12 year clinical experience with the Greenfield venacaval filter. *Surgery* 1988, **104**: 706–712.

64. Schulman S, Rhedin A. A comparison of 6 weeks with 6 months of oral anti-coagulant therapy after a first episode of venous thrombo-embolism. *N. Engl. J. Med.* 1995, **332**: 1661–1665.

65. Shad AT, Magrath IT. Diagnosis and treatment of NHL in childhood. In Wernik PH (ed.) *Neoplastic Diseases of the Blood*, 3rd edn. Edinburgh: Churchill Livingstone, 1995, pp. 925–962.

66. Lynch E. Uric acid metabolism in proliferative disease after marrow. *Arch. Intern. Med.* 1962, **9**: 43–47.

67. Braylan RC, Jaffe ES, Triche TJ, et al. Structural and functional properties of the hairy leukemic cells reticuloendotheliosis. *Cancer* 1978, **41**: 210–227.

68. Murphy SB, Melvin SL, Mauer AM, et al. Correlation of tumor cell kinetic studies with surface marker results in childhood NHL. *Cancer Res.* 1979, **39**: 1534–1538.

69. Veenstra J, Krediet RT, Somers R, et al. Tumor lysis syndrome and acute renal failure in Burkitts lymphoma: Description of 2 cases and review of the literature on prevention and management. *Netherlands J. Med.* 1994, **45**: 211–216.

70. Fleming DR, Doukas MA. Acute tumor lysis syndrome in hematological malignancies. *Leukemia Lymphoma* 1992, **8**: 315–318.

71. Hande KR, Garrow GC. Acute tumor lysis syndrome in patients with high-grade NHL. *Am. J. Med.* 1993, **94**: 133–139.

72. Chasty RC, Luin-Yin JA. Acute tumor lysis syndrome. *Br. J. Hosp. Med.* 1993, **49**: 488–492.

73. Primikirios N, Stutzman L, Sandberg A. Uric acid excretion in patients with malignant lymphoma. *Blood* 1961, **17**: 701.

74. Hande KR. Hyperuricaemia uric acid nephropathy – the tumor lysis syndrome. In McKinney TD (ed.) *Renal Complications of Neoplasia.* New York: Praeger Scientific, 1986, pp. 134–156.

75. Krakoff I, Meyer RL. Prevention of hyperuricemia in leukemia and lymphoma. *J. Am. Med. Assoc.* 1965, **193**: 89–93.

76. Cohen LF, Balow J E, Magrath IT, et al. Acute tumor lysis syndrome: A review of 37 cases. *Am. J. Med.* 1980, **68**: 486–491.

77. Tsokos G, Balow JE, Spiegel RJ, et al. Renal and metabolic complications of undifferentiated and lymphoblastic lymphomas. *Medicine* 1981, **60**: 218–229.

78. Patte C, Philip T, Rodary C, et al. Improved survival rate in patients with stage III and IV B-cell NHL and leukemias using multi-agent chemotherapy. *J. Clin. Oncol.* 1985, **4**: 1219–1226.

79. Patte C, Philip T, Rodary C, et al. High survival rate in advanced stage B-cell lymphomas and leukemias without CNS involvement with short intensive poly-chemotherapy. *J. Clin. Oncol.* 1991, **9**: 123–132S.

80. Hande KR, Hixson CL, Chabner BA, et al. Post chemotherapy purine excretion in lymphoma patients receiving allopurinol. *Cancer Res.* 1981, **41**: 2273–2279.

81. Ablin A, Stephens B. Nephropathy, xanthinurea and orotic acidurea complicating Burkitts lymphoma treated with chemotherapy and allopurinol. *Metab. Clin. Exp.* 1972, **21**: 771–778.

82. Hebert LA, Lemann J, Petersen JR, et al. Studies of the mechanism by which phosphate infusion lowers serum calcium concentration. *J. Clin. Invest.* 1966, **12**: 1886–1894.

83. Macher MA, Loirat C, Pillion G, et al. Acute kidney failure caused by hyperphosphoremia in tumor lysis. *Arch. Fr. Pediatr.* 1988, **45**: 271–274.

83a. Bajorunas DR. Clinical manifestations of cancer related hypercalcemia. *Semin. Oncol.* 1990, **17**: 16–25.

83b. Speigel A, Greene M, Magrath I, et al. Hypercalcemia with suppressed growth hormone in Burkitts lymphoma. *Am. J. Med.* 1978, **64**: 691–695.

83c. Leblanc A, Caillaud JM, Hartmann O, et al. Hypercalcemia usually occurs in unusual forms of childhood NHL, rhabdomyosarcomas and Wilms tumor. *Cancer* 1984, **54**: 2132–2136.

83d. Bull FE. Hypercalcaemia in cancer. In Yarbro JW, Bornstein RS (eds) *Oncologic Emergencies.* New York: Grune and Stratton, 1981, pp. 197–214.

84. Raisz LG, Kream BE. Regulation of bone formation. *N. Engl. J. Med.* 1983, **309**: 29–35.

85. Pimentel L. Medical complications of oncologic disease. *Emer. Med. Clin. North Am.* 1993, **11**: 407–419.

86. Muggia FM, Heinemann HO. Hypercalcaemia associated with neoplastic disease. *Ann. Intern. Med.* 1970, **73**: 281–290.

87. Mundy GR, Rick ME, Turcotte R, et. al. Pathogenesis of hypercalcemia in lymphosarcoma cell leukemia. *Am. J. Med.* 1978, **65**: 600–606.

88. Klee GG, Kao PC, Heath H. Hypercalcemia. *Endocrinol. Metab. Clin. North Am.* 1988, **17**: 573–600.

89. Ralston SH. The pathogenesis of hypercalcemia of malignancy. *Lancet* 1987, **19**: 1443–1446.

90. Mundy GR, Luben RA, Raisz LG, et al. Bone resorbing activity in supernatants from lymphoid cell lines. *N. Engl. J. Med.* 1974, **290**: 867–871.

91. Mundy GR, Raisz LG, Cooper RA, et al. Evidence for the secretion of an osteoclast stimulating factor in myeloma. *N. Engl. J. Med.* 1974, **291**: 1041–1046.

92. Besarab A, Caro JF. Mechanisms of hypercalcemia in malignancy. *Cancer* 1978, **41**: 2276–2285.

93. Suki WN, Yium JJ, Von Minden M, et al. Acute treatment of hypercalcemia with furosemide. *N. Engl. J. Med.* 1970, **283**: 836–840.

94. Ralston SH, Gallacher SJ, Patel U, et al. *Cancer* associated hypercalcemia: Morbidity and mortality. *Ann. Intern. Med.* 1990, **112**: 499–504.

95. Jacobs TP, Gordon AC, Silverberg ST, et al. Neoplastic hypercalcemia: Physiological response to IV etidronate disodium. *Am. J. Med.* 1987, **82**: 42–50.

96. Bilezikian JP. Management of acute hypercalcemia. *N. Engl. J. Med.* 1992, **326**: 1196–1203.

97. Abramowitz M. Pamidronate. *Med. Lett. Drugs Ther.* 1992, **34**: 1–2.

98. Gucalp R, Rich P. Comparative study of pamidronate sodium and etidronate disodium in the treatment of cancer related hypercalcemia. *J. Clin. Oncol.* 1992, **10**: 134–142.

99. Warrell RP, Israel R. Gallium nitrate for acute treatment of calcium related hypercalcemia. *Ann. Intern. Med.* 1988, **108**: 669–674.

100. Glover D. Metabolic emergencies. In Wittes RE (ed.) *Manual of Oncologic Therapeutics.* Philadelphia: J.B. Lippincott 1989, p. 320.

101. Chubachi A, Miura I, Hatano Y, et al. SIADH in patients with lymphoma associated hemophagocytic syndrome. *Ann. Hematol.* 1995, **70**: 53–55.

102. Moses AM. Diabetes insipidus and ADH regulation. *Hosp. Pract.* 1977, **12**: 37–44.

103. Narins RJ. Therapy of hyponatremia: Does haste make waste? *N. Engl. J. Med.* 1986, **314**: 1573–1574.

104. Abdi EA, Bishop S. SIADH with carcinoma of the tongue. *Med. Pediatr. Oncol.* 1988, **16**: 210–214.

105. Odell WD, Wolfsen AR. Humoral syndromes associated with cancer. *Ann. Rev. Med.* 1978, **29**: 379–406.

106. Blackman MR, Rosen SW, Weintraub BD. Ectopic hormones. *Adv. Intern. Med.* 1978, **23**: 85–113.

107. Walter EG, Tavare JM, Denton RM, et al. Hypoglycemia due to an insulin receptor antibody in Hodgkin's disease. *Lancet* 1987, **i**: 241–243.

108. Braund WJ, Naylor BA, Williamson DH, et al. Autoimmunity to insulin receptor and hypoglycemia in patients with Hodgkin's disease. *Lancet* 1987, **i**: 237–240.

109. Marks V, Teale JD. Tumors producing hypoglycemia. *Diabetes/Metabolism Rev.*, 1991, **2**: 79–91.

110. Taylor SI, Barbetti F, Accili D, et al. Syndromes of autoimmunity and hypoglycemia. *Endocrinol. Metab. Clin. North Am.* 1989, **18**: 123–143.

111. Gordon P, Hendricks CM, Kahn CR, et al. Hypoglycemia associated with non islet-cell tumor and insulin like growth factors. A study of the tumor types. *N. Engl. J. Med.* 1981, **305**: 1452–1455.

112. Kemeny MM, Magrath IT, Brennan MF, et al. The role of surgery in the management of American Burkitt's lymphoma and its treatment. *Ann. Surg.* 1982, **196**: 82–86.

113. Weingrad DN, Decosse DJ, Sherlock P, et al. Primary GI lymphoma: A 30 year review. *Cancer* 1982, **49**: 1258–1265.

114. Fleming ID, Mitchell S, Dilawari RA. The role of surgery in the management of gastric lymphoma. *Cancer* 1982, **49**: 1135–1141.

115. Sheridan WP, Medley G, Brodie GM. NHL of the stomach: A pilot prospective study of surgery and chemotherapy in early and advanced disease. *J. Clin. Oncol.* 1985, **3**: 495–500.

116. Paulson S, Sheehan RG, Stone MJ, et al. Large cell lymphomas of the stomach: Improved prognosis with complete resection of all GI lesions. *J. Clin. Oncol.* 1983, **1**: 263–269.

117. Ferrari LR, Bedford RF. General anaesthesia prior to treatment of anterior mediastinal masses in pediatric cancer patients. *Anaesthesiology* 1990, **72**: 991–995.

118. Langstein HN, Norton JA. Mechanisms of cancer cachexia. *Hematol. Oncol. Clin. North Am.* 1991, **5**: 103–123.

119. McNamara MJ, Alexander RH, Norton JA. Cytokines and their role in the pathophysiology of cancer cachexia. *J. Parenteral Enteral Nutr.* 1992, **16**: 50S–55S.

120. Keller U. Pathophysiology of cancer cachexia. *Support Care Cancer* 1993, **1**: 290–294.

121. Nelson KA, Walsh D, Sheehan FA. The cancer anorexia–cachexia syndrome. *J. Clin. Oncol.* 1994, **12**: 213–225.

122. Ottery FD. Cancer cachexia. *Cancer Pract.* 1994, **2**: 123–131.

123. Rabinowe SN, Soiffer RJ, Tarbell NJ, et al. Hemolytic-uremic syndrome following BMT in hematological malignancies. *Blood* 1991, **77**: 1837–1844.

124. Sierna RD. Coomb's positive hemolytic anemia in Hodgkin's disease: Case presentation and review of the literature. *Militiary Med.* 1991, **156**: 691–692.

125. Pizzo PA. Management of fever in patients with cancer and treatment-induced neutropenia. *N. Engl. J. Med.* 1993, **328**: 1323–1332.

126. Rubin M, Walsh TJ, Pizza PA, et al. Clinical approach to infections in the immunocompromised host. In Hoffman R, Benz EJ, et al. (eds) *Hematology: Basic Principles and Practice.* New York: Churchill Livingstone, 1991, pp. 1063–1114.

127. Pizzo PA, Rubin M, Freifeld A, et al. The child with cancer and infection 1. Emperic therapy for fever and neutropenia and preventive strategies. *J. Pediatr.* 1991, **119**: 679–694.

128. Pizzo PA, Rubin M, Freifeld A, et al. The child with cancer and infection 11. Non bacterial infections. *J. Pediatr.* 1991, **119**: 845–857.

129. Schimpff SC, Young VM, Greene WH, et al. Origin of infection in acute non-lymphocytic leukemia: Significance of hospital acquisition of potential pathogens. *Ann. Intern. Med.* 1972, **77**: 707–714.

130. Ladisch SL, Pizzo PA. *Staph. Aureus* sepsis in children with cancer. *Pediatrics* 1978, **61**: 231–234.

131. Cudmore MA, Silva J, Fekety R, et al. *C. difficile* colitis associated with cancer chemotherapy. *Arch. Int. Med.* 1982, **142**: 333–335.

132. Feusner J, Cohen R, O'Leary M, et al. Use of routine chest radiography in the evaluation of fever in neutropenic oncology patients. *J. Clin. Oncol.* 1988, **25**: S9–S16.

133. Pizzo PA. Evaluation of fever in the patient with cancer. *Eur. J. Cancer Clin. Oncol.* 1989, **25**: S9–S16.

134. Pizzo PA, Hathorn JW, Hiemenz J, et al. A randomized trial comparing combination antibiotic therapy to monotherapy in cancer patients with fever and neutropenia. *N. Engl. J. Med.* 1986, **315**: 552–558.

135. Huijgens PC, Ossenkoppele GJ, Weijers TF, et al. Imipenem cilastatin for empirical therapy in neutropenic patients with fever: An open study in patients with hematological malignancies. *Eur. J. Hematol.* 1991, **46**: 42–46.

136. Pizzo PA. After emperic therapy: What to do until the granulocyte comes back. *Rev. Infect. Dis.* 1987, **9**: 214–219.

137. Lieschke GJ, Burgess AW. Granulocyte colony stimulating factor and granulocyte macrophage colony stimulating factor. *N. Engl. J. Med.* 1992, **327**: 28–35, 99–106.

138. Nemunaitis J, Rabinowe SN, Singer JW, et al. Recombinant GM-CSF after autologous bone marrow transplantation for lymphoid cancer. *N. Engl. J. Med.* 1991, **324**: 1773–1778.

139. Magrath I, Adde M, Shad A, et al. Adults and children with small non-cleaved cell lymphoma have a similiar outcome when treated with the same chemotherapy regimen. *J. Clin. Oncol.* 1996, **3**: 925–934.

140. Groopman J, Molina JM, Scadden DT, et al. Hemopetic growth factors: Biology and clinical applications. *N. Engl. J. Med.* 1989, **321**: 1449–1459.

141. Weintraub M, Adde M, Venzon D, et al. Profound peripheral neuropathy associated with the administration of colony stimulating factors. *J. Clin. Oncol.* 1996, **3**: 935–937.

142. Karp JE, Merz WG, Hendricksen S, et al. Infection management during anti-leukemia treatment-induced granulocytopenia: The role for oral norfloxacin prophylaxis against infections arising from the gastro intestinal tract. *Scand. J. Inf. Dis.* (Suppl.) 1986, **48**: 66–78.

143. Dekker AW, Rosenberg-Arska M, Verhoef J. Infection prophylaxis in acute leukemia: A comparison of ciprofloxacin with trimethoprim-sulphamethoxazole and colistin. *Ann. Intern. Med.* 1987, **107**: 7–11.

144. Kotilainen P, Nikoskelainen J, Huovinen P. Emergence of ciprofloxacin resistant coagulase-negative staphylococcal skin flora in immunocompromised patients receiving ciprofloxacin. *J. Inf. Dis.* 1990, **161**: 41–44.

145. Trucksis M, Hooper DC, Wolfson JS. Emerging resistance to flouroquinolones in staphylococci: An alert. *Ann. Intern. Med.* 1991, **114**: 424–426.

146. Gilbert C, Meisenberg B, Vredenburgh J, et al. Sequential prophylactic oral and empiric once daily parenteral antibiotics for neutropenia and fever after high dose chemotherapy and autologous bone marrow support. *J. Clin. Oncol.* 1994, **12**: 1005–1011.

147. Saral R, Burns WH, Laskin OL, et al. Acyclovir prophylaxis of herpes simplex virus infections: A randomized, double blind, controlled trial in bone marrow transplant recipients. *N. Engl. J. Med.* 1981, **305**: 63–67.

148. Goodman JL, Winston DJ, Greenfield RA, et al. A controlled trial of fluconazole to prevent fungal infections in patients undergoing bone marrow transplantation. *N. Engl. J. Med.* 1992, **326**: 845–851.

149. Hughes WT, Rivera GK, Schell MJ, et al. Successful intermittent chemoprophylaxis for *Pneumocystis carinii* pneumonitis. *N. Engl. J. Med.* 1987, **316**: 1627–1632.

150. Spivak J. Recombinant human erythropoetin and the anemia of cancer. *Blood* 1994, **84**: 997–1004.

151. Case DC, Bukowski RM, Carey RW, et al. Recombinant human erythropoetin therapy for anemic cancer patients on combination chemotherapy. *J. Natl. Cancer Inst.* 1993, **85**: 801–806.

152. Henry DH, Abels RI. Recombinant human erythropoetin in the treatment of cancer and chemotherapy induced anemia. *Semin. Oncol.* 1994, **21**: 21–28.

152a. Vose JM, Armitage JO. Clinical applications of hematopoetic factors. *J. Clin. Oncol.* 1995, **13**: 1023–1035.

153. Hopkins DJ, Kusner JP. Clostridial species in the pathogenesis of necrotizing enterocolitis in patients with neutropenia. *Am. J. Hematol.* 1983, **14**: 289–295.

154. Shamberger RC, Weinstein HC, Delorey MJ, et al. The medical and surgical management of typhlitis in children with acute non-lymphocytic leukemia. *Cancer* 1986, **57**: 603–609.

155. Paulino AFG, Kenney R, Forman EN, et al. Typhlitis in a patient with acute lymphoblastic leukemia prior to the administration of chemotherapy. *Am. J. Pediatr. Hematol. Oncol.* 1994, **16**: 348–351.

156. Amrorin GD, Solomon RD. Necrotizing enteropathy: A complication of treated leukemia or lymphoma patients. *J. Am. Med. Assoc.* 1962, **182**: 23–29.

157. Mulholland MW, Delaney JP. Neutropenic colitis with aplastic anemia: A new association. *Ann. Surg.* 1983, **197**: 84–90.

158. Foucar E, Mukai K, Foucar K, et al. Colon ulceration in lethal cytomegalovirus infection. *Am. J. Clin. Path.* 1981, **76**: 788–801.

159. Keidan RD, Fanning J, Gatenby F, et al. Recurrent typhlitis, a disease resulting from aggressive chemotherapy. *Dis. Col. Rectum* 1989, **32**: 206–209.

160. Pestalozzi BC, Sotos AG, Choyke PL, et al. Typhlitis

resulting from treatment with Taxol and Doxorubicin in patients with metastatic breast cancer. *Cancer* 1993, **71**: 1797–1800.

161. Balthazar EJ, Megibow AJ, Fazzini M, et al. Cytomegalovirus colitis in AIDS: Radiological findings in 11 patients. *Radiology* 1985, **155**: 585–589.

162. Merine D, Nussbaum A, Fishman EK, et al. Sonographic observations in a patient with typhlitis. *Clin. Pediatr.* 1989, **28**: 377–379.

163. Merine D, Fishman EK, Jones B, et al. Right lower quadrant pain in the immunocompromised patient: CT findings in 10 cases. *Am. J. Roentgenol.* 1987, **149**: 1177–1179.

164. Moir CR, Scudamore CH, Benny WB. Typhlitis: Selective surgical management. *Am. J. Surg.* 1986, **151**: 563–566.

165. Resar LM, Philips PC, Kastan MB, et al. Acute neurotoxicity after intrathecal cytosine arabinoside in two adolescents with acute lymphoblastic leukemia of B-cell type. *Cancer* 1993, **71**: 117–123.

166. Werner RA. Paraplegia and quadraplegia after intrathecal therapy. *Arch. Phys. Med. Rehab.* 1988, **69**: 1054–1056.

167. Bates SE, Raphaelson MI, Price RA, et al. Ascending myelopathy after chemotherapy for CNS acute lymphoblastic leukemia: Correlation with CSF myelin basic protein. *Med. Pediatr. Oncol.* 1985, **13**: 4–8.

168. Garcia-Tena J, Lopez-Andreu JA, Ferris J, et al. Intrathecal chemotherapy related myeloencephalopathy in a young child with acute lymphoblastic leukemia. *Pediatr. Hematol. Oncol.* 1995. **12**: 377–385.

169. Gangji D, Reaman GH, Cohen SR, et al. Leukoencephalopathy and elevated levels of myelin basic protein in the CSF of patients with acute lymphoblastic leukemia. *N. Engl. J. Med.* 1980, **303**: 19–21.

170. Nicholson RJ, Feldman W. Hyponetremia in association with vincristine therapy. *Cancer Med. Assoc. J.* 1972, **106**: 356–357.

171. Harlow PJ, DeClerk YA, Shore NA, et al. A fatal case of inappropriate ADH secretion induced by cyclophosphamide therapy. *Cancer* 1979, **44**: 896–898.

171a. Doroshaw JA, Locker GY, Myers CE. The enzymatic defenses of the mouse heart against reactive oxygen metabolites. Alterations produced by doxorubicin. *J. Clin. Invest.* 1980, **65**: 128–135.

171b. Myers CE, Kinsella TJ. Cardiac and pulmonary toxicity. In DeVita VT, Hellman S, et al. (eds) *Cancer: Practice and Principles of Oncology.* Philadelphia: J.B. Lippincott, 1985, pp. 2022–2032.

172. Del Favero A, Roila F, Tonato M. Reducing chemotherapy induced nausea and vomiting: Current perspectives and future possibilities. *Drug Safety* 1993, **9**: 410–428.

173. Markman M, Scheidler V, Ettinger DS, et al. Anti emetic efficacy of dexamethasone: Randomised, double blind crossover study with prochlorperazine in patients receiving cancer therapy. *N. Engl. J. Med.* 1984, **311**: 549–552.

174. The Italian Group for Anti-emetic Research. Dexamethasone, granisetron, or both for the prevention of nausea and vomiting during chemotherapy for cancer. *N. Engl. J. Med.* 1995, **332**: 1–5.

175. Wright WE. Peridontium destruction associated with oncology therapy: 5 case reports. *J. Peridontol.* 1986, **58**: 559–563.

176. Weisdorf DJ, Bostrom B, Raether D, et al. Oropharygeal mucositis complicating bone marrow transplantation: Prognostic factors and the effect of chlorhexidine mouth rinse. *Bone Marrow Transplant.* 1989, **4**: 89–95.

177. Berger AM, Bartoshuk LM, et al. Capsacain for the treatment of oral mucositis pain. *PPO Updates* 1995, **9**: 1–11.

178. Uziely B, Jeffers S, Isacson R, et al. Liposomal doxorubicin: Antitumor activity and unique toxicities during two complementary phase 1 studies. *J. Clin. Oncol.* 1995, **13**: 1777–1785.

179. Reykdal S, Sham R, Kouides P. Cytarabine induced pericarditis. A case report and review of the literature of the cardio-pulmonary complications of cytarabine therapy. *Leukemia Res.* 1995, **19**: 141–144.

180. Aractingi S, Briant E, Marolleau JP, et al. Methotrexate induced skin detachment. *Presse Med.* 1992, **21**: 1668–1670.

181. Ghosh K, Sivakumaran M, Murphy P, et al. Visual hallucinations following treatment with vincristine. *Clin. Lab. Hematol.* 1994, **16**: 355–357.

182. Antmann KS, Griffin JD, Elias A, et al. Effect of rh-GM-CSF on chemotherapy induced myelosuppression. *N. Engl. J. Med.* 1988, **319**: 593–598.

183. Kanz L, Lindemann A, et al. Hemopoetins in clinical oncology. *Am. J. Clin. Onc.* 1995, **14** (Suppl. 1): 527–533.

184. Schwartzberg LS, Holbert JM. Hemorrhagic and thrombotic abnormalities in cancer. *Crit. Care Clinics* 1988, **4**: 107–128.

185. Ross AH, Griffith CD, Anderson JR, et al. Thromboembolic complications with silicone subclavian catheters. *J. Parenter. Enteral Nutr.* 1982, **6**: 61–65.

186. Glynn MF, Langer B, Jeejeebhoy KN, et al. Therapy for thrombotic occlusion of long term intravenous alimentation catheters. *J. Parenter. Enteral Nutr.* 1980, **4**: 387–390.

187. Hung SS. Deep vein thrombosis of the arm associated with malignancy. *Cancer* 1989, **64**: 531–535.

188. Menzoian JO, Sequira JC, Doyle JE, et al. Therapeutic and clinical course of deep vein thrombosis. *Am. J. Surg.* 1983, **146**: 581–585.

of chemotherapeutic agents, i.e., cycle active drugs. This concept provides a partial explanation for the resistance of some lymphomas to treatment. For example, the inverse correlation that is observed between growth fraction and tumor volume may account in part for the prognostic significance of tumor burden and for the lower curability of advanced-stage lymphomas [2]. A similar mechanism of drug resistance may also be operable in low-grade lymphomas where the tumor cell population has a lower growth fraction compared to the more curable aggressive lymphomas.

The greater sensitivity of proliferating tumor cells to chemotherapy could have practical significance, if methods were developed to increase the tumor growth fraction prior to its administration. Potential approaches include the selection of appropriate drugs and administration schedules, which synchronize the tumor cells and deliver chemotherapy at the height of a new round of tumor replication, and/or the use of mitogenic agents, which stimulate tumor cells to divide. It should be noted, however, that such approaches are theoretical and no clinical data exist to substantiate their efficacy.

A second important concept, emerging from the L1210 model, is that the number of tumor cells killed by a single cycle of chemotherapy is limited by first-order kinetics, i.e., a given drug dose kills a constant fraction of cells, regardless of the total cell number [1,2]. Of course, the actual fraction of cells killed is dependent on the sensitivity of the tumor to the chemotherapy agents and this fraction may change during the course of treatment. This finding implies that a single cycle of chemotherapy at standard dosage is unlikely to achieve a cure except in the most sensitive tumors, such as Burkitt's lymphoma, which, when the tumor burden is low, can occasionally be cured by a single dose of cyclophosphamide [3]. This concept also does not, apparently, apply to settings in which a single cycle of very intensive chemotherapy is administered with autologous stem cell support, since this can result in cure in relapsed aggressive lymphomas, albeit in the presence of a minimal tumor burden. The concept of fractional cell kill also implies that surgical resection of tumor, if of sufficient degree, may be beneficial, as illustrated by the excellent prognosis of patients with Burkitt's lymphoma in whom abdominal tumor can be essentially completely resected [4]. In general, however, surgical resection does not appear to improve upon the outcome of other therapeutic modalities and is not recommended unless medically necessary, for example, to prevent or deal with tumor-related bowel or stomach perforation (see Chapter 31). For the majority of clinical situations, the concept of fractional cell kill suggests that optimal results are likely to be obtained by using intensive doses of chemotherapy administered over multiple cycles.

DOSE INTENSITY

The association between the amount of drug administered per unit time, termed dose intensity (DI), and cell kill is one of the more important principles relevant to the treatment of lymphomas. In animal models of high growth rate tumors, a linear-log relationship between drug dose and tumor cell kill has been demonstrated. For example, doubling drug doses may increase cell kill by as much as ten-fold, while reductions by as little as 20% may decrease the cure rate by 50% [5]. Since fractional cell kill is rarely, if ever, 100%, it is not surprising that the dose per unit time is important to the ultimate outcome, at least in terms of achieving a complete response (CR). The importance of dose intensity in diffuse aggressive lymphomas was suggested by an analysis performed by DeVita et al., which showed a significant relation ($P < 0.001$) between the average relative dose intensity (RDI) of the major chemotherapy regimens and disease-free survival [6]. Kwak et al. performed a more specific analysis of the RDI of the individual drugs in CHOP (cyclophosphamide, doxorubicin, vincristine and prednisone), [M]BACOD (methotrexate, bleomycin, doxorubicin, cyclophosphamide, vincristine and prednisone) and MACOP-B (methotrexate, doxorubicin, cyclophosphamide, vincristine, prednisone and bleomycin) chemotherapy in 115 previously untreated patients with diffuse large-cell lymphomas and found a correlation with survival as well [7]. Interestingly, a multivariant analysis of prognostic factors performed in this analysis showed that the most important predictor of survival was an actual RDI of doxorubicin >75%, adjusted to CHOP doses.

Although the results from these studies strongly suggested the importance of DI, randomized trials comparing regimens that only differ in DI are necessary to confirm these conclusions. Meyer et al. performed such a study in 238 patients with untreated advanced-stage intermediate- or high-grade non-Hodgkin's lymphoma [8]. Patients were randomized to receive either standard (s) BACOP (bleomycin, doxorubicin, cyclophosphamide, vincristine and prednisone) or escalated (esc) BACOP with higher doses of doxorubicin. In this trial, patients in the (s)BACOP group received 80% of the projected dose of doxorubicin, compared to 108% in the (esc)BACOP group. With a median follow-up of 65 months, the trial failed to show a benefit of escalated doxorubicin doses on tumor response or patient survival. In another trial, the first-generation lymphoma regimen,

CHOP, was compared in a randomized design to the second- and third-generation regimens, m-BACOD, ProMACE-CytaBOM (prednisone, methotrexate, doxorubicin, cyclophosphamide, etoposide, cytosine arabinoside, bleomycin and vincristine) and MACOP-B [9]. Despite the increased dose intensity of the later generation regimens, none were superior to CHOP in relapse rates or disease-free survival at 3 years. Other investigators have tested the efficacy of even more dose-intense therapies in patients with previously untreated aggressive non-Hodgkin's lymphomas. In two separate trials, patients were randomized to receive high-dose therapy with autologous bone marrow rescue, if they were either slowly responding to CHOP chemotherapy or as consolidation in first complete remission [10,11]. Although the results are early, neither trial has shown a benefit for high-dose therapy, thus questioning the value of single cycles of high-dose therapy in this setting.

The results of these trials challenge the concept of DI in the design of treatment strategies for non-Hodgkin's lymphomas. However, these results should not be interpreted as suggesting that drug dose is not important. All drugs have a specific dose–response curve, dependent on both the type of drug and the patient, which may become relatively flat above a threshold dose. Because we do not know where the threshold lies for any single drug or patient, the clinician should always attempt to administer as close to full doses as possible when using a chemotherapy regimen that has proven efficacy. However, when applying the concept of dose intensity to the design of new therapies, it is important to understand the implications of these recent clinical trials. They lead to several preliminary but important conclusions. First, the increases in dose intensity of from 0.5–2-fold achieved in the second- and third-generation lymphoma regimens do not increase patient survival. Second, major increases in dose intensity in the range of 5–10-fold, achieved with single cycles of high-dose therapy and autologous bone marrow support, have not shown benefit.

The concept of dose intensity, however, should not be entirely abandoned when designing a new regimen. The aforementioned trials have not addressed all aspects of the dose intensity question and several approaches remain to be tested: (1) drugs with steep dose–response curves should be specifically chosen for escalation, such as the alkylating agents, which are relatively well tolerated at high doses; (2) significant increases in the dose intensity of selected (i.e., the most effective) drugs, of the order of 3–7-fold, should be the goal and delivered over multiple cycles of therapy; (3) continuous infusion administration schedules may allow more dose-intense administration of the natural products

(e.g., doxorubicin, etoposide and vincristine) with lower toxicity and may partially overcome multidrug resistance [12,13]. Protocols incorporating these approaches are currently undergoing testing in a number of institutions.

The achievement of a high dose intensity is not only dependent on the dose but also on the dosing interval. The randomized trials which have assessed the benefit of dose intensity have generally focused on drug doses and not on dosing interval. However, shortening the interval between treatments may be particularly important for lymphomas with high proliferation rates, such as the small noncleaved cell lymphomas. The minimal interval that can be achieved between chemotherapy cycles is dependent upon the rate at which the bone marrow recovers, and delays in drug administration may allow regrowth of the surviving fraction of tumor cells, even though they may not necessarily be drug resistant. The use, in this setting, of recombinant colony-stimulating factors, granulocyte–macrophage colony-stimulating factor (GM-CSF), granulocyte colony-stimulating factor (G-CSF), interleukin-3 (IL-3) and IL-3/GM-CSF fusion protein (Pixy), which are necessary for the normal proliferation and differentiation of hematopoietic cells, may hasten hematopoietic recovery and hence increase dose intensity (see Chapter 29) [14,15].

Pharmacology

A summary of the basic pharmacological properties of the commonly used drugs in non-Hodgkin's lymphomas is presented in Table 28.1. Most of these agents are members of four different drug classes: topoisomerase II inhibitors, tubulin binding agents, alkylating agents and antimetabolites. In this section, we will also briefly discuss two new drug classes, taxanes and topoisomerase I inhibitors, which have been tested in lymphomas in recent phase II studies [16,17].

TOPOISOMERASE INHIBITORS

Topoisomerase inhibitors are among the most important drugs for the treatment of lymphomas. The primary agents in this class are the anthracycline antibiotics and analogs and the epipodophyllotoxins, both topoisomerase II (topo II) inhibitors. Mechanistically, these drugs form a complex with DNA and the DNA repair enzyme, topoisomerase II, and produce a break in both DNA strands. Additionally, the anthracycline antibiotics may generate free radicals

Table 28.1 Principal cytotoxic drugs used for lymphomas

Class	Dose Range (mg/m²)	Frequency	Neutrophil	Platelet	Mucositis	Nausea/ vomiting	Other toxicity
Topoisomerase II inhibitors							
Doxorubicin	25–75 i.v.	q 3–4 wk	***	***	*	**	Alopecia, cardiomyopathy
Idarubicin	10–15 i.v.	q 3–4 wk	***	***	*	**	Alopecia, cardiomyopathy
Mitoxantrone	12–14 i.v.	q 3–4 wk	***	**	*	*	Cholestasis, cardiomyopathy
Etoposide	100–200 i.v.	q 3–4 wk	**	*	*	*	Leukemia
Tubulin binding agents							
Vincristine	1–1.4 i.v.	q wk	*	*	—	*	Distal neuropathy, inappropriate ADH
Vinblastine	4–6 i.v.	q wk	***	**	*	*	Jaw pain
Paclitaxel	130–250 i.v.	q 3 wk	***	**	**	*	Anaphylactoid reaction, sensory neuropathy, alopecia
Alklyating agents							
Mechlorethamine	6 i.v.	q 2–4 wk	***	**	—	**	Leukemia
Chlorambucil	1–3 p.o.	qd	**	**	—	*	Leukemia
Cyclophosphamide	350–1500 i.v.	q 3–4 wk	***	*	—	**	Cystitis, pulmonary fibrosis, water retention
Ifosfamide	4000–5000 i.v.	q 3–4 wk	***	**	—	*	Nephrotoxicity, cystitis, neurotoxicity
Procarbazine	100 p.o.	qd × 7–14d	**	**	—	*	Sensitivity to amines, sterility, leukemia
Darcarbazine	150 i.v.	qd × 5	*	*	—	***	Flu-like syndrome
CCNU	100–150 p.o.	q 4 wk	***	***	—	**	Leukemia, pulmonary fibrosis, renal failure
Antimetabolites							
Cytosine arabinoside	300–4000 i.v.	q 3–4 wk	***	***	**	**	Cholestasis, neurotoxicity
Fludarabine	20–25 i.v.	qd × 5	***	*	**	*	Neurotoxicity, hepatitis
2-Chlorodeoxyadenosine	4 i.v.	qd × 7	*	**	—	*	Immune suppression
Methotrexate	100–400 i.v.	q 3–4 wk	**	**	***	*	Renal toxicity, hepetitis
Miscellaneous							
Cisplatin	50–100 i.v.	q 3–4 wk	*	**	—	**	Renal failure, Mg²⁺ wasting, peripheral neuropathy
Bleomycin	5–10 i.v.	q 2–4 wk	*	*	—	*	Skin, pulmonary fibrosis, fever, hyper-sensitivity reactions

* Mild; ** moderate; *** marked.
ADH, Antidiuretic hormone; CCNU, 1-(2-chloroethyl)-3-cyclohexyl-nitrosourea.

by oxidation and reduction of their quinone groups, a probable cause of their cardiac toxicity. The epipodo-phyllotoxins are significantly more active against cycling cells than noncycling cells, whereas the anthracyclines are active against both cycling and quiescent cells.

The anthracycline antibiotics and analogs commonly used in lymphomas are doxorubicin, idarubicin and mitoxantrone. In lymphomas, these agents are generally administered in combination with other cytotoxic agents. Doxorubicin is usually administered at a dose of 25–75 mg/m² every 3–4 weeks, although weekly doses (e.g., 25 mg/m^2) or continuous infusions over 96 hours are used in some regimens. Schedules in which lower doses are administered over an extended period may be less cardiotoxic owing to lower peak plasma concentrations of doxorubicin. In some combination regimens, mitoxantrone or idarubicin is used in place of doxorubicin, although clinical trials have shown some significant difference in efficacy among these drugs [18,19].

Etoposide (VP-16), a semisynthetic derivative of podophyllotoxin, has significant activity against a broad range of hematologic malignancies. Etoposide has been incorporated into a number of combination chemotherapy regimens for non-Hodgkin's lymphomas and is also frequently included in high-dose chemotherapy regimens. Occasionally, etoposide is administered as a single agent, but in this case usually in the setting of relapsed disease. Etoposide has a wide therapeutic window so that drug doses are variable. In combination chemotherapy regimens, it is usually administered at 100–200 mg/m^2 every 2–3 weeks, although significantly higher doses are also well tolerated. Etoposide may be administered either orally or intravenously. When administered orally, only approximately 50% is bioavailable, so that the dose should be twice as high as the intravenous dose. The activity of etoposide is schedule-dependent and the drug is most effective when administered over a prolonged period, so that oral dosing is usually over a 7–14-day period. The dose of etoposide should be modified in patients with significant renal dysfunction, since 30–40% of unchanged drug is normally excreted in the urine [20]. The primary toxicity of etoposide is neutropenia, but mucositis can be quite prominent at higher doses. Although infrequent, etoposide has been associated with secondary acute myelogenous leukemia in children treated for acute lymphoblastic leukemia (ALL), and in adults treated for testicular cancer [21,22]. These leukemias frequently contain chromosomal translocations involving 11q23. Available information suggests that the cumulative dose and schedule of administration influence the relative risk for this toxicity.

All of the topoisomerase II (topo II) inhibitors are substrates for the P-170 glycoprotein (Pgp) membrane efflux pump, a mechanism of multidrug resistance (mdr-1). However, both idarubicin and etoposide are poorer substrates *in vitro* than doxorubicin or mitoxantrone and, thus, should be less susceptible to mdr-1 resistance [23,24].

Recently, several topoisomerase I (topo I) inhibitors have become available for clinical testing. These drugs are analogs of camptothecin and include hycamptamine (topotecan), camptothecin 11 (CPT-11) and 9-aminocamptothecin (9-AC). In an early phase II study of CPT-11 in 29 patients with relapsed lymphomas, 24% responded and four patients had complete responses [17]. Preliminary results of a recent phase II trial of 9-AC in relapsed non-Hodgkin's lymphomas at the National Cancer Institute (NCI), Bethesda, USA, showed a 25% partial response rate in 20 evaluable patients (W.H. Wilson, unpublished data). This class of drugs is potentially noncross-resistant with topo II inhibitors. Unlike topo II, topo I levels do not significantly fall in resting cells, and mutations of topo II will not affect the binding of topo I inhibitors. Moreover, topo I inhibitors are less susceptible to efflux by Pgp than topo II inhibitors; *in vitro*, 9-AC is active in mdr-1-resistant cell lines [25]. These preliminary results indicate that further studies are warranted to define the role of topo I inhibitors as single agents and in combination chemotherapy regimens for the treatment of lymphomas.

TUBULIN BINDING AGENTS

The vinca alkaloids, vincristine and vinblastine, are commonly used in the treatment of lymphomas. Mechanistically, these agents bind to tubulin and inhibit polymerization of the subunits necessary for the formation of microtubules. Consequently, assembly of the mitotic spindle is inhibited and the cells arrest in metaphase [26]. Thus, these agents are more effective against cycling cells. Clinically, vincristine is a component of most combination chemotherapy regimens for non-Hodgkin's lymphomas, whereas vinblastine is more commonly used in Hodgkin's lymphoma. Vincristine is administered intravenously, every 2–3 weeks. It is unusual for vincristine to be used as a single agent, although one trial of infusional vincristine in patients with recurrent lymphomas achieved a 36% objective response rate [27]. Neurotoxicity is a dose-limiting side-effect of vincristine, which is initially manifested as paresthesiae of the feet and hands, and loss of deep tendon reflexes. If loss of motor strength in the dorsiflexors of the feet and/or extensors of the wrists occur, the drug should be discontinued. Some clinicians advocate capping the vincristine dose at 2 mg per administration to reduce the incidence and severity of neurotoxicity, but this policy is arbitrary and is not recommended, since some patients may be underdosed, and the effect of dose on the cure rate is unknown. The vinca alkaloids are excellent substrates for Pgp and are, therefore, susceptible to mdr-1 resistance.

Recently, a new class of drugs, called taxanes, has been developed. These drugs also bind to microtubules but, unlike the vinca alkaloids, promote polymerization of the subunits. Among the drugs in this class, paclitaxel has been most extensively studied. A phase II study of paclitaxel administered as a 96-hour infusion in relapsed lymphomas was recently completed [16]. Of 29 evaluable patients, nine had low-grade, and 20 had intermediate- or high-grade lymphoma. Although most patients were heavily pretreated, having received a median of three (range 1–5) prior regimens, 68% had chemotherapy-sensitive disease, i.e., they responded to the last chemotherapy administered. However, paclitaxel was only modestly active, producing five (17%) partial responses. Although the clinical experience with paclitaxel is limited, these results suggest that patients who have received several prior regimens will probably be resistant to paclitaxel.

ALKYLATING AGENTS

Alkylating agents are among the most commonly used agents for the treatment of lymphomas. These drugs act by forming covalent bonds with electron-rich sites on DNA and cross-linking the DNA strand. They are active during all phases of the cell cycle and are therefore cycle-independent. Mechanisms of drug resistance may be alkylator-specific, e.g., impaired transport of nitrogen mustard, or non-specific, such as increased conjugation of reactive intermediates by glutathione [28]. As a group, alkylating agents produce significant hematopoietic toxicity but relatively little extramedullary toxicity. This toxicity profile has made them attractive for use in high-dose chemotherapy regimens.

In intermediate- and high-grade lymphomas, alkylating agents are usually used in combination with other drugs, while in low-grade lymphomas, single agent therapy is frequently used. Chlorambucil and cyclophosphamide are available orally and are often administered by mouth to patients with low-grade lymphomas, whereas intravenous cyclophosphamide is used in most combination regimens. Ifosfamide is more commonly employed in regimens designed for high-grade lymphomas or for salvage chemotherapy. In general, the alkylating agents, mechlorethamine, dacarbazine, procarbazine and 1-(2-chloroethyl)-3-cyclohexyl-nitrosourea (CCNU), are more often used in regimens for Hodgkin's lymphomas, although these agents have been incorporated into regimens for non-Hodgkin's lymphomas as well.

Alkylating agents do not share the schedule dependency of a number of natural products and, thus, are usually administered as short intravenous infusions. An exception to this is the oral administration of chlorambucil or cyclophosphamide, where extended daily dosing is used. At conventional doses, alkylating agents commonly cause moderate to marked hematological toxicity, and mild to moderate nausea and vomiting. Both cyclophosphamide and ifosfamide may cause severe cystitis unless adequate hydration or mercaptoethane-sulfonate (Mesna) is administered to inactivate the toxic metabolite, acrolein [29]. Most of these agents have the potential to cause secondary leukemia, the frequency of which appears to be related to total dose and to extended low-dose drug administration.

Alkylating agents are an important component of high-dose chemotherapy regimens. Experimentally, these agents have steep dose–response relationships and, when administered with stem cell rescue, their dose can be escalated from 2- to 18-fold above standard doses before extramedullary toxicity becomes dose-limiting [30–33]. Because alkylators differ in their preferred sites of DNA alkylation, and mechanisms of transport and DNA repair, they are not completely cross-resistant with one another [28]. Thus, there is a rationale for combining multiple alkylators in high-dose regimens [34]. When selecting agents for inclusion in high-dose regimens, attention should be paid to overlapping extramedullary toxicities in order to avoid additive or synergistic toxicities, which may require a reduction in the dose of all agents in the chemotherapy regimen.

ANTIMETABOLITES

Within this drug class are several important agents including methotrexate, cytosine arabinoside, 2-chlorodeoxyadenosine (2-CDA) and fludarabine phosphate. Cytosine arabinoside is an analog of deoxycytidine, which is converted intracellularly to the active metabolite, ara-cytosine triphosphate (ara-CTP). Ara-CTP inhibits DNA polymerase and terminates DNA strand elongation when incorporated into DNA [35]. Thus, these agents are significantly more active against cycling cells. Clinically, cytosine arabinoside is a component of several combination regimens for intermediate- and high-grade lymphomas as well as for several salvage chemotherapy regimens. The contribution of cytosine arabinoside, however, to the curative potential of these regimens is unclear [9,36–39]. A commonly used salvage regimen, DHAP (dexamethasone, cytosine arabinoside and cisplatin), effectively combined cytosine arabinoside and cisplatin and has been reported to give an objective response rate of 56% in patients with relapsed lymphomas [40]. In these regimens, cytosine arabinoside is administered in a variety of intravenous schedules including single or repetitive doses, or as a continuous infusion. Because of the drug's short plasma $t_{1/2}$ of 7–20 minutes, bolus doses up to 5 g/m^2 cause significantly less hematological toxicity than doses of 1g/m^2 administered over 48 hours [41]. At standard doses, myelosuppression is dose-limiting, whereas at high doses (3 g/m^2 Q12 hours), neurologic, gastrointestinal and hepatic toxicity occurs [28]. With high-dose administration, cerebellar toxicity with ataxia and slurred speech may occur, particularly in patients over 50 years old and in patients with reduced renal function [42].

Methotrexate is a folate antagonist, which inhibits the enzyme dihydrofolate reductase (DHFR), leading to the depletion of intracellular folate coenzymes, and the inhibition of thymidylate and purine biosynthesis. As a result, DNA synthesis and cell replication are blocked. Like cytosine arabinoside, methotrexate is a component of many combination chemotherapy regimens. Combination regimens for intermediate-grade lymphomas generally employ lower doses (<500 mg/m^2) whereas high-dose methotrexate (>500 mg/m^2) has been incorporated into high-grade lymphoma regimens [9,43]. For all but the lowest doses (<50 mg/m^2), leucovorin rescue must be administered within 24–42 hours after the commencement of the methotrexate infusion and continued until plasma concentrations are <5 × 10^{-7} M in order to prevent life-threatening gastrointestinal and hematologic toxicity [44]. Because methotrexate is principally eliminated by the kidney, patients with markedly decreased renal function should not be treated with this drug. The most common toxicities are hematologic and mucositis, although renal failure, skin rash and hepatitis may occasionally occur.

The contribution of methotrexate to the efficacy of intermediate-grade regimens is uncertain. Methotrexate-containing regimens such as m-BACOD, MACOP-B and ProMACE-CytaBOM were recently shown to be no better than CHOP in efficacy [9]. In regimens for high-grade lymphomas, the contribution of methotrexate to their efficacy is unclear owing to a lack of randomized studies. However, high-dose methotrexate is a component of a number of regimens which have produced promising results [43].

Two deamination-resistant purine analogs, fludarabine phosphate and 2-CDA, have demonstrated good single-agent activity in low-grade lymphomas and are currently used in patients with relapsed disease [45–48]. Fludarabine phosphate undergoes several metabolic steps to form the triphosphate, which is incorporated into DNA and RNA, and inhibits DNA polymerase [49]. It is usually administered daily for 5 days at a dose of 20–30 mg/m^2, and repeated every 3–4 weeks. Acute hematologic toxicity is moderate at these doses, but prolonged and severe myelosuppression may occur in some patients after multiple cycles [46]. Furthermore, owing to the sensitivity of normal B- and T-lymphocytes to the cytotoxic effects of fludarabine phosphate resulting in a loss of CD4 lymphocytes, patients often develop prolonged immunosuppression and an increased incidence of opportunistic infections [47]. Mild neurological toxicity, usually reported as lethargy, is quite common at these doses, although severe neurological toxicity such as seizures, coma and optic neuritis may be observed at high doses (125 mg/m^2/day × 5) [50].

Clinically, fludarabine phosphate has excellent activity against low-grade lymphomas. In two studies of fludarabine phosphate in recurrent low-grade lymphomas, 13/25 (52%) and 23/40 (58%) of patients achieved an objective response [45,46]. However, fludarabine phosphate is less active in relapsed intermediate-grade lymphomas where it had a 14% response rate in the former and a 5% response rate in the latter study.

Normal and malignant lymphocytes are also extremely sensitive to the cytotoxic effects of 2-CDA [48]. Like fludarabine phosphate, 2-CDA is converted to a triphosphate, which is incorporated into DNA [51]. It is usually administered at a dose of 4 mg/m^2 intravenously (i.v.) daily × 7 and repeated every 5 weeks. Myelosuppression is usually mild early in the treatment course, but frequently worsens after four cycles of therapy. Like fludarabine phosphate, 2-CDA causes severe immunosuppression resulting in an increased incidence of severe bacterial and opportunistic infections [52]. This drug has been shown to be effective in patients with low-grade lymphomas. In 40 patients with previously treated low-grade lymphomas, 43% achieved a response, of which half were complete [50]. These results have been confirmed by a more recent study [53].

CISPLATIN AND BLEOMYCIN

Cisplatin is a component of several effective salvage regimens, DHAP and ESAP (etoposide, solumedrol, cytosine arabinoside and cisplatin), for the treatment of lymphomas [39,54]. Mechanistically, cisplatin forms covalent bonds preferentially at the N-7 position of guanine and adenine nucleosides, forming interstrand cross-links and DNA adducts, and thereby disrupting DNA function [55]. Like classical alkylating agents, cisplatin is cycle-independent. Cisplatin is usually administered at a dose of 50–100 mg/m^2 as a bolus or 24-hour continuous infusion every 3–4 weeks. It causes mild neutropenia and moderate thrombocytopenia. Peripheral neuropathy may occur after high cumulative doses. Patients should be well hydrated before receiving cisplatin in order to reduce the incidence of renal failure.

Bleomycin is an effective antitumor agent, which has been incorporated into numerous combination chemotherapy regimens, in part because it has minimal hematopoietic toxicity. It is composed of a mixture of peptides isolated from the fungus *Streptomyces vesticillis*, which form a bleomycin:Fe(II) complex on DNA. This produces single- and double-strand breaks in the DNA and is, therefore, more cytotoxic to cycling cells [56]. Bleomycin is usually administered as an i.v. bolus of 5–10 mg/m^2 every 2–4 weeks. The incidence of pulmonary toxicity, characterized by interstitial infiltrates with cough and dyspnea, increases as cumulative bleomycin dose increases, and has a higher frequency in patients with pre-existent lung disease, patients who have received prior pulmonary irradiation, and patients exposed to high oxygen concentrations [57,58]. Other toxicities include skin changes with erythema and hyperpigmentation, and fever and malaise. Clinically, there is little evidence that bleomycin improves the efficacy of combination chemotherapy regimens. A randomized comparison of three bleomycin-containing regimens (MACOP-B, Pro-MACE-CytaBOM and m-BACOD) and CHOP in patients with previously untreated intermediate-grade lymphomas showed no advantage to the bleomycin-containing regimens [9].

Drug resistance

The inability to eradicate all tumor with chemotherapy results from a failure of the drug to reach the tumor cells, and/or to the presence or emergence of resistant tumor cells. In 1979, Goldie and Coldman proposed a hypothesis to explain the spontaneous development of resistance of cancer cells to chemotherapeutic agents [59]. This hypothesis was derived from the observation, made originally by bacterial geneticists, that the development of resistance by *E. coli* to infection by bacteriophage occurs through the preferential expansion of bacterial clones that have undergone spontaneous mutation to a resistant phenotype [60]. Goldie and Coldman extrapolated this concept to human tumors and correlated the emergence of resistant tumor cells with their spontaneous mutation rate. For example, the model predicts that, if the mutation rate for a drug resistance gene is in the range of 10^{-6} or higher, the possibility of the emergence of a least one resistant cell to a given drug is high, even before the cell population reaches 10^6 cells, a tumor size which is orders of magnitude less than can be clinically detected. Other events such as nonrandom cytogenetic alterations found in many cancers may also contribute to their intrinsic resistance to anticancer drugs [61]. Eventually, resistant subclones predominate in the tumor cell population as a result of the selective pressure of

anticancer drug treatment; that is, resistant cells are able to proliferate under conditions which lead to the death of nonresistant cells. Furthermore, the Goldie and Coldman formula predicts that resistance may emerge within a two log increment in cell number, which, in the case of rapidly proliferating lymphomas, may occur within several weeks. Consequently, prolonged delays in starting therapy and delays between cycles of therapy may reduce the chance of cure.

By providing an hypothesis for the emergence of resistant subclones the Goldie–Coldman model offers an explanation for the inverse relationship observed between curability and cell number, independent of tumor growth kinetics and fractional cell kill [59]. This model has important theoretical implications for the design of chemotherapy protocols and provides explanations for some of the principles already established through empiric observation. Firstly, the probability that cells which are resistant to one or more drugs are present in patients with large tumor burdens is high, providing one explanation for the greater efficacy of combination chemotherapy over single agents. However, combination chemotherapy has not completely overcome the problem of drug resistance, partly because the likelihood of the emergence of simultaneous resistance to two different classes of drugs is greater than the product of the mutation rate conferring resistance to each individual drug. This is because a single mutation is capable of inducing resistance to more than one class of drugs [62,63]. Therefore, although combination chemotherapy may induce a CR in the majority of lymphoma patients, the presence of even a small number of resistant cells in a large tumor mass is sufficient to account for the high relapse rate observed in some clinical circumstances. Secondly, the growth fraction of a tumor mass will increase as the tumor cells sensitive to the administered chemotherapy are killed, resulting in an increase in the mitotic rate of the remaining tumor cells, including drug-resistant subclones. Thus, the Goldie–Coldman hypothesis implies that not only is it important to minimize delays between chemotherapy cycles, but that the use of noncross-resistant drug combinations is more likely to result in a successful outcome.

An important obstacle to the cure of lymphomas is the development of simultaneous resistance to multiple classes of anticancer drugs, a phenomenon termed pleiotropic drug resistance [64,65]. Such resistance may occur spontaneously, or it may be induced by exposure to a single drug. One mechanism of pleiotropic drug resistance, which is associated with resistance to the anthracyclines, epipodophyllotoxins, vinca alkaloids, taxane and camptothecins, results from the increased expression of the multidrug resistance gene (mdr-1) [63,66]. The product of this gene, Pgp, functions as a membrane efflux pump, which, when overexpressed in tumor cells *in vitro*, results in decreased intracellular drug levels and resistance to a broad spectrum of unrelated cancer drugs. In normal cells, the function of Pgp may be to eliminate toxic compounds. Thus, it is of interest that most chemotherapeutic agents susceptible to multidrug resistance are natural products and could be encountered in small quantities during everyday life. Cells such as colonic epithelium, renal tubules and bile canaliculi, which are involved in excretion and would be predicted to encounter higher levels of such toxins, express this gene in increased amounts [67].

Increased expression of mdr-1 RNA and Pgp have been found both in untreated leukemias and in lymphomas exposed to chemotherapy, suggesting that multidrug resistance plays a role in the development of clinical drug resistance in at least some of these tumors. An analysis of tumor samples from untreated lymphoma patients showed increased expression of mdr-1 RNA in 4 out of 18 (22%) samples, and increased Pgp immunoreactivity in 28 out of 57 (49%) samples [68,69]. Of interest, however, is that no correlation was found between the increased expression of Pgp, and either response to chemotherapy or overall survival in this study [69]. In another study, increased Pgp immunoreactivity was only rarely found in untreated patients (1 out of 39) but commonly found in recurrent tumors from previously treated patients (5 out of 9), suggesting that it may play a role in the emergence of clinical drug resistance in these tumors [70].

There is sufficient evidence of increased expression of mdr-1 in relapsed lymphomas to justify the exploration of strategies designed to reverse Pgp-related drug resistance. Clinically, such strategies are made possible by the availability of noncytotoxic drugs that inhibit Pgp, such as verapamil, amiodarone, quinidine and cyclosporin [71–73]. These drugs have undergone limited testing in combination with chemotherapy in patients with solid tumors, leukemias and lymphomas [71,72,74,75]. Unfortunately, the design of most of these trials precludes an assessment of the efficacy of the Pgp blocker in overcoming drug resistance owing to the lack of adequate controls. In one trial, Miller et al. administered verapamil by intravenous infusion with cyclophosphamide and dexamethasone, and infusional vincristine and doxorubicin (C-VAD), in 18 patients with relapsed non-Hodgkin's lymphomas [70]. Unfortunately, no patient had previously received the C-VAD regimen alone, as administered in this trial, so it was not established that all patients were resistant to C-VAD. All patients, however, had obtained only an incomplete response or had pro-

gressed within 3 months of a vincristine/doxorubicin-containing regimen. The response rate to C-VAD/verapamil was high, with objective responses being observed in 11 out of 14 (79%) patients with non-Hodgkin's lymphomas, but there was no significant correlation between response rate and the presence of P-170 in the tumor cells. This suggests that the infusional C-VAD regimen itself might have been responsible for some of the responses, independent of the inhibition of Pgp by verapamil.

The disadvantages of the trial design used by Miller et al. can be overcome by using a crossover strategy in which patients receive the reversal agent only after demonstrating persistent or progressive disease on the same chemotherapy regimen. This approach was employed by Wilson et al. in a trial of dexverapamil, the dextrorotatory isomer of racemic verapamil, and EPOCH chemotherapy (intravenous infusions of vincristine, etoposide and doxorubicin with bolus cyclophosphamide and prednisone) in patients with drug-resistant lymphomas [12,76]. A schedule of administration by prolonged intravenous infusion was chosen because experimental studies in an mdr-1-resistant colon cell line suggested that resistance to doxorubicin or vincristine could be better overcome, if only partially, by using continuous low-dose exposure, rather than short high-dose exposure [13]. In this trial patients served as their own control. One hundred and one patients who had relapsed or refractory non-Hodgkin's lymphoma following a doxorubicin/vincristine-containing regimen were treated with EPOCH chemotherapy alone. EPOCH proved to be very active, and 87% of patients had either a complete or partial response [76]. Those patients with stable disease over two cycles of EPOCH alone or disease progression were crossed over to receive dexverapamil on their next and subsequent cycles of EPOCH. Of 41 evaluable patients who were crossed over, there were three complete, two partial and five minor responses following the addition of dexverapamil. Although the response rate after crossover was modest, it is important to recognize that the crossover trial design may have mitigated against a response to dexverapamil. By requiring a tumor to fail a regimen before the addition of a Pgp blocker, selection for multiple mechanisms of drug resistance, among them mdr-1, must occur. Mdr-1 expression, analyzed by quantitative polymerase chain reaction (PCR), was found to be low in 17 pretreatment biopsies, but was high in 8 out of 16 patients at the time of crossover to dexverapamil [76]. Of interest was the finding that of six patients with high mdr-1 levels at crossover, three responded to dexverapamil while only one out of eight patients with low mdr-1 levels responded.

These preliminary data provide several insights

into clinical drug resistance in lymphomas. Firstly, mdr-1 expression may be present at low levels in untreated patients but is readily detected after treatment failure in some patients. However, other mechanisms of drug resistance are clearly present, since most drug-resistant patients do not express high levels of mdr-1. Secondly, the high response rates achieved with EPOCH alone in heavily pre-treated patients suggest that infusional schedules may overcome drug resistance to some extent. Thirdly, the results of the crossover study suggest that dexverapamil can partially overcome Pgp in some drug-resistant patients. Further study will be necessary to determine the role of infusional chemotherapy and Pgp inhibition in reversing drug resistance. Ultimately, such approaches need to be tested in untreated patients with potentially curable lymphomas to determine whether reversal of mdr-1 drug resistance can increase the rate of cure.

Frequently, increased expression of Pgp is not the explanation for clinically demonstrable multidrug resistance, nor is it likely that other drug transport proteins such as the multidrug resistance-associated protein (MRP) will account for most pleiotropic drug resistance in refractory lymphomas [77]. Recent observations, however, suggest that the cellular response to chemotherapy-induced damage plays an important role in drug resistance. Following chemotherapy-induced damage to cellular proteins and DNA, a cell can either repair potentially fatal cytotoxic damage or undergo cell death by cellular necrosis or programmed cell death (apoptosis) [78]. The desired effect of cytotoxic therapy, of course, is tumor cell death. Accumulating evidence suggests that the cellular apparatus which controls the cell cycle and apoptosis is an essential component of the final common pathways through which cytotoxic drugs exert their lethal effects, and their deregulation could lead to drug resistance [79–81]. Indeed, some of the most common oncogene and/or tumor suppressor gene mutations found in lymphoid neoplasms occur in genes involved in the cell cycle or its regulation, including *bcl-1*, p53 and c-*myc* [82–84]. Among the best studied of these is p53, a tumor suppressor gene that controls the cellular responses to DNA damage by arresting cells in G_1 of the cell cycle so that repair of DNA damage may occur before the cells proceeds through DNA synthesis and mitosis [85]. If essential cellular repairs are not completed, p53 can trigger apoptosis. *In vitro*, mutations of p53 lead to increased cellular resistance to both radiation and chemotherapy [86, 87]. A recent clinical study of p53 in high-grade B-cell lymphomas found a positive correlation of p53 mutations with decreased survival time, suggesting that tumors with p53 mutations may be more drug resistant [88]. Furthermore, a study of p53 over-expression, which usually signifies mutation in the gene, in relapsed non-Hodgkin's lymphomas revealed an independent association with resistance to EPOCH chemotherapy and decreased survival [89]. Thus, mutations involving check point genes, which regulate the cell cycle and apoptosis, such as p53, may play a central role in pleiotropic drug resistance. If such pathways are important in drug resistance, the notion that alternating 'noncross-resistant' combination chemotherapy will be more effective than single regimens becomes unlikely. In fact, clinical experience with intermediate-grade non-Hodgkin's lymphomas confirms that at least some alternating 'noncross-resistant' combinations of chemotherapy do not improve patient survival [9]. Indeed, enough evidence has emerged to warrant the development of strategies to overcome the deregulation of cell cycle control and apoptosis.

Protocol design

Even before the basic principles of chemotherapy design were fully appreciated, combination drug therapy empirically evolved from a need to develop more effective treatment than was provided by single agents. It is now clear that combination therapy is markedly superior to monotherapy for the majority of drug-responsive tumors. However, its success is dependent both on the application of the principles of chemotherapy to protocol design and on the use of effective anticancer drugs. Although early combination chemotherapy protocols were developed in an era when many of these principles were not appreciated, their success can now be partly understood within the context of these principles. For example, the Goldie–Coldman hypothesis provides one explanation for why combination therapy, compared to monotherapy, more effectively overcomes tumor cell resistance and slows down or prevents the emergence of additional populations of resistant cells. Furthermore, the fact that combination therapy allows a greater dose rate to be achieved compared to monotherapy, because of its higher therapeutic ratio, is a major contributor to its effectiveness.

The development of an effective combination chemotherapy regimen is dependent on the appropriate selection of drugs and administration schedules, and on the application of the aforementioned principles [5]. Firstly, only drugs which have significant single-agent activity should be chosen and, although clinically unproven, the selection of drugs which have synergistic activity *in vitro* has theoretical appeal. It should be emphasized that, although it is not always possible to identify the most active drugs, the use of drugs which have poorer activity against the tumor being treated will add toxicity and usually lead to a reduction in the dose rate for the effective drugs. Secondly, drugs with minimal overlapping toxicity should be used whenever possible in order to avoid dose reductions of other drugs with similar toxicities and to minimize unacceptable organ toxicity. Thirdly, the choice of dose, rate and route of drug administration (e.g., oral, intravenous bolus or infusion) should be based on the pharmacokinetics of the drug(s) in question and on existing information regarding the maximal tolerated dose(s) for any given schedule. For example, *in vitro*, the natural products, doxorubicin, vincristine and etoposide, are more cytotoxic when administered at low dose over a 48-hour period than when administered at a higher dose over a short 1-hour period [13]. This suggests that these agents may be more effective when administered as continuous infusions than as a bolus. During the initial development of a new combination regimen, pharmacokinetic monitoring may allow the investigator to adjust drug doses to optimize the plasma concentrations, based on *in vitro* dose–response curves, and to characterize the pharmacodynamics of the regimen. However, pharmacokinetic monitoring may not be practical or even necessary once the regimen has been developed and is in use by the oncology community. Fourthly, combining drugs with various mechanisms of actions has theoretical appeal. For example, certain drug combinations may be synergistic (e.g., cisplatin and etoposide), and combining drugs that are cell cycle-dependent, such as antimetabolites, vinca alkaloids and epipodophyllotoxins, with cell cycle-independent drugs, such as alkylating agents and anthracyclines, may theoretically target both cycling and noncycling cells. These principles must clearly be applied within the context of both the natural history of the disease and empiric observations made from the results of previous treatment protocols. Ultimately, treatment regimens are judged by results and since there are so many variables that impact upon the outcome of chemotherapy, it must be recognized that there still remains a large element of empiricism in protocol design.

In specific situations, radiotherapy is used in combination with chemotherapy in protocols written with curative intent. Of course, with the exception of total body irradiation (TBI), radiation is a locoregional modality. Thus, its principal role in combined modality approaches is to treat local sites of bulky disease, which may be relatively chemotherapy resistant. When radiotherapy is incorporated into a regimen, it may be viewed as a treatment modality which is generally noncross-resistant with chemotherapy. It adds a specific spectrum of toxicities, whose severity and quality will depend on the type of chemotherapy administered to the patient. It should be pointed out that, with the possible exception of a small number of specific types and stages of lymphomas, the value of radiation therapy as a complement to combination chemotherapy administered for curative intent remains controversial.

Chemotherapy of lymphomas

For the purposes of treatment, the non-Hodgkin's lymphomas can be classified into a number of clinically distinct groups which are principally defined by histology, despite a rapidly expanding understanding of the immunobiology of lymphomas. Although there are several clinically equivalent classifications, the Working Formulation provides a useful division of the non-Hodgkin's lymphomas into low-, intermediate- and high-grade groups [90]. For the purposes of this chapter, we shall discuss the therapy of lymphomas within the context of these three divisions, although subtypes within these divisions may require significantly different treatment approaches (Table 28.2).

LOW-GRADE LYMPHOMAS

The low-grade lymphomas are unique among the non-Hodgkin's lymphomas because they can be effectively treated, often for years, with nonaggressive treatment approaches, such as single alkylating agents. In fact, response rates up to 80% have been reported with single agents, although the majority of responses are only partial [91]. Predictably, combination chemotherapy regimens such as cyclophosphamide, vincristine and prednisone (CVP) produce higher CR rates than single agents (37% versus 13%, respectively), but without an improvement in overall patient survival [92,93]. In the 1970s, the efficacy of a variety of therapeutic approaches were evaluated in advanced stage low-grade lymphomas, including total nodal irradiation (TNI), combined modality therapy and aggressive combination chemotherapy. Despite these more aggressive approaches, no survival benefit was found when compared to single agent therapy or CVP [94–97]. Clinical trials such as these demonstrated that durable CRs were not only uncommon but, perhaps surprisingly, did not have great prognostic significance. It is the paradoxically excellent response of these tumors to a variety of treatment approaches and yet their resistance to cure, which is so perplexing.

This paradoxical response of the low-grade lym-

Table 28.2 Standard treatment approaches for advanced-stage non-Hodgkin's lymphomas

Lymphoma subtype	Clinical setting	Approach	Regimen
Low grade (FSC, FM, DSC, SL)	Asymptomatic	Observation	None
	Symptomatic – local	Radiation	None
	Symptomatic – disseminated	Chemotherapy	Chlorambucil or Fludarabine
	Symptomatic – relapsed or histological progression	Chemotherapy	CHOP BMT
Intermediate grade (FL,DL,IBL,DM)	Advanced stage	Chemotherapy	CHOP or derivative
High grade (DI – childhood LBL,SNC)	LBL (childhood)	Chemotherapy	LSA2-L2 A-COP
	LBL (adult)	Chemotherapy	LSA2-L2 High-dose CHOP
	SNC, DL (childhood)	Chemotherapy	CODOX-M/IVAC [43]
	SNC (adult)	Chemotherapy	CODOX-M/IVAC [43]

See specific chapters for more detailed information.
FSC, follicular small cell; FM, follicular mixed; DSC, diffuse small cell; SL, small lymphocytic; FL, follicular lymphoma; DL, diffuse large cell; IBL, immunoblastic lymphoma; DM, diffuse mixed small and large cell; DI, diffuse, intermediate differentiation; LBL, lymphoblastic lymphoma; BMT, bone marrow transplantation.

phomas has been met with two radically different treatment approaches over the past 20 years. In a conservative approach, investigators at Stanford University managed a selected group of asymptomatic, advanced-stage patients by withholding therapy until medically necessary (watch and wait) [98,99]. The Stanford group found that by watching and waiting, the patient median survival of 11 years was not significantly different from that found in two prospective trials involving similar patients treated at Stanford with standard chemotherapy approaches. Although this study provided a persuasive argument for the conservative management of low-grade lymphomas, its nonrandomized design and use of historical or parallel controls treated with a variety of nonaggressive therapies left the optimal management of these diseases in doubt.

The benefit of aggressive therapy was addressed in a recently completed randomized clinical trial conducted at the NCI, Bethesda, USA. In this study, previously untreated, asymptomatic and advanced-stage patients were randomized to receive either initial therapy with intensive multimodality therapy, ProMACE-MOPP (methotrexate, doxorubicin, cyclophosphamide, etoposide, mechlorethamine, vincristine, procarbazine and prednisone) flexitherapy followed by 2200–2500 cGy TNI or watch and wait until disease progression, at which time the same intensive multimodality therapy was begun [100]. A total of 89 patients were randomized to the two treatment arms; 45 (51%) to aggressive therapy and 44 (49%) to watchful waiting. Seventy-eight per cent of patients randomized to aggressive therapy achieved a CR with a median disease-free survival (DFS) exceeding 45 months. In contrast, of 18 patients on the watchful waiting arm who crossed over to chemotherapy, only 43% achieved a CR. However, despite the difference in CR between the two arms, there was no difference in overall survival, suggesting that early aggressive intervention does not improve survival.

With the failure of aggressive 'conventional' dose therapy to cure advanced-stage patients, investigators began to study the efficacy of high-dose therapy with autologous bone marrow rescue. In a study at the Dana–Farber Cancer Institute, patients in first CR or partial remission (PR) were treated with high-dose cyclophosphamide and total body irradiation, followed by autologous bone marrow purged with a cocktail of anti-B-cell antibodies and complement [101,102]. When last reported, 48 (62%) out of 77 patients were in unmaintained CR with a median of 22 months follow-up, a result which is not significantly different from that achieved in the NCI study. Although longer follow-up is necessary to determine whether any of these patients have been cured, at present, high-dose therapy for low-grade lymphomas should be considered experimental and without proven benefit over conventional approaches.

INTERMEDIATE-GRADE LYMPHOMAS

Unlike patients with low-grade lymphomas, those with intermediate- and high-grade lymphomas do poorly when treated with nonaggressive chemotherapy, such as CVP or single agents. At best, regimens like CVP only produce CRs in 25–30% of patients, and most patients eventually relapse and die [103,104]. The first chemotherapy regimen which produced a significant rate of cure was CHOP [105]. It was basically derived from CVP by the addition of doxorubicin and by changes in drug dose and schedule. Compared to CVP, it was a major advance and improved the overall survival and cure of intermediate-grade lymphomas. Minor variations, however, such as CHOP–bleomycin and BACOP (CHOP and bleomycin with different doses and schedules) did not significantly improve upon the results obtained with CHOP [106,107]. Second-generation regimens were developed by adding noncross-resistant drugs to CHOP and by administering the drugs in shorter, alternating cycles. This was accomplished in several different ways. For example, with the m-BACOD (see Chapter 42) regimen, drugs were administered on day 1 and 14, and repeated every 3 weeks for ten cycles [108]. NCI investigators developed a more radical approach based on the Goldie–Coldman model; called ProMACE-MOPP 'flexitherapy' [109]. They reasoned that if the rate of fractional cell kill by a regimen decreased over time because of the emergence of resistant clones, then the use of a second noncross-resistant regimen at that time should result in an increased fractional cell kill. Thus, ProMACE was administered until the rate of tumor shrinkage stabilized, at which time patients crossed over to receive MOPP. However, despite the theoretical appeal of this approach, there was little evidence that it improved efficacy.

The design of third-generation regimens was not conceptually different from the second-generation regimens, with the exception of MACOP-B developed at the University of British Columbia [110]. This regimen has several features that are theoretically appealing. Firstly, drugs are administered weekly for the duration of therapy by alternating myelosuppressive and myelosparing drugs. With this schedule, the period between drug cycles, during which time tumor DNA can be repaired and growth of tumor recommenced, is minimized. In addition, the expansion of resistant clones, in theory, should be reduced by alternating noncross-resistant drugs every week. Secondly, by rapidly alternating cycle specific and nonspecific drugs, this regimen may potentially increase the number of cells in cycle, thereby increasing the fractional cell kill of the cycle specific drugs.

The second- and third-generation regimens appeared to have improved CR rates and lower relapse rates compared to first-generation regimens such as CHOP [103,104,110], and became the standard of care for many oncologists. However, the perceived improvement in efficacy of these later-generation regimens was based on nonrandomized studies with rather short follow-up durations from single institutions. Apparent advantages may well have been the result of patient selection, maximizing dose intensity, improved supportive care and short follow-up. Because the newer generation regimens were more costly and toxic than CHOP and some recent studies raised questions about their apparent advantages, the Southwest Oncology Group of the USA initiated a phase III randomized comparison of CHOP, m-BACOD, ProMACE-CytaBOM and MACOP-B in patients with advanced-stage, intermediate-grade non-Hodgkin's lymphomas [9]. A total of 899 patients were randomized among the four groups. At three years, 44% of all patients were alive without disease and there were no significant differences among the groups in disease free or overall survival. This clinical trial is important because it convincingly demonstrated that the newer-generation regimens are no more effective than CHOP. This result challenges a number of principles of chemotherapy design, as applied in these regimens, including the use of multiple noncross-resistant drugs and dose intensity. It would appear that, in order to improve upon CHOP chemotherapy, other approaches will need to be investigated, such as drug resistance modulation, optimization of administration schedules, the use of new drugs with unique mechanisms of action, immunomodulation and antibody-directed therapies. All of these approaches are currently under investigation and may ultimately be integrated into treatment approaches for newly diagnosed patients.

An important variable which must be considered when interpreting the results of chemotherapy trials in intermediate-grade lymphomas is the diverse biology of these tumors. For example, up to 30% of diffuse large-cell lymphomas carry a translocation of bcl-2, located on chromosome 18, to the immunoglobulin heavy chain locus on chromosome 14 (t(14;18)), suggesting that some of these tumors are biologically related to follicular center cell tumors [111]. Clinically, it has been shown that the diffuse large-cell lymphomas that carry this translocation have a higher chance of relapse than those without it, a not unexpected finding [112]. In another study it was observed that large-cell lymphomas which have a rearrangement of the bcl-6 gene have a more favorable prognosis [113]. Since biologically different tumors appear to have differing responses, it will be important to characterize responses in different biological subtypes in future clinical trials.

HIGH-GRADE LYMPHOMAS

High-grade lymphomas are heterogenous in their cells of origin, being principally of T-cell origin in lymphoblastic lymphomas (LBL), B-cell origin in small noncleaved lymphomas (SNCL), and of either B- or T-cell origin in immunoblastic lymphomas (IBL) [114,115]. Clinically, this diversity is reflected by their different patterns of presentation, prognosis and response to chemotherapy [35,116,117]. As such, different treatment approaches have been developed for the various subtypes. Generally, regimens developed for intermediate-grade lymphomas are used for the treatment of IBL, a subtype of diffuse large-cell lymphoma, while more dose-intensive regimens are employed for the treatment of LBL and SNCL. Numerous aggressive regimens have been developed for LBL and SNCL, and are modeled on both 'lymphoma' and 'leukemia' treatment approaches.

Although different regimens have been targeted for use in LBL and SNC subtypes and for children and adults, it is unclear if these pathological and age distinctions are significant variables for the design of therapy. Analysis of early chemotherapy trials in pediatric patients suggested that LBL responded better to 'leukemia-like' regimens in which a complex array of drugs were administered over an extended period, while SNCL responded better to intensive 'lymphoma-like' regimens in which fewer drugs were administered over a shorter period and placed a greater emphasis on alkylators. In 1976, Wollner reported a 73% long-term DFS in pediatric lymphomas treated with a ten-drug combination called LSA2-L2 [cyclophosphamide, vincristine, daunomycin, vincristine, prednisone, cytosine arabinoside, L-asparaginase, methotrexate, thioguanine, 1, 3 bis(2-chloroethyl)-1-nitrosourea (BCNU) and hydroxyurea] [36]. This regimen was based on a leukemia treatment approach in which patients received intensive induction and consolidation chemotherapy followed by maintenance for one year. The LSA2-L2 regimen was subsequently tested in patients with disseminated LBL, where it achieved good results (76% two-year DFS in one trial). However, patients with nonlymphoblastic lymphomas did poorly (26% two-year DFS) [37,116]. When it was compared in a randomized study to COMP (cyclophosphamide, vincristine, methotrexate and prednisone), a 'lymphoma' regimen, LSA2-L2 was significantly less effective in patients with nonlymphoblastic lymphomas (28% versus 57%) [116]. Further trials indicated that the success of 'leukemia'

approaches in LBL was probably not the result of the 'induction–consolidation–maintenance' design of these protocols. In fact, the Pediatric Oncology Group demonstrated no difference in therapeutic outcome in patients with LBL randomized to receive either a five-drug combination lymphoma regimen called A-COP (doxorubicin, cyclophosphamide, vincristine, prednisone) or the LSA2-L2 regimen [37]. Furthermore, in a study conducted at the NCI, there was no difference in treatment outcome between patients with LBL and SNC lymphoma treated with a 'lymphoma' regimen, which contained cyclophosphamide, doxorubicin, vincristine, methotrexate and prednisone [38].

Several conclusions regarding the choice of drugs and schedules for high-grade lymphomas can be made from these and other trials. Firstly, anthracyclines are important drugs for the treatment of LBL, while more complex and toxic 'leukemia' approaches may not be necessary. These trials also suggest that L-asparaginase is probably not essential for the treatment of LBL, at least in patients without bone marrow involvement. Secondly, cyclophosphamide, administered in a dose-intensive fashion, appears to be essential for the treatment of SNCL, as illustrated by the poor results obtained with regimens such as LSA2-L2 in which vincristine, prednisone and anthracyclines comprise the backbone of the induction phase. Agents such as methotrexate, cytosine arabinoside and etoposide have significant activity and should be considered for inclusion in protocols for the treatment of high-grade lymphomas. Clearly, there is significant overlap in the treatment approaches for LBL and SNCL and, in fact, they can probably be treated with similar regimens if properly selected. Such regimens should at least include cyclophosphamide or ifosfamide, anthracyclines, vincristine and prednisone, which are among the most effective drugs for both LBL and SNCL. One issue that remains to be determined is the duration of therapy. Lymphomas require only a few cycles of an appropriate regimen, but it is not known whether LBL, which is usually treated for longer periods, 18 months or more in most pediatric protocols – can be treated effectively in this way.

Although most of these observations are based on trials in pediatric lymphomas, the conclusions are also relevant to the treatment of high-grade lymphomas in adults. Unfortunately in adults, there is little clinical information on the differential response of LBL and SNCL to these different therapeutic approaches because of the paucity of clinical trials which include sufficient numbers of uniformly treated patients.

References

1. Skipper H, Schabel F, Wilcox W. Experimental evaluation of potential anticancer agents. XIII. On the criteria and kinetics associated with 'curability' of experimental leukemia. *Cancer Chemother. Rep.* 1964, **35**: 1–111.

2. Schabel F, Simpson-Herren L. Some variables in experimental tumor systems which complicate interpretation of data from *in vivo* kinetic and pharmacologic studies with anticancer drugs. *Fund. Cancer Chemother. Antibiotics Chemother.* 1978, **23**: 113–127.

3. Burkitt D. Long-term remissions following one and two-dose chemotherapy for African lymphoma. *Cancer* 1967, **20**: 756–759.

4. Magrath I, Lwanga S, Carswell W, et al. Surgical reduction of tumor bulk in management of abdominal Burkitt's lymphoma. *Br. Med. J.* 1974, **2**: 308–312.

5. DeVita V. In Principles of chemotherapy. DeVita V, Hellman S, Rosenberg S (eds) *Cancer: Principles and Practice of Oncology*, 2nd edn. Philedelphia: Lippincott Co., 1982, pp. 257–285.

6. DeVita V, Hubbard S, Longo D. The chemotherapy of lymphomas: Looking back, moving forward. *Cancer Res.* 1987, **47**: 5810–5824.

7. Kwak L, Halpern J, Olshen R, et al. Prognostic significance of actual dose intensity in diffuse large-cell lymphoma: Results of a tree-structured survival analysis. *J. Clin. Oncol.* 1990, **8**: 963–977.

8. Meyer R, Quirt I, Skillings J, et al. Escalated as compared with standard doses of doxorubicin in BACOP therapy for patients with non-Hodgkin's lymphoma. *N. Engl. J. Med.* 1993, **329**: 1770–1776.

9. Fisher R, Gaynor E, Dahlberg S, et al. Comparison of a standard regimen (CHOP) with three intensive chemotherapy regimens for advanced non-Hodgkin's lymphoma. *N. Engl. J. Med.* 1993, **328**: 1002–1006.

10. Verdonck LF, van Putten WLJ, Hagenbeek A, et al. Comparison of CHOP chemotherapy with autologous bone marrow transplantation for slowly responding patients with aggressive non-Hodgkin's lymphoma. *N. Engl. J. Med.* 1995, **332**: 1045–1051.

11. Haioun C, Lepage C, Gisselbrecht B, et al. Comparison of autologous bone marrow transplantation with sequential chemotherapy for aggressive non-Hodgkin's lymphoma in first complete remission: A study on 464 pateints. Group d'Etude des Lymphomes de l'Adulte. *J. Clin. Oncol.* 1994, **12**: 2543–2551.

12. Wilson W, Bryant G, Bates S, et al. EPOCH chemotherapy: Toxicity and efficacy in relapsed and refractory non-Hodgkin's lymphoma. *J. Clin. Oncol.* 1993, **11**: 1573–1582.

13. Lai G, Chen Y, Mickley L, et al. P-Glycoprotein expression and schedule dependence of Adriamycin cytotoxicity in human colon carcinoma cell lines. *Int. J. Cancer* 1991, **49**: 697–703.

14. Ema H, Suda T, Sakamoto S, et al. Effects of the *in vivo* administration of recombinant human granulocyte colony-stimulating factor following cytotoxic chemotherapy on granulocytic precursors in patients with malignant lymphoma. *Japn J. Cancer Res.* 1989, **80**: 577–582.

15. Gerhartz H, Engelhard M, Meusers P, et al. Randomized, double-blind, placebo-controlled, phase III study of recombinant human granulocyte–macrophage colony-stimulating factor as adjunct to induction treatment of high-grade malignant non-Hodgkin's lymphomas. *Blood* 1993, **82**: 2329–2339.

16. Wilson W, Chabner B, Bryant G, et al. Phase II study of paclitaxel in relapsed non-Hodgkin's lymphomas. *J. Clin. Oncol.* 1995, **13**: 381–386.

17. Ohno R, Okada K, Masaoka T, et al. An early phase II study of CPT-11: A new derivative of camptothecin for the treatment of leukemia and lymphoma. *J. Clin. Oncol.* 1990, **8**: 1907–1912.

18. Pavlovsky S, Santarelli MT, Erazo A, et al. Results of a randomized study of previously-untreated intermediate and high-grade lymphomas using CHOP versus CNOP. *Ann. Oncol.* 1992, **3**: 205–209.

19. Case DC, Gerber MC, Gams RA, et al. Phase II study of intravenous idarubicin in unfavorable non-Hodgkin's lymphoma. *Cancer Res.* 1992, **52**: 3871–3874.

20. Stewart CF, Arbuck SG, Fleming RA, et al. Changes in the clearance of total and unbound etoposide in patients with liver dysfunction. *J. Clin. Oncol.* 1990, **8**: 1874–1879.

21. Murphy SB. Secondary acute myeloid leukemia following treatment with epipodophyllotoxins. *J. Clin. Oncol.* 1993, **11**: 199–201.

22. Ratain MJ, Kaminer LS, Bitran JD, et al. Acute nonlymphocytic leukemia following etoposide and cis-platin combination chemotherapy for advanced non-small-cell carcinoma of the lung. *Blood* 1987, **70**: 1412.

23. Berman E, McBride M. Comparative cellular pharmacology of daunorubicin and idarubicin in human multidrug-resistant leukemia cells. *Blood* 1992, **79**: 3267–3273.

24. Endicott JA, Ling V. The biochemistry of P-Glycoprotein-mediated multidrug resistance. *Ann. Rev. Biochem.* 1989, **58**: 137.

25. Chen A, Yu C, Potmesil M. Camptothecin overcomes MDR-1 mediated resistance in human KB carcinoma cells. *Cancer Res.* 1991, **51**: 6039–6044.

26. Madoc-Jones H, Mauro F. Interphase action of vinblastine and vincristine: Differences in their lethal action through the mitotic cycle of cultured mammalian cells. *J. Cell Physiol.* 1968, **72**: 185–196.

27. Jackson DV, Pashold EH, Spurr CL, et al. Treatment of advanced non-Hodgkin's lymphoma with vincristine infusion. *Cancer* 1984, **76**: 2601–2606.

28. Chabner BA, Collin JM (eds). *Cancer Chemotherapy: Principles and Practice*. Philadelphia: J.B. Lippincott Co., 1990, pp. 276–313.

29. Shaw IC, Graham MI. Mesna – a short review. *Cancer Treat. Rep.* 1987, **14**: 67–86.

30. Lazarus HM, Herzig RH, Graham-Pole J, et al. Intensive melphalan chemotherapy and cryoperserved autologous bone marrow transplantation for the treatment of refractory cancer. *J. Clin. Oncol.* 1983, **1**: 359.

31. Lazarus HM, Reed MD, Spitzer TR, et al. High-dose

IV thiotepa and cryopreserved autologous bone marrow transplantation for therapy of refractory cancer. *Cancer Treat. Rep.* 1987, **71**: 689–695.

32. Peters WP, Henner WD, Grochow LB, et al. Clinical and pharmacologic effects of high dose single agent busulfan with autologous marrow support in the treatment of solid tumors. *Cancer Res.* 1987, **47**: 6402–6406.

33. Wilson WH, Jain V, Bryant G, et al. Phase I and II study of high-dose ifosfamide, carboplatin and etoposide with autologous bone marrow rescue in lymphomas and solid tumors. *J. Clin. Oncol.* 1992, **10**: 1712–1722.

34. Eder JP, Elias A, Shea TC, et al. A phase I–II study of cyclophosphamide, thiotepa, and carboplatin with autologous bone marrow transplantation in solid tumors. *J. Clin. Oncol.* 1990, **8**: 1239–1245.

35. Kufe DW, Munroe D, Herrick D, et al. Effects of 1-β-D-arabinofuranosylcytosine incorporation on eukaryotic DNA template function. *Mol. Pharmacol.* 1984, **26**: 128–134.

36. Coleman N, Cohen J, Burke J, et al. Lymphoblastic lymphoma in adults. Results of a pilot protocol. *Blood* 1981, **57**: 679–684.

37. Wollner N, Exelby P, Lieberman P. Non-Hodgkin's lymphoma in children. A progress report on the original patients treated with LSA$_2$-L$_2$ protocol. *Cancer* 1979, **44**: 1990–1999.

38. Hvizdala E, Berard C, Callihan T, et al. Lymphoblastic lymphoma in children – A randomized trial comparing LSA$_2$-L$_2$ with the A-COP + therapeutic regimen: A pediatric oncology group study. *J. Clin. Oncol.* 1988, **6**: 26–33.

39. Magrath I, Janus C, Edwards B, et al. An effective therapy for both undifferentiated (including Burkitt's) lymphomas and lymphoblastic lymphomas in children and young adults. *Blood* 1984, **63**: 1102–1111.

40. Velasquez WS, Cabanillas F, Salvador P, et al. Effective salvage therapy for lymphoma with cisplatin in combination with high-dose Ara-C and dexamethasone (DHAP). *Blood* 1988, **71**: 117–122.

41. Capizzi RL, Powell BL. Sequential high-dose ara-C and asparaginase versus high-dose ara-C alone in the treatment of patients with relapsed and refractory acute leukemias. *Semin. Oncol.* 1987, **14** (Suppl. 1): 40–50.

42. Herzig RH, Hines JD, Herzig GP, et al. Cerebellar toxicity with high-dose cytosine arabinoside. *J. Clin. Oncol.* 1987, **5**: 927–932.

43. Magrath I, Adde M, Shad A, et al. A new short duration chemotherapy protocol for the treatment of small noncleaved cell (SNCC) and large cell (LC) lymphomas. *Proc. Am. Soc. Clin. Oncol.* 1993, **12**: 1313 (abstract).

44. Stoller RG, Hande KR, Jacobs SA, et al. Use of plasma pharmacokinetics to predict and prevent methotrexate toxicity. *N. Engl. J. Med.* 1977, **297**: 630–634.

45. Hachster H, Kim K, Green M, et al. Activity of fludarabine in previously treated non-Hodgkin's low-grade lymphoma: Results of an eastern cooperative oncology group study. *J. Clin. Oncol.* 1992, **10**: 28–32.

46. Redman J, Cabanillas F, Velasquez W, et al. Phase II trial of fludarabine phosphate in lymphoma: An effective new agent in low-grade lymphoma. *J. Clin. Oncol.* 1992, **10**: 790–794.

47. O'Brien S, Kantarjian H, Beran M, et al. Results of fludarabine and prednisone therapy in 264 patients with chronic lymphocytic leukemia with multivariate analysis-derived prognostic model for response to treatment. *Blood* 1993, **82**: 1695–1700.

48. Kay A, Saven A, Carrera C, et al. 2-Chlorodeoxyadenosine treatment of low-grade lymphomas. *J. Clin. Oncol.* 1992, **10**: 371–377.

49. Brockman RW, Cheng Y-C, Schabel FM, et al. Metabolism and chemotherapeutic activity of 9-β-D-arabinofuranosyl-2-fluoroadenine against murine leukemia L1210 and evidence for its phosphorylation by deoxycytidine kinase. *Cancer Res.* 1980, **40**: 3610–3615.

50. Warrell RP and Berman E. Phase I and II study of fludarabine phosphate in leukemia: Therapeutic efficacy with delays in central nervous system toxicity. *J. Clin. Oncol.* 1986, **4**: 74–79.

51. Beutler E. Cladribine (2-chlorodeoxyadenosine). *Lancet* 1992, **340**: 952–956.

52. Seymour JF, Kurzrock R, Freireich EJ, Estey EH. 2-Chlorodeoxyadenosine induces durable remissions and prolonged suppression of CD4+ lymphocyte counts in patients with hairy cell leukemia. *Blood* 1994, **83**: 2906–2911.

53. Hickish T, Serafinowski P, Cunningham D, et al. 2'-Chlorodeoxyadenosine: Evaluation of a novel predominantly lymphocyte selective agent in lymphoid malignancies. *Br. J. Cancer* 1993, **67**: 139–143.

54. Velasquez W, Hagemeister F, McLaughlin P, et al. E-SHAP: An effective treatment for refractory and relapsed lymphoma. A long follow-up. *Proc. Ann. Meet. Am. Soc. Clin. Oncol.* 1992, **11**: A1111 (abstract).

55. Pinto AL and Lippard SJ. Binding of the antitumor drug cis-diammine-dichloroplatinum(II) (cisplatin) to DNA. *Biochem. Biophys. Acta* 1985, **780**: 167–188.

56. Umezawa H, Maeda K, Takeuchi T, et al. New antibiotics, bleomycin A and B. *J. Antibiot. Ser. A* 1966, **19**: 200–209.

57. Blum RH, Carter SK, Agre K. A clinical review of bleomycin – a new antineoplastic agent. *Cancer* 1973, **31**: 903–914.

58. Comis RL. Detecting bleomycin pulmonary toxicity: A continued conundrum. *J. Clin. Oncol.* 1990, **8**: 765–767.

59. Goldie J, Coldman A. A mathematic model for relating the drug sensitivity of tumors to their spontaneous mutation rate. *Cancer Treat. Rep.* 1979, **63**: 1727–1731.

60. Luria S, Delbruck M. Mutations of bacteria from virus sensitivity to virus resistance. *Genetics* 1943, **28**: 491–496.

61. Yunis J. The chromosomal basis of human neoplasia. *Science* 1983, **221**: 227–236.

62. Moscow J, Cowan K. Multidrug resistance. *J. Natl Cancer Inst.* 1988, **80**: 14–20.

63. Gros P, Ben Neriah Y, Croop J, et al. Isolation and expression of a complementary DNA that confers

multidrug resistance. *Nature* 1986, **323**: 728–731.

64. Ling V, Thompson L. Reduced permeability in CHO cells as a mechanism of resistance to colchicine. *J. Cell Physiol.* 1974, **83**: 103–116.

65. Bech-Hansen N, Till J, Ling V. Pleiotropic phenotype of colchicine-resistant CHO cells: Cross-resistance and collateral sensitivity. *J. Cell Physiol.* 1976, **88**: 23–31.

66. Gros P, Croop J, Housman D. Mammalian multidrug resistance gene: Complete cDNA sequence indicates strong homology to bacterial transport proteins. *Cell* 1986, **47**: 371–380.

67. Fojo A, Ueda K, Slamon D, et al. Expression of a multidrug-resistance gene in human tumors and tissues. *Proc. Natl Acad. Sci.* 1987, **84**: 265–269.

68. Goldstein L, Galski H, Fojo A, et al. Expression of a multidrug resistance gene in human cancers. *J. Natl Cancer Inst.* 1989, **81**: 116–124.

69. Niehans G, Jaszcz W, Brunetto V, et al. Immunohisto-chemical identification of P-glycoprotein in previously untreated, diffuse large cell and immunoblastic lymphomas. *Cancer Res.* 1992, **52**: 3768–3775.

70. Miller T, Grogan T, Dalton W, et al. P-Glycoprotein expression in malignant lymphoma and reversal of clinical drug resistance with chemotherapy plus high-dose verapamil. *J. Clin. Oncol.* 1991, **9**: 17–24.

71. Bates S, Denicoff A, Cowan K, et al. A study of MDR-1 expression and pharmacologic reversal in human breast cancer. *Proc. Am. Soc. Clin. Oncol.* 1991, **10**: 68 (abstract).

72. Fojo T, McAtee N, Allegra C, et al. Use of quinidine and amiodarone to modulate multidrug resistance mediated by the mdr-1 gene. *Proc. Am. Assoc. Clin. Oncol.* 1989, **8**: 68 (abstract).

73. Eliason J, Ramuz H, Kaufman F. Human multi-drug-resistant cancer cells exhibit a high degree of selectivity for stereoisomers of verapamil and quinidine. *Int. J. Cancer* 1990, **46**: 113–117.

74. Dalton W, Grogan T, Meltzer P, et al. Drug-resistance in multiple myeloma and non-Hodgkin's lymphoma: Detection of P-Glycoprotein and potential circumvention by addition of verapamil to chemotherapy. *J. Clin. Oncol.* 1989, **7**: 415–424.

75. List A, Spier C, Greer J, et al. Phase I/II trial of cyclosporine as a chemotherapy-resistance modifier in acute leukemia. *J. Clin. Oncol.* 1993, **11**: 1652–1660.

76. Wilson W, Bates S, Fojo A, et al. A controlled trial of dexverapamil, a modulator of multidrug resistance, in lymphomas refractory to EPOCH chemotherapy. *J. Clin. Oncol.* 1995, **13**: 1995–2004.

77. Cole SPC, Bhardwaj G, Gerlack JH, et al. Over-expression of a transporter gene in a multidrug-resistant human lung cancer cell line. *Science* 1992, **258**: 1650–1654.

78. Sachs L, Lotem J. Control of programmed cell death in normal and leukemic cells: New implications for therapy. *Blood* 1993, **82**: 15–21.

79. Walton MI, Whysong D, O'Connor PM, et al. Constitutive expression of human bcl-2 modulates nitrogen mustard and camptothecin-induced apoptosis. *Cancer Res.* 1993, **53**: 1853–1861.

80. Gaidano G, Ballerini P, Gong JZ, et al. P53 mutations in human lymphoid malignancies: Association with Burkitt lymphoma and chronic lymphocytic leukemia. *Proc. Natl Acad. Sci. USA* 1991, **88**: 5413–5417.

81. Hockenberry D, Nunez G, Milliman C, et al. Bcl-2 is an inner mitochondrial membrane protein that blocks programmed cell death. *Nature* 1990, **348**: 334–336.

82. Zutter M, Hockenberry D, Silverman GA, Korsmeyer SJ. Immunolocalization of the bcl-2 protein within hematopoietic neoplasms. *Blood* 1991, **78**: 1062–1068.

83. Farrugia MM, Duan L-J, Reis MD, et al. Alterations of the p53 tumor suppressor gene in diffuse large-cell lymphomas with translocations of the c-myc and bcl-2 proto-oncogenes. *Blood* 1994, **83**: 191–198.

84. Lotem J, Sachs L. Regulation of bcl-2, c-myc and p53 of susceptibility to induction of apoptosis by heat shock and cancer chemotherapy compounds in differentiation competent and defective myeloid leukemic cells. *Cell Growth Differ.* 1993, **4**: 41.

85. Harris CC, Hollstein M. Clinical implications of the p53 tumor-suppressor gene. *N. Engl. J. Med.* 1993, **329**: 1318–1327.

86. Rouby EL, Thomas A, Costin D, et al. P53 gene mutation in B-cell chronic lymphocytic leukemia is associated with drug resistance and is independent of MDR1/MDR3 gene expression. *Blood* 1993, **82**: 3452–3459.

87. O'Connor PM, Jackman J, Jondle D, et al. Role of the p53 tumor suppressor gene in cell cycle arrest and radiosensitivity of Burkitt's lymphoma cell lines. *Cancer Res.* 1993, **53**: 4776–4780.

88. Piris MA, Pezella F, Marinez-Montero JC, et al. P53 and bcl-2 expression in high-grade B-cell lymphomas: Correlation with survival time. *Br. J. Cancer* 1994, **69**: 337–341.

89. Wilson WH, Teruya-Feldstein J, Harris C, et al. P53, but not bcl-2, overexpression is independently associated with drug resistance in relapsed non-Hodgkin's lymphomas treated with EPOCH chemotherapy. *Proc. Am. Soc. Clin. Oncol.* 1995 (abstract).

90. Rosenberg S, Berard C, Brown B, et al. National Cancer Institute sponsored study of classifications of non-Hodgkin's lymphomas. Summary and description of a working formulation for clinical usage. *Cancer* 1982, **49**: 2112–2135.

91. Jones S, Rosenberg S, Kaplan H, et al. Non-Hodgkin's lymphomas. II. Single agent chemotherapy. *Cancer* 1972, **30**: 31–38.

92. Lister T, Cullen M, Beard M, et al. Comparison of combined and single-agent chemotherapy in non-Hodgkin's lymphoma of favorable histological type. *Br. Med. J.* 1978, **1**: 533–537.

93. Bagley C, DeVita V, Berard C, et al. Advanced lymphosarcoma: Intensive cyclical combination chemotherapy with cyclophosphamide, vincristine, and prednisone. *Ann. Intern. Med.* 1972, **76**: 227–234.

94. Brereton H, Young R, Longo D, et al. A comparison between combination chemotherapy and total body irradiation plus combination chemotherapy in non-Hodgkin's lymphoma. *Cancer* 1979, **43**: 2227–2231.

95. Ezdinli E, Anderson J, Melvin F, et al. Moderate versus aggressive chemotherapy of nodular lym-

phocytic poorly differentiated lymphoma. *J. Clin. Oncol.* 1985, **3**: 769–775.

96. Young R, Johnson R, Canellos G, et al. Advanced lymphocytic lymphoma: Randomized comparisons of chemotherapy and radiotherapy, alone or in combination. *Cancer Treat. Rep.* 1977, **61**: 1153–1159.

97. Hoppe R, Kushlan P, Kaplan H, et al. The treatment of advanced stage favorable histology non-Hodgkin's lymphoma: A preliminary report of a randomized trial comparing single agent chemotherapy, combination chemotherapy, and whole body irradiation. *Blood* 1981, **58**: 592–598.

98. Portlock C, Rosenberg S. No initial therapy for stage III and IV non-Hodgkin's lymphomas of favorable histologic types. *Ann. Intern. Med.* 1979, **90**: 10–13.

99. Horning S, Rosenberg S. The natural history of initially untreated low-grade non-Hodgkin's lymphomas. *N. Engl. J. Med.* 1984, **311**: 1471–1475.

100. Young R, Longo D, Glatstein E, et al. The treatment of indolent lymphomas: Watchful waiting V aggressive combined modality treatment. *Semin. Hematol.* 1988, **25**: 11–16.

101. Freedman A, Takvorian T, Anderson K, et al. Autologous bone marrow transplantation in B-cell non-Hodgkin's lymphoma: Very low treatment-related mortality in 100 patients in sensitive relapse. *J. Clin. Oncol.* 1990, **8**: 784–791.

102. Freedman A, Gribben J, Rabinowe S, et al. Autologous bone marrow transplantation in advanced low-grade B-cell non-Hodgkin's lymphoma in first remission. *Am. Soc. Hem.* 1993, **82**: 1313 (abstract).

103. Shipp M, Yeap B, Harrington D, et al. The m-BACOD combination chemotherapy regimen in large-cell lymphoma: Analysis of the completed trial and comparison with the M-BACOD regimen. *J. Clin. Oncol.* 1990, **8**: 84–93.

104. Longo D, DeVita V, Duffey P, et al. Superiority of ProMACE-CytaBOM over ProMACE-MOPP in the treatment of advanced diffuse aggressive lymphoma: Results of a prospective randomized trial. *J. Clin. Oncol.* 1991, **9**: 25–38.

105. Jones SE, Grozea PN, Metz EN, et al. Superiority of adriamycin-containing combination chemotherapy in the treatment of diffuse lymphoma. A Southwest Oncology Group Study. *Cancer* 1979, **43**: 417–425.

106. Schein P, DeVita V, Hubbard S, et al. Bleomycin, adriamycin, cyclophosphamide, vincristine, and prednisone (BACOP) combination chemotherapy in the treatment of advanced diffuse histiocytic lymphoma. *Ann. Intern. Med.* 1976, **85**: 417–422.

107. Rodriquez V, Cabanillas F, Burgess M, et al. Combination chemotherapy (CHOP-Bleo) in advanced (non-Hodgkin's) malignant lymphoma. *Blood* 1977, **49**: 325–333.

108. Skarin A, Canellos G, Rosenthal D, et al. Improved prognosis of diffuse histiocytic and undifferentiated lymphoma by use of high dose methotrexate alternating with standard agents (M-BACOD). *J. Clin. Oncol.* 1983, **1**: 91–98.

109. Fisher R, DeVita V, Hubbard S, et al: Diffuse aggressive lymphomas: Increased survival after alternating flexible sequences of ProMACE and MOPP chemotherapy. *Ann. Intern. Med.* 1983, **98**: 304–309.

110. Klimo P, Connors J. MACOP-B chemotherapy for the treatment of diffuse large-cell lymphoma. *Ann. Intern. Med.* 1985, **102**: 596–602.

111. Weiss L, Warnke R, Sklar J, et al. Molecular analysis of the t(14;18) chromosomal translocation in malignant lymphomas. *N. Engl. J. Med.* 1987, **317**: 1185.

112. Tang SC, Visser L, Hepperle B, et al. Clinical significance of bcl-2-MBR gene rearrangement and protein expression in diffuse large-cell non-Hodgkin's lymphoma: An analysis of 83 cases. *J. Clin. Oncol.* 1994, **12**: 149–154.

113. Offit K, Lo Coco F, Louie DC, et al. Rearrangement of the bcl-6 gene as a prognostic marker in diffuse large-cell lymphoma. *N. Engl. J. Med.* 1994, **331**: 74–80.

114. Foon K, Tood R. Immunologic classification of leukemia and lymphoma. *Blood* 1986, **68**: 1–31.

115. Jaffe, E. Relationship of classification to biologic behavior of non-Hodgkin's lymphomas. *Semin. Oncol.* 1986, **13**: 3–9.

116. Anderson J, Wilson J, Jenkin D, et al. The results of randomized therapeutic trial comparing a 4-drug regimen (COMP) with a 10-drug regimen (LSA$_2$-L$_2$). *N. Engl. J. Med.* 1983, **308**: 559–565.

117. Ziegler J. Burkitt's lymphoma. *N. Engl. J. Med.* 1981, **305**: 735–744.

CHAPTER 29

Role of colony-stimulating factors in therapy

REINHARD HENSCHLER, WOLFRAM BRUGGER, ROLAND MERTELSMANN
AND LOTHAR KANZ

Introduction

Colony-stimulating factors (CSFs) entered clinical hematology less than a decade ago. Now, they have not only been incorporated into standard therapy but have also made possible the wider use of new treatment modalities, such as high-dose chemotherapy. It was through the use of CSFs that the feasibility of mobilizing stem cells into the peripheral blood was established and its therapeutic use developed. This chapter will try to review important aspects of CSF biology relevant to the treatment of neoplastic disorders, with special reference to the non-Hodgkin's lymphomas, and including *in vitro* and animal data on possible CSF and cytokine combination treatment regimens, as well as experimental forms of cellular therapy.

CSFs have been defined as polypeptide growth factors affecting the survival, proliferation, differentiation and functional activation of hematopoietic cells [1–3]. In addition to the four factors characterized and molecularly cloned by the mid-1980s: granulocyte CSF (G-CSF), granulocyte–macrophage CSF (GM-CSF), macrophage CSF (M-CSF) and interleukin-3 (IL-3) [1–3], another two factors capable of stimulating colony growth on their own (and therefore representing 'true' CSFs) have been described: erythropoietin (EPO) [4] and stem cell factor (SCF) [5]. All of these factors have been used clinically; three are approved by the Federal Drug Agency (FDA) of the USA for therapeutic use: G-CSF, GM-CSF [6] and EPO [7].

A range of factors (interleukins-1, 2, 4–13, interferon-γ, transforming growth factors and others) have been found to modulate colony formation when used with CSFs *in vitro*. Although they do not directly stimulate hematopoietic colony growth, and therefore do not represent true CSFs, their potential therapeutic use will be evaluated in the near future, e.g., as adjuncts to CSFs in combination therapies. Also, they may prove to have an important role in the *ex vivo* processing of transplantable hematopoietic stem cell grafts, as discussed later in this chapter.

During extensive phase I and II trials with CSFs over recent years, optimal dosing regimens have been worked out and CSFs are now conveniently administered by, at most, once daily subcutaneous (s.c.) administration. In most cases, the approved CSFs can be reliably self-administered by patients. Some side-effects have been documented, including skin rashes and bone pain, but generally this has not been a dose-limiting problem and no permanent effects have been reported [7,8].

Role of CSFs in amelioration of the cytotoxicity of standard dose chemotherapy

Improvement in the rate of recovery of peripheral blood neutrophil counts following chemotherapy has been, to date, the most intensively studied parameter in patients receiving CSF treatment, and has become one of the single most important beneficial effects of CSF treatment in clinical oncology. The first randomized, placebo-controlled double-blind CSF trial by Crawford et al. [9] in patients with small-cell lung cancer receiving once-daily G-CSF for 14 days after standard dose chemotherapy demonstrated a significant reduction of the period of absolute neutropenia, as well as reduced white blood cell (WBC) nadirs. Concomitantly, there was a reduced frequency of documented infections, and decreases in the number of episodes of fever, days on antibiotics and days in hospital. A number of studies in which G-CSF was used after chemotherapy have been reported in a variety of neoplasms [10–17]. In all studies reduction in absolute neutropenia and in some decreases in white blood cell nadirs were reported. In a more recent randomized trial in patients with non-Hodgkin's lymphomas, G-CSF has been documented to reduce the percentage of patients developing neutropenia after vincristine, adriamycin, prednisolone, etoposide, cyclophosphamide (VAPEC-B) chemotherapy, to decrease the number of episodes of fever and to result in fewer treatment delays [18]. No significant changes were noted in antibiotic usage, days of hospitalization or overall treatment results between the G-CSF and the control groups. A number of questions remain open

with respect to the potential of CSFs to contribute to treatment outcome in terms of improved prognosis for patients undergoing standard dose chemotherapy.

Like G-CSF, GM-CSF turned out to be an effective agent for suppressing neutropenia in a variety of neoplastic diseases in the context of standard dose chemotherapy [19–23]. In addition to a decrease in the degree of neutropenia, some groups have reported a decrease in therapy-induced thrombocytopenia with GM-CSF [6,22], an observation which has not been confirmed by most investigators. GM-CSF will also stimulate the production of monocytes and eosinophils, and functionally activate these cell types [24]. It is apparent that these factors have become widely accepted as an indispensable adjunctive tool in antitumor chemotherapy.

In addition to G-CSF and GM-CSF, trials have been conducted with IL-3 [25], or combinations of IL-3 and GM-CSF or G-CSF, postchemotherapy. In patients with solid tumors, sequential IL-3/GM-CSF administration has been reported to lessen neutropenia compared to controls, or compared to patients receiving IL-3 alone [26].

These data indicate that various CSFs, alone or in combination, are capable of alleviating chemotherapy-related toxicities, and that this translates into direct benefits for patients. Until long-term evaluations have been completed, it remains uncertain whether remission and survival rates will be influenced by the addition of CSFs to chemotherapy regimens.

CSFs and escalation of chemotherapy dose intensity

Since CSFs are able to overcome bone marrow toxicity from standard dose chemotherapy to a substantial degree, it has become possible to further escalate chemotherapy doses in an attempt to achieve more effective tumor cell kill, a higher proportion of complete remissions and, possibly, increased survival. The basis for this approach is experimental evidence for a tight correlation between chemotherapy dose and tumor response, especially with alkylating agents. In animal tumor models even a relatively small reduction in the intended chemotherapy dose abrogates the curative potential [27]. Prior to the advent of CSFs, high-dose chemotherapy regimens have been associated with an incidence of hemorrhage and infection as high as 5–20%, leading to treatment-related death [28].

GM-CSF has been used successfully to accelerate neutrophil and platelet recovery after a dose-intensified regimen using 5000 mg/m^2 of cyclophosphamide, 1500 mg/m^2 of etoposide and 150 mg/m^2 of cisplatinum by Neidhart et al. [29]. This included a group of patients with non-Hodgkin's lymphomas [30]. Also, GM-CSF has been able to reduce neutropenia induced by combination chemotherapy with etoposide, ifosfamide and doxorubicin in patients with small-cell lung cancer [31], although it was noted that the frequency of episodes of febrile neutropenia was unchanged in treatment cycles with and without GM-CSF. GM-CSF has also been used in comparable high-dose protocols with similar efficiency [32–34]. In the BCNU, etoposide, ara-C, melphalan (BEAM) protocol using 300 mg/m^2 carmustine, 1200 mg/m^2 etoposide, 800 mg/m^2 cytarabine and 140 mg/m^2 melphalan, Laporte et al. [35] went as far as to use GM-CSF instead of autologous bone marrow transplantation, leading to similar recoveries in some cases. A similar study, by Sheridan et al., but using G-CSF instead of GM-CSF, demonstrated a profound shortening of neutropenia as well as thrombopenia after busulfan and cyclophosphamide chemotherapy [36].

There are presently no data to indicate whether CSF administration is harmful or beneficial with respect to tumor response rates. However, other benefits of CSF application have been reported in recent publications. Gebbia et al. conducted a prospective trial with 86 patients with a diagnosis of ovarian cancer undergoing high-dose chemotherapy [37]. The study revealed a statistically significant increase in planned dose intensity, as well as a (non-significant) decrease in oral fungal disease in the G-CSF-treated patients compared to controls. In a randomized trial of patients with a diagnosis of limited disease, or European Cooperative Oncology Group (ECOG) stage 0 or 1 extensive disease small-cell lung cancer, dose reductions as a result of leukopenia were significantly higher in the control arm [38]. However, G-CSF administration did not decrease dose reductions or treatment delays to a level that would allow an increase in received dose intensity. Ardizzoni and colleages [39] have reported a randomized trial showing that GM-CSF can accelerate the rate of delivery of chemotherapy in breast cancer patients receiving high-dose combination chemotherapy.

These studies give assurance that CSFs are of benefit to patients undergoing therapy for neoplasia. Data regarding the potential of CSFs to ameliorate toxicity in the setting of high-dose chemotherapy comes from studies in which autologous stem cell support is used after high-dose chemotherapy.

CSFs in high-dose chemotherapy with autologous stem cell support

Myelotoxicity from high-dose chemotherapy regimens has been efficiently overcome by the reinfusion of autologous bone marrow [40]. The administration of GM-CSF after autologous bone marrow transplantation has been shown to result in accelerated engraftment in a number of studies in which comparison was made between reinfusion of autologous marrow with and without concomitant growth factors [41–46], including a randomized trial in patients with non-Hodgkin's lymphoma [41] and after conditioning regimens ranging from high-dose chemotherapy to total body irradiation (TBI). Neutrophil recovery was found to be accelerated in all studies. Interestingly, whereas no reduction in the time required for platelet recovery was reported in studies using G-CSF, two groups report accelerated platelet recovery after GM-CSF [45,46]. However, this has not been confirmed in most other studies. The enhanced engraftment rates observed after GM-CSF have been interpreted as a reflection of the effect of GM-CSF on enforced differentiation of a limited number of stem cells repopulating the bone marrow, rather than enlargement of marrow stem cell and early progenitor population sizes [47]. In a recent study, no long-term deleterious effects on bone marrow function by GM-CSF were reported in a series of 128 patients with diagnoses of non-Hodgkin's lymphoma, Hodgkin's disease and acute lymphoblastic leukemia undergoing a phase III trial with autologous bone marrow transplantation (ABMT) [48]. However, previous exposure to agents that deplete stem cells did lead to significant delays in neutrophil recovery in spite of the administration of GM-CSF. Thus, GM-CSF was a safe drug in the long term and even heavily pretreated patients benefitted. Kennedy et al. treated breast cancer patients with G-CSF after ABMT [49]. In addition to a more rapid neutrophil recovery, they found that the number of days with fever was reduced and also the duration of hospitalization.

Growth factors other than G-CSF or GM-CSF have also been used in the context of ABMT. Nemunaitis and colleagues used recombinant human (rh) IL-3 in lymphoma patients after ABMT and saw no evidence of earlier hematopoietic cell recovery compared with historical controls who received GM-CSF [50]. Gianni et al. found accelerated neutrophil, platelet and reticulocyte recovery in patients receiving high-dose cyclophosphamide therapy and rhIL-3 [51]. In another study which included both melanoma and breast cancer patients, a number of cytokines and CSFs (rhIL-1, rhIL-2, rhG-CSF, rhGM-CSF and rhM-CSF) were administered after high-dose chemotherapy and ABMT. Only G-CSF and GM-CSF were reported to improve neutrophil recovery, although IL-1 administration led to accelerated recovery of CFU-GM and burst-forming units – erythrocytes (BFU-E) in bone marrow [52].

A combination of GM-CSF and EPO has been studied in patients undergoing ABMT. More rapid recovery of absolute neutrophil counts was observed with the combination (median 12.5 days) compared with GM-CSF alone (median 18 days) [53]. No effect on platelet or red cell transfusion requirements was noted.

The use of G-CSF has been effectively extended to hematopoietic recovery after radiotherapy [54].

CYTOKINES FOR MOBILIZATION OF PERIPHERAL BLOOD STEM CELLS

Following the observation that, in the recovery phase after chemotherapy, not only mature cells but also a range of immature hematopoietic precursors circulate in peripheral blood and may be harvested for transplant purposes [55], it was only a short time until the action of CSFs on peripheral blood progenitor cell (PBPC) mobilization and their synergism with chemotherapy had been demonstrated [56–62]. Nowadays, PBPC autotransplantation using CSF administration for mobilization of stem cells into peripheral blood has become a safe procedure that is sometimes used routinely as a supportive measure after chemotherapy. Arguments that support PBPC transplantation as an ideal support modality for chemotherapy dose intensification have been the relatively easy access via leukapheresis, feasible in an outpatient setting, and the observation that hematopoietic recovery is more rapid when compared with bone marrow cells [63–66].

Although PBPC may be mobilized solely by chemotherapy [67,68], there have been ongoing considerations and worries about the predictability and reliability of engraftment mediated by chemotherapy-induced precursor cells. To [69] has observed lower numbers of nucleated cells in CFU-GM derived from chemotherapy-primed PBPC as compared to PBPC primed by combined chemotherapy and CSF. In our own group, we have noted that chemotherapy alone resulted in smaller and later peaks of mobilized progenitors in peripheral blood than chemotherapy in combination with CSFs [70].

The mobilization of PBPC has been observed in humans after the administration of GM-CSF [56,70], G-CSF [58,71], and sequential administration of IL-3 plus GM-CSF [70]. In mice, mobilization of PBPC has been reported with the administration of G-CSF alone (i.e., without previous chemotherapy) [72], with SCF and with a combination of both [73–75]. Similar results have been obtained in baboons [76]. In our own group, we have compared the ability of GM-CSF alone, sequential IL-3/GM-CSF and G-CSF alone to mobilize PBPC after standard dose chemotherapy in patients with solid tumors [70,71] (Figure 29.1). Interestingly, IL-3/GM-CSF resulted in the highest absolute numbers of progenitor cells harvested. However, use of G-CSF produced an earlier peak than did either GM-CSF or sequential IL-3/GM-CSF.

PRETREATMENT STATUS AND MOBILIZATION OF PBPC

Using a standard mobilizing regimen consisting of standard dose VP-16/etoposide, ifosfamide and cis-platinum (VIP) chemotherapy followed by sub-cutaneous administration of G-CSF, the highest numbers of CD34+ cells and clonogenic progenitors are harvested from previously untreated patients. In mildly to moderately pretreated patients (less than six chemotherapy cycles), significantly fewer presursor cells can be mobilized per apheresis and, in some patients, repetitive aphereses have to be performed. In intensively pretreated patients, i.e., patients with previous radiotherapy to more than 20% of their bone marrow in addition to more than six chemotherapy cycles, only low numbers of PBPC can be recruited. Thus, PBPC collection should be timed as early in the course of the disease as possible.

TREATMENT WITH PBPC

It has been shown that autologous PBPC, mobilized by either G-CSF or GM-CSF, and with or without chemotherapy, mediate reliable and safe recovery from a number of combination chemotherapy regimens of varying dose intensity [63,77,78]. In a group of patients with solid tumors from our institution, high-dose chemotherapy with etoposide (1500 mg/m^2), ifosfamide (12000 mg/m^2) and cisplatinum (150 mg/m^2) produced severe neutropenia. G-CSF mobilized stem cells administered in the recovery phase resulted in an accelerated recovery of neutrophils (median: 6.5 days below 0.1×10^9 neutrophils as compared to 10.5 days in control patients receiving no PBPC) and platelets (median: 3 days below 20×10^9/l platelets as compared to 8 days in patients receiving no PBPC) [71]. Whereas our trials have been conducted using historical controls, Shea et al. [79] compared recovery in sequential treatment

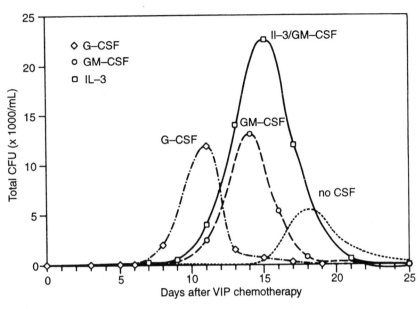

Figure 29.1 Mobilization of clonogenic cells in groups of representative patients with solid tumors after one day of combination chemotherapy with etoposide, ifosfamide and cisplatin: differential effects of various colony-stimulating factors.

cycles of high-dose carboplatin in the presence or absence of PBPC administration. They showed that the addition of PBSC led to significant reductions in neutropenia and thrombocytopenia. Other reports in which the value of PBSC after high-dose chemotherapy has been examined yielded similar results [80,81]. These studies have included defined patient populations with breast cancer receiving GM-CSF mobilized PBSC [82], and patients with advanced urothelial cancer and G-CSF-mobilized PBSC [83].

PBSC transplantation has been employed to permit the intensification of chemotherapy regimens. Kessinger et al., for example, effectively used autologous PBSC for rescue after high-dose cyclophosphamide, carmustine and etoposide in patients with relapsed Hodgkin's disease [77]. In another study, PBSC rescue resulted in faster neutrophil as well as platelet recovery in retrospective comparison to conventional ABMT in a group of 31 poor prognosis NHL patients, 12 Hodgkin's disease and 11 ALL patients [78]. Similarly, PBPC proved superior to autologous bone marrow in a another group of patients with various malignancies, including non-Hodgkin's lymphomas (NHLs), after busulfan/cyclophosphamide, with no graft failures reported during a follow-up period of 4–12 months [84].

Currently, a number of studies are under way in which high-dose chemotherapy is being used as part of the initial treatment for high-risk patients with NHL. In our own center, we pursue a high-dose chemotherapy approach with BEAM chemotherapy plus subsequent reinfusion of G-CSF-mobilized PBPC as first-line therapy in high-risk NHL patients (see Figure 29.2). Figure 29.3 shows the neutrophil and platelet recovery of a representative patient treated at our institution with busulfan/cyclophosphamide. In all our patients, we have added CSFs as supportive agents after high-dose chemotherapy.

Role of CSFs in mobilization of tumor cells into peripheral blood and possible strategies to deplete tumor cells in PBPC transplants

In a variety of neoplastic disease states, including certain NHLs, bone marrow involvement has been demonstrated. Thus, there is a possibility that concomitant mobilization of tumor cells and PBPC into the circulation will occur after chemotherapy with or without CSF. In one study, *in vitro* culture of PBPC and bone marrow showed significantly fewer cytogenetically suspicious cells in PBPC than in autologous bone marrow cells in patients with Hodgkin's disease [85]. Other investigators, including our own group, have reported similar findings, but the possibility of contamination of PBPC has been repeatedly demonstrated [86–91]. Since marrow repopulating stem cells reside in the CD34+ compartment, and most tumors do not express CD34, we have employed CD34+ selection via an immunoaffinity column system (Ceprate[TM], CellPro) to deplete possible tumor cell contaminations in PBPC collections from our patients with NHL. Engraftment data from a pilot

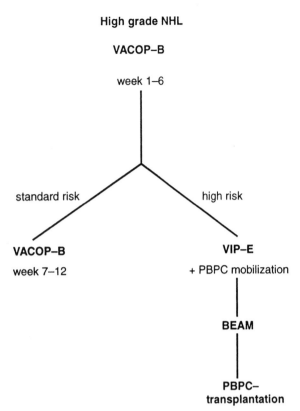

Figure 29.2 First-line therapy protocol for patients with aggressive NHL, including cytokine-mobilized peripheral blood stem cell support for high-risk patients. VACOP-B, cyclophosphamide, vincristine, prednisone, bleomycin, doxorubicin, procarbazine; VIP-E, VP-16/etoposide, ifosfamide, *cis*-platinum, epirubicin; BEAM, BCNU, etoposide, cytosine arabinoside, melphalan; NHL, non-Hodgkin's lymphoma.

study in 15 patients with solid tumors showed identical hematopoietic reconstitution with CD34+ cells compared to patients from a historical control group in which unseparated PBPCs were used [92]. This is in contrast to a delayed engraftment after purging with 4-hydroxy cyclophosphamide or amifostine [93].

It has not yet been formally shown whether tumor cell depletion by CD34+ selection will result in clinical benefit to patients with a diagnosis of non-Hodgkin's lymphoma. Gene marking studies have demonstrated that recurrent tumor cells in childhood AML patients as well as in neuroblastoma patients may contain transplanted cells [94]. It may, therefore, be inferred that, possibly in any kind of tumor, wherever chemotherapy is given with curative intent, emphasis should be given to eliminating tumor cells from hematopoietic stem cell transplants. In an effort to achieve additional tumor cell depletion, we decided to optimize growth factor conditions for *ex*

vivo liquid culture of C34+-enriched PBPC cells. We found that using CD34+-enriched cells as a starting population, a five-factor combination of SCF, IL-1β, IL-3, IL-6 and EPO resulted in optimal increases in total cell number by 2 logs in the course of an *ex vivo* culture period of 2 weeks [95]. At the same time, committed progenitor cells were also expanded by 2 logs. Optimized growth conditions for hematopoietic progenitor cells should, on the other hand, be disadvantageous for tumor cells and we are currently investigating the possible use of this system to deplete neoplastic cells present in leukapheresis preparations.

Thus, as well as depleting tumor cells from stem cell preparations, these *ex vivo* expansion cultures might permit the transplantation of higher numbers of progenitors. This may be of importance, since in patients with NHL, Hodgkin's disease or acute lymphoblastic leukemia (ALL) the engraftment time inversely correlates with the total number of progenitor cells reinfused [78]. Also, a higher threshold of stem cells required to ensure engraftment has been reported for heavily pretreated patients or patients with disorders involving the stem cell such as leukemia [59,69]. It would appear that significantly accelerated recoveries may be achieved by *ex vivo* expansion of the leukapheresis product. Furthermore, when the number of colony-forming cells is amplified by a factor of 2 logs, less than 100 ml of blood drawn into a syringe, instead of a 7 liter leukapheresis, may be sufficient to provide adequate numbers of progenitor cells for standard hematopoietic reconstitution. Thus, CSFs may be of importance not only when applied to patients as drugs, but also during *ex vivo* processing procedures of hematopoietic transplants.

Role of CSFs in allogeneic transplantation

The possible useful applications of CSFs after allogeneic transplantation include acceleration of recovery and rapid engraftment of all cell lineages posttransplantation, as well as potential effects on graft-versus-host disease (GVHD), and improved viability and even expansion of precursor cells incubated *in vitro* during purging procedures. These effects should translate into reduced infection rates posttransplant, and a reduction in the incidence of graft failure. CSFs may also permit transplantation in the presence of established infection.

Neutrophil recovery appears to have been improved by G-CSF, GM-CSF or GM-CSF/IL-3 administration in most studies reported so far, whether grafts

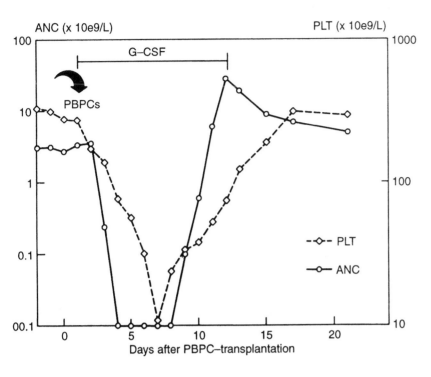

Figure 29.3 Typical recovery of absolute neutrophil count (ANC) and platelet counts (PLT) in a representative patient after conditioning with BEAM and subsequent reinfusion of G-CSF-mobilized peripheral blood stem cells. G-CSF was applied during the recovery phase.

were received from human leukocyte antigen (HLA)-matched siblings, from unrelated donors or cord blood cells were used [96–105]. To a lesser degree, neutrophil recovery was shown to be enhanced by M-CSF [106,107]. GM-CSF was not effective, however, in accelerating neutrophil recovery in patients receiving methothrexate for GVHD prophylaxis [98,108,109]. Even so, these studies showed positive effects of GM-CSF on infection and toxicity-related mortality rates. Platelet recovery was improved only in some of these studies.

CSFs are also being used in allogeneic transplantation of peripheral blood stem cells. However, reports on allogeneic PBSC transplantations are sparse up to now. A few pilot patients treated at our institution with CD34+-selected PBSC and posttransplant rhG-CSF showed comparable engraftment rates to patients receiving autologous PBPC.

As a general statement, the incidence of GVHD seemed to be unaffected, if reduced at all, by CSF treatment in the studies reported using either G-CSF, GM-CSF or M-CSF [96–109]. However, randomized trials have not yet been reported. In patients treated with GM-CSF, relapse rates seem to be either unaltered or reduced [96]. As with GVHD, conclusive evidence from randomized trials is not available to date.

In one study, the influence of the *in vitro* incubation of allogeneic bone marrow before infusion was studied. Rapid neutrophil and platelet recovery was observed [101].

Patients receiving partially mismatched bone marrow or T-cell depleted bone marrow have increased rates of graft rejection. Nemunaitis et al. first used GM-CSF in a phase I study [110], and subsequently report significantly increased survival rates (35% instead of 20% in historical controls) [96]. The study is ongoing at a multicenter level.

Since residential macrophage-derived cell populations including Kupffer cells, dermal Langerhans cells, pleural, synovial, peritoneal and lymphoid macrophages are generally of host origin in the first month after transplantation, cytokines that are able to stimulate macrophage function are of potential benefit in patients devoid of neutrophil production. In some studies, patients treated with GM-CSF posttransplant showed reduced infection rates. A similar reduction in infection rates was also noted, however, in some G-CSF studies [96]. Phase I and II trials with M-CSF indicated that patients with Karnofsky performance levels higher than 20% and invasive *Candida* infection showed dramatic improvement in survival (from 15% to 50%) when treated with rhM-CSF [96,111,112].

There seems little doubt that CSFs will be of major advantage in coping with a range of post-bone marrow transplantation (BMT) complications. However, the early results, although promising, need to be substantiated by controlled, randomized trials. A great deal of hope rests on the clinical use of other hematopoietic growth factors, including PIXY-321 or SCF, especially when used in combination with effective existing agents. Effects on platelet or erythrocyte recovery after BMT will be described in the following two sections.

CSFs in treatment-related and tumor-associated anemia

Although a transient rise in serum erythropoietin levels over approximately 7 days is observed post-chemotherapy, serum EPO levels are low for at least the following 4 weeks [113]. Similarly, in chronic anemia associated with cancer, low EPO serum levels have been reported [114,115]. Exogenous EPO has been found to provide substantial benefit in a large number of patients with endogenous EPO deficiency [113,116]. For example, in a large placebo-controlled trial [116], 30–50% of patients with either chronic anemia of cancer or chemotherapy-related anemia had responded after an 8-week course of EPO. Other studies with EPO in patients with anemia associated with neoplastic disease [117–123], including patients with low-grade non-Hodgkin's lymphomas, produced similar results [122, 123]. The role of EPO after BMT is currently under investigation. Although a group of patients conditioned with high-dose chemotherapy and irradiation showed increased serum EPO levels for at least 3–4 weeks posttransplantation [124], early reports provide evidence for a role of EPO in posttransplant engraftment [125,126]. For example, blood transfusion requirements were noted in one randomized, double-blind study with high-dose erythropoietin [127]. Since EPO receptors are present not only on committed erythroid progenitor cells, but also on primitive hematopoietic stem cells, EPO may have a previously underestimated role in stem cell transplantation.

CSFs and therapeutic effect on thrombopoiesis

In contrast to the other hematopoietic lineages, the search for a specific thrombopoietic CSF has proved elusive for a long time [128]. Very recently, however, the molecular cloning of a specific thrombopoietic CSF has been reported [129–131]. Factors synergizing with known molecules or with as yet undefined thrombopoietic activities which are under clinical evaluation for their effects on cells of the megakaryocytic lineage include SCF, IL-1, IL-3, IL-6,

IL-11 and leukemia-inhibiting factor (LIF) [128].

The most primitive megakaryocytic progenitor cell arising from pluripotent hematopoietic stem cells has been defined as the BFU-megakaryocyte (MK) [132]. BFU-MKs are thought to produce numerous colony-forming units (CFU)-MKs, derived from the direct precursors of bone marrow megakaryocytes [133]. Megakaryocytes developing through endoreplication ultimately release platelets via a poorly defined process of membrane evagination [134]. All the above-mentioned processes, as well as alterations in platelet survival, have to be considered when investigating the mechanisms whereby growth factors increase blood platelet levels [135]. It remains to be clarified where and to what extent the recently cloned factor, thrombopoietin, will be working in these steps. If thrombopoietin is applicable on a clinical scale and has acceptable side-effects, its application will probably revolutionize attempts to improve thrombobopoiesis.

Whereas EPO has known effects on megakaryocyte maturation in an *in vivo* mouse model [136], only insignificant peripheral blood platelet increases were evident in patients with chronic renal failure treated in a large phase III EPO study [137]. Most other single factor trials, including trials using G- or GM-CSF in humans, also yielded negative results with respect to improved recovery of thrombopoiesis after chemotherapy. This included patients with bone marrow failure resulting from neoplasia of the hematopoietic system [138–141] and postchemotherapy myelosuppression in patients with solid tumors [142,143]. However, possible positive effects of GM-CSF, given after chemotherapy, on thrombopoiesis have been outlined above [22,33,34]. These studies hinted at the possibility of thrombopoietic reconstitution by means of CSF therapy. Interestingly, a study using IL-1 after high-dose carboplatin treatment demonstrated accelerated platelet recovery, although at levels where substantial systemic toxocity begins [144]. Animal studies with SCF, LIF and IL-11 have also, at least in part, yielded relatively encouraging results [145–147]. In nonhuman primates, chronic IL-6 was tolerated at levels that increased blood platelet levels [148]. Platelet increases have been seen in clinical studies with IL-6 [128,149,150], although these results are insufficient to define a clinical role for IL-6 in stimulating platelet regeneration postchemotherapy.

Results from patient studies in which growth factors have been combined in order to alleviate thrombocytopenia have been sparse up to now. Geissler et al. have described the synergistic interaction of IL-3 and IL-6 on platelet recovery in a primate model [151]. It would appear that growth factor combination therapies, using several factors acting various levels of megakaryocytic maturation, represent the first step in an effort to influence thrombopoiesis more substantially. Our own studies, using IL-3 plus GM-CSF after standard dose chemotherapy, showed that platelet recovery was enhanced in intensively pretreated patients [26]. The successful search for a thrombopoietic CSF should lead to the second step and add a new dimension to the use of CSFs in modern clinical medicine.

Future prospects

Colony-stimulating factors have now, after only a few years of clinical studies, been accepted as playing a supporting role in tumor therapy. CSFs have demonstrable efficiency in alleviating postchemotherapy neutropenia and, partially, thrombopenia. Moreover, no substantial toxic or long-lasting side-effects have been reported. CSFs have made alternative approaches to high-dose chemotherapy possible – for example, through the mobilization of stem cells into peripheral blood and their subsequent use for myeloid replacement.

Peripheral blood stem cells are about to enter the field of allogeneic transplantation. New techniques such as immunoselection of CD34+ cells and *ex vivo* expansion are being tested for their clinical feasibility and usefulness in avoiding the transfusion of tumor cells in autologous transplants. EPO has successfully ameliorated tumor-related anemias, reducing the need for red cell transfusions as well as engraftment in some studies and its role may be expanded in the future. Thrombocytopenia has been difficult to treat so far. The identification and molecular cloning of thrombopoietin will, hopefully, reverse this situation within a short period of time. Perhaps the greatest potential exists in the use of combinations of CSFs, although to date, rather few clinical trials with CSF combinations have been performed. The results of animal experiments suggest that major clinical benefit may be expected from appropriate combinations.

In addition to their value as stimulators of *in vivo* hematopoiesis, the CSFs will, by providing easy access to peripheral blood stem cells, make possible a whole array of potential new therapeutic approaches. The ability to induce maturation and expansion of various cell lineages already exists and may be ready for clinical use within a short time. For example, very powerful antigen-presenting dendritic cells can be used to induce improved immune responses to microbial or cellular (e.g., tumor) targets. A creative example is given by Tao et al. [152], who developed an idiotype/GM-CSF fusion protein and demonstrated its use as an efficient vaccine for B-cell lymphoma in an animal model.

References

1. Metcalf D. The molecular control of cell division, differentiation commitment and maturation in haemopoietic cells. *Nature* 1989, **339**: 27–30.
2. Clark SC, Kamen R. The human hematopoietic colony-stimulating factors. *Science* 1987, **236**: 1229–1237.
3. Mertelsmann R. Hematopoietins: Biology, pathophysiology and potential as therapeutic agents. *Ann. Oncol.* 1991, **2**: 251–263.
4. Krantz SB. Erythropoietin. *Blood* 1991, **77**: 419–434.
5. Witte O. Steel locus defines new multipotent growth factor. *Cell* 1990, **63**: 5–6.
6. Lieschke G, Burgess AW. Granulocyte colony-stimulating factor and granulocyte–macrophage colony-stimulating factor. *N. Engl. J. Med.* 1992, **327**: 28–35, 99–106.
7. McGuire MJ, Spivak JL. Erythropoietin, erythropoiesis, and erythrocytosis. *Curr. Opin. Hematol.* 1993, **1**: 36–44.
8. Walter AS. The role of cytokines in the treatment of neutropenia. *Curr. Opin. Hematol.* 1993, **1**: 93–99.
9. Crawford J, Ozer H, Stoller R, et al. Reduction by granulocyte colony-stimulating factor of fever and neutropenia induced by chemotherapy in patients with small-cell lung cancer. *N. Engl. J. Med.* 1991, **325**: 164–170.
10. Bronchud MH, Scarffe JH, Thatcher N, et al. Phase I/II study of recombinant human granulocyte colony-stimulating factor in patients receiving intensive chemotherapy for small-cell lung cancer. *Br. J. Cancer* 1987, **56**: 809–813.
11. Morstyn G, Campbell L, Souza LM, et al. Effect of granulocyte colony stimulating factor on neutropenia induced by cytotoxic chemotherapy. *Lancet* 1988, **1**: 667–672.
12. Morstyn G, Campbell L, Lieschke G, et al. Treatment of chemotherapy-induced neutropenia by subcutaneously administered granulocyte colony-stimulating factor with optimization of dose and duration of therapy. *J. Clin. Oncol.* 1989, **7**: 1554–1562.
13. Gabrilove JL, Jakubowski A, Scher H, et al Effect of granulocyte colony-stimulating factor on neutropenia and associated morbidity due to chemotherapy for transitional-cell carcinoma of the urothelium. *N. Engl. J. Med.* 1988, **318**: 1414–1422.
14. Kotake T, Miki T, Akaza H, et al. Effect of recombinant granulocyte colony-stimulating factor (rG-CSF) on chemotherapy-induced neutropenia in patients with urogenital cancer. *Cancer Chemother. Pharmacol.* 1991, **27**: 253–257.
15. Bronchud MH, Howell A, Crowther D, et al. The use of granulocyte colony-stimulating factor to increase

the intensity of treatment with doxorubicin in patients with advanced breast and ovarian cancer. *Br. J. Cancer* 1989, **60**: 121–125.

16. Yoshida T, Nakamura S, Ohtake S, et al. Effect of granulocyte colony-stimulating factor on neutropenia due to chemotherapy for Non-Hodgkin's lymphoma. *Cancer* 1990, **66**: 1904–1909.

17. Trillet-Lenoir V, Green J, Manegold C, et al. Recombinant granulocyte colony stimulating factor reduces the infectious complications of cytotoxic chemotherapy. *Eur. J. Cancer* 1993, **29A**: 319–324.

18. Pettengell R, Gurney H, Radford JA, et al. Granulocyte colony-stimulating factor to prevent dose-limiting neutropenia in non-Hodgkin's lymphoma: A randomized controlled trial. *Blood* 1992, **80**: 1430–1436.

19. Antman KS, Griffin JD, Elias A, et al. Effect of recombinant human granulocyte–macrophage colony-stimulating factor on chemotherapy-induced myelo-suppression. *N. Engl. J. Med.* 1988, **319**: 593–598.

20. Logothetis CJ, Dexeus FH, Sella A, et al. Escalated therapy for refractory urothelial tumors: Methotrexate–vinblastine–doxorubicin–cisplatin plus unglycosylated recombinant human granulocyte–macrophage colony-stimulating factor. *J. Natl Cancer Inst.* 1990, **82**: 667–672.

21. De Vries EGE, Biesma B, Willemse PHB, et al. A double-blind placebo-controlled study with granulocyte–macrophage colony-stimulating factor during chemotherapy for ovarian carcinoma. *Cancer Res.* 1991, **51**: 116–122.

22. Steward WP, Scarffe JH, Dirix LY, et al. Granulocyte–macrophage colony-stimulating factor (GM-CSF) after high-dose melphalan in patients with advanced colon cancer. *Br. J. Cancer* 1990, **61**: 749–754.

23. Ho AD, Del Valle F, Engelhard M, et al. Mitoxanthrone/high-dose Ara-C and recombinant human GM-CSF in the treatment of refractory non-Hodgkin's lymphoma: A pilot study. *Cancer* 1990, **66**: 423–430.

24. Gasson JC. The molecular physiology of GM-CSF. *Blood* 1991, **77**: 1131–1145.

25. List A, Hersh E, Taetle R, et al. Phase I/II trial of subcutaneous recombinant interleukin-3 in patients with bone marrow failure. *Proc. Am. Soc. Clin. Oncol.* 1992, **33**: 1456a (abstract).

26. Brugger W, Schulz JFG, Pressler K, et al. Sequential administration of interleukin-3 and granulocyte–macrophage colony-stimulating factor following standard dose combination chemotherapy with etoposide, ifosfamide and cisplatin. *J. Clin. Oncol.* 1992, **10**: 1452–1459.

27. Schabel FJ, Griswold DP, Corbett TH, et al. Increasing the therapeutic response rates to anticancer drugs by applying the basic principles of pharmacology. *Cancer* 1994, **54**: 1160–1167.

28. Zorsky PE, Perkins JB. Optimizing high-dose chemotherapy using pharmacokinetic principles. *Semin. Oncol.* 1993, **5**: 2–18.

29. Neidhart JA, Mangalik A, Stidley CA, et al. Optimum dosing regimen of granulocyte–macrophage colony-stimulating factor (GM-CSF) to support dose-intensive chemotherapy. *J. Clin. Oncol.* 1992, **10**: 1460–1469.

30. Neidhart J, Kubica R, Stidley C, et al. Multiple cycles of dose-intensive cyclophosphamide etoposide and cisplatin (DICEP) produce durable responses in refractory non-Hodgkin's lymphoma. *Cancer Invest.* 1994, **12**: 1–11.

31. Gurney H, Anderson H, Radford J, et al. Infection risk in patients with small cell lung cancer receiving intensive chemotherapy and recombinant human granulocyte–macrophage colony-stimulating factor. *Eur. J. Cancer* 1992, **28**: 105–112.

32. Gulati SC, Bennett CL. Granulocyte-macrophage colony-stimulating factor (GM-CSF) as adjunct therapy in relapsed Hodgkin disease. *Ann. Intern. Med.* 1992, **116**(3): 177–182.

33. Gianni AM, Bregni M, Siena S, et al. Recombinant human granulocyte–macrophage colony-stimulating factor reduces hematologic toxicity and widens clinical applicability of high-dose cyclophosphamide treatment in breast cancer and non-Hodgkin's lymphoma. *J. Clin. Oncol.* 1990, **8**: 768–778.

34. Barlogie B, Jagannath S, Dixon DO, et al. High-dose melphalan and granulocyte–macrophage colony-stimulating factor for refractory multiple myeloma. *Blood* 1990, **76**: 677–680.

35. Laporte JP, Fouillard L, Douay L, et al. GM-CSF instead of autologous bone-marrow transplantation after the BEAM regimen. *Lancet* 1991, **338**: 601–602.

36. Sheridan WP, Morstyn G, Wolf M, et al. Granulocyte colony-stimulating factor and neutrophil recovery after high-dose chemotherapy and autologous bone marrow transplantation. *Lancet* 1989, **2**: 891–895.

37. Gebbia V, Testa A, Valenza R, et al. A prospective evaluation of the activity of human granulocyte colony-stimulating factor on the prevention of chemotherapy-related neutropenia in patients with advanced carcinoma. *J. Chemother.* 1993, **5**: 186–190.

38. Miles DW, Fogarty O, Ash CM, et al. Received dose-intensity: A randomized trial of weekly chemotherapy with and without granulocyte colony-stimulating factor in small-cell lung cancer. *J. Clin. Oncol.* 1994, **12**: 77–82.

39. Ardizzoni A, Venturini M, Sertoli MR, et al. Granulocyte–macrophage colony-stimulating factor allows acceleration and dose-intensity increase of CEF chemotherapy: A randomized in patients with advanced breast cancer. *Br. J. Cancer* 1994, **69**: 385–391.

40. DeVita VT. *Cancer, Principles and Practice of Oncology*, 3rd edn. New York: J.B. Lippincott, 1990.

41. Gorin NC, Coiffier B, Hayat M, et al. Recombinant human granulocyte–macrophage colony stimulating factor after high dose chemotherapy and autologous bone marrow transplantantion with unpurged and purged marrow in non-Hodgkin's lymphoma: A double-blind placebo-controlled trial. *Blood* 1992, **80**: 1149–1157.

42. Advani R, Chao NJ, Horning SJ, et al. Granulocyte–macrophage colony-stimulating factor (GM-CSF) as an adjunct to autologous hematopoietic stem cell transplantation for lymphoma. *Ann. Intern. Med.* 1992, **116**: 183–189.

43. Link H, Boogaerts MA, Crella AM, et al. A controlled trial of recombinant human granulocyte–macrophage colony stimulating factor after total body irradiation,

high-dose chemotherapy, and autologous bone marrow transplantation for acute lymphoblastic leukemia or malignant melanoma. *Blood* 1992, **80**: 2188–2195.

44. Clark DA, Neidhart JA. Granulocyte–macrophage colony-stimulating factor with dose-intensified treatment of cancer. *Semin. Hematol.* 1992, **4**: 27–32.

45. Brandt SJ, Peters WP, Atwater SK, et al. Effect of recombinant human granulocyte–macrophage colony-stimulating factor on hematopoietic reconstitution after high-dose chemotherapy and autologous bone marrow transplantation. *N. Engl. J. Med.* 1988, **318**: 860–876.

46. Gulati S, Bennett C, Toia M, et al. Role of granulocyte–macrophage colony-stimulating factor after autologous bone marrow transplantation for Hodgkin's disease. *Anti-Cancer Drugs* 1993, **4**(Suppl. 1): 13–16.

47. Lazarus HM, Andersen J, Chen MG, et al. Recombinant granulocyte–macrophage colony-stimulating factor after autologous bone marrow transplantation for relapsed non-Hodgkin's lymphoma: Blood and bone marrow progenitor growth studies. A phase II Eastern Cooperative Oncology Group trial. *Blood* 1991, **78**: 830–837.

48. Rabinowe SN, Neuberg D, Bierman PJ, et al. Long-term follow-up of a phase III study of recombinant human granulocyte–macrophage colony-stimulating factor after autologous bone marrow transplantation for lymphoid malignancies. *Blood* 1993, **81**: 1903–1908.

49. Kennedy MJ, Davis J, Passos-Coelho J, et al. Administration of human recombinant granulocyte colony-stimulating factor (filgrastim) accelerates granulocyte recovery following high-dose chemotherapy and autologous marrow transplantation with 4-hydroperoxycyclophosphamide-purged marrow in women with metastatic breast cancer. *Cancer Res.* 1993, **53**: 5424–5428.

50. Nemunaitis J, Appelbaum FR, Singer J, et al. Phase I trial with recombinant human interleukin-3 in patients with lymphoma undergoing autologous bone-marrow transplantation. *Blood* 1993, **82**: 3273–3278.

51. Gianni AM, Siena S, Bregni M, et al. Recombinant human interleukin-3 hastens trilineage hematopoietic recovery folliing high-dose ($7g/m^2$) cyclophosphamide therapy. *Ann. Oncol.* 1993, **4**: 759–766.

52. Laughlin MJ, Kirkpatrick G, Sabiston N, et al. Hematopoietic recovery following high-dose combined alkylating-agent chemotherapy and autologous bone-marrow support in patients with phase-I clinical trials of colony-stimulating factors: G-CSF, GM-CSF, IL-1, IL-2, M-CSF. *Ann. Hematol.* 1993, **67**: 267–276.

53. Pene R, Appelbaum FR, Fisher L, et al. Use of granulocyte–macrophage colony-stimulating factor and erythropoietin in combination after autologous marrow transplantation. *Bone Marrow Transplant.* 1993, **11**: 219–222.

54. Schmidberger H, Hess CF, Hoffmann W, et al. Granulocyte colony-stimulating factor treatment of leukopenia during fractionated radiotherapy. *Eur. J. Cancer* 1993, **29A**: 1927–1931.

55. Socinski MA, Cannistra SA, Sullivan R, et al. Granulocyte–macrophage colony-stimulating factor expands the circulating haemopoietic progenitor cell compartment in man. *Lancet* 1988, **1**: 1194–1198.

56. Gianni AM, Bregni M, Siena S, et al. Recombinant human granulocyte–macrophage colony-stimulating factor reduces hematologic toxicity and widens clinical applicability of high-dose cyclophosphamide treatment in breast cancer. *J. Clin. Oncol.* 1990, **8**: 768–778.

57. Gabrilove JL, Jakubowski A, Fain K, et al. Phase I study of granulocyte colony-stimulating factor in patients with transitional-cell carcinoma of the urothelium. *J. Clin. Invest.* 1988, **82**: 1454–1461.

58. Dührsen U, Villeval JL, Boyd J, et al. Effects of recombinant human granulocyte colony-stimulating factor on hematopoietic progenitor cells in cancer patients. *Blood* 1988, **72**: 2074–2081.

59. Lowry PA, Tabbara IA. Peripheral hematopoietic stem cell transplantation: Current concepts. *Exp. Hematol.* 1992, **20**: 937–942.

60. Eaves CJ. Peripheral blood stem cells reach new heights. *Blood* 1993, **82**: 1957–1959.

61. Gianni AM, Siena S, Bregni M, et al. Granulocyte–macrophage colony-stimulating factor to harvest circulating hematotopoietic stem cells for autotransplantation. *Lancet* 1989, **2**: 580–585.

62. Kessinger A, Armitage JO. The evolving role of autologous peripheral stem cell transplantation following high-dose therapy for malignancies. *Blood* 1991, **77**: 211–213.

63. Sheridan WP, Begley G, Juttner CA, et al. Effect of peripheral-blood progenitor cells mobilised by filgrastim (G-CSF) on platelet recovery after high-dose chemotherapy. *Lancet* 1992, **339**: 640–644.

64. Juttner CA, To LB, Ho JQ, et al. Early lympho-hemopoietic recovery after autografting using peripheral blood stem cells. *Transplantation* 1988, **44**: 585–588.

65. Kessinger A, Armitage JO, Landmark JD, et al. Autologous peripheral hematopoietic stem cell transplantation restores hematopoietic function following marrow ablation. *Blood* 1988, **71**: 723–727.

66. Kessinger A, Armitage JO, Smith DM, et al. High dose therapy and peripheral blood stem cell transplantation for patients with lymphoma. *Blood* 1989, **74**: 1260–1265.

67. Richman CM, Weiner RS, Yankee RA. Increase in circulating stem cells following chemotherapy in man. *Blood* 1976, **47**: 1031–1039.

68. To LB, Juttner CA. Peripheral blood stem cell autografting: A new therapeutic option for AML? *Br. J. Haematol.* 1987, **66**: 285–288.

69. To LB. Assaying the CFU-GM in blood: Correlation between cell dose and hematopoietic reconstitution. *Bone Marrow Transplant.* 1990, **5**(Suppl. 1): 16.

70. Brugger W, Bross KJ, Frisch J, et al. Mobilization of peripheral blood progenitor cells by sequential administration of IL-3 and GM-CSF following chemotherapy with etoposide, ifosfamide, and cisplatin. *Blood* 1992, **79**: 1193–2000.

71. Brugger W, Birken R, Bertz H, et al. Peripheral blood progenitor cells mobilized by chemotherapy + G-CSF accelerate both neutrophil and platelet recovery after high dose VP16, ifosfamide and cisplatin. *Br. J.*

Haematol. 1993, **84**: 402–407.

72. Molineux G, Pojda Z, Hampson IN, et al. Transplantation potential of peripheral blood stem cells induced by granulocyte colony-stimulating factor. *Blood* 1990, **76**: 2153–2158.

73. Bodine DM, Seidel NE, Zsebo KM, et al. In vivo administration of stem cell factor to mice increases the absolute number of pluripotent hematopoietic stem cells. *Blood* 1993, **82**: 445–455.

74. Fleming WH, Alpern EJ, Uchida N, et al. Steel factor influences the distribution and activity of murine hematopoietic stem cells in vivo. *Proc. Natl Acad. Sci. USA* 1993, **90**: 3760–3764.

75. Molineux G, Migdalska A, Szmitkovski M, et al. The effect on hematopoiesis of recombinant stem cell factor (ligand for c-kit) administered in vivo to mice either alone or in combination with granulocyte colony-stimulating factor. *Blood* 1991, **78**: 961–966.

76. Andrews RG, Bensinger WI, Knitter GH, et al. The ligand for c-kit, stem cell factor, stimulates the circulation of cells that engraft irradiated baboons. *Blood* 1992, **80**: 2715–2720.

77. Kessinger A, Armitage JO, Landmark JD, et al. High-dose therapy and autologous peripheral blood stem cell transplantation for patients with lymphoma. *Blood* 1989, **74**: 1260–1265.

78. Pettengell R, Morgenstern GR, Woll P, et al. Peripheral blood progenitor cell transplantation in lymphoma and leukemia using a single apheresis. *Blood* 1993, **82**: 3770–3777.

79. Shea TC, Mason JR, Storniolo AM, et al. High-dose carboplatin chemotherapy with GM-CSF and peripheral blood progenitor cell support: A model for delivering reperted cycles of dose-intensive therapy. *Cancer Treat. Rev.* 1993, **19**(Suppl. C): 11–20.

80. Tepler I, Cannistra SA, Frei E, et al. Use of peripheral-blood progenitor cells abrogates the myelotoxicity of repetititve high-dose carboplatin and cyclophosphamide chemotherapy. *J. Clin. Oncol.* 1993, **11**: 1583–1591.

81. Peters WP, Rosner G, Ross M, et al. Comparative effects of granulocyte–macrophage colony-stimulating factor (GM-CSF) and granulocyte colony-stimulating factor (G-CSF) on priming peripheral blood progenitor cells for use with autologous bone marrow after high dose chemotherapy. *Blood* 1993, **81**: 1709–1719.

82. Kritz A, Cron JP, Motzer RJ. Beneficial impact of peripheral blood progenitor cells in patients with metastatic breast cancer treated with high-dose chemotherapy plus granulocyte–macrophage colony-stimulating factor. *Cancer* 1993, **71**: 2515–2521.

83. Seidman AD, Scher HI, Gabrilove JL, et al. Dose-intensification of MVAC with recombinant granulocyte colony-stimulating factor as initial therapy in advanced urothelial cancers. *J. Clin. Oncol.* 1993, **11**: 408–414.

84. Bensinger W, Singer J, Appelbaum F, et al. Autologous transplantation with peripheral blood mononuclear cells collected after administration of recombinant granulocyte colony stimulating factor. *Blood* 1993, **81**: 3158–3163.

85. Weisenburger DD, Armitage JO, Kessinger A, et al. Culture of Reed–Sternberg-like cells from peripheral blood stem cell and bone marrow harvests of patients with Hodgkin's disease. *Exp. Hematol.* 1990, **18**: 65 (abstract).

86. Sharp J, Kessinger A, Armitage JO, et al. Clinical significance of occult tumor cell contamination of hematopoietic harvests in non-Hodgkin's lymphoma and Hodgkin's disease. *Proceedings of the International Symposium on ABMT in Lymphoma, Hodgkin's Disease, and Multiple Myeloma*, Wilsede, Germany, 1991.

87. Ross AA, Cooper BW, Lazarus HM, et al. Detection and viability of tumor cells in peripheral blood stem cell collections from breast cancer patients using immunocytochemical and clonogenic techniques. *Blood* 1993, **82**: 2605.

88. Sharp JG, Kessinger A, Vaughan WP, et al. Detection and clinical significance of minimal tumor cell contamination of peripheral blood stem cell harvests. *Int. J. Cell Cloning* 1992, **10**: 92–98.

89. Brugger W, Bross KJ, Glatt M, et al. Mobilization of tumor cells and hematopoietic progenitor cells into peripheral blood of patients with solid tumors. *Blood* 1994, **83**: 636–640.

90. Gribben JG, Freedman AS, Neuberg D, et al. Immunologic purging of marrow assessed by PCR before autologous bone marrow transplantation for B-cell lymphoma. *N. Engl. J. Med.* 1991, **325**: 1525–1533.

91. Shpall EJ, Jones RB. Release of tumor cells from bone marrow. *Blood* 1994, **83**: 623–625.

92. Brugger W, Henschler R, Heimfeld S, et al. Hematoietic recovery after high-dose chemotherapy is identical with positively selected peripheral blood CD34+ cells and unseparated peripheral blood progenitor cells. *Blood*, 1993, **84**: 1421–1426.

93. Shpall EJ, Stemmer SM, Hami L, et al. Amifostine (WR-2721) shortens the engraftment period of 4-hydroxycyclophosphamide-purged bone marrow in breast cancer patients receiving high-dose chemotherapy with autologous bone marrow support. *Blood* 1994, **83**: 3132–3137.

94. Brenner MK, Rill DR, Holladay MS, et al. Gene marking to determine whether marrow infusion restores long-term haemopoiesis in cancer patients. *Lancet* 1993, **342**: 1134–1137.

95. Brugger W, Moecklin W, Heimfeld S, et al. *Ex vivo* expansion of peripheral blood CD34+ progenitor cells by stem cell factor, interleukin-1beta (IL-1beta), IL-6, IL-3, interferon-gamma, and erythropoietin. *Blood* 1993, **81**: 2579–2584.

96. Nemunaitis J. Growth factors in allogeneic transplantation. *Semin. Oncol.* 1993, **20**: 96–101.

97. Masaoka T, Takaku F, Kato S, et al. Recombinant human granulocyte colony-stimulating factor in allogeneic bone marrow transplantation. *Exp. Hematol.* 1989, **17**: 1047–1050.

98. Nemunaitis J, Buckner CD, Appelbaum FR, et al. Phase I/II trial of recombinant human granulocyte–macrophage colony-stimulating factor following allogeneic bone marrow transplantation. *Blood* 1991, **77**: 2065–2071.

99. Dewitte T, Gratohl A, Vanderley N, et al. Recombinant

human granulocyte–macrophage colony-stimulating factor (rhGM-CSF) reduces infection-related mortality after allogeneic T-depleted bone marrow transplantation. *Bone Marrow Transplant.* 1991, **7**: 83–89.

100. Powles R, Smith G, Milan S, et al. Human recombinant GM-CSF in allogeneic bone marrow transplantation for leukemia: A double-blind, placebo-controlled trial. *Lancet* 1990, **336**: 1417–1420.

101. Naparstek E, Hardan Y, Ben-Shahar M, et al. Enhanced marrow recovery by short term preincubation of bone marrow allografts with human recombinant IL-3 and GM-CSF. *Blood* 1992, **80**: 1673–1678.

102. Hiraoka A, Masaoka T, Moriyama Y, et al. A double blind placebo controlled test of recombinant human nonglycosylated GM-CSF for allogeneic bone marrow transplantation. *Blood* 1993, **83**: 2086–2092.

103. Chap L, Schiller G, Nimer SD. The use of recombinant GM-CSF following allogeneic bone marrow transplants for aplastic anemia. *Bone Marrow Transplant.* 1993, **12**: 173–175.

104. Nemunaitis J, Albo V, Zeigler Z, et al. Reduction of allogeneic transplant morbidity by combining peripheral blood and bone marrow progenitor cells. *Leuk. Lymph.* 1993, **10**: 405–406.

105. Vowels M, Tang RLP, Berdoukas V, et al. Correction of x-linked lymphoproliferative disease by transplantation of cord blood stem cells. *N. Engl. J. Med.* 1992, **329**: 1623–1625.

106. Masaoka T, Motoyoshi K, Takaku F, et al. Administration of human urinary colony-stimulating factor after bone marrow transplantation. *Bone Marrow Transplant.* 1988, **3**: 121–127.

107. Masaoka T, Shibata H, Ohno R, et al. Double-blind test of human macrophage colony-stimulating factor for allogeneic and syngeneic bone marrow transplantation: Effectiveness of treatment and two-year followup for relapse of leukemia. *Br. J. Haematol.* 1990, **76**: 501–505.

108. Nemunaitis J, Anasetti C, Buckner CD, et al. Long-term follow-up of 103 patients who received rhGM-CSF after unrelated donor bone marrow transplant. *Blood* 1993, **81**: 865–869.

109. Nemunaitis J, Anasetti C, Storb R, et al. Phase II trial of recombinant human granulocyte–macrophage colony-stimulating factor (rhGM-CSF) in patients undergoing allogeneic bone marrow transplantation from unrelated donors. *Blood* 1992, **79**: 2572–2577.

110. Nemunaitis J, Singer J, Buckner CD, et al. The use of recombinant human granulocyte–macrophage colony-stimulating factor in graft failure following bone marrow transplantation. *Blood* 1990, **76**: 245–253.

111. Nemunaitis J, Myers JD, Buckner CD, et al. Phase I trial of recombinant human macrophage colony-stimulating factor in patients with invasive fungal infections. *Blood* 1991, **78**: 907–913.

112. Nemunaitis J, Shannon-Dorcy K, Appelbaum FR, et al. Long-term followup of patients with invasive fungal disease who received adjunctive therapy with recombinant human macrophage colony-stimulating factor (rhM-CSF). *Blood* 1993, **82**: 1422–1427.

113. Bunn HF. Recombinant erythropoietin therapy in cancer patients. *J. Clin. Oncol.* 1990, **8**: 949–951.

114. Boyd HK, Lappin TRJ. Erythropoietin deficiency in the anemia of chronic disorders. *Eur. J. Haematol.* 1991, **46**: 198–201.

115. Miller CB, Platanias LC, Mills SR, et al. Phase I–II trial of erythropoietin in the treatment of cisplatin-associated anemia. *J. Natl Cancer Inst.* 1992, **84**: 98–103.

116. Case DC, Bukowski RM, Carey R, et al. Recombinant human erythropoietin therapy for anemic cancer patients on combination chemotherapy. *J. Natl Cancer Inst.* 1993, **85**: 801–806.

117. Oster W, Herrmann F, Gamm H, et al. Erythropoietin for the treatment of the anemia associated with neoplastic bone marrow infiltration. *J. Clin. Oncol.* 1990, **8**: 956–962.

118. Abes R, Larholt K, Nelson R, et al. Prediction of response to recombinant human erythropoietin therapy in anemic cancer patients. *Blood* 1993, **82**(Suppl.1): 92 (abstract).

119. Ludwig H, Fritz E, Leitgeb C, et al. Erythropoietin treatment for chronic anemia of selected hematological malignancies and solid tumors. *Ann. Oncol.* 1993, **44**: 161–167.

120. Miller CB, Jones RJ, Piantadosi S, et al. Decreased erythropoietin response in patients with the anemia of cancer. *N. Engl. J. Med.* 1990, **322**: 1689–1692.

121. Platanias LC, Miller CB, Mick R, et al. Treatment of chemotherapy-induced anemia with recombinant human erythropoietin in cancer patients. *J. Clin. Oncol.* 1991, **9**: 2021–2026.

122. Cazzola M, Ponchio L, Beguin Y, et al. Subcutaneous erythropoietin for treatment of refractory anemia in hematologic disorders. Results of a phase I/II trial. *Blood* 1992, **79**: 29–37.

123. Pangalis GA, Poziopoulos CH, Panayiotidis P, et al. Treatment of anemia in B-chronic lymphocytic leukemia (B-CLL) with recombinant human erythropoietin. *Blood* 1993, **82**(Suppl.1): 574 (abstract).

124. Lazarus HM, Goodnough LT, Goldasser E, et al. Serum erythropoietin levels and blood component therapy after autologous bone marrow transplantation: Implications for erythropoietin therapy in this setting. *Bone Marrow Transplant.* 1992, **10**: 71–75.

125. Locatelli F, Pedrazzoli, Barosi G, et al. Recombinant human erythropoietin is effective in correcting erythropoietin-deficient anemia after allogeneic bone marrow transplantation. *Br. J. Haematol.* 1992, **80**: 545–549.

126. Vanucchi AM, Bosi A, Grossi A, et al. Stimulation of erythroid engraftment by recombinant human erythropoietin in ABO-compatible, HLA-identical, allogeneic bone marrow transplant patients. *Leukemia* 1992, **6**: 215–219.

127. Klaesson S, Ringdén O, Ljungman P, et al. Reduced blood transfusion requirements after allogeneic bone marrow transplantation: Results of a randomised, double-blind study with high-dose erythropoietin. *Bone Marrow Transplant.* 1994, **13**: 397–402.

128. Gordon MS, Hoffman R. Growth factors affecting human thrombocytopoiesis: Potential agents for the treatment of thrombocytopenia. *Blood* 1992, **80**: 302–307.

129. Bartley TD, Bogenberger J, Hunt P, et al. Identification and cloning of a megakaryocyte growth and develop-

ment factor that is a ligand for the cytokine receptor mpl. *Cell* 1994, **77**: 1117–1124.

130. Lok S, Kaushansky K, Holly D, et al. Cloning and expression of murine thrombopoietin cDNA and stimulation of platelet production in vivo. *Nature* 1994, **369**: 565–568.

131. Wendling F, Maraskovsky E, Debili N, et al. c-Mpl ligand is a humoral regulator of megakaryocytopoiesis. *Nature* 1994, **369**: 571–574.

132. Long MW, Gragowski LL, Heffner CH, et al. Phorbol diesters stimulate the development of an early murine progenitor cell: The burst forming unit-megakaryocyte. *J. Clin. Invest.* 1985, **76**: 431–438.

133. Hoffman R. Regulation of megakaryocytopoiesis. *Blood* 1989, **74**: 1196–1212.

134. Radley GM, Scurfield D. The mechanisms of platelet release. *Blood* 1980, **56**: 996–999.

135. Williams N, Jackson H, Walker T, et al. Multiple levels of regulation of megakaryocytopoiesis. *Blood Cells* 1989, **15**: 123–133.

136. McDonald TP, Cottrell MB, Clift RE, et al. High doses of recombinant erythropoietin stimulate platelet production in mice. *Exp. Hematol.* 1987, **15**: 719–721.

137. Eschbach J, Abdulhadi MH, Brone JK, et al. Recombinant human erthropoietin in anemic patients with end-stage renal disease. Results of a phase-III multicenter trial. *Ann. Intern. Med.* 1989, **111**: 992–1000.

138. Ganser A, Volkers B, Hoelzer D. Recombinant human granulocyte–macrophage colony-stimulating factor in patients ith myelodysplastic syndromes – a phase I/II trial. *Blood* 1989, **73**: 31–37.

139. Vadhan-Raj S, Keating M, Le Maitre A, et al. Effects of recombinant human granulocyte–macrophage colony-stimulating factor in patients with myelodysplastic syndromes. *N. Engl. J. Med.* 1987, **317**: 1545–1552.

140. Ganser A, Seipelt G, Lindemann A, et al. Effects of human recombinant interleukin-3 in patients with myelodysplastic syndromes. *Blood* 1990, **76**: 455–462.

141. Gillio A, Castro-Malaspina H, Gasparetto C, et al. Human recombinant interleukin-3 treatment in patients with myelodysplastic syndrome and aplastic anemia. *Blood* 1991, **78**(Suppl.): 372a (abstract).

142. Nemumaitis J, Rabinowe S, Singer JW, et al. Recombinant granulocyte–macrophage colony stimulating factor after autologous bone marrow transplantation for lymphoid cancer. *N. Engl. J. Med.* 1991, **324**: 1773–1778.

143. Crown J, Jakubowski A, Kemeny N, et al. Phase I trial of recombinant human interleukin-1 beta with and without 5-fluorouracil in patients with gastrointestinal cancer. *Blood* 1991, **78**: 1420–1427.

144. Smith JW, Longo DL, Gregory Alvord W, et al. The effects of treatment with interleukin-1alpha on platelet recovery after high-dose carboplatin. *N. Engl. J. Med.* 1993, **328**: 756–761.

145. Andrews RG, Bensinger WI, Knitter GH, et al. The ligand for c-kit, stem cell factor, stimulates the circulation of cells that engraft lethally irradiated baboons. *Blood* 1992, **80**: 2715–2720.

146. Leonhard JP, Quinto CM, Kozotza MK, et al. Recombinant human interleukin-11 stimulates multilineage hematopoietic recovery in mice after a myelosuppressive regimen of sublethal irradiation and carboplatin. *Blood* 1994, **83**: 1499–1506.

147. Du XX, Neben T, Goldman S, et al. Effects of recombinant human interleukin-11 on hematopoietic reconstitution in transplant mice: Acceleration of recovery of peripheral blood neutrophils and platelets. *Blood* 1993, **81**: 27–34.

148. Zeidler C, Kanz L, Hurkuck F, et al. In vivo effects of interleukin-6 on thrombopoiesis in healthy and irradiated primates. *Blood* 1992, **80**: 2740–2745.

149. Demetri GD, Bukowski RM, Samuels B, et al. Stimulation of thrombopoiesis by recombinant human interleukin-6 pre- and post-chemotherapy in previously untreated sarcoma patients with normal hematopoiesis. *Blood* 1993, **82**: 367a.

150. Ritch PS, Schiller J, Rivkin S, et al. Phase I evaluation of recombinant human interleukin-6. *Blood* 1993, **82**: 367a.

151. Geissler K, Valent P, Bettelheim P, et al. In vivo synergism of recombinant human interleukin-3 and recombinant human interleukin-6 on thrombopoiesis in primates. *Blood* 1992, **79**: 1155–1160.

152. Tao MH, Levy R. Idiotype/granulocyte/macrophage colony-stimulating factor fusion protein as a vaccine for B-cell lymphoma. *Nature* 1993, **362**: 755–758.

CHAPTER 30

Radiation therapy in the non-Hodgkin's lymphomas

JAMES R. GRAY AND ELI GLATSTEIN

Introduction

Ionizing radiation has been an important therapeutic agent in the treatment of the non-Hodgkin's lymphomas for many decades. Data from patients treated as early as the 1930s with orthovoltage equipment suggest that 'some lymphoma patients may have been cured by adequate radiation therapy' [1]. Indeed, until the advent of modern multiagent chemotherapy over the last 10–20 years, radiation therapy represented the only significant curative hope for lymphoma patients, and then only for those with earlier stages of the disease. More recently, the application of multiagent chemotherapy to the malignant lymphomas has resulted in dramatic responses. The use of combination chemotherapy in the non-Hodgkin's lymphomas now appears to offer the potential for cure to many patients with disseminated disease, at least to those with aggressive histologies.

In the 1980s the prevailing emphasis on combined modality therapy led to efforts to integrate radiation therapy and chemotherapy in the curative therapeutic approaches to malignant lymphomas. However, the enthusiasm for even more aggressive treatment regimens must be tempered by the potential for late complications and second malignancies. The deleterious as well as beneficial effects of combined modality therapy make it critical to establish the roles of radiation therapy and chemotherapy in the treatment of the non-Hodgkin's lymphomas through prospective, carefully controlled clinical trials.

This chapter will deal only with the role (past and present) of radiation therapy in the treatment of non-Hodgkin's lymphomas in adults. In childhood, the results of multiagent chemotherapy are sufficiently good that radiation therapy is usually used today only for local palliation or as part of transplantation programs in which total body irradiation is given.

Hodgkin's disease and the non-Hodgkin's lymphomas

The current temporary terminology of 'non-Hodgkin's lymphomas' reflects somehow the contemporary provisional concepts in terms of natural history and correct approach to therapeutic problems. [2]

Unfortunately, nearly two decades after this statement, significant confusion still remains regarding the classification, staging and treatment of the non-Hodgkin's lymphomas. Even the designation of this heterogeneous group of malignant lymphoid tumors as non-Hodgkin's lymphomas reflects the confusion of earlier investigators. Most of our treatment strategies for the non-Hodgkin's lymphomas were extrapolated from the successful therapy of Hodgkin's disease. However, investigators soon realized that significant differences exist between the non-Hodgkin's lymphomas and Hodgkin's disease with respect to their natural histories and response to therapy.

In the 1950s and 1960s, the conceptual basis for the treatment of Hodgkin's disease was established. Patients with Hodgkin's disease were generally young and otherwise healthy. The disease had a predictable mode of lymphatic spread and relatively infrequent extranodal extension [3]. Epitrochlear, mesenteric and Waldeyer's ring nodes were infrequently involved. This led to the concept of 'prophylactic irradiation', i.e., the irradiation of the uninvolved nodal groups adjacent to involved nodal regions. The pioneering studies of Dr Henry Kaplan and his colleagues at Stanford University helped to define treatment strategies for patients with Hodgkin's disease in the era of megavoltage radiation therapy. Their treatment philosophy evolved from the demonstration that high-dose irradiation resulted in greater than 90% local control [4] and that irradiation of large volumes of nodal tissue (i.e., beyond the confines of overt disease) in continuity (so-called extended-field irradiation) resulted in the cure of many patients with early-stage disease. The concepts of staging which evolved at the Rye [5] and Ann Arbor [6] meetings were also based on the understanding of the patterns of spread of Hodgkin's disease.

Unfortunately, the malignant lymphomas other than Hodgkin's disease did not demonstrate the same high rate of curability when treated with involved or extended-field radiation therapy. Investigators became aware that the natural histories of Hodgkin's disease and the non-Hodgkin's lymphomas were markedly different, and that central nodal irradiation did not yield the same probability of cure in the non-Hodgkin's lymphomas as it did in Hodgkin's disease.

The non-Hodgkin's lymphomas differ in many ways from Hodgkin's disease. An understanding of these differences is essential to an understanding of the relative importance of radiation in the treatment of these two groups of diseases. As a group, the NHLs, in contrast to Hodgkin's disease, have a remarkable propensity to spread beyond the lymphatic system. There are marked increases in the frequency of involvement of bone marrow, mesenteric nodes, Waldeyer's ring and central nervous system (CNS). Although the most common sites of recurrence are in lymph nodes, extranodal involvement at the time of relapse is almost as frequent. Patients with non-Hodgkin's lymphomas tend to be two to three decades older than Hodgkin's disease patients. As a consequence they manifest more organ dysfunction unrelated to lymphoma. In contrast, they are less likely to have systemic symptoms at diagnosis related to their malignancy (B symptoms) than Hodgkin's patients (10–15% versus 30–35%). Patients with Hodgkin's disease frequently present when the disease is still localized; 60–70% have stage I or II lymphoma at presentation. In contrast, the vast majority of non-Hodgkin's lymphoma patients present with advanced-stage disease (III or IV). In patients with nodular histology, fewer than 20% of patients present with pathological stage I or II disease. In patients with diffuse histology lymphomas, between 30% and 50% of patients have early-stage disease, but less than 15% are classified as stage I [7–10]. An additional difference is the much wider range of histological subtypes of NHL. Unfortunately, the subjective nature of histological classification leads to rather poor agreement among pathologists – even highly experienced hematopathologists – with respect to histological categorization. Over the past three decades, at least six major histopathological classification systems for the non-Hodgkin's lymphomas have been proposed, which has resulted in considerable confusion. Comparison of the results of various clinical studies is complicated and often impossible.

The development of the Working Formulation for Clinical Usage of the Non-Hodgkin's Lymphomas Pathologic Classification Project [11] was an important step in encouraging communication among pathologists. It has provided a means for translating clinical trials from different institutions into common terminology and, by dividing lymphomas into low, intermediate and high grade, helped in emphasizing the prognostic relevance of the major categories in the context of modern therapeutic modalities. The study which led to the development of the formulation demonstrated that the recognition of a follicular pattern, one of the major prognostic variables in predicting natural history and determining therapy, was highly reproducible (95% probability) [12]. There was considerable variation in identification of many of the other histological subtypes. This wide range in reproducibility applied both to individual pathologists reviewing a single slide twice, and to multiple pathologists evaluating the same slide. It is apparent that there is still a need for improvement in the classification of the non-Hodgkin's lymphomas. The application of new immunological and molecular data should ultimately help to distinguish further the subtypes of malignant lymphomas.

In addition to the inherent difficulties in reproducibility of histological classification is the problem of multiple subtypes existing in the same patient. Divergent histologies may be present during the initial staging either in the same or different lymph nodes [13,14]. In a study performed at the National Cancer Institute in which 101 patients had multiple tissue sites biopsied at presentation [15], 33 had more than one histological subtype identified. Sometimes a different histology is documented at the time of a repeat biopsy months after the initial diagnosis, or at autopsy [16–18].

All of these issues add to the confusion regarding the classification of the non-Hodgkin's lymphomas and to difficulty in planning optimal therapy. It is important that clinicians have realistic expectations and appreciate the uncertainties involved.

Radiation dose and local control

The era of megavoltage radiation therapy began in the 1950s. Radiation oncologists were no longer limited by the toxicity associated with kilovoltage irradiation where maximal dose was delivered to the skin surface. The devices capable of providing beams with energies of millions of electron volts included Van de Graaff generators, radioactive cobalt-60 teletherapy units, Betatrons and linear accelerators. These high-energy machines allowed for treatment of all lymphoid tissue in the body with acceptable normal tissue toxicity. This led to encouraging results in the treatment of Hodgkin's disease.

The curative potential of radiation therapy in Hodgkin's disease has been recognized by several groups prior to the 1950s [19,20]. However, the depth–dose characteristics of kilovoltage X-ray beams with maximal surface dose and rapid attenuation in tissue hampered these early investigators' attempts to deliver curative doses to adequate volumes. Modern radiation therapy techniques utilizing high-energy machines and complex multifield treatment planning have optimized dose distribution. This allows for tumoricidal doses to be delivered to involved areas with tolerable doses to normal tissues. Skin dose is minimized through the use of multiple field arrangements and the skin-sparing characteristic of megavoltage X-rays (maximum tissue dose absorption occurs deep to the dermis). Additionally, dose fractionation is now recognized as a highly significant factor in tumor control and normal tissue damage. Early radiation oncologists often employed single-fraction high-dose therapy. Trial and error, plus unacceptable normal tissue complications, eventually led to protracted fractionation schemes. A daily dose of 180–200 cGy delivered in five fractions per week has ultimately proven to be highly effective and to have tolerable side-effects.

Another major issue for the radiation oncologist, related to both tumor control and complications, is the volume to be irradiated. If irradiation is to be used as a single agent, the irradiated field must include clinically apparent tumor as well as occult microscopic disease. When defining a course of radiation therapy for a specific patient, the probability of acute and chronic complications must be weighed against tumor control. Optimal therapy is that which provides maximal probability of cure with minimal adverse effects.

The deposition of energy in tissue from radiation is a random event, as is the cell injury which results. The dose–cell death relationship is exponential, i.e., for every increment of radiation dose, the same proportion, not the same number, of cells are killed. Therefore, the total number of surviving cells after a given dose of radiation will be proportional to the initial number present and the fraction killed with that dose of radiation. Thus, various total doses of radiation (assuming comparable fractionation) will result in differing probabilities of local tumor control based on the inherent radiosensitivity of the tumor, the number of clonogenic cells present in each tumor, and the number of sites involved in each patient.

Curves can be generated describing tumor control as a function of radiation dose. Likewise, similarly shaped curves define the probability of normal tissue damage as a function of radiation dose. The dose–response relationship can be described as a three-part sigmoid-shaped curve of probability. At low doses, a gradual improvement in response is gained with progressive increments of radiation. As the dose is increased, the slope of the curve becomes steep, with dramatic changes in response for small dose increments. Finally, a region of diminishing returns is seen as the curve flattens asymptotically, at dose levels close to 100% certainty of response. Such a dose–response curve can be described for both malignant tissues ('tumor control curve') and normal tissues ('complication curve') as shown in Figure 30.1. The therapeutic ratio is the comparison between tumor control and complication frequency.

Fortunately for most of the lymphomas, the therapeutic ratio is relatively favorable, i.e., the curve for tumor control is to the left of that for normal tissue damage, meaning that a given dose of radiation will produce a higher probability of tumor control than of normal tissue complications. Optimally, radiation dose is selected within this 'window' between the curves as shown in Figure 30.1. Dose B represents a compromise between an acceptable normal tissue complication rate and a good level of tumor control. By contrast, dose A sacrifices tumor control for an inconsequential reduction in the complication rate, and dose C results in an unacceptable complication rate for a small gain in tumor control.

Kaplan compiled data from numerous studies on the recurrence rates of Hodgkin's disease as a function of radiation dose. At a dose of approximately 4400 cGy delivered in 4–4.5 weeks, the rate of true local recurrence was 1.3%, whereas at 1000 cGy or less, there was an 80% probability of local recurrence [21]. There appeared to be no relationship between the risk of failure and the histological subtype of Hodgkin's disease. In contrast, with the non-Hodgkin's lymphomas, dose–response relationships vary with histology. Even the early report of Peters [1], based on kilovoltage as well as megavoltage data documented that the diffuse lymphomas, particularly diffuse histiocytic lymphomas, required a considerably higher dose for local control than follicular lymphomas. Peters reported the tumor dose ranges which were successful in preventing local recurrence as follows:

1. 2500 cGy in 2 weeks to 3000 cGy in 4 weeks for 'giant follicular lymphoma'.
2. 1500 cGy in 1 week to 4500 cGy in 4 weeks for 'lymphosarcoma'.
3. 5000 cGy in 4 weeks for 'reticulum cell sarcoma'.

A substantial body of data has been published since that time confirming many of these early observations. Dose–response relationships for the non-Hodgkin's lymphomas have been reviewed by numerous authors [22–24]. Fuks and Kaplan [25] at Stanford University reported on dose–response relationships in all of the subtypes of the non-Hodgkin's lymphomas using the histopathological classification of Rappaport. Recurrence was defined as 'the appearance of lymphadenopathy or other evidence of tumor growth in a previously treated involved field as the first new manifestation of lymphoma following an initial course of radiotherapy'. Evaluating the nodular histologies, at doses of 1500–3500 cGy, recurrence rates were 50% for nodular lymphocytic, poorly differentiated (NLPD), 15% for nodular mixed lymphoma (NML) and 45% for nodular histiocytic lymphoma. At ≥ 4400 cGy, the control was excellent for all of the nodular lymphomas: 94% for NLPD, 97% for NML, and 100% for nodular histiocytic lymphoma. Dose–response data for all the nodular lymphomas are shown in Figure 30.2.

Bush and Gospodarowicz [26,27] confirmed the excellent local control rates in nodular lymphomas. In their pooled data for indolent histology lymphomas treated at the Princess Margaret Hospital, Toronto, local control was compared for fields receiving doses ≤ 3450 cGy (average 2715 cGy) and > 3450 cGy (average 3787 cGy). The control rate was 90% in both low- and high-dose subgroups except in patients aged 60 years or older with a tumor

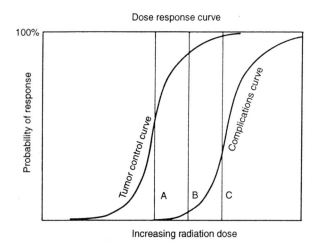

Figure 30.1 Model of dose–response curve (not based on actual data).

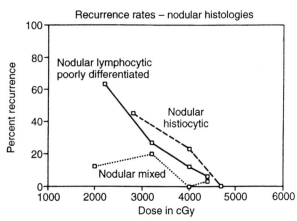

Figure 30.2 Recurrence rates within irradiated areas as a function of dose in the nodular lymphomas. Adapted from Fuks and Kaplan [25].

mass of 2.5 cm or more. Because of the small numbers of failures at any dose level, dose–response curves were not constructed. It is difficult to compare these data with the Stanford University data, since very few patients at the Princess Margaret Hospital were treated with less than 2000 cGy.

The Stanford University data for local control in diffuse lymphomas are shown in Figure 30.3 [25]. Fuks and Kaplan could not demonstrate a clear dose–response curve in the diffuse histiocytic lymphomas (DHL) – perhaps because of the heterogeneity of this 'entity'. With doses ranging between 1500 and 6500 cGy, recurrence rates were between 21 and 37%. However, most of these patients had advanced disease (stage III and IV). In patients with stages I and II DHL, the recurrence rate was still 19.2% with high dose radiation (greater than 3500 cGy). This was caused by a group of particularly unresponsive tumors which were given additional radiation treatment despite failure to respond at 4000 cGy. The majority of such 'self-selected' cases were controlled by administering doses up to 6500 cGy; in chemotherapeutic parlance, they were non-responders. Data from the Princess Margaret Hospital [26,27] show a dose–response curve for DHL with a suggestion of a plateau above 4000–4500 cGy. In stages IA–IIA, they reported control rates of 75–80% with doses of 4000 cGy or greater. It is apparent that DHLs require higher doses for local control, and there are clearly some tumors that are not controlled even with radiation doses greater than 6000 cGy.

Fuks and Kaplan [25], in diffuse lymphocytic, poorly differentiated (DLPD) lymphoma, were able to discern a dose–response curve, with a relatively low recurrence rate at 4400 cGy or greater (15%). This finding was consistent with the Bush and Gospodarowicz data on DLPD, which was included with their indolent lymphoma group [27]. Bush and

Gospodarowicz suggested that although 2500–3000 cGy result in 90% local control in the involved site, the chance of tumor control falls to 81% ($0.9 \times 0.9 \times 100$) when two regions are involved with lymphoma. They therefore recommended a higher dose, approaching normal tissue tolerance, to maximize the chance of control of multiple sites in each patient. This is consistent with the theoretical arguments of Kaplan in his discussion of Hodgkin's disease [21].

In light of the above information on dose–response relationships in the non-Hodgkin's lymphomas, one can better evaluate published data on local control of these tumors when treated with radiation therapy. Fuks et al. [29] were able to achieve a high percentage of local control in all histological subtypes except DHL (69%) and nodular histiocytic lymphomas (74%) (Table 30.1). This study involved a review of patients with stages I, II and III lymphomas, all of whom were treated with radiation alone as initial therapy. There are a number of other studies in which early-stage patients have been reviewed, from which one can estimate the risk of local failure after irradiation. The results of many series in which stages I and II nodular lymphomas were treated with radiation therapy confirmed the high rate of local control. In six major studies, which included a total of 493 patients with early stage nodular lymphomas [27,29–33], the frequency of local recurrence was only 7% in areas treated with doses ranging from 2000 to 5000 cGy. The majority of patients were treated with 3500 cGy or greater. Six studies in which a total of 614 patients with stages IA and IIA DHL and DML were included [27,29,34–37]; the local failure rate was 21% with doses ranging from 2500 to 5600 cGy. In 323 patients who received treatment with 4000 cGy or greater, local failure occurred in approximately 11%.

Several papers address the issue of bulky disease and the probability of local control in areas of massive tumor treated with radiation therapy alone. In patients with intermediate- or high-grade tumors, predominantly DHL, several studies suggest that relapse after radiation therapy is strongly related to the size of the tumor. Bush and Gospodarowicz [27] reported that local recurrence in DHL when tumor sizes were less than 2.5 cm was approximately 17%, in contrast to a 45% control rate in tumors greater than 2.5 cm. Mauch et al. [35] reported no local failures in patients with tumors less than 10 cm in contrast to 43.5% (10/23) failure rate in tumors of larger size. Patients in this study received 3500–5600 cGy, with a median of 5000 cGy. There is still considerable controversy about the issue of bulk of tumor as a prognostic factor for survival in DHL patients treated with chemotherapy [38], but most investigators believe that there is an inverse correla-

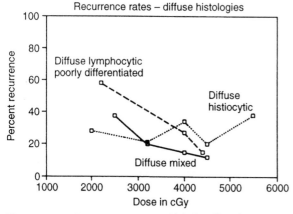

Figure 30.3 Recurrence rates within irradiated areas as a function of dose in the diffuse lymphomas. Adapted from Fuks and Kaplan [25].

Table 30.1 Local control of lymph node involvement in patients with malignant non-Hodgkin's lymphoma treated with radiation therapy (3500 cGy or more)

Lymphoma	No. of patients				No. of failures in irradiated nodes	Local control of nodal disease (%)
	I	II	III	Total		
NLPD	11	16	22	49	1	98
NM	9	16	31	56	3	95
NH	4	10	5	19	5	74
DLPD	6	12	7	25	5	89
DM	5	9	6	20		
DH	13	33	19	65	20	69

NLPD, nodular lymphocytic poorly differentiated; NM, nodular mixed; NH, nodular histiocytic; DLPD, diffuse lymphocytic poorly differentiated; DM, diffuse mixed; DH, diffuse histiocytic.
Adapted from Fuks et al. [29].

tion between the size of a tumor mass and outcome in the aggressive lymphomas.

A correlation between tumor bulk and local recurrence is more difficult to discern in the favorable histology non-Hodgkin's lymphomas. In a series reported from Princess Margaret Hospital [27], relapse-free survival was different in patients with tumors less than or greater than 2.5 cm ((diffuse lymphocytic, well differentiated (DLWD), diffuse lymphoma, intermediate differentiation (DLID), NLPD, mixed cell (MC), nodular histiocytic (NH)). However, there appeared to be minimal impact on local control. A review of nodular and favorable histology lymphomas, stages I and II, treated with megavoltage irradiation at Stanford University Hospital [33], reported no difference in survival or freedom from relapse at 5 years between patients

with tumors greater than or less than 5 cm.

The issues of dose–response, local control, number of sites of disease and bulk of tumor are all critical factors to be taken into account when planning radiation therapy for patients with non-Hodgkin's lymphomas, and must also be considered when comparing the results of specific protocols. In contrast, the ability of multiagent chemotherapy to achieve local control of lymph node involvement is a subject that has been neglected by most medical oncologists. Making some assumptions which appear to be reasonable, and using the data of Anderson et al. [38], it is possible to make an estimate of local control rates achieved by chemotherapy. This estimate is projected to be approximately 35% of all patients who were treated (Table 30.2). While it must be acknowledged that the regimens used belonged to

Table 30.2 Local control of lymph node involvement in patients with malignant lymphoma treated with C-MOPP, CVP or BACOP

Lymphoma	No.	No. in CR	No. not relapsed	
NLPD	49	33	12	81% of relapses (37 of 46)
NM	31	24	20	occurred only in lymph nodes,
NH	4	3	0	virtually always previously
DLWD	11	7	2	involved.
DLPD	25	7	1	
DM	10	1	1	Estimate of local lymph node
DH	62	29	23	control in this series is
DU	7	3	2	61+9=70 out of 199 patients (35%).
Total	199	107 (54%)	61	

NLPD, nodular lymphocytic poorly differentiated; NM, nodular mixed; NH, nodular histiocytic; DLWD, diffuse lymphocytic, well differentiated; DLPD, diffuse lymphocytic, poorly differentiated; DM, diffuse mixed; DH, diffuse histiocytic; DU, diffuse undifferentiated; C-MOPP, cyclophosphamide, vincristine, procarbazine, prednisone; CVP, cyclophosphamide, vincristine, procarbazine; BACOP, bleomycin, adriamycin, cyclophosphamide, vincristine, prednisone.
Adapted from Anderson et al. [38].

the first and second generations of chemotherapy protocols for non-Hodgkin's lymphomas, long-term data showing a clear superiority for today's regimens over these earlier regimens are lacking. It is precisely because local control with drugs alone is so low and because the typical sites of failure in irradiated patients are outside the portals of treatment that we believe more studies of combined modality treatment are indicated.

Dose fractionation

Dose fractionation has been studied in many patients with Hodgkin's disease [39–41]. Several groups have reported similar results. The method used involved plotting a scatter diagram on which each point represented an instance of local control or recurrence of lymphoma in a field treated with a specified dose in a specified number of days. From such diagrams, regression curves may be derived to obtain an estimate of the lowest total dose of irradiation, delivered over a defined time interval, at which few local recurrences would be expected. The curves for Hodgkin's disease indicate greater than 95% probability for local control with doses of 4000–4300 cGy in 40 days. Other fractionation schemes yielded the same probability of control with 2500–3200 cGy in 10 days or 2900–3900 in 30 days. These data were consistent with clinical studies demonstrating high rates of local control with 4000–4400 cGy.

There are fewer dose fractionation data available for the non-Hodgkin's lymphomas. Time–dose scattergrams were reported by Cox et al. [42] for 131 patients with lymphoreticular malignancies. They described isoeffect lines as essentially flat at 2200 cGy for the nodular and 4200 cGy for diffuse lymphomas. They noted that small tumors were as likely to recur as large at a given dose level and that fractionation did appear to be critical. These and other time–dose data on the non-Hodgkin's lymphomas suggest that total dose was the most important variable in the control of these malignancies. The problems in determining optimal dose from these retrospective data are as follows:

1. Fractionation schemes have generally been disregarded.
2. Lower doses have generally been used only when regression of the tumor mass was marked, such that it seemed reasonable to discontinue radiation.
3. Quantification of tumor bulk has generally been neglected – obviously persistent disease has usually received additional doses.

Local control has been reported with radiation schemes ranging from single fractions of 800–1000 cGy, to multiple 15 cGy fractions for a total of 150 cGy as delivered with total body irradiation. One of the major issues in deciding on a fractionation scheme is normal tissue tolerance. Normal tissue damage is greatly influenced by the fractionation scheme. Late sequelae appear to be substantially more severe in patients receiving a large dose per fraction. Again, considering the therapeutic window described with sigmoid dose–response curves, the use of large doses per fraction moves the normal tissue complication risk curve to the left and closer to the tumor control curve. This will result in a higher incidence of complications for the same degree of tumor control. Standard therapy regimens utilize 180–200 cGy per fraction delivered five times per week, representing a reasonable compromise between duration of treatment and acceptable risk of complications. Such fractionation schemes have proved to be highly effective in the treatment of the non-Hodgkin's lymphomas, especially of non-large-cell histologies, with excellent local control and acceptable normal tissue toxicity.

Radiation volume

The non-Hodgkin's lymphomas have been treated with radiation therapy fields ranging from small fields confined to sites of clinically apparent disease to total body irradiation. One must consider the histological subtype, the stage of disease, and obviously whether the goal is curative or palliative when determining the extent of the treatment fields.

As a palliative modality, radiation may be extremely effective when delivered to sites of tumor involvement which are causing symptoms. In this circumstance it is necessary to decide whether contiguous sites of disease will require palliative radiation therapy in the future and plan for potential match areas between radiation fields. If the prior treatment dose has been low, one can also consider re-irradiation of previous fields. This is important, since a commonly used palliative dose is 3000 cGy in 200 cGy fractions, leaving 'room' for additional palliative radiation: retreatment with another 3000 cGy is possible in most sites, except when normal tissue tolerance is lower than the combined total dose as, for example, applies to the spinal cord. An additional 1500–2000 cGy (depending upon the elapsed time interval since the prior palliative treatment), however, can be delivered to the spinal cord and provide effective palliation.

When the goal of radiation therapy of the non-

Hodgkin's lymphomas is curative, there remains considerable controversy with respect to the volume to be treated. The definition of terms is essential in evaluating the literature in this respect. Involved field radiation therapy refers to treatment limited only to involved lymph node chains. Extended-field radiation includes treatment of any apparently uninvolved lymphatic regions which are contiguous to sites of involvement. Therapy to all major lymph node areas is referred to as total nodal irradiation. Total lymphoid irradiation includes additional areas such as Waldeyer's ring, the spleen and mesenteric nodes. This may include treatment of the whole abdomen, as described by Goffinet et al. at Stanford [28]. Total body irradiation, whichever of the several techniques of delivery are used, implies the irradiation of all body tissues. Only low doses of radiation, given as a 'spray', can be delivered to so large a volume.

Critical to the determination of optimal field size is the evaluation of sites of relapse in the non-Hodgkin's lymphomas. Fuks et al. [29] reviewed 234 patients with stages I, II and III non-Hodgkin's lymphomas treated initially with radiation therapy alone. Patients received either involved-field or extended-field irradiation for stages I and II disease. Total nodal irradiation was most commonly used in the management of stage III disease. In spite of a conspicuous pattern of involvement of contiguous lymph node areas at presentation (79%), relatively few patients failed only in adjacent nodal sites (32%). Eighty per cent of initial failures of the stages I and II nodular lymphoma patients were in lymph nodes; 47% failed in noncontiguous nodes and 33% in contiguous nodes. Thirteen per cent failed in extralymphatic sites and 7% of failures involved both lymphatic and extralymphatic extension. In the lymphomas of diffuse histology, 43% of patients failed in extralymphatic sites: 21% failed in extralymphatic sites alone, 57% in lymphatic sites and 22% failed at both extralymphatic and lymphatic sites. Thirty per cent of all patients failed in contiguous nodal areas and 27% in noncontiguous areas without involvement of extralymphatic sites. Thus, unlike Hodgkin's disease, where 80% of nodal relapses occurred in contiguous nodal areas, non-Hodgkin's lymphomas showed a more irregular pattern of relapse, including a significant proportion of patients with extranodal spread.

The relatively moderate risk of contiguous spread in patients treated with radiation therapy has been confirmed in other studies. In data from Yale University, Chen et al. [30] reported on 114 patients with clinically staged I and II non-Hodgkin's lymphoma. Contiguous nodal relapse was not documented in any patient with nodular histology. There were four true recurrences in the patients with diffuse histologies and no other contiguous nodal relapses. Noncontiguous nodal disease accounted for 75% (six of eight) of the relapses in nodular lymphoma patients and 13% (four of 30) in diffuse histology patients. Sixty-three per cent of all failures involved extralymphatic sites. The apparent discrepancies in these data may be partly explained by the fact that transdiaphragmatic spread via the thoracic duct was considered noncontiguous by Chen et al. and contiguous by Fuks et al., if the left neck was involved. Nevertheless, the critical issue to the radiation oncologist is whether increasing the volume of irradiated nodal tissue is likely to result in improved survival rates. To a large degree, the answer depends on histology, because chemotherapeutic efficacy with curative intent is dependent on histology.

Early-stage low-grade lymphomas

The so-called low-grade or 'indolent' lymphomas have, on average, a longer natural history and a tendency to 'smolder' (remain stable or progresses very slowly) or even spontaneously regress. However, these low-grade lymphomas can be very frustrating for the clinician to manage since, even when they respond to treatment, relapse at a later date is usual. It is therefore tempting to lump all of these patients into an 'untreatable' category, on the grounds that treatment is futile until symptoms demand it. Approximately 10–20% of these patients, however, may truly have localized disease and can be rendered disease-free through relatively low-risk radiation therapy.

In a retrospective review, Paryani et al. [33] evaluated 124 patients with stages I and II favorable histology (low-grade) lymphomas who were treated at Stanford University with involved, extended or total lymphoid irradiation. Doses ranged from 3500 to 5000 cGy. With a median follow-up of 5.5 years, there were no significant differences in survival among the three treatment groups, although patients treated with total lymphoid irradiation (TLI) had significantly better 'freedom from relapse' than patients treated with either involved field or extended field. The actuarial freedom from relapse at 10 years is approximately 85% in the TLI group versus 40–50% in the involved- or extended-field group. However, further follow-up indicates more convergence of these curves, with approximately 50% of patients overall achieving cure. Attempting more precisely to define optimal treatment volume in early-stage favorable histology patients, investigators at Stanford are presently conducting a prospective randomized study. Patients in this trial have stages I and II NLPD or NML, and are surgically staged. They are randomized to receive involved field or TLI. Data on the first 20 patients entered into this protocol reveal no statistical difference in survival or freedom from relapse.

A number of reports in which patients with pathologic stage (through exploratory laparotomy) I and II nodular lymphoma were treated with radiation therapy to only one side of the diaphragm describe similar 5-year survival rates (62–87%) to those obtained in Stanford (Table 30.3). In clinically staged patients with stage I and II low-grade lymphomas, results are very similar (Table 30.3). Because of the retrospective nature of most of these reports, the variability in staging procedures, the differences in treatment fields and dose, and the limited follow-up, it is difficult to determine the optimal treatment volume for radiation in the low-grade lymphomas. Nonetheless, there are data that suggest that treatment of involved nodal regions and contiguous, clinically uninvolved areas is curative in approximately one-half of the patients with low-grade lymphomas of stage I and II. In a review of the experience of the National Cancer Institute, Lawrence et al. [32] noted that 71% of recurrences occurring after radiation therapy alone in low-grade lymphomas were within previously untreated nodal groups. With a median follow-up of 9 years, the latest relapse among 27 stage I patients was at 6.5 years. The authors suggest that these findings imply a role for total lymphoid irradiation.

Given these data, it is reasonable to treat early-stage patients with low-grade lymphomas with curative intent radiotherapy, using either involved-field irradiation or more comprehensive central or total lymphatic irradiation. This patient group may well benefit from relatively aggressive radiation therapy. It is important to realize that, at present, no chemotherapeutic regimen has been demonstrated to be curative for patients with low-grade lymphomas, regardless of stage.

Early-stage intermediate- and high-grade lymphomas

Unlike the low-grade lymphomas, almost half of patients diagnosed with the more aggressive intermediate- and high-grade lymphomas will present with localized (Ann Arbor stage I, IE, II and IIE) disease. Although a large fraction of these patients can be cured with local treatment only, there is a high probability that many patients have occult disseminated disease. Paradoxically, even patients with disseminated disease are curable.

There is some controversy over the appropriate management for patients with diffuse aggressive lymphomas: should these patients receive aggressive chemotherapy similar to that used for patients with advanced disease, or should a more conservative approach be used to minimize the risk of toxicities associated with such regimens? And if chemotherapy is used, is there a role for radiation to disease sites in the hope of destroying tumor cell clones which have survived multiagent chemotherapy? Such an approach would only be logical if resistant cells were confined to sites of known disease. For stage I patients this may often be the case, but the poor results with involved field radiation in stage II patients indicate that this is usually not the case in patients with more extensive disease. Sweet et al. [36] from the University of Chicago initially reported their results with radiation treatment of pathologically staged (staging laparotomy) localized aggressive lymphoma in 1981. This has subsequently been updated by Vokes et al. [43] in 1985 and Hallahan et al. [44] in 1989. Thirty-six patients with pathologic stage I (22) and pathologic stage II disease (14) were treated with extended-field radiation (27 patients) or involved-field radiation (nine patients). With a median follow-up of 7 years, the 10-year actuarial relapse-free survival was 91% for stage I patients and 35% for stage II patients. Toonkel et al. [37] reviewed a small number of pathologically staged patients: nine of 12 patients with stage I or IE DHL remained disease free in contrast to one of three with stage II or IIE disease. Because of the apparent differences between stage I and stage II patients, it is more difficult to interpret data in which these patients are considered

Table 30.3 Stage I–II low-grade lymphomas: 5-year survival when treated with radiation therapy alone

Pathologic staging:

Paryani et al.[33]	84%
Toonkel et al.[37]	87%
Mclaughlin et al. [45]	74%
Lawrence et al.[32]	78%
Monfardini et al.[46]	62%

Clinical staging:

Chen et al.[30]	83%
Bush et al.[26]	72%
Reddy et al.[47]	91%
Timothy et al.[48]	77%
Peckham et al.[49]	75%

as a single group. In a recent report from the MD Anderson Hospital, Lester et al. [50] reviewed 31 patients with large-cell lymphoma (23 with stage I or IE, eight with II or IIE) who were treated with radiation therapy alone. Disease-free survival was 62% and overall survival after salvage therapy was 88%. A small series reported by Levitt et al. [51] revealed no failures among nine pathologic stage I patients and one pathologic stage II patient treated with extended-field technique, with a median follow-up of 56 months. Kaminski et al. [52] reviewed the Stanford experience of 121 patients treated with primary radiation therapy; 38% had stage I or IE and 62% had stage II or IIE disease. In this series, 72 patients received limited-field irradiation, defined as treatment to one side of the diaphragm, either involved or extended field. Five-year survival in this group was 35% and 5-year freedom from relapse was 25%. In patients who received extensive irradiation (either subtotal or total lymphoid), 5-year survival and freedom from relapse were both 67%. The latter results are similar to comparable patients treated at Stanford during the same time period who received limited irradiation plus adjuvant chemotherapy. Survival and freedom from relapse in the latter group were 68% and 65% respectively.

There are numerous reports which give survival rates in clinically staged patients with aggressive lymphomas, predominantly diffuse histiocytic lymphoma, treated with radiation therapy alone. In six studies in which stage I and stage II patients were evaluated separately [30,31,34,48,50,53], relapse-free survival in stage I patients ranged from 35% to 65%, with an average of approximately 58%. In stage II patients, the data revealed relapse-free survival ranging from 0% to 47% with an average of 26%. These data must be compared with studies evaluating chemotherapy alone or in combination with radiation. Three studies have addressed this in a randomized fashion with a mixed population of stage I and II patients, and reported improvement in relapse-free as well as survival data in patients treated with a combination of radiation and chemotherapy compared to radiation alone [46,53,54]. Several studies have also demonstrated excellent disease-free and overall survival in patients treated with chemotherapy alone [55,56].

Most recent trials have emphasized the integration of chemotherapy, now considered a staple in the therapeutic armamentarium, with radiation. Prestidge et al. [57] reported their results in 94 patients treated at Stanford with combined modality therapy. After a median follow-up of 33 months, relapse-free survival at 5 years for stage I and II were 78% and 70%, respectively. Among 21 patients treated with two to three cycles of chemotherapy 'sandwiched' around radiation, no relapses have been observed. Jones et

al. [58] have combined the experience of Arizona and Vancouver. One hundred and forty-two patients have been followed for a median of 4.8 years. Virtually all of the patients in Vancouver were treated with three cycles of CHOP (see Chapter 42) followed by involved-field irradiation, while patients in Arizona had radiation therapy added to their treatment at the discretion of the treating physicians. The entire group of patients have a 5-year relapse-free survival of 82%. Although no significant difference in relapse-free survival was noted between the group that received combined modality therapy and the group that received chemotherapy alone, a trend favoring those whose treatment included radiation therapy was noted. When radiation was included, patients were usually given fewer courses of chemotherapy. It is possible that patients who were given radiotherapy in Arizona were selected because of slow response to chemotherapy or bulkier disease, but this is not commented upon by the authors. Tondini et al. [59] have treated 183 consecutive patients at the Milan Cancer Institute with four cycles of CHOP followed by irradiation. With a median follow-up of 4 years, they report a 5-year relapse-free survival of 83% among stage I and II patients. Finally, impressive results in stage I patients have been noted at the National Cancer Institute using 75% dose ProMACE-MOPP followed by involved field irradiation. Originally reported in 1989 by Longo et al. [60], this series has been updated with a median follow-up of 7.4 years. Sullivan et al. [61] now report a 10-year actuarial disease-free survival of 95%. They advocate limiting the radiation field to the involved site, since using fields which cover adjacent uninvolved nodal regions led to a higher rate of chronic complications (45% versus 14%) with no noticeable improvement in disease control. Certainly, these results will be virtually impossible to improve upon and have set the standard that newer regimens must match. It remains to be seen whether these results can be extended to patients with stage II disease.

With uncertainty over the most important prognostic factors, the difficulty in stratifying patients, and the ever-present possibility of selection biases, comparison of different series is difficult. Most investigators now agree that the optimal treatment for localized presentations should include doxorubicin-containing chemotherapy, but there is no general agreement on the role of radiation. Ongoing trials may help to answer this question. Among these is an Eastern Cooperative Oncology Group study in which patients with early-stage diffuse aggressive lymphomas receive eight cycles of CHOP chemotherapy and are randomized to receive or not to receive radiation. The Southwestern Oncology Group is randomizing patients between two arms, one of which consists of eight cycles of CHOP, and the other, three cycles of CHOP followed by irradiation. Until the results of these trials are reported, it appears reasonable to treat adult patients with stage I or II lymphomas of diffuse aggressive histology with 3–8 cycles of CHOP or similar chemotherapy, followed by involved-field irradiation to a dose of approximately 4000 cGy.

Advanced-stage low-grade lymphomas

Defining the radiation volume has been of primary concern in the early-stage non-Hodgkin's lymphomas where irradiation has played a major role in the development of a curative approach to treatment. However, for the nodular lymphomas, a significant percentage of patients with advanced-stage disease relapse exclusively in nodal sites. In patients with stage III disease, this raised the question whether irradiation of the majority of lymph node areas could have curative potential. In 1976, Glatstein et al. [62] and later Cox et al. [22] evaluated the role of total lymphoid irradiation in patients with stage III low-grade lymphomas. With a median follow-up of 80 months, Glatstein et al. reported survival rates of 75% at 5 years and 68% at 10 years. The relapse-free survival rates were 43% and 33% at 5 and 10 years respectively. Cox reported survival and relapse-free survival rates of 78% and 61%, respectively, with a median period of observation of 6 years. These figures compare favorably with the results obtained with chemotherapy, although 10-year figures relapse-free survival rates have rarely been reported. Interestingly, of the 28 patients with nodular lymphomas who relapsed after total nodal irradiation, 64% (18/28) had their initial relapse confined to lymph nodes; five were intra-abdominal and six were epitrochlear or brachial. This would suggest that increasing the volume of treatment to include these areas might improve results. Cox's total central lymphatic irradiation included the whole abdomen but not epitrochlear nodes. As in the report by Glatstein, Waldeyer's ring was treated in most of the patients. Recently Jacobs et al. reported a disease-free survival rate of 40% at 15 years after central lymphatic irradiation (similar to Cox's technique) for stage III nodular lymphoma in 34 patients, with a median follow-up of almost 10 years [63]. Because of the prolonged period during which relapses can occur in patients with these lymphomas (median survival of 8 years), additional follow-up is necessary to determine if central lymphatic irradiation will result in the cure of some patients with stage III nodular lymphoma. Certainly, excellent complete response (100% and 97%) and local control rates can be obtained with radiation therapy, and new treatment approaches for this subset of patients should be able to offer comparable quality of life to patients as that offered by total lymphoid irradiation.

It remains to be established whether chemotherapy combined with total nodal irradiation, as suggested by several authors, will improve the survival with advanced-stage follicular lymphomas. Many advocate a more conservative approach with treatment reserved for obvious disease progression or for the alleviation of symptoms directly attributed to the lymphoma (see Chapter 41). Investigators at Stanford have reviewed their experience with 83 advanced-stage patients managed without therapy at initial presentation [64,65]. Treatment was initiated at a median time of 3 years. With a median follow-up of 4 years, actuarial survival was 73% at 10 years. Obviously, patients had to meet certain criteria to be eligible for this study which must be taken into consideration when comparing this result with other published data. Observation after initial diagnosis does represent, however, a reasonable approach in carefully selected patients, especially the elderly.

Advanced-stage intermediate- and high-grade lymphomas

For patients with stages III and IV diffuse aggressive lymphomas, the main treatment modality is chemotherapy. Radiation therapy is presently reserved for dealing with symptomatic local problems that do not respond to multiagent drug therapy. However, the use of radiation therapy as an adjunct to chemotherapy has been considered. Advanced-stage patients with local sites of bulky disease (generally defined as disease equal to or greater than 10 cm) may benefit from the use of adjuvant radiation therapy. Shipp et al. [66], however, in a review from the Dana–Farber Cancer Institute reported that relapse does not occur consistently in sites of prior bulk disease. Consequently, they contend that radiation therapy would have little impact upon the outcome of therapy. Although this applies to stage IV patients, it should be noted that a significant fraction of stage III patients relapse exclusively in nodal regions, whether previously involved or not. Since radiation therapy is not dependent upon cell membrane transport mechanisms, radiation therapy represents a potentially noncross-resistant therapy, and total nodal or total lymphatic irradiation could significantly improve the results achieved with multiagent chemotherapy alone. Unfortunately, the combined marrow toxicity of this approach renders it prohibitively toxic, although progress in the development of hematopoietic growth factors would ultimately permit sufficient hematopoietic support to be achieved for this to be a feasible approach. Until that time, only selected patients with advanced-stage aggressive lymphomas will benefit from irradiation as part of their curative regimen.

Specific localized sites

Some sites of involvement in patients with early-stage disease deserve special mention. Although overall management of NHL at these sites is discussed in other chapters, the role of radiation therapy in these situations will be discussed here. Some of these sites have been reported from institutions with long-term experience, which may predate modern multiagent chemotherapy, and emphasized radiation therapy as the most effective treatment at the time.

GASTROINTESTINAL LYMPHOMAS

The gastrointestinal tract is the most common site of extranodal lymphomas, and the gastric lymphomas account for approximately half of these. The historical approach to patients with gastric lymphoma has been to perform partial or total gastrectomy followed by irradiation and/or systemic chemotherapy [67–69]. Most patients receive doxorubicin-containing chemotherapy. This has resulted in 5-year relapse-free survival rates of approximately 60%. Clinical evaluation of these patients should include the entire gastrointestinal tract and Waldeyer's ring for involvement, particularly if radiation only is to be used after surgery. It should be noted, however, that only patients with small-sized localized disease have been successfully treated with surgery and irradiation alone.

Today, the most pressing question is whether gastrectomy is necessary. There is little evidence that surgical debulking is useful in the treatment of lymphoma, although surgical excision of all or some of the disease has been the standard of care in gastric lymphoma. Since the diagnosis is often made at the time of exploratory laparotomy, surgery may have been done in many patients without it being part of an overall treatment plan. The fear of gastric perforation resulting from dissolution of transmural plaque of lymphoma in response to cytotoxic therapy

has been an additional reason that resection has been advocated. However, modern endoscopic evaluation and biopsy has allowed the diagnosis of most gastric lesions without laparotomy (and without the questionable additive value of surgical staging). In addition, although the risk of spontaneous gastric perforation after cytotoxic therapy has been noted [70], this is an uncommon occurrence. Maor et al. [71] from the MD Anderson Hospital have treated 34 patients with localized gastric lymphoma without gastrectomy. In general, these patients received CHOP–Bleo followed by regional irradiation. None of the patients experienced a gastric perforation or hemorrhage, and the 5-year relapse-free survival of 62% is similar to that reported in patients who have had surgery as part of their treatment. Since the potential morbidity (including malabsorption syndromes) of gastrectomy appears to be avoidable, it may be the preferred therapy in many patients. The extent and also the role of radiation in patients treated with chemotherapy after biopsy remains to be established, but in general the entire gastric silhouette and the immediate surrounding lymphatics plus other identified abdominal disease is irradiated to a dose of approximately 4000 cGy.

Primary central nervous system lymphomas

Malignant lymphoma arising in the CNS has a particularly virulent clinical course, with median survival times being usually of the order of 15 –18 months. Rarely do patients survive for 5 years. The traditional treatment for these patients has generally been cranial irradiation, since few have disease outside of the CNS and the majority progress only within the CNS. In addition, the blood–brain barrier is a significant impediment to the delivery of effective cytotoxic drugs to intraparenchymal lesions, although it does not hinder the physicochemical damage inflicted by ionizing radiation. Many investigators have begun using systemic and intrathecal chemotherapy in addition to irradiation. DeAngelis et al. [72] at Memorial Sloan–Kettering Cancer Center have reported their results in 31 patients treated with an aggressive regimen using intrathecal (via an Ommaya reservoir) and systemic methotrexate, high-dose systemic cytarabine (ara-C), and cranial irradiation consisting of 4000 cGy to the whole brain plus a 1440 cGy local boost. The median relapse-free survival time in this study was 41 months. This and other studies have confirmed the contribution of intrathecal and/or systemic chemotherapy to the treatment of intraparenchymal lymphoma. Similar results have been obtained with the use of blood–brain barrier disruption prior to chemotherapy and reserving cranial irradiation only for patients who progress [73]. While local control remains poor (70–90% of patients ultimately progressing in the brain) the potential contribution of radiation to treatment in this situation remains unclear.

TESTICULAR LYMPHOMAS

Primary testicular non-Hodgkin's lymphoma is rare and unusual in that it may be associated with occult involvement of the CNS and Waldeyer's ring. Systemic chemotherapy should always be given after diagnostic orchiectomy but there may be a role for scrotal irradiation since penetration of some chemotherapeutic agents into the testis is suboptimal [74]. The use of radiation therapy to the pelvic or retroperitoneal lymph nodes should be governed by the presence of disease in those sites. CNS prophylaxis may also be appropriate in these patients.

ORBITAL LYMPHOMAS

Lymphoma localized to the orbit may be treated with radiation alone if it is of low or intermediate grade. Orbital lymphoma must be distinguished from the polyclonal pseudolymphomas which are not true lymphomas. Other orbital presentations include conjunctival lymphoma, which can be easily treated with a local electron field [75], and ocular lymphoma, which often serves as a marker for primary CNS lymphoma. Local control of pseudolymphomas can be achieved with 2000 cGy; the low-grade lymphomas require higher doses of radiation but can probably be effectively treated with 2400–3000 cGy [76]. High- and intermediate-grade orbital lymphomas should be treated with chemotherapy, with or without radiation.

THYROID LYMPHOMAS

Treatment of lymphoma originating in the thyroid has generally included thyroidectomy and regional irradiation. Radiation therapy alone has resulted in 5 year relapse-free survivals of 49–78% [77–80]. Although direct comparisons of radiation with combined modality have not been made, it is possible that the combined use of chemotherapy and radiation together for these predominantly high-grade lymphomas will result in higher relapse-free survivals.

LYMPHOMA OF BONE

There is insufficient experience with doxorubicin-containing chemotherapy to assess the impact of combined modality therapy on these generally aggressive lesions. Five-year survival has been reported as 56–64% if aggressive noncleaved histologies are excluded [81–84]. This is similar to the earlier reports with nodal and extranodal nonosseous aggressive lymphomas yet falls short of results obtained with more recent series. Perhaps similar aggressive treatment of these lesions will yield higher success. Whether the use of local field radiation therapy will improve outcome is yet to be determined.

Total body irradiation

The largest volume that can be irradiated is the entire body, i.e., total body irradiation. Although single-dose exposure of the entire body to approximately 400 cGy will lead to death in 50% of human subjects, the tolerance of fractionated irradiation is much higher. The most frequent use of TBI today is as part of the marrow ablation regimen preceding bone marrow transplantation, but the necessity of including TBI as part of the preparatory regimen has been questioned. This issue is discussed in other chapters. Here, we shall discuss the use of TBI as a therapeutic modality in its own right outside the context of bone marrow transplantation.

The extreme sensitivity of the lymphomas to radiation led to the concept of using radiation as a 'systemic agent', i.e., irradiating all body tissues. Early reports of response of lymphomas to this therapy [85] led the National Cancer Institute in 1968 to initiate a prospective randomized study in poorly differentiated lymphocytic lymphomas in which extensive radiation therapy (11/49 having extended total nodal irradiation and 38/49 having total body irradiation) was compared to combination chemotherapy [cyclophosphamide, vincristine, prednisone (CVP) or cyclophosphamide, vincristine, procarbazine, prednisone (C-MOPP)]. The complete response rate for nodular lymphomas treated with radiation (33 patients: 25 NPDL, eight NML) was 85% and for diffuse lymphomas (eight DPDL), 69%. For chemotherapy-treated patients, the complete response rates for nodular and diffuse lymphomas were 62% and 13%, respectively. Long-term survival and relapse-free survival were almost identical for patients treated with either radiation or with chemotherapy. In spite of the excellent response of these tumors to radiation, only 20% of patients remained continuously free of disease at 4 years. In a second NCI trial, C-MOPP alone was compared to C-MOPP and total body irradiation. In both regimens, similar, excellent response rates were observed, but only 50% of patients remained disease free at 2 years – data which are similar to most reports of multiagent chemotherapy used without TBI.

In numerous other studies TBI has been evaluated as treatment for advanced non-Hodgkin's lymphoma. The usual dose is 10–15 cGy given 2–3 times per week to a total dose of 150–200 cGy. In order to include the entire patient in the field, the patient is treated at a distance of approximately 3 m from the collimator, which results in lowering the dose rate to less than 10 cGy/min. The results obtained in all these studies were similar. The complete response rate was approximately 81% in nodular lymphomas and 70% in diffuse lymphomas [86–89, 91–93]. Five-year survival rate was 68% in the nodular lymphoma patients and 50% in diffuse lymphoma patients, and the corresponding relapse-free survival rates were 25% and 16%. In a study conducted at Stanford University [90] in which TBI was compared with either single-agent or combination chemotherapy, there was no significant advantage to either approach in lymphomas with favorable histology. Two recent reports in which long-term survival rates were described [94,95] showed a relative plateau in the survival curves with 10–20% of patients remaining relapse free at 10 years.

It is unlikely that TBI can result in a cure for any except a small fraction of patients with non-Hodgkin's lymphoma, regardless of histology. In indolent lymphomas, however, the complete response and survival rates obtained are comparable to those achieved with chemotherapy regimens. Dose escalation of TBI may be possible with the use of radioprotective agents such as WR-2721: this could result in a prolongation of response in some patients [96], such that TBI may have a role in the initial treatment of patients with low-grade lymphomas who are not good candidates for chemotherapy or who decline chemotherapy.

Emergencies

Certain presentations of lymphoma lead to an urgent need for therapy in order to alleviate life-threatening symptoms or to prevent long-term consequences of tissue damage. The most common emergencies are spinal cord compression, superior vena cava syndrome and airway compression.

Spinal cord compression generally occurs as a result of anterior epidural encroachment upon the spinal canal. Although surgical decompression is frequently indicated in radioresistant lesions with a rapid onset of neurologic compromise, the overall results of surgery versus radiation therapy are equivalent with respect to the effective palliation of symptoms and prevention of permanent cord dysfunction. Surgery is rarely used when lymphoma causes cord compression, since these masses quickly respond to radiation therapy and/or chemotherapy.

Immediate decompression of the spinal cord is best achieved with high-dose bolus intravenous dexamethasone (25–100 mg) followed by regular intravenous maintenance doses (4–25 mg every 6 hrs). One important effect of this therapy is analgesia, since virtually every patient with cord compression has a history of recent worsening back pain, with or without associated neurological signs. Once the diagnosis of lymphoma has been made, all efforts should be made to identify the histologic subtype (if not already done) and stage the patient in order to determine the appropriate therapy for the systemic disease, since even with this presentation, many patients will be cured of their disease. Even though steroids are cytotoxic to lymphoma cells and chemotherapy may be started soon thereafter, there should usually be no delay in initiating radiation therapy to the spinal lesion in order to bring to bear the most intensive treatment to the site of the compression. In the very chemoresponsive high-grade lymphomas, particularly the small non-cleaved cell lymphomas, this policy should be modified, since rapid decompression can be achieved by chemotherapy alone.

Superior vena cava syndrome can be part of the presentation of lymphoma in the chest at initial diagnosis or at relapse. Although benign causes of SVC obstruction may be present, such as thrombus (particularly in a patient with intravascular monitoring devices), the majority of cases will be the result of extraluminal compression by tumor. Most cases of SVC syndrome are caused by non-small cell lung cancer and are best managed with radiation therapy. However, management of SVC syndrome in the lymphoma patient should always take into consideration the entire disease process. Although cerebral or laryngeal edema can be life-threatening, this is rarely the case and therapy can generally be delayed for 1 or 2 days. Tissue diagnosis should always be obtained, and basic staging studies should be performed in order to determine the appropriate therapeutic approach.

Unlike most malignant causes of SVC syndrome, lymphoma is quite sensitive to chemotherapy and reasonably prompt initiation of a curative regimen will alleviate most symptoms. However, these patients must be monitored closely during the first days of treatment and, if they do not improve, treatment with radiation therapy may be indicated. The radiation oncologist must be cognizant of the potential contribution of radiation therapy to the definitive treatment regimen and design the urgent treatment appropriately, using involved field or mantle fields as indicated. Although some have advocated 300–400 cGy fractions initially, this is probably not necessary with lymphoma and in fact may be contraindicated. The vast majority of these patients should respond quickly with improvement or elimination of their symptoms within days.

Airway obstruction can be present or develop at relapse with lymphoma. In addition to compromising air flow, this frequently puts the patient at risk for postobstructive pneumonia – a major risk in patients receiving myelosuppressive chemotherapy. Radiation therapy may be useful in reducing the restricting mass and alleviating or preventing obstructive symptoms. This rarely, however, constitutes a radiotherapeutic emergency and the decision to irradiate should be made in conjunction with the overall treatment plan.

References

1. Peters MV. The contribution of radiation therapy in the control of early lymphomas. *Am. J. Roentgenol.* 1963, **5**: 956–967.
2. Veronesi U, Musumeci R, Pizzetti F, et al. Proceedings: The value of staging laparotomy in non-Hodgkin's lymphomas (with emphasis on the histiocytic type). *Cancer* 1974, **33**: 446–459.
3. Rosenberg SA, Kaplan HS. Evidence for an orderly progression in the spread of Hodgkin's disease. *Cancer Res.* 1966, **31**: 1225–1231.
4. Kaplan HS. Evidence of a tumoricidal dose level in the radiotherapy of Hodgkin's disease. *Cancer Res.* 1966, **26**: 1221–1224.
5. Rosenberg SA. Report of the Committee on the Staging of Hodgkin's Disease. *Cancer Res.* 1966, **26**: 1310.
6. Carbone PP, Kaplan HS, Smithers DW, et al. Report of the committee on Hodgkin's disease staging classification. *Cancer Res.* 1971, **31**: 1860–1861.
7. Castellani R, Bonadonna G, Spinelli P, et al. Sequential pathologic staging of untreated non-Hodgkin's lymphomas by laparoscopy and laparotomy combined with marrow biopsy. *Cancer* 1977, **40**: 2322–2328.
8. Chabner BA, Johnson RE, Young RC, et al. Sequential nonsurgical and surgical staging of non-Hodgkin's lymphoma. *Ann. Intern. Med.* 1976, **85**: 149–154.
9. Goffinet DR, Castellino RA, Kim H, et al. Staging laparotomies in unselected previously untreated patients with non-Hodgkin's lymphomas. *Cancer* 1973, **32**: 672–681.
10. National Cancer Institute sponsored study of classifications of non-Hodgkin's lymphomas: Summary and description of a formulation for clinical usage. The non-Hodgkin's Lymphoma Pathologic Classification Project. *Cancer* 1982, **49**: 2112–2135.
11. National Cancer Institute Non-Hodgkin's Classification Project Writing Committee. *Cancer* 1985, **55**: 91–95.
12. Kim H, Hendrickson MR, Dorfman RF. Composite lymphoma. *Cancer* 1977, **40**: 959–976.
13. Mead GM, Kushlan P, O'Neil M, et al. Clinical aspects of non-Hodgkin's lymphomas presenting with discordant histologic subtypes. *Cancer* 1983, **52**: 1496–1501.
14. Warnke RA, Kim H, Fuks Z, et al. The coexistence of nodular and diffuse patterns in nodular non-Hodgkin's lymphomas: Significance and clinicopathologic correlation. *Cancer* 1977, **40**: 1229–1233.
15. Fisher RI, Jones RB, DeVita VT, et al. Natural history of malignant lymphomas with divergent histologies at staging evaluation. *Cancer* 1981, **47**: 2022–2025.
16. Acker B, Hoppe RT, Colby TV, et al. Histologic conversion in the non-Hodgkin's lymphomas. *J. Clin. Oncol.* 1983, **1**: 11–16.
17. Garvin AJ, Simon RM, Osborne CK, et al. An autopsy study of histologic progression in non-Hodgkin's lymphomas. 192 cases from the National Cancer Institute. *Cancer* 1983, **52**: 393–398.
18. Hubbard SM, Chabner BA, DeVita VT, et al. Histologic progression in non-Hodgkin's lymphoma. *Blood* 1982, **59**: 258–264.
19. Easson EC, Russell MH. The cure of Hodgkin's disease. *Br. Med. J.* 1963, **1**: 1704–1797.
20. Peters MV. A study of survivals in Hodgkin's disease treated radiologically. *Am. J. Roentgenol.* 1950, **63**: 299–311.
21. Kaplan HS. On the natural history, treatment, and prognosis of Hodgkin's disease. In *Harvey Lectures 1968–1969*. New York: Academic Press, 1970, pp. 215–259.
22. Cox JD, Komaki R, Kun LE, et al. Stage III nodular lymphoreticular tumors (non-Hodgkin's lymphoma): Results of central lymphatic irradiation. *Cancer* 1981, **47**: 2247–2252.
23. Newall J, Friedman M. Reticulum-cell sarcoma. II. Radiation dosage for each type. *Radiology* 1970, **94**: 643–647.
24. Seydel HG, Bloedorn FG, Wizenberg M. et al. Time–dose relationships in radiation therapy of lymphosarcoma and giant follicle lymphoma. *Radiology* 1971, **98**: 411–418.
25. Fuks Z, Kaplan HS. Recurrence rates following radiation therapy of nodular and diffuse lymphomas. *Radiology* 1973, **108**: 675–684.
26. Bush RS, Gospodarowicz M, Sturgeon J, et al. Radiation therapy of localized non-Hodgkin's lymphoma. *Cancer Treat. Rep.* 1977, **61**: 1129–1136.
27. Bush RS, Gospodarowicz M. The place of radiation therapy in the management of patients with localized non-Hodgkin's lymphomas. In Rosenberg SA, Kaplan HS (eds) *Malignant Lymphomas.* New York: Academic Press, 1982, pp. 485–502.
28. Goffinet DR, Glatstein E, Fuks Z, et al. Abdominal irradiation of non-Hodgkin's lymphomas. *Cancer* 1976, **37**: 2797–2806.

29. Fuks Z, Glatstein E, Kaplan HS. Patterns of presentation and relapse in the non-Hodgkin's lymphomata. *Br. J. Cancer* 1975, **31**(Suppl.II): 286–297.
30. Chen MG, Prosnitz LR, Gonzalez-Serva A, et al. Results of radiotherapy in control of stage I and II non-Hodgkin's lymphomas. *Cancer* 1979, **43**: 1245–1254.
31. Hagberg H, Glimelius B, Sundstrom C. Radiation therapy of non-Hodgkin's lymphoma stages I and II. *Acta Radiol. Oncol.* 1982, **21**: 145–150.
32. Lawrence TS, Urba WJ, Steinberg SM, et al. Retrospective analysis of stage I and II indolent lymphomas at the National Cancer Institute. *Int. J. Radiat. Oncol. Biol. Physics* 1988, **14**: 417–424.
33. Paryani SB, Hoppe RT, Cox RS, et al. Analysis of non-Hodgkin's lymphomas with nodular and favorable histologies, stages I and II. *Cancer* 1983, **52**: 2300–2307.
34. Kun LE, Cox JD, Komaki R. Patterns of failure in treatment of stage I and II diffuse malignant lymphoid tumors. *Radiology* 1981, **141**: 791–794.
35. Mauch P, Leonard R, Skarin A, et al. Improved survival following combined radiation therapy and chemotherapy for unfavorable prognosis stage I-II non-Hodgkin's lymphomas. *J. Clin. Oncol.* 1985, **3**(10): 1301–1308.
36. Sweet DL, Kinzie J, Gacke ME, et al. Survival of patients with localized diffuse histiocytic lymphoma. *Blood* 1981, **58**: 1218–1223.
37. Toonkel LM, Fuller LM, Gamble JF, et al. Laparotomy staged I and II non-Hodgkin's lymphomas: Preliminary results of radiotherapy and adjunctive chemotherapy. *Cancer* 1980, **45**: 249–260.
38. Anderson T, Bender RA, Fisher RI, et al. Combination chemotherapy in non-Hodgkin's lymphoma: Results of a long-term follow-up. *Cancer Treat. Rep.* 1977, **61**:1057–1066.
39. Friedman M, Pearlman AW, Turgeon L. Hodgkin's disease: Tumor lethal dose and iso-effect recovery curve. *Am. J. Roentgenol.* 1967, **99**: 843–850.
40. Scott RM, Brizel HE. Time-dose relationships in Hodgkin's disease. *Radiology* 1964, **52**: 1043–1049.
41. Seydel HG, Bloedorn FG, Wizenberg MJ. Time–dose–volume relationships in Hodgkin's disease. *Radiology* 1967, **89**: 919–922.
42. Cox JD, Koehl RH, Turner WM, et al. Irradiation in the local control of malignant lymphoreticular tumors (non-Hodgkin's malignant lymphoma). *Radiology* 1974, **112**: 179–185.
43. Vokes EE, Ultmann JE, Golomb HM, et al. Long-term survival of patients with localized diffuse histiocytic lymphoma. *J. Clin. Oncol.* 1985, **3**: 1309–1317.
44. Hallahan DE, Farah R, Vokes EE, et al. The patterns of failure in patients with pathological stage I and II diffuse histiocytic lymphoma treated with radiation therapy alone. *Int. J. Radiat. Oncol. Biol. Physics* 1989, **17**: 767–771.
45. McLaughlin P, Fuller LM, Velasquez WS, et al. Stage I–II follicular lymphoma. Treatment results for 76 patients. *Cancer* 1986, **58**: 1596–1602.
46. Monfardini S, Banfi A, Bonadonna G, et al. Improved 5-year survival after combined radiotherapy for stage I–II non-Hodgkin's lymphoma. *Int. J. Radiat. Oncol. Biol. Physics* 1980, **6**: 125–134.
47. Reddy S, Saxena VS, Pellettiere EV, et al. Early nodal and extra-nodal non-Hodgkin's lymphomas. *Cancer* 1977, **40**: 98–104.
48. Timothy AR, Lister TA, Katz D, et al. Localized non-Hodgkin's lymphoma. *Eur. J. Cancer* 1980, **16**: 799–807.
49. Peckham MJ, Guay JP, Hamlin ME, et al. Survival in localized nodal and extranodal non-Hodgkin's lymphoma. *Br. J. Cancer* 1975, **31**: 413–424.
50. Lester JN, Fuller LM, Conrad FG, et al. The role of staging laparotomy, chemotherapy, and radiotherapy in the management of localized diffuse large cell lymphoma. *Cancer* 1982, **49**: 1746–1753.
51. Levitt SH, Bloomfield CD, Frizzera G, et al. Curative radiotherapy for localized diffuse histiocytic lymphoma. *Cancer Treat. Rep.* 1980, **64**: 175–177.
52. Kaminski MS, Coleman CN, Colby TV, et al. Factors predicting survival in adults with stage I and II large-cell lymphoma treated with primary radiation therapy. *Ann. Intern. Med.* 1986, **104**: 747–756.
53. Nissen NI, Ersboll J, Hansen HS, et al. A randomized study of radiotherapy versus radiotherapy plus chemotherapy in stage I–II non-Hodgkin's lymphoma. *Cancer* 1983, **52**: 1–7.
54. Landberg TG, Hakansson LG, Moller TR, et al. CVP-remission-maintenance in stage I or II non-Hodgkin's lymphomas: Preliminary results of a randomized study. *Cancer* 1979, **44**: 831–838.
55. Cabanillas F, Bodey GP, Freireich EJ. Management with chemotherapy only of stage I and II malignant lymphoma of aggressive histologic types. *Cancer* 1980, **46**: 2356–2359.
56. Miller TP, Jones SE. Initial chemotherapy for clinically localized lymphomas of unfavorable histology. *Blood* 1983, **62**: 413–418.
57. Prestidge BR, Horning SJ, Hoppe RT. Combined modality therapy for stage I–II large cell lymphoma. *Int. J. Radiat. Oncol. Biol. Physics* 1988, **15**: 633–639.
58. Jones SE, Miller TP, Connors JM. Long-term follow-up and analysis for prognostic factors for patients with limited-stage diffuse large-cell lymphoma treated with initial chemotherapy with or without adjuvant radiotherapy. *J. Clin. Oncol.* 1989, **7**: 1186–1191.
59. Tondini C, Zanini M, Lombardi F, et al. Combined modality treatment with primary CHOP chemotherapy followed by locoregional irradiation in stage I or II histologically aggressive non-Hodgkin's lymphomas. *J. Clin. Oncol.* 1993, **11**: 720–725.
60. Longo DL, Glatstein E, Duffey PL, et al. Treatment of localized aggressive lymphomas with combination chemotherapy followed by involved-field radiation therapy. *J. Clin. Oncol.* 1989, **7**: 1295–1302.
61. Sullivan FJ, Hahn SM, Johnstone PA, et al. Radiation therapy in the National Cancer Institute combined modality trial of localized aggressive non-Hodgkin's lymphoma: What constitutes the involved field? (Submitted).
62. Glatstein E, Fuks Z, Goffinet RD, et al. Non-Hodgkin's lymphoma of stage III extent: Is total lymphoid irradiation appropriate treatment? *Cancer* 1976, **37**: 2806–2812.

63. Jacobs JP, Murray KJ, Schultz CJ, et al. Central lymphatic irradiation for stage III nodular lymphomas: Long-term results. *J. Clin. Oncol.* 1993, **11**: 233–238.

64. Horning SJ, Rosenberg SA. The natural history of initially untreated low-grade non-Hodgkin's lymphomas. *N. Engl. J. Med.* 1984, **311**: 1471–1475.

65. Portlock CS, Rosenberg SA. No initial therapy for stage III and IV non-Hodgkin's lymphomas of favorable histologic types. *Ann. Intern. Med.* 1979, **90**: 10–13.

66. Shipp MA, Klatt MW, Yeap B, et al. Patterns of relapse in large-cell lymphoma patients with bulk disease: Implications for the use of adjuvant radiation therapy. *J. Clin. Oncol.* 1989, **7** 613–618.

67. Shimm DS, Dosoretz DE, Anderson T, et al. Primary gastric lymphoma: An analysis with emphasis on prognostic factors and radiation therapy. *Cancer* 1983, **52**: 2044–2048.

68. Mittal B, Wasserman TH, Griffith RC. Non-Hodgkin's lymphoma of the stomach. *Am. J. Gastroenterol.* 1983, **78**: 781–787.

69. Shiu MH, Nisce LZ, Pinna A, et al. Recent results of multimodal therapy of gastric lymphoma. *Cancer* 1986, **58**: 1389–1399.

70. Ricci JL, Turnbull ADM. Spontaneous gastroduodenal perforation in cancer patients receiving cytotoxic therapy. *J. Surg. Oncol.* 1989, **41**: 219–221.

71. Maor MH, Velasquez WS, Fuller LM, et al. Stomach conservation in stages IE and IIE gastric non-Hodgkin's lymphoma. *J. Clin. Oncol.* 1990, **8**: 266–271.

72. DeAngelis LM, Yahalom J, Thaler HT, et al. Combined modality therapy for primary CNS lymphoma. *J. Clin. Oncol.* 1992, **10**: 635–643.

73. Neuwelt EA, Goldman DL, Dahlborg SA, et al. Primary CNS lymphoma treated with osmotic blood–brain barrier disruption: Prolonged survival and preservation of cognitive function. *J. Clin. Oncol.* 1992, **9**: 1580–1590.

74. Connors JM, Klimo P, Voss N, et al. Testicular lymphoma: Improved outcome with early brief chemotherapy. *J. Clin. Oncol.* 1988, **6**: 776–781.

75. Dunbar SF, Linggood RM, Doppke KP, et al. Conjunctival lymphoma: Results and treatment with a single anterior electron field. A lens sparing approach. *Int. J. Radiat. Oncol. Biol. Physics* 1990, **19**: 249–257.

76. Minehan KJ, Martenson JA, Garrity JA, et al. Local control and complications after radiation therapy for primary orbital lymphoma: A case for low-dose treatment. *Int. J. Radiat. Oncol. Biol. Physics* 1991, **20**: 791–796.

77. Vigliotti A, Kong JS, Fuller LM, et al. Thyroid lymphomas stages IE and IIE: Comparative results for radiotherapy only, combination chemotherapy only, and multimodality treatment. *Int. J. Radiat. Oncol. Biol. Physics* 1986, **12**: 1807–1812.

78. Blair TJ, Evans RG, Buskirk SJ, et al. Radiotherapeutic management of primary thyroid lymphoma. *Int. J. Radiat. Oncol. Biol. Physics* 1985, **11**: 365–370.

79. Logue JP, Hale RJ, Stewart AL, et al. Primary malignant lymphoma of the thyroid: A clinicopathological analysis. *Int. J. Radiat. Oncol. Biol. Physics* 1992, **22**: 929–933.

80. Tupchong L, Hughes F, Harmer CL. Primary lymphoma of the thyroid: Clinical features, prognostic factors, and results of treatment. *Int. J. Radiat. Oncol. Biol. Physics* 1986, **12**: 1813–1821.

81. Dosoretz DE, Raymond AK, Murphy GF, et al. Primary lymphoma of bone: The relationship of morphologic diversity to clinical behavior. *Cancer* 1982, **50**: 1009–1014.

82. Ostrowski ML, Unni KK, Banks PM, et al. Malignant lymphoma of bone. *Cancer* **58**: 2646–2655.

83. Mendenhall NP, Jones JJ, Kramer BS, et al. The management of primary lymphoma of bone. *Radiother. Oncol.* 1987, **9**: 137–145.

84. Clayton F, Butler JJ, Ayala AG, et al. Non-Hodgkin's lymphoma in bone: Pathologic and radiologic features with clinical correlates. *Cancer* 1987, **60**: 2494–2501.

85. Cox JD. Total central lymphatic irradiation for stage III nodular malignant lymphoreticular tumors. *Int. J. Radiat. Oncol. Biol. Physics* 1976, **1**: 491–496.

86. Young RC, Johnson RE, Cannellos GP, et al. Advanced lymphocytic lymphoma: Randomized comparisons of chemotherapy and radiotherapy, alone or in combination. *Cancer Treat. Rep.* 1977, **61**: 1153–1159.

87. Brereton HD, Young RC, Longo DL, et al. A comparison between combination chemotherapy and total body irradiation plus combination chemotherapy in non-Hodgkin's lymphoma. *Cancer* 1979, **43**: 2227–2231.

88. Chaffey JT, Hellman S. Rosenthal DS, et al. Total-body irradiation in the treatment of lymphoreticular lymphoma. *Cancer Treat. Rep.* 1977, **61**: 1149–1152.

89. Chaffey JT, Rosenthal DS, Moloney WC, et al. Total body irradiation as treatment for lymphosarcoma. *Int. J. Radiat. Oncol. Biol. Physics* 1976, **1**: 399–405.

90. Hoppe RT, Kushlan P, Kaplan HS, et al. The treatment of advanced stage favorable histology non-Hodgkin's lymphoma: A preliminary report of a randomized trial comparing single agent chemotherapy, combination chemotherapy, and whole body irradiation. *Blood* 1981, **58** (3): 592–598.

91. Thar TL, Million RR, Noyes WD. Total body irradiation in non-Hodgkin's lymphoma. *Int. J. Radiat. Oncol. Biol. Physics* 1979, **5**: 171–176.

92. Choi NC, Timothy AR, Kaufman SD, et al. Low dose fractionated whole body irradiation in the treatment of advanced non-Hodgkin's lymphoma. *Cancer* 1979, **43**: 1636–1642.

93. Glatstein E, Donaldson SS, Rosenberg SA, et al. Combined modality therapy in malignant lymphomas. *Cancer Treat. Rep.* 1977, **61**: 1199–1207.

94. Mendenhall NP, Noyes WD, Million RR. Total body irradiation for stage II–IV non-Hodgkin's lymphoma: Ten-year follow-up. *J. Clin. Oncol.* 1989, **7**: 67–74.

95. Lybeert MLM, Meerwaldt JH, Deneve W. Long-term results of low dose total body irradiation for advanced non-Hodgkin's lymphoma. *Int. J. Radiat. Oncol. Biol. Physics* 1987, **13**: 1167–1172.

96. Coia L, Krigel R, Hanks G, et al. A phase I study of WR-2721 in combination with total body irradiation (TBI) in patients with refractory lymphoid malignancies. *Int. J. Radiat. Oncol. Biol. Physics* 1992, **22**: 791–794.

CHAPTER 31

The role of surgery

JONATHAN J. LEWIS AND MURRAY F. BRENNAN

Introduction

The role of the surgeon in the management of the non-Hodgkin's lymphomas extends to both diagnosis and treatment. Surgery will frequently provide the tissue on which the pathologist will make a diagnosis. Thereafter, in consultation with medical and radiation oncologists, the most appropriate therapy can be chosen. The role of surgery as a primary therapeutic modality in abdominal non-Hodgkin's lymphoma other than in the context of a surgical emergency is an area of controversy. Evolution in our understanding of the biology of non-Hodgkin's lymphomas, together with improvements in chemotherapy and radiation therapy, have undoubtedly reduced the role of primary therapeutic surgery, but the surgeon is frequently called upon to evaluate and treat some of the complications of non-Hodgkin's lymphoma. Thus, surgery may still play a significant part in the management of these patients.

In this chapter we review the literature and outline the surgeon's role in the management of the non-Hodgkin's lymphomas, encompassing diagnostic procedures, surgical emergencies, and surgical resection and reduction of tumor bulk. We approach this on an anatomic basis.

Asymptomatic lymphadenopathy is the most frequent presentation for patients with non-Hodgkin's lymphoma. We discuss the principles and technique of lymph node biopsy to establish the diagnosis of lymphoma. Beyond a role in establishing a diagnosis, the principal area of involvement of the surgeon in non-Hodgkin's lymphoma is in the management of abdominal lymphomas, a topic that will constitute the majority of this chapter. In addition, we discuss the role of surgery in the management of specific gastrointestinal complications of non-Hodgkin's lymphomas *per se*, or of non-surgical primary treatment. We also include a brief discussion of some of the rarer sites of involvement of non-Hodgkin's lymphoma (thyroid, breast, salivary gland, testicle) which may lead to the patient presenting initially to the surgeon.

Principles of lymph node biopsy

Approximately 66% of patients with non-Hodgkin's lymphoma present with asymptomatic lymphadenopathy. The most common site of lymph node involvement is the cervical area (65–80%) with axillary (10–15%) and inguinal (6–12%) being much

Table 31.2 Five-year survival data for patients undergoing surgery and combined modality treatment for gastric lymphoma

Treatment	Year	N	Survival (%) Stage IE	Survival (%) stage IIE
Surgery alone				
Lim et al. [21]	1977	36	88	32
Herrmann et al. [2]	1980	10	60	40
Weingrad et al. [4]	1982	24	85	45
Paulson et al. [26]	1983	16	100	37
Maor et al. [27]	1984	12	67	40
MSKCC (unpublished)	1994	17	100 (N=14)	100 (IIE$_1$, N=3)
Surgery + RT				
Herrmann et al. [2]	1980	10	100	70
Shiu et al. [25]	1982	21	50	67
Weingrad et al. [4]	1982	32	83	62
Maor et al. [27]	1984	12	80	28
MSKCC (unpublished)	1994	4	100	100 (IIE$_1$)
Surgery + chemotherapy				
Weingrad et al. [4]	1982	10	100	70
Maor et al. [27]	1984	5	100	100
Sheridan et al. [45]	1985	14	100	75
Shiu et al. [46]	1986	4	100	50
MSKCC (unpublished)	1994	11	100	82 (IIE$_1$)
Surgery + RT + chemotherapy				
Maor et al. [27]	1984	13	60	62
Shiu et al. [46]	1986	4	50	50
MSKCC (unpublished)	1994	5	—	81 (IIE$_1$)
RT alone				
Weingrad et al. [4]	1982	9	85	—
Paulson et al. [26]	1983	3	—	0
Mittal et al. [47]	1983	10	67	55
Chemotherapy + RT				
Mittal et al. [47]	1983	10	100	75
Maor et al. [48]	1990	34	79	73

RT, Radiation therapy; MSKCC, Memorial Sloan–Kettering Cancer Center.

resection using a standard surgical pathology definition [10,11,21,24–26,31–36]. In a multivariate analysis of 106 patients, Azab et al. [31], for example, found surgical resection to be the most significant variable affecting prognosis, while Dragosics et al. [10] found that radical resection significantly increased 2-year survival. Similarly, Steward et al. [36] demonstrated that complete surgical resection is an independent favorable prognostic factor. Rosen et al. [24] observed a 5-year survival of 75% in patients in whom complete excision was performed compared to 32% with partial excision or biopsy and nonsurgical treatment. Of course, these results are dependent upon both the possibility of accomplishing complete resection (something which, at least in part, depends upon the individual surgeon) and the quality of the nonsurgical treatment administered.

Gastric lymphomas are frequently large or involve the stomach diffusely (Figure 31.1). Thus, subtotal and, occasionally, total gastrectomy are required to excise the tumor completely. When there is invasion into adjacent organs, including liver, pancreas, spleen and transverse colon, the entire tumor can sometimes be resected *en bloc*, although the advantage of performing such radical surgery is unclear. In deciding how much to resect, it is important to consider the site of the tumor, the patient's age, general medical condition and consequent surgical

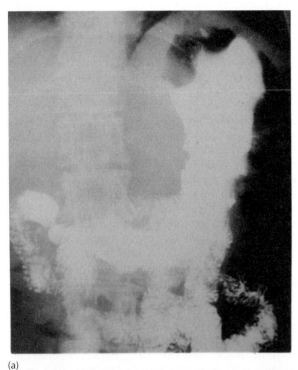

(a)

Figure 31.1 Upper GI barium study (a) and CT scan (b) of a patient with diffuse histiocytic lymphoma of the stomach. Gastric lymphomas may frequently be large or involve the stomach diffusely and near-total gastrectomy may be required for complete excision. Our practice is to avoid total and proximal-subtotal gastrectomy for this disease, and patients requiring this would be treated by primary nonsurgical therapy.

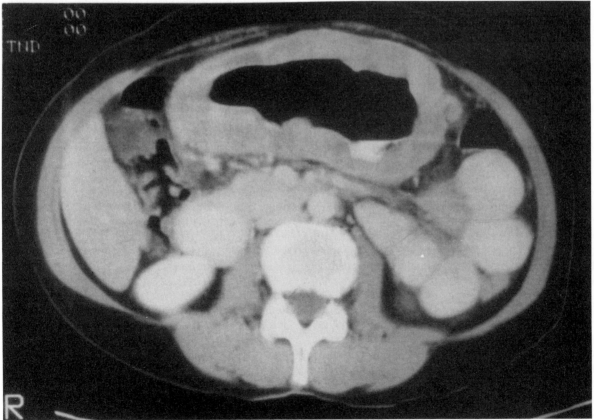

(b)

risk, as well as the potential local complications of leaving the tumor *in situ*. Although some benefit has been demonstrated for tumor-free margins [24,25], both univariate and multivariate analyses have demonstrated that patients with positive margins who receive postoperative radiation therapy have similar disease-free survival to those with complete resection [4,37]. Thus, in deciding how much to resect, it is also important to take into consideration the functional outcome and potential morbidity of the procedure. Distal subtotal gastrectomy, in appropriately selected patients, is generally very well tolerated. Proximal subtotal or total gastrectomy has a much greater incidence of 'postgastrectomy' sequelae, and adversely affects both nutritional status and quality of life. This may also be associated with poor compliance with aggressive postoperative chemotherapy, which in turn, may lead to a poor outcome [38].

Perigastric and periaortic lymph nodes should be sampled as part of the procedure, for operative staging. A thorough sampling of all abdominal nodes is not required, although any suspicious nodes should be biopsied. Similarly, involvement of the spleen or liver is usually grossly apparent so that routine splenectomy and liver biopsy are not necessary.

Because of the absence of comparative trials, it is difficult to rigorously compare survival rates with and without surgery. The operative mortality rate for elective subtotal or total gastrectomy is less than 5% for patients operated on in the decade 1980–1990 [14]. The treatment-related death for recent chemotherapy protocols for nodal non-Hodgkin's lymphoma ranges from 1% to 10% [39–41]. In addition, acute nonlymphocytic leukemia, carcinoma of the bladder, myelodysplastic syndrome and Hodgkin's disease may occur as dose-dependent treatment complications, although these late complications vary greatly with different treatment regimens [42–44].

While no definitive data are available, it appears that in some patients with stage IE disease, the addition of postoperative chemotherapy to surgery may further improve prognosis [4,27,45]. For stage IIE disease, prognosis is significantly improved by postoperative chemotherapy with or without radiation [2,4,25,27,45,46]. Until recently, the results of primary radiation therapy with or without primary chemotherapy have been believed to be the same as, or inferior to, surgery alone [4,47]. In contrast, recent data from the MD Anderson Cancer Center [48] suggests that primary surgery is not necessary and that favorable results (see Table 31.2) can be achieved by combining effective chemotherapy and local radiation.

Our approach to these patients is individualized. Once the diagnosis is established patients are staged by CT scan and endoscopic ultrasound. Patients with an equivocal diagnosis initially undergo either diagnostic laparoscopy or exploratory laparotomy. Patients who have a lesion in the distal stomach, have early-stage disease (IE and IIE$_1$) and are a good operative risk, are offered the option of exploratory laparotomy and distal gastrectomy. They are then staged both intraoperatively and by histopathologic evaluation. Patients with stage IE, low-grade and small (< 10 cm) lesions receive surgery alone. Patients with intermediate- or high-grade histology, receive, in addition, postoperative chemotherapy with or without radiation. Radiation is only given, in addition to chemotherapy, to patients with positive margins, unresectable disease or large (> 10 cm) lesions. The timing of adjuvant radiation or chemotherapy is important. Too great a delay will permit regrowth of tumor, while immediate adjuvant therapy is associated with impaired wound healing. There is no evidence that waiting more than 7 days after surgery is beneficial to wound healing and thus no reason (from this perspective) to wait longer. However, circumstances will dictate the management of individual patients and sometimes compromises must be made. We do not generally operate on patients with proximal lesions (necessitating near-total or total gastrectomy) or with late-stage disease (IIE$_2$, III and IV), unless they present with or develop a surgical complication.

PRESENTATION WITH AN ACUTE ABDOMEN: THE ROLE OF EMERGENCY SURGERY

Emergency surgical intervention may be required for patients who present with bleeding, perforation or obstruction. The prevalence of bleeding is 2–43% in the literature, with generally lower rates for perforation and obstruction (see Table 31.3) [49–51]. These data vary markedly from one series to another because of the different criteria used for reporting, nor do they indicate the proportion of patients who require operative intervention.

Patients presenting with upper gastrointestinal bleeding should be evaluated and managed in the standard manner. Thus, appropriate fluid resuscitation together with hemodynamic monitoring should be routinely initiated. The source of bleeding is confirmed with upper gastrointestinal endoscopy and, if possible, biopsies taken. Initial local endoscopic control using electrocoagulation or laser coagulation should be attempted. Endoscopic control of bleeding from a necrotic or ulcerated tumor will, however, usually be transient and surgical control of bleeding is frequently required.

Table 31.3   Prevalence of bleeding, perforation and obstruction at presentation in gastric lymphoma

Reference	N	Bleeding (%)	Perforation (%)	Obstruction (%)
Orlando et al. [54]	42	30	8	—
Paulson et al. [26]	37	16	—	3.0
Thorling [55]	48	25	—	2.0
Skudder et al. [49]	46	43	—	7.0
Gobbi et al. [12]	56	2.6	—	1.3
Shutze et al. [56]	35	33	—	40.0

The preoperative diagnosis of perforation is usually based on the clinical and radiologic findings. Perforation requires surgical intervention. These patients should receive preoperative resuscitation and appropriate antibiotic therapy. The etiology of perforation is commonly not made until the time of surgery, and the primary diagnosis may not be known preoperatively. In contrast, patients presenting with gastric outlet obstruction will frequently have a histopathologic diagnosis preoperatively. These patients also require careful fluid, electrolyte and nutritional correction prior to performing surgery.

In patients taken for emergency exploration, the diagnosis is confirmed and the disease staged. The choice of operation will be dictated by the patient's overall medical condition together with the stage of disease. In general, if the patient's condition and the tumor extent permits, subtotal gastrectomy is the optimal procedure in the emergency setting. It should be borne in mind that healing will be impaired by radiation and chemotherapy, but that significant delays in the initiation of adjuvant therapy may also permit tumor progression. Simple repair and patching of a perforation or ligation of bleeding vessels are performed if the tumor is unresectable or if the patient's overall poor medical condition precludes resectional surgery. Similarly, in gastric outlet obstruction, resection is preferred to bypass. Gastrectomy may afford a cure in early-stage disease and reduces the risk of bleeding and perforation during medical therapy.

COMPLICATIONS OF PRIMARY RADIATION AND CHEMOTHERAPY REQUIRING EMERGENCY SURGERY

Data on the prevalence of hemorrhage and perforation occurring during radiation and chemotherapy are provided in Table 31.4. Risk factors for the development of these complications have not been defined, although perforation probably occurs more

Table 31.4   Emergency surgery required during primary radiation or chemotherapy for gastric lymphoma

Complication	Year	N	Surgery (%)	Pre-existing therapy
Hemorrhage				
Fleming et al. [11]	1982	15	60	CHOP
Mittal et al. [47]	1983	9	0	RT
Economopolous et al. [53]	1985	9	11	CHOP
Sheridan et al. [45]	1985	5	20	CHOP
Burgers et al. [22]	1988	32	6	CHOP + RT
Maor et al. [48]	1990	34	0	Chemo + RT
Bozzetti et al. [52]	1991	52	0	Chemo + RT
Perforation				
Fleming et al. [11]	1982	15	0	CHOP
Mittal et al. [47]	1983	9	0	RT
Sheridan et al. [45]	1985	5	20	CHOP
Maor et al. [48]	1990	34	0	Chemo + RT
Bozzetti et al. [52]	1991	52	2	Chemo + RT

CHOP, Cyclophosphamide, doxorubicin, vincristine and prednisone; Chemo, chemotherapy; RT, radiation therapy.

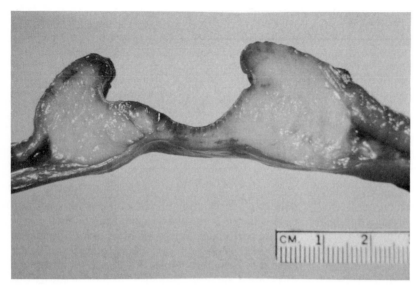

Figure 31.2 Gross pathology specimen of resected gastric lymphoma involving full thickness of the stomach wall. Perforation, as a complication of chemotherapy or radiation therapy, is more likely to occur when the entire thickness of the gastric wall is involved [52].

commonly when the entire thickness of the gastric wall is involved (Figure 32.2) [52]. Both hemorrhage and perforation may occur with chemotherapy or radiation alone, or in combination. Perforation, when it does occur, usually presents 7–10 days after administration of chemotherapy, and this may be after the first or subsequent cycles. The reported prevalence of some degree of hemorrhage is from 11% to 20%, although not all patients who bleed require operation [11,22,45,47,48,52–56]. Perforation has been reported to occur in 0–20% of patients (Figure 31.3) [11,45,47,48,52,55]. Several authors advocate primary surgery to obviate these risks [2,4,32,57]. This argument is in part the result of the substantial mortality associated with emergency operations performed on these patients – often 5–10-fold higher than in the elective setting [14]. In contrast, recent experience with stomach conservation, and combined primary chemotherapy and radiation therapy, by Maor et al. [48] at the MD Anderson Cancer Center suggests that, in their hands, the need for emergency surgery is extremely rare. In their series, no patient developed bleeding or perforation as a result of therapy. One patient required a subtotal gastrectomy for gastric outlet obstruction from a chronic benign cicatrizing ulcer in the antrum.

Patients presenting with complications during treatment require standard evaluation and treatment as outlined above. When these complications do occur, they often require surgical intervention. A thorough diagnostic evaluation is required, in particular for upper gastrointestinal bleeding, since bleeding is often related to causes other than the tumor itself. Hemorrhagic gastritis and peptic ulceration are the two most common causes of gastrointestinal bleeding in lymphoma patients [58]. In addi-

tion, Mallory–Weiss tears, esophageal varices and *Candida* esophagitis may be causal in patients treated with chemotherapy [59]. The presence of thrombocytopenia necessitates specific supportive measures, and if surgery can safely be delayed, it is better performed during or after recovery from neutropenia. The operative technique will depend on the patient's general condition and specific findings at surgery. In contrast to patients operated on electively or presenting *de novo* with a surgical complication, patients who subsequently develop complications are frequently seriously ill, and as already mentioned, have significant mortality associated with surgery.

Intestinal lymphoma

Lymphomas make up about 20% of primary small bowel tumors and 0.4% of primary colon tumors [11]. Virtually all of these are non-Hodgkin's lymphomas. Between 30% and 50% of these patients present with an abdominal emergency [60,61]. Preoperative diagnosis of intestinal lymphoma is rare and misdiagnoses include intestinal obstruction from other causes, appendicitis, diverticulitis and inflammatory bowel disease (Figure 31.4 and 31.5) [60]. A frequent presentation, particularly in children, is ileocolic intussusception.

Laparotomy, either emergency or elective, is performed as a diagnostic procedure in up to 80% of reported cases [62]. Any abdominal emergency, if present, needs to be surgically managed. Enough tissue must be obtained to establish an accurate

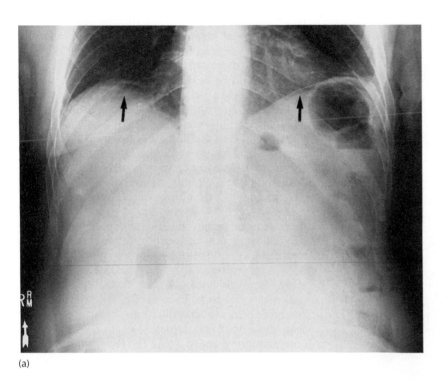

(a)

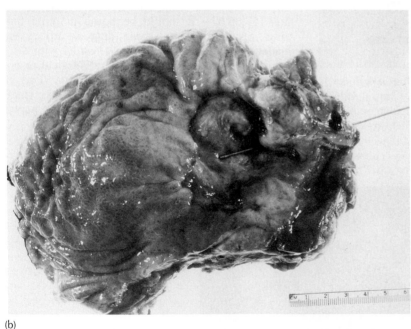

(b)

Figure 31.3 Chest X-ray (a) and resected stomach (b) of a patient with gastric lymphoma complicated by perforation subsequent to undergoing a second cycle of CHOP chemotherapy. The arrows illustrate free air under the diaphragm (a) and the site of perforation is marked by the probe (b). Perforation has been reported in 0–20% of patients undergoing primary nonsurgical therapy.

histopathologic diagnosis. The surgeon must carefully explore the entire abdomen and biopsy any suspicious lymph nodes or viscera for reliable staging, as this may be crucial to planning subsequent therapy.

Surgical resection of the tumor is mandated as part of the management of any intestinal surgical complication including obstruction, perforation or bleed-ing. In addition, resection plus chemotherapy may offer a survival advantage compared to chemotherapy alone [11,57,63–65], although this will vary with the efficacy of chemotherapy. Resection should leave bowel margins negative for tumor and include sufficient mesentery to encompass gross disease. Bowel continuity is re-established with an anastomosis except when resecting an unprepared colon,

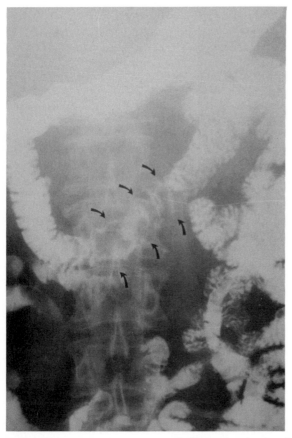

Figure 31.4 Upper GI contrast study illustrating duodenal changes consistent with inflammatory bowel disease, carcinoma or lymphoma. This patient had intestinal lymphoma involving the duodenum, confirmed at exploratory laparotomy.

when a temporary colostomy may be required.

The surgical management of extensive, unresectable tumors depends on the associated conditions. If there is obstruction, perforation or bleeding, the tumor should be biopsied and the abdomen staged. Bleeding should be controlled whenever possible and unresectable tumors that are obstructing or have caused perforation can be managed by exclusion and intestinal bypass. Radiopaque clips should be placed around the tumor to guide the radiation therapist, if subsequent radiation therapy is planned.

Despite the systemic nature of intestinal lymphoma and the development of effective chemotherapy, virtually every series reported to date demonstrates improved survival in patients in whom surgical resection is accomplished compared to treatment with the primary tumor in place [57,60,65, 66]. While resectability may reflect biology and stage, the experience has been that, stage for stage, patients with stage IE and IIE disease who are resected prior to combination therapy do better than those with incomplete resection followed by combination therapy [65,67]. In addition, complications of bleeding, perforation and obstruction have been reported as frequently as 25% of the time, in intestinal lymphoma treated without resection [57,66,67]. It should be borne in mind that these results may, to some degree, reflect the inadequacy of chemotherapy. As results with drug combinations improve, the value of surgical resection is likely to become less apparent. This is illustrated by a specific lymphoma subtype, small noncleaved cell lymphoma (see below and Chapter 37).

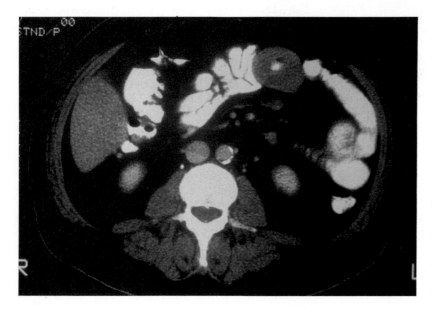

Figure 31.5 Small bowel tumor illustrated on CT scan. The differential diagnosis included adenocarcinoma, carcinoid tumor and lymphoma, with the diagnosis of lymphoma being made at exploratory laparotomy.

Childhood abdominal non-Hodgkin's lymphoma and abdominal Burkitt's lymphoma

Non-Hodgkin's lymphoma is the third most common childhood neoplasm and occurs in the abdomen in approximately 35% of cases [60,68]. The most common cell types in childhood abdominal non-Hodgkin's lymphoma are small noncleaved Burkitt's and small noncleaved non-Burkitt's [69]. The prognosis for childhood non-Hodgkin's lymphoma improved significantly with the advent of systemic therapy in the mid-1970s. In patients with primary presentation in the abdomen, the role of surgical debulking, in an era when only approximately one half of patients with extensive disease were curable with chemotherapy, was controversial. Magrath et al. supported aggressive operative debulking (> 90% tumor removal) prior to chemotherapy, after analysis of a large single institution series of patients with Burkitt's lymphoma from Uganda [64,70]. Kemeny et al. also suggested a survival advantage in patients with Burkitt's lymphoma undergoing complete resection, but noted that this may reflect the fact that less disease is more easily resected [65]. In contrast, others have cautioned against extensive initial surgery which may delay institution of systemic therapy [71–73].

In a multivariate analysis of patients with abdominal non-Hodgkin's lymphoma in the CCG-551 study (Childrens Cancer Study Group), LaQuaglia et al. attempted to define a rational surgical approach [74]. They found that these patients can be divided into two groups: those with localized disease, often involving bowel wall, and those with extensive disease including bulky mesenteric and retroperitoneal tumor. While it was noted that on univariate analysis complete excision favorably affects outcome, none of the patients with extensive disease underwent complete resection. When tumor burden was compared with resectability on multivariate analysis, only the extent of disease remained an independent predictor of event-free survival. Thus, resectability appeared to be biologically predetermined. Furthermore, in this series, attempts at complete resection in extensive disease were associated with significant postoperative complications.

Appropriate surgical management depends on the stage of the disease at presentation and has evolved as the results of chemotherapy have improved. Localized disease should be completely resected as this may affect a reduction in intensity and duration of chemotherapy without sacrificing survival [75].

This minimizes the early and late complications of curative therapy including growth failure, sterility, cardiomyopathy and second neoplasms. Bulky abdominal tumors, whether intestinal or extraintestinal in origin, are usually unresectable. While aggressive debulking has, in the past, been advocated prior to chemotherapy, it is only of any proven value in Burkitt's lymphoma, and even then, only in patients in whom resection can be readily accomplished [64,70]. Attempts at complete resection may result in significant postoperative complications, particularly when surgery is extensive. While hemorrhage and perforation may occur in Burkitt's lymphoma, these complications are relatively uncommon and do not constitute a sufficient problem to justify more frequent surgical intervention. Finally, since the results of treatment with chemotherapy alone have greatly improved, such that patients with extensive intra-abdominal tumor now have an excellent prognosis, a policy of aggressive debulking can no longer be advocated.

Primary lymphoma of the spleen

While the spleen is found to be involved in 50–80% of patients with non-Hodgkin's lymphoma at autopsy, splenomegaly is the presenting feature in less than 1% of cases [76–78]. This 'entity' is termed lymphoma with prominent splenic involvement (LPS). Associated involvement of abdominal lymph nodes, liver and bone marrow is frequent, and at least 75% of patients with LPS are cytopenic [79,80]. The role of the surgeon in this setting is to perform splenectomy, when indicated, to correct the hypersplenism and related cytopenia.

The response rate to splenectomy is excellent, and 82–96% of patients with LPS will reverse their cytopenia [79,81–84]. While there are no criteria predictive of response, it appears that patients who present with cytopenia at the time of diagnosis will have a good response [81]. Patients who respond with increased cell counts have prolonged survival, possibly because they are better able to tolerate aggressive chemotherapy [79]. In contrast, patients who fail to correct thrombocytopenia after splenectomy have a poorer prognosis. The advent of cytokine hematopoietic support of leukopenia during chemotherapy, with granulocyte colony-stimulating factor (G-CSF) and granulocyte–macrophage colony-stimulating factor (GM-CSF), may negate the necessity to perform splenectomy. There are, however, no data comparing their use with splenectomy.

34. List AF, Greer JP, Cousar JC, et al. Non-Hodgkin's lymphoma of the gastrointestinal tract: An analysis of clinical and pathological features affecting outcome. *J. Clin. Oncol.* 1988, **6**: 1125–1131.

35. Shepherd FA, Evans WK, Kutas G, et al. Chemotherapy following surgery for stages IE and IIE non-Hodgkin's lymphoma of the gastrointestinal tract. *J. Clin. Oncol.* 1988, **6**: 253–260.

36. Steward WP, Harris M, Wagstaff J, et al. A prospective study of the treatment of high-grade non-Hodgkin's lymphoma involving the gastrointestinal tract. *Eur. J. Cancer Clin. Oncol.* 1985, **21**: 1195–2001.

37. Shimm DS, Dosoretz DE, Anderson T, et al. Primary gastric lymphoma. An analysis with emphasis on prognostic factors and radiation therapy. *Cancer* 1983, **52**: 2044–2048.

38. ReMine SG. Abdominal lymphoma. Role of surgery. *Surg. Clin. North Am.* 1985, **65**: 301–313.

39. Coiffier B, Byron PA, Berger F, et al. Intensive and sequential combination chemotherapy for aggressive malignant lymphomas (protocol LNH-80). *J. Clin. Oncol.* 1986, **4**: 147–153.

40. Boyd DB, Coleman M, Papish SW, et al. COPBLAM III: Infusional combination chemotherapy for diffuse large-cell lymphoma. *J. Clin. Oncol.* 1988, **6**: 425–433.

41. Steinke B, Bross K, Reinhold H, et al. Cyclic alternating chemotherapy of high-grade malignant non-Hodgkin's lymphoma with VIM-Bleo and CHOP. *Eur. J. Cancer* 1992, **28**: 100–104.

42. Pedersen-Bjergaard J, Ersboll J, Sorensen HM, et al. Risk of acute non-lymphocytic leukemia and preleukemia in patients treated with cyclophosphamide for non-Hodgkin's lymphoma. *Ann. Intern Med.* 1985, **103**: 195–200.

43. Pedersen-Bjergaard J, Ersboll J, Hansen VL, et al. Carcinoma of the urinary bladder after treatment with cyclophosphamide for non-Hodgkin's lymphoma. *N. Engl. J. Med.* 1988, **318**: 1028–1032.

44. Carrato A, Filippa D, Koziner B. Hodgkin's disease after treatment of non-Hodgkin's lymphoma. *Cancer* 1987, **60**: 887–896.

45. Sheridan WP, Medley G, Brodie GN. Non-Hodgkin's lymphoma of the stomach: A prospective pilot study of surgery plus chemotherapy in early and advanced disease. *J. Clin. Oncol.* 1985, **3**: 495–500.

46. Shiu MH, Nisce LZ, Pinna A, et al. Recent results of multimodal therapy of gastric lymphoma. *Cancer* 1986, **58**: 1389–1399.

47. Mittal B, Wasserman TH, Griffith RC. Non-Hodgkin's lymphoma of the stomach. *Am. J. Gastroenterol.* 1983, **78**: 780–787.

48. Maor MH, Velasquez WS, Fuller LM, et al. Stomach conservation in stages IE and IIE gastric non-Hodgkin's lymphoma. *J. Clin. Oncol.* 1990, **8**: 266–271.

49. Skudder PA Jr, Schwartz SI. Primary lymphoma of the gastrointestinal tract. *Surg. Gynecol. Obstet.* 1985, **160**: 5–8.

50. Bailey RL, Laws HL. Lymphoma of the stomach. *Am. Surg.* 1989, **55**: 665–668.

51. Solidoro A, Payet C, Sanchez-Lihon J, et al. Gastric lymphomas: Chemotherapy as a primary treatment. *Semin. Surg. Oncol.* 1990, **6**: 218–225.

52. Bozzetti F, Audisio RA, Fissi S, et al. Ruolo della chirurgia nel trattamento del linfoma gastrico primitivo. *Argomenti Oncol.* 1991, **12**: 413–422.

53. Economopoulos T, Alexopoulos C, Stathakis N, et al. Primary gastric lymphoma – the experience of a general hospital. *Br. J. Cancer* 1985, **52**: 391–397.

54. Orlando R, Pastuszak W, Preissler PL, et al. Gastric lymphoma: A clinicopathologic reappraisal. *Am. J. Surg.* 1982, **143**: 450–455.

55. Thorling K. Gastric lymphomas. Clinical features, treatment and prognosis. *Acta Radiol. Oncol.* 1984, **23**: 193–197.

56. Shutze WP, Halpern NB. Gastric lymphoma. *Surg. Gynecol. Obstet.* 1991, **172**: 33–38.

57. Bellesi G, Alterini R, Messori A, et al. Combined surgery and chemotherapy for the treatment of primary gastrointestinal intermediate- or high-grade non-Hodgkin's lymphomas. *Br. J. Cancer* 1989, **60**: 244–248.

58. Lightdale CJ, Kurtz RC, Boyle CC, et al. *Cancer* and upper gastrointestinal tract hemorrhage. *JAMA* 1973, **226**: 139–144.

59. Kemeny MM, Brennan MF. The surgical complications of chemotherapy in the cancer patient. *Curr. Prob. Surg.* 1987, **24**: 607–614.

60. Fleming ID, Turk PS, Murphy SB, et al. Surgical implications of primary gastrointestinal lymphoma of childhood. *Arch. Surg.* 1990, **125**: 252–256.

61. Freeman C, Berg J, Culter S. Occurrence and prognosis of extra-nodal lymphomas. *Cancer* 1972, **29**: 252–257.

62. Fleming ID. Primary malignant lymphoma of the intestinal tract. *Surg. Oncol. Clin. North Am.* 1993, **2**: 233–242.

63. Baildam AD, Williams GT, Schofield PF. Abdominal lymphoma – the place for surgery. *J. R. Soc. Med.* 1989, **82**: 657–660.

64. Magrath IT, Lwanga S, Carswell W, et al. Surgical reduction of tumor bulk in management of abdominal Burkitt's lymphoma. *Br. Med. J.* 1974, **2**: 308–312.

65. Kemeny MM, Magrath IT, Brennan MF. The role of surgery in the management of American Burkitt's lymphoma and its treatment. *Ann. Surg.* 1982, **196**: 82–86.

66. Salles G, Herbrecht R, Tilly H, et al. Aggressive primary gastrointestinal lymphomas: Review of 91 patients treated with the LNH-84 regimen. A study of the Groupe d'Etude des Lymphomes Agressifs. *Am. J. Med.* 1991, **90**: 77–84.

67. Rackner VL, Thirlby RC, Ryan JA Jr. Role of surgery in multimodality therapy for gastrointestinal lymphoma. *Am. J. Surg.* 1991, **161**: 570–575.

68. Murphy SB. Management of childhood non-Hodgkin's lymphoma. *Cancer Treat. Rep.* 1977, **61**: 1161–1173.

69. Murphy SB, Fairclough DL, Hutchinson RE, et al. Non-Hodgkin's lymphomas of childhood: An analysis of the histology, staging, and response to treatment of 338 cases at a single institution. *J. Clin. Oncol.* 1989, **7**: 186–193.

70. Janus C, Edwards BK, Sariban E, et al. Surgical resection and limited chemotherapy for abdominal undifferentiated lymphomas. *Cancer Treat. Rep.* 1984, **68**: 599–605.

71. Kaufman BH, Burgert EO Jr, Banks PM. Abdominal Burkitt's lymphoma: Role of early aggressive surgery. *J. Pediatr. Surg.* 1987, **22**: 671–674.

72. Zea JM, Exelby PR, Wollner N. Abdominal non-Hodgkin's lymphoma in childhood. *J. Pediatr. Surg.* 1976, **11**: 363–369.

73. Hoppe RT. The non-Hodgkin's lymphomas: Pathology, staging, treatment. *Curr. Prob. Cancer* 1987, **11**: 359–447.

74. LaQuaglia MP, Stolar CJ, Krailo M, et al. The role of surgery in abdominal non-Hodgkin's lymphoma: Experience from the Childrens Cancer Study Group. *J. Pediatr. Surg.* 1992, **27**: 230–235.

75. Murphy SB, Hustu HO, Rivera G, et al. End results of treating children with localized non-Hodgkin's lymphomas with a combined modality approach of lessened intensity. *J. Clin. Oncol.* 1983, **1**: 326–330.

76. Strauss DJ, Filippa DA, Lieberman PH. The non-Hodgkin's lymphomas: A retrospective clinical and pathological analysis of 499 cases diagnosed between 1958 and 1969. *Cancer* 1983, **51**: 101–109.

77. Risdall R, Hoppe RT, Warnke R. Non-Hodgkin's lymphoma: A study of the evolution of the disease based upon 92 autopsied cases. *Cancer* 1979, **44**: 529–542.

78. Ahmann DL, Kiely JM, Harrison EG. Malignant lymphoma of the spleen: A review of 49 cases in which the diagnosis was made at splenectomy. *Cancer* 1966, **19**: 461–469.

79. Kehoe J, Strauss DJ. Primary lymphoma of the spleen: Clinical features and outcome after splenectomy. *Cancer* 1988, **62**: 1433–1438.

80. Spier CM, Kjeldsberg CR, Eyre HJ, et al. Malignant lymphoma with primary presentation in the spleen: A study of 20 patients. *Arch. Pathol. Lab. Med.* 1985, **109**: 1076–1080.

81. Morel P, Dupriez B, Gosselin B, et al. Role of early splenectomy in malignant lymphomas with prominent splenic involvement (primary lymphomas of the spleen). A study of 59 cases. *Cancer* 1993, **71**: 207–215.

82. Kehoe JE, Daly JM, Straus DJ, et al. Value of splenectomy in non-Hodgkin's lymphoma. *Cancer* 1985, **55**: 1256–1264.

83. Delpero JR, Houvenaeghel G, Gastaut JA, et al. Splenectomy for hypersplenism in chronic lymphocytic leukemia and malignant non-Hodgkin's lymphoma. *Br. J. Surg.* 1990, **77**: 443–449.

84. Gill PG, Souter RG, Morris PJ. Splenectomy for hypersplenism in malignant lymphomas. *Br. J. Surg.* 1981, **68**: 29–33.

85. Vlasveld LT, Zwaan FE, Fibbe WE. Neutropenic enterocolitis following treatment with cytosine arabinoside regimens for hematological malignancies. A potentiating role for amsacrine. *Ann. Hematol.* 1991, **62**: 129–134.

86. Alt B, Glass NR, Sollinger H. Neutropenic enterocolitis in adults. Review of the literature and assessment of surgical intervention. *Am. J. Surg.* 1985, **149**: 405–408.

87. Starnes HF, Moore FD, Mentzer S, et al. Abdominal pain in neutropenic cancer patients. *Cancer* 1985, **57**: 616–622.

88. Haddad GK, Gradsinsky C, Allen H. The spectrum of radiation enteritis: Surgical considerations. *Dis. Colon. Rectum* 1983, **26**: 590–596.

89. Swan RW, Fowler WC, Boronow RC. Surgical management of radiation injury to the small intestine. *Surg. Gynecol. Obstet.* 1976, **43**: 325–331.

90. Heimann R, Vannineuse A, DeSloover C, et al. Malignant lymphoma and undifferentiated small cell carcinoma of the thyroid; a clinicopathological review in light of the Kiel classification for malignant lymphomas. *Histopathology* 1978, **2**: 201–211.

91. Tupchong L, Hughes F, Harmer CL. Primary lymphomas of the thyroid: Clinical features, prognostic factors and results of treatment. *Int. J. Radiat. Oncol. Biol. Phys.* 1986, **12**: 1813–1820.

92. Vigliotti A, Kong JS, Fulle LM, et al. Thyroid lymphomas stages IE and IIE: Comparative results for radiotherapy only, combination chemotherapy only, and multi-modality treatment. *Int. J. Radiat. Oncol. Biol. Phys.* 1986, **12**: 1807–1812.

93. Doria R, Jekel JF, Cooper DL. Thyroid lymphoma. *Cancer* 1994, **73**: 200–206.

94. Lamovec J, Jancar J. Primary malignant lymphomas of the breast. *Cancer* 1987, **60**: 3033–3036.

95. Brustein S, Kimmel M, Lieberman PH, et al. Malignant lymphoma of the breast: A study of 53 patients. *Am. Surg.* 1987, **205**: 144–150.

96. Eby NL, Grufferman S, Flannelly CM, et al. Increasing incidence of primary brain lymphoma in the US. *Cancer* 1988, **62**: 2461–2465.

97. McLaughlin P, Velasquez WS, Redman JR, et al. Chemotherapy with dexamethasone, high-dose cytarabine, and cisplatin for parenchymal brain lymphoma. *J. Natl Cancer Inst.* 1988, **80**: 1408–1412.

98. Kawakami Y, Tabuchi K, Ohnishi R, et al. Primary central nervous system lymphoma. *J. Neurosurg.* 1985, **62**: 522–527.

CHAPTER 32

Biological response modifiers

LARRY W. KWAK AND DAN L. LONGO

Introduction

The probability that biologic agents work by mechanisms entirely different from chemotherapeutic agents makes them very attractive for potential combination with other forms of therapy. In principle, biologic agents would be optimally used when the host immune system is minimally compromised, either early in the course of a disease, and/or in the setting of minimal residual disease achieved by cytotoxic agents. Unfortunately, as is evident by their nonillustrious 20-year track record in cancer therapy, biologic therapies have failed to fulfill their enormous theoretical promise. Indeed, in 1994 there is no biologic therapy that has a role in the primary treatment of any non-Hodgkin's lymphoma. Nevertheless, novel biologic therapies are being developed which are just now beginning to bring the above principles to reality. In this chapter we will provide a review of the field from a historical perspective and highlight some of the newer biologic agents that hold promise for eventual introduction into the primary treatment of lymphoma.

The history of biological therapy can be divided into two eras. Prior to 1975, the available tools were crude mixtures and extracts of a variety of substances, mainly bacteria or bacterial products, reflecting the relative state of unsophistication of the field

at that time. However, with the advent of hybridoma technology and recombinant DNA techniques introduced in the mid-1970s, the spectrum of what is possible in biologic therapy has been greatly expanded.

Many studies of nonspecific immune stimulation were conducted in patients with lymphoma during the initial era. Yet the considerable number of clinical trials undertaken with *Corynebacterium parvum*, bacille Calmette–Guérin (BCG) and levamisole, including well-designed prospective randomized studies, have failed to demonstrate positive effects of these agents on complete remission rates or remission durations [1–3]. The Southwest Oncology Group Study 7426 remains the only trial suggesting that the addition of BCG to chemotherapy as induction therapy may improve the complete response rate in patients with follicular or diffuse large-cell lymphoma, and the overall survival of patients with indolent histologies [4]. In this study, patients with advanced-stage lymphoma were randomized to receive COP–bleo (cyclophosphamide, vincristine, prednisone, bleomycin), CHOP–bleo (COP–bleo + doxorubicin), or CHOP–BCG, with BCG given by scarification on days 8 and 15 of each 21-day cycle. For the entire group of patients there were no significant differences in complete response rate or remission duration between CHOP–bleo and CHOP–BCG; however, the subgroup of follicular and diffuse large-cell lymphoma patients had a significantly higher complete response rate to CHOP–BCG (68%) than to CHOP–bleo (48%). This subgroup of CHOP-BCG-treated patients with follicular or diffuse large-cell lymphoma were also observed to have a significant survival advantage over those treated with CHOP–bleo. Patients with indolent lymphomas also had a significant survival advantage ($P = 0.05$) but in the absence of significant differences in complete response rate or remission duration. It is difficult to interpret prolongation of survival in the absence of any impact on response rate or duration.

The use of nonspecific stimulants to maintain chemotherapy-induced complete responses has been equally disappointing [3,5,6]. The only positive study was that reported by the Fondation Bergonie, an update of which recently appeared [6]. These investigators reported on the long-term follow-up of 43 patients with non-Hodgkin's lymphomas of all stages and histologies who received one of three different induction chemotherapy regimens, and were then randomized to receive BCG maintenance therapy or no further therapy. Patients received BCG weekly by scarification for 3 years. Nine out of 21 BCG-treated patients relapsed, compared with 15 of 22 control patients ($P = 0.03$). Seven BCG-treated patients have died compared with 11 control patients. It is difficult to draw conclusions from this small study because it includes so few patients of any particular histological subtype. However, it appears that nearly all of the benefits from BCG (if any) were in aggressive histology patients with localized disease, a group in which modern therapy would be expected to cure 85–90% of patients.

Since the vast majority of patients with indolent lymphoma can be expected to relapse, this group is a reasonable one in which to test the value of maintenance therapy. However, single or multiagent chemotherapy programs, and levamisole or BCG immunotherapy have all failed to improve disease-free survival in this disease setting. Thus, the weight of evidence does not provide a compelling reason to recommend further study of nonspecific immune stimulants in combination with modern third-generation chemotherapeutic regimens, either as induction or as maintenance therapy, in the management of any histologic subset of lymphoma.

Interferons

The biology of the interferons and the application of interferon therapy to the lymphomas have been extensively reviewed [7–9]. Interferon has little significant antitumor activity in lymphomas of aggressive histology. However, there has been considerable effort to evaluate the role of interferon in the treatment of indolent lymphomas and cutaneous T-cell lymphomas. Three preparations of interferon-α (lymphoblastoid, α2a, α2b) have been used at doses ranging from 1 million units (MU) daily to 50 MU/m^2 three times weekly. In general, the highest response rates have been reported at the highest doses. Foon and colleagues [10] reported 13 responses (four complete, nine partial) among 24 patients treated with 50 MU/m^2 interferon-α2a intramuscularly (IM) three times a week. However, the responses were short-lived once therapy was stopped and were maintained only by continuing therapy at doses that were too toxic to continue indefinitely. Mantovani and colleagues [11] reported a 52% response rate using six MU/m^2 interferon-α2a three times a week, a dose nearly ten-fold lower than that reported by Foon and colleagues. At the National Cancer Instutute (NCI), we performed a small prospective randomized trial to evaluate the dose dependency of the response rate of indolent lymphoma patients treated with interferon [12]. Patients received either 3 MU interferon-α2a daily or 50 MU/m^2 twice weekly. Patients randomized to the low-dose arm could receive the high-dose therapy if they did not respond within the first 3 months. Only 5 out of 19 (26%) patients treated with low-dose interferon responded, and all were partial responses lasting a median of only 3 months. Eight patients who did not respond within 3 months had their doses escalated. None of these responded. Seven of 20 (35%) patients treated on the high-dose arm responded. Two patients had complete responses. Of the 20 patients randomized to the high-dose therapy, 17 (85%) required at least one dose reduction and seven required two dose reductions. Of the ten patients who were able to receive the high-dose therapy for at least 2 months without dose reduction, six responded. Unfortunately, the majority of patients required dose reductions before the time at which responses were most often seen. However, the responses were generally of greater magnitude and more prolonged duration on the high-dose arm.

Thus, up to one-half of the patients with indolent lymphoma treated with interferon respond for a few months. The duration of the response is short if therapy is discontinued, although patients responding initially often respond to subsequent retreatment courses. The major problem, though, remains that the toxicity of this therapy is greater than most patients can tolerate. Virtually all patients treated with any of the interferon preparations experience acute toxicities consisting of fever, chills, myalgia and headache. Tachyphylaxis to these acute toxicities commonly occurs. However, chronic toxicities of fatigue and anorexia generally appear after about 2 weeks of therapy and persist as long as interferon is administered. These are the usual dose-limiting toxicities. A minority of patients may suffer serious central nervous system, cardiac, hepatic or hematopoietic toxicity.

Several studies aimed at adding interferon to chemotherapy in indolent lymphoma patients have been reported or are in progress. Although the addition of interferon-α to chemotherapy probably does not improve complete response rates [13,14], there may be a role for interferon as maintenance therapy in the treatment of low-grade lymphoma. For example, Smalley et al. [15] reported on an Eastern Cooperative Oncology Group randomized trial of patients with advanced low-grade non-Hodgkin's lymphoma treated either with COPA (cyclophosphamide, vincristine, prednisone and doxorubicin) or COPA combined with interferon-α2a administered at a dose of 6 MU/m^2 i.m. on days 22–26 of each 28-day cycle. All patients received 8–10 cycles of treatment. The patients enrolled in this study were selected for poor prognostic clinical factors and were eligible only if they had either B symptoms or signs of 'aggressive disease'. Approximately 30% of the patients also had diffuse small cleaved cell or follicular large-cell histologies, formally classified as intermediate-grade lymphomas in the Working Formulation. One hundred and twenty-seven patients were enrolled on the COPA arm and 122 patients on the interferon–COPA arm, and both regimens produced comparable complete response rates of 29% and 32%, respectively. However, among those patients achieving a complete response, the median disease-free survival for the interferon–COPA group was superior (median not reached) compared with the COPA group (median 1.7 years). Interestingly, with a median follow-up 3.2 years, there was a significant advantage in overall survival for the interferon–COPA group, with 2-year survival figures of 87% for interferon-COPA and 79% for COPA. In addition, interferon treatment emerged as an independent predictor of survival when tested with other known prognostic factors. Hiddemann et al. [16] reported on a phase II study of 19 patients with relapsed advanced-stage low-grade non-Hodgkin's lymphoma who had received prednimustine and mitoxantrone in combination followed by interferon-α2b, 5 MU subcutaneously three times weekly as maintenance therapy. Thirteen of the 19 patients achieved a complete (four patients) or partial (nine patients) remission and were eligible for maintenance therapy. With a very limited median remission duration of 14.5 months, there was a tendency toward superior survival without progression when compared with unmaintained historical controls.

There are several ongoing multicenter randomized trials comparing initial chemotherapy with initial chemotherapy plus interferon-α maintenance therapy in previously untreated patients. Chisesi et al., on behalf of the Italian Non-Hodgkin's Lymphoma Cooperative Study Group [17], published an interim report of a prospective randomized study comparing chlorambucil alone to a combined schedule of chlorambucil and interferon induction. Seventy patients with low-grade non-Hodgkin's lymphoma enrolled on this study received either chlorambucil 10 mg per day on days 1–21 or chlorambucil 5 mg per day on days 1–21 plus interferon-α2b (5 MU/m^2 subcutaneously three times per week) on days 1–21 of each 28-day cycle. Among 63 evaluable patients, similar response rates of 62.1% and 64.7%, respectively, were observed for each treatment arm. Then, of particular interest, patients who achieved a complete or partial remission were again randomized to receive interferon maintenance therapy (2 MU/m^2 3 weeks per month for 6 months) or to no further therapy. At this early timepoint, there is a suggestion that maintenance therapy with α-interferon is associated with superior disease-free survival, with 2-year actuarial disease-free survival rates of 70% for those receiving interferon maintenance therapy and 55% for those receiving no maintenance therapy. Preliminary results are also available from another multicenter study in which patients are initially randomized to receive chlorambucil alone or chlorambucil with interferon-α, and those achieving an excellent response to induction therapy are randomized a second time to receive interferon-α or no maintenance therapy [18]. With a median follow-up of 32 months, the group randomized to receive interferon-α as part of induction and maintenance has the best disease-free survival (80% at 3 years). There are no survival differences among the treatment arms as yet.

Solal-Celigny and colleagues in the Groupe d'Etude des Lymphomes de l'Adulte [19] reported their results using CHVP (cyclophosphamide, doxorubicin, teniposide and prednisone) given for six monthly cycles followed by six bimonthly cycles followed by randomization to receive maintenance interferon-α2b or no further therapy. Patients receiving interferon maintenance had a significantly higher overall response rate, a longer median event-free survival (34 months versus 19 months) and a higher 3-year survival rate (86% versus 69%).

In general, patients whose remissions are maintained with chronic interferon therapy relapse within about a year of discontinuing the treatment. Thus, the data are most consistent with a role for interferon in suppressing the growth of subclinical disease. Whether this effect will be found to be sufficiently valuable, in terms of symptomatic relief and survival, to counterbalance the chronic fatigue and malaise that usually accompanies chronic interferon therapy will require longer periods of follow-up to ascertain. However, there is no hint that the addition of interferon produces long-term disease-free survival off therapy. It is of interest, however, that anecdotal evidence suggests that the rate of histologic progression to aggressive-histology lymphoma may be decreased by chronic interferon treatment. Clearly the large numbers of patients who have received interferon maintenance therapy will be a useful group in whom to examine this important question more closely.

Interferon has also produced responses in most patients with cutaneous T-cell lymphoma. Bunn and colleagues [20] reported two complete and seven partial responses among 20 previously treated patients receiving 50 MU/m^2 interferon-α2a i.m. three times weekly. Covelli and colleagues [21] reported even higher response rates in previously untreated patients. In an effort to preserve the high response rate but diminish toxicity, Kohn and colleagues [22] treated 24 patients with advanced refractory disease with 10 MU/m^2 interferon-α2a IM on day 1 followed by 50 MU/m^2 on days 2–5 every 3 weeks. One complete and six partial responses were observed (29% response rate) and toxicity was reduced as compared with the thrice-weekly schedule. Papa et al. [23] demonstrated that recombinant interferon-α was very effective as a single agent for early stage disease. They treated 28 previously untreated patients with escalating doses of interferon-α and observed an overall response rate of 79% (36% complete responses, 43% partial responses), with an estimated event-free survival of 40%.

More recently, several investigators have also reported pilot studies of interferon-α in combination with retinoids to treat patients with cutaneous T-cell lymphoma with equally encouraging results [24,25]. Finally, a remarkable pilot study suggests that the dose of interferon may be reduced when it is combined with phototherapy for cutaneous lymphoma. Kuzel and colleagues [26] reported 12 complete and two partial responses in 15 patients treated with 6–30 MU/m^2 interferon-α2a i.m. three times weekly, together with psoralen and ultraviolet light. The median response duration exceeded 13 months. Fevers and malaise were encountered in more than 90% of patients. However, refinements of this treatment approach hold enormous promise in the management of this difficult clinical problem.

There is considerably less experience using interferon-α and interferon-β in lymphoma patients. Interferon-β is highly likely to be similar to interferon-α in its activities. Interferon-γ is more potent in its effects on the immune system and it is more

difficult to predict its efficacy when tested at the optimal biological dose. One pilot study of interferon-γ reported a 31% partial response rate in cutaneous T-cell lymphoma [27].

Interleukin-2

Disappointing results have been observed with interleukin-2 (IL-2) therapy in patients with either Hodgkin's or non-Hodgkin's lymphoma. IL-2 was administered at a dose of 3 MU/m^2 per day as a continuous infusion for 5 days by Lim and colleagues in a phase II trial of seven patients [28]. The best response observed was stable disease in two patients. The Surgery Branch of the National Cancer Institute reported on its experience of 19 patients with low- or intermediate-grade lymphomas treated with bolus high-dose IL-2 alone (11 patients) or IL-2 with lymphokine activated killer (LAK) cells (eight patients) [29]. IL-2 was administered by intravenous bolus infusion at 120 000 Cetus units per kilogram every 8 hours. Only one complete response was observed, although three partial responses were documented and all four responses were observed in patients with follicular histologies who had received LAK cells. Bernstein and colleagues [30] treated 19 patients with non-Hodgkin's lymphoma or Hodgkin's disease with combination IL-2 plus LAK cells and administered the IL-2 as a 24-hour continuous intravenous infusion (three million units/m^2 per day). They observed no complete responses and only two partial remissions. Duggan et al. [31] for the Cancer and Leukemia Group B reported on a randomized phase II trial of IL-2 with or without interferon-β in 49 patients with relapsed or refractory non-Hodgkin's lymphoma. They observed severe toxicity, with three treatment-related deaths and 17 additional patients experiencing life-threatening toxicity. Responses were noted in only seven patients overall (17%). No significant differences were observed between the two treatment arms in toxicity profile or response rate, or in modulation of *in vivo* natural killer or LAK activity. The authors concluded that IL-2 (with or without interferon-β) is not effective therapy for non-Hodgkin's lymphoma. Certainly, the single-agent response rate of IL-2 appears to be lower than what one would expect to see with chemotherapy in the same patients.

Monoclonal antibody therapy

The use of monoclonal antibodies in the treatment of hematologic malignancies continues to be an area of intense investigation. It was recently reviewed by Grossbard et al. [32]. The first trial of monoclonal antibody therapy using an antibody to a lymphoma-associated antigen (Ab 89) was reported by Nadler and his colleagues in 1980 [33]. Reports of the use of monoclonal antibodies directed against the CD5 antigen soon followed [34,35], and these reports demonstrated that antibodies could produce transient antitumor responses in patients with cutaneous T-cell lymphoma, and less impressive responses in CLL. In these early studies, a number of observations were made that are still valid today. Firstly, large quantities (up to 1500 mg) of mouse immunoglobulin can be infused into patients repeatedly if the infusion is slow (one hour or longer). Secondly, a rapid drop in circulating cells that bear the target antigen can be observed after a single antibody injection, but the response usually lasts only for a few hours. When antibody is infused every 3–4 days over several weeks, a sustained decrement may be achieved. Thirdly, cells coated with antibody are not always removed by the immune system. For example, cells coated with antibody may be found in the marrow for a prolonged period after the infusion. Fourthly, over time, tumor cells may become refractory to further treatment by modulating the target antigen from the surface of the tumor. Finally, other mechanisms by which patients become refractory to antibody therapy are the development of antimouse antibodies and the blocking of the antibody by circulating target antigen.

There is little evidence that the mouse antibodies that have been used have acted by complement-mediated lysis mechanisms. There are four major classes of mechanisms by which monoclonal antibodies are more likely to kill tumor cells: (1) by activating host immune effector mechanisms (e.g., antibody-dependent cellular cytotoxicity); (2) by triggering or interfering with the function of physiologically important receptors; (3) by targeting biologically active moieties to tumor cells (e.g., toxins, isotopes, drugs, cytokines); and (4) by eliciting an antitumor response indirectly by inducing autoantibodies or by activating cellular responses to the tumor antigen (i.e., antibody functioning as a biologic response modifier).

Patients with B-cell lymphoma have been treated with murine or rat monoclonal antibodies directed against the idiotype of the surface immunoglobulin [36–39], a panlymphoid cell antigen (CAMPATH) [40], CD20 [41] and the Epstein–Barr virus receptor [42]. With the exception of the first patient treated with anti-idiotype antibody, only a minority of patients treated with 'naked' antibody have experienced tumor regressions that meet criteria for complete responses and such responses are generally short lived. The major obstacles limiting further success with monoclonal antibodies in this disease remain the inability of antibodies to activate tumor cell killing mechanisms, downmodulation of the target antigen, circulating target antigen and the induction of a host xenogeneic neutralizing antibody response.

Until now, a total of approximately 40 patients have been treated with customized anti-idiotype monoclonal antibodies. The complete response rate is approximately 15%, with a median duration of remission of 6 months or less. However, a large proportion of partial remissions can be achieved with this therapy (approximately 50%). The main obstacle limiting the success of this elegant approach to monoclonal antibody therapy has been the emergence of idiotype-negative tumors that express a clonally related immunoglobulin molecule, which has somatically mutated its variable regions such that it is no longer susceptible to anti-idiotype therapy. The results of the Stanford group's most recent clinical trial were published recently [43]. In an attempt to address the problem of idiotype-negative tumor variants, monoclonal anti-idiotype antibody therapy was combined with a short course of cell cycle-active chemotherapy (chlorambucil) at a time when idiotype-negative cells were presumed to be proliferating. Thirteen patients with relapsed lymphomas were treated with two courses of monoclonal anti-idiotype antibody therapy, first alone, and then in combination with a pulse dose of chlorambucil. One complete remission and eight partial remissions were observed. However, analysis of pre- and posttherapy biopsies revealed the persistence of idiotype-negative tumor variants in approximately one-half of the relapsed specimens.

One strategy to overcome the problem of antigenic heterogeneity is to use a monoclonal antibody armed with an effector molecule, e.g., radioisotope or toxin. This approach is reasonable because the radiation emitted by the isotope may kill target antigen-negative cells present in close promixity (several cell diameters) to target antigen-positive cells. There have been several studies using radiolabeled antibodies to treat lymphoma in humans. Press et al. [44] administered ^{131}I-labeled anti-CD37 antibody to patients with relapsed lymphoma. With initial tracer doses of antibody, they found that in five patients with splenomegaly the antibody did not distribute to tumor in a way that would result in the tumor receiving more radioactivity than normal organs. However, in four other patients who showed good tumor localization of the tracer, subsequent administration of therapeutic doses of labeled antibody delivered 850–4260 Gy of radiation to sites of tumor. All four patients achieved a complete remission, and two remained in remission at 8+ and 11+ months. Kaminski et al. [45] treated 12 patients with the same ^{131}I-labeled monoclonal antibody (MB-1). Eleven of these patients had positive tumor imaging after a tracer dose, although the overall sensitivity for the detection of known tumor sites was only 39%. Furthermore, the dose to tumor exceeded that of any normal organ in only three patients. Ten patients went on to receive radioimmunotherapy at whole body doses projected to be 20–50 cGy on the basis of tracer studies. Only one complete response of 2 months duration, one partial response and one minor response were observed. DeNardo and colleagues [46,47] treated 20 B-cell lymphoma patients with ^{131}I-labeled Lym-1 antibody. They observed three complete responses, and the response rate was dose-related. Patients receiving 100 mCi or greater doses of ^{131}I were more likely to respond.

In what may be the most promising results to date, Kaminski et al. [48] used ^{131}I-labeled anti-B1 (anti-CD20) antibody in ten patients with relapsed B-cell lymphomas with extraordinary results. Tracer doses of radiolabeled antibody were given intravenously, first without pretreatment with unlabeled anti-B1 antibody, then subsequently with pretreatment with unlabeled antibody in an attempt to enhance subsequent access of radiolabeled antibody to tumors through presaturation of nonspecific binding sites. However, after pretreatment only three of the patients experienced an increase of more than 20% in the tumor to whole-body dose ratio compared with the ratio after a previous tracer dose without pretreatment. Significantly, all known disease sites larger than 2 cm could be imaged. Nine patients went on to receive radioimmunotherapeutic doses intended to deliver 25–45 cGy to the whole body. Remarkably, six of the nine patients had substantial tumor responses, four complete remissions and two partial responses. In three of these patients responses began after they received tracer doses, even before the administration of radioimmunotherapeutic doses. Of the four patients with complete remissions, one was of 8 months duration, and the other three were still in complete remission at 8, 9 and 11 months at the time of the report. At the current dose levels reached in this ongoing phase I trial, only mild myelosuppression was observed. A second experience with this radiolabeled antibody was reported recently with similarly encouraging results. Press et al. [49] selected 19 patients with B-cell lymphoma with favorable distribution of test doses of radiolabeled anti-CD20 or anti-CD37 antibodies prior to therapy with much higher doses of the same radiolabeled antibodies. The infusion of autologous marrow in 15 patients was used to circumvent the myelotoxicity of the therapy. Sixteen (84%) complete responses and two partial responses were reported. An important feature of both of these studies was the observation that the majority of the responses occurred in patients with small tumor burdens of less than 500 ml.

None of the published studies have sufficient follow-up times to evaluate the durability of responses. However, in light of the sensitivity of follicular lymphoma to radiation therapy, these novel radio-therapy delivery systems show promise and are worthy of further attempts at clinical development.

Several clinical studies describing the use of immunotoxins in B-cell lymphoma have been published. Grossbard et al. [50] reported on three sequential studies with anti-B4-blocked ricin immunotoxin. This novel immunotoxin combines the anti-B4 monoclonal antibody, which recognizes the CD19 molecule on B-cells, with a modified plant toxin ricin, in which the nonspecific binding of ricin has been attenuated by attaching affinity ligands to the galactose binding sites that mediate nonspecific binding. In the initial phase I dose escalation trial of daily bolus infusion in patients with relapsed and refractory B-cell neoplasms, a maximum tolerated dose of 50 μg/kg/day was established for a consecutive 5-day course. Dose-limiting toxicity was defined by reversible grade II elevations in hepatic enzymes. Despite what was believed to be inadequate serum levels of immunotoxin with bolus injections, one complete response, two partial responses and several transient responses were observed. Based on preclinical *in vitro* studies indicating that administration of anti-B4-blocked ricin by continuous infusion could yield greater cytotoxicity than equivalent doses administered by bolus injection, a second phase I trial was undertaken to determine the maximum tolerated dose of the immunotoxin when it was administered as a 7-day continuous infusion. Thirty-four patients with relapsed and refractory B-cell neoplasms were treated on this second phase I study [51]. Successive cohorts of at least three patients each were treated at doses of 10–70 μg/kg/day for 7 days with the dose increased by 10 μg/kg/day for each cohort. The maximum tolerated dose was reached at 50 μg/kg/day. Dose-limiting toxicities were grade IV reversible increases in hepatic enzymes and grade IV thrombocytopenia. Other adverse reactions included fevers, nausea, headaches, myalgias, dyspnea, edema and capillary leak syndrome. A pharmacokinetic profile was achieved whereby potentially therapeutic serum levels of anti-B4-blocked ricin could be sustained for 4 days at the maximum tolerated dose. Two complete responses three partial responses, and 11 transient responses were recorded. The testing of anti-B4-blocked ricin in patients with smaller tumor burdens was evaluated in the third phase I trial by Grossbard et al. [52], in which anti-B4-blocked ricin was administered by 7-day continuous infusion as adjuvant therapy to autologous bone marrow transplantation (ABMT) in 12 patients. All 12 patients had been in complete remission for at least 60 days following conditioning with total body irradiation and high-dose cyclophosphamide with purged autologous marrow reinfusion (range 61–208 days post-ABMT). Patients were treated at 20, 40 or 50 μg/kg/day for 7 days, and the maximum tolerated dose in this trial was 40 μg/kg/day. Dose-limiting toxicity was again reversible grade IV thrombocytopenia and elevation of hepatic transaminases. A somewhat surprising finding was the observation that 7 of the 12 patients developed anti-immunotoxin antibodies, even though most of these patients were treated in the early posttransplant period ($\leq$ 100 days), at a time when host immunologic recovery would not have been expected to be complete. Eleven of the 12 patients remain in complete remission with a limited median follow-up period of 17 months. Of particular interest was the observation that three of the four patients whose marrows remained positive, using the polymerase chain reaction (PCR), for the rearranged *bcl*-2 oncogene post-bone marrow transplantation (BMT) were found to be negative for this translocation by PCR analysis following anti-B4-blocked ricin immunotherapy. Amlot et al. [53] treated 26 relapsed B-cell lymphoma patients with an anti-CD22 antibody conjugated to a ricin A chain. Five partial responses and one complete response lasting only 30–78 days were recorded. Nine of the 24 evaluable patients developed either antimouse or antitoxin antibodies.

Although immunotoxins also have therapeutic potential, their development is unlikely to progress until the human antitoxin and antimouse antibody response of the host can be safely and chronically inhibited.

Progress has also been made in the treatment of T-cell lymphomas with monoclonal antibodies. Patients with T-cell lymphoma have been treated with murine or rat monoclonal antibodies directed against CD5 (T101 and Leu-1) [54,55], a panlymphoid cell antigen (CAMPATH-1) [40], the IL-2 receptor (anti-Tac) [56] and CD4 [57]. A chimeric (humanized) anti-CD4 antibody was used to treat patients with cutaneous T-cell lymphoma, and some partial responses were observed [57]. Rosen and colleagues [58] treated five patients with cutaneous T-cell lymphoma with ^{131}I-labeled T101. Patients had subjective improvement in pruritus and objective responses lasting 3 weeks to 3 months. At the highest doses, myelosuppression was dose limiting. In a novel approach, Waldmann and colleagues [56,59] have used antibodies directed against the IL-2 receptor α-chain (anti-Tac) to treat adult T-cell leukemias (ATL), which constitutively express large numbers of high-affinity IL-2 receptors. Anti-IL-2 receptor antibodies have been shown to prevent the growth of certain cell lines *in vitro*, even in the absence of complement, by blocking the IL-2 from gaining access to its receptor. Unfortunately, there is not much evidence that ATL T-cells respond to IL-2 or use the cell surface receptor for IL-2. In addition, large amounts of IL-2 receptor are shed into the serum of ATL patients. Waldmann et al. [59] recently described their experience administering anti-Tac intravenously to 19 patients with ATL. Two complete and four partial remissions were observed, lasting from 9 weeks to greater than 3 years, and one mixed response was recorded. Toxicity was minimal, and 18 of 19 patients did not suffer any reduction in normal formed elements of the blood. The initial experience of this same group of investigators with yttrium-90-labeled antibodies for the treatment of ATL has shown more significant antitumor effects. At the 5–15 mCi doses used, two complete responses and eight partial responses in a group of 15 patients have been recorded to date.

IL-2 receptor-targeted therapy

Another approach designed to achieve selective targeting of the IL-2 receptor has been described by LeMaistre et al. [60], who used a novel recombinant fusion toxin in which the receptor binding domain of diphtheria toxin had been replaced by human IL-2 by genetic engineering. This chimeric protein, consisting of diphtheria toxin linked to IL-2 (DAB$_{486}$ IL-2) was used in a phase I trial of 18 patients with IL-2 receptor-positive hematologic malignancies. In the course of establishing the maximal tolerated dose, one complete response and two partial responses were observed; interestingly, all three patients had low-grade lymphomas of B-cell origin. Approximately 50% of the patients treated in this study developed an antibody response either to the diphtheria toxin or chimeric protein. These investigators extended the clinical experience with this novel ligand fusion toxin to 23 other patients who were treated with escalating doses of DAB$_{486}$IL-2 adminstered as an infusion over 90 minutes in an attempt to achieve more sustained blood levels [61]. A maximum tolerated dose of 0.3 mg/kg per day was defined by renal insufficiency associated with hemolysis and thrombocytopenia. Two partial responses were recorded and four additional patients had tumor reduction not sufficient to be recorded as an objective response. Expression of the p55 subunit of the IL-2 receptor appeared to be necessary but not sufficient to achieve a tumor response.

Immunoglobulin idiotype antigen vaccines

This section is devoted to an in-depth discussion of the novel use of the idiotype of the surface immunoglobulin of a human B-cell lymphoma as a tumor-specific antigen for vaccine development. The development of a therapeutic vaccine against human malignancies in general has been a long-sought goal, which is just now beginning to be realized. Historically, many of the efforts towards this end have been frustrated by the lack of identification of tumor-specific antigens that would allow tumor cells to be distinguished from all other normal cells. Conceptually, such an antigen could be used as an immunogen to activate host antitumor immunity.

B-Cell malignancies of humans are composed of clonal proliferations of cells arising at various stages of normal B-cell differentiation, each synthesizing a single rearranged immunoglobulin gene product with unique variable regions [62–64]. For example, most cases of acute lymphocytic leukemia are the neoplastic counterparts of precursor B-cells, and either fail to express immunoglobulin or express cytoplasmic μ-chains, while B-cell lymphomas are neoplasms of mature, resting and reactive lymphocytes, which generally express immunoglobulin on the cell surface. To complete the spectrum, the normal counterpart of multiple myeloma is the plasma cell. The variable regions of immunoglobulin molecules contain unique determinants or *idiotypes*, which can themselves be recognized as antigens. The idiotypic determinants of the surface immunoglobulin of a B-cell lymphoma can thus serve as a tumor-specific marker for the malignant clone and can serve as a target for therapeutic approaches. The use of idiotype as a form of *active* immunotherapy (immunization of a human host with human tumor antigen), should be distinguished from *passive* immunotherapy, in which murine antibodies with specificity for idiotype are used as the immunotherapeutic agent or targeting vehicle. Active immunization of the host might be expected to produce both humoral and cellular immunity against tumor cells bearing the unique idiotype antigen. These responses would be of host origin and might therefore be long lasting. Active immunization with immunoglobulin idiotype, because it should result in the induction of a *polyclonal* immune response

directed against multiple idiotypic determinants on the molecule, may overcome the problem of tumor heterogeneity and the emergence of tumor cell variants that express mutated surface immunoglobulin, which limits the success of monoclonal anti-idiotype antibody therapy. This approach should also be distinguished from anti-idiotype vaccines, in which host immunization is achieved with a murine anti-idiotype monoclonal antibody that bears the internal image of the antigen rather than the human antigen itself.

The discoveries providing the rationale for this approach were initially made in the 1970s. First, Sirisinha and Eisen [65] made the observation that inbred mice could be induced to make antibodies against idiotypic determinants on myeloma proteins from mice of the same strain (syngeneic), thus establishing that idiotypic determinants could be recognized as autoantigens. Soon thereafter, Lynch et al. demonstrated that immunization of syngeneic mice against a myeloma protein resulted in protection from subsequent lethal challenge with myeloma cells from which the protein had been derived [66]. Subsequent studies in a number of syngeneic experimental tumor models confirmed that active immunization against idiotypic determinants on malignant B-cells produced resistance to tumor growth, as well as specific antitumor therapy against established tumors [67–77]. These studies also demonstrated that optimal immunization with lymphoma-derived idiotype required conjugation of the protein to an immunogenic protein carrier (keyhole limpet hemocyanin; KLH) and emulsification in an adjuvant.

PRODUCTION OF HUMAN IDIOTYPE VACCINES AND PHASE I CLINICAL TRIAL

The strategy used to isolate immunoglobulin from the surface of human B-cell lymphomas involves the formation of a somatic cell hybrid between the lymphoma cell and a modified mouse myeloma cell that grows *in vitro*, and has the cellular machinery to synthesize and secrete large quantities of immunoglobulin [78]. Such myeloma fusion partners have been engineered not to secrete any immunoglobulin of their own; therefore, the immunoglobulin that is secreted is purely derived from the human tumor.

The production of idiotype protein begins with the isolation of malignant cells from tumor biopsy specimens, most commonly involved lymph nodes. However, tumor cells can also be isolated from peripheral blood, bone marrow or spleen. The minimum starting material is about 10–50 million tumor cells. Lymphoma cells are fused with a hypoxanthine–aminopterin–thymidine (HAT)-sensitive fusion partner and heteromyelomas selected from HAT medium. Those that secrete immunoglobulin (Ig) with the type of heavy and light chains corresponding to the known immunophenotype of the tumor specimen are identified. Heteromyelomas identified in this way are expanded, and idiotype protein is then purified from collected culture supernatants by affinity chromatography using Sepharose–anti-human IgM or Sepharose–protein A, depending on the isotype of the lymphoma immunoglobulin. Finally, each idiotype is conjugated to KLH and it is this idiotype–KLH conjugate that is used to immunize the patient from whose tumor it was originally isolated. Under optimal conditions, approximately 3 months are required for production of the final product. This time period is not usually a limitation, since in the initial Phase II studies the vaccine will be used only after 6–8 months of cytoreduction by conventional chemotherapy.

Kwak et al. [79], performed an initial pilot study of autologous idiotype immunization in nine patients with B-cell lymphoma, using idiotype isolated in this way. The characteristics of the nine patients immunized with autologous idiotype protein are shown in Table 32.1. None of these patients received antitumor therapy during the time of the study. All were either in complete remission or had achieved minimal residual disease status following conventional chemotherapy. The primary objective of this study was to determine whether immune responses against this autologous antigen could be induced in such patients. In addition, three patients with rapidly progressive recurrent lymphoma were enrolled in a separate safety study. All three required reinstitution of chemotherapy shortly after enrolment, did not complete the immunization series and were not studied further. They received intramuscular injections of 0.5 mg of idiotype conjugated to KLH at 0, 2, 6, 10 and 14 weeks, followed by two booster injections at 24 and 28 weeks. Patients in the first cohort (five patients) of the nine patients with minimal residual disease received idiotype–KLH alone for the first three immunizations, then idiotype–KLH emulsified in a Pluronic polymer-based adjuvant vehicle formulation for all subsequent immunizations. Because no idiotype-specific immune responses were observed before the addition of the adjuvant to the vaccine in this first group of patients, patients in the second cohort (four patients) received the entire series of immunizations with adjuvant. The KLH carrier provided a convenient internal control for the immunocompetence of the patients, and all except one patient demonstrated both humoral and lymphoproliferative responses to the KLH protein. One patient developed only lymphoproliferative responses to KLH.

In all, seven of the nine patients demonstrated either a humoral ($N = 2$) or a cell-mediated ($N = 4$) anti-idiotypic immunological response, or both

Table 32.1 Characteristics of patients with B-cell lymphoma treated with autologous idiotype vaccines

Patient no. (sex/age)	Histologic subtype	Surface immunoglobulin	Prior therapy (no. of cycles)*	Months since last therapy	Site of measurable disease
Group 1					
1 (F/41)	FM	IgM lambda	CVP (8)	9	Submandibular lymph node
2 (M/56)	FM	IgA lambda	CVP (10)	8	None
3 (M/47)	FSC	IgM kappa	Chl/P (12)	6	None
4 (F/43)	FSC→DM	IgM kappa	mAb, CEPP (4), ABMT	7	Cutaneous mass
5 (M/59)	FSC	IgM kappa	CVP (9)	8	None
Group 2					
6 (M/45)	FSC	IgM kappa	CVP (10)	6	None
7 (M/50)	FM	IgM kappa	CVP (8)	18	None
8 (F/25)	FSC	IgM kappa	CVP (9)	20	None
9 (M/56)	FLC	IgG kappa	[131I]anti-CD20, ABMT	12	None

* CVP, cyclophosphamide, vincristine and prednisone; Chl/P, pulsed chlorambucil and prednisone; mAb, anti-idiotype monoclonal antibody; CEPP, cyclophosphamide, etoposide, prednisone and procarbazine; ABMT, autologous bone marrow transplantation; [131I]anti-CD20, radiolabeled monoclonal antibody; FM, follicular, mixed; FSC, follicular, small cell; FLC, follicular, large cell; DM, diffuse, mixed.

Adapted from Kwak et al. [79] and reprinted with permission.

($N = 1$). The anti-idiotypic antibodies produced by one of the responding patients were purified by affinity chromatography and were shown to contain heterogenous light chains as well as IgG heavy chains, suggesting a polyclonal immune response. The ability of the idiotype-specific humoral response to bind autologous *tumor* cells was also demonstrated by the inhibition of binding of a labeled murine anti-idiotype monoclonal antibody (mAb) to tumor cells from a pretreatment lymph node tumor specimen by hyperimmune, but not by preimmune, serum.

All patients were also closely monitored for disease activity and toxicity. Of the two patients with measurable tumor at the initiation of idiotype immunization, one (patient 1) experienced complete regression of a single 2.5 cm left submandibular lymph node, and the other (patient 4) experienced complete regression of a 4.5 cm cutaneous lymphomatous mass on the right arm. This clinical response in patient 4 correlated with an idiotype-specific peripheral blood mononuclear cell (PBMC) proliferative response *in vitro*. At the time of the report, the clinical responses in both patients had lasted 24 and 10 months, respectively, after completion of the immunization series. Moreover, with a median follow-up time of 10 months, the only case of tumor recurrence that had been observed among those patients who were in remission and completed the immunization series occurred in one of the two patients who failed to demonstrate an idiotype-specific immunological response. Toxicity was minimal in all 12 patients and was characterized by transient local reactions at the injection sites.

These results demonstrate that patients with B-cell lymphoma can be induced to develop sustained humoral and cellular idiotype-specific immune responses. Although relatively weak in magnitude, these responses have been shown to be highly specific for idiotype, demonstrating that autologous idiotype, made immunogenic by conjugation to KLH, can serve as an immunogen (antigen) to elicit host immunological responses.

PHASE II CLINICAL TRIALS OF IDIOTYPE VACCINATION

We continue to pursue a therapeutic vaccine approach to B-cell lymphomas in the setting of a minimal tumor burden. Our hypothesis is that the best candidates for demonstration of an immune response to components of autologous tumor are patients whose tumors are in remission and whose previous therapy has been limited. Building on the promising results of the phase I trial, idiotype vaccine development in the Division of Clinical Sciences of the NCI

is focused on the following two goals: (1) the development of more potent vaccine formulations; and (2) the development of formulations that are more effective in activating the cellular arm of the immune system. There is a growing body of evidence from experimental model systems suggesting that T-cells can recognize idiotypic determinants that have been processed and presented as peptides in combination with MHC molecules on the surface of antigen presenting cells [80–86]. Most idiotype-specific T-cell lines or clones isolated from immunized mice have been of the CD4 phenotype but, at least in one case, MHC class I-restricted CD8+ T-cells specific for idiotype were described. These findings should encourage the design of vaccine formulations capable of eliciting such T-cell responses in patients. Figure 32.1 shows the design of the first phase II trial currently in progress. It is a single arm prospective clinical trial open to patients with follicular low-grade lymphomas. It represents an advance over the pilot study, described above in the following aspects: (1) idiotype vaccination is administered in first complete remission, which means that only previously untreated patients are eligible for this trial; (2) uniform induction chemotherapy with a modified ProMACE regimen (prednisone, doxorubicin, cyclophosphamide and etoposide) is being adminstered to all patients; and (3) low-dose subcutaneous GM-CSF is being administered together with autologous idiotype–KLH as the adjuvant. Since the phase I study established the requirement for an immunological adjuvant, the identification and testing of novel, more potent, adjuvants may be worthwhile. The effect of GM-CSF in enhancing cellular immune responses to idiotype has been demonstrated in an experimental model system (unpublished data).

In addition to clinical end-points, patients on this trial are being monitored for the induction of idiotype-specific immune responses and for eradication of minimal residual disease as assessed by PCR amplification of the rearranged *bcl*-2 oncogene, which is associated with the characteristic t(14;18) present in 80–85% of follicular lymphomas [87], from bone marrow cells. In addition, host peripheral blood T-cells are being monitored prospectively for the expression of a functional T-cell receptor ζ-chain, impairment of which may need to be overcome by any active immunotherapy approach against human cancer [88]. Already, 35 patients have been enrolled on this study.

FUTURE DIRECTIONS

If tumor-specific vaccines directed against idiotypes are to become an effective form of therapy, one task

CLINICAL TRIAL SCHEMA

Study design: Single-arm prospective

Lymphoma type: Follicular, low-grade

Patients: Previously untreated (vaccination in first CR)

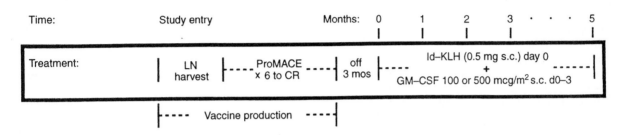

Figure 32.1   Design of the first NCI phase II idiotype vaccine clinical trial. Id-KLH, idiotype–KLH conjugate; LN, lymph node (containing tumor); TCR, T-cell receptor.

which must be accomplished is the enhancement of the immunogenicity of an otherwise weakly immunogenic, autologous, tumor-specific antigen. Table 32.2 lists the experimental strategies our laboratory is currently exploring to accomplish the goals above. Live recombinant vaccine delivery vehicles and viral vectors have shown promise for their ability to prime an MHC class I- or II-restricted T-cell immune response [89–92]. Using techniques of polymerase chain reaction (PCR) amplification and rapid sequencing of variable region genes, we have constructed Ig heavy and light chain variable region gene fragments linked together by a short oligonucleotide linker

Table 32.2   NCI strategies for second-generation idiotype vaccine development

---

Novel immunological adjuvants

Live delivery systems/vectors
  Recombinant BCG
  Recombinant vaccinia or canarypox viruses

sFv-cytokine/chemokine fusion proteins

DNA vaccine

Liposome encapsulation

Combinations with engineered cellular vaccines

NCI, National Cancer Institute; BCG, bacille Calmette–Guérin; sFv, single chain Fv.

(sFv) and expressed them in recombinant BCG and pox viruses. We are also exploring the expression of sFv–cytokine or sFv–chemokine fusion proteins in prokaryotic expression systems, and testing their ability to prime for a T-cell response in mouse tumor models. This is similar to the approach described by Tao et al. [93], who generated a whole immunoglobulin–GM-CSF fusion protein expressed in myeloma cells. This proved to be efficient at priming mice to develop an antibody response to idiotype. Liposome encapsulation of protein antigens appears to be particularly effective at rendering nonimmunogenic (or weakly immunogenic) antigens immunogenic [94–96] and, in some cases liposomal-based proteins can prime for MHC class I-restricted CD8+ T-cell antigen-specific responses [97–100]. We are currently experimenting with whole immunoglobulin as well as immunoglobulin fragments incorporated into liposomes of various compositions. Finally, preclinical studies exploring a strategy of priming with irradiated cellular vaccines, followed by boost immunizations with refined antigen (idiotype), have been very effective in inducing a cellular immune response to idiotype. If more potent vaccines can be formulated, it might even be possible to extend the idiotype vaccine approach to patients with greater tumor burdens.

These studies also have important implications for the development or refinement of therapeutic vaccines for other B-cell malignancies, most notably multiple myeloma, in which the convenience of isolating idiotype protein from the plasma or urine of patients would be technically appealing. Although the early work from Eisen's group was done in murine myelomas [66], the theoretical barrier to the application of an idiotype vaccine to myeloma has been the huge amount of circulating antigen in the patient, which would be expected to block any anti-idiotype response induced. However, anti-idiotypic T-cells may not be blocked at all by soluble idiotype, as T-cells recognize only membrane-bound antigen, which has been processed and presented in the form of peptides in association with MHC molecules. Our initial results in a single patient with myeloma who underwent allogeneic bone marrow transplantation may bear out this prediction. We isolated idiotype protein from the patient's plasma, chemically conjugated it to KLH and formulated it with the adjuvant used in the phase I trial described above before using it to immunize an human leukocyte antigen (HLA)-matched sibling who was also the donor of the bone marrow allograft [101]. An idiotype-specific T-cell line of donor origin was established from the patient's peripheral blood after the bone marrow transplant, despite the persistence of circulating paraprotein in the recipient.

The application of idiotype vaccination to other clinical settings of lymphoma, such as intermediate- and high-grade tumors, and as post-BMT immuno-therapy can also be envisaged [102]. It must, however, be acknowledged that immunoglobulin idiotype antigen vaccines must be produced individually for each patient. Whichever idiotype vaccine formulation shows the most potency and promise for testing in phase III clinical trials must also be technically feasible to produce.

Activation-induced cell killing

Something of a paradox has been discovered about lymphoma cells that express receptors through which normal lymphocytes may be stimulated or costimulated. Signal transduction through antigen receptors [the T-cell antigen receptor on T-cells, surface immunoglobulin (IgM or IgD) on B-cells] and/or any of a host of co-stimulatory receptors (such as CD2 and CD26 in T-cells, and CD40, CD19 and class II MHC in B-cells) that are associated with stimulation and proliferation of normal lymphocytes induces irreversible growth arrest with or without apoptosis in lymphoma cells [103–108]. There are antibodies to a number of these activation-associated receptors but, perhaps even more importantly, some of these receptors have known physiologic ligands.

Since these ligands are autologous human proteins, it seems unlikely that they will induce an induced immune response. It is attractive to speculate that chronic administration of CD40 ligand may be a superior method of treating, for example, acquired immunodeficiency syndrome-associated B-cell lymphoma or lymphoma in very old people than combination chemotherapy, which may be associated with serious and life-threatening toxicity in certain groups of patients. In addition, the bacterial superantigens that activate all T-cells-bearing receptors derived from particular $V\beta$ gene families are also candidates for therapy of T-cell lymphoma. Indeed, there is already evidence that at least some antibodies may work via activation of receptor pathways in lymphoma cells. Vuist and colleagues, for example, recently reported that the induction of lymphoma regression by monoclonal anti-idiotypic antibodies *in vivo* was related to the ability of the antibodies to induce signal transduction *in vitro* [109]. Thus, it seems likely that lymphoma treatment in the future may include physiologic ligands or ligand mimetics that activate the lymphoma cells and induce cell death via apoptosis.

References

1. Plaumann L, Havemann K, Diehl V, et al. Results of a study on the treatment of non-Hodgkin's lymphoma using a combined modality approach. *J. Cancer Res. Clin. Oncol.* 1982, **103**(Suppl.): A15.
2. Hryniuk W. A randomized trial of BCG in poor prognosis non-Hodgkin's lymphoma. *Proc. Am. Assoc. Cancer Res.* 1982, **23**: 112.
3. Jones SE, Grozea PN, Miller TP, et al. Chemotherapy with cyclophosphamide, doxorubicin, vincristine, and prednisone or with levamisole or with levamisole plus BCG for malignant lymphoma: A Southwest Oncology Group study. *J. Clin. Oncol.* 1985, **3**: 1318–1324.
4. Jones SE, Grozea PN, Metz EN, et al. Improved complete remission rates and survival for patients with large cell lymphoma treated with chemoimmunotherapy: A Southwest Oncology Group study. *Cancer* 1983, **51**: 1083–1090.
5. Thomas JW, Plenderleith IH, Landi S, et al. Bacille Calmette–Guerin as maintenance therapy for non-Hodgkin's lymphoma. *Can. Med. Assoc. J.* 1983, **129**: 439–442.
6. Rabaud A, Eghbali H, Trojani M, et al. Adjuvant bacillus Calmette–Guerin therapy in non-Hodgkin's malignant lymphomas: Long-term results of a randomized trial in a single institution. *J. Clin. Oncol.* 1990, **8**: 608–614.
7. Goldstein D, Laszlo J. Interferon therapy in cancer: from imaginon to interferon. *Cancer Res.* 1986, **46**: 4315–4329.

8. Urba WJ, Longo DL. α-interferon in the treatment of nodular lymphomas. *Semin. Oncol.* 1986, **13**: 40–47.

9. Gilewski TA, Richards JM. Biologic response modifiers in non-Hodgkin's lymphomas. *Semin. Oncol.* 1990, **17**: 74–87.

10. Foon KA, Sherwin SA, Abrama PG, et al. Treatment of advanced non-Hodgkin's lymphoma with recombinant leukocyte A interferon. *N. Engl. J. Med.* 1984, **311**: 1148–1152.

11. Mantovani L, Guglielmi C, Martelli M, et al. Recombinant alpha interferon in the treatment of low-grade non-Hodgkin's lymphoma: Results of a cooperative phase II trial in 313 patients. Haematologica 1990, **74**: 571–575.

12. VanderMolen LA, Steis RG, Duffey PL, et al. Low-versus high-dose interferon alfa-2a in relapsed indolent non-Hodgkin's lymphoma. *J. Natl Cancer Inst.* 1990, **82**: 235–238.

13. Rohatiner AZS, Richards MA, Barnett MJ, et al. Chlorambucil and interferon for low-grade non-Hodgkin's lymphoma. *Br. J. Cancer* 1987, **55**: 225–226.

14. Clark RH, Dimitrov NV, Axelson JA, et al. A phase II trial of intermittent leukocyte interferon and high dose chlorambucil in the treatment of non-Hodgkin's lymphoma resistant to conventional therapy. *Am. J. Clin. Oncol.* 1989, **12**: 75–77.

15. Smalley RV, Andersen JW, Hawkins MJ, et al. Interferon alfa combined with cytotoxic chemotherapy for patients with non-Hodgkin's lymphoma. *N. Engl. J. Med.* 1992, **327**: 1336–1341.

16. Hiddemann W, Unterhalt M, Koch P, et al. Alpha interferon maintenance therapy in patients with low-grade non-Hodgkin's lymphomas after cytoreductive chemotherapy with prednimustine and mitoxantrone. *Eur. J. Cancer* 1991, **27**(Suppl. 4): S37–S39.

17. Non-Hodgkin's Lymphoma Cooperative Study Group. Randomized study of chlorambucil (CB) compared to interferon (alfa-2b) combined with CB in low-grade non-Hodgkin's lymphoma: An interim report of a randomized study. *Eur. J. Cancer* 1991, **27**(Suppl 4): 31–33.

18. Price CGA, Rohatiner AZS, Steward W, et al. Interferon-α_{2b} in the treatment of follicular lymphoma: Preliminary results of a trial in progress. *Ann. Oncol.* 1991, **2**(Suppl. 2): 141–145.

19. Solal-Celigny P, Lepage E, Brousse N, et al. Recombinant interferon alfa-2b combined with a regimen containing doxorubicin in patients with advanced follicular lymphoma. *N. Engl. J. Med.* 1993, **329**: 1608–1614.

20. Bunn PA, Foon KA, Ihde DC, et al. Recombinant leukocyte A interferon: An active agent in advanced cutaneous T-cell lymphomas. *J. Exp. Med.* 1984, **101**: 2153–2157.

21. Covelli A, Papa G, Vegna M, et al. Recombinant alpha-2a interferon as initial therapy in mycosis fungoides: Results of a 3-year follow-up. *Proc. Am. Soc. Clin. Oncol.* 1989, **8**: 251.

22. Kohn EC, Steis RG, Sausville EA, et al. Phase II trial of intermittent high-dose recombinant interferon alfa-2a in mycosis fungoides and the Sezary syndrome. *J. Clin. Oncol.* 1990, **8**: 155–160.

23. Papa G, Tura S, Mandelli F, et al. Is interferon alpha in cutaneous T-cell lymphoma a treatment of choice? *Crit. J. Hematol.* 1991, **79**: 48–51.

24. Knobler RM, Trautinger F, Radaszkiewicz T, et al. Treatment of cutaneous T-cell lymphoma with a combination of low-dose interferon alfa-2b and retinoids. *J. Am. Acad. Dermatol.* 1991, **24**: 247–252.

25. Dreno B, Claudy A, Meynadier J, et al. The treatment of 45 patients with cutaneous T-cell lymphoma with low doses of interferon-α and etretinate. *Br. J. Dermatol.* 1991, **125**: 456–459.

26. Kuzel TM, Gilyon K, Springer E, et al. Interferon alfa-2a combined with phototherapy in the treatment of cutaneous T-cell lymphoma. *J. Natl Cancer Inst.* 1990, **82**: 203–207.

27. Kaplan EH, Rosen ST, Norris DB, et al. Phase II study of recombinant human interferon gamma for treatment of cutaneous T-cell lymphoma. *J. Natl Cancer Inst.* 1990, **82**: 208–212.

28. Lim SH, Worman CP, Callaghan T, et al. Continuous intravenous infusion of high-dose recombinant interleukin-2 for advanced lymphomas: A phase II study. *Leukemia Res.* 1991, **15**: 435–440.

29. Weber JS, Yang JC, Topalian SL, et al. The use of interleukin-2 and lymphokine-activated killer cells for the treatment of patients with non-Hodgkin's lymphoma. *J. Clin. Oncol.* 1991, **10**: 33–40.

30. Bernstein ZP, Friedman N, Vaickus L, et al. IL-2 LAK therapy of non-Hodgkin's lymphoma and Hodgkin's disease. *J. Immunother.* 1991, **10**: 141–146.

31. Duggan DB, Santarelli MT, Zamkoff K, et al. A phase II study of recombinant interleukin-2 with or without recombinant interferon-beta in non-Hodgkin's lymphoma. A study of the Cancer and Leukemia Group B. *J. Immunother.* 1992, **12**: 115–122.

32. Grossbard ML, Press OW, Appelbaum FR, et al. Monoclonal antibody-based therapies of leukemia and lymphoma. *Blood* 1992, **80**: 863–878.

33. Nadler LM, Stashenko P, Hardy R, et al. Serotherapy of a patient with a monoclonal antibody directed against a human lymphoma-associated antigen. *Cancer Res.* 1980, **40**: 3147–3154.

34. Miller RA, Levy R. Response of cutaneous T-cell lymphoma to therapy with hybridoma monoclonal antibody. *Lancet* 1981, **2**: 226–230.

35. Foon KA, Schroff RW, Bunn PA, et al. Effects of monoclonal antibody therapy in patients with chronic lymphocytic leukemia. *Blood* 1984, **64**: 1085–1093.

36. Miller RA, Maloney DG, Warnke R, et al. Treatment of B-cell lymphoma with monoclonal anti-idiotype antibody. *N. Engl. J. Med.* 1982, **306**: 517–522.

37. Meeker T, Lowder J, Maloney DG, et al. A clinical trial of anti-idiotype therapy for B-cell malignancy. *Blood* 1985, **65**: 1349–1363.

38. Rankin EM, Hekman A, Sowers R, et al. Treatment of two patients with B-cell lymphoma with monoclonal anti-idiotype antibodies. *Blood* 1985, **65**: 1373–1381.

39. Brown SL, Miller RA, Horning SJ, et al. Treatment of B-cell lymphoma with anti-idiotype antibodies alone and in combination with alpha interferon. *Blood* 1989, **73**: 651–661.

40. Dyer MJS, Hale G, Hayhoe FGJ, et al. Effects of CAMPATH-1 antibodies in vivo in patients with lymphoid malignancies: Influence of antibody isotype. *Blood* 1989, **73**: 1431–1439.

41. Press OW, Applebaum F, Ledbetter JA, et al. Monoclonal antibody 1F5 (anti-CD20) serotherapy of human B-cell lymphomas. *Blood* 1987, **69**: 584–591.

42. Scheinberg SA, Straus DJ, Yeh SD, et al. A phase I toxicity, pharmacology, and dosimetry trial of monoclonal antibody OKB7 in patients with non-Hodgkin's lymphoma: Effects of tumor burden and antigen expression. *J. Clin. Oncol.* 1990, **8**: 792–803.

43. Maloney DG, Brown S, Czerwinski DK, et al. Monoclonal anti-idiotype therapy of B-cell lymphoma: The addition of a short course of chemotherapy does not interfere with the antitumor effect nor prevent the emergence of idiotype-negative variant cells. *Blood* 1992, **80**: 1502–1510.

44. Press OW, Eary JF, Badger CC, et al. Treatment of refractory non-Hodgkin's lymphoma with radiolabeled MB-1 (anti-CD37) antibody. *J. Clin. Oncol.* 1989, **7**: 1027–1038.

45. Kaminski MS, Fig LM, Zasadny KR, et al. Imaging, dosimetry, and radioimmunotherapy with iodine 131-labeled anti-CD37 antibody in B-cell lymphoma. *J. Clin. Oncol.* 1992, **10**: 1696–1711.

46. DeNardo GL, DeNardo SJ, O'Grady LF, et al. Fractionated radioimmunotherapy of B-cell malignancies with ^{131}I-Lym-1. *Cancer Res.* 1990, **50**: 1014S–1016S.

47. O'Grady L, DeNardo S, Lewis J, et al. Radioimmunotherapy of lymphoma. *Blood* 1990, **76** (Suppl.): 365a.

48. Kaminski MS, Zasadny KR, Francis IR, et al. Radioimmunotherapy of B-cell lymphoma with ^{131}I-Anti-B1 (anti-CD20) antibody. *N. Engl. J. Med.* 1993, **329**: 459–465.

49. Press OW, Eary JF, Appelbaum FR, et al. Radiolabeled-antibody therapy of B-cell lymphoma with autologous bone marrow support. *N. Engl. J. Med.* 1993, **329**: 1219–1224.

50. Grossbard ML, Freedman AS, Ritz J, et al. Serotherapy of B-cell neoplasms with anti-B4-blocked ricin: A phase I trial of daily bolus infusion. *Blood* 1992, **79**: 576–585.

51. Grossbard ML, Lambert JM, Goldmacher VS, et al. Anti-B4-blocked ricin: A phase I trial of 7-day continuous infusion in patients with B-cell neoplasms. *J. Clin. Oncol.* 1993, **11**: 726–737.

52. Grossbard ML, Gribben JG, Freedman AS, et al. Adjuvant immunotoxin therapy with anti-B4-blocked ricin after autologous bone marrow transplantation for patients with B-cell non-Hodgkin's lymphoma. *Blood* 1993, **81**: 2263–2271.

53. Amlot PL, Stone MJ, Cunningham D, et al. A phase I study of an anti-CD22-deglycosylated ricin A chain immunotoxin in the treatment of B-cell lymphomas resistant to conventional therapy. *Blood* 1993, **9**: 2624–2633.

54. Dillman RO, Shawler DL, Dillman JB, et al. Therapy of chronic lymphocytic leukemia with T101 monoclonal antibody. *J. Clin. Oncol.* 1984, **2**: 881–891.

55. Miller RA, Oseroff AR, Stratte PT, et al. Monoclonal antibody therapeutic trials in seven patients with T-cell lymphoma. *Blood* 1983, **62**: 988–995.

56. Waldmann TA, Goldman CK, Bongiovanni KF, et al. Therapy of patients with human T-cell lymphotropic virus-I-induced adult T-cell leukemia with anti-Tac, a monoclonal antibody to the receptor for interleukin 2. *Blood* 1988, **72**: 1805–1816.

57. Knox SJ, Levy R, Hodgkinson S, et al. Observations on the effect of chimeric anti-CD4 monoclonal antibody in patients with mycosis fungoides. *Blood* 1991, **77**: 20–30.

58. Rosen ST, Zimmer AM, Goldman-Leikin R, et al. Radioimmunodetection and radioimmunotherapy of cutaneous T-cell lymphomas using ^{131}I-labeled monoclonal antibody: An Illinois *Cancer* Council study. *J. Clin. Oncol.* 1987, **5**: 562–573.

59. Waldmann TA, White JD, Goldman CK, et al. The interleukin-2 receptor: A target for monoclonal antibody treatment of human T-cell lymphotropic virus-I-induced adult T-cell leukemia. *Blood* 1993, **82**: 1701–1712.

60. LeMaistre CF, Meneghetti C, Rosenblum M, et al. Phase I trial of an interleukin-2 (IL-2) fusion toxin (DAB_{486}IL-2) in hematologic malignancies expressing the IL-2 receptor. *Blood* 1992, **79**: 2547–2554.

61. LeMaistre CF, Craig FE, Meneghetti C, et al. Phase I trial of a 90-minute infusion of the fusion toxin DAB_{486} IL-2 in hematological cancers. *Cancer Res.* 1993, **53**: 3930–3934.

62. Fialkow PJ, Klein E, Klein G, et al. Immunoglobulin and glucose-6-phosphate dehydrogenase as markers of cellular origin in Burkitt lymphoma. *J. Exp. Med.* 1973, **138**: 89–102.

63. Salmon SE, Seligmann M. B-Cell neoplasia in man. *Lancet* 1974, **23**: 1230–1233.

64. Preud'homme JL, Seligmann M. Surface bound immunoglobulins as a cell marker in human lymphoproliferative diseases. *Blood* 1972, **40**: 777–794.

65. Sirisinha S, Eisen HN. Autoimmune-like antibodies to the ligand-binding sites of myeloma proteins. *Proc. Natl Acad. Sci. USA* 1971, **68**: 3130–3135.

66. Lynch RG, Graff RJ, Sirisinha S, et al. Myeloma proteins as tumor-specific transplantation antigens. *Proc. Natl Acad. Sci. USA* 1972, **69**: 1540–1544.

67. Jorgensen T, Gaudernack G, Hannestad K. Immunization with the light chain and the V_L domain of the isologous myeloma protein 315 inhibits growth of mouse plasmacytoma MOPC315. *Scand. J. Immunol.* 1980, **11**: 29–35.

68. Daley MJ, Gebel HM, Lynch RG. Idiotype-specific transplantation resistance to MOPC-315: Abrogation by post-immunization thymectomy. *J. Immunol.* 1978, **120**: 1620–1624.

69. Bridges SH. Participation of the humoral immune system in the myeloma-specific transplantation resistance. *J. Immunol.* 1978, **121**: 479–483.

70. Freedman PM, Autry JR, Tokuda S, et al. Tumor immunity induced by preimmunization with BALB/c mouse myeloma protein. *J. Natl Cancer Inst.* 1976, **56**: 735–740.

71. Sugai S, Palmer DW, Talal N, et al. Protective and cellular immune responses to idiotypic determinants on cells from a spontaneous lymphoma of NZB-NZW

F1 mice. *J. Exp. Med.* 1974, **140**: 1547–1558.

72. Stevenson FK, Gordon J. Immunization with idiotypic immunoglobulin protects against development of B lymphocytic leukemia, but emerging tumor cells can evade antibody attack by modulation. *J. Immunol.* 1983, **130**: 970–973.

73. George AJT, Tutt AL, Stevenson FK. Anti-idiotypic mechanisms involved in the suppression of a mouse B-cell lymphoma, BCL₁. *J. Immunol.* 1987, **138**: 628–634.

74. Kaminski MS, Kitamura K, Maloney DG, et al. Idiotype vaccination against murine B-cell lymphoma: Inhibition of tumor immunity by free idiotype protein. *J. Immunol.* 1987, **138**: 1289–1296.

75. Campbell MJ, Esserman L, Byars NE, et al. Idiotype vaccination against murine B-cell lymphoma: Humoral and cellular requirements for the full expression of antitumor immunity. *J. Immunol.* 1990, **145**: 1029–1036.

76. George AJT, Folkard SG, Hamblin TJ, et al. Idiotypic vaccination as a treatment for a B-cell lymphoma. *J. Immunol.* 1990, **141**: 2168–2174.

77. Campbell MJ, Esserman L, Levy R. Immunotherapy of established murine B-cell lymphoma: Combination of idiotype immunization and cyclophosphamide. *J. Immunol.* 1988, **141**: 3227–3233.

78. Carroll WL, Thielmans K, Dilley J, et al. Mouse x human heterohybridomas as fusion partners with human B cell tumors. *J. Immunol. Meth.* 1986, **89**: 61–72.

79. Kwak LW, Campbell MJ, Czerwinski DK, et al. Induction of immune responses in patients with B cell lymphoma against the surface immunoglobulin idiotype expressed by their tumors. *N. Engl. J. Med.* 1992, **327**: 1209–1215.

80. Bogen B, Malissen B, Haas W. Idiotope-specific T-cell clones that recognize syngeneic immunoglobulin fragments in the context of class II molecules. *Eur. J. Immunol.* 1986, **16**: 1373–1378.

81. Waters SJ, Bona CA. Characterization of a T-cell clone recognizing idiotypes as tumor-associated antigens. *Cell. Immunol.* 1988, **111**: 87–93.

82. Wright A, Lee JE, Link MP, et al. Cytotoxic T lymphocytes specific for self tumor immunoglobulin express T-cell receptor δ chain. *J. Exp. Med.* 1989, **169**: 1557–1564.

83. Wilson A, George AJT, King CA, et al. Recognition of a B-cell lymphoma by anti-idiotypic T-cells. *J. Immunol.* 1990, **145**: 3937–3943.

84. Weiss S, Bogen B. MHC class-II-restricted presentation of intracellular antigen. *Cell* 1991, **64**: 767–776.

85. Chakrabarti D, Ghosh SK. Induction of syngeneic T lymphocytes against a B-cell tumor. *Cell. Immunol.* 1992, **144**: 443–454.

86. Cao W, Myers-Powell BA, Braciale TJ. Recognition of an immunoglobulin V_H epitope by influenza virus-specific class I major histocompatibility complex-restricted cytolytic T lymphocytes. *J. Exp. Med.* 1994, **179**: 195–202.

87. Offit K, Chaganti RSK. Chromosomal aberrations in non-Hodgkin's lymphoma: Biologic and clinical correlations. *Hematol. Oncol. Clin. North Am.* 1991, **5**: 853–869.

88. Mizoguchi H, O'Shea JJ, Longo DL, et al. Alterations in signal transduction molecules in T lymphocytes from tumor-bearing mice. *Science* 1992, **258**: 1795–1798.

89. Stover CK, de la Cruz VF, Fuerst TR, et al. New use of BCG for recombinant vaccines. *Nature* 1991, **351**: 456–460.

90. Aldovini A, Young RA. Humoral and cell-mediated immune responses to live recombinant BCG-HIV vaccines. *Nature* 1991, **351**: 479–482.

91. Jacobs WR Jr, Snapper SB, Lugosi L, et al. Development of BCG as a recombinant vaccine vehicle. *Curr. Top. Microbiol. Immunol.* 1990, **155**: 153–160.

92. Cox WI, Tartaglia J, Paoletti E. In Binns MM, Smith GL (eds) *Poxvirus Recombinants as Live Vaccines*. Boca Raton: CRC Press, Inc., 1992, pp. 123–162.

93. Tao M-H, Levy R. Idiotype/granulocyte-macrophage colony-stimulating factor fusion protein as a vaccine for B-cell lymphoma. *Nature* 1993, **362**: 755–758.

94. Gregoriadis G, Panagiotidi C. Immunoadjuvant action of liposomes: Comparison with other adjuvants. *Immunol. Lett.* 1989, **20**: 237–240.

95. Alving CR. Liposomes as carriers of antigens and adjuvants. *J. Immunol. Meth.* 1991, **140**: 1–13.

96. Brynestad K, Babbitt B, Huang L, et al. Influence of peptide acylation, liposome incorporation, and synthetic immunomodulators on the immunogenicity of a 1–23 peptide of glycoprotein D of herpes simplex virus: Implications for subunit vaccines. *J. Virol.* 1990, **64**: 680–685.

97. Reddy R, Zhou F, Nair S, et al. In vivo cytotoxic T lymphocyte induction with soluble proteins administered in liposomes. *J. Immunol.* 1992, **148**: 1585–1589.

98. Harding CV, Collins DS, Kanagawa O, et al. Liposome-encapsulated antigens engender lysosomal processing for class II MHC presentation and cytosolic processing for class I presentation. *J. Immunol.* 1991, **147**: 2860–2863.

99. Noguchi Y, Noguchi T, Sato T, et al. Priming for in vitro and in vivo anti-human T lymphotropic virus type 1 cellular immunity by virus-related protein reconstituted into liposome. *J. Immunol.* 1991, **146**: 3599–3603.

100. White K, Krzych U, Gordon DM, et al. Induction of cytolytic and antibody responses using plasmodium falciparum repeatless circumsporozoite protein encapsulated in liposomes. *Vaccine* 1993, **11**: 1341–1346.

101. Kwak LW, Taub DD, Duffey PL, et al. Transfer of myeloma idiotype-specific immunity from an actively immunized marrow donor. *Lancet* 1995, **345**: 1016–1020.

102. Kwak LW, Campbell MJ, Zelenetz AD, et al. Combined syngeneic bone marrow transplantation and immunotherapy of a murine B-cell lymphoma: Active immunization with tumor-derived idiotypic IgM. *Blood* 1990, **76**: 2411–2417.

103. Ashwell JD, Longo DL, Bridges SH. T-cell tumor elimination as a result of T-cell receptor-mediated activation. *Science* 1987, **237**: 61–64.

104. Bridges SH, Kruisbeek AM, Longo DL. Selective in vivo antitumor effects of monoclonal anti-I-A antibody

on B-cell lymphoma. *J. Immunol.* 1987, **139**: 4242–4249.

105. Page DM, Defranco A. Role of phosphoinositide-derived second messengers in mediation of anti-IgM-induced growth arrest of WEHI-231 B lymphoma cells. *J. Immunol.* 1988, **140**: 3717–3724.

106. Arasi VE, Lieberman R, Sandlund J, et al. Anti-immunoglobulin inhibition of Burkitt's lymphoma cell proliferation and concurrent reduction of c-myc and μ heavy chain gene expression. *Cancer Res.* 1989, **49**: 3235–3241.

107. Beckwith M, Urba WJ, Ferris DK, et al. Anti-IgM-mediated growth inhibition of a human B lymphoma cell line is independent of phosphatidylinositol turnover and protein kinase C activation and involves tyrosine phosphorylation. *J. Immunol.* 1991, **147**: 2411–2418.

108. Funakoshi S, Longo DL, Beckwith M, et al. Inhibition of human B-cell lymphoma growth by CD40 stimulation. *Blood* 1994, **83**: 2787–2794.

109. Vuist WMJ, Levy R, Maloney DG. Lymphoma regression induced by monoclonal anti-idiotypic antibodies correlates with their ability to induce Ig signal transduction and is not prevented by tumor expression of high levels of bcl-2 protein. *Blood* 1994, **83**: 899–906.

CHAPTER 33

Management of recurrent or refractory lymphomas

ALEJANDRO PRETI AND FERNANDO CABANILLAS

Introduction

Malignant lymphomas are biologically heterogeneous neoplastic disorders considered to be among the most sensitive to chemotherapy and radiation therapy. In spite of this, frontline chemotherapy fails or disease relapses in a significant fraction of patients. The prognosis of such patients varies according to the biologic characteristics of their disease. Patients with low-grade lymphoma can sometimes survive for many years with recurrent disease, but the prognosis of patients with intermediate- or high-grade lymphoma is poor after relapse, particularly when salvage therapy fails. Chemotherapeutic agents such as ifosfamide and etoposide, used in combination, have proved to be relatively effective in this setting, resulting in a second, clinically complete remission in a significant fraction of patients who relapse. Similarly, advances in the areas of bone marrow transplantation, peripheral stem cell collection, purging techniques and high-dose chemotherapy have resulted in high response rates and cures in a small, selected subgroup of patients. Finally, immunotoxins or radioimmunotherapy targeted against T- and B-cell-specific antigens, discussed in Chapters 25 and 32, have provided a promising alternative treatment strategy.

The purpose of this chapter is to review the status of both single-agent and combination chemotherapies used for recurrent or refractory lymphoma.

Refractory lymphoma

Patients who achieve a partial response, or less than a partial response, to frontline chemotherapy regimens are normally considered to have refractory disease because subsequent progression is inevitable if the same drug regimen is continued. Patients who initially respond completely to frontline regimens but subsequently relapse while still undergoing treatment can also be considered to have refractory lymphoma or, in this instance, 'acquired' resistance. The occurrence of relapse within 6 months after chemotherapy is discontinued can also be considered acquired refractoriness to treatment. It is important, whenever possible, to recognize partial sensitivity to chemotherapy before the onset of disease progression because, if such patients are identified at the time of the plateau of their response, a change in the chemotherapy regimen can frequently result in a complete response.

ESTABLISHING THE PRESENCE OF RECURRENT OR RESIDUAL LYMPHOMA

Before undertaking treatment for recurrent or refractory lymphoma, it is mandatory to confirm its existence histologically since a number of clinical situations can mimic the presence of lymphoma while persistently abnormal imaging studies do not always indicate residual disease. Bulky abdominal or mediastinal masses at presentation, in particular, are often reduced in size by chemotherapy but do not always completely disappear. Specimens from repeat biopsies show that such residual masses frequently consist of only fibrotic tissue and fatty changes, but do not contain any viable tumor. This phenomenon is more frequent in patients with sclerosing lymphoma in which the collagen matrix is not affected by treatment. When radiation therapy is given to residual masses without histological confirmation, the situation can become even more confusing because of radiation-induced fibrosis, particularly in lung tissue adjacent to the mediastinum. When evaluating the response to therapy in patients with intermediate-grade lymphoma, the gallium scan may help to localize disease activity and to guide the biopsy.

Pleural effusions may also represent a diagnostic problem. An exhaustive investigation of the pleural fluid should be carried out in patients whose effusion does not reveal cytological evidence of malignancy. Surface markers of contained cells and, if possible, cytogenetics should be used wherever possible to assist in the establishment of a diagnosis in these circumstances. Benign processes such as constrictive pericarditis secondary to radiation therapy can also closely mimic malignancy by presenting with recurrent pleural effusions, but most of the time in such cases the fluid will show the characteristics of a transudate. However, second malignancies such as carcinoma of the lung can complicate the picture and need to be included in the differential diagnosis.

A serious effort to obtain tissue to establish the presence of tumor should always be made, either by an excisional biopsy or, in cases of deep-seated abdominal masses, by fine-needle aspirate. Repeat biopsy is also mandatory in patients with recurrent low-grade lymphoma to rule out transformation to a large-cell lymphoma.

MANAGEMENT OF RECURRENT OR REFRACTORY LYMPHOMA IN ADULTS

Clinical problems of the adult patient with recurrent lymphoma

The patient with recurrent lymphoma usually tolerates salvage chemotherapy less well than the patient who presents with lymphoma *de novo*. This is largely because most of these patients have had a considerable amount of prior chemotherapy and many of them may also have received radiation therapy to abdominal or pelvic fields (i.e., to a significant

portion of the bone marrow). Also, bone marrow invasion by lymphoma occurs more frequently in patients with recurrent lymphoma than at the time of initial presentation. Nevertheless, administration of maximumally tolerated doses is necessary to achieve a maximal response and provision should be made for adequate supportive management of infections or febrile neutropenic episodes, which occur most often in patients with recurrent disease.

The potential problems of myelosuppression are not the only problems likely to be encountered: metabolic abnormalities are also more common. Biliary and ureteral obstruction are common in the presence of intra-abdominal lymphoma, while renal failure and hyperbilirubinemia complicate the use of some drugs that are metabolized by the liver and kidneys. In such cases, it may be necessary to perform biliary or ureteral decompression by means of a percutaneous catheter or stents until an anti-tumor response is obtained.

CLINICAL FEATURES ASSOCIATED WITH SURVIVAL AFTER RELAPSE OF ADULT LYMPHOMA

Usually the response to salvage therapy correlates well with the degree of response to frontline chemotherapy. Patients who achieved a complete response with frontline chemotherapy have a higher likelihood of response after relapse than those who failed to respond or who only achieved a partial response. Another important variable that correlates with response to therapy in this setting is the serum lactic dehydrogenase (LDH) level; the higher the LDH level, the worse the response to treatment and the shorter the survival [1]. In general, the more relapses a patient has experienced in the past, the more unfavorable the outcome in terms of both response to treatment and survival. Patients with indolent lymphoma will frequently survive for several years, even after multiple relapses [2]. In our patient series, the median survival of patients with low-grade lymphoma after a first or second relapse was 36 months, and after a third relapse was 14 months. Features that were associated with short median survival after relapse were the presence of B symptoms, bulky tumor mass, more than two relapses, LDH > 400 μg/ml (normal= 225 μg/ml), and hemoglobin < 1.5 mmol/l (10 g/dl). Whenever one of these variables was present, the median survival was 28 months, and when two or more were present, it was 8.5 months. On the other hand, when none of these adverse features was present, the median survival had not been reached at 6 years. Another feature associated with a very short median survival was the transformation from low-grade follicular lymphoma to an intermediate-grade type [1].

SINGLE-AGENT CHEMOTHERAPY RESULTS FOR RECURRENT OR REFRACTORY LYMPHOMA IN ADULTS

Before being included as part of combination chemotherapy programs, new agents are offered to patients with relapsing lymphoma and tested individually in phase I and II trials (Table 33.1). Responses obtained in this setting of heavily pretreated patients are usually partial and short lived, resulting only in palliation.

Etoposide (VP-16)

Etoposide is one of the most active agents used to treat recurrent lymphoma. Response rates have varied from 5% in a study performed by the Southwest Oncology Group to 60% in a study conducted in South Africa [3,4]. In a total of 116 patients treated in four different series in which etoposide was used as a single agent, the combined response rate was 22% [5,6]. The broad range of responses observed was due to differences in the prognostic features in each series. Some patients, e.g., those in the Southwest Oncology Group series, were very heavily pretreated. In addition, the dose of etoposide used in the latter study was half of the generally accepted optimal dose, providing good reasons for the worse response rate in this series. The combined response rate in the remaining 60 patients from the three other series was 37%.

In a phase II study of chronic oral etoposide given at 50 mg/m^2 daily for 21 days, 21 patients with refractory lymphoma were evaluable. Fifteen patients had low-grade histologies and 10 had intermediate-grade lymphoma. The overall response rate was 67% for patients with low-grade histologies and 50% for patients with higher-grade malignancies. The median duration of response was 8 and 3 months for patients with low- and intermediate-grade lymphomas respectively [7].

Mitoxantrone

Mitoxantrone is one of the drugs most recently identified as being active against lymphoma. In a collaborative multi-institutional trial in which a dose of 14 mg/m^2 of mitoxantrone was administered every 3 weeks, an overall response rate of 40% was obtained in 122 patients [8]. Of these responses, 32% were partial and 8% were complete. Patients with

Table 33.1 Single-agent activity in lymphomas

Drug	No. of patients	CR (%)	CR+PR (%)	Duration (weeks)	References
Etoposide					
i.v.	116	NA	22	NA	3–6
p.o.	25	NA	60	22	7
Mitoxantrone	122	8	40	NA	8
Ifosfamide	41	NA	68	NA	9
Platinum	19	NA	26	4	13
Methotrexate	26	19	50		14
High dose Ara-C	28	NA	29	10	15
Bleomycin	190	14	41	10	16–18
5-Fluorouracil	21	NA	26	NA	19–23
Fludarabine					
LGL	63	16	54	NA	25–27
IGL	53	8	14	NA	28
2-CDA, LGL	40	20	43	5	29
Pentostatin					
LGL	40	8	28	NA	30
IGL	26	0	8	NA	
Camptothecin	76	16	42	NA	31
Idarubicin	31	10	43	10	12–15
Paclitaxel	6	NA	50	NA	32

CR, complete response; PR, partial response; i.v., intravenous; p.o., oral; NA, not available; Ara-C, cytosine arabinoside; IGL, intermediate-grade lymphomas; LGL, low-grade lymphomas; 2-CDA, 2-chlorodeoxyadenosine.

follicular lymphoma had an overall response rate of 56%, whereas the response rate in patients with large-cell lymphoma was 25%. Median response durations were 8 months in responding patients with low-grade follicular lymphoma, and 6 months in patients with large-cell lymphoma. This median duration of response compares well with that observed in other relapse patients treated with other single agents. Apparently, the schedule of mitoxantrone administration has an important bearing on the response rate. When a weekly schedule of 5 mg/m² for 6 weeks was utilized in a Southeastern Group study, the response rate was only 10% (three of 29 patients) [8].

Ifosfamide

Four independent studies of ifosfamide carried out in the United States and Europe in which a total of 41 patients were treated achieved a combined response rate of 68% [9]. Most of these responses were partial. Some patients who were resistant to cyclophosphamide, however, did respond to ifosfamide. The major dose-limiting toxic effect caused by ifosfamide is hemorrhagic cystitis. With the use of mesna, this complication practically disappears. Another phase II study with ifosfamide, at a dose of 1200 mg/m²/day given for 5 days, incuded 13 patients with high-grade lymphoma refractory to high-dose chemotherapy and total body irradiation [10,11].

Idarubicin

Idarubicin, a relatively new anthracycline with both oral and parenteral activity, has been tested in lymphoma in four clinical trials [12–15]. In two trials, oral idarubicin was used in patients with refractory lymphoma. In the first trial, which included seven patients, no activity was observed, whereas in the second trial a 58% response rate was observed in patients with low-grade lymphoma [13,14]. In the third trial intravenous idarubicin was administered to 14 patients with intermediate- or high-grade lymphoma and several patients with low-grade lymphoma, but none responded to therapy [15]. Finally, 15 mg/m² of idarubicin was administered to 31 patients previously treated with doxorubicin. A median of five cycles of idarubicin cycles were administered. The response rate in this trial was 43% (ten partial and three complete responses), and the median duration of remission was 10+ months (2–29+ months) [12].

Platinum

In early phase I studies, platinum was found to have some activity against lymphoma, but the doses used in those studies were very variable. In a phase II trial carried out by the Cancer and Leukemia Group B, 27 patients, 19 with lymphoma and eight with Hodgkin's disease were accrued [16]. All responses were partial (26%), and the median duration of response was only 6 weeks. The dose used in this study was 70 mg/m² once every 3 weeks.

Methotrexate

As a single agent, high-dose methotrexate with leucovorin rescue has been associated with high response rates, but reponses are usually short lived. In a study in which the dose ranged from 3 to 7 g/m², 26 patients with lymphoma were entered; responses were seen in 13, giving an overall response rate of 50%. Of these responses, five (19%) were complete [17]. The short median duration of responses in this study suggests that as a single agent, this drug is at best of marginal benefit for the treatment of relapsed or refractory lymphoma.

High-dose cytosine arabinoside

In one study in which cytosine arabinoside was administered as a single agent at a dose of 2 g/m² over 3 h every 12 h for a total of 4–8 g/m² per course, the response rate in 28 evaluable patients with malignant lymphoma was 29% (25% in the 32 patients entered). The median response duration, however, was relatively short (10 weeks), ranging from 6 to 33 weeks. None of the responses were complete [18].

Bleomycin

Bleomycin has been extensively studied as a single agent in patients with lymphoma because it was found to be active during its initial clinical trials. Although the contribution of bleomycin to CHOP (see Chapter 42) has been questioned, its activity as a single agent is documented in several studies with a total of 190 patients showing an overall response rate of 41%. Several doses and schedules have been used, which has caused some confusion. It is important to bear in mind that most single-agent trials conducted in patients with lymphoma have used doses of bleomycin that are higher than those used in combination regimens [19,20].

5-Fluorouracil

Traditionally considered to be an effective drug against carcinomas, 5-fluorouracil was shown to give a combined response rate of 28% when used as a single agent in studies conducted during the 1960s [21–24]. This drug, however, has never been tested in combination regimens against lymphoma.

Fludarabine

Fludarabine is an adenine nucleoside analog that has recently been studied in the management of indolent lymphomas. The most prominent activity has been noted in patients with chronic lymphocytic leukemia, but in patients with indolent lymphoma, a 25–30% partial response rate was observed in phase I studies [25]. Subsequent phase II studies have reported complete and partial response rates of more than 50% in several series that included patients with low-grade lymphoma [26–28]. Patients with follicular lymphoma appear to have higher response rates than patients with intermediate-grade lymphoma, for which the response rate from fludarabine treatment appears to be 10% at best.

2-Chlorodeoxyadenosine

2-Cholorodeoxyadenosine is an adenosine deaminase-resistant purine nucleoside that is effective in treating lymphoid malignancies. In patients with low-grade lymphoma the overall response rate observed with doses of 0.1 mg/kg/day fludarabine for 7 days was 43%, 20% of patients achieving complete remissions. The drug has not been tested in more aggressive histologic entities [29].

Deoxycoformycin

Pentostatin or 2'-deoxycoformycin, an adenosine deaminase inhibitor with activity against a variety of hematological malignancies, was studied in 25 patients with refractory lymphoma at a dose of 5 mg/m^2 intravenously for three consecutive days of every 3-week cycle. Seven of these patients had low-grade lymphoma and the rest had unfavorable histologic profiles. The response rate was 20% with no complete remissions. Interestingly, 10 of 31 and two of six patients with cutaneous T-cell lymphoma or low-grade lymphoma, respectively, had responses in this study. All patients had received at least two prior chemotherapy regimens [30]. Pentostatin has been regarded as T-cell-specific chemotherapy because of the promising activity against this lymphoma subset.

Camptothecin analogs

The camptothecin analogs (Camptothecin, Topotecan) are a family of topoisomerase I inhibitors with activity against a variety of solid tumors and lymphoid malignancies. Major responses were observed by Japanese investigators in 49% of 47 patients with recurrent or refractory non-Hodgkin's lymphoma who received CPT-11 for 3 consecutive days each week [31].

Taxol

Taxol (Paclitaxel), a new alkaloid ester that enhances tubulin polymerization and has noncross-resistant activity against a variety of malignancies, was evaluated at the National Cancer Institute in six patients with refractory lymphoma at a dose of 140 mg/m^2 infused over 96 h. Three patients had partial responses, two had minimal responses, and two had progressive disease. All patients had been heavily pretreated less than 6 months before receiving Paclitaxel therapy [32]. This compound is being formally investigated in two other phase II single-agent trials in patients with recurrent lymphoma by the Southwest Oncology Group and The University of Texas MD Anderson Cancer Center.

COMBINATION CHEMOTHERAPY RESULTS

Complete remissions obtained with single agents are scarce and responses are usually short lived. Nevertheless, the observation of some complete responses with different drugs provides the first step in the development of new combinations. If proven effective, regimens tested in recurrent disease can then be incorporated into frontline treatment.

The rationale for combining different chemotherapeutic agents has been based on the single-agent activity of individual components and on the synergism identified between drugs. At the MD Anderson Cancer Center, the first-generation salvage regimens were built on the demonstration of noncross-resistant activities [1] of ifosfamide and etoposide used as single agents. The resultant drug combination, MIME (methyl-GAG, ifosfamide, methotrexate and etoposide) was associated with an overall response rate of 60% and a complete response rate of 25% [33]. Numerous ifosfamide–etoposide trials have been conducted in Europe and the United States with similar complete and overall response rates [33–36] (Table 33.2).

The next generation of salvage regimens resulted from the observed synergism between cytarabine and platinum; the resultant regimen, DHAP (dexamethasone, cytarabine and platinum) [37], gave a response rate similar to MIME. Long-term follow-up showed that close to 10% of patients with intermediate-grade lymphoma are cured with these regimens. Modification of MIME resulted in a combination known as MINE (mesna, ifosfamide, mitoxantrone and etoposide) in which methyl-GAG was replaced by mitoxantrone and methotrexate was deleted. A protocol was developed in which a response-adapted consolidation phase, ESHAP (etoposide, methyl-

Table 33.2   Combination chemotherapy in relapsing or refractory lymphoma

Drugs	Center	No. of patients	CR (%)	CR+PR (%)	References
IM-VP16	MD Anderson	52	37	62	44
MIME	MD Anderson	208	24	60	1
VIM-Bleo	Essen/Germany	30	30	53	34
VIM	Vienna LSG	30	17	33	37
BMV-VIP	Westminster	29	28	NA	36
DHAP	MD Anderson	90	31	55	39
MINE/ESHAP	MD Anderson	42	43	68	40
CEPP-Bleo	Stanford	61	34	70	45
EPOCH	NCI	70	27	87	34
DICE	Toronto	32	22	69	46
IDA/Ara-C	Strasbourg	23	60	64	42
PROMACE/MOPP	Utrecht	31	16	90	47

CR, complete response; PR, partial response; IM-VP16, ifosfamide, methotrexate, etoposide; MIME; methyl-GAG, ifosfamide, methotrexate, etoposide; VIM-Bleo, etoposide, ifosfamide, methotrexate, bleomycin; VIM, etoposide, ifosfamide, mitoxantrone, prednisone; BMV-VIP, bleomycin, methylprednisolone, vindesine, ifosfamide, etoposide; DHAP, dexamethasone, high-dose cytosine arabninoside, platinum; MINE, mesna, ifosfamide, novantrone, etoposide; ESHAP, etoposide, solumedrol (methylprednisolone), high-dose cytosine arabinoside, platinum; CEPP-Bleo, cyclophosphamide, etoposide, procarbazine, prednisone, bleomycin; EPOCH, infusional etoposide, platinum, vincristine, cyclophosphamide, adriamycin; DICE, dexamethasone, ifosfamide, cisplatinum, etoposide; IDA/Ara-C, idarubicin, cytosine arabinoside; PROMACE/MOPP, procarbazine, methotrexate, cytosine arabinoside, etoposide, meclorethamine, vincristine, procarbazine, prednisone; LSG, Lymphoma Study Group, Vienna, Austria; NCI, National Cancer Institute, USA.

prednisolone, cytarabine and cisplatin) was added after best response to MINE was achieved. MINE-ESHAP constitutes the third generation of salvage regimens to be used at MD Anderson. With 42 patients treated, the overall and complete response rates were 69% and 48%, respectively, with a median survival of 24 months and a 2-year disease-free survival of 43% and 37% for patients with low- and intermediate-grade lymphomas respectively [38].

Based on *in vitro* evidence that tumor cells are less resistant to prolonged exposure to low concentrations of drugs derived from natural products than to brief exposure to higher concentrations, a 96-h infusional regimen called EPOCH (etoposide, prednisone, vincristine, cyclophosphamide and doxorubicin) was developed at the National Cancer Institute, Bethesda, USA [39]. Fifty of 74 treated patients had intermediate-grade lymphomas and were evaluable for response. Eighteen (36%) of these patients achieved a complete response and 26 (52%) a partial response, giving an overall response rate of 87%. Interestingly, 71% of the patients had previously received all the drugs contained in the regimen, and 92% had received at least four of the drugs. Since patients in this study who responded received autologous bone marrow transplants, longer-term results will not be available.

In three European studies, the efficacies of the combinations of ifosfamide and mitoxantrone, and idarubicin and cytosine arabinoside was examined. The Yorkshire Regional Lymphoma and Central Lymphoma groups administered ifosfamide at 6 g/m^2 and mitoxantrone at 12 mg/m^2 in 33 patients with recurrent high-grade lymphoma who could be evaluated for response. They observed ten (30%) complete responses and six (18%) partial responses with an overall response rate of 48% [40]. A similar regimen but with an attenuated 1.2 g/m^2 ifosfamide dose was used by investigators at Bari Oncologic Institute. Twenty-two patients with relapsed or refractory lymphoma were treated, and complete and overall response rates of 38% and 57%, respectively, were observed. Only two patients in the trial had low-grade lymphoma; all others had intermediate-grade lymphomas [41]. The combination of idarubicin and cytosine arabinoside was evaluated in a phase II study for relapsed or refractory high- or intermediate-grade lymphoma by Dufour et al [42]. Among 22 patients who could be evaluated, 13 had a complete response and one a partial response giving a 63% overall response rate. The median time to progression was 340 days (60+ to 1348+).

Current treatment strategies for patients younger than 60 years who have relapsed or have refractory intermediate-grade lymphoma include consolidation with high-dose chemotherapy and autologous bone marrow support, or continued therapy with standard-dose chemotherapy. To compare the results of these very different appproaches – conventional therapy versus massive chemotherapy plus autologous bone marrow transplant in patients with relapsed non-Hodgkin's lymphoma, a randomized multicentre study was initiated by the Parma group [43]. Between July 1987 and November 1992, 200 consecutive patients from 49 worldwide institutions were included in the study. All patients with intermediate- or high-grade lymphoma had previously achieved a complete remission, and were included in the study at the time of first or second relapse. All patients received the same rescue protocol, DHAP, for two consecutive courses at 3–4 week intervals. One hundred and eleven patients were in complete or partial remission after two courses of DHAP, and were randomized to receive four additional courses of DHAP or massive chemotherapy with BEAC (carmustine, etoposide, cytarabine and cyclophosphamide) and autologous bone marrow transplantation. With a median follow-up of 63 months the response rate was 84% after bone marrow transplantation and 44% after chemotherapy without transplantation. At five years, the rate of event-free survival was 46% in the transplantation group and 12% in the group receiving chemotherapy without transplantation ($P = 0.001$). The rate of overall survival was 53 and 32% respectively ($P = 0.038$). Based on the PARMA Study treatment with high-dose chemotherapy and bone marrow transplantation is considered today the standard of care in chemotherapy-sensitive relapsing lymphoma.

HIGH-DOSE CHEMOTHERAPY AND AUTOLOGOUS BONE MARROW SUPPORT

Considerable experimental and clinical data support the relevance of dose intensity in chemotherapy-sensitive tumors. The steepness of the dose–response curves is different for drugs and tumors. Although hematopoietic cells can be manipulated to avoid long-term or permanent bone marrow suppression, anticipated toxicity to other organs limits high-dose chemotherapy such that, with present regimens, there is at least a 10% mortality rate. Over the past 20 years the use of high-dose chemotherapy with autologous bone marrow support, which is discussed in detail in Chapter 34, has contributed to our understanding of relapsed and refractory lymphomas. In the first stages of the development, investigators realized that the response to frontline and previous salvage chemotherapy was critical in determining the outcome for patients receiving autologous bone marrow transplantation. Ideally, patients should be in a state of minimal residual disease or clinical complete remission to make cure possible. This is achievable through the use of cytoreductive standard-dose chemotherapy before the administration of high-dose chemotherapy. The ideal combination chemotherapy regimen in this setting has yet to be defined.

DHAP is the most commonly used combination and, although effective, is probably not the best. Finally, with the advent of new purging techniques in bone marrow and peripheral stem cell progenitors, and the availability of molecular probes to detect minimal residual lymphoma, chances for cure may increase in this patient population.

References

1. Cabanillas F, Hagemeister FB, McLaughlin P. Results of MIME salvage regimen for recurrent or refractory lymphoma. *J. Clin. Oncol.* 1987, **5**: 407–412.
2. Spinolo J, Cabanillas F, Dixon DO, et al. Therapy of relapsed or refractory low-grade follicular lymphomas: Factors associated with complete remission, survival and time to treatment failure. *Ann. Oncol.* 1992, **3**: 227–32.
3. Cecil JW, Quagliana JM, Coltman, CA, et al. Evaluation of VP-16–213 in malignant lymphoma and melanoma. *Cancer Treat. Rep.* 1978, **62**: 801–803.
4. Jacobs P, King HS, Cassidy F, et al. VP-16–213 in the treatment of stage III and IV diffuse lymphocytic lymphoma of the large cell (hysticotic) variety: An interim report. *Cancer Treat. Rep.* 1981, **65**: 987–993.
5. Bender R, Anderson T, Fisher RI, et al. Activity of the epipodophyllotoxin VP-16 in the treatment of combination chemotherapy-resistant non-Hodgkin's lymphoma. *Am. J. Hematol.* 1978, **5**(3): 203–209.
6. Dombernowsky P, Nissen N, Larsen V. Clinical investigation of a new podophyllum derivative, epipodophyllotoxin, 4'-demethyl-9-(4,6-O-2-thenylidene-D-glucopyranoside) (NSC-122819), in patients with malignant lymphomas and solid tumors. *Cancer Chemother. Rep.* 1972, **56**: 71–82.
7. Hainsworth JD, Johnson DH, Greco A. Chronic etoposide schedules in the treatment of non-Hodgkin's lymphoma. *Semin. Oncol.* 1992, **6**: 13–18.
8. Gams RA, Bryan S, Dukart G, et al. Mitoxantrone in malignant lymphoma. *Investigational New Drugs* 1985, **3**: 219–222.
9. Brade W, Herdrich K, Varini M. Ifosfamide-pharmacology, safety and therapeutic potential. *Cancer Treat. Rev.* 1985, **12**: 1–47.
10. Case DC Jr, Anderson J, Ervin TJ, et al. Phase II trial of ifosfamide and mesna in previously treated patients with non-Hodgkin's lymphoma: Cancer and leukemia Group B study 8552. *Hematol. Oncol.* 1991, **9**: 189–196.
11. Magrath I, Adde M, Sandlund J, et al. Ifosfamide in the treatment of high-grade recurrent non-Hodgkin's lymphomas. *Hematol. Oncol.* 1991. 9: 267–274.
12. Case DC, Hayes DM, Gerber M. Phase II study of oral idarubicin in favorable histology non-Hodgkin's lymphoma. *Cancer Res.* 1990, **50**: 6833–6835.
13. Coonley CJ, Warrell RP Jr, Straus DJ, et al. Clinical evaluation of 4-demethoxydaunorubicin in patients with advanced malignant lymphoma. *Cancer Treat. Rep.*, 1983, **67**: 949–950.
14. Lopez M, DiLauro L, Papaldo P. Oral idarubicin in non-Hodgkin's lymphoma. *Investigational New Drugs*

1986, **4**: 263–267.

15. Case DC, Gerber MC, Gams RA. Phase II study of intravenous idarubicin in unfavorable non-Hodgkin's lymphoma. *Leukemia Lymphoma* 1993, **10**: 73–79.

16. Cavalli F, Jungi WF, Nissen NI, et al. Phase II trial of cis-dichlorodiamminoplatinum (II) in advanced malignant lymphoma: A study of the Cancer and Leukemia Group B. *Cancer*, 1981, **48**: 1927–1930.

17. Frei E, Blum RH, Pitman SW, et al. High-dose methotrexate with leucovorin rescue. Rationale and spectrum of antitumor activity. *Am. J. Med.* 1980, **68**: 370–376.

18. Kantarjian H, Barlogie B, Plunkett W, et al. High-dose cytosine arabinoside in non-Hodgkin's lymphoma. *J. Clin. Oncol.* 1983, **1**: 689–694.

19. Haas CD, Coltman CA, Gottlieb JA. Phase II evaluation of bleomycin. A Southwest Oncology Group Study. *Cancer* 1976, **38**: 8–12.

20. Rudders RA. Treatment of advanced malignant lymphomas with bleomycin. *Blood* 1972, **40**: 317–332.

21. Olson K, Greene J. Evaluation of 5-fluorouracil in the treatment of cancer. *J. Natl Cancer Inst.* 1960, **25**: 133.

22. Kennedy B, Theologides A. Uracil mustard, a new alkylating agent for oral administration in the management of patients with leukemia and lymphoma. *N. Engl. J. Med.* 1961, **263**: 790–793.

23. Ansfield F, Schroeder J, Curreri A. Five years clinical experience with 5-fluorouracil. *JAMA* 1962, **181**: 295–299.

24. Moore G, Bross I, Ausman R. Effects of 5-fluorouracil (NSC-19893) in 389 patients with cancer. Eastern Clinical Drug Evaluation Program. *Cancer Chemother. Rep.* 1968, **52**: 641.

25. Hochster H, Cassileth P. Fludarabine phosphate therapy of non-Hodgkin's lymphoma. *Semin. Oncol.* 1990, **17**: 63–65.

26. Chun HG, Leyland-Jones B, Cheson BD. Fludarabine phosphate: A synthetic purine antimetabolite with significant activity against lymphoid malignancies. *J. Clin. Oncol.* 1991, **9**: 175–188.

27. Redman JR, Cabanillas F, Velasquez WS, et al. Phase II trial of fludarabine phosphate in lymphoma: An effective new agent in low-grade lymphoma. *J. Clin. Oncol.* 1992, **10**(5): 790–794.

28. Keating MJ. Fludarabine in malignant lymphoma: Present status and future possibilities. *Fifth International Conference on Malignant Lymphoma* 1993, Lugano, Switzerland.

29. Saven A, Piro LD. 2-Chlorodeoxyadenosine: A new nucleoside agent effective in the treatment of lymphoid malignancies. *Leukemia Lymphoma* 1993, **10**: 43–49.

30. Cummings FJ, Kim K, Neiman RS, et al. Phase II trial of Pentostatin in refractory lymphomas and cutaneous T-cell disease. *J. Clin. Oncol.* 1991, **9**: 565–571.

31. Slichenmyer WJ, Rowinsky EK, Donehower RC, et al. The current status of Camptothecin analogues as antitumor agents. *J. Natl Cancer Inst.* 1993, **85**: 271–293.

32. Wilson WH, Chabner B, Bryant G, et al. Phase II study of Paclitaxel in relapsed non-Hodgkin's lymphoma. *J. Clin. Oncol.* 1995, **13**: 381–386.

33. Cabanillas F, Velasquez WS, McLaughlin P, et al. Results of recent salvage chemotherapy regimens for lymphoma and Hodgkin's disease. *Semin. Hematol.* 1988, **25**(2 Suppl. 2): 47–50.

34. Nowrousian M, Anders C, Niederle N. Etoposide, ifosfamide, and methotrexate with or without bleomycin in refractory or recurrent lymphomas. *Ann. Oncol.* 1991, **2**: 25–30.

35. Heinz R, Dittric H, Ludwig H. Results of a new drug combination (VP-16-ifosfamide–mitoxatrone–bleomicin) VIM-Bleo in advanced non-Hodgkin's lymphomas. *Contrib. Oncol.* 1987, **?**: 438–445.

36. Retsas S, Baughan C. The BMV-VIP regimen in the treatment of refractory lymphomata. *Contrib. Oncol.* 1987, **26**: 400–407.

37. Velazquez W, Cabanillas F, Salvador P. Effective salvage therapy for lymphoma with cisplatin in combinations with high dose Ara-C and dexamethasone (DHAP). *Blood* 1988, **71**: 117–122.

38. Rodriguez MA, Cabanillas FC, Velazquez WS. Results of a salvage treatment program for relapsing lymphoma: MESNA/ifosfamide, novantrone, and etoposide (MINE), consolidated with etoposide, solumedrol, high dose arabinoside and cisplatinum (ESHAP). *J. Clin. Oncol.* 1995, **13**: 1734–1741.

39. Wilson WH, Bryant G, Bates S, et al. EPOCH chemotherapy: Toxicity and efficacy in relapsed and refractory non-Hodgkin's lymphoma. *J. Clin. Oncol.* 1993, **11**: 1573–1582.

40. Child JA, Simmons AV, Barnard DL. Twin-track studies of ifosfamide and mitoxantrone (I-M) in recurrent high-grade non-Hodgkin's lymphoma and Hodgkin's disease. *Hematol. Oncol.* 1991, **9**: 235–244.

41. Lorusso V, Paradiso A, Guida M, et al. Ifosfamide plus mitoxantrone as salvage treatment in Non-Hodgkin's lymphomas. *Am. J. Clin. Oncol.* 1991, **14**: 492–495.

42. Dufour P, Mors R, Lamy T. Idarubicin (IDA) and high dose aracytine (HD-ara-C): A new promising salvage treatment in relapsed or refractory non Hodgkin's lymphoma. *Proceedings of the American Society for Clinical Oncology* 1993.

43. Guglielmi C, et al. The PARMA International randomized prospective study in relapsed non Hodgkins lymphoma: Second interim analysis of 172 patients and update (at 20/11/92: 200 patients). *Fifth International Conference on Malignant Lymphoma* 1993. Kluwer Academic Publishers.

44. Cabanillas F, Hagemeister FB, Bodey GP, et al. IMVP-16, an effective regimen for patients with lymphoma who have relapsed after initial combination chemotherapy. *Blood* 1982, **60**: 693–697.

45. Chao NJ, Rosenberg SA, Horning SJ. CEPP(B): An effective and well-tolerated regimen in poor-risk, aggressive non-Hodgkin's lymphoma. *Blood* 1990, **76**: 1293–1298.

46. Goss P. New perspectives in the treatment of non-Hodgkin's lymphoma. *Semin. Oncol.* 1992, **19**: 23–30.

47. Verdonck L, Dekker AW, de Gast GC, Salvage therapy with ProMACE-MOPP followed by intensive chemoradiotherapy and autologous bone marrow transplantation for patients with non-Hodgkin's lymphoma who failed to respond to first-line CHOP. *J. Clin. Oncol.* 1992, **12**: 1949–1954.

48. Philip T, Guglielmi C, Hagenbeek A, et al. Autologous bone marrow transplantation as compared with salvage chemotherapy in relapses of chemotherapy-sensitive non-Hodgkin's lymphoma. *N. Engl. J. Med.* 1995, **333**: 1540–1545.

CHAPTER 34

Bone marrow transplantation for non-Hodgkin's lymphomas

JULIE M. VOSE AND JAMES O. ARMITAGE

Introduction

Significant advances have been made in the development of combination chemotherapy for the treatment of the non-Hodgkin's lymphomas (NHLs) over the past two decades. However, only 30–50% of the patients receiving third-generation chemotherapy regimens will achieve long-term disease-free survival [1–4]. Although numerous regimens have been designed, which include using new, active drugs, increasing the dose intensity of the drugs, or administering drugs with alternative schedules, a clearly superior regimen has yet to be identified [5].

The use of salvage chemotherapy after the failure of frontline chemotherapy for intermediate- or high-grade NHL has been disappointing; less than 5–10% of patients achieve long-term, disease-free survival with this therapy [6–10]. Following the principles of the dose–response effect established by Frei and Canellos, very intensive high-dose chemo-/radiotherapy regimens were designed for the treatment of the patients who had failed frontline chemotherapy. The chemotherapy and/or radiotherapy used in such regimens was designed to have myelosuppression as the major toxicity while limiting nonmyelosuppressive toxicity as much as possible. Although not all such regimens were expected to induce permanent myelosuppression, hematopoietic rescue was included in order to shorten the duration of pancytopenia. As will be discussed in this chapter, the use of high-dose chemo-/radiotherapy and hematopoietic stem cell transplantation has become very well established as treatment for patients with NHL who have failed frontline therapy. In addition, its use as part of the primary therapy of patients with high-risk NHL is currently being extensively evaluated. The use of hematopoietic growth factors has greatly decreased the infectious complications associated with this procedure and allowed its use in a wider range of patient populations.

Rationale for high-dose chemo-/radiotherapy and transplantation

The basic principles of dose escalation were first proposed by Skipper et al. [11] from experiments on the transplantable mouse leukemia, L1210. They proposed that, for a given tumor, a particular dose of an alkylating agent drug would result in a specific number of logs reduction in the tumor cell burden. Therefore, the amount of tumor present and the size of the dose would determine whether the subject was curable. As the intensity of chemotherapy is increased, many agents cause myelosuppression which at some point is fatal in the absence of hematopoietic reconstitution. If myelosuppression could be ignored as a factor in selecting therapy, the intensity of the treatment could be increased significantly with the aim of overcoming the chemotherapy resistance of the malignant clone. The choice of the drugs used in the regimen, however, cannot be based exclusively on their efficacy in conventional doses for treatment of NHL. For example, intercalating agents such as adriamycin when given at conventional doses are very valuable for the treatment of NHL, but are of limited value in dose escalation therapy owing to other organ toxicities which become dose limiting, such as cardiotoxicity.

Because of these limitations in the use of certain chemotherapeutic agents, the noncycle-specific agents such as the alkylating agents and nitrosoureas have become the most commonly used for dose escalation. Unlike patients with Hodgkin's disease, most patients with NHLs have not received extensive radiotherapy as part of their initial treatment. Therefore, total body irradiation (TBI) is frequently also used as part of the conditioning regimen. There are theoretical reasons for believing that the addition of TBI would be beneficial. Like the alkylating agents and nitrosoureas, it is not dependent on the cell cycle for tumor destruction, and many (NHLs) are relatively radiosensitive. However, TBI is not without nonmyelosuppressive toxicity, and evaluation of the relative outcomes with TBI- and non-TBI containing regimens is ongoing.

The dose intensity of any preparative regimen must be based on the 'window of opportunity'. In other words, the doses of the agents used must be high enough to effectively treat the NHLs but should not result in severe nonhematologic toxicity. Hematologic toxicity must be sufficiently ameliorated, by the use of hematopoietic stem cells from an autologous, allogeneic or syngeneic source, that the treatment has an acceptable morbidity and mortality rate. Each

optimal source of hematopoietic stem cells has advantages and disadvantages but, as yet, randomized trials designed to identify the optimal source have not been conducted.

Clinical studies in transplantation

INTERMEDIATE-GRADE NHLS AND IMMUNOBLASTIC NHL

Historical perspectives

The development of combination drug regimens for induction therapy of patients with newly diagnosed intermediate-grade NHLs has been one of the greatest successes of oncology over the past two decades. The development of the original CHOP regimen (cyclophosphamide, doxorubicin, vincristine and prednisone) for the treatment of patients with NHLs produced a 45–55% complete response rate with a 30–35% long-term disease-free survival rate [1]. Various strategies were explored in attempting to increase the long-term disease-free survival rate including the addition of other agents to the original CHOP regimen and the use of alternating noncross-resistant therapies. Regimens such as m-BACOD (methotrexate, bleomycin, doxorubicin, cyclophosphamide, vincristine and dexamethasone), MACOP-B (methotrexate, doxorubicin, cyclophosphamide, vincristine and bleomycin), and ProMACE-CytaBOM (prednisone, doxorubicin, cyclophosphamide and etoposide, followed by cytarabine, bleomycin, vincristine and methotrexate) initially appeared to produce improved complete response rates of 60–80% [2–4], but in a prospective randomized trial the long-term disease-free survival of patients treated with the newer regimens was similar to that of patients treated with the original CHOP regimen [5]. Subset analysis of this study failed to identify any group that benefited from a particular regimen [5].

Just as progress in the primary therapy of patients with NHL appears to have stalled, the treatment of relapsed NHL with conventional salvage chemotherapy has, not surprisingly, been disappointing. Many salvage regimens have been formulated over the last two decades, including DHAP (dexamethasone, cytarabine and cisplatin), MIME (ifosfamide, methyl-GAG and etoposide), and IMVP-16 (ifosfamide, methotrexate and etoposide) [6–8]. Although patients often have partial responses to these agents, complete responses are reported in only 20–30% of cases and are usually of short duration [6–10]. In a review of 16 studies, Singer and Goldstone found that only 12 of 398 relapsed patients treated with a variety of different chemotherapeutic programs were in continuous complete remission at 2 years [12]. The poor results of conventional salvage chemotherapy prompted the investigation of high-dose chemotherapy with hematopoietic rescue in this patient population.

Patient selection for transplantation

Because high-dose chemotherapy and autologous transplantation is highly toxic, most studies have limited the use of this therapy to patients under age 60, who have good end-organ function and performance status. Allogeneic transplantation is usually limited to patients under the age of 45–50 . Most reported studies have focused on patients who have either never achieved complete remission or have relapsed after an initial complete remission and have subsequently been treated with high-dose chemotherapy. Within this group of patients, several categories have been evaluated, which are outlined below.

Refractory to induction therapy

Most studies of high-dose chemotherapy and autologous bone marrow transplantation in this group of

patients show a 0–10% long-term disease-free survival rate at 2–3 years posttransplant (Table 34.1) [13–15]. These patients are highly chemotherapy resistant and an alternative approach may be necessary to increase the chance of survival in this patient population.

Resistant relapse

Patients who have relapsed after initial complete remission following induction chemotherapy and are not responsive to salvage chemotherapy have been reported to have a long-term disease-free survival of 14–25% in most series (Table 34.1) [13–18].

Sensitive relapse

Patients who have relapsed after initial complete remission following induction chemotherapy and are responsive to further salvage chemotherapy have been reported to have a long-term disease-free survival of 35–60% in several publications (Table 34.1) [13–18].

Many centers will now only accept patients for high-dose chemotherapy and autologous bone marrow transplant if their recurrent disease has been to be sensitive to salvage chemotherapy. However, some centers are continuing to evaluate the use of alternative preparative regimens or other adjuvant

Table 34.1 Results of high-dose chemotherapy and transplantation for relapsed intermediate-grade non-Hodgkin's lymphomas

Reference	Status at BMT	Regimen	Results (survival in months)
13	Never in CR Resistant relapse Sensitive relapse	Variable	0% (12) 14% (54) 36% (75)
14	Induction failure Refractory relapse Sensitive relapse	Cy/TBI	10% (48) 28% (36) 50% (72)
15	Induction failure Refractory relapse Sensitive relapse	Variable	0% (3) 10% (36) 45% (62)
16	Resistant relapse Sensitive relapse	BEP	3/9 pts (57) 12/18 pts (56)
17	Resistant relapse Sensitive relapse	Variable	10% (28) 50% (75)
18	Complete remission Sensitive relapse Progressive disease	VP/Cy/TBI	80% (70) 60% (84) 11% (14)

BMT, Bone marrow transplantation; CR, complete remission; Cy, cyclophosphamide; TBI, total body irradiation; BEP, bleomycin, etoposide, cis-platinum; VP, etoposide (VP16).

The future of bone marrow transplantation for NHLs

TIMING ISSUES

With the clarification of prognostic factors that may affect the long-term outcome of patients receiving standard induction chemotherapy for NHL, the use of high-dose chemotherapy and transplantation in first CR or partial response (PR) has been suggested as a possible alternative for high-risk patients. Several pilot trials have now demonstrated a possible improvement in the outcome for high-risk patients treated with this modality [25–28]. No randomized trials in high-risk patients have been initiated to test this hypothesis in the United States, but a few trials conducted in Europe have demonstrated an advantage for high-risk patients treated with high-dose chemotherapy and ABMT compared to conventional therapy [109–110]. One large trial by Haion et al, using high-dose chemotherapy with the CVB regimen and ABMT compared to an intensive consolidation therapy, demonstrated no overall difference in disease-free survival between the two groups [111]. However, when the international prognostic factor index was applied to these patients, those in the index 3 groups had a 20% improvement in disease-free survival (DFS) in the ABMT group (*P*=0.07) [111]. Further analysis of the use of high-dose chemotherapy and ABMT in high-risk patients is warranted.

IMMUNOMODULATION

Another area of intensive investigation involves the use of immunomodulating agent following transplantation to decrease the risk of relapse in those patients with minimal residual disease remaining after transplant. Agents such as interferon-α, interleukin-2 (IL-2), Bestatin, and anti-B4 (CD19)-blocked ricin are currently undergoing preliminary trials [112–115]. Manipulation of the hematopoietic graft product with agents such as IL-2 in order to increase the natural killer cell activity infused may also be another method to investigate as a means of increasing the antitumor effect of the transplant.

RADIOIMMUNOCONJUGATES WITH ABMT

Some promising results in the use of radioimmunoconjugates for the treatment of relapsed NHL

have recently been obtained [116,117]. Kaminski et al. [116] administered ^{131}I-labeled anti-CD20 to nine patients with relapsed B-cell NHLs. Six of the nine patients had tumor responses, and four patients remained in complete remission at 8, 8+, 9+ and 11+ months. If these initial studies can be confirmed, one possible way to increase the antilymphoma effect of high-dose chemotherapy and ABMT would be to add radioimmunoconjugate therapy to this procedure as part of the preparative regimen. Because the major toxicity associated with radioimmunoconjugate therapy is myelosuppression, the use of this therapy with high-dose chemotherapy and ABMT could have additive antitumor benefits without additional nonhematopoietic toxicities. This concept has been tested in a phase I trial for the treatment of Hodgkin's disease and found to be feasible [118]. Further analysis of the use of radioimmunoconjugates with transplantation is continuing.

MULTIPLE HIGH-DOSE CHEMOTHERAPY CYCLES

With the advent of mobilized peripheral blood progenitors and hematopoietic growth factors, high-dose chemotherapy and autologous transplant is now associated with less morbidity and mortality than in previous years. It is also one of the few areas in medicine where the cost of the procedure has decreased over the past years instead of increased [86]. This progress has led to the development of another approach to high-dose therapy – the use of multiple high-dose chemotherapy cycles supported by peripheral blood progenitors. This therapy is feasible in some but not all patients; in heavily pretreated patients there may be difficulty in achieving stem cell mobilization, there may be excessive morbidity associated with the first cycle, or financial concerns may preclude this approach. The overall improvement in long-term disease-free survival using 'tandem transplants' has yet to be demonstrated, but further analysis of this and other techniques to improve the outcome of patients undergoing high-dose therapy and transplantation is ongoing.

Conclusions

Following relapse from standard induction chemotherapy, treatment with conventional dose chemotherapy salvages fewer than 10% of the patients (6–8). The use of high-dose chemotherapy and transplant in the setting of relapsed NHL can offer the possibility of an improvement in these results to 25–50% [13–15]. The correlation between chemotherapy sensitivity [13,17] and other prognostic factors present at the time of transplant and the patient's response to transplant is now well recognized [30]. With improvements in supportive care measures, such as hematopoietic growth factors, this technology has now expanded to high-risk NHL patients as an integrated part of their induction therapy while they are in first PR/CR. The optimal timing for this therapy and its advantages and disadvantages need to be further evaluated in prospective randomized trials.

There are a number of issues regarding transplantation which continue to be debated. These include the optimal high-dose ablative regimen, the optimal source of hematopoietic stem cells, and the need for additional post-transplant therapy such as immunomodulating agents or monoclonal antibody therapy.

The choice of the ablative regimen continues to be a matter of significant debate. To date, no preparative regimen has been shown to be superior to any other. A successful regimen must have maximum dose intensity and tumoricidal activity with minimal nonhematopoietic toxicity. The use of TBI may be of concern because of increased short- and long-term toxicity. Although an increase in secondary MDS and AML has been noted in those patients receiving TBI in one study, the overall outcome was not affected by this incidence [66]. Certain histologic subtypes, such as follicular NHL may benefit from the use of TBI as compared to intermediate NHL.

The optimal source of hematopoietic stem cells also has not been adequately studied. There is a definite theoretical advantage for the use of allogeneic bone marrow with the 'graft-versus-lymphoma' effect. However, the lack of HLA-identical sibling donors, and the increased toxicities associated with this procedure, have not allowed a statistical benefit to be seen in clinical trials comparing allogeneic transplants to autologous transplants, with the possible exception of lymphoblastic NHL [40]. The concern over occult tumor cells in autologous bone marrow or peripheral blood progenitors is appropriate since lymphoma cells have been detected in autologous hematopoietic cell sources in a number of trials [78]. However, the contribution of these cells to the eventual relapse is unknown in lymphoma patients. There is some evidence that for intermediate-grade NHL there is less tumor cell contamination in the peripheral blood compared to the bone marrow [80]. Along with the ease of collection of peripheral blood progenitors with modern mobilization techniques, this has popularized their use for transplantation over the past few years. Randomized trials will be necessary to confirm any differences that may exist between the two techniques.

Now that the ability of high-dose chemotherapy and transplantation to produce long-term disease-free survival in a percentage of patients has been defined in multiple studies, the next frontier concerning transplantation will include the investigation of newer chemotherapeutic agents or additional agents such as immunomodulating agents and monoclonal antibodies to add antitumor activity to the transplant regimen. It will not be possible to further escalate dose to any great extent in the currently available ablative regimens owing to the non-hematologic toxicities of the agents. Therefore, additional tumoricidal activity must be added by agents which have little or no toxicity other than hematologic toxicity, such as radioimmunoconjugates, or by stimulating endogenous host immune responses such as T-cell-mediated functions and natural killer activity. These techniques doubtless will be evaluated in the near future for their impact on disease-free survival for patients undergoing high-dose chemotherapy and transplantation for lymphoma.

References

1. DeVita VT Jr, Canellos GP, Chabner B, Schein P, Hubbard SP, Young RC. Advanced diffuse histiocytic lymphoma, a potentially curable disease. *Lancet* 1975, **1**: 248–250.
2. Shipp MA, Harrington DP, Klatt MM, et al. Identification of major prognostic subgroups of patients with large-cell lymphoma treated with m-BACOD or M-BACOD. *Ann. Intern. Med.* 1986, **104**: 757–765.
3. Klimo P, Connors JM. MACOP-B chemotherapy for the treatment of diffuse large-cell lymphoma. *Ann. Intern. Med.* 1985, **102**: 596–602.
4. Fisher RI, DeVita VT, Hubbard SM, et al. Randomized trial of ProMACE-MOPP vs. ProMACE-CytaBOM in previously untreated, advanced stage, diffuse aggressive lymphomas. *Proc. Am. Soc. Clin. Oncol.* 1984, **3**: 242.
5. Fisher RI, Gaynor ER, Dahlberg S, Oken MM, Grogan TM, et al. Comparison of a standard regimen (CHOP) with three intensive chemotherapy regimens for advanced non-Hodgkin's lymphoma. *N. Engl. J. Med.* 1993, **328**: 1002–1006.
6. Cabanillas F, Hagemeister FB, Bodey GP, Freireich EJ. IMVP-16: An effective regimen for patients with lymphoma who have relapsed after initial combination chemotherapy. *Blood* 1982, **60**: 693–697.
7. Velasquez WS, Cabanillas F, Salvador P, et al. Effective salvage therapy for lymphoma with cisplatin in combination with high-dose Ara C and dexamethasone (DHAP). *Blood* 1988, **71**: 117–122.
8. Cabanillas F, Hagemeister FB, McLaughlin P, et al. Results of MIME salvage regimen for recurrent or

logous stem cell transplantation for lymphoid malignancy: Characterization and relative risk. *Proceedings of the Fifth International Conference on Lymphoma.* 1993, p. 42a. Kluwer Academic Publishers.

67. Appelbaum FR, Fefer A, Cheever MA, et al. Treatment of non-Hodgkin's lymphoma with marrow transplantation in identical twins. *Blood* 1981, **58**: 509–513.

68. Appelbaum FR, Sullivan KM, Buckner CD, et al. Treatment of malignant lymphoma in 100 patients with chemotherapy, total body irradiation, and marrow transplantation. *J. Clin. Oncol.* 1987, **5**: 1340–1347.

69. Jones RJ, Ambinder RF, Piantadosi S, Santos GW. Evidence of a graft-versus-lymphoma effect associated with allogeneic bone marrow transplantation. *Blood* 1991, **77**: 649–653.

70. Shepherd JD, Barnett MJ, Connors JM, et al. Allogeneic bone marrow transplantation for poor-prognosis non-Hodgkin's lymphoma. *Bone Marrow Transplant.* 1993, **12**: 591–596.

71. Phillips GL, Herzig RH, Lazarus HM, et al. High-dose chemotherapy, fractionated total-body irradiation and allogeneic marrow transplantation for malignant lymphoma. *J. Clin. Oncol.* 1986, **4**: 480–488.

72. Baro J, Richard C, Sierra J, et al. Autologous bone marrow transplantation in 22 adult patients with lymphoblastic lymphoma responsive to conventional dose chemotherapy. *Bone Marrow Transplant.* 1992, **10**: 33–38.

73. Kessinger A, Armitage JO, Smith DM, et al. High-dose therapy and autologous peripheral blood stem cell transplantation for patients with lymphoma. *Blood* 1989, **74**: 1260–1265.

74. Brice P Marolleua JP, Dombret H, et al. Autologous peripheral blood stem cell transplantation after high dose therapy in patients with advanced lymphomas. *Bone Marrow Transplant.* 1992, **9**: 337–342.

75. Klumpp TR, Mangan KF, Glenn LD, et al. Phase I/II study of high-dose cyclophosphamide, etoposide and cisplatin followed by autologous bone marrow or peripheral blood stem cell transplantation in patients with poor prognosis Hodgkin's disease or non-Hodgkin's lymphoma. *Bone Marrow Transplant.* 1993, **12**: 337–345.

76. Pettengell R, Testa NG, Swindell R, et al. Transplantation potential of hematopoietic cells released into the circulation during routine chemotherapy for non-Hodgkin's lymphoma. *Blood* 1993, **82**: 2239–2248.

77. Vose JM, Anderson JR, Kessinger A, et al. High-dose chemotherapy and autologous hematopoietic stem-cell transplantation for aggressive non-Hodgkin's lymphoma. *J. Clin. Oncol.* 1993, **11**: 1846–1851.

78. Sharp JG, Joshi SS, Armitage JO, et al. Significance of detection of occult non-Hodgkin's lymphoma in histologically uninvolved bone marrow by a culture technique. *Blood* 1992, **79**: 1074–1080.

79. Treleaven JG, Kemshead JT. Removal of tumor cells from bone marrow: An evaluation of the available techniques. *Hematol. Oncol.* 1985, **3**: 65–75.

80. Sharp JG, Crouse DA. Marrow contamination Detection and significance. In Armitage J, Antman K (eds) *High-dose Cancer Therapy Pharmacology, Hematopoietins, Stem Cells.* Baltimore: Williams & Wilkins, 1992, pp. 226–248.

81. Berenson RJ, Shpall EJ, Franklin W, et al. Transplantation of CD34 positive (+) marrow and/or peripheral blood progenitor cells (PBPC) into breast cancer patients following high-dose chemotherapy (HDC). *Blood* 1993, 678a.

82. Wagner JE, Broxmeyer JE, Byrd RL, et al. Transplantation of umbilical cord blood after myeloablative therapy: Analysis of engraftment. *Blood* 1992, **79**: 1874–1881.

83. Koller MR, Emerson SG, Palsson BO. Large-scale expansion of human stem and progenitor cells from bone marrow mononuclear cells in continuous perfusion cultures. *Blood* 1993, **82**: 378–384.

84. Link H, Boogaerts MA, Carella AM, et al. A controlled trial of recombinant human granulocyte–macrophage colony-stimulating factor after total body irradiation, high-dose chemotherapy, and autologous bone marrow transplantation for acute lymphoblastic leukemia or malignant lymphoma. *Blood* 1992, **80**: 2188–2195.

85. Nemunaitis J, Rabinowe SN, Singer JW, et al. Recombinant granulocyte macrophage colony-stimulating factor after autologous bone marrow transplantation for lymphoid cancer. *N. Engl. J. Med.* 1991, **324**: 1773–1778.

86. Bennett CL, Armitage JL, Armitage GO, et al. A 'learning curve' exists in autologous transplantation for Hodgkin's disease and non-Hodgkin's lymphoma as evidenced by improvements in cost and in-hospital mortality. *Blood* 1993, **82**: 571a.

87. Gorin NC, Coiffier B, Hayat M, et al. Recombinant human granulocyte–macrophage colony-stimulating factor after high-dose chemotherapy and autologous bone marrow transplantation with unpurged and purged marrow in non-Hodgkin's lymphoma: A double-blind placebo-controlled trial. *Blood* 1992, **80**: 1149–1157.

88. Nemunaitis J, Buckner CD, Appelbaum FR, et al. Phase I trial with recombinant human interleukin-3 (IL-3) in patients with lymphoid cancer undergoing autologous bone marrow transplantation (ABMT). *Blood* 1992, **80**: 331a.

89. Lazarus HM, Winton EF, Williams SF, et al. Phase I study of recombinant human interleukin-6 (IL-6) after autologous bone marrow transplant (ABMT) in patients with poor-prognosis breast cancer. *Blood* 1993, **82**: 677a.

90. Gordon MS, Battiato L, Hoffman R, et al. Subcutaneously (SC) administered recombinant human interleukin-11 prevents thrombocytopenia following chemotherapy (CT) with cyclophosphamide (C) and doxorubicin (A) in women with breast cancer (BC). *Blood* 1993, **82**: 1258a.

91. Vose JM, Anderson J, Bierman PJ, et al. Initial trial of PIXY321 (GM-CSF/IL-3) fusion protein following high-dose chemotherapy and autologous bone marrow transplantation (ABMT) for lymphoid malignancy. *Proceedings of the ASCO* 1993, p. 1237a. W.B. Saunders.

92. Link H, Fauser A, Hubner G, et al. Recombinant human erythropoietin after bone marrow transplantation: A prospective placebo controlled trial in Europe. *Blood* 1993, **82**: 1123a.

93. Miller CB, Mills SR, Barnett AG, et al. A randomized trial of recombinant human erthropoietin (rHuEPO) after purged autologous bone marrow transplant (BMT). *Blood* 1993, **82**: 1124a.

94. Peters WP, Stuart A, Affronti ML, et al. Neutrophil migration is defective during recombinant human granulocyte–macrophage colony-stimulating factor infusion after autologous bone marrow transplantation in humans. *Blood* 1988, **72**: 1310–1315.

95. Nemunaitis J, Meyers JD, Buckner CD, et al. Phase I trial of recombinant human macrophage colony-stimulating factor in patients with invasive fungal infections. *Blood* 1991, **78**: 907–913.

96. Gurwitz MJ, Brunton JL, Lank BA, et al. A prospective controlled investigation of prophylaxis in patients with cancer: A double-blind randomized placebo-controlled trial. *J. Pediatr.* 1983, **102**: 125–129.

97. Schmidt GM, Horak DA, Niland JC, et al. A randomized, controlled trial of prophylactic ganciclovir for cytomegalovirus pulmonary infection in recipients of allogeneic bone marrow transplants. *N. Engl. J. Med.* 1991, **324**: 1005–1009.

98. Vose J, Kennedy BC, Bierman PJ, et al. Long-term sequelae of autologous bone marrow transplantation or peripheral stem cell transplantation for lymphoid malignancies. *Cancer* 1992, **69**: 784–788.

99. Sullivan KM, Kopeck KJ, Jocom J, et al. Immuno-modulatory and antimicrobial efficacy of intravenous immunoglobulin in bone marrow transplantation. *N. Engl. J. Med.* 1990, **323**: 705–712.

100. Graham-Pole J, Camitta B, Casper J, et al. Intravenous immunoglobulin may lessen all forms of infection in patients receiving allogeneic bone marrow transplantation for acute lymphoblastic leukemia: A Pediatric Oncology Group study. *Bone Marrow Transplant.* 1988, **3**: 559–563.

101. Winick NJ, McKenna RW, Shuster JJ, et al. Secondary acute myeloid leukemia in children with acute lymphoblastic leukemia treated with etoposide. *J. Clin. Oncol.* 1993, **11**: 209–217.

102. van Leeuwen FE, Somers R, Taal BG, et al. Increased risk of lung cancer, non-Hodgkin's lymphoma, and leukemia following Hodgkin's disease. *J. Clin. Oncol.* 1989, **7**: 1046–1058.

103. Miller JS, Arthur DC, Litz CE, et al. Myelodysplastic syndrome following autologous bone marrow transplantation: An additional late complication of curative cancer therapy. *Blood* 1993, **82**: 1804a.

104. Traweek ST, Slovak ML, Nademanee AP, et al. Myelodysplasia occurring after autolgous bone marrow transplantation (ABMT) for Hodgkin's disease (HD) and non-Hodgkin's lymphoma (NHL). *Blood* 1993, **82**: 1805a.

105. Chao NJ, Tierney K, Bloom JR, et al. Dynamic assessment of quality of life after autologous bone marrow transplantation. *Blood* 1992, **80**: 825–830.

106. Winer EP, Sutton LM. Quality of life after bone marrow transplantation. *Oncology* 1994, **8**: 19–27.

107. Syrjala KL, Chapko MK, Vitaliano PP, et al. Recovery after allogeneic marrow transplantation: Prospective study of predictors of long-term physical and psychosocial functioning. *Bone Marrow Transplant.* 1993, **11**: 319–327.

108. Sullivan KM, Agura E, Anasetti C, et al. Chronic graft-versus-host disease and other late complications after marrow transplantation. *Semin. Hematol.* 1991, **28**: 250–259.

109. Zinzani PL, Tura S, Mazza P, et al. ABMT vs. DHAP in residual disease following third generation regimens for aggressive non-Hodgkin's lymphoma. *Proceedings of the Fifth International Conference on Malignant Lymphoma* 1993, p. 41a. Kluwer Academic Publishers.

110. Sweetenham JW, Proctor SJ, Blaise D, et al. High dose therapy and autologous bone marrow transplantation (ABMT) in first complete remission for adult patients with high-grade non-Hodgkin's lymphoma: The EBMT experience. *Ann. Oncol.* 1994, **5** (Suppl. 2): s155–s159.

111. Haioun C, Lepage E, Gisselbrecht C, et al. Comparison of autologous bone marrow transplantation (ABMT) with sequential chemotherapy for aggressive non-Hodgkin's lymphoma (NHL) in first complete remission: A study on 464 patients (LNH 87 protocol). *Blood* 1993, **82**: 334a.

112. Smalley RV, Andersen JW, Hawkins MJ, et al. Interferon alfa combined with cytotoxic chemotherapy for patients with non-Hodgkin's lymphoma. *N. Engl. J. Med.* 1992, **327**: 1336–1341.

113. Lauria F, Raspadori D, Zinzani PL, et al. Clinical and immunologic effects of IL-2 in non-Hodgkin's lymphoma patients after autologous bone marrow transplantation. *Blood* 1993, **82**: 566a.

114. Urabe A, Mutoh Y, Mizoguchi H, et al. Ubenimex in the treatment of acute nonlymphocytic leukemia in adults. *Ann. Hematol.* 1993, **67**: 63–66.

115. Grossbard ML, Gribben JG, Freedman AS, et al. Adjuvant immunotoxin therapy with anti-B4-blocked ricin after autologous bone marrow transplantation for patients with B-cell non-Hodgkin's lymphoma. *Blood* 1993, **81**: 2263–2271.

116. Kaminski MS, Zasadny KR, Francis IR, et al. Radioimmunotherapy of B-cell lymphoma with [131I] Anti-B1 (Anti-CD-20) antibody. *N. Engl. J. Med.* 1993, **329**: 459–465.

117. Press OW, Eary JF, Appelbaum FR, et al. Radiolabeled-antibody therapy of B-cell lymphoma with autologous bone marrow support. *N. Engl. J. Med.* 1993, **329**: 1219–1224.

118. Bierman PJ, Vose JM, Leichner PK, et al. Yttrium 90-labeled antiferritin followed by high-dose chemotherapy and autologous bone marrow transplantation for poor-prognosis Hodgkin's disease. *J. Clin. Oncol.* 1993, **11**: 698–703.

CHAPTER 35

Prognostic factors in non-Hodgkin's lymphomas

BERTRAND COIFFIER, GILLES SALLES AND YVES BASTION

What is the main interest of prognostic factors?

Every disease, and particularly non-Hodgkin's lymphoma (NHL), is heterogenous. In NHL, the major reasons for this heterogeneity come from the numerous different histologic subtypes, the possibility that the lymphoma may arise from either nodal or extranodal sites, and its capacity to remain localized or to disseminate throughout the body. This heterogeneity is further complicated by the patient's age and associated diseases. In proposing the best therapeutic options to patients, a physician must take into account the prognostic implications of this heterogeneity. Because of the multiplicity of histologic subtypes and of the possible manifestations of a lymphoma, it is impossible to predict the outcome of therapy accurately in individual patients. Descriptions of subgroups based on large numbers of patients with histologically similar lymphomas and similar clinical manifestations, however, are likely to lead to the identification of meaningful prognostic indicators.

The first step in the description of such subgroups was the application to NHL patients of the Ann Arbor staging system [1] described for Hodgkin's disease patients. This staging system has been applied to lymphoma patients for more than 20 years but its limitations have become more apparent as therapeutic results have improved, an improvement that has been associated with more intensive chemotherapy regimens. During the years 1980–1990, new prognostic parameters were described and some of them were more useful than the Ann Arbor staging system [2]. The description of these new prognostic indicators has permitted the development of prognostic indexes that combine the more useful prognostic parameters. Finally, major centers involved in the treatment of patients with NHL have decided to work together, a collaboration that has led to the development of an International Prognostic Index [3].

The new emphasis on prognostic factors should permit the identification of meaningful subgroups amidst the heterogeneity, should lead to an understanding of why some patients do not respond to therapy as well as expected, should allow better stratification of patients before entry into clinical trials such that results from different trials around the world can be compared and, finally, should lead to significant improvement in decision making relevant to the treatment of lymphoma patients.

In this chapter, we will review all parameters associated with outcome in all lymphoma subtypes, emphasize the most important ones, and describe the major indexes used to stratify patients before treatment. We will then describe recent studies designed to identify new biologically based prognostic parameters. Finally, we will outline how prognostic parameters may influence routine practice in the management of lymphoma patients.

Description of major prognostic parameters

Numerous clinical or biological abnormalities have been associated with treatment outcome in lymphomas. We have classified such abnormalities into several subgroups: (1) morphologic lymphoma subtypes; (2) parameters related to the patient which are independent of the lymphoma, e.g., age; (3) parameters associated with the tumor burden, e.g., number of involved sites or largest diameter of tumor mass; (4) parameters related to the patient–tumor relationship, e.g., performance status; (5) parameters related to the physician(s) in charge of this patient, e.g., choice of therapeutic regimen.

A variety of clinical features have been identified as being associated with response to treatment and survival. The features that have most frequently been associated with the ability to achieve a complete remission after treatment and with a long overall survival are listed in Table 35.1. These clinical features reflect the tumor growth and the tumor invasive potential [serum lactic dehydrogenase (LDH) level, Ann Arbor stage, tumor size, number of extranodal sites of disease, presence of bone marrow involvement, and serum β_2-microglobulin level], the

Table 35.1 Prognostic factors associated with achievement of complete remission, time to treatment failure and long-term survival in univariate analyses in all lymphoma subtypes

---

Age (<60 years versus ≥60 years)
Performance status (ECOG scale 0 or 1 versus ≥2)
B symptoms (absence versus presence)
Stage [local (I or II) versus disseminated (III or IV)]
Tumor size (<10 cm versus ≥10 cm)
Number of extranodal sites of disease (0 or 1 versus ≥2)
Bone marrow involvement (absence versus presence)
Serum LDH level (normal versus increased)
Serum β_2-microglobulin level (<3 mg/l versus ≥3 mg/l)
Serum albumin level (<35 g/l versus ≥35 g/l)

ECOG, Eastern Clinical Oncology Group; LDH, lactic dehydrogenase.

patient's response to the tumor (performance status, B symptoms), and the patient's ability to tolerate intensive therapy (performance status, age).

HISTOLOGIC SUBTYPES

A substantial tissue specimen of the tumor should be obtained in order to establish the diagnosis of lymphoma and its subtype formerly. Additional studies may be useful to obtain or confirm the diagnosis, and to establish biological and molecular prognostic factors.

Numerous subtypes of lymphomas are described in Part 2 of this book [4–6]. The patient course associated with each of these subtypes varies from being indolent to aggressive and histologic subtypes have been divided into subgroups with a low, intermediate or high risk of progression. However, clinical outcome changes with time as therapeutic strategies improve and some histological subtypes now have a better prognosis than was the case years ago. The prognosis of other subtypes, however, has not improved and the prognosis has remained relatively poor. The cases, for instance, with mantle cell lymphoma [7,8] and low-grade lymphomas in general are usually considered to be incurable at the present time while children with high-grade lymphomas have an excellent prognosis when treated with modern therapy. Because of this, it is probably better not to include prognostic implications in histologic designations; the best lymphoma classification describes histologic subtypes based only on morphology, immunology and genotype alone, i.e., will aim to describe discrete disease entities without taking prognosis into consideration as proposed recently with the Revised American–European Lymphoma (REAL) classification [6]. Therefore, our descriptions of prognostic factors are not linked to the prognostic groups of the Working Formulation for Clinical Usage or the Kiel classification. Of course, it must also be borne in mind that the value of prognostic factors derived from disease or host characteristics other than histology are also likely to change with different treatment approaches.

Histologic entities

Follicular lymphomas

Patients with follicular lymphoma have long been considered as having an indolent disease that may not require any therapy for a long period of time [9]. However, while this is true for 50% of follicular lymphoma patients, the other half have clinical or biological abnormalities associated with a high tumor burden and these patients require treatment at the time of diagnosis [10]. Follicular lymphomas are composed of a mixture of centrocytes and centroblastes associated with follicular dendritic cells. According to the number of centroblastic cells, these lymphomas are subdivided into three classes in the Working Formulation for Clinical Usage [4,11]. However, the reproducibility of this subdivision has been greatly discussed [12,13]. Indeed, follicular lymphomas represent a continuum which ranges from tumors which contain mostly small cells to those which contain only large cells. Moreover, the number of centroblastic (large) cells may change from one follicle to another in the same patient.

In the original description of the Working Formulation for Clinical Usage, follicular large-cell lymphoma patients had a significantly shorter survival than those with a small-cell or mixed subtype [4]. This poorer outcome in large-cell follicular lymphoma patients has been confirmed in some but not all retrospective analyses [13–17]. Today, most physicians agree that this subdivision is not of clinical value and that treatment should not be decided on the percentage of large cells, but, rather, according to whether or not adverse clinical or biological prognostic factors are present [18].

Patients in whom the histology shows both follicular and diffuse patterns and in whom the diffuse areas account for more than 25% of the available histologic material have been reported to have a median survival of 40 months compared to 68 months for patients with a pure follicular pattern [19]. However, this finding has not been confirmed by more recent studies [16,17,20].

Diffuse large-cell lymphomas (B-cell or T-cell subtypes)

Diffuse large-cell lymphomas comprise diffuse mixed lymphomas (F subtype in the Working Formulation for Clinical Usage [4]), large-cell lymphomas (G subtype), and immunoblastic lymphomas (H subtype) and may have either a B-cell or a T-cell phenotype. In the Kiel classification, they are described as centroblastic or immunoblastic subtypes. No difference has been observed in the prognosis of these subtypes in several studies [3,21].

Since the description of the Working Formulation and the Kiel classification, new subtypes of large-cell lymphomas have been described [22]: anaplastic large-cell lymphomas [23,24] and mediastinal clear cell lymphoma [25]. Anaplastic large-cell lymphomas were initially characterized by their expression of the CD30 or Ki-1 antigen, but CD30 positivity is not associated with a specific histological appearance or with a specific phenotype [26–30]. No prognostic value has been associated with these

different lymphoma subtypes. Patients with cutaneous anaplastic large-cell lymphoma have been reported to have a longer survival than patients with systemic CD30-positive lymphoma [31–33] but this better outcome is consistent with the good prognosis observed with all cutaneous large-cell lymphoma patients, whether CD30-positive or not [34]. In our experience [35] as well as that of others [36], patients with CD30-positive lymphomas of T-cell, B-cell or undetermined origin have a prognosis similar to that of patients with CD30-negative large-cell lymphomas when matched for clinico-biologic prognostic parameters.

Mediastinal B-cell lymphoma with sclerosis was originally associated with a poor outcome [37,38] but larger series of patients have shown that cure can be achieved in this disease with the same frequency as in other patients with large-cell lymphoma of the mediastinum [39,40]. Prognostic indicators in these patients are no different from those found in other patients with a large-cell lymphoma, and include the presence of tumor outside the thorax, the number of extranodal sites and the serum LDH level (see below). In fact, at present, there seems to be no good reason to treat patients with mediastinal cell lymphoma with sclerosis differently from patients with other types of large-cell lymphoma [41].

Patients with immunoblastic lymphoma seemed to have a worse prognosis a few years ago and thus were individualized and classified as high grade in the Working Formulation for Clinical Usage. However, more recent studies have not found a worse outcome for these patients when compared to centroblastic lymphoma or other subtypes of large-cell lymphoma [21,42,43]. Similarly, no significant difference in prognosis has been observed between diffuse large-cell cases additionally subclassified as large cleaved cell and those with large noncleaved cell lymphoma [42]. The diagnosis of large-cell subtypes is often difficult and sufficiently nonreproducible that in the REAL classification it has been proposed that they are grouped together [6].

Small lymphocytic/lymphoplasmacytoid lymphomas (immunocytomas)

This category of lymphomas is not yet well defined. It was originally related to chronic lymphocytic leukemia (CLL) but its frequent tumoral mass in lymph nodes distinguish it from CLL. Differing degrees of cellular differentiation and percentages of large cells have led to the description of three subtypes (small lymphocytic lymphoma, lymphoplasmacytoid lymphoma and immunocytoma), each with a distinctive prognosis. However, earlier descriptions

outcome associated with the T-cell phenotype observed in some series is related to the immunologic phenotype of lymphoma cells *per se*, or arises from the fact that T-cell lymphomas are more frequently associated with poor prognostic factors, although at least one multiparametric analysis, including more than 300 patients, indicated that T immunophenotye was independently associated with a poor outcome [64].

True histiocytic lymphomas have been described [72,73] but patient numbers are too low to be able to identify prognostic indicators within this group.

Karyotypic abnormalities associated with prognosis

Major karyotypic changes related to particular histological subtypes

Certain chromosomal translocations have been closely associated with specific histological subtypes (see Chapter 11 of this book). It is currently unknown whether the presence or absence of these characteristic translocations has a prognostic value that transcends histology.

The t(8;14)(q24;q32) and variant translocations [t(2;8) and t(8;22)], which result in juxtaposition of the proto-oncogene c-*myc*, situated on chromosome 8q24, with immunoglobulin genes, causes deregulation of the expression of c-*myc* messenger RNA and protein. These abnormalities were first identified in small noncleaved cell (SNCC) Burkitt's lymphomas and were thought to be associated with the poorer prognosis of this histological subtype. The presence of the t(8;14)(q24;q32) translocation, however, has also been reported in large-cell lymphomas and follicular lymphomas [74], and, interestingly, in the few follicular lymphomas that have been reported with this translocation, the c-*myc* gene does not seem to be rearranged or dysregulated, indicating that the breakpoint may lie in a different genetic region than the breakpoint encountered in SNCC lymphomas [75]. This may explain the lack of prognosis significance attributed to this translocation when encountered in follicular lymphomas [74] and underlines the need for careful molecular genetic examination when attempting to interpret the prognostic significance of karyotypic changes.

The t(14;18)(q32;q21) and variant translocations t(2;18) and t(18;22) juxtapose the *bcl*-2 gene with the immunoglobulin genes. This abnormality is present in 70–90% of follicular lymphomas, and in 15–30% of large-cell lymphomas [74]. The prognostic value of t(14;18) in large-cell lymphomas is controversial, different series reporting either an adverse outcome [74,76,77] or no difference [78]. Some studies may

have been confounded by the fact that a fraction of these large-cell lymphomas with a t(14;18) arise from histologic transformation of a pre-existing low-grade follicular lymphoma, a situation known to be associated with a poor outcome. However, whether apparently *de novo* large-cell lymphomas associated with a t(14;18) arise from subclinical follicular lymphomas or whether these tumors are biologically distinct from transformed follicular lymphomas is not known.

Other cytogenetic abnormalities associated with prognosis (Table 35.3)

Frequently, the karyotypic aberrations in non-Hodgkin's lymphomas turn out to be complex: multiple abnormalities are often encountered in the same tumor, some of them are present in all tumor cells and some only in a subset of clones; certain abnormalities are present from the onset of the disease and other seem to be acquired during its evolution.

A number of karyotypic aberrations have been associated with a poor prognosis. For example, abnormalities of either the long (1q21–23) or short (1p32–36) arms of chromosome 1 have been associated with an adverse outcome in intermediate- and low-grade lymphomas [74,79]. Multiple chromosomal abnormalities involving chromosome 6 have been reported in up to one-third of lymphomas and may be associated with adverse outcome in large-cell lymphomas [74,79–81]. Recent molecular analyses indicate, however, that distinct breakpoints in 6q21–27 may be implicated in different histological subtypes, and further analysis is needed to determine whether these abnormalities are really of prognostic significance [82]. Structural abnormalities or monosomy of chromosomes 7 and 17 have also been reported to confer an adverse prognostic [74,79,83, 84], as well as trisomy 7 [74]. Trisomy 12 has been associated with adverse prognosis in low-grade lymphomas [74] and a small multiparametric analysis showed that trisomy 5, 6 or 8, chromosome 5 abnormalities, and 14q11–12 aberrations were significantly associated with an adverse prognosis [85]. A larger multivariate analysis performed on a cohort of 205 large-cell lymphoma patients demonstrated that breaks at 1q21–23 or the presence of four marker chromosomes were significantly and independently associated with shortened survival [74].

The most frequent example of disease progression is transformation of follicular lymphomas, and several chromosomal changes (del 6q, chromosome 17 abnormalities, 8q24 rearrangements and others) have been reported to be superimposed on t(14;18) in association with histologic transformation or even to precede it [81,86,87].

Table 35.3 Prognostic value of karyotypic abnormalities related to different morphological subtypes in which they are encountered

Chromosomal change	Predominant histology	Prognostic value
t(14;18)(q32;q21)	Follicular	No
	Diffuse large cell	Unknown (conflicting results)
t(8;14)(q24;q32)	Small noncleaved	No
	Other subtypes	Unknown (various breakpoints?)
t(11;14)(q24;q32)	Mantle cell lymphoma	No
t(2;5)(p23;q35)	Anaplastic large cell	Unknown
More than four marker chromosomes	Diffuse large cell	Adverse
1q21–23	Diffuse large cell	Adverse
1p32–36	Low grade and diffuse large cell	Adverse ?
3q27	Diffuse large cell	Unknown
6q21–27	Various	Adverse
Chromosome 7 (trisomy or monosomy)	Various	Adverse
Chromosome 17	Various	Adverse (p53 allelic loss?)
Trisomy 12	Low grade	Adverse
Abnormalities associated with t(14;18)(q32;q21)	Follicular	Adverse

Rearrangement of the *bcl*-6 gene located on 3q27 has been recently identified in 15–35% of diffuse large-cell lymphomas. The prognostic significance of this is uncertain, since in one series it has been suggested that it is associated with a good prognosis [88] and in another that it is not [89].

Finally, the presence of karyotypic abnormalities in addition to the abovementioned aberrations appears to be of adverse prognostic significance, i.e., the number of different chromosomal aberrations identified is important [74,79,81,85].

Other genetic changes

As outlined already, recurrent karyotypic abnormalities result in altered gene structure or expression that dramatically influences the biology of lymphoma cells. Therefore, the molecular lesions encountered in NHLs may profoundly influence the clinical behavior of the disease and outcome of therapy. Given the complexity of karyotypic changes, the identification of the genes that are affected and the elucidation of the functional consequences is slow, although many such genes have been characterized over the past 10 years. This – and the difficulty of routine molecular investigations – explains the paucity of clinical data correlating prognosis with molecular abnormalities. However, to date, the clinical correlates of rearrangements of three genes have been studied (Table 35.3).

c-myc
c-*myc* rearrangement is more frequent in primary extranodal lymphomas than in primary nodal lymphomas [90]. Abnormalities of c-*myc* have been well documented to occur in association with histologic progression in follicular lymphomas but these cases seem to be infrequent [91,92].

bcl-2
Expression of the *bcl*-2 protein has no influence on prognosis follicular lymphoma [93] but, in large-cell lymphomas, expression of the *bcl*-2 protein has been associated with a poor outcome [94].

p53
Recent data suggest that mutations of the p53 gene, a tumor suppressor gene located on chromosome 17, may occur in a subset of NHL and that such mutations confer a poor prognosis. Mutations of p53 in NHL were first detected in a significant fraction (38%) of Burkitt's lymphomas [95]. p53 mutations were also reported to be more frequently found in more advanced tumors [96]. Other reports have suggested that the occurrence of p53 mutations is frequently associated with histologic transformation of follicular lymphomas, and may even precede, in some cases, the clinical occurrence of transformation [97,98]. These findings need to be confirmed in a larger series but it may turn out that p53 mutations will be relevant to prognosis in some subsets of lymphoma patients.

In summary, chromosomal and genetic changes in non-Hodgkin's lymphomas are likely to be of considerable relevance to prognosis, and may substantially improve histologically and clinically based prognostic indexes. However, cytogenetic and molecular analyses are still conducted only in highly specialized centers and more convenient tools need to be developed to more definitively establish their clinical importance and, ultimately, influence our routine practice.

PARAMETERS RELATED TO THE PATIENT

Outcome of lymphoma patients may be different according to the existence of previous diseases not related to the lymphoma and to his or her age at the time of diagnosis.

Age

The effect of age on treatment results has been analyzed differently in different published studies. In a Southwest Oncology Group (SWOG) study, older patients had a worse outcome because they responded less well to treatment and relapsed more often. This poorer outcome was related to a decrease in chemotherapy dose intensity because older patients received only 50% of the drug dosage [99]. In another study, elderly patients were observed to die more often during the first courses of treatment but those who responded did not have a higher rate of relapse [100,101]. It was then concluded that elderly patients are more likely to develop complications after chemotherapy because of their age and the

possible existence of comorbidities. Whatever the reason, age was identified as an adverse prognostic factor in all studies [54,102–105].

The cutoff between young and old patients is between 60 and 65 for patients with a large-cell lymphoma [3]. As an example, Figure 35.1 shows the survival of patients treated for an aggressive lymphoma in the Groupe d'Etude des Lymphomes de l'Adulte (GELA) showing three subgroups of patients: those younger than 50 with the best outcome, those aged between 50 and 65 with an intermediate outcome, and those older than 65 with the worst outcome.

When prognostic parameters were analyzed separately for patients younger or older than 60, few differences could be found between the groups [103,106,107]. Older patients often have a poorer performance status or a stage IV disease, but these differences are rarely statistically significant. Finally, the predictive capacity of chronological age and the tolerance to therapy are related to the poor performance status (PS), the presence of concomitant diseases, the dose intensity of chemotherapy regimen, and the patients' physiological resources. In elderly patients with a good PS, and few or no debilitative concomitant diseases, there is no reason to withhold curative treatment.

Sex

Males have been reported to have a shorter survival than females, particularly for follicular lymphomas [108–111], but this is difficult to explain and may be related to the shorter survival in males compared to females in the general population rather than differences in the disease or its impact on the patient.

Infection by HIV

The development of a non-Hodgkin's lymphoma is frequently observed in HIV-seropositive individuals. It has been suggested that the prolongation of the survival of HIV-infected individuals secondary to the use of specific antiviral therapy and to improved treatment of opportunistic infections will result in an increased frequency of NHLs in such patients [112]. The type of lymphoma that occurs relates to the patient's immune status and clinical course with respect to the underlying HIV infection. Histologically aggressive and disseminated NHLs often occur early in the disease, and may even constitute the first AIDS manifestation. Primary central nervous system (CNS) lymphomas appear later in the evolution of AIDS and have an extremely poor prognosis [55]. Several studies have identified prognostic factors in AIDS-related lymphoma patients

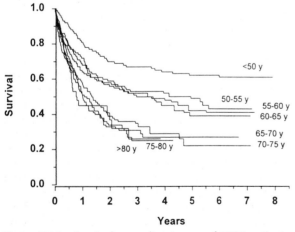

Figure 35.1 Survival according to age of 2235 patients treated with the LNH-84 and LNH-87 protocols in the Groupe d'Etude des Lymphomees de l'Adulte studies [43,232].

[113,114]. In 141 patients who were prospectively treated with an intensive chemotherapy regimen, multivariate analysis identified four major prognostic factors: (1) CD4+ lymphocyte count below 100 x 10^6/l; (2) performance status greater than 1; (3) immunoblastic histological subtype; and (4) AIDS manifestations prior to the onset of lymphoma [114]. Therefore, HIV-induced severe immunosuppression seems to be the main adverse factor affecting the outcome, although in a substantial proportion of patients without adverse prognostic factors, a durable remission can be achieved.

PROGNOSTIC PARAMETERS RELATED TO THE TUMORAL MASS

A large tumor mass has long been recognized as an

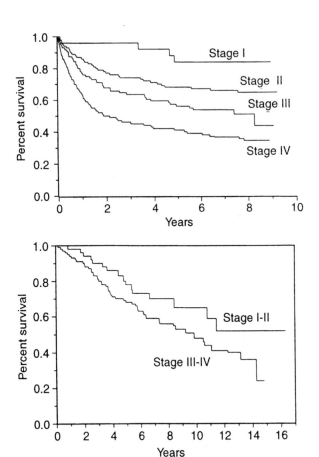

Figure 35.2 Advanced-stage patients have a poorer outcome than localized disease patients (Ann Arbor staging). (a) Overall survival of patients included in the LNH-84 regimen [21] according to disease stage ($P<10^{-4}$). (b) Overall survival of 220 follicular lymphoma patients treated in our center [17] according to disease stage (not significant).

important adverse parameter. However, the method of estimating of the total tumor mass has been quite different from one study to another. Parameters associated with a large tumor mass and with prognosis are: number of nodal sites; number of extranodal sites; location; largest diameter of the tumor; stage; LDH level; and β_2-microglobulin level. We will describe each of these factors and discuss their relative ability to distinguish poor outcome patients.

Stage

Ann Arbor stage was originally described for Hodgkin's disease patients [1] but was subsequently applied to NHL patients. However, Ann Arbor stage was described for what is essentially a nodal disease and it is somewhat difficult to apply to NHL because of the involvement of the bone marrow (particularly follicular lymphomas), because of the extranodal primary localizations in up to 40% of the large-cell subtype patients, and because of the weak correlation between extranodal diffusion and outcome in some lymphoma subtypes.

Stage is, however, in some way related to outcome and, in most studies, stage I patients have a longer survival than stage IV patients [21,105,115–117]. The results obtained in patients treated with the LNH-84 regimen [43] and in follicular lymphoma patients treated at our center [17] illustrate the poorer outcome of advanced-stage patients (Figure 35.2). After histologic subtype, stage, localized or disseminated, is one of the most predictive variables for outcome in lymphoma patients.

Number of nodal sites

The spread of a lymphoma may reflect its tumor mass and this point has been taken into account in the Ann Arbor staging system. Patients with truly localized disease (stage I) have a better outcome than patients with locally disseminated disease (stage II) or than patients with enlarged lymph nodes throughout the entire body (stage III disease). However, the number of nodal areas involved by the lymphoma has never been studied, probably because it may be done only after biopsies of all lymph node areas and because establishing a true estimate of lymphoma cell dissemination was not believed to be useful for establishing the prognosis or deciding upon treatment.

The number of lymph node areas with a lymph node larger than 2 cm has been described as a powerful prognostic parameter [104,118–120]. It is, however, dependent upon even more powerful prognostic parameters and disappears in multivariate analyses.

Today, the number of involved nodal sites is not considered a prominent prognostic indicator. The estimation of clinical stage, either localized or disseminated, is easier to accomplish and appears to be more useful.

Number of extranodal sites

The number of lymphoma localizations found depends on the specialized examinations used to detect them (i.e., CT scans, endoscopy, serous fluid examinations, biological examinations, etc.).

Patients with extranodal sites of disease may have either lymphoma localized to a single site, with or without regional dissemination or disseminated disease. The number of extranodal localizations is probably a reflection of the propensity of the disease to disseminate throughout the whole body. The presence of more than one extranodal site of disease has been associated with a poor prognosis [21,104,119–123]. Indeed, the number of extranodal sites of disease is one of the strongest prognostic factors in aggressive (large-cell) lymphomas and in follicular lymphoma, and it retains its prognostic value in multivariate analyses [2,3,17,21,124].

Largest diameter of the tumor

One other means of expressing the aggressivity of a lymphoma is to measure the largest diameter of the largest (nodal) tumor on a CT scan. A poor outcome has been associated with larger tumors, but the cutoff in various studies varies from 5 to 10 cm [21,104, 110,119,121,123,125]. Large tumors are thought be associated with an increased risk of the development of more aggressive clones of lymphoma cells, but in fact this adverse risk does not persist in some multiparametric analyses [3] because it is highly related to other adverse parameters.

Specific extranodal localizations

Lymphoma cells may arise in every organ or lymph node of the body and thus the extranodal sites may be as diverse as the number of body parts. The most frequent localizations of lymphomatous masses are based on information from: (1) a Danish NHL Registry; and (2) a large series of aggressive lymphomas (listed in Table 35.4). Some of these extranodal sites may be associated with a poorer outcome in retrospective studies. However, multiparametric analyses have uniformly shown that the poorer outcome was a function of the number of extranodal sites rather than the specific location [3,21,119,121,123,125].

Bone marrow involvement

Patients with bone marrow involvement have disseminated disease and thus have a poorer outcome than those without bone marrow involvement. However, bone marrow involvement is present in more than

Table 35.4 Frequency of extranodal sites of disease in newly diagnosed patients included in the LNH-84 regimen, aggressive lymphoma patients with primary and secondary involvement [43], and in the Danish NHL Registry [233]

Extranodal sites of disease	LNH-84 regimen patients		Danish NHL registry patients	
	N (%)	Prognostic value	(%)	Prognostic value
Bone marrow	173 (23)	0.001	89 (19)	0.031
Spleen	158 (21)	0.01		
GI tract	124 (17)			
Stomach			87 (19)	
Intestine			52 (11)	
Liver	117 (16)	0.01	27 (6)	0.001
Pleura	98 (13)	0.01		
Head and neck	85 (12)			
Bone	68 (9)		41 (9)	
Lung	64 (9)		24 (5)	
Skin	46 (6)		56 (12)	
CNS	37 (5)		33 (7)	
Salivary glands			17 (4)	
Thyroid			25 (5)	
Testes			15 (3)	0.015

NHL, non-Hodgkin's lymphoma; GI, gastrointestinal; CNS, central nervous system.

70% of patients with follicular lymphoma, immunocytoma or mantle cell lymphoma and, in these tumors at least, may not alter the prognosis [126]. Patients with Burkitt's lymphoma or lymphoblastic lymphoma with bone marrow involvement, however, have a considerably worse prognosis than those without marrow involvement. Patients with lymphoblastic lymphoma are generally treated as leukemia patients [57,127,128], but patients with Burkitt's lymphoma do best with short duration, intensive chemotherapy [129].

Only 20–25% of patients with large-cell lymphoma have bone marrow involvement at the time of diagnosis, but these patients have a poorer response to therapy and shorter survival [110,130,131]. This poorer outcome has not, however, always been found and its prognostic significance has rarely been conserved in multiparametric analysis [3,21,121,126]. Recently, bone marrow infiltration was subdivided into infiltration by large cells similar to those seen in the lymph node and infiltration by small cells. Patients with a large-cell lymphoma and bone marrow infiltrate of small-cell lymphoma have a higher risk of relapse but a longer survival than patients with involvement by large cells [132–134].

Blood involvement

A leukemic phase is uncommon in large-cell lymphoma, particularly when the disease is first diagnosed, but patients with peripheral blood involvement have a very poor outcome [135]. In one study, the presence of putative lymphoma cells in peripheral blood, as evidenced by a clonal excess, was not associated with an adverse outcome, particularly in follicular lymphomas [136].

Gastrointestinal localizations

Gastrointestinal localization is the most frequent extranodal site in lymphomas but its prognostic significance as well as its therapy have been discussed for more than 30 years without reaching firm conclusions [137]. Sometimes, gastrointestinal involvement is confounded with MALT lymphoma but large-cell lymphoma is more frequent than MALT subtypes and it carries a poorer prognosis.

MALT lymphoma is more frequent in the stomach, is often localized, and is associated with a good response to treatment and long survival. Large-cell lymphomas represent 50–60% of gastrointestinal localizations and are more frequent in the stomach, intestine and colon. At these sites the prognosis is related to the usual clinico-biologic parameters [138]. Mantle cell lymphoma is the third most frequently observed subtype in the gastrointestinal

tract. It occurs particularly in the colon and is always associated with a poor survival [7,8].

The idea that a more favorable outcome is associated with gastrointestinal tract lymphomas may be related to the fact that 80% of them are gastric lymphomas, and that 30–40% of gastric lymphomas have a MALT subtype. Furthermore, half of the large-cell lymphomas from gastric or intestinal sites are localized. Patients with localized gastrointestinal lymphomas have a similar prognosis to patients with localized disease in other sites [139] (Figure 35.3).

Central nervous system localization

Central nervous system lymphomas have always been thought to be a special case for which different treatment is required. In fact, CNS lymphomas comprise four different subgroups of patients: those with meningeal localization; those with a spinal extradural location with cord compression; those with primary large-cell lymphoma of a cerebral hemispheric or nonhemispheric site; and immunocompromised patients with a lymphoma as secondary manifestation, particularly HIV-positive patients.

Meningeal involvement may be seen in small-cell lymphomas or large cell lymphomas, but is more frequent in lymphoblastic or Burkitt's subtypes [140, 141]. This involvement reflects disseminated disease and is always associated with a worse outcome. However, patients with CNS disease do not appear to have a worse prognosis than patients without CNS involvement who have similar degrees of LDH elevation or who have bone marrow involvement, suggesting that extensive disease rather than CNS involvement is responsible for the poor prognosis [52].

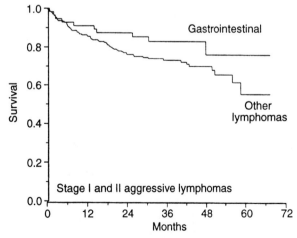

Figure 35.3 Overall survival of patients with diffuse aggressive lymphomas; localized gastrointestinal lymphomas compared to localized nodal or other extranodal lymphomas treated with the LNH-84 regimen [139].

Lymphoma of the extradural spinal space associated with a spinal cord compression has been associated with a worse outcome, but this localization has never been studied in large series or by multiparametric analysis [142].

Primary CNS lymphomas are usually large-cell lymphomas and are rarely associated with nodal or other extranodal sites of lymphoma [143,144]. Adverse prognostic factors associated with these lymphomas are identical to those identified in non-CNS lymphoma patients: high LDH level, poor PS and age older than 60. Specific adverse prognostic parameters have been identified in large series of patients: high CSF protein at diagnosis, impaired neurologic function, particularly memory dysfunction, and a nonhemispheric tumor site [144,145]. High-dose methotrexate in the treatment has been associated with a longer survival [144,146]. Intraocular lymphoma is frequently associated with primary CNS lymphomas [147].

Pleural effusion

Pleural effusion is the most frequent manifestation of serous involvement in lymphoma patients is more frequently observed in patients with a large thoracic tumor burden. It has been associated with a poorer outcome whatever the histologic type [39,148].

Skin localizations

Primary cutaneous lymphomas are polymorphic in appearance, clinical manifestations, histological subtypes and outcome. While the cutaneous T-cell lymphoma of mycosis fungoides subtype, with its characteristic epidermoid infiltration, is well recognized, all other subtypes may occur as a primary cutaneous lymphoma. The most frequent subtypes are large B-cell lymphomas and CD30-positive lymphomas [149].

Large B-cell lymphomas of the skin are often localized, indolent in their evolution and associated with a good prognosis [34,150]. They may, however, disseminate to noncutaneous sites after some months or years. Because of this favorable outcome they have been compared to MALT lymphoma of the skin [151].

The most common cutaneous lymphoma is a large-cell, CD30-positive, lymphoma with a T-cell or null phenotype [30]. These patients have often several cutaneous sites of disease that may appear or disappear over time before becoming larger. This lymphoma has a favorable outcome [31], although the better survival of cutaneous CD30-positive cell patients has not, to date, been ascribed to differences in age, stage or the initial mode of treatment [152].

Testis

Lymphomas localized to the testis are often of lymphoblastic or Burkitt's subtype and carry the adverse prognosis associated with disseminated disease in these diseases [153,154]. However, the numbers of patients in published series are too low to determine whether large-cell lymphomas of the testis have a worse outcome.

Lactic dehydrogenase level

LDH is a cytoplasmic enzyme whose level increases in blood when cell are lysed by any mechanism (viral hepatitis, infarction, spontaneous death). In neoplastic diseases, the serum LDH level is a marker of increased cell turnover and a surrogate for tumor mass [155]. Increased serum LDH has been identified as a prognostic factor in lymphoma patients since the first prognostic factor studies [156–158] and in nearly all published prognostic analyses [2,21,54,104,115,119,130,159]. Moreover, the higher the LDH level, the poorer the outcome of treatment [2,21]. An elevated LDH level is one of the most important prognostic factor, as has recently been recognized in multivariate analyses [2,3,21].

β_2-Microglobulin level

The adverse prognostic associated with high serum level of β_2-microglobulin was recognized in lymphoma patients as well as myeloma patients years ago [160,161] but this parameter has not been widely used for 15 years, particularly in the United States.

A high serum β_2-microglobulin level is defined as greater than 3 mg/ml, that is, between 1.25 and 1.4 times the normal value (2.1–2.4 mg/ml). The putative importance of the β_2-microglobulin level has been recognized and applied to prognostic analyses in several centers [17,162–164]. In the MD Anderson Cancer Center (Houston, TX), the serum LDH and β_2-microglobulin levels are the two most important parameters for predicting the outcome of large-cell and follicular lymphoma patients [163,164]. This has been confirmed in Europe in several studies which included all lymphoma subtypes [7,17,162]. The overall survival of follicular and nonfollicular, small-cell lymphoma patients treated at our center according to serum β_2-microglobulin levels is shown in Figure 35.4a and b. Like LDH level, β_2-microglobulin level seems to be one of the parameters that may predict the risk of relapse for patients in complete remission [165]. The real importance of β_2-microglobulin level compared to other prognostic indicators will only be known when

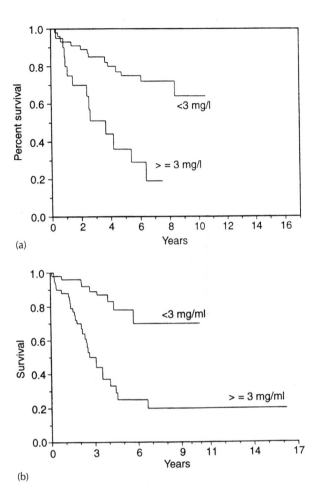

(a)

(b)

Figure 35.4   Prognostic value of β_2-microglobulin level. (a) Overall survival in follicular lymphoma patients ($P<0.0001$) [124] and (b) in nonfollicular small-cell lymphoma patients ($P=0.0001$) [7].

multiparametric analyses are conducted in large series of patients with prospective determination of major prognostic parameters as well as serum β_2-microglobulin levels.

PROGNOSTIC PARAMETERS RELATED TO THE PATIENT–TUMOR RELATIONSHIP

Under this heading, we have assembled parameters not directly related to tumor burden. These include B symptoms, performance status, albumin and hemoglobin levels. These parameters are well correlated with each other and any given study of prognostic factors may identify only one of them as being highly significant correlate of outcome. They probably reflect the same phenomenon – cytokine secretion by either tumor cells or, more likely, by the patient's immune cells in response to the tumor (see below). Earlier studies focused on B symptoms, more recent ones, such as the International Prognostic Index, on performance status, and statisticians will select serum albumin or hemoglobin level because it is more easily measurable.

B symptoms

B symptoms were originally described in patients with Hodgkin's disease [1]. They are defined as either weight loss greater than 10%, fever greater than 38°C for more than one week, or abundant night sweats, i.e., necessitating a change of bedclothes two or three times a night. Fever or night sweats are indirect manifestations of interleukin secretion which may be difficult to define (see below). They are not related to tumor burden. While B symptoms were extensively used in earlier studies [20,110] they have now been supplanted either by the major B symptom, significant weight loss, or by performance status. We propose to abandon the use of fever and night sweats as prognostic indicators. Weight loss may also be related to interleukin secretion, but can also be secondary to gastrointestinal (GI) tract location, age of the patient or poor PS. It has *per se* prognostic implications [21,43].

Performance status

The ability to lead a normal life may be measured by performance status, as defined by the Eastern Clinical Oncology Group (ECOG) or by DA Karnovsky [166] (Table 35.5). This assessment of functional status has been widely used in oncology to measure the loss of normal functions caused by the physiological and psychological effects of cancer. The ECOG scale is simpler and more widely used, but both scales, though somewhat subjective, have been validated in a prospective study which included a large number of patients, and in which PS was independently assessed by two physicians and by the patient [167]. Patients with a PS equal to or greater than two are nonambulatory and unable to do everyday things by themselves. Lymphoma patients with B symptoms, older age, weight loss, or a high tumor burden lymphoma frequently have a PS greater than or equal to two.

Poor PS has been associated with an adverse prognosis in nearly all the analyses in which it was included as a potential prognostic parameter [2,3, 105,121,125].

Table 35.5   Equivalence of performance status as defined originally by the Eastern Cooperative Oncology Group (ECOG) and Karnovsky's index

	ECOG scale		Karnovsky's index
0	No symptoms	90–100%	Normal activity
1	Symptoms but continued ability to ambulate	80%	Decreased capacity to work
2	Bedridden status less than 50% of the day	70%	Home work possible but significant effort impossible
3	Bedridden status greater than 50% of the day	50–60%	Limited home work with need of help
4	Chronic bedridden status and requirement for daily maintenance	10–40%	Chronic bedridden status and requirement for daily maintenance

Serum albumin level

Four recent analyses of potential prognostic factors [21,111,115,168] demonstrated that the serum albumin level is a powerful prognostic indicator in large-cell lymphomas. Patients with a serum albumin lower than 35 g/l have a high death rate during treatment (Figure 35.5). This was associated with a greater treatment-related toxicity, particularly hematologic, and a higher failure rate. In our own analyses, serum albumin level is highly correlated with B symptoms, weight loss and poor PS. We also found serum albumin level to be a major prognostic indicator in other lymphoma subtypes [7]. This parameter was not taken into account in the International Prognostic Index study because it was not measured in a sufficient number of patients.

Hemoglobin level

Hemoglobin level at diagnosis, like serum albumin level, has been shown to correlate with the death rate during treatment and also the response rate [54,111]. Anemia is usually defined as a hemoglobin level of less than 12 g/dl. The shorter survival of anemic patients is independent of the presence of bone marrow infiltration by lymphoma cells [169]. In our

analyses based on a large number of patients, we observed that anemia was correlated with the serum level of tumor necrosis factor-α (TNF-α) (see below) and with survival (Figure 35.6).

PROGNOSTIC PARAMETERS RELATED TO THE PHYSICIAN IN CHARGE OF THAT PATIENT

Although somewhat controversial, the outcome of treatment has also been related to the physician who treats that patient. Non-Hodgkin's lymphoma is a complicated disease; optimal therapy has to be delivered by physicians experienced in the field. It has been suggested that full awareness of the clinical aspects, treatment-related complications and range of therapeutic interventions requires that a physician sees at least 40 patients a year (a goal that cannot always be accomplished and is belied, somewhat, by the situation in pediatric lymphomas). An association with a large cooperative lymphoma group may be useful and is recommended. In addition, increasing experience with a treatment regimen (whatever

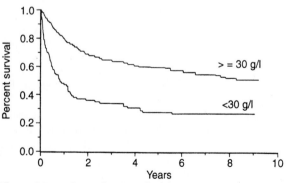

Figure 35.5   Overall survival of the patients treated with the LNH-84 regimen [43] according to serum albumin level (*P*<0.0001).

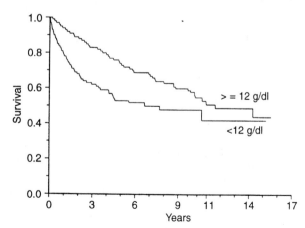

Figure 35.6   Overall survival of 990 lymphoma patients treated in our center according to hemoglobin level at diagnosis (*P*<0.0001).

the regimen) seems to be associated with improved treatment results, largely through a decrease in treatment-related mortality [101,170,171].

Choice of treatment

The various therapeutic modalities and most widely used protocols are described in specific chapters of this book and only general aspects of treatment relevant to outcome will be presented here. The treatment employed and the quality of the necessary supportive care are, ultimately, the most important determinants of prognosis. Treatment must be adapted to the patient and to the aggressiveness of the lymphoma. As such, it must take into account all the most important prognostic parameters described in this chapter.

The ultimate objective of treatment must be to reach a complete remission as quickly as possible. Whatever the lymphoma subtypes and the treatment, patients who reach only a partial response have a poorer outcome than patients who achieve a complete remission [17,115]. Moreover, the speed at which complete remission is attained may be important [172].

Involvement of the CNS was frequent in patients with recurrent large-cell lymphoma, or another aggressive subtype treated with either the cyclophosphamide, vincristine and prednisone (CVP) or cyclophosphamide, doxorubicin, vincristine and prednisone (CHOP) regimen which contain no effective CNS prophylactic therapy. In one SWOG study, 5% of 1039 patients had a CNS relapse [173], 10% had CNS relapse in a trial, which included 174 patients, conducted at the MD Anderson Cancer Center [174], and 9% of 592 patients from Boston developed this complication [140]. Since high-dose intravenous methotrexate is very effective for treating CNS lymphoma, the use of high-dose methotrexate (greater than 200 mg/m^2) in frontline chemotherapy regimens has dramatically decreased recurrence at this site and has probably increased the cure rate. For example, less than 1% of patients without initial CNS disease included in the LNH-84 regimen recurred in the CNS (meningeal or hemispheric sites) [43].

Importance of dose intensity

The dose intensity (DI) of a regimen can be modified by increasing individual drug doses or adding new drugs [175]. Several regimens containing 4–5 drugs have been reported with complete response (CR) and survival rates comparable to regimens using smaller numbers of drugs [176,177]. The identical results obtained with ProMACE–MOPP (see Chapter 42) and ProMACE–MOPP 'flexitherapy' (in which MOPP sequences were delivered later) also suggest

that the number of noncross-resistant drugs administered over a short induction period is not a determinant factor for outcome [178]. Attempts to increase CHOP or MACOP-B (see Chapter 42) 'dose intensity' with the addition of bleomycin or etoposide also did not improve CR rates or survival [179]. In most cases, the addition of new drugs into a regimen results in decreased doses of the drugs already administered in this regimen to avoid unacceptable toxicity. The resulting decreased DI of drugs such as doxorubicin and cyclophosphamide may affect the final outcome.

Although it has been suggested that increased DI may improve the survival of patients with aggressive lymphoma [175,180], no randomized study has been conducted in which a combination regimen has been compared with the same regimen used at an increased DI. However, many studies have shown that patients receiving low doses of therapy because of old age or other adverse factors (such as bone marrow involvement) have a very poor outcome [99]. Several retrospective analyses conducted in patients who received CHOP, CHOP-like or high-dose CHOP regimens have suggested that delivered DI could influence survival [181,182]. In the largest of these studies, the outcome of 311 patients included in the prospective LNH-87 trial according to the received relative DI of doxorubicin and cyclophosphamide was analyzed [181]. Significantly decreased response rate (65% versus 79%) and survival rate (61% versus 72%) were observed in patients receiving a DI below 70% of the planned dose, and this difference remained significant in multiparametric analysis ($P=0.004$). However, in several phase II SWOG studies, relative DI of the first 12 weeks of treatment was associated with CR and survival, but was not found to be an independent prognostic variable. The retrospective character of all these studies is an important limitation since the physician's decision to administer drugs at high DI is heavily influenced by pretreatment prognostic factors such as age, performance status or B symptoms such that DI could simply become a surrogate for these recognized prognostic indicators.

Taken together, these data suggest that the number of drugs administered is less important than the DI of 'standard' drugs such as cyclophosphamide and doxorubicin. These data, however, do suggest that increased DI may improve the outcome of patients with aggressive lymphoma. Regimens with a high DI (especially a high DI of cyclophosphamide) have been used for selected patients who have a predicted poor outcome with promising preliminary results [183]. Unfortunately, the definition of 'high-risk' patients in these studies is quite heterogeneous. A consensus definition of poor-prognosis patients will facilitate the interpretation of further studies of this kind [3]. We may also conclude from the published data that therapeutic innovations based on small alterations of prior existing regimens are unlikely to result in significant differences in outcome and may, in the event that dose reductions in the most effective agents are made, actually lead to a worse outcome.

Prognostic indexes

A number of investigators have utilized the subset of clinical features that retained independent significance in multivariate analysis of their patients to develop prognostic factor models predictive of an individual patient's risk of shortened survival. Although the specific clinical features utilized in the prognostic factor models differs, each model incorporates features that reflect the volume of disease and the extent of tumor involvement at diagnosis, confirming the primary importance of these factors [2].

PREVIOUS INDEXES

Large-cell lymphomas

The Dana–Farber Cancer Institute (Boston, MA) developed a prognostic factor model in aggressive lymphoma patients treated with M-BACOD or m-BACOD (see Chapter 42) regimens based on pretreatment performance status, tumor size and the number of extranodal sites of disease [121,125]. Investigators at the MD Anderson Cancer Center have developed several prognostic factor models [104,119,164], including one based on pretreatment serum LDH level and the assessment of tumor burden (number of extranodal and extensive nodal sites of involvement). Investigators at the Memorial Sloan–Kettering Cancer Center (New York) defined a prognostic factor model based on pretreatment serum LDH level, and an assessment of the location and size of nodal and extranodal sites of disease (level of site involvement) [123].

Recently the GELA group compared the predictive value of these prognostic factor models and found that they were equally predictive of survival in the 737 aggressive-lymphoma patients treated with the LNH-84 regimen [2]. This group also developed its own prognostic factor model which incorporated an assessment of pretreatment serum LDH level, Ann Arbor stage, the number of extranodal sites of disease and tumor bulk [21].

In addition to identifying clinical prognostic features that predict the likelihood of large-cell

lymphoma patients achieving a complete remission and surviving 5 years, attempts have also been made to identify the clinical characteristics associated with the risk of relapse. This parameter is important because patients who are at high risk of relapse may benefit from more intensive consolidation chemotherapy. In several independent studies, increased pretreatment serum LDH level and disseminated disease (Ann Arbor stage III or IV) have been associated with the likelihood of relapse [21,184].

Follicular lymphomas

Several centers have tried to describe prognostic indexes for follicular lymphoma patients [185–187]. Leonard [185] has presented an index based on performance status, age, stage, sex and hemoglobin level. Even if this index can really separate patients into three distinct groups it is rather complicated and for this reason alone may not be widely used. In addition the index does not include the more recently identified, and probably more reliable, prognostic parameters (see above). Romaguera has presented an index based on sex and tumor burden [108]. The tumor burden assessment was calculated according to the number of extranodal sites and the size of nodal masses. This index has not been validated in another set of patients. We have applied our own index for patients with aggressive lymphoma, the LNH-84 [21] index, that was developed from retrospective analysis and prospectively validated on other sets of patients with aggressive lymphoma, to patients with follicular lymphoma treated in our center. This index appears to successfully divide them into three different groups [17,18].

However, this index has not been prospectively evaluated in patients with follicular lymphoma. Overall, prognostic indexes for patients with follicular lymphoma remain unsatisfactory. Patients with follicular large-cell lymphoma were often excluded from these analyses and the type of therapy administered differed from one study to another. The fact that the biology of the follicular lymphomas differs from diffuse aggressive lymphomas, and the incurability of most patients increases the difficulty of developing a useful prognostic index.

THE INTERNATIONAL NON-HODGKIN'S LYMPHOMA PROGNOSTIC INDEX (IPI)

In 1990, there was a consensus that an international classification system based on clinically relevant prognostic factors in large-cell lymphoma should be developed and utilized in this disease [188]. For this reason, 16 single institutions and cooperative groups in the United States, Europe and Canada participated in the International Non-Hodgkin's Lymphoma Prognostic Factor Project [3]. In 2031 patients of all ages, this model, based on age, tumor stage, serum LDH concentration, performance status and number of extranodal disease sites, led to the identification of four risk groups with predicted 5-year survival rates of 73%, 51%, 43% and 26% (Table 35.6). In 1274 patients aged 60 or younger, an age-adjusted model based on tumor stage, serum LDH level and performance status identified four risk groups with predicted 5-year survival rates of 83%, 69%, 46% and 32%. In both models, the increased risk of death was a result of both a lower rate of complete responses and a higher rate of relapse.

· These two indexes, the IPI and the age-adjusted international index, have been shown to be significantly more accurate than the Ann Arbor classification in predicting long-term survival. The expectation is that the international index and the age-adjusted international index will be used in the design of future therapeutic trials in patients with aggressive non-Hodgkin's lymphoma and in the selection of appropriate therapeutic approaches for individual patients.

It is probable that the International Index may also be effectively applied to patients presenting with lymphoma subtypes other than large-cell lymphoma. We have applied the IPI to retrospective cohorts of patients with follicular lymphoma or nonfollicular small-cell lymphomas treated in our department in the course of the last 15 years. Figure 35.7a,b show that the IPI allows patients with both diffuse large-cell lymphoma and follicular lymphoma to be stratified into groups with different treatment outcomes.

LDH PLUS β₂-MICROGLOBULIN-BASED INDEX

Because serum β_2-microglobulin level was measured in very few centers at the time of diagnosis in patients included in the IPI project, ten years ago, the IPI could not incorporate this important prognostic indicator into multivariate analyses. However, the MD Anderson Cancer Center team has developed multivariate models which include the β_2-microglobulin level and other important parameters [164, 189]. An index based on LDH and β_2-microglobulin level has been proposed and it was shown to be effective in discriminating patients with good or poor risk whatever the lymphoma subtype (Figure 35.8). It seems likely that both of these parameters are surrogate markers for the total tumor burden.

Table 35.6 The International Non-Hodgkin's Lymphoma Prognostic Factors Index. Adapted from Shipp and Coll [3].

Model	Age-adjusted model	
Age		
Ann Arbor Stage	Ann Arbor Stage	
Performance status	Performance status	
Serum LDH	Serum LDH	
Number of extranodal sites of disease		
Number of factors and percentage of patients	5-year DFS	5-year survival
Survival according to risk group		
0 or 1 (35)	70	73
2 (27)	50	51
3 (22)	49	43
4 or 5 (16)	40	26
Age-adjusted index in patients below 60		
0 (22)	86	83
1 (32)	66	69
2 (32)	53	46
3 (14)	58	32

LDH, Lactate dehydrogenase; DFS, disease-free survival.

Parameters influencing the relapse rate in CR patients

PARAMETERS ASSOCIATED WITH RELAPSE IN CR PATIENTS

Depending upon their histologic subtype, 30–100% of patients who achieve CR will ultimately relapse. If patients with a high risk of relapse could be recognized, treatment might be modified to try to decrease their risk of relapse after CR. The previously described prognostic indicators are as good at predicting the patients who will relapse as they are at predicting the survival of the whole population. This is probably because relapse is correlated with LDH level and other, as yet unknown, parameters.

Large-cell lymphomas

Cabanillas et al. [190] have studied relapses that arose after 30 months of CR in 503 patients. The overall risk was 6.8% and a greater risk was

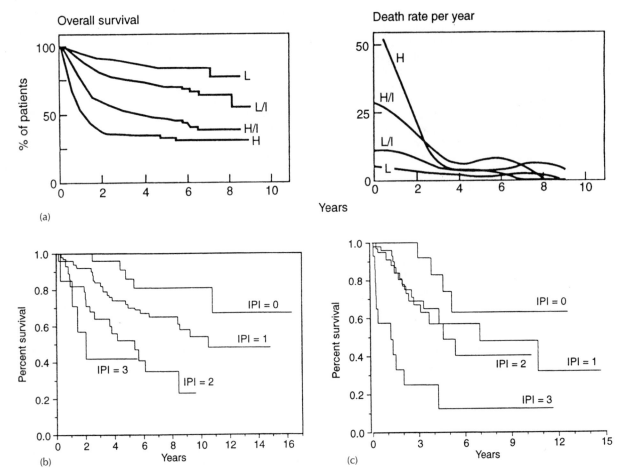

Figure 35.7 (a) Original description of the International Non-Hodgkin's Lymphoma Prognostic Index for lymphoma patients: Large-cell lymphoma patients from the original description. Reprinted with permission from [3]. Application of this index to (b) follicular lymphoma patients treated in our center (*P* = 0.0001) [18]. (c) Nonfollicular small-cell lymphoma patients treated in our center (*P*<0.001) [7].

associated with divergent histology (large cells in nodes and small cells in bone marrow), sclerosing large-cell lymphoma, or a diagnosis based on biopsy of an extranodal site. When none of these features were present, the risk of relapse was only 3%. When any of these features was present, the risk was 14%. Patients with divergent histology had a 43% late relapse rate. Five of the eight B-cell lymphoma patients with late relapse had a low S phase, suggesting that chemotherapy had eliminated rapidly proliferating clones, i.e., resulted in the selection of a cell clone with low proliferative potential that could have given rise to the late relapse. Immuno-phenotypic analysis of three cases at diagnosis and after relapse failed to support the hypothesis of a second *de novo* lymphoma, and were consistent with a true recurrence of the original tumor.

In our analysis of prognostic factors in patients treated with the LNH-84 regimen, the only initial parameters that were associated with a higher relapse rate were high LDH level, advanced stage, nonlarge-cell subtype and T-cell phenotype. However, these parameters were only associated with relapse during the first 2 or 3 years after treatment, and we were not able to find specific indicators of late relapses [191]. For CR patients at the end of their treatment, no indicator of early relapse has yet been found (see below).

Follicular lymphomas

Nearly all disseminated follicular patients relapse. As previously described [124], the risk of progression is higher and the progression-free survival is shorter in non-CR patients. High initial LDH and β_2-microglobulin levels are also associated with a higher relapse rate and a shorter time to treatment failure.

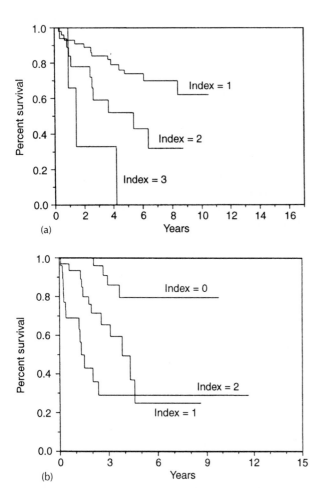

(a)

(b)

Figure 35.8 Application of the LDH-β_2-microglobulin index described in the MD Anderson Cancer Center [164] to patients treated in our center. (a) Overall survival of follicular lymphoma patients (*P*<0.01) and (b) nonfollicular small-cell lymphoma patients (*P*<0.001).

RESIDUAL DISEASE

Radiologically detectable masses

With modern radiologic examinations, nearly all patients with an initial bulky tumor had persistent radiologic abnormalities at the end of their treatment. These patients may either be in true CR with persistent fibronecrotic masses, or may have persistent lymphoma cells. The problem is particularly important for patients with persistent masses larger than 3 cm. In larger tumors, cytologic or histologic examination of residual masses must be performed, particularly in young patients, because intensive therapy in these truely PR patients, may permit CR and even a cure to be achieved [170].

For patients treated with the LNH-84 regimen

[43], 518 of the 553 who achieved CR patients were evaluated for persistent masses seen on imaging studies and 150 patients were found to have a so-called persisting fibronecrotic mass. Thirty-seven percent of the patients with a persistent mass relapsed compared to 35% of those without persisting radiologic abnormalities. Disease-free survival was no different for the two patient subgroups (Figure 35.9). This observation was confirmed in studies from the Dana–Farber Cancer Institute (Boston) and the National Cancer Institute [184,192]. Patients with persistent radiologic abnormalities may relapse but in these studies they did not relapse more frequently than patients without these abnormalities. Moreover, the site of relapse did not necessarily, or even frequently, involve the persistent abnormal mass.

Gallium-67 imaging

Gallium-67 imaging has been proposed to separate patients with persistent fibronecrotic mass from those with a persistent lymphoma mass [193]. Persisting lymphoma cells take up gallium-67 and, therefore, a persistent mass that can be imaged with gallium-67 is believed to have a higher relapse risk than one that cannot be imaged. However, few prospective studies exist which demonstrate that gallium imaging is useful in all patients. The special case of abnormal mediastinal gallium-67 uptake in the absence of relapse is worthy of mention. This is due to immunological 'thymic rebound' and occurs particularly in children [194].

Minimal residual disease

The assessment of minimal residual disease (MRD) requires characteristic molecular markers. Although antigen–receptor gene rearrangement and karyotypic abnormalities are present in almost every lymphoma

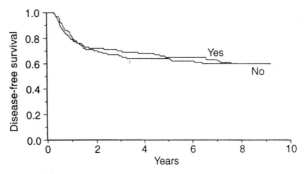

Figure 35.9 Freedom-from-relapse survival in aggressive-lymphoma patients treated with the LNH-84 regimen [43] according to the presence or absence of a persisting tumor mass after completion of chemotherapy (not significant).

sample, their use for detection of MRD has not been assessed in large series until recently. The use of the polymerase chain reaction (PCR) to detect lymphoma cells carrying the t(14;18) in the bone marrow of patients who received autologous purged bone marrow transplant has recently been reported [195]. This study shows that the presence or absence of t(14;18) PCR-positive cells after transplant is a strong predictor of disease-free survival. Although this analysis did not include a specific comparison of t(14;18) PCR positivity with other known and validated prognostic variables (stage, β_2-microglobulin, LDH, PS, etc.), it suggests that molecular monitoring of minimal residual disease may constitute a powerful tool to predict patient outcome after bonemarrow transplant. Further studies need to be undertaken to validate these important data.

Future prognostic indicators

PARAMETERS RELATED TO THE PROLIFERATION RATE OF LYMPHOMA CELLS

Tumor proliferation rate should still be considered a potential prognostic parameter because the best means of measuring this proliferation rate have not yet been determined. To date, very few large studies have demonstrated a correlation between measurements of proliferative rate and survival in multivariate analysis. The proliferative activity of lymphoma cells may be measured by assessing the S or $S+G_2M$ fractions (S-phase fraction or SPF) in representative samples. Lymphomas with a high number of cells in the SPF are thought to be actively expanding and, thus, to have a worse prognosis. However, no convincing evidence exists that demonstrates a direct relationship between the cell proliferation rate and stage, B symptoms or tumor bulk [196]. In follicular lymphoma or small lymphocytic lymphomas, three studies have documented a worse prognosis for patients with a high SPF (>5%) [197,198], and in large-cell lymphomas or other high-grade lymphomas, there is a strong suggestion that high proliferative activity (SPF >15–20%) adversely affects survival [197,199,200].

Recently, the proliferative activity of lymphoma cells has been measured by detection of the proliferation-associated nuclear antigens [201,202]. The percentage of cells expressing Ki-67 is a strong predictor of survival [201]. For example, Grogan [203] analyzed 105 patients for Ki-67 positivity;

patients with >60% of Ki-67-positive cells had a poor median survival (8 months) compared to patients with <60% Ki-67-positive cells (39 months); this poor prognosis persisted in multivariate analysis (Figure 35.10). Other parameters such as the number of proliferating cell nuclear antigen (PCNA)-positive cells or AgNOR(s) number (nuclear organizer regions) have also been associated with outcome [204–206]. Patients with >50% PCNA-positive lymphoma cells or a high number of AgNORs have a shorter survival.

Thymidine kinase (TK) is a cellular enzyme which is activated in the G_1/S phase of the cell cycle and its activity has been shown to correlate with the proliferative activity of tumor cells [207]. TK seems to correlate with clinical stage and provides significant information on progression-free or overall survival. This prognostic information seems to be more important in small-cell lymphomas where it was found to be predictive of relapse or histologic progression [208].

PARAMETERS RELATED TO LYMPHOMA CELLS AND THEIR ENVIRONMENT

Adhesion molecules

Normal and pathological lymphocytes intimately adhere to surrounding cells and to extracellular matrix components through the mediation of various cell surface receptors. The expression of some of these adhesion molecules has been associated with a particular pattern of spread of lymphoma cells. For instance, ICAM-1 (CD54) expression has been reported to be expressed in 64% of B-cell lymphomas, and the lack of ICAM-1 expression seems to be associated with bone marrow [209] or peripheral

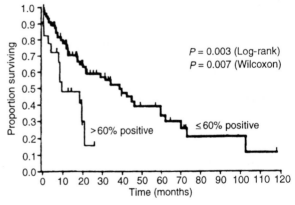

Figure 35.10 Survival of large-cell lymphoma patients according to expression of Ki-67 antigen. Data from Miller et al. [202] (reprinted with permission)

blood involvement [210]. N-CAM expression has been found in T-cell lymphomas involving unusual anatomic sites, such as the CNS, muscle, GI tract and nasopharynx, suggesting a role for this molecule in the extranodal extension of these lymphomas [211]. LAM-1 (LECAM-1), or L-selectin, was also found to be predominantly expressed on nodal lymphomas, whereas GI tract lymphomas were negative for this antigen [212]. Although these data suggest that adhesion molecules play a role in lymphoma cell localization, they do not indicate how this relates to prognosis.

Expression of the LFA-1 $\beta2$ chain (CD18) has been reported to be associated with a better patient outcome, although most studies have not compared its predictive value to other prognostic parameters and included relatively low numbers of patients [213]. In another study, the prognostic advantage conferred by CD18 was found to be limited to a patient subgroup whose tumors were negative for another adhesion molecule, CD44 [214].

Expression of the CD44 antigen (hyaluronate receptor) has been associated, in two different studies, to advanced stage disease [215] and CD44 expression has been reported to be an independent adverse prognostic parameter (for survival) [214]. Molecular isoforms of the CD44 molecule involved in solid tumor metastasis and in tumor progression have been described [216]. Interestingly, a CD44 isoform containing the central part of the protein, which is associated with metastasis in rats and humans, has recently been identified on lymphoma cells [217,218]. Experimental data also suggest that CD44 may contribute to the tendency of lymphoma cells to spread [219]. Taken altogether, these results suggest that the expression of certain CD44 isoforms may be associated with lymphoma spread and prognosis, a possibility which deserves further investigation.

Enzymes modifying the extracellular matrix

Aberrant expression of secreted proteinases and their inhibitors is thought to play a role in tumor spread and, hence, possibly survival. Expression of the 92 kD gelatinase (type IV collagenase) mRNA, for example, has been correlated with survival in a small series of immunoblastic lymphoma patients [220].

CYTOKINE PRODUCTION AND PATIENT OUTCOME

Cytokines can be produced by tumor cells or by reactive cells, and may influence tumor growth and the host immune system. In addition, soluble cytokine receptors are thought to modulate the activity of the cytokines themselves. Although multiple cytokines can be produced by lymphoma cells *in vitro*, the production of a cytokine *in vivo* is difficult to assess [221]. In few studies have cytokines or cytokine receptor levels in lymphoma patients been studied in relationship to clinical outcome. In serum from pediatric and adult NHL patients, however, higher levels of soluble interleukin-2 (IL-2) receptors have been observed in patients with advanced-stage disease [222–224]. In children with high-grade lymphomas, soluble IL-2 receptor levels were found to be an independent prognostic variable for disease-free survival, with a stronger predictive value than serum LDH or disease stage [222,223].

Recent studies have found serum IL-6 to be elevated in a substantial portion of lymphoma patients, and elevated levels to be correlated with the presence of B symptoms and patient survival [225]. Other studies have also indicated that TNFα and soluble TNF receptors are also elevated in a substantial proportion of lymphoma patients at diagnosis [226]. High levels correlate with B symptoms and altered performance status, as well as abnormal LDH and β_2-microglobulin levels. In addition, soluble TNF receptors were found to be an independent adverse prognostic factor for progression-free survival. Both IL-6 and TNFα play an important role in inflammatory reactions, but their origin and significance in lymphoma patients and their relationship to clinical presentation and outcome remain to be confirmed in larger studies.

Recently, serum IL-10 was detected in 47 of 101 lymphoma patients with active disease [227]. Elevated IL-10 was an independent adverse prognostic factor for survival and progression-free survival in aggressive lymphoma patients. Patients with stage IV disease and elevated IL-10 had an extremely poor outcome. These observations are noteworthy since IL-10 has been identified as a B-cell growth-promoting factor. However, it is possible that elevated serum levels of this and other cytokines, when produced by the lymphoma cells, simply reflect the total tumor burden.

DRUG RESTANCE OF TUMOR CELLS

The *mdr*-1 gene encodes the multidrug transporter P-glycoprotein (P-gp) which is the principal mediator of multidrug resistance (MDR) in cancer cells. There is now a lot of evidence that *mdr*-1 is highly expressed in many tumors that are clinically resistant to chemotherapy and, in some cancers, *mdr*-1 expression constitutes an adverse prognostic factor. Several non-cytotoxic drugs competitively inhibit P-gp and sensitize MDR cells *in vitro*. Combined therapy with

MDR-related cytotoxics and inhibitors reduces tumor size and prolongs life span in some animal models [228]. Lymphoma cells tend to be negative for *mdr*-1 expression at diagnosis and sensitive to MDR-related chemotherapy drugs (anthracyclins, vinca alkaloids, podophyllotoxins and taxanes). The high incidence of tumor *mdr*-1 expression in patients who relapse or who are resistant to initial therapy indicates that MDR induction may be an important clinical mechanism of resistance to treatment. Patients with more than 30% MDR-positive cells at diagnosis have a worse prognosis [229,230].

Prognostic factors in clinical practice

PROGNOSTIC FACTORS AT THE PATIENT'S BEDSIDE

Basic information

At the present time, the first piece of information required for the selection of appropriate treatment is the precise histologic subtype of lymphoma. The presence of prognostic factors described by the International Non-Hodgkin's Lymphoma Prognostic Factor Index is then determined in order to assign the patient to a prognostic group (Table 35.6). This will require a detailed clinical examination, computed tomography scans and bone marrow examinations should be performed to assess the clinical stage and the number of extranodal sites of disease. Performance status should be carefully assessed according to the objective criteria described in this index (Table 35.5). Serum LDH should be measured, using correct sampling technique and transfer to the laboratory in order to avoid hemolysis, which can result in overestimated results. Measurement of tumor masses is not required for prognostic estimates but provides information essential to the accurate assessment of treatment response. Special examinations of extranodal sites are recommended in particular circumstances: CSF examination in aggressive lymphomas (large cells, T-cell lymphomas, small noncleaved and lymphoblastic cells); GI tract exploration in the presence of clinical symptoms or oropharyngeal involvement and in specific histologic subtypes (mucosa-associated lymphoid tissue lymphomas and mantle cell lymphomas).

Useful, but not essential, information

Although β_2-microglobulin is not a prognostic factor included in the IPI, its measurement provides useful information and can be used in addition to it (see page 755).

Most of the other prognostic factors are provided by further analysis of the lymphoma specimen. Their routine evaluation cannot be recommended, and they have not, so far, been better at predicting outcome than histology or added discriminatory power to the International Index. However, large studies in which the predictive value of these new parameters is analyzed should be performed; such studies could, for example, provide new insights into the influence of biological parameters on clinical outcome. Immunophenotyping usually helps the histologic diagnosis (e.g., discriminating between B- or T-cell lymphomas and subtypes within these categories) and is therefore recommended as a means of more objectively classifying histologic subtypes. Further, the examination of the expression of other markers such as adhesion molecules may provide new biological insights. Karyotypic analysis also provides important information but is only available in highly specialized centers. The preservation of a tumor specimen frozen in liquid nitrogen should be strongly promoted to allow further immunohistologic investigations, molecular examinations, to assess the presence of PCR amplifiable markers useful for monitoring minimal residual disease and for other biological studies. Similarly, the preservation of frozen plasma or serum samples is to be encouraged since it is highly likely that new serologic markers will be identified in the future. The ready availability of serum samples, particularly a pretreatment sample, will greatly increase the speed at which such markers can be evaluated.

FUTURE IMPROVEMENT

Prognostic parameters are variables measured in individual patients which offer a partial explanation of the heterogeneity observed in the outcome of lymphoma patients. Studies of prognostic factors are important for at least two reasons. Firstly, prognostic factors may be used to predict, with some accuracy, the outcome of the disease for a patient or a group of patients. Combinations of such factors may be used to construct prognostic indexes and risk groups, and may have an important role in the selection of treatment. Secondly, the study of some prognostic factors may help us to understand the mechanisms of lymphoma and, thus, they may provide new directions for further studies. However, it is important to note that major prognostic parameters in one treatment era may subsequently become less important, or even irrelevant, because they have helped to define new treatment strategies adapted to the poor-risk patients. Alternatively, descriptions of new and more precise prognostic parameters may super-cede previous 'surrogate' markers of underlying biology.

The definition of prognostic factors and of prog-nostic indexes has allowed us to propose treatment strategies adapted to patient status, and thus to increase the number of patients who tolerate treat-ment, respond to treatment, and are cured by treat-ment [231]. While not a true therapeutic advance, prognostic factors have improved the efficiency of patient care.

References

1. Carbone PP, Kaplan HS, Musshoff K, et al. Report of the Committee on Hodgkin's disease staging clas-sification. *Cancer Res.* 1971, **31**: 1860–1861.
2. Coiffier B, Lepage E. Prognosis of aggressive lym-phoma: A study of five prognostic models with patients included in the LNH-84 regimen. *Blood* 1989, **74**: 558–564.
3. The International Non-Hodgkin's Lymphoma Prog-nostic Factors Project: A predictive model for aggres-sive non-Hodgkin's lymphoma. *N. Engl. J. Med.* 1993, **329**: 987–994.
4. The Non-Hodgkin's Lymphoma Pathologic Classifi-cation Project. National Cancer Institute sponsored study of classifications of non-Hodgkin's lymphomas. Summary and description of a Working Formulation for Clinical Usage. *Cancer* 1982, **49**: 2112–2135.
5. Lennert K, Mohri N, Sein H, et al. The histopathology of malignant lymphoma. *Br. J. Haematol.* 1975, **31**: 193–203.
6. Harris NL, Jaffe ES, Stein H, et al. A revised European–American Classification of lymphoid neo-plasms. A proposal from the International Lymphoma Study Group. *Blood* 1994, **84**: 1361–1392.
7. Berger F, Felman P, Sonet A, et al. Nonfollicular small B-cell lymphomas: A heterogeous group of patients with distinct clinical features and outcome. *Blood* 1994, **83**: 2829–2835.
8. Banks PM, Chan J, Cleary ML, et al. Mantle cell lymphoma. A proposal for unification of morphologic, immunologic, and molecular data. *Am. J. Surg. Pathol.* 1992, **16**: 637–640.
9. Horning SJ, Rosenberg SA. The natural history of initially untreated low-grade non-Hodgkin's lym-phomas. *N. Engl. J. Med.* 1984, **311**: 1471–1475.
10. Coiffier B. How should prognostic factors influence therapy in follicular lymphomas? *Ann. Oncol.* 1991, **2**: 619–620.
11. Mann R, Berard C. Criteria for the cytologic subclas-sification of follicular lymphomas: A proposed alter-native method. *Hematol. Oncol.* 1982, **1**: 187–195.
12. Nathwani BN, Metter GE, Miller TP, et al. What should be the morphologic criteria for the subdivision of follicular lymphomas? *Blood* 1986, **68**: 837–845.
13. Dardick I, Caldwell DR. Follicular center cell lym-phoma. Morphologic data relating to observer repro-ducibility. *Cancer* 1986, **58**: 2477–2484.
14. Gospodarowicz MK, Bush RS, Brown TC, et al. Prognostic factors in nodular lymphomas: A multi-variate analysis based on the Princess Margaret Hospital experience. *Int. J. Radiat. Oncol. Biol. Physics* 1984, **10**: 489–497.
15. Paryani SB, Hoppe RT, Cox RS, et al. Analysis of non-Hodgkin's lymphomas with nodular and favorable histologies, stages I and II. *Cancer* 1983, **52**: 2300–2307.
16. Anderson JR, Vose JM, Bierman PJ, et al. Clinical features and prognosis of follicular large-cell lym-phoma. A report from the Nebraska Lymphoma Study Group. *J. Clin. Oncol.* 1993, **11**: 218–224.
17. Bastion Y, Berger F, Bryon PA, et al. Follicular lymphomas: Assessment of prognostic factors in 127 patients followed for 10 years. *Ann. Oncol.* 1991, **9**: 123–129.
18. Bastion Y, Coiffier B. Is the international prognostic index for aggressive lymphoma patients useful for follicular lymphoma patients? *J. Clin. Oncol.* 1994, **12**: 1340–1342.
19. Ezdinli EZ, Costello WG, Kucuk O, et al. Effect of the degree of nodularity on the survival of patients with nodular lymphomas. *J. Clin. Oncol.* 1987, **5**: 413–418.
20. Anderson T, DeVita VT, Simon RM, et al. Malignant lymphoma. II. Prognostic factors and response to treatment of 473 patients at the National Cancer Institute. *Cancer* 1982, **50**: 2708–2721.
21. Coiffier B, Gisselbrecht C, Vose JM, et al. Prognostic factors in aggressive malignant lymphomas. Descrip-tion and validation of a prognostic index that could identify patients requiring a more intensive therapy. *J. Clin. Oncol.* 1991, **9**: 211–219.
22. Burke JS. The histopathologic classification of non-Hodgkin's lymphomas. Ambiguities in the Working Formulation and two newly reported categories. *Semin. Oncol.* 1990, **17**: 3–10.
23. Penny RJ, Blaustein JC, Longtine JA, Pinkus GS: Ki-1-positive large cell lymphomas, a heterogenous group of neoplasms. Morphologic, immunophenotypic, genotypic, and clinical features of 24 cases. *Cancer* 1991, **68**: 362–373.
24. Kadin ME. Ki-1 positive anaplastic large-cell lym-phoma: A clinicopathologic entity. *J. Clin. Oncol.* 1991, **9**: 533–536.
25. Moller P, Lammler B, Eberlein-Gonska M, et al. Primary mediastinal clear cell lymphoma of B-cell type. *Virchows Arch. Pathol. Anat.* 1986, **409**: 79–92.
26. Bitter MA, Franklin WA, Larson RA, et al. Morphology in Ki-1 (CD30)-positive non-Hodgkin's lymphoma is correlated with clinical features and the presence of a unique chromosomal abnormality, t(2, 5)(p23, q35). *Am. J. Surg. Pathol.* 1990, **14**: 305–316.
27. Feller AC, Sterry W: Large cell anaplastic lymphoma

tissue (SALT)-related B-cell lymphoma (primary cutaneous B-cell lymphoma). A concept and a clinicopathologic entity. *Arch. Dermatol.* 1993, **129**: 353–355.

152. De Bruin PC, Beljaards RC, Van Heerde P, et al. Differences in clinical behavior and immunophenotype between primary cutaneous and primary nodal anaplastic large cell lymphoma of T-cell or null cell phenotype. *Histopathology* 1993, **23**: 127–135.

153. Liang R, Chiu E, Loke SL. An analysis of 12 cases of non-Hodgkin's lymphomas involving the testis. *Ann. Oncol.* 1990, **1**: 383.

154. Doll DC, Weiss RB. Malignant lymphoma of the testis. *Am. J. Med.* 1986, **81**: 515–524.

155. Pan L, Beverley PCL, Isaacson PG. Lactate dehydrogenase (LDH) isoenzymes and proliferative activity of lymphoid cells. An immunocytochemical study. *Clin. Exp. Immunol.* 1991, **86**: 240–245.

156. Ferraris AM, Giuntini P, Gaetani GF. Serum lactic dehydrogenase as a prognostic tool for non-Hodgkin lymphomas. *Blood* 1979, **54**: 928–932.

157. Csako G, Magrath IT, Elin RJ. Serum total and isoenzyme lactate dehydrogenase activity in American Burkitt's lymphoma patients. *Am. J. Clin. Pathol.* 1982, **78**: 712–717.

158. Koziner B, Little C, Passe S, et al. Treatment of advanced diffuse histiocytic lymphoma. An analysis of prognostic variables. *Cancer* 1982, **49**: 1571–1579.

159. Shimamoto Y, Suga K, Nishimura J, et al. Major prognostic factors of Japanese patients with lymphoma-type adult T-cell leukemia. *Am. J. Hematol.* 1990, **35**: 232–237.

160. Cassuto JP, Krebs BP, Viot G, et al. β2-Microglobulin, a tumor marker of lymphoproliferative disorders. *Lancet* 1978, **ii**: 108–109.

161. Hagberg H, Killander A, Simonsson B. Serum β2-microglobulin in malignant lymphoma. *Cancer* 1983, **51**: 2220–2225.

162. Johnson PWM, Whelan J, Longhurst S, et al. β2-Microglobulin. A prognostic factor in diffuse aggressive non-Hodgkin's lymphomas. *Br. J. Cancer* 1993, **67**: 792–797.

163. Litam P, Swan F, Cabanillas F. Prognostic value of serum β2-microglobulin in low-grade lymphoma. *Ann. Intern. Med.* 1991, **114**: 855–860.

164. Swan F, Velasquez WS, Tucker S, et al. A new serologic staging system for large-cell lymphomas based on initial β2-microglobulin and lactate dehydrogenase levels. *J. Clin. Oncol.* 1989, **7**: 1518–1527.

165. Aviles A, Narvaez BR, Diaz-Maqueo JC, et al. Value of serum beta 2 microglobulin as an indicator of early relapse in diffuse large cell lymphoma. *Leuk. Lymph.* 1993, **9**: 377–380.

166. Karnovsky DA, Abelmann WH, Craver LF, et al. The use of nitrogen mustards in the palliative treatment of cancer. *Cancer* 1948, **1**: 634–656.

167. Conill C, Verger E, Salamero M. Performance status assessment in cancer patients. *Cancer* 1990, **65**: 1864–1866.

168. Mackintosh JF, Cowan RA, Jones M, et al. Prognostic factors in stage I and II high and intermediate grade non-Hodgkin's lymphoma. *Eur. J. Cancer Clin. Oncol.* 1988, **24**: 1617–1622.

169. Conlan MG, Armitage JO, Bast M, et al. Clinical significance of hematologic parameters in non-Hodgkin's lymphoma at diagnosis. *Cancer* 1991, **67**: 1389–1395.

170. Armitage JO. Treatment of non-Hodgkin's lymphoma. *N. Engl. J. Med.* 1993, **328**: 1023–1030.

171. Brown MJ, Hubbard SM, Longo DL, et al. Excess prevalence of pneumocystis carinii pneumonia in patients treated for lymphoma with combination chemotherapy. *Ann. Intern. Med.* 1986, **104**: 338–344.

172. Armitage JO, Weisenburger DD, Hutchins M, et al. Chemotherapy for diffuse large-cell lymphoma. Rapidly responding patients have more durable remissions. *J. Clin. Oncol.* 1986, **4**: 160–164.

173. Herman TS, Hammond N, Jones SE, et al. Involvement of the central nervous system by non-Hodgkin's lymphoma. The Southwest Oncology Group experience. *Cancer* 1979, **43**: 390–397.

174. Litam JP, Cabanillas F, Smith TL, et al. Central nervous system relapse in malignant lymphomas. Risk factors and implications for prophylaxis. *Blood* 1979, **54**: 1249–1257.

175. DeVita VT, Hubbard SM, Longo DL. The chemotherapy of lymphomas. Looking back, moving forward. The Richard and Hinda Rosenthal Foundation award lecture. *Cancer Res.* 1987, **47**: 5810–5824.

176. Zuckerman KS, LoBuglio AF, Reeves JA. Chemotherapy of intermediate grade and high-grade non-Hodgkin's lymphomas with a high-dose doxorubicin-containing regimen. *J. Clin. Oncol.* 1990, **8**: 248–256.

177. Lee R, Cabanillas F, Bodey GP, et al. A 10-year update of CHOP-Bleo in the treatment of diffuse large-cell lymphoma. *J. Clin. Oncol.* 1986, **4**: 1455–1461.

178. Longo DL, Duffey PL, Devita VT, et al. The calculation of actual or received dose intensity. A comparison of published methods. *J. Clin. Oncol.* 1991, **9**: 2042–2051.

179. Gottlieb AJ, Anderson JR, Ginsberg SJ. A randomized comparison of methotrexate dose and the addition of bleomycin to CHOP therapy for diffuse large cell lymphoma and other non-Hodgkin's lymphomas. Cancer and Leukemia Group B Study 7851. *Cancer* 1990, **66**: 1888–1896.

180. Meyer RM, Hryniuk WM, Goodyear MDE. The role of dose intensity in determining outcome in intermediate-grade non-Hodgkin's lymphoma. *J. Clin. Oncol.* 1991, **9**: 339–347.

181. Lepage E, Gisselbrecht C, Haioun C, et al. Prognostic significance of received relative dose intensity in non-Hodgkin's lymphoma patients: Application to LNH-87 protocol. *Ann. Oncol.* 1993, **4**: 651–656.

182. Kwak LW, Halpern J, Olshen RA, et al. Prognostic significance of actual dose intensity in diffuse large cell lymphoma. Results of a tree structured survival analysis. *J. Clin. Oncol.* 1990, **8**: 963–977.

183. McMaster ML, Greer JP, Wolff SN, et al. Results of treatment with high intensity, brief duration chemotherapy in poor prognosis non-Hodgkin's lymphoma. *Cancer* 1991, **68**: 233–241.

183a. Shipp MA, Neuberg D, Janicek M, et al. High-dose CHOP as initial therapy for patients with poor-prognosis aggressive non-Hodgkin's lymphoma – a dose-finding pilot study. *J. Clin. Oncol.* 1995, **13**: 2916–2923.

184. Shipp MA, Klatt MM, Yeap B, et al. Patterns of relapse in large-cell lymphoma patients with bulk disease: Implications for use of adjuvant radiation therapy. *J. Clin. Oncol.* 1989, **7**: 613–618.

185. Leonard RCF, Hayward RL, Prescott RJ, et al. The identification of discrete prognostic groups in low-grade non-Hodgkin's lymphoma. *Ann. Oncol.* 1991, **2**: 655–662.

186. Lepage E, Sebban C, Gisselbrecht C, et al. Treatment of low-grade non-Hodgkin's lymphomas: Assessment of doxorubicin in a controlled trial. *Hematol. Oncol.* 1990, **8**: 31–39.

187. Soubeyran P, Eghbali H, Bonichon F, et al. Low-grade follicular lymphomas: Analysis of prognosis in a series of 281 patients. *Eur. J. Cancer* 1991, **27**: 1606–1613.

188. Coiffier B, Shipp MA, Cabanillas F, et al. Report of the first workshop on prognostic factors in large-cell lymphomas. *Ann. Oncol.* 1991, **2**: 213–217.

189. Rodriguez J, Cabanillas F, McLaughlin P, et al. A proposal for a simple staging system for intermediate grade lymphoma and immunoblastic lymphoma based on the 'tumor score'. *Ann. Oncol.* 1992, **3**: 711–717.

190. Cabanillas F, Velasquez WS, Hagemeister FB, et al. Clinical, biological, and histologic features of late relapses in diffuse large cell lymphoma. *Blood* 1992, **79**: 1024–1028.

191. Coiffier B, Tilly H, Bosly A, et al. Long term follow-up of the 737 aggressive lymphoma patients treated in the LNH-84 protocol: Very few late relapses after 5 years. *Thirty-fifth Meeting of the American Society of Hematology*, 1993, St Louis, MO, Vol. 82, p. 444a (Abstract 1760).

192. Surbone A, Longo DL, DeVita VT, et al. Residual abdominal masses in aggressive non-Hodgkin's lymphoma after combination chemotherapy: Significance and management. *J. Clin. Oncol.* 1988, **6**: 1832–1837.

193. Kaplan WD, Jochelson MS, Herman TS, et al. Gallium-67 imaging: A predictor of residual tumor viability and clinical outcome in patients with diffuse large-cell lymphoma. *J. Clin. Oncol.* 1990, **8**: 1966–1970.

194. Peylan-Ramu N, Haddy TB, Jones E, et al. High frequency of benign mediastinal uptake of Gallium-67 after completion of chemotherapy in children with high-grade non-Hodgkin's lymphoma. *J. Clin. Oncol.* 1989, **7**: 1800–1806.

195. Gribben JG, Neuberg D, Freedman AS, et al. Detection by polymerase chain reaction of residual cells with the bcl-2 translocation is associated with increased risk of relapse after autologous bone marrow transplantation for B-cell lymphoma. *Blood* 1993, **81**: 3449–3457.

196. Macartney JC, Camplejohn RS. DNA flow cytometry of non-Hodgkin's lymphomas. *Eur. J. Cancer* 1990, **26**: 635–637.

197. Rehn S, Glimelius B, Strang P, et al. Prognostic significance of flow cytometry studies in B-cell non-Hodgkin lymphoma. *Hematol. Oncol.* 1990, **8**: 1–12.

198. Macartney JC, Camplejohn RS, Alder J, et al. Prognostic importance of DNA flow cytometry in non-Hodgkin's lymphoma. *J. Clin. Pathol.* 1986, **39**: 542–546.

199. Cowan RA, Harris M, Jones M, et al. DNA content in high and intermediate grade non-Hodgkin's lymphoma. Prognostic significance and clinicopathological correlations. *Br. J. Cancer* 1989, **60**: 904–910.

200. Akerman M, Brandt L, Johnson A, et al. Mitotic activity in non-Hodgkin's lymphoma. Relation to the Kiel classification and to prognosis. *Br. J. Cancer* 1987, **55**: 219–223.

201. Slymen DJ, Miller TP, Lippman SM, et al. Immuno-biologic factors predictive of clinical outcome in diffuse large-cell lymphoma. *J. Clin. Oncol.* 1990, **8**: 986–993.

202. Miller TP, Grogan TM, Dahlberg S, et al. Prognostic significance of the Ki-67 associated proliferative antigen in aggressive non-Hodgkin's lymphomas: A prospective Southwest Oncology Group trial. *Blood* 1994, **83**: 1460–1466.

203. Grogan TM, Lippman SM, Spier CM, et al. Independent prognostic significance of a nuclear proliferation antigen in diffuse large cell lymphomas as determined by the monoclonal antibody Ki-67. *Blood* 1988, **71**: 1157–1160.

204. Jakic-Razumovic J, Tentor D, Petrovecki M, et al. Nucleolar organiser regions and survival in patients with non-Hodgkin's lymphomas classified by the working formulation. *J. Clin. Pathol.* 1993, **46**: 943–947.

205. Klemi PJ, Alanen K, Jalkanen S, et al. Proliferating cell nuclear antigen (PCNA) as a prognostic factor in non-Hodgkin's lymphoma. *Br. J. Cancer* 1992, **66**: 739–743.

206. Kamel OW, Lebrun DP, Davis RE, et al. Growth fraction estimation of malignant lymphomas in formalin-fixed paraffin-embedded tissue using anti-PCNA/cyclin 19A2. Correlation with Ki-67 labeling. *Am. J. Pathol.* 1991, **138**: 1471–1477.

207. Hallek M, Wanders L, Strohmeyer S, et al. Thymidine kinase: A tumor marker with prognostic value for non-Hodgkin's lymphoma and a broad range of potential clinical applications. *Ann. Hematol.* 1992, **65**: 1–5.

208. Martinsson U, Glimelius B, Hagberg H, et al. Prognostic relevance of serum-markers in relation to histopathology, stage, and initial symptoms in advanced low-grade non-Hodgkin lymphomas. *Eur. J. Haematol.* 1988, **40**: 289–298.

209. Nozawa Y, Yamaguchi Y, Tominaga K, et al. Expression of leukocyte adhesion molecules (ICAM-1/LFA-1) related to clinical behavior in B-cell lymphomas. *Hematol. Oncol.* 1992, **10**: 189–194.

210. Horst E, Radaszkiewicz T, den Otter AH, et al. Expression of the leucocyte integrin LFA-1 (CD11a/CD18) and its ligand ICAM-1 (CD54) in lymphoid malignancies is related to lineage derivation and stage of differentiation but not to tumor grade. *Leukemia* 1991, **5**: 848–853.

211. Kern WF, Spier CM, Hanneman EH, et al. Neural cell

has become a larger component of the overall number of deaths recorded amongst patients treated for NHL [4], although most of these occur at or soon after diagnosis. Nevertheless, the number attributable to cardiotoxicity and second malignant tumours is a measurable cause for concern and must represent a target for reduction in the future.

Adverse effects appear with time and the true incidence of late effects following treatment with current multiagent chemotherapy strategies is not yet known. Survival to 3 years in first remission (certainly to 5 years) is evidence of cure for patients with childhood non-Hodgkin's lymphoma [5] and implies that there is opportunity for early definition of the population at risk for serious adverse effects of treatment. These survivors must remain under long-term surveillance, if the true cost of cure is to be defined. It is possible that the risk of late effects carried by survivors can be stratified not only by exposure to certain forms of therapy, but also by underlying individual biology – for example, some patients with second malignant tumours may carry a predisposing germline mutation [6].

Strategies for the surveillance of survivors must be based on the treatment received and a record of cumulative drug and radiation exposure should be compiled for each patient at the end of treatment. A summary of the known major sequelae is given in Table 36.1.

Second tumours

Much of the data about the risk of second cancer in survivors of cancer in childhood comes from patients treated in the prechemotherapy era. This will, therefore, involve a bias towards the effects of radiotherapy and represent the natural history of diseases where long-term survival has been achieved for many years. In this context, Hodgkin's disease has been studied in detail. The risk of both haematological and nonhaematological malignancy after treatment for Hodgkin's disease is well recognized. Acute non-lymphoblastic leukemia (ANLL) is reported in as many as 5% of those receiving combined chemo-radiotherapy at a median of 5–7 years from first diagnosis [7,8]. The risk of leukemia seems to increase with increasing exposure to alkylating agents (for example after treatment for relapse) [9]. It is suggested that ANLL is rare after radiation therapy alone, but under these circumstances, there is a much clearer association with nonhematological second

Table 36.1   Late effects from cancer treatment

Therapy risk factor	Sequelae	References
All chemotherapy	Dental caries	87
	Increased benign naevi (children)	88
Alkylating agents	Gonadal damage	40, 43, 44, 45, 46, 48
	Hemorrhagic cystitis/bladder fibrosis (prevented by mesna?)	76
	Second malignancy	9, 13
Cyclophosphamide	Possible cardiotoxicity (potentiates anthracycline risk?)	60
Ifosfamide	Renal tubular and glomerular toxicity	53, 73, 74, 75
BCNU and busulphan	Pulmonary toxicity	70, 71
Anthracyclines	Cardiotoxicity	57, 58, 59, 63
Doxorubicin	Possible risk factor for second malignancy	13, 14
Epipodophyllotoxins	Secondary leukaemia	15–17
Methotrexate	Neuropsychological damage	81
	Liver dysfunction?	86
Steroids	Cataract	84
	Osteoporosis	
Radiotherapy	Second malignancy	10, 11, 18, 19
Cranial RT	Neuropsychological damage	77, 78, 80
	Hypothalamic–pituitary damage	21, 22
TBI	Multiple endocrinopathy	34, 35, 39
	Infertility	51
	Cardiotoxicity	60, 65, 66
	Pulmonary toxicity	67–69
Surgery	Consequences are site- and procedure-dependent	

BCNU, carmustine.

cancer [10]. Such tumours usually occur in the radiation field, are usually bone or soft tissue sarcomas, skin and thyroid carcinomas, and appear to have a longer latency than treatment-induced ANLL [11].

These data are likely to be applicable to risk of second malignancy after treatment for NHL and, indeed, the occurrence of ANLL after exposure of patients with NHL to combined modality therapy has been described [12]. Whilst most of the chemotherapy risks have been attributed to the use of alkylating agents, for which a clear dose relationship can be identified [13], there is now some concern about the role of other agents including anthracyclines and epipodophyllotoxins. The Late Effects Study Group identified doxorubicin as a possible risk factor in secondary leukemia [13] and in one study of patients with secondary bone sarcoma, a history of exposure to anthracyclines appeared to reduce the latent interval of occurrence of the second tumour from the time of first diagnosis [14]. The evidence that exposure to epidophyllotoxin increases the risk of secondary leukemia is now generally accepted but, interestingly, the risk may relate to the scheduling of drug administration as much as to the cumulative dose given [15,16]. There also appear to be characteristic clinical and biological differences between the secondary leukemia related to alkylating agents and to epipodophyllotoxins, which may be important in understanding the biological basis of the leukemogenesis. These include a longer latent interval for leukemia induced by alkylating agents and the frequent finding of a chromosome abnormality involving 11q23 amongst those induced by epipodophyllotoxins [17].

These groups of drugs have a role in current multiagent chemotherapy strategies for both lymphoblastic and nonlymphoblastic lymphoma. Their therapeutic contribution, together with a better assessment of the safe dose threshold of alkylator therapy, must be evaluated.

The role for radiotherapy is now considerably reduced, even for central nervous system (CNS)-directed therapy, although there are many survivors who have received such treatment in the past. Nevertheless, it will retain a place as total body irradiation (TBI) in the management of a high-risk patients treated with myeloablative therapy and autologous bone marrow transplantation (ABMT), or peripheral blood stem cell support (PBSC). This represents an additive risk for second malignancy, particularly ANLL and myelodysplasia (MDS) [18]. Although the treatment given prior to myeloablative therapy for NHL would almost always include an alkylating agent, there is evidence to suggest that high-dose treatment itself is implicated as a risk factor. Patients receiving TBI and those aged over

40 years may have the highest risk [19].

One small but nevertheless important factor is the evidence that inherited genetic abnormalities relate to the pathogenesis of some cases of NHL. For example, patients with immunodeficiency syndromes have an increased risk of lymphoproliferative malignancy and this predisposition could transmit an increased risk of second cancer in such survivors. Patients with germline p53 mutations cannot be identified solely on the basis of family history and it is likely that this unrecognized risk factor contributes to some second malignancies. While p53 mutations have been described in several NHLs, particularly Burkitt's lymphoma [20], there is only one report of a patient with NHL who has developed a second malignancy and who has been shown to have a germline p53 mutation [6].

Growth and endocrine sequelae

The risk of abnormal growth as a result of endocrine consequences of therapy is well recognized, particularly following radiotherapy to the pituitary, thyroid and gonads [21]. Patients with obvious endocrine insufficiency can be successfully managed with endocrine replacement therapy but other issues including poor nutrition, corticosteroids and factors that influence the timing and pace of puberty, may also have important influence on growth and achievement of final adult height. Furthermore, direct damage to bone and soft tissues within radiation fields may make a significant impact on final height, or induce limb or spinal asymmetry. Major effects on endocrine function should now be unusual in patients treated with current multiagent chemotherapy – the avoidance of radiotherapy in both systemic therapy and as a component of CNS protection will have significantly improved the quality of outcome for more recent survivors.

GROWTH HORMONE DEFICIENCY

Growth hormone (GH) deficiency is the most common cause of growth abnormality in patients who have received cranial radiotherapy, either as part of previous strategies for CNS protection or as TBI for bone marrow transplantation (BMT) conditioning. Growth hormone deficiency is often the only endocrine abnormality following cranial irradiation, and there is a strong correlation between the pituitary dose received and both the risk and time of onset of symptomatic GH deficiency [22]. Young age at treatment may also increase the risk of damage [23]. It is probable that most cases of induced GH deficiency result from a disruption of the GH-releasing hormone/somatostatin feedback mechanism with dysfunction at the level of the hypothalamus rather than the pituitary [24].

Previous protocols for the treatment of lymphoblastic lymphoma have included a combination of cytotoxic drugs, corticosteroids and, for some, radiotherapy, a treatment strategy similar to that used for acute lymphoblastic leukemia for which more data are available. Each of these therapy elements may have an influence on growth [25]. Some studies have suggested that the chemotherapy used in acute lymphoblastic leukemia (ALL) has no effect on growth [26,27] but clinical observations often demonstrate treatment-related growth impairment followed by catch-up growth [28]. The intensity of chemotherapy may matter and growth performance of children with ALL receiving chemotherapy according to the more intensive LSA_2L_2 protocol [29] was worse than a similar group of patients treated on a conventional leukemia strategy (UKALL VIII) [28], although both groups received equivalent cranial radiation therapy. It is possible therefore that the intensity of chemotherapy does have an impact on growth [30] and studies of more recently treated patients receiving multiagent chemotherapy without cranial radiotherapy will be of interest.

Although GH-induced growth failure can be successfully treated by GH supplementation with achievement of satisfactory final adult height, it is important to recognize that GH is involved in a number of other physiological processes. Individuals who are GH deficient may be lethargic, show increased fat-to-lean body mass, have raised cholesterol and triglyceride levels, and have increased mortality [31,32]. They may also experience premature osteoporosis [33].

There is now adequate experience with the outcome of growth and development in children undergoing TBI for BMT conditioning. Most patients experience significant growth retardation after 1000 cGy given as a single fraction [34] but fractionation of the dose may reduce this risk. Other factors implicated in the growth problems of these children include thyroid dysfunction, radiation-induced skeletal dysplasia and chronic graft versus host disease (GVHD) and its treatment [35].

THYROID DYSFUNCTION

There is no evidence that chemotherapy alone is toxic to the thyroid in the absence of radiotherapy [36,37] and few patients with NHL would now be expected to receive radiotherapy to the neck. Previously, however, even scatter dose from cranial radiotherapy fields has been implicated as a cause of thyroid damage [38] and all patients receiving radiotherapy to a field incorporating or bordering on the thyroid (including TBI) must be monitored for the onset of compensated (normal T4, increased thyroid stimulating hormone) or true primary hypothyroidism. Monitoring must include careful clinical examination of the thyroid as these patients are also at risk of thyroid carcinoma [39].

PUBERTY AND FERTILITY

The risk of damage to gonadal function by both chemotherapy and radiation therapy is well recognized [40]. Depending on the type of damage to gonadal tissue, it may be necessary to intervene medically to allow children to achieve normal sexual development but most drugs that induce gonadal toxicity, including the alkylating agents, have a major effect against fertility rather than gonadal steroidogenesis. Fertility is also more likely to be damaged by radiotherapy, but children who receive direct gonadal irradiation are likely to also require lifelong sex hormone replacement therapy to maintain progress in puberty and induce secondary sexual characteristics [41,42].

Cyclophosphamide is the most common alkylating agent used in NHL protocols and its effects on male fertility are well recognized. The risk is dose-dependent and age or pubertal status at time of exposure seem unimportant [43]. Recovery over a period of years has been reported occasionally [44] and children treated prepubertally show normal progression through puberty as steroidogenesis is unaffected. The effects of other alkylating agents are probably the same, although long-term follow-up data for ifosfamide are not yet available. In adults, loss of libido and impairment of Leydig cell function is sometimes reported after exposure to chemotherapy such as mustine, oncovin, procarbazine, prednisone (MOPP) or mustine, vinblastine, procarbazine, prednisone (MVPP) [45].

The threshold dose at which radiotherapy damages the testis is uncertain, and most boys who receive TBI for conditioning prior to BMT are likely to retain hormone production and experience normal puberty. However, direct radiotherapy to the testes (e.g., for relapse in ALL) will result in damage to androgen production for which replacement therapy is required. In contrast, even scatter doses to the testes (e.g., from abdominal radiation fields) are likely to result in germ cell damage and reduced fertility [41].

The effects of chemotherapy on fertility in girls

are less certain but appear to be less severe than in boys [40,46]. Transient disturbance of established menstrual pattern is common during and immediately after treatment, but most prepubertal girls achieve normal puberty [47]. Female survivors of chemotherapy strategies containing alkylating agents are likely to be fertile (in contrast to boys) [48], despite evidence for changes in ovarian development [49]. Normal fertility has been reported in survivors of Burkitt's lymphoma who received doses of cyclophosphamide up to 9 g/m^2 [50].

Radiation doses in excess of 20 Gy are sterilizing [51] and lower doses may result in disturbances of ovarian endocrine function [42,46]. There is concern that patients exposed to doses less than 20 Gy may experience premature menopause, but the size of this risk is unknown. Patients who experience complete ovarian failure require oestrogen replacement not merely to induce development of secondary sexual characteristics, but also to relieve symptoms of estrogen deficiency, and to protect against premature onset of osteoporosis and ischemic heart disease.

SKELETAL DAMAGE

The risk of direct damage to skeletal growth is confined to structures directly within radiation fields [52]. This should be a rare occurrence in current management but recent reports of metabolic bone damage following ifosfamide-induced renal tubular toxicity are a reason for caution, particularly in young children treated with this drug [53].

Risk for pregnancy and offspring

Despite reports of high fetal loss in some survivors, outcome of pregnancy is likely to be normal for all women except those who have received radiation to the abdomen [54]. These are, of course, likely to be women at high risk of infertility in which case there is also concern that structural and vascular changes induced by radiation to the uterus would also limit potential for successful pregnancy after *in vitro* fertilization and embryo re-implantation [55].

There is no current evidence that any potential for germ cell mutagenesis induced by treatment is exhibited as cancer or congenital abnormality in the offspring of survivors [56], but detailed studies of more recently diagnosed patients, especially those treated with aggressive therapies, are required to confirm this.

Cardiac toxicity

The cardiotoxic effects of anthracycline drugs have been recognized for some years. Acute toxicity is rare and is usually characterized by benign supraventricular arrhythmia. Subacute toxicity can occur within days or weeks of exposure. This may evolve into chronic cardiomyopathy but, perhaps of greater concern, is the risk that this can develop in apparently asymptomatic patients. This poses considerable uncertainties for patients exposed to anthracyclines as the onset of cardiac failure may occur after an interval of many years beyond completion of therapy and may be unheralded by any previous symptoms. The risk is dose related and rises steeply with increasing dose exposure beyond 500 mg/m^2 [57]. The precise incidence of subclinical myocardial damage is less certain but the risk of clinical symptoms may increase with length of follow-up [58]. One study indicated that 65% of patients exposed to doses of anthracycline ranging from 228 to 550 mg/m^2 (median 360 mg/m^2) showed late echocardiogram abnormalities [59]. Evidence suggests that the risk is enhanced by young age at first treatment with anthracycline, mediastinal radiation and, perhaps, by exposure to other drugs – cyclophosphamide has been implicated [60], particularly at higher doses (>120 mg/kg in one week) [61], although these data rest on relatively small experience. There is also indirect evidence to implicate the role of ifosfamide [62]. This combination of risk factors places survivors of the more intensive strategies used in the treatment of NHL at some risk, and also the survivors of BMT. Schedule of administration seems to be important and risk may be reduced by prolonging infusion times [63].

The implications of such serious toxicity are, first, the necessity to follow all survivors who have received anthracyclines with appropriate monitoring of cardiac function and, second, the need to offer advice about exercise and life style. For girls there may be particular risk of cardiac decompensation during pregnancy. The best approach to the treatment of asymptomatic myocardial dysfunction is unclear but there is some interest in the use of angiotensin-converting enzyme (ACE) inhibitor drugs in this setting. Treatment of established cardiac failure requires conventional management but some patients have required cardiac transplantation for irreversible cardiomyopathy.

Prevention of anthracycline cardiotoxicity currently depends on a cautious approach to cumulative dose and the use of longer infusion times. Interest in anthracycline analogues with less intrinsic cardiotoxic potential and in the development of cardioprotective medications are important areas for future development, although the risk that therapeutic efficacy may be lessened by cardioprotective agents must be considered and explored [64].

Several reports suggest that mediastinal irradiation may not only potentiate anthracycline toxicity but may also predispose to premature coronary artery disease [65]. In addition, radiation can cause constrictive pericarditis although this is unusual at doses less than 40 Gy [66].

Pulmonary function

Pulmonary fibrosis and pneumonitis are well recognized after radiation and, in adults, late changes are more likely to occur in patients who have shown acute pulmonary toxicity. This rarely occurs at doses below 30 Gy [67,68]. The physiological changes noted in patients damaged by radiotherapy during adolescence or adult life are largely those of fibrosis with loss of lung volume and reduced compliance. In contrast the problems experienced by survivors of treatment during childhood will represent a restriction in the growth of the whole chest, as well as the specific effects on the lung. Furthermore, damage probably occurs at a lower dose of radiation in children [69].

A number of chemotherapy agents have been associated with pulmonary damage, of which BCNU is likely to be of most concern to survivors of therapy for NHL. Toxicity to bis(2-chloroethyl)-nitrosurea (BCNU, carmustine) is dose related and evidence of fibrosis has been reported in over 50% of patients receiving cumulative doses greater than 1500 mg/m^2 [70,71]. There are also reports of toxicity with other alkylating agents, including cyclophosphamide, busulfan and melphalan, and with methotrexate [72]. Damage from methotrexate, although rare, may occur at relatively low doses and suggests that an element of individual idiosyncrasy is involved.

There are no data addressing the potential additive role of environmental factors (smoking or occupational exposures) but it would be sensible to advise patients at risk particularly to avoid such additional hazards.

Renal function

One of the few reasons for patients with NHL to receive irradiation to the kidney is during TBI for BMT. Although this is an obvious additional risk for nephrotoxicity, significant problems are rarely encountered. Toxicity induced by chemotherapy is of greater concern, particularly as this may impose additional damage to renal function already compromised by tumor lysis at the time of diagnosis and/or by nephrotoxic antimicrobial therapy during treatment. Ifosfamide, the nitrosureas and methotrexate are all potential concerns [73,74]. Ifosfamide has been incorporated into strategies for treatment of NHL only recently and long-term follow-up is limited. Nevertheless, its use introduces a new element of nephrotoxicity, which may be manifest by early clinical or subclinical renal tubular damage. This may progress to cause serious metabolic problems as well as reduced glomerular function [75].

Acute bladder toxicity from the use of cyclophosphamide and ifosfamide is rare with the now widespread use of mesna and aggressive hydration schedules. Late-onset bladder bleeding can occur from telangiectatic changes to bladder mucosa [76] but persistent symptoms merit investigation to exclude secondary malignant disease.

Neuropsychological and psychosocial sequelae

Cranial irradiation for CNS prophylaxis has been part of earlier treatments for lymphoblastic lymphoma but, as adequate control can be achieved utilizing chemotherapy strategies, it is likely that radiotherapy will be used in the future only for the small number of patients who present with CNS disease at diagnosis or relapse. Experience of large numbers of children treated for ALL has provided a good insight into the risk of neuropsychological damage after cranial radiation at doses up to 24 Gy [77]. Although many children who receive a course of cranial radiation appear to function in the normal range, formal testing shows neuropsychological test scores below those of control groups, including other patients with cancer not receiving CNS therapy. Deficits are generally greater in terms of attention span and nonverbal cognitive processing skills, rather than in verbal skills [78], hence many such children may demonstrate specific difficulties with educational tasks, such as math and spelling, whilst otherwise showing normal performance. Young age at treatment is probably the most important risk factor at a given dose range [79] but dose itself is important as indicated by the outcome for children receiving higher doses for treatment of brain tumours – such patients are undoubtedly more severely damaged. The effect on neuropsychological performance of a reduction in prophylactic radiation dose from 24 to 18 Gy has not yet been adequately assessed and at least one report has concluded that the doses are equally neurotoxic [80]. Most chemotherapy strategies now incorporate intrathecal and high-dose intravenous methotrexate, and there is insufficient evidence to prove that alternative strategies to protect the CNS with chemotherapy alone are less damaging than radiation, although it is hoped that this will be the case [81].

Chronic neurotoxicity may represent a spectrum of disease and, whilst most affected children demonstrate educational difficulties of varying severity, a minority go on to manifest evidence of leukoencephalopathy with severe intellectual, sensory and physical handicaps. The risk is greatest in those who have received more than one course of cranial radiotherapy, usually in combination with intrathecal and systemic methotrexate [82]. Correlation of neurological outcome with structural abnormalities seen on computed tomography or magnetic resonance imaging scans is notoriously difficult [83]. Additional neurological problems may relate to visual impairment from steroid- or radiation-induced cataracts, and this will include patients undergoing BMT [84].

Although measurable neuropsychological damage from CNS prophylaxis is the most obvious adverse outcome of therapy, there is good evidence that some survivors experience difficulties in adult life, including problems with employment, insurability and in establishing close relationships [85]. Children and adolescents are especially vulnerable to disruption of their education and to difficulties with the development of normal peer relationships. Awareness of such issues has encouraged cancer centers to offer a wide range of strategies for personal and family support.

Miscellaneous late effects

BOWEL

The use of radiation therapy to the abdomen is unusual in the context of treatment for NHL (except as TBI in conditioning for BMT) and, as the role of chemotherapy in inducing important late effects of therapy in the gastrointestinal tract is largely to potentiate the long-term effects of radiotherapy, the incidence of chronic gastrointestinal problems is low. Patients who require surgery for intestinal lymphoma are at risk of intestinal obstruction from adhesions. Resection of the distal small bowel is theoretically associated with vitamin B_{12} malabsorption but, as current strategies for the management of advanced intra-abdominal B-cell NHL do not advocate debulking or tumor resection, the problem should be rarely encountered.

LIVER

Radiation damage to the liver is recognized but the need for such therapy in the treatment of NHL is remote. Hepatic fibrosis from administration of methotrexate is greatest in relation to chronic oral administration for prolonged periods and the risk of this from intravenous methotrexate seems small [86]. There is no evidence to suggest that the transient acute changes in liver function encountered during chemotherapy are relevant to late sequelae if normal liver function tests are documented at the end of therapy.

TEETH

Direct irradiation of developing teeth is damaging but unlikely to be encountered in this group of patients. Nevertheless, the generally deleterious effect of chemotherapy is recognized, including an increased risk of dental caries [87].

SKIN AND HAIR

Alopecia induced by chemotherapy is almost always reversible but hair loss after radiation therapy may be incomplete, although this is unusual at the doses used for CNS prophylaxis. Skin pigmentation induced by chemotherapy may be prolonged but usually resolves slowly with time. Children receiving chemotherapy are reported to develop increased numbers of benign naevi, the significance of which is uncertain [88].

Conclusion

The declining role for radiotherapy as part of the treatment for NHL has reduced or eliminated the risk of certain important late effects in more recently diagnosed patients. The greater challenge to the long-term health of survivors treated with current multi-agent chemotherapy schedules lies in the risks imposed by exposure to anthracycline and alkylating drugs. The elimination of such agents from treatment schedules may not yet be possible, but it would remove the risk of cardiotoxicity, avoid male infertility and significantly reduce the risk of second malignancy. Conversely, the introduction of newer chemotherapy agents presents new risks, for example, ifosfamide-induced nephrotoxicity and secondary leukemia after exposure to etoposide.

Survivors need to be monitored for potential complications, and they and their other medical attendants must be fully informed of their treatment and its risks. Continuing and indefinite follow-up is required to provide such support and to document the development of late toxicity with accuracy, for the benefit of the planners of future treatment.

References

1. Stiller CA, Bunch KJ. Trends in survival for childhood cancer in Britain diagnosed 1971–1985. *Br. J. Cancer* 1990, **62**: 806–815.
2. Link MP, Donaldson SS, Berard CW, et al. Results of treatment of childhood non-Hodgkin's lymphoma with combination chemotherapy with or without radiotherapy. *N. Engl. J. Med.* 1990, **322**: 1169–1174.
3. Hawkins MM, Kingston JE, Kinnier Wilson LM. Late deaths after treatment for childhood cancer. *Arch. Dis. Child.* 1990, **65**: 1356–1363.
4. Robertson CM, Stiller CA, Kingston JE. Causes of death in children with non-Hodgkin's lymphoma between 1974 and 1985. *Arch. Dis. Child.* 1992, **67**: 1378–1383.
5. Hawkins MM. Long term survival and cure after childhood cancer. *Arch. Dis. Child.* 1989, **64**: 798–807.
6. Malkin D, Jolly KW, Barbier N, et al. Germline mutations of the p53 suppressor gene in children and young adults with second malignant neoplasms. *N. Engl. J. Med.* 1992, **326**: 1309–1315.
7. Coleman CN. Secondary malignancies after treatment for Hodgkin's disease: An evolving picture. *J. Clin. Oncol.* 1986, **4**: 821–826.
8. Valagussa P, Santoro A, Fossati-Bellini F, et al. Second acute leukaemia and other malignancies following treatment for Hodgkin's disease. *J. Clin. Oncol.* 1983, **4**: 830–837.
9. Meadows AT, Obringer AC, Marrero O, et al. Second malignant neoplasms following childhood Hodgkin's disease: Treatment and splenectomy as risk factors. *Med. Pediatr. Oncol.* 1989, **17**: 477–484.
10. Coltman CA, Dixon DO. Second malignancies complicating Hodgkin's disease: A South West Oncology Group 10 year follow up. *Cancer Treat. Rep.* 1982, **66**: 1023–1033.
11. Tucker MA, Coleman CN, Cox RS, et al. Risk of second cancers after treatment for Hodgkin's disease. *N. Engl. J. Med.* 1988, **318**: 76–81.
12. Ingram L, Mott M, Mann JR, et al. Second malignancies in children treated for non-Hodgkin's lymphoma and T cell leukaemia with UKCCSG regimens. *Br. J. Cancer* 1987, **55**: 463–466.
13. Tucker MA, Meadows AT, Boice JD, et al. Leukemia after therapy with alkylating agents for childhood cancer. *J. Natl. Cancer Inst.* 1978, **78**: 459–464.
14. Newton WA Jr, Meadows AT, Shimada H, et al. Bone sarcomas as second malignant neoplasms following childhood cancer. *Cancer.* 1991, **67**: 193–201.
15. Pui CH, Ribiero RC, Hancock ML, et al. Acute myeloid leukemia in children treated with epipodophyllotoxins for acute lymphoblastic leukemia. *N. Engl. J. Med.* 1991, **325**: 1682–1687.
16. Hawkins MM, Kinnier Wilson LM, Stovall MA, et al. Epipodophyllotoxins, alkylating agents and radiation and risk of secondary leukaemia after childhood cancer. *Br. Med. J.* 1992, **304**: 951–958.
17. Whitlock JA, Greer JP, Lukens JN. Epipodophyllotoxin related leukemia. Identification of a new subset of secondary leukemia. *Cancer* 1991, **68**: 600–604.
18. Rohatiner A. Myelodysplasia and acute myelogenous leukemia after myeloablative therapy with autologous stem cell transplantation. *J. Clin. Oncol.* 1994, **12**: 2521–2523.
19. Darrington DL, Vose JM, Anderson JR, et al. Incidence and characterisation of secondary myelodysplastic syndrome and acute myelogenous leukemia following high dose chemoradiotherapy and autologous stem cell transplantation for lymphoid malignancies. *J. Clin. Oncol.* 1994, **12**: 2527–2534.
20. Gaidano G, Ballerine P, Gong JZ, et al. p53 mutations in human lymphoid malignancies: Association with Burkitt's lymphoma and chronic lymphocytic leukemia. *Proc. Natl Acad. Sci. USA* 1991, **88**: 5413–5417.
21. Rappaport R, Brauner R. Growth and endocrine disorders secondary to cranial irradiation. *Pediatr. Res.* 1989, **25**: 561–567.
22. Shalet SM, Clayton PE. Factors influencing the development of irradiation induced growth hormone deficiency. *Horm. Res.* 1990, **33**: 99.
23. Berry DH, Elders MJ, Crist W, et al. Growth in children with acute lymphoblastic leukaemia. *Med. Pediatr. Oncol.* 1983, **11**: 39–45.
24. Lannering B, Albertson-Wikland K. Growth hormone release in children after cranial irradiation. *Horm. Res.* 1987, **27**: 13–22.
25. Blatt J, Bercu BB, Gillin JC, et al. Reduced pulsatile growth hormone secretion in children after therapy for acute lymphoblastic leukaemia. *J. Pediatr.* 1984, **104**: 182–186.
26. Sunderman PA, Pearson HA. Growth effects of long term anti leukaemic therapy. *J. Pediatr.* 1969, **75**: 1058–1062.
27. Wells RJ, Foster MB, D'Ercole J, et al. The impact of cranial irradiation on the growth of children with acute lymphoblastic leukaemia. *Am. J. Dis. Child.* 1983, **137**: 37–39.
28. Clayton PE, Shalet SM, Morris Jones PH, et al. Growth

in children treated for acute lymphoblastic leukaemia. *Lancet* 1988, **i**: 460–462.

29. Kirk JA, Raghupathy P, Stevens MM, et al. Growth failure and growth hormone deficiency after treatment for acute lymphoblastic leukaemia. *Lancet* 1987, **i**: 190–193.

30. Shalet SM, Clayton PE, Price DA. Growth and pituitary function in children treated for brain tumours or acute lymphoblastic leukaemia. *Horm. Res.* 1988, **30**: 53–61.

31. Blackett PR, Weech PK, McConathy WJ, et al. Growth hormone in the regulation of hyperlipidemia. *Metabolism* 1982, **31**: 117–120.

32. Salomon F, Cuneo RC, Hesp R, et al. Growth hormone deficiency in adults. *Acta Pediatr. Scand.* 1989, **356**: 69.

33. Gilsanz V, Carlson ME, Roe TF, et al. Osteoporosis after cranial irradiation for acute lymphoblastic leukemia. *J. Pediatr.* 1990, **117**: 238–244.

34. Kolb HJ, Bender-Gotze C. Late complications of allogeneic bone marrow transplantation for leukemia. *Bone Marrow Transplant.* 1990, **6**: 61–72.

35. Sanders JE, Buckner CD, Sullivan KM, et al. Growth and development in children after bone marrow transplantation. *Horm. Res.* 1988, **30**: 92–97.

36. Nygaard R, Bjerve KS, Kolmannskog S, et al. Thyroid function in children after cytostatic treatment for acute leukemia. *Pediatr. Hematol. Oncol.* 1988, **5**: 35–38.

37. Devney RB, Sklar CA, Nesbit ME Jr, et al. Serial thyroid function measurements in children with Hodgkin's disease. *J. Pediatr.* 1984, **105**: 223–227.

38. Rogers PC, Fryer CJ, Hussein S. Radiation dose to the thyroid in the treament of acute lymphoblastic leukaemia. *Med. Pediatr. Oncol.* 1982, **10**: 385–388.

39. Barnes ND. Effects of external irradiation on the thyroid gland in childhood. *Horm. Res.* 1988, **30**: 84–89.

40. Shalet SM. Disorders of gonadal function due to radiation and cytotoxic chemotherapy in children. *Adv. Intern. Med. Pediatr.* 1989, **58**: 1–21.

41. Shalet SM, Horner A, Ahmed SR, et al. Leydig cell damage after testicular irradiation for lymphoblastic leukaemia. *Med. Pediatr. Oncol.* 1985, **13**: 65–68.

42. Hamre MR, Robison LL, Nesbit ME, et al. Effects of radiation on ovarian function in long term survivors of childhood acute lymphoblastic leukemia: A report from the Children's Cancer Study Group. *J. Clin. Oncol.* 1987, **5**: 1759–1765.

43. Watson AR, Rance CP, Bain J. Long term effects of cyclophosphamide on testicular function. *Br. Med. J.* 1985, **291**: 1457–1460.

44. Wallace WHB, Shalet SM, Lendon M, et al. Male fertility in long term survivors of acute lymphoblastic leukaemia in childhood. *Int. J. Androl.* 1991, **14**: 312–319.

45. Byrne J, Mulvihill JJ, Myers MH, et al. Effects of treatment on fertility in long term survivors of childhood or adolescent cancer. *N. Engl. J. Med.* 1987, **317**: 1315–1321.

46. Clayton PE, Shalet SM, Price DA, Morris Jones PH. Ovarian function following chemotherapy for childhood brain tumours. *Med. Pediatr. Oncol.* 1989, **17**: 92–96.

47. Quigley C, Cowell C, Jiminez M, et al. Normal or early development of puberty despite gonadal damage in children treated for acute lymphoblastic leukemia. *N. Engl. J. Med.* 1989, **321**: 143–151.

48. Wallace WHB, Shalet SM, Tetlow LJ, et al. Ovarian function following treatment of childhood acute lymphoblastic leukaemia. *Med. Pediatr. Oncol.* 1993, **21**: 333–339.

49. Himmelstein-Braw R, Peters H, Faber M. Morphological study of the ovaries of leukaemic children. *Br. J. Cancer* 1978, **38**: 82–87.

50. Neequaye JE, Byrne J, Levine PH. Menarche and reproduction after treatment for African Burkitt's lymphoma. *Br. Med. J.* 1991, **303**: 1033.

51. Wallace WHB, Shalet SM, Crowne EC, et al. Ovarian failure following abdominal radiation in childhood: Natural history and prognosis. *Clin. Oncol.* 1989, **1**: 75–79.

52. Butler MS, Robertson WW Jr, Rate W, et al. Skeletal sequelae of radiation therapy for malignant childhood tumours. *Clin. Orthop. Rel. Res.* 1990, **251**: 235–240.

53. Pratt CB, Meyer WH, Jenkins JJ, et al. Ifosfamide, Fanconi's syndrome and rickets. *J. Clin. Oncol.* 1991, **9**: 1495–1499.

54. Hawkins MM, Smith RA. Pregnancy outcomes in childhood cancer survivors: Probable effects of abdominal irradiation. *Intl. J. Cancer* 1989, **43**: 399–402.

55. Critchley HOD, Wallace WHB, Mamtora H, et al. Ovarian failure after whole abdominal radiotherapy: The potential for pregnancy. *Br. J. Obstet. Gynaecol.* 1992, **99**: 392–394.

56. Hawkins MM. Is there evidence of a therapy related increase in germ cell mutation among childhood cancer survivors? *J. Natl Cancer Inst.* 1991, **83**: 1643–1650.

57. Von Hoff DD, Rozencweig M, Layard M, et al. Daunomycin induced cardiotoxicity in children and adults. *Am. J. Med.* 1977, **62**: 200–208.

58. Steinherz LJ, Steinherz PG, Tan CT, et al. Cardiac toxicity 4–20 years after completing anthracycline therapy. *JAMA.* 1991, **266**: 1672–1677.

59. Lipshultz SE, Colan SD, Gelber RD, et al. Late cardiac effects of doxorubicin therapy for acute lymphoblastic leukaemia in childhood. *N. Engl. J. Med.* 1991, **324**: 808–815.

60. Watts RG. Severe and fatal anthracycline cardiotoxicity at cumulative doses below 400mg/m^2: Evidence for enhanced toxicity with multiagent chemotherapy. *Am. J. Hematol.* 1991, **36**: 217–218.

61. Steinherz LJ, Steinherz PG, Mangiacasale D, et al. Cardiac changes with cyclophosphamide. *Med. Pediatr. Oncol.* 1981, **9**: 417–422.

62. Oberlin O, Habrand J-L, Zucker JM, et al. No benefit of ifosfamide in Ewing's sarcoma: A nonrandomised study of the French Society of Pediatric Oncology. *J. Clin. Oncol.* 1992, **10**: 1407–1412.

63. Legha SS, Benjamin RS, Mackay B, et al. Reduction of doxorubicin cardiotoxicity by prolonged continuous intravenous infusion. *Ann. Intern. Med.* 1982, **96**: 133–139.

64. Speyer JL, Green MD, Kramer E, et al. Protective effect of the bispiperazinedione ICRF-187 against

different degrees of differentiation – probably a consequence, in part, of differences in the genetic abnormalities in the tumor cells, and possibly also of subtle differences in their cellular origins. The likelihood that SNCC lymphoma is predominantly of MALT origin, for example, is supported by its similar distribution to low-grade MALT lympomas.

Incongruency of a different kind between histology and cytogenetics is demonstrated by the observation that a proportion of SNCC lymphomas (up to 50%) in adults, generally above the age of 40 years, have been reported to contain 14;18 translocations [13], a translocation that occurs predominantly in follicular lymphomas [9], but which is also observed in perhaps a third of large B-cell lymphomas [9,10]. Rare tumors, and at least one derived cell line, containing both c-*myc*/Ig and 14;18 translocations, have also been described [9, 14–16]. These data probably indicate that there is a subset of SNCC lymphoma, which tend to arise in older individuals, that are closely related to follicular lymphoma and may represent transformation of subclinical follicular lymphoma into a more aggressive (high-grade) lymphoma through acquisition of additional genetic changes, including, in some cases, a c-*myc*/Ig translocation. Indeed, several cases of overt follicular lymphoma transforming into a Burkitt's or Burkitt-like lymphoma/leukemia, sometimes with and sometimes without the acquisition of a c-*myc*/Ig translocation have been reported [15,17–19]. A paradigm for the relationship between these various histological and cytogenetic entities is depicted in Figure 37.1.

It seems likely, as discussed in Chapter 16, that the chromosomal translocations with which the SNCC lymphomas are associated arise in precursor B-cells, but that the translocation-containing cell clone must undergo further differentiation before being manifested as a neoplasm. In spite of the phenotypic resemblance to follicular center cells, however, the aggressive clinical behavior of small noncleaved cell lymphomas is quite distinct from the much more slowly progressive follicular lymphomas and, although 'homing' of Burkitt's lymphoma cells to germinal centers in mesenteric nodes adjacent to a bowel mass has been described [20], SNCC lymphomas are always diffuse and never have a follicular architecture. When transformation occurs in a pre-existing follicular lymphoma, it is probable that an 8;14 translocation develops in an immature B-cell that already contains a 14;18 translocation, dramatically altering the behavior of the neoplastic cells (Figure 37.1).

While it is apparent that the histological category of 'SNCC lymphoma' is heterogeneous – both with respect to histology and cytogenetics – there is probably less heterogeneity in children and young adults, who normally have Burkitt's lymphomas with a c-*myc*/Ig translocation, than in older individuals [13]. A more precise diagnosis is possible when phenotype and karyotype are examined in addition to histology, and their routine employment is strongly recommended. However, at the present time there is no evidence that patients with cytogenetically different tumors within the histological category of SNCC lymphoma have a different

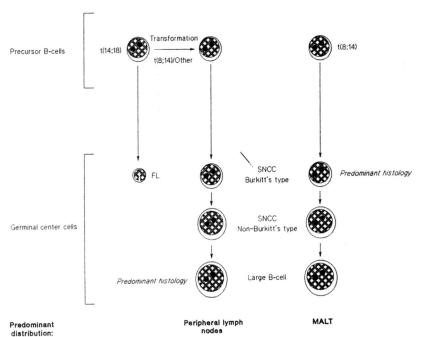

Figure 37.1 Diagrammatic depiction of the probable relationships between SNCC lymphomas of Burkitt's and non-Burkitt's subtypes and large-cell lymphomas. The development of genetic changes in precursor B-cells is shown, including the occasional transformation of a pre-existing follicular lymphoma (FL) by acquisition of additional genetic changes, e.g., a p53 mutation, unknown genetic lesions or, occasionally, a c-*myc*/Ig translocation (8;14 or variant).

prognosis when treated with the same drug regimens. Adult patients with small noncleaved cell lymphomas have, in the past, frequently been included in the category of diffuse aggressive lymphoma, and treated with the same regimens used for diffuse large-cell lymphoma. In recent years, however, there has been a trend towards managing the SNCC lymphomas separately – a practice that has resulted in improved survival rates (see below) in contrast to the lack of progress that has been observed in large B-cell lymphomas. It may now be appropriate, therefore, to determine whether patients with large B-cell lymphomas – particularly that subset which is associated with c-*myc*/Ig translocations – might not be better treated with regimens used for patients with SNCC.

HISTOLOGICAL BOUNDARIES

A detailed description of the histological appearance of SNCC has been given in Chapter 3. The essential features of Burkitt's lymphoma are a lack of evidence of differentiation towards plasma cells or mature lymphocytes, a high nuclear to cytoplasmic ratio, a round or oval nucleus with a coarse or 'open' chromatin pattern (i.e., giving the appearance of being able to see through the chromatin network) and multiple (usually 2–5), readily discernible nucleoli (occasionally a single large nucleolus – see below). The narrow rim of cytoplasm is very basophilic (also staining intensely with methyl-green pyronine) because of the abundant free ribosomes, which are seen readily on electron microscopy. The cytoplasm contains, almost invariably, lipid vacuoles, which stain with Oil Red O, the significance of which is unknown. Histological sections usually demonstrate the presence of macrophages scattered among the tumor cells in which nuclear debris is discernible, and which give rise to the often-quoted 'starry-sky' appearance. This pattern is not pathognomonic and may be seen in any rapidly proliferating tumor. Burkitt-like (small noncleaved, non-Burkitt's lymphomas) lymphomas are distinguished in American classification schemes [3,4,21] by a greater degree of pleomorphism and a higher frequency of cells with a single large nucleolus in the neoplastic population. This is suggestive of a degree of differentiation towards B-immunoblasts or plasmacytoid cells. The degree of pleomorphism, or the required proportion of cells with single nucleoli that distinguishes these two categories of SNCC lymphoma is not defined, so that there is considerable subjectivity and rather poor reproducibility with respect to the distinction between these histological categories. In some classification schemes, notably the Kiel classification [22], such a division is not made. In addition to the blurred

boundary between Burkitt's and Burkitt-like lymphomas, the latter merge imperceptibly with large B-cell lymphoma, the distinction being based on the proportion of cells with a nucleus larger than a macrophage nucleus. The nuclei of Burkitt's lymphoma cells, by arbitrary definition, may not be larger than a macrophage nucleus. Burkitt-like lymphomas contain some cells with larger nuclei, while, in large B-cell lymphomas, most neoplastic nuclei are larger than macrophage nuclei. Clearly, there is a gradual merging, histologically, of Burkitt's lymphoma with large B-cell lymphoma, with Burkitt-like lymphomas at the interface [4,23]. For this reason, in the REAL classification, Burkitt-like lymphoma is a provisional entity – i.e., it is recognized that it could be a mixture of Burkitt's lymphomas and large B-cell lymphomas rather than a truly discrete entity. There is some evidence that Burkitt-like lymphomas are more likely to have an unrearranged c-*myc* gene or a 14;18 translocation, and such tumors are also more likely to occur in older individuals, all of which could be interpreted as indicating that most of these tumors would be better classified as large B-cell lymphomas [13]. Interestingly, in children, and in adults treated with intensive regimens, there appears to be no prognostic significance to the histological categories within SNCC lymphoma – a further argument for studying the efficacy of treatment regimens used in these tumors in large B-cell lymphomas [24,25].

RELATIONSHIP TO ACUTE LYMPHOBLASTIC LEUKEMIA

While the SNCC lymphomas almost invariably fail to express TdT, rare cases of acute lymphoblastic leukemia (ALL) of the French–American–British L3 type, which express TdT, some of which have been documented to contain 8;14 translocations, have been reported [26,27]. Similarly, other patients have been described in which an acute leukemia of pre-B-cell phenotype has been associated with L3 morphology, sometimes with documentation of a c-*myc*/Ig translocation [28–32]. In such patients it would appear that genetic differences have obviated the more usual need for the neoplastic cell to differentiate to the phenotypic level of a follicular center cell in order, presumably, to achieve full neoplastic transformation. Most L3 ALLs, however, are TdT-negative, and of B-cell immunophenotype – i.e., they express surface Ig, usually IgM and more often λ than κ [31], and only occasionally is the absence of a c-*myc*/Ig translocation demonstrated. Thus, the majority of L3 leukemias appear to represent SNCC lymphomas which present with diffuse bone marrow infiltration [31–34]. Such patients may or may not have solid masses elsewhere, for example in the abdomen. As such, the use of the term 'acute B-cell leukemia' is confusing and might better be dropped – at least in the context of SNCC lymphoma. At present, an arbitrary dividing line of 25% tumor cells in the bone marrow is used in pediatric oncology, and 30%, by many adult oncologists to distinguish between acute B-cell leukemia (above these levels) and SNCC lymphoma (below these levels). However, since SNCC neoplasms in both groups should be treated with regimens designed for SNCC lymphoma, and *not* with regimens designed for ALL (see below), there is little point in making this distinction, particularly since it does not appear to have prognostic significance. Because of the heterogeneity of FAB L3 ALL, it would be appropriate to require the expression of surface Ig as a minimum and, if possible, evidence for a c-*myc*/Ig translocation (cytogenetic or molecular genetic) in patients with L3 ALL before making a diagnosis of SNCC lymphoma/leukemia. The optimal therapy for the rare acute B-cell leukemias that lack a c-*myc*/Ig translocation is unknown.

EPIDEMIOLOGY

In the USA and Europe, SNCC lymphomas account for 3–4% of all non-Hodgkin's lymphomas [35] but 40–50% of childhood lymphomas. The incidence is age-dependent, being much higher in the first two decades of life, but occurring at all ages, although the disease is essentially unknown in children less than the age of 2. In the USA, the average annual incidence rate of SNCC lymphoma reported by the National Cancer Institute's Surveillance, Epidemiology and End Results Program (SEER) was 6 per million (all races, all ages) between 1987 and 1991, and approximately 3–5 per million in the age group 0–19 years [36]. Thus, more adults (who represent some 85% of the population) than children develop this disease each year in the USA. The incidence of SNCC lymphomas, however, differs dramatically in different parts of the world, although information in this respect is much better for children than for adults. In so-called 'endemic' regions for Burkitt's lymphoma, which include equatorial Africa and Papua New Guinea, estimates made some 30 years ago suggest a relatively high incidence rate of some 5–10 cases per 100 000 children below the age of 16 years (higher than that of ALL in the USA and Europe). In Nigeria, incidence rates of 22 and 10 per 100 000 in males and females, respectively, were reported in 5–9-year-olds (the age group in which the incidence rate peaks) in 1964 [37]. In equatorial Africa, the incidence of ALL appears to be low, and

represents only some 5% of all childhood cancers, while Burkitt's lymphoma accounts for between 30% and 70% [37]. North Africa and South America appear to be regions of intermediate incidence, but precise figures are difficult to obtain because of the lack of population-based registries. In both endemic and sporadic regions the male:female ratio is between 2 and 3 to 1.

There is accumulating evidence that childhood Burkitt's lymphoma differs biologically in different world regions. Although all tumors appear to have c-*myc*/Ig translocations, the chromosomal breakpoints associated with these translocations differ (see Chapter 16), as does the fraction of tumors that are associated with Epstein–Barr virus (EBV) DNA [12,38]. EBV DNA has been shown to be present in the tumor cells of some 95% of the SNCC lymphomas in endemic regions, but only about 15–20% of tumors in the USA and Europe. The frequency of EBV association in South America appears to be intermediate – some 50–60% [38,39]. EBV and other environmental factors, such as malaria, the ingestion of medicinal plants and possibly other environmental factors, however, clearly have varying degrees of importance in the pathogenesis of the disease in different world regions. It does seem that malaria and early infection with EBV account for the very high incidence of Burkitt's lymphoma in equatorial Africa and New Guinea. The pathogenesis of Burkitt's lymphoma is discussed in detail in Chapter 16.

SNCC lymphomas also occur at increased frequency in patients with an underlying immunodeficiency, particularly in individuals infected with the human immunodeficiency virus (HIV) (see Chapters 19 and 20, this volume) and occasionally in families with the X-linked lymphoproliferative syndrome [40]. It seems probable that immunodeficiency is responsible for increasing the size of B-cell populations in which genetic changes occur, with a resultant increased likelihood that chromosomal translocations will develop.

TUMOR CELL PROLIFERATION KINETICS

SNCC lymphomas are rapidly growing neoplasms with very high growth fractions (approaching 100% in some cases). Potential doubling times (i.e., calculated doubling times, which do not take into account spontaneous cell death in the neoplasm) range from 12 hours to a few days [41]. In practice the measured (actual) doubling time is several days, the mean for three skin tumors being 66 hours in one study [41], although there is considerable variation from patient to patient and between different tumor sites in the same patient. The actual doubling time depends upon the spontaneous cell death rate, which in turn varies according to tumor size (being greater in larger tumors). The spontaneous cell death rate has been measured in African Burkitt's lymphoma to be about 70% of all progeny cells [41]. Up to 27% of the cells may be in S-phase (measured by flow cytometry) [42,43]. These observations have relevance to management. The high spontaneous cell turnover rate in untreated tumors is the immediate cause of pretreatment hyperuricemia, which occurs frequently in patients with a high tumor cell burden. The short actual doubling times, and consequent rapid growth rates, mean that treatment should be commenced at the earliest possible time. Any delay will increase the chance of complications and, theoretically, could worsen the prognosis, since tumor burden, after treatment, is perhaps the single most important prognostic factor [44–46]. The high growth fraction of SNCC lymphomas is, however, also beneficial once treatment has been initiated, since it is probable that this is an important factor in the excellent response and frequent cure of these lymphomas when treated with chemotherapy.

Table 37.1 Relative frequency of involvement of different sites at presentation in endemic Burkitt's lymphoma (Uganda Cancer Institute series) versus sporadic Burkitt's lymphoma (USA National Cancer Institute series)

Site*	Uganda (224 patients) (%)	USA (135 patients) (%)
Jaw	58	14
Abdomen/pelvis	58	80
CSF/cranial nerves	19	11
Paraspinal	17	2
Orbit	11	5
Bones	9	24
Thyroid	8	0
Bone marrow	7	21
Salivary glands	5	0
Peripheral lymph nodes	4	42
Pleura/effusion	3	26
Skin/soft tissues	3	5
Testis	2	6
Breast	2	4
Mediastinal nodes	1	12
Sinus	<1	3
Pharynx	0	10

* Detection of sites differed in the two series. In Africa, clinical examination was supplemented by chest X-ray, intravenous pyelogram, bone marrow and CSF examination. In the USA series, CT and nuclear medicine scans were performed as well as CSF and bone marrow examination.

CSF, Cerebrospinal fluid; CT, computed tomography.

Clinical features and staging

PRESENTATION AND ANATOMICAL DISTRIBUTION OF TUMOR

The SNCC lymphomas can involve almost any organ or tissue in the body, but patients generally present with one of a number of clinical patterns of disease, which vary according to age and geographical region. There are general differences in these patterns between endemic (equatorial African) tumors and tumors in Western countries (sporadic) (Table 37.1) and, although they overlap considerably, e.g., with respect to abdominal involvement, it appears that in other world regions (e.g., the Middle East and some regions in South America), the clinical pattern is intermediate, particularly with respect to the frequency of jaw tumors (Table 37.2) and bone marrow involvement. The possibility that patients with marrow involvement are not included as SNCC lymphomas but are diagnosed as ALL in some world regions must, however, be considered.

Endemic Burkitt's lymphoma

The jaw is the most frequently involved site of Burkitt's lymphoma and the most common presenting feature in patients with Burkitt's lymphoma in equatorial Africa and New Guinea [47,48]. It characteristically effects multiple jaw quadrants (Figure 37.2) and tends to be age-dependent, occurring much more frequently in young children (Figure 37.3), since it arises in close proximity to the developing molar tooth buds. This is rarely observed in sporadic tumors (Figure 37.4). In Burkitt's own series from Uganda, 70% of children below 5 years with Burkitt's lymphoma had jaw involvement compared to 25% of patients above 14 years [47,48]. In very young children, orbital involvement is often present in patients who do not have overt jaw tumors, although at least some of these orbital tumors arise in the maxilla (Figure 37.5). Jaw involvement appears to be more frequent, even within equatorial Africa, in regions of higher incidence. Patients from highland regions, for example, in which the incidence of Burkitt's lymphoma is much lower, have a higher median age – probably accounting for the difference in the frequency of jaw tumors [49].

Abdominal involvement is also frequent in endemic Burkitt's lymphoma, being present in almost 60% of the patients at presentation, although the intra-abdominal sites of involvement differ to some extent in endemic versus sporadic disease. Presentation

Table 37.2 Relative frequency of jaw tumors in various world regions

Country or region	Total patients	Percentage with jaw tumors	Reference
Uganda	291	72	163
Ghana	110	60	164
Cape Province (South Africa) and Namibia	22	59*	65
Sudan	7	71	66
Algiers	40	18	72
Egypt	21	·14	170
Jordan	24	8	190
Middle East†	34	24	67
Israel	112	15	172
Mexico	30	13	71
Colombia	9	22	183
Thailand	25	38	68
Japan ·	14	36	74
Turkey	81	26	70
Singapore	14	36	184
France	47	4	185
Norway‡	8	0	186
Denmark	13	0	187
USA	135	14	§
Papua New Guinea	37	43	188
Papua New Guinea	35	31	189¶

* Frequency similar in White (4 out of 6) and non-White patients (9 out of 16).
† This series consisted of patients referred to the American University Medical Center in Beirut from several Middle Eastern countries.
‡ Cases with bone marrow involvement were excluded.
§ Updated information from the National Cancer Institute series.
¶ Some of these cases are also included in the previous series.

with a resectable right iliac fossa mass or with intussusception, for example, is uncommon in African patients (Wright reported that no case of intussusception was observed in Uganda in over 500 cases [50]), but involvement of the mesentery and omentum are common and ascites may be present. Renal involvement is common, as is ovarian involvement in girls, while liver and spleen are less often involved. Unfortunately, precise figures for involvement of various intra-abdominal and retroperitoneal structures are not available as relatively few centers in Africa possess a computed tomography scanner. A high fraction of patients present with clinically obvious or even massive abdominal disease, but do not have laparotomies, either because disease present at extra-abdominal tumor sites is more readily biopsied for diagnostic purposes, or because the diagnosis is less traumatically, less expensively and more rapidly established by needle biopsy rather than by a surgical procedure.

Central nervous system (CNS) involvement – including cerebrospinal fluid (CSF) pleocytosis, cranial nerve palsies and paraplegia from paraspinal

disease – is relatively common in the African patient, being present in approximately 40% of patients at presentation [51]. Interestingly, cranial nerve involvement is frequently unassociated with CSF pleocytosis at presentation, but malignant cells are nearly always detectable in the CSF in patients with cranial nerve palsies at relapse [48]. Cranial nerve palsies and meningeal involvement have been described as the only sites of disease [52]. Paraplegia is the presenting feature in approximately one in six patients, and is quite frequently the only site of disease, such that laminectomy is required to make a diagnosis. Intracerebral disease is very uncommon and usually occurs in patients who have had persistent or multiply relapsed cranial nerve palsies/CSF pleocytosis [53].

Salivary glands and endocrine organs (thyroid particularly, adrenal occasionally) as well as breast (in pubertal girls or lactating women), testis, bone, pleura and occasionally heart (either involvement of the cardiac muscle or pericardium) may be involved. Bone marrow involvement, as assessed by aspiration biopsy, occurs in some 7–8% of patients

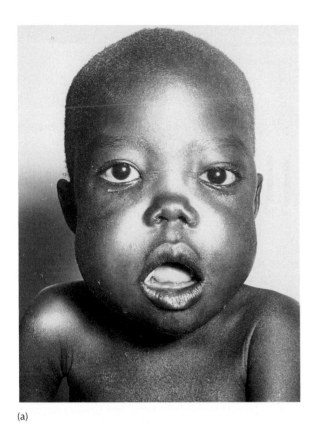
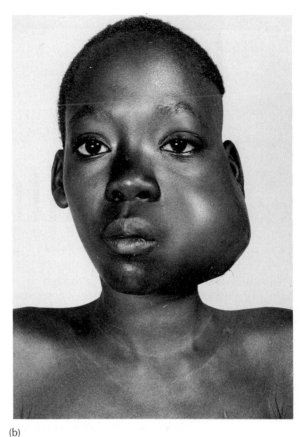

(a)   (b)

Figure 37.2   Multiple jaw tumors (a) maxillary, and (b) maxillary and mandibular in children with Burkitt's lymphoma.

(and is no more often involved at relapse). Naso-pharyngeal involvement and peripheral lymphadeno-pathy are rare in the African patient.

Sporadic Burkitt's lymphoma

In the USA and Europe a high proportion of patients (80–90%) have abdominal tumor at the time of presentation [54], providing strong support for the possibility that the tumor is a high-grade lymphoma of MALT. Abdominal disease is usually manifested as abdominal pain and/or swelling (more rapid if ascites is present), frequently accompanied by a change in bowel habits or nausea and vomiting, and sometimes by overt intestinal obstruction. Gastro-intestinal bleeding occurs, but is relatively uncom-mon, and intestinal perforation is seen only occasion-ally, although a relatively high frequency (9 in 147 patients) has been reported from Mexico [55]. In some of the latter patients the perforation was associated with prior biopsy at the site, or incomplete resection. The infrequency of bleeding and perfora-tion probably results from the tendency of the lymphoma cells to diffusely infiltrate the bowel wall (like normal mucosa-associated lymphoid tissue

lymphoid cells) rather than erode it. Presentation with a right iliac fossa mass – sometimes mistaken for an appendix mass – is quite common, and was the sole site of disease in some 25% of patients in the National Cancer Institute (NCI) series [56]. In all, perhaps 40% of patients have disease at this site.

Children with intussusception usually have a very low tumor burden; this is one of the few situations in which a tumor mass of less than 1 cm diameter may precipitate severe pain, and rapidly lead to a correc-tive and diagnostic laparotomy. Similarly, many patients with a right iliac fossa tumor prove, at surgery, to have readily resectable disease [56]. Such patients have an excellent prognosis, even when less intensive chemotherapy regimens are administered, but the risk of tumor regrowth is very high if chemotherapy is not given very soon (within days) after surgery. Abdominal involvement is frequently associated with disease at other sites, such as pleural effusions, bone marrow involvement, skin, bone, peripheral lymphadenopathy, breast (most often in pubertal girls or lactating women, as in endemic patients), pharyngeal disease or testicular involve-ment [57–62]. These sites may also be involved in the absence of abdominal disease. At presentation,

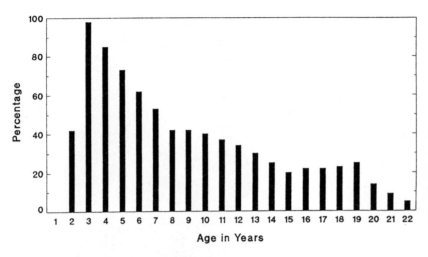

Figure 37.3 Relationship between age and the likelihood of the presence of a jaw tumor at presentation in African patients with Burkitt's lymphoma. Based on data provided in reference 47 from over 600 cases of Burkitt's lymphoma recorded in Uganda.

CNS involvement is uncommon, although it is distinctly more common in the presence of bone marrow disease [33]. In the absence of CNS prophylactic therapy, however, CNS spread will occur in a high proportion of patients, particularly those with extensive disease or head and neck primaries. Any cranial nerve can be affected by tumor, but ophthalmic and facial palsies are the most common. Paraplegia, in contrast to endemic Burkitt's lymphoma, occurs in only some 2% of patients.

Jaw involvement in sporadic Burkitt's lymphoma occurs in 15% or less of patients at presentation, usually involves a single jaw quadrant and, in contrast to endemic tumors, is not age related [63]. It is frequently associated with multiple bony sites of disease outside the head and neck, as well as bone marrow disease (which is uncommon in endemic Burkitt's lymphoma) and thus, in most patients with sporadic Burkitt's lymphoma, is simply a site of bone involvement. Jaw tumors that resemble those seen in endemic patients, either clinically or radiologically (Figure 37.4), however, are occasionally seen [64].

A curious and not infrequent physical sign is the occurrence in some patients of numbness of the chin. This is caused by compression of the mental branch of the inferior alveolar nerve and is probably the result of tumor infiltration of the marrow of the mandible, through which the nerve passes. It most often occurs in patients with diffuse marrow involvement.

Intermediate geographic regions

In some developing countries, the incidence of Burkitt's lymphoma appears to be intermediate between that of endemic and sporadic regions (although precise incidence rates are usually not available because of the lack of population-based

cancer registries). The clinical pattern of disease in such regions also appears to be intermediate between that of classical endemic and sporadic regions, but it is not clear whether this is because there is a mixture of endemic and sporadic types of Burkitt's lymphoma, or whether the disease in these regions is biologically homogeneous, but is different from either sporadic or endemic Burkitt's lymphoma. For example, in South Africa, Turkey, some Asian countries, including the Middle East, and Latin America, typical 'endemic-type' jaw tumors occur at higher frequency that in the USA or Europe [65–71] (Table 37.2), but the frequency of bone marrow disease, at least in some of these countries, is similar to that observed in Western countries – i.e., approximately 20% [70,71]. It is difficult to provide meaningful figures for the clinical spectrum, with respect to disease sites at presentation, in entire developing countries, since the clinical pattern differs in different socioeconomic groups and/or different geographic regions within such countries. Patients in North Africa appear to have a spectrum of organ involvement which more closely approximates that of the sporadic disease rather than the endemic form [72], but jaw tumors are observed more frequently in the Sudan and Ethiopia [66,73]. Unexpectedly, jaw tumors also appear to be common in Japanese patients [74].

Unfortunately, information on clinical patterns of disease in various world regions is incomplete, and published data can be misleading since diagnostic criteria (or quality of diagnosis) are variable, the pattern of disease may vary in different regions or in patient series collected at different centers in the same region (e.g., because different centers cater to different sectors of the population), thus giving apparently conflicting data, while some series may be collected because of involvement of specific sites (e.g., jaw or abdomen) [72,75]. In addition to

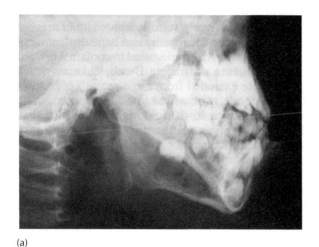

(a)

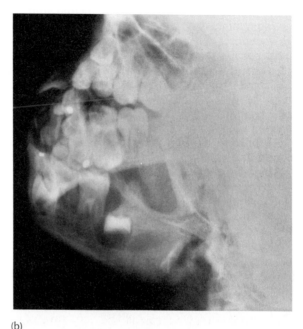

(b)

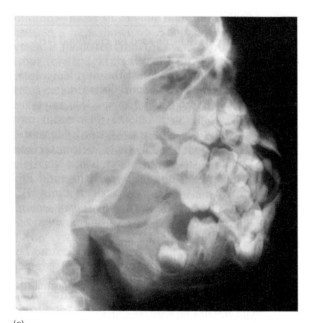

(c)

Figure 37.4 (a) Oblique radiograph of the jaw in an African child showing lytic lesions adjacent to an unerupted molar tooth. Note loss of the lamina dura. (b) Oblique radiograph of the jaw in a child from the USA with a similar appearance. (c) Oblique radiograph of normal jaw from the same patient shown in (b). Note normal lamina dura surrounding the developing teeth.

differences in the clinical pattern, the incidence of the disease differs in different populations. In Israel, for example, it was reported in 1970 that Burkitt's lymphoma showed a striking predilection for Arab children and Sephardic Jews, being uncommon in Jewish children of European ancestry [76].

Frequency of bone marrow involvement in SNCC lymphoma

In sporadic Burkitt's lymphoma, bone marrow involvement occurs in about 20% of patients at presentation [33,54], although there is evidence from the culture and karyotyping of microscopically uninvolved bone marrow that occult involvement occurs in approximately another 20% of patients [77]. Some patients

prognosis and, consequently, to the design of risk-adapted chemotherapy regimens. As treatment results improve, the value of these factors as predictors of outcome is lost, since most patients are cured – even those who formally fell into a very high-risk group. They are likely, however, to retain importance as determinants of the type or intensity of therapy that will be used.

Treatment and prognosis

COMPLICATIONS CONSEQUENT UPON SITE OR VOLUME OF TUMOR

Patients with SNCC lymphomas are prone to develop a number of the complications described in Chapter 27 and these frequently require urgent attention at the time of presentation. They include intestinal obstruction (most commonly from intussusception), perforation or hemorrhage, airway obstruction from pharyngeal tumor, and respiratory or cardiac insufficiency from pleural effusions and pericardial effusions. Among the most common complications at presentation, however, are biochemical abnormalities related to the high proliferative rate of SNCC lymphomas. The likelihood of uric acid nephropathy prior to the commencement of chemotherapy, or of the development of biochemical abnormalities immediately after chemotherapy, known as the 'acute tumor lysis syndrome', correlates directly with the tumor burden [91,92,92a]. This syndrome, which was first recognized when sudden death occurred as a consequence of posttreatment hyperkalemia [93], most commonly presents as oliguric renal failure occurring immediately postchemotherapy. The sensitivity of the tumor to chemotherapy and, conversely, the therapy used, is also relevant to the development of this syndrome, but is less important than the tumor burden, since primary chemotherapy resistance is rare.

Because of the short doubling time of SNCC lymphomas and the considerable risks associated with rapid tumor lysis, the initiation of therapy should be considered a medical emergency, and staging procedures should be completed as expeditiously as possible. Prior to commencing therapy, however, it is essential to ensure that the serum uric acid level is not elevated, and that the patient is well hydrated and able to maintain a high urine flow. If a period of biochemical correction is necessary, it should be limited, wherever possible, to 24–48 hours. The reduction of serum uric acid to normal levels can

usually be accomplished within this period by alkaline diuresis and high-dose allopurinol administration (e.g., initially 10 mg/kg). Uricase can also be used, if available. Only in patients with long-standing renal compromise, outlet tract obstruction, or less commonly, massive involvement of the kidneys by tumor, will require hemodialysis (or in some circumstances, the placement of bilateral nephrostomies) prior to chemotherapy. In such patients, the administration of chemotherapy without prior correction of biochemical abnormalities would compound the problem and risk fatal acute tumor lysis. When hemodialysis is performed before treatment is initiated, chemotherapy is usually commenced after the completion of a period of hemodialysis when biochemical parameters are close to normal. Dialysis must be continued as indicated by biochemical indicators of renal function and urine flow rates.

The tumor lysis syndrome can nearly always be avoided in patients with good urine flow rates in whom correction of biochemical abnormalities has been accomplished prior to chemotherapy. All patients with a large tumor burden are best managed in a critical care unit where frequent monitoring can be performed. It is imperative to maintain a high urine flow (150–350 ml/m^2 per hour, higher rates being used in patients with higher tumor burdens), for the first few days after the initiation of chemotherapy to ensure that the high solute burden from tumor lysis is accommodated without the onset of potentially fatal hyperkalemia or the development of acute renal failure from intratubular deposition of oxypurines and/or phosphates; a consequence of exceeding their solubility in urine. In patients with serous effusions or inferior vena caval obstruction, vigorous use of diuretics will be required to prevent 'third spacing' of infused fluids. Potassium should not normally be included in the intravenous solutions, and it is preferable not to administer bicarbonate during chemotherapy because of the relatively poor solubility of phosphate in an alkaline urine and the increased risk of symptoms when hypocalcemia is accompanied by alkalosis. Intravenous calcium chloride should be avoided because of the risk of extraosseous calcification in the presence of a high serum phosphate level. Further information on the acute tumor lysis syndrome is provided in Chapter 27.

CHOICE OF THERAPEUTIC MODALITIES

The primary therapeutic modality for SNCC lymphomas is chemotherapy. This is based not only on the belief that these lymphomas are generalized diseases, but also on clinical experience, which has demonstrated that the majority of patients can be cured by chemotherapy alone. Local or locoregional therapy alone has been shown to provide inadequate therapy, by modern standards, even for patients with localized disease. In a review of eight series of patients with localized non-Hodgkin's lymphomas (one, containing 221 patients, was a literature review) treated with radiation therapy, with or without surgical resection and single-agent chemotherapy, published between 1966 and 1978 [94–101], Jenkin et al. reported a combined long-term survival rate of 18% in 370 patients [102]. In only one of these series did more than 50% of children achieve long-term survival, and that series contained only eight patients [96]. In two of these series, in which only patients with gastrointestinal disease were included, 15 of 37 patients achieved prolonged survival [96–97]. These results contrast dramatically with those obtained when children with localized disease are treated with combination chemotherapy. With more recent protocols, 90% or more of patients can be expected to enjoy long-term survival [25,103–107]. Further, a randomized study has shown that radiation adds no therapeutic benefit to chemotherapy in patients with limited disease, but does increase toxicity [104]. There is also no evidence that radiotherapy to sites of bulk disease adds benefit to chemotherapy in patients with extensive disease, and one small study showed that it adds only toxicity [108]. Even in patients with residual tumor after chemotherapy, local radiation appears to have been of no benefit [105]. Thus, at best, radiation subserves an ancillary role, i.e., as emergency treatment for sanctuary sites, such as the CNS or testis, and even in these circumstances its use is controversial and has not been shown, in retrospective comparisons, to provide added therapeutic benefit [62,109]. Randomized clinical trials, however, of radiation versus chemotherapy alone in these situations, have not been conducted. The absence of demonstrable added value of local irradiation to chemotherapy is consistent with the marked radioresistance of African Burkitt's lymphoma to conventionally fractionated radiation therapy [110]. The suggestion that hyperfractionation of radiation dose may be effective [110] has not been systematically explored.

Although local irradiation may be of no therapeutic benefit, there is evidence that surgical resection, in some circumstances, may be beneficial. Patients with abdominal disease in whom tumor can be completely resected prior to chemotherapy have an excellent prognosis, which at one time, in both endemic and sporadic Burkitt's lymphoma, was clearly better than that of patients with unresected abdominal disease, although patients with very small tumor burdens, and hence the best prognosis, are also those that are most readily resected [56,78,111–114].

Evidence that major debulking (greater than 90%) can be advantageous comes, however, from complete resection of massive ovarian disease in African pateints treated subsequently with very simple chemotherapy [78]. The advantage of complete resection no longer applies when patients are to be treated with one of the highly successful protocols presently being used in the industrial nations (although one argument for attempting resection in selected cases is that patients in whom complete resection is successfully accomplished require less intensive, and therefore less toxic and less expensive, chemotherapy). However, when patients present with an acute abdominal emergency, or with an abdominal mass that on laparotomy proves to be completely resectable with minimal impact on organ function (e.g., resection of intussuscepted bowel), diagnosis is made with an excisional biopsy. Surgical resection could decrease the risk of gastrointestinal bleeding and bowel perforation, but these complications are sufficiently uncommon that surgery is not indicated for this purpose. Moreover, in the previously mentioned Mexican series, surgery in patients in whom complete resection could not be accomplished may have increased the risk of perforation [55]. Reduction of the risk of tumor lysis is also not an indication for surgery, since the majority of patients with a high tumor burden do not have completely resectable disease. This does not apply to patients with massive ovarian involvement as the sole site of disease – this can sometimes be readily resected – although the advantages of bilateral oophorectomy must be weighed against sterility [78]. In all, when a highly effective chemotherapy protocol with acceptable toxicity is to be used, there is rarely sufficient reason to attempt surgical resection in order to improve survival (bearing in mind that partial resection is never of benefit in this regard [78]), although surgery remains important in the establishment of a diagnosis, and, rarely, in the management of specific complications, such as perforation, fistula or bleeding. Nonetheless, in some world regions (e.g., Africa), where intensive therapy is not possible, or is of limited availability, it appears reasonable to recommend complete surgical resection, where feasible, in order to improve outcome after chemotherapy.

Finally, even in patients with a residual mass after chemotherapy, surgical resection does not appear to be advantageous – in a recently reported Berlin, Frankfurt, Munster (BFM) study, patients in whom the resected material contained no viable tumor had an excellent prognosis, and it is unlikely that surgery was a contributing factor to this outcome. Patients in whom residual tumor was documented, however, had a poor prognosis in spite of local therapy [105].

CHEMOTHERAPY OF SNCC LYMPHOMAS IN THE USA AND EUROPE

SNCC lymphomas respond to a wide range of chemotherapeutic agents, in part due, no doubt, to the high growth fraction. Response rates in African Burkitt's lymphoma to a series of single agents are shown in Table 37.4, and sporadic tumors appear to have a similar spectrum of sensitivity to chemotherapeutic agents (although very few studies of single agent activities have been published), as well as a demonstrable response to high-dose methotrexate [115]. Previous experience has clearly indicated that the results of drug combination therapy are far superior to treatment with single agents, although a small fraction of patients with SNCC lymphomas, generally those with limited disease, can be cured by single agents – an almost unique situation in oncology, which highlights the extreme chemosensitivity of this tumor [48,116–119]. Another feature of treatment protocols for the SNCC lymphomas is that there appears to be no indication for prolonged therapy. In early trials at the NCI as few as three cycles of a combination of cyclophosphamide, methotrexate and vincristine resulted in long-term disease-free survival in 82% of patients with limited disease and 41% with advanced disease [120–122]. While improved survival was probably obtained in a subsequent protocol that had a treatment duration of 15 months [45], even better results are now being obtained with more intensive protocols that last for only 12–15 weeks [25,105]. Although the therapy duration need not be prolonged, it is important, because of the rapid tumor cell doubling time and the potential for tumor regrowth before bone marrow recovery, to ensure that cycles are delivered with as short an intercycle interval as possible. In most modern protocols, successive cycles of chemotherapy are initiated as soon as the absolute granulocyte count has reached 200–1000 per mm^3 [25,105,123].

It has been clearly shown in several different studies that treatment protocols based upon the principles shown to be effective for ALL, such as the LSA$_2$L$_2$ (see Chapter 38), the BFM 75 and 81, or the APO (adriamycin, prednisone, oncovin) regimens are suboptimal for the treatment of small noncleaved cell lymphomas [124–128]. Better results have been obtained (50–75% long-term survival rates) using even only a two-drug regimen [129], or with combinations of cyclophosphamide, vincristine, prednisone, intermediate- or high-dose methotrexate, and in some cases additional drugs, such as adriamycin or Ara-C [25,106,107,120–127,130,131]. All these protocols are clearly suboptimal for patients with extensive tumor, particularly in patients with bone marrow and/or CNS disease and some may give worse results for patients with localized disease (Table 37.5). The best results in patients with extensive disease have been obtained with regimens that include additional drugs – particularly high-dose Ara-C, high-dose methotrexate, and in some cases, ifosfamide and etoposide [25,105,132–134].

Comparison of outcome in adults versus children

In spite of a sense, on the part of many oncologists, that SNCC lymphoma in adults has a particularly poor prognosis, adult patients treated with suitably intensive treatment protocols have had a good outcome [106,107]. In protocol 77–04, used at the NCI, Bethesda, patients above and below 18 years had a similar prognosis [25,45], while a modified version of this protocol used in adult patients at Stanford University Medical Center gave very similar results to those achieved at the NCI [135]. Most adult patients with SNCC lymphoma, however, have been treated with chemotherapy regimens designed for diffuse aggressive lymphomas (primarily of intermediate grade). Whether they have a worse prognosis than patients with large B-cell lymphoma treated with the same regimens is unclear because the number of patients with SNCC lymphomas included in such studies is small, and the disease extent is often not provided. In the LNH80 protocol, the results for SNCC lymphoma, although inferior to the most recently reported results with protocols designed for SNCC lymphomas, appear to be similar to those obtained with the earlier combination regimens used in children (53% of 19 patients with SNCC lymphoma were alive at 5 years) [136]. Even if the prognosis for patients with SNCC lymphoma is the same as that for large B-cell lymphomas, the results achieved for the latter patients with standard regimens are clearly much worse than those achieved in children with SNCC lymphoma today. Moreover with the most recently reported protocols that have been used in both adults and children there is, as with NCI 77–04, no difference between the disease-free survival rates in adults and children (Figure 37.6) [25,137]. Thus, it would appear that, if treated similarly, adult patients – at least those less than 60 years – have the same, excellent prognosis as children and standard protocols for intermediate-grade lymphomas should not be used for patients with SNCC lymphoma.

Results in patient subsets

Limited disease

Patients with limited SNCC lymphoma (in children,

Table 37.4 Single-agent activity in African Burkitt's lymphoma*

Drug	No. of patients tested	Complete response	Complete and partial responses	Patients responding (%)
Cyclophosphamide	163	43	132	81
Nitrogen mustard	61	10	44	72
Melphalan	26	8	16	61
Chlorambucil	12	3	10	83
Procarbazine	6	0	0	0
Orthomerphalan	14	?	14	100
BCNU	5	0	4	80
Vincristine	21	10	17	81
Vinblastine	2	0	0	—
Methotrexate	45	11	26	58
6-Mercaptopurine	3	0	0	—
Cytosine arabinoside	3	2	2	—
Epipodophyllotoxin	2	2	2	—
Actinomycin D	4	1	4	—
Terephthalanilide	18	1	14	78

* See [48,116,157–160].

BCNU, bis-(2-chloroethyl)nitrosourea.

all B-cell lymphomas), i.e., localized, or completely resected small volume intra-abdominal disease (stages I and II, St Jude) currently have an excellent prognosis (90–100% cure rate) (Table 37.5) and require less intensive treatment than patients with more extensive disease (all other stages). Combination regimens including only four or five drugs – cyclophosphamide, vincristine, prednisone and methotrexate or adriamycin – provide adequate therapy if the dose intensity is high enough (some protocols give rather low event-free survival rates (EFS) for stages I or II of less than 80% at 2 years and beyond). Whether or not prednisone is important in these regimens has not been studied, although in the most

Table 37.5 Event-free survival rates in limited-stage childhood B-cell NHL (predominantly SNCC lymphoma) with current regimens

Protocol	No. of patients	Stages I and II (%)	Reference
NCI 74–0/75–6*	17	82	121
CCG 551; COMP	115	86	138
CCG 501; COMP	96	98	138
POG ACOP+	51	78	126
NCI 77–04†	17	78	‡
BFM 81	18	100	127
POG 83–87§	129	87	139
BFM 86	42	98	105
NCI 89–C–41¶	12	100	25
LMB 84/86 – adults	12	92	137

* Stages A, B and AR.
† Includes both children and adults. Some patients who had extensive abdominal disease resected are included.
‡ Updated information as of December 1994.
§ Includes small noncleaved cell (56), large cell (21), lymphoblastic lymphomas (17) and 'other' (7) lymphomas, and a randomization to receive or not to receive radiation. No significant differences were observed in any of these groups.
¶ Includes both children and adults.

NHL, Non-Hodgkin's lymphomas; SNCC, small noncleaved cell.

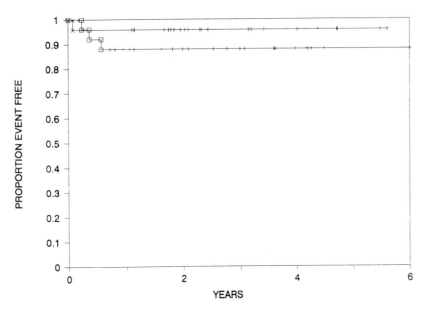

Figure 37.6 Event-free survival in adults (24 patients) and children (26 patients) with small noncleaved cell lymphoma treated according to NCI protocol 89–C–41. Upper curve (×) > 18 years, lower curve (□) < 18 years.

recent NCI protocol (89-C-41), this drug is not administered, with no apparent detriment – all 'low-risk' patients have survived, disease free, to date, but the number of patients treated is small – 12 [25]. The same question could be raised, of course, in the context of other drugs, and it is possible that only two or three drugs would be sufficient if given in adequate dosage.

Patients with limited disease present either with extra-abdominal disease, e.g., pharyngeal tumor or localized peripheral lymphadenopathy, or with completely resectable intra-abdominal disease. The main question in this patient group is how little therapy can be given without compromising the cure rate. The CCSG initially gave 18 months of COMP (cyclophosphamide, vincristine, methotrexate and prednisone) therapy with local radiation (including patients with a gastrointestinal site), but subsequently showed that 6 months of therapy (also with radiation) gave identical results [138]. The long-term disease-free survival rates for protocols 551 and 501 were 86% and 98%, and survival rates of 91% and 98% (*P*<0.01), respectively. These protocols differed only with respect to the timing and doses of intrathecal therapy (this was omitted for patients with localized abdominal disease) and the dose of radiation and volume irradiated (both were less in protocol 501), and the reasons for the difference in survival are not clear. The Pediatric Oncology Group (POG), having first demonstrated the lack of benefit of local radiation [104], subsequently showed that after 9 weeks of therapy with cyclophosphamide, vincristine, adriamycin and prednisone, an additional 24 weeks of continuation therapy with daily oral 6-mercaptopurine and weekly oral methotrexate

made no difference to outcome [139]. In this study, 5-year event-free survival was 85% and overall survival 94% (although most relapses occurred in the 15% of lymphoblastic lymphoma patients, who were also included in the study).

Others have for long been using very short duration therapies without radiation. For example, in the BFM 86 protocol patients with limited B-cell lymphoma (stages I and II) received only three courses of therapy lasting a total of 7 weeks [105] but this resulted in an EFS at 7 years of 98%. Similar results have been obtained with the SFOP (French Society of Pediatric Oncology) LMB 89 protocol, in which patients with completely resected abdominal disease (group A) are given only two cycles of therapy [134]. In NCI protocol 89-C-41, patients with localized disease receive three cycles of therapy and currently have a disease-free survival rate of 100% at greater than 2 years [25].

Abdominal disease

The tumor burden in patients with abdominal disease can vary markedly. Some patients may present with less than a few grams of tumor as a result of intussusception, while others may have kilograms of tumor – occasionally relatively localized, e.g., ovarian involvement – but more often widespread throughout the abdomen. In patients in whom the tumor burden is small, all tumor is usually completely resected at the time of diagnosis, since this entails laparotomy anyway. Such patients fall into the category of limited disease, and their therapy has already been dealt with. However, it is clear, from the strong association of prognosis with tumor

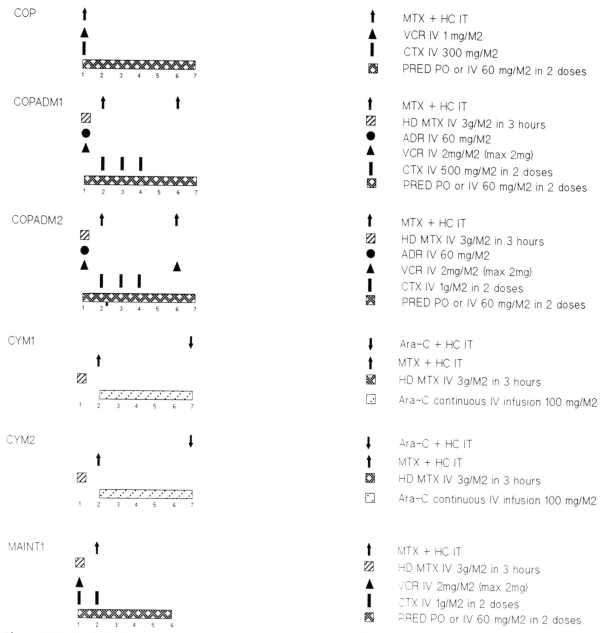

Figure 37.7 The LMB-86 protocol of the Société Francaise d'Oncologie Pediatrique (SFOP) for B-cell lymphomas. This is the protocol used for group B patients, i.e., those with more than completely resected disease (group A), but less than 70% of blast cells in the bone marrow (group C). The former receive two courses of COPAD (similar to COPADM but without high-dose methotrexate) and the latter a higher dose of MTX in COPADM (8 g/m²), consolidation cycles that contain VP16 (CYVE) and a second type of maintenance cycle. A total of four monthly maintenance cycles are given compared to the single cycle that group B patients receive. In maintenance cycle 1, group C patients also receive cranial irradiation (24 cG), high-dose methotrexate (8 g/m²) and triple IT drugs. Maintenance cycle 3 is similar to 1 except that high-dose MTX is not given. Prepared from information provided by Dr Catherine Patte.

volume [44,45] and the improved results of treatment in patients in whom large reductions in tumor volume can be accomplished surgically before chemotherapy [56,78], that the prognosis (in the context of treatment with the 4–5 drug combinations used in the 1980s) in patients with unresected abdominal disease varies markedly according to the extent of disease. This has been confirmed by the identification of prognostic subgroups within stage III, based on whether or not tumor extends beyond

Table 37.6 Results (event-free survival rate at 2 years or greater) of various protocols used in the treatment of patients (children and adults) with advanced small noncleaved cell lymphoma*

Protocol	No. of patients†	Stage III (%)	Stage IV‡ (%)	Reference
NCI 74–0 and 75–6	37	41		121
CCSG COMP	93	50		125
CCSG LSA$_2$L$_2$	44	29		125
POG ACOP+	16	17		126
NCI 77–04	55	61	18	¶
Total B	29	81[ll]	37,17[ll]	131
SFOP LMB 02	114	73	48	130
BFM 81	37	63[a]	49[b]	127
POG 9317	68	87	63,83	145
HiC-Com	20	92	50	123
SFOP LMB 84[c]	201	80	68	133
BFM 86	150	73	75	105
SFOP 89	181	87	85,87	134
NCI 89–C–41	38	92	81	25
81–01/84–30[e] – adults	44	91[f]	24	106
LMB 84/86 – adults	53[g]	76	57	137
Vanderbilt[e] – adults	20	—	60[h]	107

* Some protocols include large B-cell lymphoma, which has generally a similar prognosis to small noncleaved cell lymphoma in children when treated identically.
† Children unless indicated.
‡ If only a single percentage is given, both stage IV and patients with greater than 25% of blast cells in the bone marrow (frequently referred to as 'acute B-cell leukemia' or acute lymphoblastic leukemia of L3 type) are included. If two percentages are given, the first is for stage IV patients, the second for acute B-cell leukemia.
§ Includes children and adults.
¶ Updated information as of December 1994.
[ll] Disease-free survival, i.e., based on the 27 (93%) of patients who achieved a complete response.
[a] Includes stages IINR (unresected) to IV.
[b] Includes only patients with acute B-cell leukemia.
[c] Excludes patients with CNS disease at presentation.
[d] Includes children and adults.
[e] Ann Arbor staging.
[f] Includes stages I and II.
[g] Includes 13 patients who had bone marrow transplantation in first CR. These 13 patients had a worse outcome – 54% remain alive in first remission.
[h] Includes all stages – 16 were stage IV.

An issue that remains controversial is the influence of the extent of bone marrow involvement on prognosis. In the SFOP LMB-0281 protocol, 76% of 21 patients with bone marrow disease (but without CNS involvement) achieved long-term survival, but no difference in survival was apparent between patients with less than or more than 25% of tumor cells in the bone marrow [130]. More recently the SFOP has adopted a three-tier risk-adapted approach to chemotherapy in which group C patients (those with the highest risk) have more than 70% of tumor cells in the bone marrow [134]. It would seem more likely that prognosis relates to the total tumor burden, taking into consideration disease sites outside the bone marrow, rather than simply the degree of involvement of the marrow, but it is possible that the latter reflects the former. More data are required before this issue can be resolved. In the meanwhile, most of the more recently designed protocols achieve at least 60% EFS rates in patients with stage IV disease – comparable to the results achieved for stage III patients in earlier protocols – and some have reported considerably better results [25,105,134, 147] (Table 37.6).

Although CNS disease, at one time, was considered to be an obstacle to cure [98], this assumption has undergone revision. Fifty per cent of African patients with CNS disease – which is often associated with small-volume systemic disease – achieve long-term DFS with relatively simple therapy [48]. Thus, the evidence that the CNS is not as protected a sanctuary as had been supposed has existed for some time. Moreover, the association of CNS disease with bone marrow involvement in sporadic

SNCC has also long been recognized [34,148,149], and CNS disease may be associated with a particularly high tumor burden. This suggests that it was not the CNS disease *per se* that resulted in a poor outcome, but the extent of systemic disease [150], which in turn, may be related to the likelihood of the presence of resistance-inducing mutations in tumor cells. The markedly improved results of treatment in patients with CNS disease that have been achieved by the intensification of systemic therapy – including the use of high-dose systemic methotrexate and Ara-C – support this interpretation [25,134].

It would appear that the earlier suggestion that patients with CNS disease might best be treated with high-dose therapy followed by autologous bone marrow rescue [132] has been superceded by the improved results being obtained with conventional therapy. Indeed, a retrospective analysis of adult patients (by no means exclusively patients with CNS disease) treated by SFOP LMB 84 or 86 protocols or by autologous bone marrow transplantation after the induction of remission showed a worse survival rate in the transplanted group [137].

The role of radiation therapy in patients with CNS disease is coming increasingly into question. A retrospective examination of NCI patients with CNS disease did not reveal a clear advantage to radiation [109], and presently patients treated with NCI protocol 89-C-41 are treated without radiation, except when there is intracerebral disease – with, to date, excellent results, although more patients will need to be successfully treated before there are sufficient data to put this matter to rest. In contrast, in SFOP trials, patients with CNS disease presently receive radiation after the completion of chemotherapy, although this policy, which is not supported by data from clinical trials, may change.

Paraplegia at presentation is a rare occurrence except in endemic Burkitt's lymphoma. Until recently, radiation was unavailable in equatorial Africa and most patients there still do not have access to it. Thus, the majority of patients with paraplegia have been treated with chemotherapy alone. Excellent results, both with regard to survival (such patients often have disease confined to the paraspinal region, and therefore low tumor volume and an excellent prognosis), and ambulation are obtained, except in the circumstance that paraplegia is long standing, or vascular occlusion has caused infarction of the spinal cord [151]. As with meningeal and cranial nerve involvement, there is no reason to believe that patients would have been better treated had radiotherapy been available, and it is unlikely that controlled clinical trails can be feasibly performed in the USA or Europe, to examine this question. While it has been traditional to irradiate the spinal cord in the presence of documented spinal cord compression, the lack of evidence that radiation provides an effective therapeutic modality in Burkitt's lymphoma, and the potential for increased toxicity, particularly in small children, suggests that a more rational perspective would be not to use radiation unless it can be shown by clinical studies to be of benefit.

Other 'special' sites of disease

Specific treatment approaches are not required for patients with other sites of disease except insofar as this has an impact upon emergency management. This applies to the treatment of patients with disease sites traditionally treated with local therapy in addition to chemotherapy, such as those with localized bone or testicular involvement.

Two retrospective reviews of patients with bone disease (including both single and multiple lesions) in which radiotherapy was not used have indicated that bone lesions respond well to chemotherapy alone [59,60]. In the NCI series, in which the earlier protocol, 77–04 was used, even in patients with multiple lesions, overall survival was approximately 70% in patients treated with chemotherapy alone, except in the presence of bone marrow involvement – a result that was similar to that achieved in patients with similar tumor burdens but without bone involvement. There is thus no evidence that radiation is required for the treatment of bony sites of disease and, because of the potential for added toxicity, it is not recommended. In this respect, it is worth noting that in one series of patients with primary lymphoma of bone, two of ten who received local radiation (5000 and 5400 rads) in addition to chemotherapy subsequently developed sarcomas within the radiation field [152].

For patients with testicular disease at presentation, there is a paucity of data regarding the optimal approach. In patients treated according to NCI protocol 77–04, there was some evidence that this regimen did not provide adequate therapy for testicular disease [61], although the literature does not provide evidence that radiotherapy would have been beneficial [62]. In the absence of controlled clinical studies, it seems reasonable to conclude that testicular disease may be treated adequately with chemotherapy alone, but that not all chemotherapy regimens are equivalent in this regard. There seems little doubt that the most recent protocols, which include high-dose S-phase agents, will provide adequate therapy for testicular disease, and there is no good argument for adding radiation to chemotherapy in this clinical context – particularly in light of the evidence that radiation is not a highly effective modality in SNCC lymphoma.

CNS prophylactic therapy

CNS prophylaxis is indicated in the majority of patients with SNCC lymphomas, but there is good evidence that cranial or craniospinal radiation are not indicated. Firstly, the rate of isolated CNS recurrence is very low with protocols that do not include radiation. Secondly, radiation does not appear, on the basis of published results, to provide effective CNS prophylaxis. Craniospinal irradiation, for example, was shown to have no value in preventing CNS disease in African patients [153] or in patients with 'acute B-cell leukemia' [147]. Effective prophylaxis can clearly be provided, however, by intrathecal therapy reinforced in high-risk patients by high-dose methotrexate, and often high-dose ara-C as well.

There is good evidence that patients with completely resected abdominal disease (who fall into St Jude stage II) do not require intrathecal prophylaxis; among 32 patients with gastrointestinal primaries in the POG study of low-risk patients, in which intrathecal therapy (methotrexate) was given only to patients with head and neck primaries, none relapsed [104]. Similarly, in CCSG trials in patients with localized disease, in which intrathecal therapy was also omitted for patients with gastrointestinal primaries (there were 55 such patients with SNCC lymphoma) none developed a CNS relapse [138]. The latter patients, in contrast to those entered into the POG study, received intermediate dose methotrexate intravenously. Whether this was an element in the prevention of CNS disease is unknown, but multiple courses of 2.7 g or more of methotrexate infused over 42 hours did not prevent isolated CNS relapse in NCI protocol 77-04 [45]. Irrespective of this, because of the very small, but significant risk of severe myelopathy with intrathecal therapy, it would appear appropriate to avoid intrathecal therapy in patients with small-volume gastrointestinal disease that has been completely resected, although it would be prudent, in the absence of definitive information, to continue to provide CNS prophylaxis to patients with extensive, but completely resected abdominal disease. The latter patients will be uncommonly encountered, but occasionally complete resection is performed at diagnostic laparotomy. All other patients, in whom the risk of developing CNS relapse is significant, should receive CNS prophylactic therapy with intrathecal therapy and, in patients with a high tumor burden, high-dose systemic S-phase specific agents in addition.

CHEMOTHERAPY OF BURKITT'S LYMPHOMA OUTSIDE THE USA AND EUROPE

Equatorial Africa

In the early 1970s, the majority of children with advanced SNCC lymphoma in the USA and Europe died from their disease; survival rates ranged from 5% to 10% [98,154,155]; only patients with limited disease, usually treated with local irradiation with or without chemotherapy, had a significant chance of survival (ranging up to 50% in various series [94–98]). In contrast, in a series of 119 patients with Burkitt's lymphoma reported from Uganda in 1972 [156], in which all patients had been followed for at least 18 months, the survival rate at 3 years was 50% in children with stage III disease (intrathoracic, intra-abdominal, paraspinal or osseous tumor, excluding facial bones), 44% in stage IV (CNS or bone marrow involvement) and 73% in children with stage I and II disease (single or multiple jaw tumors). All patients were treated with single-agent cyclophosphamide (1–6 doses at 40 mg/kg) and no radiation was given (it was unavailable in Uganda at the time).

These early results suggested that endemic SNCC was much more responsive to chemotherapy than sporadic SNCC, although treatment tended to be more variable in the USA and Europe, and emphasis on chemotherapy may have been delayed by the traditional emphasis on radiation therapy, such that chemotherapy was initially considered an adjunctive modality. Although extensive single-agent data were collected in African patients [116,157–162], little information of this kind existed (or exists) for patients outside Africa. There is some evidence, however, that a fraction of patients with sporadic SNCC can achieve long-term survival with single agents. In one series of 22 patients treated at the NCI with cyclophosphamide alone, for example, although an apparently lower overall response rate in comparison to African patients was observed (59% of 22 patients compared to 81%) [117], 9 of the 22 patients achieved long-term survival (the majority had received six doses of cyclophosphamide at 40 mg/kg). Unfortunately, the size of the tumor burdens in these patients is difficult to discern since some had extensive surgical resection.

One remarkable difference between endemic and sporadic Burkitt's lymphoma is the difference in the prognosis of patients who relapse. African children treated with one or two doses of cyclophosphamide (Burkitt had earlier suggested that further therapy could be deleterious through suppression of a host antitumor response [116]) often suffered one or several relapses, which frequently responded either to cyclophosphamide again, or to other drugs, such as methotrexate, Ara-C and vincristine. Patients would then frequently go on to achieve long-term survival. In the Uganda Cancer Institute series, some 40% of patients who survived disease free for between 4 and 10 years had had a relapse, and many had had more than one relapse [118]. Even patients with limited or surgically resected disease, almost 90% of whom achieved long-term survival, had a high relapse rate – approximately 40% after one or two doses of cyclophosphamide [78,156]. In sporadic SNCC, prior to the advent of high-dose chemotherapy, relapse nearly always heralded rapid demise in spite of chemotherapy. Whether this difference was the result of the type of therapy administered (e.g., the much more prolonged therapy given to patients in the USA, after the model of ALL), or to biological differences is unclear. Perhaps moderate- to high-dose pulse therapy is less likely to induce drug resistance than continuous lower-dose therapy – particularly if the latter includes multiple agents. Indeed, relapses that occurred on therapy in Uganda were generally unresponsive to further treatment with cyclophosphamide, but would respond to other drugs [156]. Similarly, patients who relapsed early (less than 12 weeks), had a significantly worse prognosis than those who relapsed later [156,163], and tended to occur at the same site rather than at a previously uninvolved site. Very similar results were obtained, using the same treatment approaches, in Ghana [164].

The high response rate of African patients who relapse suggests that they were simply being undertreated, and did not have chemotherapy-resistant disease *de novo*. It also seems probable that the vigorous treatment of the usually sensitive relapses, including the use of intrathecal therapy [165], is the reason for the improved results of the Uganda Cancer Institute series compared to earlier African series [161,162,166], and for the apparent lack of a survival advantage to multiple doses of cyclophosphamide (a planned six) [167] – the high fraction of patients who relapsed after a single dose would be effectively treated with additional cyclophosphamide or other drugs.

Because patients who relapsed during treatment with multiple doses of cyclophosphamide responded to other drugs, a clinical trial was designed in Uganda to compare primary treatment with cyclophosphamide with an alternating sequence of cyclophosphamide, vincristine and methotrexate, and Ara-C (TRIKE). Although initially there appeared to be no difference in the pattern of relapses between these two arms [156], a survival advantage to the sequential regimen was eventually observed [163]. Subsequently, a simultaneous combination of cyclophosphamide, vincristine and methotrexate (COM) was also compared to cyclophosphamide in Uganda. Interestingly, the relapse pattern observed with COM was dramatically different in that the majority (eight out of ten) patients had their first relapse in the CNS alone [167]. In contrast, seven out of eight patients treated with cyclophosphamide alone relapsed at both systemic (usually the same site as the presenting tumor) and CNS sites, and only one patient had an isolated CNS relapse. Fortunately, six out of eight patients who relapsed in the CNS alone following COM therapy subsequently survived for 9–22 months, confirming earlier studies that indicated that isolated CNS relapse is not a poor prognostic sign (55% of patients who presented with, or subsequently developed, meningeal involvement became long-term survivors [156,167]), and leading to the eventual demonstration of a survival advantage to the combination regimen compared to cyclophosphamide alone [163]. Surprisingly, an earlier, randomized comparison of no CNS prophylaxis with alternating intrathecal methotrexate and Ara-C over 4 days had not appeared to prevent CNS recurrence (perhaps because systemic therapy was inadequate), and patients treated with COM were therefore not given intrathecal prophylaxis, but were randomized to receive craniospinal irradiation after the induction of complete remission. As already mentioned, this proved unsuccessful but, unfortunately, further studies of intrathecal prophylactic therapy could not be completed because of political circumstances in Uganda.

These studies, although including small numbers of patients, did suggest that drug combinations were preferable to single-agent therapy in African Burkitt's lymphoma. In Ghana, a combination of cyclophosphamide, Ara-C and vincristine, with intrathecal methotrexate also appeared to be superior to cyclophosphamide alone in patients with abdominal disease, insofar as patients who achieved remission had a significantly greater chance of remaining in remission compared to patients treated with cyclophosphamide alone (63% versus 30%) [168]. There were also fewer CNS relapses in the combination arm (17% versus 44%). Unfortunately, this arm was also associated with an increased number of early deaths; 4 out of 42 patients died within 48 hours, probably from metabolic complications, compared to 1 out of 44 treated with cyclophosphamide alone. Seven more patients treated with the drug combination died in the first cycle of therapy, five from severe infection, compared to only one patient treated with cyclophosphamide alone. These toxic deaths were sufficient to overcome the improved antitumor effect of the combination and overall survival was not improved. Perhaps a first cycle of cyclophosphamide alone would have avoided these problems. Interestingly, an increase in early deaths was not observed with the COM regimen used in Uganda [167].

Taken as a whole, and bearing in mind the difficulties of making comparisons when the spectrum of disease, treatment facilities and protocol management are so different, these results do not suggest that endemic SNCC is significantly more responsive to therapy than sporadic SNCC lymphoma. Indeed, similar survival rates (40% for patients with extensive disease) were obtained in children from the United States treated with COM or a derivative combination, COMP [121] to African patients treated with simple drug combinations [163,168]. Because of the limited facilities for supportive care and the high cost of chemotherapeutic agents, African patients have not been treated as intensively as patients in many other countries in recent years and, in general, therapeutic approaches have advanced little beyond those used in the 1970s.

Other regions

The results of treatment of patients with SNCC in regions such as Latin America vary greatly throughout the region. In some of the major centers, similar or only slightly worse overall results to those being obtained in the USA and Europe have been reported, but in other countries results appear to be significantly worse [71,169]. In some series there appears to be a relative paucity of patients with bone marrow disease, so that the efficacy of the protocols in patients with stage IV disease (and patients with greater than 25% of marrow involvement) are difficult to discern. Many patients in Latin America suffer from malnutrition, which may lessen the chance of survival as a result of impaired immune responsiveness, possibly impaired mucosal barriers, and in some circumstances, increased drug toxicity (e.g., liver toxicity). The possibility that there is a higher rate of bowel perforation in some countries, such as Mexico, has already been mentioned, although the cause of this is not clear, and could relate to surgical practice, or possibly biological differences in tumor location or invasiveness. The anatomical distribution of tumor may even differ in different regions within the same country (e.g., equatorial versus temperate Brazil). In many Latin American countries supportive care is less than optimal. In Asia, including the Middle East, North Africa and Turkey, similar circumstances pertain, but the fraction of patients with jaw tumors and bone marrow disease varies, and it is important, as always, to examine the results by stage in different series in order to make valid comparisons [69,70, 170–172].

RECURRENT DISEASE

In the SNCC lymphomas relapse occurs predominantly in the first 8 months after presentation and in sporadic tumors is almost unknown after 10 months, regardless of the type and duration of therapy [25, 45,130,133,147]. Interestingly, in endemic tumors, late relapse – occurring after a disease-free period of up to 5 years – has been described in a small percentage of patients [173]. There is evidence that such tumors represent new tumors rather than recurrence [174]. This would explain the almost exclusive occurrence of such late relapses in endemic regions, where environmental factors are much more conducive to the development of SNCC. This explanation is consistent with the documented occurrence of second SNCC lymphomas in patients with HIV infection, who are also at very high-risk for the development of SNCC lymphoma [175].

Patients who relapse after treatment with one of the highly successful protocols reported in recent years have an extremely poor prognosis. Autologous bone marrow transplantation (ABMT) has been successful in the past, beginning with the BCNU, Ara-C, cyclophosphamide, 6-thioguamine (BACT) protocol used at the NCI [176], but patients who have demonstrably resistant disease, i.e., patients who have a poor response to a salvage regimen [177,178] have a very poor prognosis, and such patients are now rarely subjected to transplantation. This suggests that the success rate of ABMT is likely to be less when relapse occurs after today's very intensive primary therapy protocols. Occasional patients who respond to a salvage regimen, however, may still achieve prolonged survival after allogeneic transplantation – perhaps because of a graft-versus-tumor effect [25]. An optimal salvage protocol for relapse after recently reported primary treatment protocols has not been developed, although platinum compounds are worthy of exploration in this context; at least one successful protocol incorporates platinum into primary therapy [179] and one patient who relapsed after treatment with NCI protocol 89-C-41 achieved a complete response to a platinum-based regimen [25]. The possibility of a graft-versus-tumor effect makes allogeneic transplantation (even haplotype-mismatched transplantation) more attractive than ABMT in this context, even though it is associated with greater toxicity.

FUTURE DIRECTIONS

While therapy targeted at the molecular lesions, or viral sequences present in tumor cells, is attractive (see Chapter 51)[180], it will be many years before the role of such approaches in primary therapy will be defined since they are only now beginning to enter clinical trials. In the meantime, with excellent results being achieved by conventional therapy – even in patients with the highest tumor burdens – considerable focus should be placed upon the improved identification of prognostic groups in order to improve risk adaptation of chemotherapy. While tumor burden (after treatment) remains the single most useful predictor of outcome, the possibility that the presence of p53 mutations will increase the precision of prognostication is of particular interest [87,88]. This may result in both expansion of the low-risk group, thus permitting a larger fraction of patients to be treated with less toxic regimens, and could also lead to improved definition of the highest risk groups – the 20% or so of patients in stage IV who still relapse, such that new protocols could be developed for these patients. Logically, therapy in patients in whom p53 mutations have been demonstrated in tumor cells should optimize agents that do not depend, for their cytotoxicity, on DNA damage – e.g., mitotic spindle inhibitors. The identification of other mechanisms of drug resistance may also permit the development of approaches to overcoming this problem. To date, however, attempts to overcome mdr-1-mediated drug resistance in adult lymphomas have been disappointing [181].

Follow-up

Appropriate intervals between follow-up studies for SNCC lymphomas can never be optimal because of the very rapid growth rate of these tumors, such that the detection of recurrence before it has become clinically apparent would probably require weekly staging studies. Because of this, it could be argued that routine restaging studies after the cessation of treatment are of questionable value, although frequent follow-up visits are useful; the development of symptoms should precipitate appropriate investigations to determine their origin. The relatively short period during which patients with SNCC lymphomas are 'at risk' for relapse and the likelihood of relapse should also be taken into account when deciding on the timing of appropriate follow-up visits. Patients with limited disease now approach 100% EFS rates, while even patients with the most extensive tumor burdens at presentation have only a 10–20% chance of recurrence with the most successful protocols. Thus imaging studies are most unlikely to be of value in patients with limited disease, and of no value in any patient group after a period of 10 months has passed from the date of presentation

without evidence of recurrence. Given present results, it would seem reasonable to follow, with imaging studies, sites of residual abnormalities monthly for a few months after the cessation of chemotherapy to ensure that they are shrinking or stable. Although a significant fraction of patients, particularly those with extensive disease at presentation, may have such residual abnormalities on CAT or MRI scans, the majority of these will prove not to represent viable tumor. The absence of gallium-67 uptake in such areas of residual abnormality is reassuring, but not definitive evidence of the absence of residual disease [182]. A progressively rising serum LDH level is also a useful marker of recurrence, although LDH is not specific. At present, when patients are treated with one of the most effective protocols, there seems to be no indication for routine bone marrow or CSF surveillance after the completion of chemotherapy.

Should more sensitive measures of minimal residual disease based on serum measurements be developed, e.g., of tumor products or the detection, by PCR, of evidence of a tumor-associated translocation, and in the event that such measurements are shown to correlate with relapse, a case could be made for frequent surveillance, using such techniques, in the first few months of therapy. However, in the absence of effective salvage treatment, it is not clear that the early detection of recurrent disease would have significant medical advantages.

References

1. Rappaport H. *Tumors of the Hempoietic System. Atlas of Tumor Pathology*, Section III, Fascicle 8. Washington, DC: Armed Forces Institute of Pathology, 1966.
2. Lukes RJ, Collins RD. New approaches to the classification of the lymphomata. *Br. J. Cancer* 1975, **31**(Suppl. II): 1–28.
3. National Cancer Institute sponsored study of classifications of non-Hodgkin's lymphoma. Summary and description of a working formulation for clinical usage. *Cancer* 1982, **49**: 2112–2135.
4. Harris N, Jaffe E, Stein H, et al. A proposal for an international consensus on the classification of lymphoid neoplasms. *Blood* 1994, **84**: 1361–1392.
5. Gregory CD, Turtz T, Edwards CF, et al. Identification of a subset of normal B-cells with a Burkitt's lymphoma (BL)-like phenotype. *J. Immunol.* 1987, **139**: 313–318.
6. Gregory CD, Murray RF, Edwards CF, et al. Down-regulation of cell adhesion molecules LFA-3 and ICAM-1 in Epstein–Barr virus positive Burkitt's lymphoma underlies tumor cell escape from virus-specific T-cell surveillance. *J. Exp. Med.* 1988, **167**: 1811–1824.

Trop. Geogr. Med. 1990, **42**: 255–260.

74. Miyoshi I. Japanese Burkitt's lymphoma. Clinicopathological review of 14 cases. *Jap. J. Clin. Oncol.* 1983, **13**: 489–496.

75. Kamunvi F, Njino MJ. Epidemiology of jaw tumors in Nyanza province with special reference to Burkitt's lymphoma: Report of preliminary findings in the Nyanza general hospital, Kisumu, Kenya. *E. Afr. Med. J.* 1985, **62**: 122–128.

76. Hulu N, Ramot B, Sheehan W. Childhood abdominal lymphoma in Israel. *Israel J. Med. Sci.* 1970, **6**: 246–252.

77. Benjamin D, Magrath IT, Douglass EC, et al. Derivation of lymphoma cell lines from microscopically normal bone marrow in patients with undifferentiated lymphomas; evidence of occult bone marrow involvement. *Blood* 1983, **61**: 1017–1019.

78. Magrath IT, Lwanga S, Carswell W, et al. Surgical reduction of tumor bulk in management of abdominal Burkitt's lymphoma. *Br. Med. J.* 1974, **2**: 308–312.

79. Ziegler JL, Magrath IT. Burkitt's lymphoma. In Ioachim HL (ed.) *Pathobiology Annual.* New York: Appleton Century Croft, 1974, pp. 129–142.

80. Magrath IT. Malignant Non-Hodgkin's lymphomas. In Pizzo PA, Poplack DG (eds) *Principles and Practice of Pediatric Oncology.* 2nd edn. Philadelphia: J. B. Lippincott, 1993, pp. 537–575.

81. Sandrock D, Lastoria S, Magrath IT, et al. The role of gallium scintigraphy in patients with small noncleaved cell lymphoma. *Eur. J. Nucl. Med.* 1993, **20**: 119–122.

82. Krudy AD, Dunnick N, Magrath IT, et al. CT of American Burkitt's lymphoma. *Am. J. Rad.* 1981, **136**: 747–754.

83. Shawker TH, Dunnick N, Head GL, et al. Ultrasound evaluation of American Burkitt's lymphoma. *J. Clin. Ultrasound* 1979, **7**: 279–283.

84. Haddy TB, Parker RI, Magrath IT. Bone marrow involvement in young patients with non-Hodgkin's lymphoma: The importance of multiple bone marrow samples for accurate staging. *Med. Pediatr. Oncol.* 1989, **17**: 418–423.

85. Csako G, Magrath I, Elin R. Serum total and iso-enzyme lactate dehydrogenase activity in American Burkitt's lymphoma. *Am. J. Clin. Path.* 1982, **78**: 712–717.

86. Nkrumah F, Henle W, Henle G, et al. Burkitt's lymphoma: Its clinical course in relation to immunologic reactivities to Epstein–Barr virus and tumor related antigens. *J. Natl Cancer Inst.* 1976, **57**: 1051–1056.

87. Gutierrez MI, Bhatia K, Diez B, et al. Prognostic significance of p53 mutations in small noncleaved cell lymphomas. *Int. J. Oncol.* 1994, **4**: 567–571.

88. Venkatesh H, Adde M, Gutierrez M, et al. A study of the prognostic significance of p53 in small noncleaved cell lymphomas. *Proc. ASPH/O* 1995, **4**: 630 (abstract).

89. Caron de Fromentel C, May-Levin F, Mouriesse H, et al. Presence of circulating antibodies against cellular protein p53 in a notable proportion of children with B-cell lymphoma. *Int. J. Cancer* 1987, **39**: 185–189.

90. Fontanini G, Fiore L, Bigini D, et al. Levels of p53 antigen in the serum of non-small cell lung cancer patients correlate with positive p53 immunohistochemistry on tumor sections, tumor necrosis and nodal involvement. *Int. J. Oncol.* 1994, **5**: 553–558.

91. Cohen LF, Balow J, Magrath IT, et al. Acute tumor lysis syndrome: A review of 37 patients with Burkitt's lymphoma. *Am. Med.* 1980, **68**: 486–491.

92. Tsokos G, Balow J, Spiegel RJ, et al. Renal and metabolic complications of undifferentiated and lymphoblastic lymphomas. *Medicine* 1981, **60**: 218–229.

92a. Stapleton FB, Strother DR, Roy S, et al. Acute renal failure at onset of therapy for advanced stage Burkitt lymphoma and B cell acute lymphoblastic lymphoma. *Pediatrics* 1988, **82**: 863–869.

93. Arseneau JC, Bagley CM, Anderson T, et al. Hyperkalemia, a sequel to chemotherapy of Burkitt's lymphoma. *Lancet* 1973, **1**: 10–14.

94. Glatstein E, Kim H, Donaldson S, et al. Non-Hodgkin's lymphoma VI. Results of treatment in childhood. *Cancer* 1974, **34**: 204–211.

95. Aur RJ, Hustu HO, Simone JV, et al. Therapy of localized and regional lymphosarcoma of childhood. *Cancer* 1971, **27**: 1328–1331.

96. Jenkin RDT, Sonley MJ, Stephens CA, et al. Primary gastrointestinal tract lymphoma in childhood. *Radiology* 1966, **92**: 763–767.

97. Nelson DF, Cassady JR, Traggis D, et al. The role of radiation therapy in localized resectable intestinal non-Hodgkin's lymphoma in children. *Cancer* 1977, **39**: 89–97.

98. Murphy SB, Frizzera G, Evans AE, et al. A study of childhood non-Hodgkin's lymphoma. *Cancer* 1975, **36**: 2121–2131.

99. Cebrian-Bonesana A, Schvartzman E, Roca-Garcia C, et al. Non-Hodgkin's lymphoma in children. An analysis of 122 cases from Argentina. *Cancer* 1978, **41**: 2372–2378.

100. Jenkin RDT. The management of malignant lymphoma in childhood. In Deeley TJ (ed.) *Modern Radiotherapy and Oncology – Malignant Diseases in Children.* London: Butterworths, 1969, pp. 319–359.

101. Murphy SB, Hustu HO, Rivera G, et al. End results of treating children with localized non-Hodgkin's lymphoma with a combined modality approach of lessened intensity. *J. Clin. Oncol.* 1983, **1**: 326–330.

102. Jenkin RD, Anderson JR, Chilcote RR, et al. The treatment of localized non-Hodgkin's lymphoma in children: A report from the Children's Cancer Study Group. *J. Clin. Oncol.* 1984, **2**: 88–97.

103. Murphy SB, Fairclough DL, Hutchison RE, et al. Non-Hodgkin's lymphomas of childhood: An analysis of the histology, staging, and response to treatment of 338 cases at a single institution. *J. Clin. Oncol.* 1989, **7**: 186–193.

104. Link MP, Donaldson SS, Berard CW, et al. Results of treatment of childhood localized non-Hodgkin's lymphoma with combination chemotherapy with or without radiotherapy. *N. Engl. J. Med.* 1990, **322**: 1169–1174.

105. Reiter A, Schrappe M, Parwaresch R, et al. Non-Hodgkin's lymphomas of childhood and adolescence:

Results of a treatment stratified for biological subtypes and stage. A report of the BFM group. *J. Clin. Oncol.* 1995, **7**: 186–193.

106. Lopez TM, Hagemeister FB, McLaughlin P, et al. Small non-cleaved cell lymphoma in adults: Superior results for stages I–III. *J. Clin. Oncol.* 1990, **8**: 615–622.

107. McMaster ML, Greer JP, Greco A, et al. Effective treatment of small non-cleaved-cell lymphomas with high-intensity, brief-duration chemotherapy. *J. Clin. Oncol.* 1991, **9**: 941–946.

108. Murphy SB, Hustu HO. A randomised trial of combined modality therapy of childhood non-Hodgkin's lymphoma. *Cancer* 1980, **45**: 630–637.

109. Magrath IT, Haddy TB, Adde M. Treatment of patients with high-grade non-Hodgkin's lymphoma and central nervous system involvement: Is radiation an essential component of treatment. *Leuk. Lymphoma* 1996, **21**:99–105.

110. Norin T, Clifford P, Einhorn J, et al. Conventional and superfractionated radiation therapy in Burkitt's lymphoma. *Acta Radiol.* 1971: 10: 545–557.

111. Kemeny MM, Magrath IT, Brennan MF. The role of surgery in the management of American Burkitt's lymphoma and its treatment. *Ann. Surg.* 1982, **196**: 82–86.

112. Fleming ID, Turk PS, Murphy SB, et al. Surgical implications of primary gastrointestinal lymphoma of childhood. *Arch. Surg.* 1990, **125**: 252–256.

113. Stovroff MC, Coran AG, Hutchison RJ. The role of surgery in American Burkitt's lymphoma in children. *J. Pediatr. Surg.* 1991, **25**: 1235–1238.

114. LaQuaglia MP, Stolar CHJ, Krailo M, et al. The role of surgery in abdominal non-Hodgkin's lymphoma. Experience from the Children's Cancer Study Group. *J. Pediatr. Surg.* 1992, **27**: 230–235.

115. Djerassi I, Kim JS. Methotrexate and citrovorum factor rescue in the management of childhood lymphosarcoma and reticulum cell sarcoma (non-Hodgkin's lymphomas). *Cancer* 1976, **38**: 1043–1051.

116. Burkitt D. Long term remissions following one and two dose chemotherapy for African lymphoma. *Cancer* 1967, **20**: 756–759.

117. Arseneau JC, Canellos GP, Banks PM, et al. American Burkitt's lymphoma – a clinicopathological study of 30 cases. I. Clinical factors relating to long term survival. *Am. J. Med.* 1975, **58**: 314–321.

118. Ziegler J, Magrath IT, Olweny CLM. Cure of Burkitt's lymphoma: 10 year follow-up of 157 Ugandan patients. *Lancet* 1979, **2**: 936–938.

119. Olweny, CLM, Katongole-Mbidde E, Otim D, et al. Long-term experience with Burkitt's lymphoma in Uganda. *Int. J. Cancer* 1980, **26**: 261-266.

120. Ziegler JL, DeVita VT, Graw RG, et al. Combined modality treatment of American Burkitt's lymphoma. *Cancer* 1976, **38**: 2225–2231.

121. Ziegler JL. Treatment results of 54 American patients with Burkitt's lymphoma are similar to the African experience. *N. Engl. J. Med.* 1977, **297**: 75–80.

122. Ziegler JL, Magrath IT, Deisseroth AB, et al. Combined modality treatment of Burkitt's lymphoma. *Cancer Treat. Rep.* 1978, **62**: 2031–2034.

123. Schwenn M, Blattner SR, Lynch E, et al. HiC-COM: A 2 month intensive chemotherapy regimen for children with stage III and IV Burkitt's lymphoma and B-cell acute lymphoblastic leukemia. *J. Clin. Oncol.* 1991, **9**: 133–138.

124. Anderson JR, Wilson JF, Jenkin DT, et al. Childhood non-Hodgkin's lymphoma. The results of a randomized therapeutic trial comparing a 4-drug regimen (COMP) with a 10-drug regimen (LSA$_2$L$_2$). *N. Engl. J. Med.* 1983, **308**: 559–565.

125. Anderson JR, Jenkin DT, Wilson JF, et al. Long-term follow-up of patients treated with COMP or LSA$_2$L$_2$ therapy for childhood non-Hodgkin's lymphoma: A report of CCG-551 from the Childrens Cancer Group. *J. Clin. Oncol.* 1993, **11**: 1024–1032.

126. Hvizdala EV, Berard C, Callihan T, et al. Nonlymphoblastic lymphoma in children – histology and stage-related response to therapy: A Pediatric Oncology Group Study. *J. Clin. Oncol.* 1991, **9**: 1189–1195.

127. Müller-Weihrich S, Henze G, Langermann HJ, et al. Kindliche B zell-Lymphome und-Leukämien. Verbesserung der Prognose durch eine für B-Neoplasien konzipierte Therapie der BFM Studiengruppe. *Onkologie* 1984, **7**: 205–208.

128. Weinstein H, Vance Z, Jaffe N, et al. Improved prognosis for patients with mediastinal lymphoblastic lymphoma. *Blood* 1979, **53**: 687–697.

129. Sullivan M, Ramirez I. Curability of Burkitt's lymphoma with high-dose cyclophosphamide–high dose methotrexate therapy and intrathecal chemoprophylaxis. *J. Clin. Oncol.* 1985, **3**: 627–636.

130. Patte C, Philip T, Rodary C, et al. Improved survival rate in children with stage III and IV B-cell non-Hodgkin's lymphoma and leukemia using multiagent chemotherapy: Results of a study of 114 children from the French Pediatric Oncology Society. *J. Clin. Oncol.* 1986, **4**: 1219–1226.

131. Murphy S, Bowman W, Abromowitch M, et al. Results of treatment of advanced stage Burkitt's lymphoma and B-cell, (SIg+) acute lymphoblastic leukemia with high-dose fractionated cyclophosphamide and coordinated high-dose methotrexate and cytarabine. *J. Clin. Oncol.* 1986, **4**: 1732–1739.

132. Philip T, Pinkerton R, Biron P, et al. Effective multiagent chemotherapy in children with advanced B-cell lymphoma: who remains the high risk patient? *Br. J. Haematol.* 1987, **65**: 159–164.

133. Patte C, Philip T, Rodary C, et al. High survival rate in advanced-stage B-cell lymphomas and leukemias without CNS involvement with a short intensive polychemotherapy: Results from the French Pediatric Oncology Society of a randomized trial of 216 children. *J. Clin. Oncol.* 1991, **9**: 123–132.

134. Patte C, Leverger G, Rubie H, et al. High cure rate in B-cell (Burkitt's) leukemia in the LMB 89 protocol of the SFOP (French Pediatric Oncology Society). *Proc. Am. Soc. Clin. Oncol.* 1993, **12**: 1050 (Abstract).

135. Bernstein JI, Coleman CN, Strickler JG, et al. Combined modality therapy for adults with small non-cleaved cell lymphoma (Burkitt's and non-Burkitt's types). *J. Clin. Oncol.* 1988, **4**: 847–858.

136. Coiffier B, Bryon P-A, French M, et al. Intensive chemotherapy in aggressive lymphomas: Updated

results of LNH-80 protocol and prognostic factors affecting response and survival *Blood* 1987, **70**: 1394–1399.

137. Soussain C, Patte C, Ostronoff M, et al. Small non-cleaved cell lymphoma and leukemia in adults. A retrospective study of 65 adults treated with the LMB pediatric protocols. *Blood* 1995, **85**: 664–674.

138. Meadows AT, Sposto R, Jenkin RDT, et al. Similar efficacy of 6 and 18 months of therapy with four drugs (COMP) for localized non-Hodgkin's lymphoma of children: A report from the children's cancer study group. *J. Clin. Oncol.* 1989, **17**: 92–99.

139. Link MP, Shuster JJ, Berard CW, et al. Nine weeks of chemotherapy without radiotherapy is sufficient treatment for most children with localized non-Hodgkin's lymphoma (NHL). *Proc. Am. Soc. Clin. Oncol.* 1993, **12**: 1309 (abstract).

140. Sandlund JT, Crist WM, Abromowitch M, et al. Pleural effusion is associated with a poor treatment outcome in stage III small non-cleaved cell lymphoma. *Leuekmia* 1991, **5**: 71–74.

141. Jones GR, Ettinger LJ. Continuous infusion of high-dose cytosine arabinoside for treatment of childhood acute leukemia and non-Hodgkin's lymphoma in relapse. *Semin. Oncol.* 1985, **12**: 150–154.

142. Gentet JC, Patte C, Quintana E, et al. Phase II study of cytarabine and etoposide in children with refractory or relapsed non-Hodgkin's lymphoma: A study of the French Society of Pediatric Oncology. *J. Clin. Oncol.* 1990, **8**: 661–665.

143. Magrath I, Adde M, Sandlund J, et al. Ifosfamide in the treatment of high-grade recurrent non-Hodgkin's lymphomas. *Hematol. Oncol.* 1991, **9**: 267–274.

144. Chilcote M, Krailo C, Kjeldsberg C, et al. Daunomycin plus COMP vs COMP therapy in childhood non-lymphoblastic lymphomas. *Proc. Am. Soc. Clin. Oncol.* 1991, **10**: 289 (1011A).

145. Bowman PW, Shuster JJ, Cook B, et al. Improved survival for children with B cell acute lymphoblastic leukemia and stage IV small noncleaved cell lymphoma: A Pediatric Oncology Group study. *J. Clin. Oncol.* 1996, **14**: 1252–1261.

146. Vlasveld LTH, Zwaan FE, Fibbe WE, et al. Neutropenic enterocolitis following treatment with cytosine arabinoside containing regimens for hematological malignancies: A potentiating role for amsacrine. *Ann. Hematol.* 1991, **62**: 129–134.

147. Reiter A, Schrappe M, Ludwig W-D, et al. Favorable outcome of B-cell acute lymphoblastic leukemia in childhood: A report of three consecutive studies of the BFM group. *Blood* 1992, **80**: 2471–2478.

148. Wanatabe A, Sullivan MP, Sutow WW, et al. Undifferentiated lymphoma, non-Burkitt's type: Meningeal and bone marrow involvement in children. *Am. J. Dis. Child.* 1973, **125**: 57–61.

149. Hutter JJ, Favara BE, Nelson M, et al. Non-Hodgkin's lymphoma in children. Correlation of CNS disease with initial presentation. *Cancer* 1975, **36**: 2132–2137.

150. Haddy TB, Adde MA, Magrath IT. Central nervous system involvement in small non-cleaved cell lymphoma: Is CNS disease *per se* a poor prognostic sign? *J. Clin. Oncol.* 1991, **9**: 1973–1982.

151. Wright DH. Gross distribution and haematology. In Burkitt DP, Wright DH (eds) *Burkitt's Lymphoma.* Edinburgh: E and S Livingstone, 1970, pp. 64–81.

152. Loeffler JS, Tarbell NH, Kozakewich H, et al. Primary lymphoma of bone in children: Analysis of treatment results with adriamycin, prednisone, oncovin (APO), and local radiation therapy. *J. Clin. Oncol.* 1986, **4**: 496–501.

153. Olweny CLM, Atine I, Kaddu-Mukasa A, et al. Cerebrospinal irradiation of Burkitt's lymphoma. Failure in preventing central nervous system relapse. *Acta Radiol. Ther. Phys. Biol.* 1977, **16**: 225–231.

154. Sullivan MP. Non-Hodgkin's lymphoma of childhood. In Sutow WW, Vietti TJ, Fernback DJ (eds) *Clinical Pediatric Oncology.* St Louis: CV Mosby Co., 1973, pp. 313–336.

155. Lemerle M, Gerard-Marchant R, Sarrazin D, et al. Lymphosarcoma and reticulum cell sarcoma in children – retrospective study of 172 cases. *Cancer* 1973, **32**: 1499–1507.

156. Ziegler JL. Chemotherapy of Burkitt's lymphoma. *Cancer* 1972, **30**: 1534–1540.

157. Oettgen HF, Burkitt D, Burchenal JH. Malignant lymphoma involving the jaw in African children: Treatment with methotrexate. *Cancer* 1963, **16**: 616–623.

158. Burkitt D. The African lymphoma. Preliminary observations on response to therapy. *Cancer* 1965, **18**: 399–410.

159. Burkitt D. African lymphoma. Observations on response to vincristine sulphate therapy. *Cancer* 1966, **19**: 1131–1137.

160. Clifford P. Long-term survival of patients with Burkitt's lymphoma; an assessment of treatment and other factors which may relate to survival. *Cancer Res.* 1967, **27**: 2578–2615.

161. Burkitt D. Treatment. General features. In Burkitt D, Wright DH (eds) *Burkitt's Lymphoma.* Edinburgh: E and S Livingstone, 1970, pp. 43–51.

162. Clifford P. Treatment. Response to particular chemotherapeutic and other agents and treatment of CNS involvement. In Burkitt D, Wright DH (eds) *Burkitt's Lymphoma.* Edinburgh: E and S Livingstone, 1970, pp. 52–63.

163. Olweny CLM, Katongole-Mbidde E, Otim D, et al. Long term experience with Burkitt's lymphoma in Uganda. *Int. J. Cancer* 1980, **26**: 261–266.

164. Nkrumah FK, Perkins IV. Burkitt's lymphoma. A clinical study of 110 patients. *Cancer* 1976, **37**: 671–676.

165. Ziegler JL, Bluming AZ. Intrathecal chemotherapy in Burkitt's lymphoma. *Br. Med. J.* 1971, **3**: 508–512.

166. Morrow RH, Pike MC, Kisuule A. Survival of Burkitt's lymphoma patients in Mulago Hospital, Uganda. *Br. Med. J.* 1967, **4**: 323–327.

167. Olweny CLM, Katongole-Mbidde E, Kaddu-Mukasa A, et al. Treatment of Burkitt's lymphoma: Randomized clinical trials of single-agent versus combination chemotherapy. *Int. J. Cancer* 1976, **17**: 436–440.

168. Nkrumah FK, Perkins IV, Biggar RJ. Combination chemotherapy in abdominal Burkitt's lymphoma. *Cancer* 1977, **40**: 1410–1416.

169. de Andrea ML, de Camargo B, Melaragno R. A new treatment protocol for childhood non-Hodgkin's lymphoma: Preliminary evaluation. *J. Clin. Oncol.* 1990, **8**: 666–671.

170. Gad-el-Mawla N, Hussein MH, Abdel-Hadi S, et al. Childhood non-Hodgkin's lymphoma in Egypt: Preliminary results of treatment with a new ifosfamide-containing regimen. *Cancer Chemother. Pharmacol.* 1989, **24** (Suppl. 1): S20–23.

171. Al-Attar A, Pritchard J, Al-Saleem T, et al. Intensive chemotherapy for non-localised Burkitt's lymphoma. *Arch. Dis. Child.* 1986, **14**: 1013–1019.

172. Kaplinsky C, Zaizov R. Childhood B-cell non-Hodgkin's lymphoma in Israel. *Leuk. Lymph.* 1994, **14**: 49–53.

173. Biggar RJ, Nkrumah FK, Henle W, et al. Very late relapses in patients with Burkitt's lymphoma; clinical and serological studies. *J. Natl Cancer Inst.* 1981, **66**: 439–444.

174. Fialkow PJ, Klein E, Klein G et al. Immunoglobulin and glucose-6-phosphate dehydrogenase as markers of cellular origin in Burkitt's lymphoma. *J. Exp. Med.* 1973, **138**: 89–102.

175. Barriga E, Lee J, Whang-Peng C, et al. Development of a second clonally discrete Burkitt's lymphoma in a human immunodeficiency virus (HIV) positive homosexual patient. *Blood* 1988, **72**: 792–795.

176. Appelbaum FR, Deisseroth A, Graw RG Jr, et al. Prolonged complete remission following high dose chemotherapy of Burkitt's lymphoma in relapse. *Cancer* 1978, **41**: 1059–1063.

177. Philip T, Pinkerton R, Hartmann'O, et al. The role of massive therapy with autologous bone marrow transplantation in Burkitt's lymphoma. *Clin. Haematol.* 1986, **15**: 205–217.

178. Philip T, Biron P, Philip I, et al. Massive therapy and autologous bone marrow transplantation in pediatric and young adults Burkitt's lymphoma (30 courses in 28 patients: A 5-year experience). *Eur. J. Cancer Clin. Oncol.* 1986, **22**: 1015–1027.

179. Gasparini M, Rottoli L, Massimino M, et al. Curability of advanced Burkitt's lymphoma in children by intensive short-term chemotherapy. *Eur. J. Cancer* 1993, **29A**: 692–698.

180. Magrath IT, Bhatia K, Huber B. Genetic intervention in the control of neoplasia. In Hodges GM, Rowlatt C (eds) *Developmental Biology and Cancer.* Boca Raton: CRC Press, 1992, pp. 479–523.

181. Wilson WH, Bates SE, Fojo A, et al. Controlled trial of dexverapamil, a modulator of multidrug resistance, in lymphomas refractory to EPOCH chemotherapy. *J. Clin. Oncol.* 1995, **13**: 1995–2004.

182. Kaplan WD, Jochelson MS, Herman TS, et al. Gallium-67 imaging: A predictor of residual tumor viability and clinical outcome in patients with diffuse large-cell lymphoma. *J. Clin. Oncol.* 1990, **8**: 1966–1970.

183. Beltran G. Childhood lymphoma in Colombia, South America. With special mention of cases resembling Burkitt's tumor. *Cancer* 1966, **19**: 1124–1130.

184. Shanmugaratnam K, Tan KK, Lee KW. Lymphoma of the Burkitt type in Singapore. *Int. J. Cancer* 1967, **2**: 576–580.

185. Philip T, Lenoir GM, Bryon AP, et al. Burkitt-type lymphoma in France among non-Hodgkin malignant lymphomas in caucasian children. *Br. J. Cancer* 1982, **45**: 670–678.

186. Iverson, OH, Harket R. Burkitt's lymphoma in Norway. A Survey of possible cases occurring in the period 1953 and 1962. *Eur. J. Cancer* 1968, **4**: 383–389.

187. Kerndrup G, Pallesen G. A clinico-pathological study of 13 Danish cases of Burkitt's lymphoma. *Scand. J. Haematol.* 1981, **27**: 99–107.

188. Booth K. Burkitt DP, Bassett JK, et al. Burkitt lymphoma in Papua, New Guinea. *Br. J. Cancer* 1967, **21**: 657–664.

189. Ten Seldam REJ, Cooke R, Atkinson L. Childhood lymphoma in the territories of Papua and New Guinea. *Cancer* 1966, **19**: 437–446.

190. Madanat FF, Amr SS, Tarawneh MS, et al. Burkitt's lymphoma in Jordanian children: epidemiological and clincial study *J. Trop. Med. Hygiene* 1986, **89**: 189–191.

CHAPTER 38

Lymphoblastic lymphoma

JOHN T. SANDLUND AND IAN T. MAGRATH

Definitions and general description

The lymphoblastic lymphomas consist of several phenotypically similar diseases that are morphologically indistinguishable. Lymphoblastic lymphomas, as now characterized by the NCI Working Formulation [1], represent, at best, a small subset of those designated lymphoblastic in the first half of this century (see Chapter 1) and were more recently included in the diffuse, poorly differentiated category of Rappaport [2]. The characteristic morphology and clinical pattern of this lymphoma first led to its recognition as a discrete entity by Lukes and Collins in 1975 [3], who referred to it as a tumor of convoluted lymphocytes, and by Nathwani and Kim in 1976 [4], who used the term 'lymphoblastic' in describing the tumor. In European classification schemes (the Kiel classification and the British Lymphoma Investigation), the term lymphoblastic is used more broadly and originally included the small noncleaved cell lymphomas. This chapter deals only with those tumors classified as 'lymphoblastic' in the NCI Working Formulation and the recently proposed REAL classification (see Chapter 3).

LYMPHOBLASTIC LEUKEMIA VERSUS LYMPHOBLASTIC LYMPHOMA

The tumor cells of lymphoblastic lymphoma are histologically, cytologically and immunophenotypically indistinguishable from the lymphoblasts of acute lymphoblastic leukemia (ALL). Indeed, the distinction between them is arbitrary and based upon the degree of marrow involvement. In some patients there may be no bone marrow involvement at all, so that a diagnosis of leukemia cannot be entertained; in others the clinical presentation is one of marrow failure, owing to extensive lymphoblast infiltration with or without generalized lymphadenopathy, and a mediastinal mass, so that the patient falls into a clinical category of leukemia. In many patients the distinction is less clear. Most pediatric oncologists use a criterion of less than or greater than 25% of blast cells present in bone marrow aspirates to differentiate between lymphoblastic lymphoma and ALL, respectively, but this criterion is not widely used in adult patients (some adult oncologists use a dividing line of 30%). In any event, any numerical definition can only be operational and arbitrary. Clinical studies comparing disease-free survival rates among patients segregated purely on this basis must be viewed with skepticism because the observed differences could be a consequence of other variables (e.g., the total tumor volume). Moreover, the criterion itself is imperfect because of the potential for sampling error in the assessment of marrow infiltration by tumor cells. Multiple marrow samples taken at the same time or at different times from a single patient frequently vary with respect to the proportion of malignant cells present. The distinction between lymphoblastic leukemia and lymphoma, however, while of questionable biological significance, is of considerable practical importance, both with respect to the selection of treatment options and the analysis of the results of treatment protocols. Only when the criteria used for inclusion of patients are given can the results of clinical trials be compared with confidence.

It is clear that the lymphoblastic leukemias and lymphomas are neoplasms arising from precursor cells at various stages of differentiation in both the T- and B-cell lineages [5–9]. Cells at different stages of differentiation are located in different anatomical regions and their malignant counterparts tend to mirror these topographical differences in their clinical presentations. Thus, pre-B-cells reside primarily, but not exclusively, in the bone marrow, so that neoplasms of these cells predominantly present as leukemias. T-Cell precursors arise in the bone marrow, migrate to the thymus and travel to the secondary lymphoid organs, which include the bone marrow. It is not surprising, then, that T-cell neoplasms may present as either leukemias or lymphomas, and that T-cell precursor neoplasms much more frequently present without overt bone marrow disease than B-cell precursor neoplasms. Because the cells of a given tumor usually represent

more than one developmental stage, individual patients may have clinical features of both leukemia and lymphoma concurrently or consecutively in the course of the disease (e.g., bone marrow involvement at relapse of lymphoma). These considerations indicate that our concepts of leukemia and lymphoma are artificial, in that they do not designate distinct pathologic entities any more than does involvement of the bone marrow by solid tumors. These terms, however, have been in the vocabulary of clinicians and pathologists for more than a century and are unlikely to fall into disuse in the near future. This is unfortunate, as they hinder the understanding and treatment of lymphoid neoplasia, particularly those originating in T-cell precursors.

HISTOLOGY

A detailed description of the histology of lymphoblastic lymphoma has been given in Chapter 2 [1–5]. They are invariably diffuse and lack a follicular cytoarchitecture, although occasionally the patterns of adjacent normal lymphoid tissue may

Table 38.1 (See page 821 under 'Advanced stage'.) Treatment outcome for advanced-stage lymphoblastic non-Hodgkin's lymphomas

Protocol	Duration (months)	Stage	No. of patients	Outcome	Reference
LSA$_2$L$_2$ (modified)*	18	III/IV	124	5-year EFS = 64%	67
BFM 86†	24	I–IV	73	7-year EFS = 82% ± 5%	52
SJCRH-XH‡	32	III/IV	22	4-year DFS = 73%	68
APO§	24	III/IV	21	3-year DFS = 58% ± 23%	65
NCI-7704¶	15	III	16	5-year EFS = 81%	
		IV	9	5-year EFS = 11%	
A-COP+‖	24	III	33	3-year DFS = 54% ± 9%	66
	36	IV	7	3-year DFS = 14% ± 13%	
LMT 81	24	III	33	EFS = 79% ± 4%	51
		IV/ALL	43	EFS = 72% ± 4%	

DFS, Disease-free survival; EFS, event-free survival.

* Cyclophosphamide (1.2 g/m^2 × 1), vincristine, methotrexate, daunomycin (60 mg/m^2 × 2), prednisone, cytarabine, thioguanine, asparaginase, carmustine, hydroxyurea, intrathecal methotrexate; IFRT to bulk (>3 cm).

† Prednisone, vincristine, daunorubicin (40 mg/m^2 × 4), asparaginase, cyclophosphamide (1 g/m^2 × 3 courses), cytarabine, mercaptopurine, methotrexate (5 g/m^2 × 1), dexamethasone, doxorubicin (30 mg/m^2 × 4), thioguanine, intrathecal methotrexate, ± IFRT (residual disease).

‡ Prednisone, vincristine, asparaginase, cytarabine, teniposide (165 mg/m^2 × 28), methotrexate, mercaptopurine, intrathecal methotrexate.

§ Vincristine, adriamycin (75 mg/m^2 × 2, then 30 mg/m^2 q 3 weeks to 450 mg/m^2 max.), prednisone, mercaptopurine, asparaginase, intrathecal methotrexate, ± IFRT (residual disease).

¶ Cyclophosphamide (1.2 g/m^2 × 15), vincristine, adriamycin (40 mg/m^2 × 14), prednisone, methotrexate (2.7 g/m^2 × 15), cytarabine, intrathecal methotrexate, cytarabine.

‖ Vincristine, prednisone, adriamycin (60 mg/m^2 q 6 wks), cyclophosphamide, methotrexate, mercaptopurine, intrathecal methotrexate, hydrocortisone; ± IFRT (residual disease).

a Methotrexate (3 g/m^2 × 10), daunomycin (60 mg/m^2 × 2, 45 mg/m^2 × 7), cyclophosphamide (1.2 g/m^2 × 1; 600 mg/m^2 × 7), vincristine, prednisone, asparaginase, thioguanine, cytarabine, hydroxyurea, carmustine, intrathecal methotrexate, hydrocortisone.

b Some of these patients had more than 25% blasts in the bone marrow.

result in a mistaken impression of nodularity. The essential cytologic features include a high nuclear to cytoplasmic ratio, variably basophilic cytoplasm (usually less basophilic than in the small noncleaved lymphomas), a clearly discernible nuclear envelope, finely stippled nuclear chromatin, and multiple

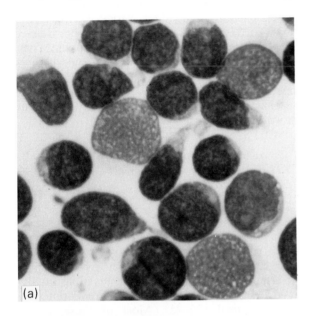

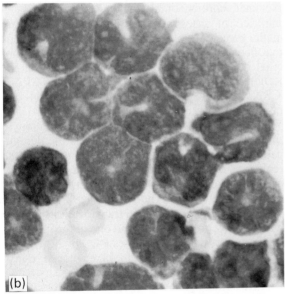

Figure 38.1 Cytological appearance of lymphoblastic lymphoma. (a) Needle aspirate from a peripheral tumor; (b) cytocentrifuge preparation of cerebrospinal fluid from the same patient showing nuclear convolutions. The tumor cells demonstrate a high nuclear to cytoplasmic ratio, variably basophilic cytoplasm, clearly discernible nuclear envelope, finely stippled nuclear chromatin and multiple nucleoli that are usually poorly discernible or imperceptible. Cytoplasmic vacuoles are occasionally seen.

nucleoli that are usually poorly discernible or imperceptible (Figure 38.1). Cytoplasmic vacuoles are occasionally seen. A subset of cells may possess an irregular nuclear outline and the appearance of nuclear 'folds' (sometimes referred to as crow's feet [5]) due to nuclear convolutions. The degree of convolution and fraction of convoluted cells varies from tumor to tumor, but this feature is not required for the diagnosis. It is often better perceived on cytocentrifuge preparations, and is readily seen by electron microscopy, which also demonstrates abundant free ribosomes but scanty rough endoplasmic reticulum. When the nuclei are predominantly convoluted, a greater variation in nuclear and cell sizes occurs. In this situation, the smallest cells have a hyperchromatic pattern of chromatin and are quite mature in appearance, but they can still be distinguished from normal lymphocytes by their nuclear convolutions. Neither the cytomorphology in general nor the nuclear convolutions in particular have been shown to correlate with phenotype or prognosis.

The most characteristic cytochemical finding other than the expression of lineage-specific or associated markers is the presence of focal areas of strong acid phosphatase activity, which are often localized in the region of the Golgi apparatus. The acid nonspecific esterase reaction and the β-glucuronide reaction give a similar staining pattern. There may occasionally be isolated clumps of periodic acid–Schiff-positive material that tends to be diastase resistant. These special stains have largely been superseded by immunophenotyping, which is strongly recommended for confirmation of the diagnosis of lymphoblastic lymphoma [5].

IMMUNOPATHOLOGY

Although lymphoblastic lymphoma encompasses both B- and T-cell lineages, the T-cell phenotype is clearly dominant [6–12]. Regardless of phenotype, almost all (perhaps 5% are negative) lymphoblastic lymphomas express the enzyme terminal deoxyribonucleotidyl transferase (TdT) [13]. This property is consistent with a lymphocyte precursor cell origin, because TdT is involved in the generation of antigen receptor diversity in both B- and T-cells (see Chapter 3).

LYMPHOBLASTIC LYMPHOMA OF THYMIC ORIGIN

The T-cell marker most frequently present on the surface of neoplasms derived from thymocytes is the glycoprotein known as gp40 (CD7, function undetermined) [14,15]. Demonstration of the presence of this antigen may be the best single test for identifying T-cell precursor neoplasms and is often present when the receptor for sheep red cells, CD2, formerly the most widely accepted marker of the T-cell lineage, is absent [14,15].

Other T-cell markers vary according to the stage of thymocyte differentiation. When cells reach intermediate stages of differentiation, they express CD1, and both CD4 and CD8, the antigens expressed by T-cells activated by antigen expressed in the context of class II and class I HLA antigens respectively [16]. As differentiation continues, thymocytes express either CD4 or CD8, as well as the T-cell receptor for antigen coupled to the CD3 molecule. The rearrangement of T-cell receptor genes also varies with stage of thymocyte differentiation [16]. The γ- and δ-chains are the first to be rearranged, followed by complete β- then α-chain rearrangement, which together form the antigen receptor molecule expressed on the cell surface in proximity to CD3 [16–20]. The ontogeny of B- and T-cells is discussed in detail in Chapters 7 and 8.

In Europe and the USA, the phenotype of T-cell lymphoblastic lymphoma corresponds, in the majority of cases, to the phenotype of intermediate or late thymocytes, although atypical patterns may be seen [7–10]. In contrast, a significant fraction of T-cell ALL cases have been reported to have either early or intermediate thymocyte marker expression. The division between intermediate and late stages however, remains controversial, and in part is a practical issue (e.g., CD3, a marker of intermediate and late thymocytes, is expressed in the cytoplasm before being inserted into the cell membrane). This problem is not of major significance, because the designations of intermediate and late are artificial, and such divisions probably do not have prognostic significance [10]. Moreover, an individual tumor may include individual cells at slightly different stages of differentiation. T-Cell lymphoblastic lymphomas also differ from T-cell ALL with respect to CD3-associated T-cell receptor (TCR) expression. TCRγ/δ expression is more common in cases of T-cell ALL in contrast to cases of T-cell lymphoblastic lymphoma, which usually express TCRγ/δ [21].

LYMPHOBLASTIC LYMPHOMA OF NON-T ORIGIN

Lymphoblastic lymphoma infrequently expresses a pre-B- (HLA-DR+, CALLA+, cytoplasmic μ-chain positive) and common ALL [HLA-DR, common acute lymphoblastic leukemia antigen (CALLA+)] phenotype [6,22–24]. Such cases usually present with peripheral lymphadenopathy, isolated bone involvement or subcutaneous tumor without mediastinal masses.

Sheibani et al. [25] reported a series of six patients with lymphoblastic lymphoma whose blast cells expressed antigens associated with natural killer (NK) cells. They all expressed CD2 receptors and reacted positively with anti-CD16 and anti-CD57 antibodies which are expressed by a subset of lymphocytes with NK activity. The most common immunophenotype in their series was CD16+, CD2+, CD57+, CD4+, HLA-DR+, without evidence of cytoplasmic or surface immunoglobulin. Their patients were primarily non-White females. Three had stage I disease and three had involvement of the bone marrow (less than 25%, i.e., stage IV). Three presented with a mediastinal mass. Only two of the six were long-term survivors.

CYTOGENETICS AND MOLECULAR CHARACTERIZATION

Nonrandom chromosomal abnormalities specific for all lymphoblastic lymphomas, or even for phenotypic subsets of lymphoblastic lymphomas, have not been observed. However, in T-cell lymphoblastic leukemias and lymphomas, a number of translocations involving genes associated with T-cell differentiation have been described [26–45]. Most of these T-cell-associated chromosomal translocations have been identified in cases of T-cell leukemia. A much smaller percentage of lymphoblastic lymphoma cells have been characterized cytogenetically. Chromosomal breakpoints are particularly frequent at the location of the TCR genes. These include the TCRα/δ, TCRβ, and TCRγ genes, located at 14q11, 7q34–q36 and 7p15, respectively.

The presumed mechanism of transformation in lymphomas with such translocations is the deregulated expression of oncogenes situated at or near the breakpoint of the partner chromosome to chromosome 7 or chromosome 14 – reminiscent of the small noncleaved cell (SNCC) non-Hodgkin's lymphomas (NHL) in which the reciprocal translocations involving c-*myc* on chromosome 8 and one of the immunoglobulin genes on chromosomes 14, 2 or 22 result in the deregulated expression of c-*myc*. Indeed, c-*myc* may be deregulated in some of these translocations (see below). The genes most commonly involved in precursor T-cell include the transcription factor genes TAL1 [38–43] and HOX11 [29,30], and the cysteine-rich (LIM) proteins RHOMB1 and RHOMB2 [31–34]. TAL1 is a member of the basic helix–loop–helix family of transcription factors and is normally expressed only in immature hematopoietic cells. It is rearranged in the t(1;14)(p32;q11), which occurs in approximately 3% of cases of T-ALL; submicroscopic deletions in the same region of

TAL1 can be detected in up to 25% of cases of T-ALL [38–43]. HOX11, a transcription factor gene containing a homeobox domain, is normally expressed only in nonhematopoietic cells during embryogenesis. It is disrupted in the t(10;14)(q24;q11) which is identified in 5–10% of cases of T-ALL [29,30]. The RHOMB1 and RHOMB2 genes code for proteins that contain a cystein-rich protein–protein interaction domain, and are not normally expressed in T-cells. The deregulation of these genes may contribute to leukemogenesis by inhibiting the function of the transcription factors to which they normally dimerise. They are abnormally expressed in the t(11;14) (p13;q11) and t(11;14)(p15;q11) chromosomal abnormalities, respectively [31–34].

c-*myc*, like TAL1, is also a number of the basic helix–loop–helix family of transcription factors. Mathieu-Mahul et al. [36] studied a cell line with an 8(q24);14(q11) translocation derived from a patient with T-cell leukemia. They demonstrated that the breakpoint on chromosome 8 was located on the 3' side of the third exon of c-*myc*. The breakpoint on chromosome 14 was located at q11, within the TCRα locus. McKeithan et al. [37] described a similar translocation in the Molt-16 cell line, which also was established from a patient with T-cell ALL. The translocation of TCRα sequences distal (3') to c-*myc* parallel the variant translocations occurring in the small noncleaved lymphomas, in which immunoglobulin light chain sequences (probably containing enhancer elements) are translocated to a similar position with respect to c-*myc*, and it is likely that they also result in c-*myc* deregulation.

Additional cases of lymphoblastic NHL need to be studied to determine whether cytogenetic differences exist between T-ALL and T-cell lymphoblastic NHL. The characterization of the genes involved in the translocations should be helpful in both establishing the diagnosis and in the development of techniques for the detection of minimal residual disease with PCR technology.

Epidemiology

Compared with information on the small noncleaved lymphomas, few epidemiologic data are available on lymphoblastic lymphomas. Lymphoblastic lymphomas occur throughout the world, but comprise a variable fraction of all NHL in different geographical regions. The statistics may, however, be somewhat misleading, because the arbitrary distinction between lymphoblastic lymphoma and ALL may vary from country to country [46].

The relative proportion of histologic subtypes of NHL observed in children is strikingly different from that observed in adults. In children, high-grade diffuse lymphomas predominate. For example, the lymphoblastic subtype comprises a much larger precentage of NHL cases among children as compared to adults. Among 338 children with NHL evaluated at St Jude Children's Research Hospital, 28.1% were classified as lymphoblastic [47]. In contrast, less than 10% of adult NHL cases are of the lymphoblastic subtype. However, in a review by Nathwani et al. [48] of 97 patients with this disease, 50% of the patients were older than 30, with a median age of 27 years in males and of 50 years in females. The male:female ratio was 2:1. Males demonstrated a bimodal age distribution, with peaks in both the second and seventh decades. These findings may be skewed, in that the patient population of the Repository Center for Lymphoma Clinical Studies, from which the data were obtained, consists primarily of adults.

Unlike the SNCC and immunoblastic lymphomas, lymphoblastic lymphoma has not been directly shown to occur at increased frequency in patients with an underlying immunodeficiency syndrome [5], nor is radiation known to play a significant role in pathogenesis. Unlike acute leukemia, there was no early lymphoma peak in children who survived the atomic bomb explosions in Nagasaki and Hiroshima. Although there was an increased incidence of NHL in individuals who were exposed to greater than 200 or 100 cGy at Nagasaki and Hiroshima, respectively, there was no significant trend for increased incidence with increased dose [49].

Clinical features and staging

Patients with lymphoblastic lymphoma most commonly present with a mediastinal mass (50–70%); in many cases a pleural effusion and sometimes a pericardial effusion may also be present (Figure 38.2) [5,47]. The associated symptoms may include dyspnea, dysphagia and pain, and, in the event of superior vena caval obstruction, swelling of the neck, face and upper extremities. Cardiac tamponade may ensue from pericardial effusions. Lymphadenopathy, usually located in the neck, axilla or supraclavicular region, occurs in 50–80% of all patients. Although the liver, spleen, kidney or para-aortic lymph nodes may be involved in more disseminated cases, isolated or prominent abdominal disease is very unusual. Other potential sites of involvement include the pharynx, bone, skin and testes [5,47].

of these. If CNS prophylaxis is not included as a component of therapy, CNS disease is likely to occur, particularly in patients with primary sites in the head and neck.

STAGING SYSTEMS AND PROCEDURES

The most common staging system for childhood lymphoblastic lymphoma is that used at St Jude Children's Research Hospital [54]. It is described in Chapter 24 and is modified from the Ann Arbor system, which was originally devised for Hodgkin's Disease to reflect the noncontiguous nature of disease spread, the predominant extranodal involvement, involvement of CNS, and the tendency for leukemic transformation in childhood NHL. There is room for improvement, however. The use of the diaphragm as a means of defining spread of disease is arbitrary, the term 'extensive intrathoracic tumor' as a criterion for stage III disease invites ambiguous interpretation.

Before starting treatment, it is imperative that a definitive tissue diagnosis be made. Generally, biopsy of an easily accessible node or examination of pleural fluid is required. A bone marrow examination may also help in making the diagnosis. If disease is limited to the mediastinum, mediastinoscopy or biopsy via a small parasternal incision is indicated. If the mediastinal mass is compressing the airway (sometimes compression occurs only in the supine position), general anesthesia or even sedation may result in respiratory distress, or arrest and cardiac arrest has also occurred in this situation. Consultation with an anesthesiologist and experienced thoracic surgeon is indicated in the setting of airway compromise prior to performing a biopsy. Low-dose involved field radiation with or without concurrent steroids is sometimes administered acutely in this setting, but there is no evidence that radiation has any advantage over chemotherapy. In patients with significant venous obstruction, consideration should be given to the best vessel in which to place an indwelling intravenous line, which may increase the risk of thrombotic occlusion. Ideally, compromised veins should be avoided.

Appropriate studies for determining the extent of tumor have been described in Chapter 12. In lymphoblastic lymphomas, a careful examination of the chest is mandatory and computed tomographic scanning is usually performed. Magnetic resonance imaging (MRI) may be helpful in examining tumor in relation to the heart. Computerized scanning of the abdomen is also usually performed but tends to be a low-yield procedure. Gallium-67 is much less avidly taken up in the lymphoblastic lymphomas than in small noncleaved cell lymphomas, but it is worth

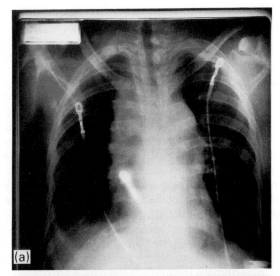

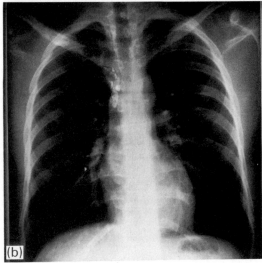

Figure 38.2 Chest X-ray demonstrating a mediastinal mass in a patient with lymphoblastic lymphoma (a) before and (b) 10 days after chemotherapy.

BONE MARROW AND CENTRAL NERVOUS SYSTEM INVOLVEMENT

Bone marrow involvement is common in lymphoblastic lymphoma [50–52], but in view of the arbitrary and controversial distinction between T-cell ALL and lymphoblastic lymphoma, estimates depend upon the parameters used to distinguish these conditions. Central nervous system (CNS) involvement is uncommon at presentation, but it is more likely in patients who have bone marrow involvement [50–53]. Central nervous system involvement is manifested by either meningeal infiltration (malignant cerebrospinal fluid pleocytosis), cranial nerve infiltration (ophthalmic or facial nerves), or some combination including in the routine scanning procedures. Bone scan should be done to detect the presence of occult bone disease and, if positive, X-rays of involved bones should be performed. Bilateral iliac crest bone marrow examination (aspirates and biopsies) is mandatory. There is evidence that multiple sampling including bone marrow biopsy, even in lymphoblastic lymphoma, increases the detection rate of marrow involvement [55]. However, bone marrow biopsies have not been performed routinely in all pediatric centers. MRI of the bone marrow may be of value in detecting occult disease in these patients, as it has been in other lymphomas.

A staging laparotomy is not indicated in patients with lymphoblastic lymphoma. Not only is intra-abdominal tumor rare but, because chemotherapy is administered for all disease stages, pathological staging is not indicated.

Treatment and prognosis

EMERGENCY MANAGEMENT

Patients with lymphoblastic lymphoma may present with tumor-associated problems, which require immediate attention. The most common complications are those which develop secondary to a large mediastinal mass, including superior vena caval syndrome, dyspnea, dysphagia and, rarely, cardiac arrhythmias or tamponade. There is also an increased risk for anesthesia-related complications, cardiac arrest and bleeding, at surgery, from engorged mediastinal vessels in patients with mediastinal primaries [56]. Pleural effusions may need immediate attention. Airway obstruction by pharyngeal tumor is a rare occurrence. Uric acid-induced nephropathy may also occur, although not as commonly as in B-cell tumors, which have a higher growth fraction. Management of these problems is dealt with in Chapter 15.

It is worth emphasizing that the role of radiation therapy (RT) in the management of superior vena caval obstruction is questionable in this disease, since radiation appears to confer no prognostic advantage and will increase toxicity, particularly if anthracyclines are used in treatment [57,58]. In the rare instance in which no response to chemotherapy is observed, RT may be indicated, although if lack of response is caused by resistant tumor, the prognosis is extremely poor. It may also be indicated if the degree of airway compromise is deemed immediately life threatening (e.g., there is also respiratory obstruction) and the added security of combined modality treatment is desired. In these situations, relatively low-dose therapy (e.g., 1200 cGy) is preferable to avoid excessive toxicity.

CNS involvement at diagnosis may require the immediate addition of RT to the therapeutic regimen although this situation has not been studied. In patients who present with cranial nerve involvement, low-dose RT to the base of the skull may be necessary if there is not an immediate response to chemotherapy, or at least stabilization. Intracerebral extension of tumor may require full doses of cranial radiation (3000 cGy). Patients with paraplegia secondary to paraspinal tumor are often treated with radiation, particularly if there is not an immediate improvement with specific chemotherapy, but once again, an advantage to this approach has not been demonstrated. However, the potential neurological consequences of an inadequate response of a paraspinal tumor persuade many oncologists to irradiate such tumors in addition to administering chemotherapy when paraparesis is advanced. If there is not a good response to combined RT and chemotherapy, neurosurgical intervention may be necessary.

SPECIFIC THERAPY

The primary treatment modality in lymphoblastic lymphoma is chemotherapy [47,51,52,58–68]. The use of radiation or surgery alone prior to the advent of combination chemotherapy yielded very poor results, although a small proportion of patients with localized disease achieved long-term survival [69]. Surgery has no role in lymphoblastic lymphoma, except in establishing the diagnosis. The role of RT (to sites of bulk disease) is presently controversial and the most recent successful treatment programs have not employed it. A prospective randomized trial conducted by the Pediatric Oncology Group demonstrated that RT provided no therapeutic benefit to patients with localized disease [St Jude Childrens Research Hospital (SJCRH) stages I and II] [58]. A similar conclusion was reached in patients with more extensive disease (SJCRH stages III and IV) studied at SJCRH, although patient numbers in this study were small [57]. The excellent treatment results achieved with modern multiagent chemotherapy regimens which do not incorporate RT further support the exclusion of RT from modern treatment regimens. The special situations in which RT may be indicated are almost exclusively limited to patients presenting or recurring with testicular tumor or with CNS involvement.

CHEMOTHERAPY

Over the last 25 years, the development of effective multiagent chemotherapy regimens has resulted in dramatic improvement in the treatment outcome over that achieved with less intensive single agent therapy [47,51,52,57–68]. Wollner et al. [70] reported no long-term survivors among patients with mediastinal NHL treated before 1976 with single-agent chemotherapy and RT. Multiagent chemotherapy regimens were subsequently developed, but for childhood NHL, the optimal strategy was unclear. The similarity of pediatric NHL to leukemia (with respect to the frequency of bone marrow involvement and histology) persuaded some investigators that treatment with 'leukemia therapy' would be the most rational approach. On the other hand, Burkitt's lymphoma had been successfully treated with a few cycles of alkylating agent-based therapy – whether or not histology was important to outcome was also unknown. The Children's Cancer Study Group (CCSG) therefore performed a randomized trial comparing these two main treatment approaches in patients with either lymphoblastic or nonlymphoblastic NHL. The precise regimens chosen were cyclophosphamide, vincristine, methotrexate and prednisone (COMP) and LSA_2L_2 (see Figure 38.3) [61, 67]. COMP, adapted from the work of Zeigler [71], and of Djerassi and Kim [72], and successful in the treatment of Burkitt's lymphoma, combined pulsed high-dose cyclophosphamide, vincristine, moderate-dose methotrexate and prednisone (see Chapter 37). LSA_2L_2, designed by Wollner (Memorial Sloan–Kettering Cancer Center) for the treatment of

acute lymphoblastic leukemia (ALL) and lymphoma, is an intensive 10-drug regimen that includes induction, consolidation and maintenance phases (Figure 38.3) [60,70]. In the CCSG trial, both regimens were administered for 18 months. The results of this study have greatly influenced the management of patients with lymphoblastic lymphoma. Patients with limited-stage disease had an excellent outcome, regardless of histologic subtype or treatment arm. The outcome for children with advanced stage disease varied with both histologic subtype and treatment arm, and favored the use of LSA_2L_2 in patients with lymphoblastic lymphoma.

LIMITED STAGE

The prognosis for long-term survival in patients with limited-stage non-Hodgkin lymphoma (SJCRH stage I or II) is excellent. In the CCSG study [61,67] in which the COMP and LSA_2L_2 regimens were compared, a 5-year event-free survival of 84% was achieved for patients with localized disease of all histologies collectively, regardless of treatment arm. Subsequent studies were focused primarily on reducing treatment intensity without compromising the high cure rate. For example, Murphy et al. designed a combined modality regimen of lessened intensity, which reduced the total number of doses of cyclophosphamide and RT, shortened treatment time and curtailed prophylactic treatment of the CNS, except in patients with a primary head or neck tumor [63]. All 28 patients attained a CR and 24 of 28 remained disease free at 4+ months to 4 years from diagnosis (median, 24+ months). However, most of these cases were of nonlymphoblastic histology. Further reductions in treatment intensity were subsequently studied.

A randomized trial performed by the Pediatric Oncology Group (POG) demonstrated that involved field radiation could be deleted from a regimen consisting of an induction/consolidation phase containing cyclophosphamide, adriamycin, vincristine and prednisone, followed by a 24-week continuation phase of daily 6-mercaptopurine (6-MP) and weekly methotrexate, without compromising cure rate for children with limited-stage NHL of all histologies [58]. A successor POG trial demonstrated that the 24-week continuation phase could be safely deleted for nonlymphoblastic cases but not for lymphoblastic NHL [59]. In these two trials, the 5-year event-free survival for patients with lymphoblastic NHL was inferior (66%, SE 9%). Overall survival (93%, SE 6%), however, was similar to that observed in other histologies because patients who frequently have a precursor B-cell phenotype can be salvaged by standard ALL therapy [59]. The fact that a high

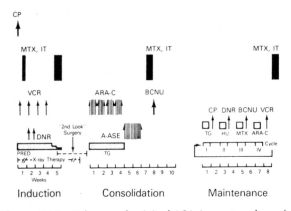

Figure 38.3 Schema of original LSA_2L_2 protocol used by the Pediatric Oncology Group for childhood non-Hodgkin's lymphoma [56]. CP, cyclophosphamide; MTX IT, intrathecal methotrexate; VCR, vincristine; DNR, daunomycin; PRED, prednisone; ARA-C, cytarabine; A-ASE, asparaginase; TG, thioguanine; BCNU, bis-(2-chloroethyl) nitrosurea; HU, hydroxyurea. Reproduced with permission from Sullivan et al. [62].

proportion of patients with limited-stage lymphoblastic lymphoma can achieve long-term remission with only 33 weeks of therapy may have implications for the treatment of ALL.

In an alternative approach, French investigators have treated patients with limited-stage disease as aggressively as those with advanced-stage disease (LMT 81 protocol) [51]. The event-free survival for the eight patients with limited-stage disease was 73% (SE 8) with a median follow-up of 57 months. Thus, the optimal initial therapy for patients with limited stage lymphoblastic NHL remains controversial, particularly in light of the ability to salvage patients who fail treatments of lessened intensity as demonstrated in the POG study.

ADVANCED STAGE

The CCSG trial comparing COMP and LSA_2L_2 demonstrated that the LSA_2L_2 was significantly more effective than the COMP regimen for children with advanced-stage lymphoblastic lymphoma (5 year event-free survival rate, 64% versus 34%, respectively, $P<0.001$) [61,67]. More recently, Patte et al. (French Society of Pediatric Oncology; SFOP) have reported an apparent improvement in the results of the LSA_2L_2 arm used in the CCSG study. In their LMT 81 protocol, which incorporates 10 courses of high-dose methotrexate into the LSA_2L_2 regimen, event-free survival was 79% (SE 4), and 72% (SE 4) for stages III and IV, respectively, with a median follow-up of 57 months [51].

Other successful multiagent regimens, delivered over 18–30 months, have also been reported (Table 38.1). One of these is the Berlin–Frankfurt–Münster (BFM) cooperative study protocol used in Germany for the treatment of patients with ALL [73]. This regimen produces excellent results regardless of ALL phenotype. Disease-free survival in patients with stage III and IV lymphoblastic lymphoma was 78%, with a 48+ month follow-up. A subsequent study (BMF 86) which included a high-dose methotrexate (5 g/m²)

consolidation phase (Figures 38.4 and 38.5) also resulted in an excellent treatment outcome (7-year event-free survival, 82 ± 5%; N=73, limited and advanced stage combined) [52]. In a study at SJCRH, the merits of 'early' and 'intermittent' use of teniposide (VM-26) plus cytarabine (ara-C) before and after remission induction with prednisone, vincristine, and asparaginase and during the first year of maintenance therapy were examined [68]. Anthracycline, high-dose methotrexate (MTX), alkylating agents and involved-field RT were not included. Excellent results were obtained: 22 (96%) of 23 evaluable patients achieved a complete remission, with a projected 4-year continuous complete remission rate of 73% for all patients and 79% for the 19 patients who presented with mediastinal involvement at diagnosis. These data appear to validate the effectiveness of adding VM-26 and ara-C to an otherwise conventional ALL protocol in the management of lymphoblastic lymphoma, but the small numbers and lack of later reports (the study was published 10 years ago) preclude drawing a definitive conclusion.

The multiagent nature of these various treatments make it difficult to determine which are the most important components and how best to build on prior results. In fact, although there is now a preference for protocols based on ALL therapy, protocols such as LSA_2L_2 may not represent optimal therapy for lymphoblastic lymphoma, or at least, for all subgroups of patients with lymphoblastic lymphoma. For example, in the POG study of a modified version of LSA_2L_2 [62], only 40% of patients with mediastinal lymphoblastic lymphoma were long-term survivors. At least one treatment regimen not based on an ALL protocol, NCI 77–04 (Figure 38.6) [64] has been successful, particularly in patients with large mediastinal masses, although the number of patients in this study is small. The estimated long-term disease-free survival for patients with lymphoblastic lymphoma without marrow involvement treated according to this protocol is 81%. This regimen, which contains both an anthracycline and a high-dose methotrexate infusion with leucovorin rescue,

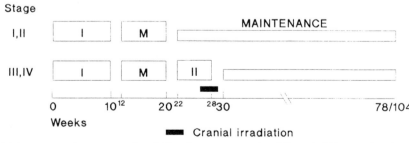

Figure 38.4 Schema of the Berlin–Frankfurt–Münster (BFM) cooperative study protocol 1986 for the treatment of patients with lymphoblastic (non-B) lymphomas [54] showing induction protocol I, consolidation protocol M and reinduction protocol II.

Maintenance therapy consisted of oral mercaptopurine (50 mg/m²/day) and oral methotrexate (20 mg/m² once per week). The duration of maintenance for patients entered on the study since March 1987 was 24 months. Schemata for protocols I, M and II are provided in Figure 38.5. Modified from reference 52.

INDUCTION PROTOCOL I

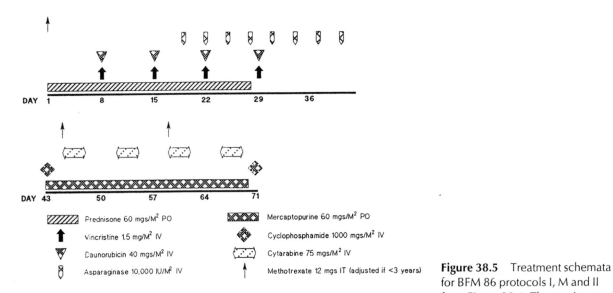

DAY 1   8   15   22   29   36

DAY 43   50   57   64   71

//// Prednisone 60 mgs/M² PO	XXXX Mercaptopurine 60 mgs/M² PO
↑ Vincristine 1.5 mg/M² IV	◆ Cyclophosphamide 1000 mgs/M² IV
▼ Daunorubicin 40 mgs/M² IV	⟨...⟩ Cytarabine 75 mgs/M² IV
8 Asparaginase 10,000 IU/M² IV	↑ Methotrexate 12 mgs IT (adjusted if <3 years)

CONSOLIDATION PROTOCOL M

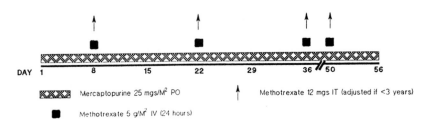

DAY 1   8   15   22   29   36 // 50   56

XXXX Mercaptopurine 25 mgs/M² PO	↑ Methotrexate 12 mgs IT (adjusted if <3 years)
■ Methotrexate 5 g/M² IV (24 hours)	

REINDUCTION PROTOCOL II

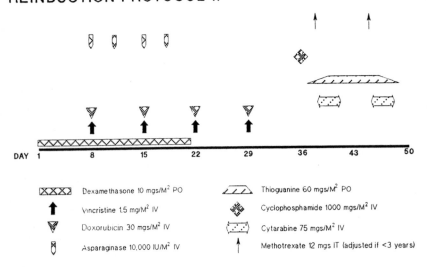

DAY 1   8   15   22   29   36   43   50

XXXX Dexamethasone 10 mgs/M² PO	⟨//⟩ Thioguanine 60 mgs/M² PO
↑ Vincristine 1.5 mg/M² IV	◆ Cyclophosphamide 1000 mgs/M² IV
▼ Doxorubicin 30 mgs/M² IV	⟨...⟩ Cytarabine 75 mgs/M² IV
8 Asparaginase 10,000 IU/M² IV	↑ Methotrexate 12 mgs IT (adjusted if <3 years)

Figure 38.5 Treatment schemata for BFM 86 protocols I, M and II from Figure 38.4. The maximum vincristine dose is 2 mg. Methotrexate infusions (5 g/m²) are followed by leucovorin rescue (75 mg/m² i.v. at hour 36 followed by five doses of 15 mg/m² i.v./per os every 3 hours and an additional four doses every 6 hours. Since October 1988, a total of six doses at 15 mg/m² every 6 hours, have been given. Cranial irradiation (12 Gy for CNS-negative patients) was performed in the second phase of reinduction protocol II. For patients with overt CNS disease, patients less than 1 year received no cranial irradiation. Patients received 18 Gy in the second year of life and 24 Gy in older children. Additional doses of IT methotrexate were given on days 8, 15, 22 and 29 for CNS-positive patients. In patients with testicular involvement, irradiation of the testes (24 Gy) was performed. Local radiation in surgical resection was performed for patients with residual disease after protocol I. Maintenance therapy is described in the legend to Figure 38.4. Based on information provided in reference 52.

also provided therapy at least as effective as COMP for patients with small noncleaved cell lymphomas, but is no longer recommended for patients with advanced small noncleaved cell lymphoma. The addition of doxorubicin to a COMP-like regimen was also shown to be effective in the A-COP+

PROTOCOL 77-04

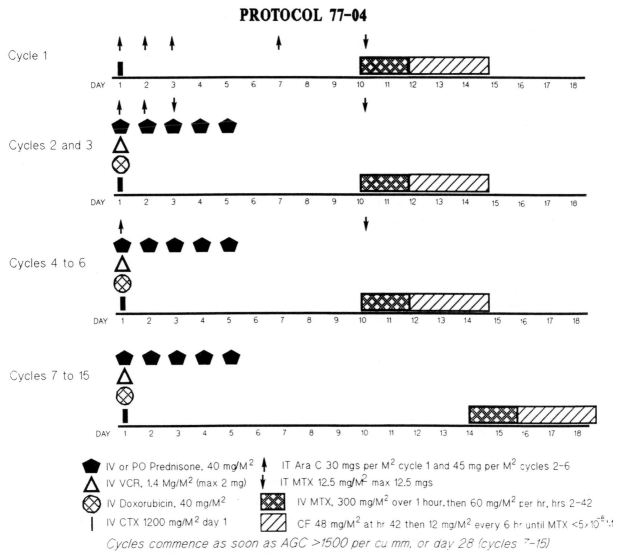

Figure 38.6 Schema of the NCI protocol (77–04) for the treatment of non-Hodgkin's lymphoma [67].

(doxorubicin, cyclophosphamide, vincristine, prednisone) regimen, which was compared to LSA$_2$L$_2$ in a randomized clinical trial conducted by the POG [66]. After adjusting for stage (I and II, III, IV), there was no statistically significant difference ($P = 0.19$) between A-COP and LSA$_2$L$_2$ regimens on the basis of 3-year survival and disease-free survival (62% versus 72%, and 53% versus 58%, respectively, for the two treatment regimens), however, the ability to detect a clinically meaningful difference in the outcome with the two regimens was limited both by the small number of patients, and by the imbalance of stage III and stage IV patients between the two arms of the study.

In a randomized CCGS trial of COMP plus daunomycin and L-asparaginase versus modified LSA$_2$L$_2$, there was no significant difference in 5-year event-free survival (64% and 74%, respectively; $P = 0.17$, adjusted for extent and site of disease) [73a].

CNS PROPHYLAXIS

The CNS is very seldom overtly involved at presentation in patients with lymphoblastic lymphoma. At one time it was a very frequent (approximately 50%) site of relapse but, since the advent of effective CNS prophylaxis, isolated CNS recurrence has been encountered only rarely [51–53].

Various methods of prophylaxis are in use [51,52, 64,67,68]. Some regimens specify cranial irradiation and intrathecal methotrexate (IT MTX); in others, IT MTX and/or intrathecal cytarabine (IT ara-C) are administered with intermediate- or high-dose MTX. The adverse effects of cranial irradiation on the CNS argue strongly against its use. Intrathecal chemotherapy (using established doses and schedules of agents) coupled with intermediate- or high-dose MTX infusions appears to be the treatment of choice for CNS prophylaxis.

TREATMENT IN ADULTS

In adults, very few long-term disease-free survivors with lymphoblastic lymphoma were documented prior to the development of intensive, continuous, multiagent treatment regimens. Levine et al. [74] treated 15 patients with lymphoblastic lymphoma using a modified LSA_2L_2 regimen (2000 cGy to the mediastinum, cranial RT and IT MTX). The relapse-free survival rate at 5 years was about 35%. Slater et al. [75] at Memorial Sloan–Kettering Cancer Center summarized the results of therapy for 51 patients with lymphoblastic lymphoma or ALL who were enrolled in one of five successive intensive chemotherapy programs for ALL since 1971. The 5-year survival rate for leukemic and nonleukemic patients was 45%. Colemen et al. [76] reported a 3-year disease-free survival rate with of 56% with two successive regimens incorporating CHOP (cyclophosphamide, doxorubicin, vincristine, prednisone), high-dose MTX, L-asparaginase, IT MTX, 6-MP and MTX treatment for Ann Arbor stage I–IV lymphoblastic lymphoma. In the second regimen, CNS prophylaxis including cranial RT and intrathecal MTX was begun earlier, resulting in a reduction in the incidence of CNS relapse from 31% to 3%. More recently, Morel et al. [77] reported similar results among 80 adult patients treated with various CHOP-based NHL and ALL protocols. The continuous complete remission and overall survival rates at 30 months were 46% and 51%, respectively.

Although more intensive chemotherapy combined with CNS prophylaxis has extended the long-term survival of patients with lymphoblastic lymphoma, the treatment results in adults fall short of those for children. This may reflect differences in the clinical and biological characteristics of adult versus pediatric lymphoblastic lymphoma as first proposed by Nathwani et al. [48] who reported differences in the incidence of mediastinal masses, numbers of mitotic figures, and incidence of leukemic conversions between younger patients and those older than 30 years.

FACTORS IN PROGNOSIS

Adults

Risk factors have been identified in various studies, which are associated with a poorer treatment outcome. Slater et al. reported that age >30 years, white blood cell count (WBC) >50 000/μl (note the lack of differentiation between leukemia and lymphoma), failure to achieve complete response (CR), and a late CR during induction were all associated with a poor prognosis [75]. Coleman et al. identified Ann Arbor Stage IV disease (bone marrow or CNS involvement) and initial serum lactic dehydrogenase (LDH) concentration of >300 IU/l (normal, <200) as high-risk features. He reported significantly different 5-year freedom from relapse rates for low- and high-risk groups (94% and 19%, respectively; P=0.0006) [76]. Morel et al. reported that failure to achieve CR, age greater than 40 years, B symptoms and LDH greater than twice the upper limit of normal were all associated with a shorter survival [77].

Children

The tumor burden at diagnosis is the most reliable indicator of treatment outcome in children with NHL – as it probably is in adults [5,47]. Clinical staging generally reflects tumor burden; however, not all staging systems are based on step-wise increments in tumor burden. Serum levels of various molecules, either secreted by tumor cells or accumulated as a result of cellular breakdown, may be more indicative of tumor burden [78–81]. Examples include LDH, β_2-microglobulin, lactic acid and the soluble interleukin-2 receptor (sIL-2R). Wagner et al. [78] performed a multivariate analyses of patients with NHL treated with the National Cancer Institute (NCI) protocol 77–04 and found that sIL-2R levels were superior to all other prognostic variables examined. A similar study done by Pui et al. [81] demonstrated a correlation between sIL-2R levels and both serum LDH levels (P = 0.0001) and disease stage. The findings of their multivariate analysis, like those of Wagner et al., identified the serum sIL-2R level as a better indicator of treatment response than either disease stage or serum LDH levels. Biochemical correlates of prognosis are important because they provide the most objective measure of tumor burden, facilitating risk-group assignment and subsequent selection of appropriate therapy. They may also have implications for the incorporation of biologic response modifiers into therapy.

Other prognostic factors associated with specific treatment protocols for T-cell lymphoblastic disease have been reported. As part of the POG study of

LSA$_2$L$_2$ in T-cell ALL patients, a multivariate analysis of potential risk factors (age at diagnosis, presenting white count, platelet count, hemoglobin level, percentage of E-rosetting cells, sex and race) indicated that only the presenting WBC, less than or greater than 50 x 10^9/l, a reflection of tumor burden, was predictive of the duration of continuous complete remission and of the duration of CNS remission. Interestingly, T-cell ALL (T-ALL) patients with less than 50 x 10^9/l WBC at diagnosis had approximately the same long-term CR rate as did mediastinal NHL patients treated with the same protocol (modified LSA$_2$L$_2$), suggesting that WBC T-ALL patients with a lower white count are more clinically similar to the T-cell non-Hodgkin's lymphoma (T-NHL) patients than are T-ALL patients with a high white count (who had a very poor prognosis) [82]. These data also suggest that, among advanced-stage patients, the degree of bone marrow involvement does not have prognostic significance. This conclusion is supported by the results of the very successful French LMT 81 protocol in which the degree of bone marrow involvement (less than 25% versus greater than 25%) did not influence treatment outcome. In the latter study, the event-free survival for the 60 children with no or less than 25% bone marrow blasts was 73% (SE 3) and that for the 24 with greater than 25% marrow blasts was 77% (SE 4) [51].

Finally, a particularly important area that needs to be addressed in lymphoblastic lymphoma is the prognostic signficance of molecular genetic lesions. Information at present is essentially nonexistent.

LATE EFFECTS

Recommendations to reduce the long-term complications of therapy for lymphoblastic lymphoma in children are evolving. With studies demonstrating no therapeutic benefit from adjuvant involved-field radiation in the treatment of patients with NHL [57, 58], RT is rarely used in current treatment regimens. This is likely to reduce the associated injury to heart, esophagus and lungs. However, with improved survival obtained with newer, more aggressive chemotherapy regimens, follow-up studies are expected to reveal additional long-term sequelae.

There are three problems areas for patients who have completed therapy: reproductive dysfunction, risk of second malignancies and the psychological implications of experiencing a life-threatening illness. These issues are dealt with in Chapter 36. It is appropriate to point out, however, that in general, late toxic effects correlate with the cumulative doses of drugs received by patients. Studies have not been performed in lymphoblastic lymphoma to assess the optimal *duration* of therapy – an important determinant of cumulative dose.

Future considerations

The development of additional active single agents or new ways of using presently available active drugs for incorporation into aggressive multiagent chemotherapy programs provides the most likely immediate possibility for improved treatment. Molecularly cloned hematopoietic growth factors (e.g., granulocyte or granulocyte–macrophage colony-stimulating factors), which minimize or eliminate myelosuppression, may permit investigators to increase the dose intensity of existing regimens, although to date there is little evidence to suggest that this will be of sufficient magnitude to result in a survival advantage. The role of autologous or allogeneic bone marrow transplantation (BMT) in lymphoblastic lymphoma, particularly as frontline therapy in high-risk patients, has yet to be clarified; the preliminary results appear promising in adult trials. In a retrospective study, Baro et al. [83] reported a 77% 2-year disease-free survival among 14 patients who received an autologous BMT in first CR. Verdonck et al. [84] treated nine poor-risk adult patients in first CR with autologous BMT. Six of these remain in first CR with a follow-up of 12–113 months (median, 53 months) after BMT. Milpied et al. [85] reported a 68 ± 9% disease-free survival for 25 adult patients treated with either autologous or allogeneic BMT in first CR. There was no difference in outcome between those treated with autologous versus allogeneic BMT.

Perhaps the best hope for improved therapy with a low toxic cost is the development of treatment approaches targeted to tumor cells (see Chapter 51). In the case of lymphoblastic lymphoma a great deal more ground work needs to be done in characterizing the molecular genetic abnormalities before such approaches can be contemplated.

References

1. National Cancer Institute Sponsored Study of classifications of Non-Hodgkin's Lymphomas: Summary and description of a working formulation for clinical usage. The Non-Hodgkin's Lymphoma Pathologic Classification Project. *Cancer* 1982, **49**: 2112–2135.
2. Rappaport H. In *Atlas of Tumor Pathology*, Section 3, Fascicle 8. Washington, D.C.: US Armed Forces Institute of Pathology, 1966.

3. Lukes RJ, Collins RD. New approaches to the classification of the lymphomata. *Br. J. Cancer* 1975, **31**: 1–28.

4. Nathwani BN, Kim H, Rappaport H. Malignant lymphoma, lymphoblastic. *Cancer* 1976, **38**: 964–983.

5. Magrath IT. Malignant non-Hodgkins lymphomas in children. In Pizzo PA, Poplack DP (eds) *Principles and Practices of Pediatric Oncology*, 2nd edn. Philadelphia: Lippincott, 1993, pp. 537–576.

6. Cossman J, Chused TM, Fisher RI, et al. Diversity of immunological phenotypes of lymphoblastic lymphoma. *Cancer Res.* 1983, **43**: 4486–4490.

7. Bernard A, Boumsell L, Reinherz EL, et al. Cell surface characterization of malignant T-cells from lymphoblastic lymphoma using monoclonal antibodies: Evidence for phenotypic differences between malignant T-cells from patients with acute lymphoblastic leukemia and lymphoblastic lymphoma. *Blood* 1981, **57**: 1105–1110.

8. Roper M, Crist WM, Metzgar R, et al. Monoclonal antibody characterization of surface antigens in childhood T-cell lymphoid malignancies. *Blood* 1983, **61**: 830–837.

9. Crist WM, Kelly DR, Ragab AH, et al. Predictive ability of Lukes–Collins classification for immunologic phenotypes of childhood non-Hodgkin lymphoma: An institutional series and literature review. *Cancer* 1981, **48**: 2070–2075.

10. Shikano T, Arioka H, Kobayashi R, et al. Acute lymphoblastic leukemia and non-Hodgkin's lymphoma with mediastinal mass – a study of 23 children; different disorders or different stages. *Leuk. Lymphoma* 1994, **13**: 161–167.

11. Link MP, Stewart SJ, Warnke RA, et al. Discordance between surface and cytoplasmic expression of the Leu-4 (T3) antigen in thymocytes and in blast cells from childhood T lymphoblastic malignancies. *J. Clin. Invest.* 1985, **76**: 248–253.

12. Mori N, Oka K, Yoda Y, et al. Leu-4 (CD3) antigen expression in the neoplastic cells from T-ALL and T-lymphoblastic lymphoma. *Am. J. Clin. Path.* 1988, **90**: 244–249.

13. Braziel RM, Keneklis T, Donlon JA, et al. Terminal deoxynucleotidyl transferase in non-Hodgkin's lymphoma. *Am. J. Clin. Path.* 1983, **80**: 655–659.

14. Vodinelich L, Tax W, Bai Y, et al. A monoclonal antibody (WT1) for detecting leukemias of T-cell precursors (T-ALL). *Blood* 1983, **62**: 1108–1113.

15. Link M, Warnke R, Finlay J, et al. A single monoclonal antibody identifies T-cell lineage of childhood lymphoid malignancies. *Blood* 1983, **62**: 722–728.

16. Reinherz EL, Kung PC, Goldstein G, et al. Discrete stages of human intrathymic differentiation: Analysis of normal thymocytes and leukemic lymphoblasts of T-cell lineage. *Proc. Natl Acad. Sci. USA* 1980, **77**: 1588–1592.

17. Royer HD, Acuto O, Fabbi M, et al. Genes encoding the Ti beta subunit of the antigen/MHC receptor undergo rearrangement during intrathymic ontogeny prior to surface T3-Ti expression. *Cell* 1984, **39**: 261–266.

18. Royer HD, Ramarli D, Acuto O, et al. Genes encoding the T-cell receptor alpha and beta subunits are transcribed in an ordered manner during intrathymic ontogeny. *Proc. Natl Acad. Sci. USA* 1985, **82**: 5510–5514.

19. Meuer SC, Acuto O, Hussey RE, et al. Evidence for the T3-associated 90K heterodimer as the T-cell antigen receptor. *Nature* 1983, **303**: 808–810.

20. Strominger JC. Developmental biology of T-cell receptors. *Science* 1989, **244**: 943–950.

21. Gouttefangeas C, Bensussan A, Boumsell L. Study of the CD3-associated T-cell receptors reveals further differences between T-cell acute lymphoblastic lymphoma and leukemia. *Blood* 1990, **75**: 931–934.

22. Bernard A, Murphy SB, Melvin S, et al. Non-T, non-B lymphomas are rare in childhood and associated with cutaneous tumor. *Blood* 1982, **59**: 549–554.

23. Link MP, Roper M, Dorfman RF, et al. Cutaneous lymphoblastic lymphoma with pre-B markers. *Blood* 1983, **61**: 838–841.

24. Grogan T, Spier C, Wirt DP, et al. Immunologic complexity of lymphoblastic lymphoma. *Diagn. Immunol.* 1986, **4**: 81–88.

25. Sheibani K, Winberg CD, Burke JS, et al. Lymphoblastic lymphoma expressing natural killer cell-associated antigens: A clinicopathologic study of six cases. *Leuk. Res.* 1987, **11**: 371–377.

26. Raimondi SC, Behm FG, Roberson PK, et al. Cytogenetics of childhood T-cell leukemia. *Blood* 1988, **72**: 1560–1566.

27. Anonymous. Correlation of chromosome abnormalities with histologic and immunologic characteristics in non-Hodgkin's lymphoma and adult T-cell leukemia-lymphoma. Fifth International Workshop on Chromosomes in Leukemia–Lymphoma. *Blood* 1987, **70**: 1554–1564.

28. Smith SD, Morgan R, Link MP, et al. Cytogenetic and immunophenotypic analysis of cell lines established from patients with T-cell leukemia/lymphoma. *Blood* 1986, **67**: 650–656.

29. Dube ID, Kamel-Reid S, Yuan CC, et al. A novel human homeobox gene lies at the chromosome 10 breakpoint in lymphoid neoplasias with chromosomal translocation t(10;14). *Blood* 1991, **78**: 2996–3003.

30. Dube ID, Raimondi SC, Pi D, Kalousek DK. A new translocation, t(10;14)(q24;q11), in T-cell neoplasia. *Blood* 1986, **67**: 1181–1184.

31. Ribeiro RC, Raimondi SC, Behm FG, et al. Clinical and biologic features of childhood T-cell leukemia with the t(11;14). *Blood* 1991, **78**: 466–470.

32. Champagne E, Takihara Y, Sagman U, et al. The T-cell receptor delta chain locus is disrupted in the T-ALL associated t(11;14)(p13;q11) translocation. *Blood* 1989, **73**: 1672–1676.

33. Yoffe G, Schneider N, Van Dyk L, et al. The chromosome translocation (11;14)(p13;q11) associated with T-cell acute lymphocytic leukemia: An 11p13 breakpoint cluster region. *Blood* 1989, **74**: 374–379.

34. Le Beau MM, McKeithan TW, Shima EA, et al. T-Cell receptor alpha-chain gene is split in a human T-cell leukemia cell line with a t(11;14)(p15;q11). *Proc. Natl Acad. Sci. USA* 1986, **83**: 9744–9748.

35. Maziarz RT, Arceci RJ, Bernstein SC, et al. A gamma delta+ T-cell leukemia bearing a novel t(8;14)(q24; q11) translocation demonstrates spontaneous in vitro

natural killer-like activity. *Blood* 1992, **79**: 1523–1531.

36. Mathieu-Mahul D, Sigaux F, Zhu C, et al. A t(8;14) (q24;q11) translocation in a T-cell leukemia (L1-ALL) with c-myc and TcR-alpha chain locus rearrangements. *Int. J. Cancer* 1986, **38**: 835–840.

37. McKeithan TW, Shima EA, Le Beau MM, et al. Molecular cloning of the breakpoint junction of a human chromosomal 8;14 translocation involving the T-cell receptor alpha-chain gene and sequences on the 3' side of MYC. *Proc. Natl Acad. Sci. USA* 1986, **83**: 6636–6640.

38. Bash RO, Crist WM, Shuster JJ, et al. Clinical features and outcome of T-cell acute lymphoblastic leukemia in childhood with respect to alterations at the TAL1 locus: A Pediatric Oncology Group study. *Blood* 1993, **81**: 2110–2117.

39. Carroll AJ, Crist WM, Link MP, et al. The t(1;14)(p34; q11) is nonrandom and restricted to T-cell acute lymphoblastic leukemia: A Pediatric Oncology Group study. *Blood* 1990, **76**: 1220–1224.

40. Kikuchi A, Hayashi Y, Kobayashi S, et al. Clinical significance of TAL1 gene alteration in childhood T-cell acute lymphoblastic leukemia and lymphoma. *Leukemia* 1993, **7**: 933–938.

41. Breit TM, Beishuizen A, Ludwig WD, et al. tal-1 deletions in T-cell acute lymphoblastic leukemia as PCR target for detection of minimal residual disease. *Leukemia* 1993, **7**: 2004–2011.

42. Breit TM, Wolvers-Tettero IL, van Dongen JJ. Lineage specific demethylation of tal-1 gene breakpoint region determines the frequency of tal-1 deletions in alpha beta lineage T-cells. *Oncogene* 1994, **9**: 1847–1853.

43. Hsu HL, Wadman I, Tsan JT, et al. Positive and negative transcriptional control by the TAL1 helix–loop–helix protein. *Proc. Natl Acad. Sci. USA* 1994, **91**: 5947–5951.

44. Fitzgerald TJ, Neale GA, Raimondi SC, et al. c-tal, a helix–loop–helix protein, is juxtaposed to the T-cell receptor-beta chain gene by a reciprocal chromosomal translocation: t(1;7)(p32;q35). *Blood* 1991, **78**: 2686–2695.

45. Westbrook CA, Rubin CM, Le Beau MM, et al. Molecular analysis of TCRB and ABL in a t(7;9)-containing cell line (SUP-T3) from a human T-cell leukemia. *Proc. Natl Acad. Sci. USA* 1987, **84**: 251–255.

46. West R: Childhood cancer mortality: International comparisons 1955–1974. *World Health Stat.* 1984, **37**: 98.

47. Murphy SB, Fairclough DL, Hutchison RE, et al. Non-Hodgkin lymphomas of childhood: an analysis of the histology, staging, and response to treatment of 338 cases at a single institution. *J. Clin. Oncol.* 1989, **7**: 186–193.

48. Nathwani BN, Diamond LW, Winberg CD, et al. Lymphoblastic lymphoma: A clinicopathologic study of 95 patients. *Cancer* 1981, **48**: 2347–2357.

49. Finch S. *Pathogenesis of Leukemias and Lymphomas: Environmental Influences.* New York: Raven Press, 1984, pp. 207–223.

50. Sandlund JT, Ribeiro R, Lin J-S, et al. Factors contributing to the prognostic significance of bone marrow involvement in childhood non-Hodgkin lymphoma. *Med. Pediatr. Oncol.* 1994, **23**: 350–353.

51. Patte C, Kalifa C, Flamant F, et al. Results of the LMT81 protocol, a modified LSA2L2 protocol with high dose methotrexate, on 84 children with non-B-cell (lymphoblastic) lymphoma. *Med. Pediatr. Oncol.* 1992, **20**: 105–113.

52. Reiter A, Schrappe M, Parwaresch R, et al. Non-Hodgkin's lymphomas of childhood and adolescence: Results of a treatment stratified for biologic subtypes and stage – a report of the Berlin–Frankfurt–Munster Group. *J. Clin. Oncol.* 1995, **13**: 359–372.

53. Hutter JJ Jr, Favara BE, Nelson M, et al. Non-hodgkin's lymphoma in children. Correlation of CNS disease with initial presentation. *Cancer* 1975, **36**: 2132–2137.

54. Murphy SB: Classification, staging and end results of treatment of childhood non-Hodgkin's lymphomas: Dissimilarities from lymphomas in adults. *Semin. Oncol.* 1980, **7**: 332.

55. Haddy TB, Parker RI, Magrath IT. Bone marrow involvement in young patients with non-Hodgkin's lymphoma: The importance of multiple bone marrow samples for accurate staging. *Med. Pediatr. Oncol.* 1989, **17**: 418–423.

56. Carabell SC, Goodman RL. In DeVita VT, Hellman S, Rosenburg SA (eds) *Principles and Practice of Oncology*, 2nd edn, Philadelphia: Lippincott, 1985, pp. 1855–1860.

57. Murphy SB, Hustu HO. A randomized trial of combined modality therapy of childhood non-Hodgkin's lymphoma. *Cancer* 1980, **45**: 630–637.

58. Link MP, Donaldson SS, Berard CW, et al. Results of treatment of childhood localized non-Hodgkin's lymphoma with combination chemotherapy with or without radiotherapy. *N. Engl. J. Med.* 1990, **322**: 1169–1174.

59. Link MP, Shuster JJ, Berard CW, et al. Nine weeks of chemotherapy without radiotherapy is sufficient treatment for most children with localized non-Hodgkin's lymphoma (NHL). *Proc. ASCO* 1993, **12**: 384.

60. Wollner N, Exelby PR, Lieberman PH. Non-Hodgkin's lymphoma in children: A progress report on the original patients treated with the LSA2-L2 protocol. *Cancer* 1979, **44**: 1990–1999.

61. Anderson JR, Wilson JF, Jenkin DT, et al. Childhood non-Hodgkin's lymphoma. The results of a randomized therapeutic trial comparing a 4-drug regimen (COMP) with a 10-drug regimen (LSA2-L2). *N. Engl. J. Med.* 1983, **308**: 559–565.

62. Sullivan MP, Boyett J, Pullen J, et al. Pediatric Oncology Group experience with modified LSA2-L2 therapy in 107 children with non-Hodgkin's lymphoma (Burkitt's lymphoma excluded). *Cancer* 1985, **55**: 323–336.

63. Murphy SB, Hustu HO, Rivera G, Berard CW. End results of treating children with localized non-Hodgkin's lymphomas with a combined modality approach of lessened intensity. *J. Clin. Oncol.* 1983, **1**: 326–330.

64. Magrath IT, Janus C, Edwards BK, et al. An effective therapy for both undifferentiated (including Burkitt's) lymphomas and lymphoblastic lymphomas in children and young adults. *Blood* 1984, **63**: 1102–1111.

65. Weinstein HJ, Cassady JR, Levey R. Long-term results of the APO protocol (vincristine, doxorubicin [adriamycin], and prednisone) for treatment of mediastinal lymphoblastic lymphoma. *J. Clin. Oncol.* 1983, **1**: 537–541.

66. Hvizdala EV, Berard C, Callihan T, et al. Lymphoblastic lymphoma in children – a randomized trial comparing LSA2-L2 with the A-COP+ therapeutic regimen: A Pediatric Oncology Group Study. *J. Clin. Oncol.* 1988, **6**: 26–33.

67. Anderson JR, Jenkin RD, Wilson JF, et al. Long-term follow-up of patients treated with COMP or LSA2L2 therapy for childhood non-Hodgkin's lymphoma: A report of CCG-551 from the Childrens Cancer Group [see comments]. *J. Clin. Oncol.* 1993, **11**: 1024–1032.

68. Dahl GV, Rivera G, Pui CH, et al. A novel treatment of childhood lymphoblastic non-Hodgkin's lymphoma: Early and intermittent use of teniposide plus cytarabine. *Blood* 1985, **66**: 1110–1114.

69. Glatstein E, Kim H, Donaldson SS, et al. Non-Hodgkin's lymphomas. VI. Results of treatment in childhood. *Cancer* 1974, **34**: 204–211.

70. Wollner N, Burchenal JH, Lieberman PH, et al. Non-Hodgkin's lymphoma in children. A comparative study of two modalities of therapy. *Cancer* 1976, **37**: 123–134.

71. Ziegler JL. Treatment results of 54 American patients with Burkitt's lymphoma are similar to the African experience. *N. Engl. J. Med.* 1977, **297**: 75–80.

72. Djerassi I, Kim JS. Methotrexate and citrovorum factor rescue in the management of childhood lymphosarcoma and reticulum cell sarcoma (non-Hodgkin's lymphomas): prolonged unmaintained remissions. *Cancer* 1976, **38**: 1043–1051.

73. Muller-Weihrich, Henze G, Odenwald E, et al. BFM trials for childhood NHL. In Cavilli F, Bonadonna G, Rozencweig M (eds) *Malignant Lymphomas and Hodgkin's Disease: Experimental and Therapeutic Advances.* Boston: Kluwer Academic Publishers, 1985, p. 633.

73a. Tubergen DG, Krailo MD, Meadows AT, et al. Comparison of treatment regimens for pediatric lymphoblastic non-Hodgkin's lymphoma: A Childrens Cancer Group Study. *J. Clin. Oncol.* 1995, **13**: 1368–1376.

74. Levine AM, Forman SJ, Meyer PR, et al. Successful therapy of convoluted T-lymphoblastic lymphoma in the adult. *Blood* 1983, **61**: 92–98.

75. Slater DE, Mertelsmann R, Koziner B, et al. Lymphoblastic lymphoma in adults. *J. Clin. Oncol.* 1986, **4**: 57–67.

76. Coleman CN, Picozzi VJ Jr, Cox RS, et al. Treatment of lymphoblastic lymphoma in adults. *J. Clin. Oncol.* 1986, **4**: 1628–1637.

77. Morel P, Lepage E, Brice P, et al. Prognosis and treatment of lymphoblastic lymphoma in adults: A report on 80 patients. *J. Clin. Oncol.* 1992, **10**: 1078–1085.

78. Wagner DK, Kiwanuka J, Edwards BK, et al. Soluble interleukin-2 receptor levels in patients with undifferentiated and lymphoblastic lymphomas: Correlation with survival. *J. Clin. Oncol.* 1987, **5**: 1262–1274.

79. Hagberg H, Killander A, Simonsson B. Serum beta 2-microglobulin in malignant lymphoma. *Cancer* 1983, **51**: 2220–2225.

80. Csako G, Magrath IT, Elin RJ. Serum total and isoenzyme lactate dehydrogenase activity in American Burkitt's lymphoma patients. *Am. J. Clin. Pathol.* 1982, **78**: 712–717.

81. Pui CH, Ip SH, Kung P, et al. High serum interleukin-2 receptor levels are related to advanced disease and a poor outcome in childhood non-Hodgkin's lymphoma. *Blood* 1987, **70**: 624–628.

82. Pullen DJ, Sullivan MP, Falletta JM, et al. Modified LSA2-L2 treatment in 53 children with E-rosette-positive T-cell leukemia: Results and prognostic factors (a Pediatric Oncology Group Study). *Blood* 1982, **60**: 1159–1168.

83. Baro J, Richard C, Sierra J, et al. Autologous bone marrow transplantation in 22 adult patients with lymphoblastic lymphoma responsive to conventional dose chemotherapy. *Bone Marrow Transplant.* 1992, **10**: 33–38.

84. Verdonck LF, Dekker AW, de Gast GC, et al. Autologous bone marrow transplantation for adult poor-risk lymphoblastic lymphoma in first remission. *J. Clin. Oncol.* 1992, **10**: 644–646.

85. Milpied N, Ifrah N, Kuentz M, et al. Bone marrow transplantation for adult poor prognosis lymphoblastic lymphoma in first complete remission. *Br. J. Haematol.* 1989, **73**: 82–87.

CHAPTER 39

Large-cell lymphomas in children

ALFRED REITER AND HANSJÖRG RIEHM

Introduction

The difference in the response to a treatment between histological subtypes of non-Hodgkin's lymphomas (NHLs) of childhood was recognized early after the development of effective chemotherapy protocols [1,2]. The distinction between lymphoblastic lymphomas and small noncleaved cell lymphomas turned out to be most important for the determination of the appropriate treatment modalities (see Chapters 37 and 38). Whereas lymphoblastic lymphomas (LBLs) and diffuse small noncleaved cell lymphomas (SNCLs) are rather homogenous clinicopathological subentities of NHL in childhood (see Chapters 37 and 38) large-cell lymphomas (LCLs) constitute a more heterogeneous group of lymphoid neoplasms. With respect to their cellular origin, most LCLs correspond to various differentiation stages of antigen-reactive B- or T-cells of the peripheral lymphoid organs (Chapters 17,18,37). In therapeutic studies on childhood NHLs, children suffering from LCLs have been included in the groups of 'B-cell lymphomas' [1,3–5], or 'nonlymphoblastic lymphomas' [1,6–10] or 'undifferentiated lymphomas' [11]. However, LCLs in children differ in many respects at the clinical and bio-

logical level from LBLs and SNCLs. Thus, the question arises whether a special therapy strategy is needed for the treatment of LCLs of childhood. Owing to the marked clinical and biological differences of the subsets of LCLs, one might ask whether even different treatment modalities are needed for different subsets.

Definitions and general description

Table 39.1 presents the distinct subsets of LCLs in children, which will be discussed in this chapter, and a comparison of their terminology in different classification schemes. Diffuse histiocytic lymphoma of the Rappaport classification [12] may be the most comprehensive term (although now known to be erroneous) used for this group of lymphomas, which includes subsets of different morphological appearance and cellular origins which are united only by the fact that all have malignant cells of 'large' size. In the National Cancer Institute Working Formulation for Clinical Usage (WF) [13] diffuse histiocytic lym-

Table 39.1 Terminology of large-cell lymphomas of childhood in different classification systems

Rappaport [12]	NCI Working Formulation [13]	Lukes and Collins [14]	Kiel classification [36]
Histiocytic Lymphoma	ML, diffuse large cell, noncleaved cell	ML of large follicle center cells, noncleaved cell	ML, centroblastic
	ML, diffuse large cell, immunoblastic	Immunoblastic Sarcoma of T- and B-cells	ML, immunoblastic of T- and B-cells
	Plasmacytoid		ML, pleomorphic T-cell, large cell
	Clear cell		
	Polymorphous		Large-cell anaplastic lymphoma (ALCL)

Mediastinal large B-cell lymphoma with sclerosis is a distinct subset of large-cell lymphoma [58,61] also occurring in children that has no corresponding term in any of the above classification schemes.

NCI, National Cancer Institute; ML, malignant lymphoma.

phomas of the Rappaport classification were subdivided into two main categories: diffuse large-cell (cleaved and noncleaved cell) malignant lymphomas (MLs) and diffuse large-cell immunoblastic MLs. The first category corresponds to the ML of follicular center cell type of the Lukes and Collins classification [14] and partly overlaps with the category ML centroblastic of the Kiel classification [15,16]. Large-cell, immunoblastic ML in the WF corresponds to the immunoblastic sarcoma of T- or B-cell type in the classification of Lukes and Collins, and immunoblastic ML of T- or B-cell type and remaining part of the category of centroblastic ML in the Kiel classification [16]. The subtypes of immunoblastic lymphoma in the WF, namely, plasmacytoid, clear cell and polymorphous, correspond to ML, immunoblastic lymphoma of the B- and T-cell type, and large-cell pleomorphic T-cell lymphoma, in the Kiel classification, respectively [16]. In this chapter the terminology of the Kiel classification and the WF will be used.

With continued improvements in immunological and molecular biological methods of lymphoma characterization, coupled to careful clinical studies, distinct clinicopathological subentities of large-cell lymphomas have recently been recognized which have no definite equivalents in any of the existing classification systems. These include peripheral (post-thymic) T-cell lymphomas, particularly anaplastic large-cell lymphoma and mediastinal large B-cell lymphoma with sclerosis.

Anaplastic large-cell lymphoma (Ki-1 ALCL) was first described by Stein et al. in 1985 [17]. This new entity was characterized by large pleomorphic cells with strong reactivity with the monoclonal antibody, Ki-1 (CD30), originally raised against the Reed–Sternberg cell line L428 [18], and the presence of activation markers such as interleukin-2 (IL-2) receptor and HLA-DR antigens [17]. The cellular origins of Ki-1 ALCL are clearly heterogeneous in

that it can originate from lymphocytes of both T- and B-lineage. In a minority of cases the tumor cells lack T- and B-cell antigens while others express both T- and B-cell antigens [17,19–23]. In most cases a clonal rearrangement of T-cell receptor chain genes or of immunoglobulin chain genes can be detected [17,19,20,23–25], and it is believed, therefore, that most Ki-1 ALCLs are neoplastic proliferations of activated T- or B-cells [17]. In a few cases, however, a germline configuration of the T-cell receptor β- and γ-chain genes as well as the immunoglobulin heavy and light chain genes has been found [26]. In a series of 62 prospectively evaluated children up to 18 years of age suffering from Ki-1 ALCL, 60% of 52 cases in whom the tumor was sufficiently well characterized by immunophenotyping were positive for the T-cell antigen CD3, 6% expressed the B-cell antigen CD20, and 29% were negative for both CD3 and CD20. Two cases lacked lymphoid features but expressed the monocyte–macrophage-associated antigen, CD68 and lysozyme [27]. The relationship between cases of Ki-1 ALCL with a monocyte–macrophage phenotype to CD30 antigen-negative neoplasms of true histiocytic origin [28] remains to be determined.

The clonal nature of ALCL has been further confirmed by the detection of the nonrandom chromosomal translocation t(2;5)(p23;q35) in the malignant cells [29,30–33]. Possible implications of this genetic aberration in the pathogenesis of Ki-1 ALCL are discussed in Chapter 18. The translocation t(2;5) (p23;q35) is not confined to Ki-1 ALCL – it has also been detected, for example, in peripheral T-cell lymphomas other than Ki-1 ALCL [34] while the breakpoint 5q35 has been detected in a case of Hodgkin's disease of the nodular sclerosis type [35].

Ki-1 ALCL is now included as a category in the updated Kiel classification for NHL as a high-grade malignant NHL [36]. Ki-1 ALCL partially corresponds to diffuse large-cell lymphoma of the immunoblastic type in the WF [37]. Characteristic morphological features are a sinus pattern of lymph node infiltration, paracortical lymph node involvement, sparing of the B-cell follicle areas, fibrosis and sclerosis, foci of necrosis and a high mitotic rate [17,20,23]. Erythrophagocytosis has been observed in some cases [23]. A distinct feature is the cellular pleomorphism ranging from bizarre multinucleated or multilobulated giant cells with abundant cytoplasm to cells with more regular, oval–round nuclei and basophilic cytoplasm [17,23,27]. The multinucleated giant cells may resemble Reed–Sternberg cells. Owing to the marked cytomorphologic pleomorphism, several subdivisions of Ki-1 ALCL have been described based on cytomorphological criteria. However, the clinical relevance of these subdivisions remains to be determined prospectively in larger series of patients [21,38–40].

Prior to its recognition, Ki-1 ALCL was misdiagnosed as a number of other diseases. In childhood, Ki-1 ALCL was especially confused with malignant histiocytosis, regressing atypical histiocytosis, Hodgkin's disease or even reactive lymphadenopathy [17,19,20,22,41–43]. In some cases a remarkable fibrohistiocytic activation can be observed so that the tumor cells are overgrown by fibroblasts and histiocytic cells expressing monocyte–macrophage-associated antigens and lysozyme. Such cases are likely to have been erroneously diagnosed as malignant histiocytosis. Ki-1 ALCL can be distinguished from malignant histiocytosis by the absence of monocyte–macrophage-associated antigens and lysozyme on the tumor cells [17,19,22,44]. Furthermore, Ki-1 ALCL cells have no ultrastructural evidence of phagolysosomes [21]. However, rare cases have been reported in which the tumor cells expressed histiocyte-associated markers in addition to CD30 and in association with clonally rearranged T-cell receptor (TCR) β- and γ-chain genes [45] or immunoglubulin (Ig) heavy chain genes [46]. The significance of this is unknown. Ki-1 ALCL differs histologically from Hodgkin's disease, which does not manifest the sinus pattern of lymph node infiltration so characteristic of ALCL. Furthermore, most cases of Ki-1 ALCL express the epithelial membrane antigen, which is rarely detected in Hodgkin's disease. In contrast, Ki-1 ALCL cells usually (but not invariably) lack the expression of the Hodgkin-cell associated antigen CD15 [41,43,47].

Ki-1 ALCL occurs either as a *de novo* malignant lymphoma or as a secondary lymphoma which evolves from a low-grade or high-grade malignant T-cell lymphoma, Hodgkin's disease or lymphomatoid papulosis [16,19,27,48,49].

The expression of the Ki-1 antigen is not restricted to anaplastic large-cell lymphomas. This antigen can also be detected on Reed–Sternberg cells of Hodgkin's disease, and various large-cell non-Hodgkin's lymphomas such as pleomorphic (peripheral) T-cell lymphoma, immunoblastic lymphoma of T- and B-cell type and centroblastic lymphoma [16,17]. Therefore, the expression of the Ki-1 antigen is not the ultimate criterion with which to define Ki-1 ALCL. While the morphological appearance is presently the major diagnostic feature, the borders of this pathologic entity are not sharply defined [16].

Apart from Ki-1 ALCL of T-cell type, peripheral T-cell lymphomas of postthymic origin are rare in childhood [34,50,51]. Pleomorphic T-cell lymphoma (PTCL), which is subdivided according to the size of the malignant cells into PTCL of small-cell type and PTCL of intermediate and large-cell type, can be distinguished from ALCL histologically [16,36,52]. Pleomorphic T-cell lymphoma may, however, be closely related to Ki-1 ALCL of T-cell type. Strong evidence for this is provided by the detection of the nonrandom chromosomal translocation t(2;5) (p23;q35) in both Ki-1 ALCL and peripheral T-cell lymphoma of mixed- and large-cell type [34]. In addition, shifts of morphology and immunophenotype from one form to the other in individual patients [16,48] has been observed. In one child a morphological change from Ki-1 ALCL towards small-cell pleomorphic T-cell lymphoma was observed at relapse. Ki-1 ALCL morphology was again observed at the time of disease progression [27].

Miller and coworkers described in 1978 'diffuse histiocytic lymphoma with sclerosis' as a clinicopathologic entity with frequent occurrence of superior vena caval obstruction [53]. Subsequent studies led to the recognition of the clinicopathological entity of primary mediastinal diffuse large-cell lymphoma with marked sclerosis, characterized by a strong tendency for local invasive growth [54–63]. The cytomorphological appearance is described as large cleaved cell, clear cell or simply large cell. Immunophenotypic and genotypic studies have revealed that this lymphoma is a neoplasm corresponding to the terminal steps of B-cell differentiation to plasma cells [64–66] and which most probably arise from B-cells resident in the thymus [58,67,68]. Although mediastinal large B-cell lymphoma with sclerosis is now recognized in the literature as a distinct clinicopathological subentity of large-cell lymphoma, it is not categorized in either the WF or the Kiel classification. The disease occurs most commonly in young adults but it is sometimes seen in children. Large B-cell lymphoma of the mediastinum may be confused with malignant thymoma, Hodgkin's disease, germ cell tumors and even T-cell lymphoblastic lymphoma if this diagnosis is not considered or if insufficient pathological material is examined [57,63,68].

Epidemiology

In a retrospective population-based study in Finland the proportion of LCL patients was only 8% among NHL patients up to 15 years of age [69], but in large multicenter studies which enrol children and adolescents up to 18 years of age with any type of NHL, LCLs account for roughly 20% of the study population [6,51]. The distributions of subtypes of LCLs in two multicenter trials are shown in Table 39.2. In a classification study of the Pediatric Oncology Group (POG) using the WF, diffuse large-cell lymphoma, (noncleaved cell) was the most frequent subtype of LCL diagnosed [70]. In the POG study, which was confined to patients 'with adequate histological material for review', the proportion of patients with LCL was relatively high (32%). In a German study, NHL-BFM 90, which included 454 children (up to 18 years) enrolled over a 3½ year period, the proportion of patients with LCLs was 20%. According to the Kiel classification, Ki-1 ALCL was the most frequent subtype diagnosed, accounting for 50% of the LCL patients and for 11% of the study population.

Owing to their heterogeneity and the limited comparability of the definitions and terminology used for subtypes of LCL in children, potentially valuable information concerning differences in the relative frequency of LCL subtypes in different ethnic groups are difficult to obtain from reports in the literature. In a retrospective study, a predominance of peripheral T-cell lymphoma other than Ki-1 ALCL was observed among children suffering from LCL in Taiwan [71] whereas, in the German Berlin, Frankfurt, Munster (BFM) studies large-cell pleomorphic T-cell lymphoma accounted for less than 1% of the study population (Table 39.2). Whether these differences are the result of differences in histological classification or of geographical differences in the incidence of these tumors is unknown.

The median age of children diagnosed as having NHL is between 9 and 10 years, and the disease is rare below the age of 3 years [6,51,72,73]. Patients diagnosed as suffering from LCLs are less frequent in the 3–5 years age group and slightly more frequent in the 10–18 years age group as compared to those with small noncleaved cell lymphomas and lymphoblastic lymphoma [51]. The age at diagnosis, however, may be different for different subsets of LCLs. Whereas children with Ki-1 ALCL were as young as 0.8 years, other subtypes of LCL – centroblastic (CB), immunoblastic (IB), mediastinal large B-cell lymphoma with sclerosis (MLBLS) – have never been diagnosed in children less than 3 years of age. In a series of the POG, patients with diffuse large noncleaved cell lymphoma were significantly younger than patients with large-cell immunoblastic ML according to the WF [70]. However, in the absence of better discrimination among pathological entitites, the latter differences are difficult to interpret.

The predominance of males is less pronounced among patients suffering from LCL (male:female ratio approximately 1.5:1) [27,51,70,74] as compared to children with lymphoblastic or small noncleaved cell lymphoma (Chapters 37 and 38). The male:female ratio is slightly different among subtypes of LCLs. In the 62 Ki-1 ALCL patients treated in BFM studies, the male:female ratio was 2:1 [27]. In contrast, females predominated among patients suffering from mediastinal large B-cell lymphoma with sclerosis in children (data of NHL-BFM studies) and in adults [57,63].

Genetic predispositions to LCL in childhood have not been identified except for the increased incidence

Table 39.2   Distribution of subtypes of large-cell lymphomas in childhood in two multicenter studies

Pediatric Oncology Group [70]			NHL-BFM 90*		
Working Formulation subtype	% of LCLs (N = 72)	% of study population (N = 227)	Kiel classification subtype	% of LCLs (N = 90)	% of study population (N = 453)
DLC, cleaved	4	1	Centroblastic	31	7
DLC, noncleaved	40	13	Immunoblastic	3	<1
IB, plasmacytoid	24	7	MLBLS†	4	1
IB, clear cell	26	8	Ki-1 ALCL	48	11
IB, polymorphous	2	1	PTCL, large cell	4	<1
IB, NOS	2	1			

* Unpublished data of the ongoing study NHL-BFM 90 based on patients enrolled from April 1990 through September 1993.
† Included in the section 'rare subtypes' in the updated Kiel classification but not an own category.

DLC, Diffuse large cell; IB, immunoblastic; NOS, not otherwise specified; MLBLS, mediastinal large B-cell lymphoma with sclerosis; ALCL, anaplastic large-cell lymphoma; PTCL, pleomorphic T-cell lymphoma.

of immunoblastic lymphoma in patients with immunodeficiency disorders (Chapter 19).

Only limited data exist regarding the potential influence of environmental factors in the pathogenesis of LCLs in children. The detection of monoclonal Epstein–Barr virus (EBV) DNA sequences and latent EBV gene products in Ki-1 ALCL cells raises the possibility that this virus is implicated in the pathogenesis of Ki-1 ALCL [75,76]. EBV DNA is most frequently detected in Ki-1 ALCL cases of B-cell type. Surprisingly, Lee and coworkers found EBV DNA in four of six cases of peripheral T-cell lymphoma (other than Ki-1 ALCL) but in none of 19 cases of other subentities, including Burkitt's lymphoma, in Taiwan [71]. The putative association of the human T-lymphotropic virus type 1 (HTLV-1) with cutaneous CD30-positive ALCL deserves further clarification [71,77].

Diagnosis and staging

The establishment of a diagnosis of large-cell lymphoma is still based on histopathology and immunophenotyping (see Chapter 3). However, a complete characterization of the lymphoma cells would necessitate the examination of their karyotype, molecular genetic analysis of Ig gene and TCR gene rearrangements, and the investigation of the presence or absence of viral DNA and viral genome products, as outlined in Chapters 4 and 11–13. Analysis of the configuration of the Ig genes and TCR genes can be of particular value in the differentiation of LCLs from reactive or other benign lymphoproliferative disorders as well as from malignancies of nonlymphoid origin (Chapter 4). Major difficulties may arise in the separation of Ki-1 ALCL from Hodgkin's disease of the nodular sclerosis type, the rare cases of true malignant histiocytosis, soft tissue sarcomas, primary bone tumors, lymphomatoid papulosis and even reactive lymphoproliferative processes. In particular, the distinction between virus-associated [78] or other hemophagocytic syndromes, and Ki-1 ALCL or peripheral T-cell lymphomas accompanied by marked hemophagocytosis in the bone marrow may also be difficult [79]. Therefore, although the diagnostic investigations should not delay chemotherapy, it is essential to obtain enough tumor tissue for a comprehensive diagnostic work-up. Apart from formalin-fixed material for routine histopathology and tumor touch print preparations for cytomorphology, fresh tissue should be obtained for cytogenetic and molecular genetic analysis as well as for studies of viral antigens and DNA sequences. Although basic immunohistochemistry studies are possible on conventional paraffin sections using the streptavidin–biotin–peroxidase complex [80] or alkaline phosphatase antialkaline phosphatase techniques for detection [81], and paraffin-resistant antibodies including anti Ki-1 (CD30) [82], the preservation of snap-frozen tumor tissue for a more complete immunophenotyping is advantageous (see Chapter 4).

Staging procedures are similar for all children with NHL. In children suffering from LCLs, however, special attention should be directed to the examination of soft tissue and skin, because of their relatively frequent involvement as discussed below. Complete peripheral blood examination (PB), bone marrow (BM) aspiration smears from at least two sites and cerebrospinal fluid (CSF) analyses are mandatory. In most instances ultrasonography is sufficient to detect involvement of abdominal and retroperitoneal organs. Adominal computed tomography (CT) may be performed in some circumstances. Chest X-ray is routinely performed, but in the case of a mediastinal mass a CT scan of the thorax gives additional information regarding possible infiltration of the lungs and other thoracic organs. This is of particular interest in patients suffering from a Ki-1 ALCL, mediastinal large B-cell lymphoma with sclerosis or a large-cell pleomorphic T-cell lymphoma. Skeletal scintigraphy is obligatory, owing to the frequent involvement of bone in LCLs. Areas of increased activity in the skeletal scintigraphy should be further examined by X-ray and magnetic resonance imagirig (MRI). In patients with an otherwise proven diagnosis of NHL, bone involvement can be diagnosed if imaging studies reveal one or more bone lesions. Additional biopsy of bone lesions to prove lymphoma infiltration are not needed except when bone lesion(s) are the only manifestations of the disease. The need for a cranial CT scan or MRI is debatable, since involvement of the CNS in patients suffering from LCLs is rare, but because of the adverse consequences for the patient if an intracerebral focus remains undetected at the time of diagnosis, a cranial CT or MRI scan would seem to be justifiable. Magnetic resonance imaging has been shown to be useful in the detection of focal lymphomatous infiltration of the bone marrow, which may escape detection by marrow aspiration [83]. It is questionable, however, whether this information is clinically useful, since relapses involving the bone marrow are rare in patients suffering from LCL (see below). Gallium-67 scintigraphy is not used by all centers for staging studies in children with lymphoma (see Chapter 25). Uptake among different subtypes varies and the radionuclide uptake is not specific for lymphoma tissue, but is also taken up by normal thymus and areas of inflammation [84,85]. Immunoscintigraphy using radionuclide-labelled monoclonal anti-CD30 antibodies has been shown to be a valuable method of visualizing tumor masses in patients with CD30-antigen-positive Hodgkin's disease and Ki-1 ALCL [86]. Further investigations are needed to determine whether this method will have a place in staging studies and monitoring of treatment response in LCLs in children.

The St Jude staging system is widely in use for staging of NHL in childhood [87] (see Chapter 24). This staging system is based on the clinico-anatomical pattern and the more frequent involvement of bone marrow and CNS in lymphoblastic lymphoma, and small noncleaved cell lymphoma and has proved useful for the stratification of therapy intensity for the treatment of these entities (see Chapters 37 and 38). Owing to the more unusual distribution pattern in most LCLs, the validity of the St Jude staging system for stratification of treatment in this context is less well defined. The staging of patients with multifocal bone lesions without bone marrow involvement, or with multiple skin or soft tissue lesions may be difficult in the St Jude staging system. Staging according to the modified Ann Arbor staging classification for Hodgkin's disease [88] may be easier to perform in such cases, although the assignment of an Ann Arbor stage is probably no more helpful for the stratification of therapy.

Serum concentrations of lactate dehydrogenase (LDH) at the time of diagnosis as a marker of tumor volume correlates with prognosis in Burkitt's lymphoma [72,89]. However, the prognostic implication of LDH levels for treatment outcome of patients suffering from LCLs is less clear. Serum LDH levels at diagnosis are lower in patients suffering from LCLs as compared to patients with lymphoblastic lymphoma and small noncleaved cell lymphoma (Table 39.3). Serum concentrations of soluble IL-2 receptor have been found to correlate with stage and prognosis in NHLs [90,91] and may be of special value in Ki-1 ALCL [92]. A even more specific parameter of the total tumor burden may be the serum concentration of the CD30 antigen which is released from Ki-1 (CD30)-antigen-positive tumor cells [93]. Prospective studies are needed to determine the value of those measurements for staging of LCLs in children.

Clinical characteristics

The clinical features of LCLs in children are compared to those of lymphoblastic and small noncleaved cell lymphomas in Table 39.3. LCLs differ from LBLs and SNCLs with respect to the lower frequency of BM and CNS involvement, a greater likelihood of a history of fever, and more frequent involvement of bone, soft tissue, skin and lungs. The distribution pattern in terms of head and neck, mediastinal or abdominal disease is not characteristic. However, apart from the rare involvement of the BM and CNS, the clinical features of the distinct subsets of LCLs in children differ considerably, as shown in Table 39.3, for the two most frequent subsets – Ki-1 ALCL and centroblastic lymphoma.

After the description of Ki-1 ALCL as a histopathological entity, several distinctive clinical features were recognized including a predilection for skin involvement in association with peripheral lymphadenopathy [19], a high frequency of extranodal involvement [21,42,43] and some unique features in the clinical history. Patients with Ki-1 ALCL may have an indolent phase consisting of mild lymphadenopathy as well as a longer history of illness characterized by fever and, most intriguingly, a waxing and waning course of adenopathy and skin lesions until finally rapid progression takes place [27,42,43,94]. Spontaneous regression appears to be mediated by cytokines such as transforming growth factor beta [95] and final progression may be the result of escape from cytokine-mediated suppressive effects [96]. In a series of 62 patients from three consecutive BFM group studies the following clinical pattern was observed [27]: 40% of patients had a history of fever (which is uncommon in patients with other subtypes of LCLs), lymphadenopathy was present in 90%, and 40% had exclusively nodal disease. A single affected node was rarely observed, while generalized lymphadenopathy was not infrequent. Peripheral nodes were most frequently involved, followed by retroperitoneal and mediastinal nodes. The pattern of spread of nodal disease is difficult to interpret in Ki-1 ALCL patients. A contiguous pattern was observed in two-thirds of patients but a noncontiguous pattern in one-third of the patients. Even such widely separated lymph node regions as cervical and inguinal nodes were sometimes affected in the same patient without a 'bridge' in between. Splenomegaly was observed in 21% and hepatomegaly in 27% of patients. Extranodal involvement was diagnosed in 60% of patients and roughly 10% had exclusively extranodal disease. Soft tissue and bone were the most frequent sites of extranodal involvement (21% of patients each) followed by the skin (14%) and lung (6%). Fourteen per cent of patients had malignant effusions. Rarely, focal infiltrations of the pancreas, the kidney, the liver and the intestinal tract were observed. Soft tissue manifestations included multiple tumors in the subcutaneous tissue and muscles, or as a single larger tumor resembling a soft tissue sarcoma. Bone

Table 39.3 Clinical characteristics of histopathological subtypes of non-Hodgkin's lymphoma in children*

| | LB-L (N=89) | SNCL (N=215 | LCL (N=90) | Subtypes of LCL | |
| | | | | Ki-ALCL (N=48) | CB (N=31) |
	% of patients	% of patients	% of patients	% of patients	% of patients
Stage†					
I	6	11	13	4	21
II	8	21	27	25	35
III	63	40	43	48	32
IV	24	9	17	23	3
B-ALL		20			
BM involved	19	26	0	0	0
CNS disease	6	11	3	6	0
Fever	11	13	27	42	13
Hepatomegaly	29	26	19	25	6
Splenomegaly	11	12	9	12	3
Localization type					
Head/neck	8	19	21	12	39
Mediastinum	68	5	32	33	19
Abdomen	9	54	20	17	26
Extranodal disease					
Intestine	3	39	11	6	23
Bone	1	6	12	19	3
Soft tissue	1	1	9	13	6
Skin	0	<1	6	11	0
Lung	4	1	12	10	6
LDH (U/l) median	458	474	272	268	238
range	135–2800	105–17000	121–4620	137–1587	121–4620

* Based on 453 patients up to 18 years of age enrolled on to the multicenter study NHL-BFM 90 from April 1990 through September 1993.
† St Jude staging system [87] with one modification: patients with multifocal bone disease without bone marrow involvement were defined as having stage IV. This modification mainly came into force for LCL patients.

LB-L, Lymphoblastic lymphoma; SNCL, small noncleaved cell lymphoma; LCL, large-cell lymphomas; Ki-1 ALCL, anaplastic large-cell lymphoma; CB, centroblastic lymphoma; B-ALL, B-cell acute lymphoblastic leukemia; BM, bone marrow; CNS, central nervous system.

manifestations varied from small osteolytic lesions to large tumors simulating bone tumors. In 5% of the patients the disease was confined to the bone. Three types of skin lesions were observed. Single or multiple bluish-colored cutaneous/subcutaneous nodules, large ulcerated lesions, and multiple or disseminated papulomatous lesions of red–yellow color. The disease was never confined to the skin; all patients had additional involvement of nodes or other extranodal sites. In only one of the 62 patients was meningeal involvement present at diagnosis. An intracerebral mass subsequently developed during the course of the disease. No patient had BM disease detected by examination of BM aspiration smears. However, marked hemophagocytosis by macrophages could be observed in the BM of some patients. According to a modified St Jude staging scheme (patients with multifocal bone disease were qualified for stage IV even without BM involvement), 6% of the 62 patients had stage I disease, 26% had stage II, 56% stage III and 11% had stage IV disease. According to the Ann Arbor staging classification, 13% of the patients had stage I, 29% stage II, 21% stage III and 37% had stage IV disease.

Some of the distinctive clinical features of Ki-1 ALCL may be caused by cytokine production of the tumor cells. Ki-1 ALCL cells have been shown to produce IL-6, which may be responsible for fever, bone lesions and thrombocytosis, IL-9, IL-4, interferon-gamma, as well as granulocyte–macrophage colony-stimulating factor (GM-CSF) and granulocyte colony-stimulating factor (G-CSF), which may induce leukocytosis [97–100]. Twelve per cent of the

48 Ki-1 ALCL patients in the NHL-BFM 90 study had a leukocyte count of more than 20 000/μl at the time of diagnosis. Thrombocytosis of more than 500 000/μl was noticed in 21% of the patients while thrombocytopenia of less than 100 000/μl was seen in 6% of patients, although none of them had detectable BM invasion.

The clinical pattern of patients suffering from centroblastic lymphomas is not characteristic. Single node disease of stage I occurs more frequently than in Ki-1 ALCL (Table 39.3). Nodes at any site may be affected, including mediastinal and retroperitoneal nodes. However, unlike Ki-1 ALCL, the disease is almost always restricted to a distinct anatomic region. Tumors of the tonsil, and large multifocal tumors of the liver and kidney were observed, and tumors of the gastrointestinal tract are rather frequent. In contrast to Ki-1 ALCL, involvement of bone, soft tissue and skin as well as hepatomegaly and splenomegaly are rare features in patients suffering from centroblastic lymphoma.

Mediastinal large B-cell lymphoma with sclerosis has characteristic clinical features in children as well as in young adults [51,57–63]. These patients have a large anterior mediastinal mass with aggressive local invasivion into the large vessels, pericardium, pleura, lungs, sternum and chest wall. Pleural and pericardial effusions are frequent. The patients often have chest pain and cough preceding the diagnosis of lymphoma, and frequently have superior vena cava syndrome and dyspnea at presentation as a result of compression and direct invasion of the mediastinal structures. Contiguous lymphomatous spread restricted to adjacent nodes predominates whereas superficial nodes are rarely involved. CNS involvement was never observed at diagnosis and BM disease was detected in few cases. A unique feature is the presence of distant metastasis in the form of large bilateral tumors of the kidneys and, less frequently, in the adrenal glands and the ovaries. According to the St Jude staging system the patients always have at least stage III disease.

Only preliminary descriptions of the clinical features of large-cell pleomorphic T-cell lymphoma in children are possible owing to its rarity in this age group. Patients suffering from that subentity may have some clinical features in common with Ki-1 ALCL patients. In the largest published series of 22 patients up to 20 years of age, 45% of the patients had B symptoms, and 55% had extranodal disease with the skin being the most frequent site of involvement followed by bone and the lungs [34]. However, the population of that retrospective study only partially corresponds to large-cell pleomorphic T-cell lymphoma discussed here, since seven cases of mixed cellularity and five cases of anaplastic large-cell lymphoma were included. More patients are needed to more clearly define the clinical characteristics of this subentity.

Similarly, a distinct clinical pattern of immunoblastic lymphomas (Kiel classification) in children cannot be defined owing to the small numbers of patients.

In contrast to patients suffering from advanced stage SNCLs or LBLs, patients with LCLs rarely present with life-threatening complications at diagnosis. Exceptions are patients with mediastinal large B-cell lymphoma with sclerosis who often have superior vena caval syndrome and dyspnea at presentation, as discussed above. Respiratory distress may also be present in patients suffering from Ki-1 ALCL or pleomorphic T-cell lymphoma with advanced lung infiltrations. Disseminated intravascular coagulation has occasionally been reported in a cases of Ki-1 ALCL [101].

Prognostic factors

In large multicenter studies as well as in a single institution series the treatment outcome in children suffering from LCL does not differ significantly from that of patients with SNCL or LBL [7,72,102]. Furthermore, no significant differences in the event-free survival estimates were seen between distinct subsets of LCLs in the two consecutive German studies, NHL-BFM 86 and 90 [102, and unpublished results] as well as in two series of patients of the St Jude Hospital and the POG [70,74]. Whether large-cell pleomorphic T-cell lymphoma represents a worse prognostic group of LCLs cannot be determined at present since number of patients is too small.

Clinical and biological variables may have a different prognostic impact in different subsets of LCL of childhood. However, after subclassification, the number of patients in most subsets is too small for meaningful evaluation of prognostic parameters. In patients suffering from Ki-1 ALCL a number of variables have been reported to be associated with the risk of treatment failure, among them involvement of the liver and lungs [103], and the presence of B symptoms [42]. In a multivariate analysis of a prospective series of 62 patients énrolled in three consecutive BFM trials with stage-adapted treatment intensity, skin involvement at diagnosis was the only negative prognostic parameter whereas stage, presence of B symptoms, hepato- and/or splenomegaly, presence and site of extranodal involvement and the immunophenotype of the tumor cells had no prognostic influence [27]. The prognostic implication of the nonrandom translocation t(2;5)(p23;q35) is yet to be determined owing to the small number of patients evaluated. Secondary Ki-1 ALCL may have a worse prognosis than primary Ki-1 ALCL. However, the evaluation of secondary Ki-1 ALCL as a 'prognostic factor' is difficult. Casual observations suggest that, at the time of diagnosis, secondary Ki-1 ALCL may coexist with components of, for example, low-grade malignant T-cell lymphoma or may already completely dominate the histopathological appearance. The issue of the identification of secondary Ki-1 ALCL and its potential prognostic relevance needs more investigation. In the series of Gordon et al., consisting of 22 patients with peripheral T-cell lymphoma, the stage of disease did not correlate with relapse-free survival, while patients older than 12 years of age did better than younger children [34]. Stage at diagnosis may be of prognostic impact in centroblastic and immunoblastic lymphomas of B-cell lineage; statistical evaluation, however, is difficult owing to the small number of patients. In the German study NHL-BFM 86, none of 11 patients with stage I or II disease failed therapy whereas three of nine patients with stage III disease failed to enter remission. Measures of the total tumor burden at the time of diagnosis such as serum LDH and soluble IL-2 receptor levels correlate with prognosis in advanced-stage Burkitt's lymphoma [72,89–91]. The prognostic implication of those parameters for children suffering from LCLs has not yet been determined. In patients with Ki-1 (CD30)-antigen-positive neoplasms, serum concentrations of CD30 antigen may be a reliable parameter of the tumor cell mass and prognosis [93]. Prospective studies are needed to determine the prognostic value of these parameters in childhood LCLs.

Treatment

Therapy protocols effective for childhood acute lymphoblastic leukemias (ALL) and those derived from the LSA_2L_2 protocol have been proven to be a successful treatment for lymphoblastic lymphoma [1–3,7,104,105] as discussed in Chapter 37. In SNCL, however, a strategy of repeated short intensive therapy courses based on cyclophosphamide and methotrexate has been found to be more effective [2–5,106–108] as shown in Chapter 38. This type of treatment strategy became known as 'B-cell lymphoma strategy'. No special treatment strategies for children with LCLs have been developed and only a few reports on treatment results confined to patients with LCL have been published. In various therapeutic studies, patients with LCLs have been included in the subgroups of 'B-cell lymphomas' [3–5], 'nonlymphoblastic lymphomas' [2,6,7–10] or 'undifferentiated lymphomas' [11]. In reports of these trials the results in patients with LCL are not always provided separately and the results for different subsets of LCLs are given even more rarely. The diversity of classification schemes used makes the comparison of results of clinical studies particularly difficult. Furthermore, Ki-1 ALCL was recognized as a clinicopathologic subentity of NHL during the recent past, but, prior to this, many of the latter patients were diagnosed as histiocytic disorders and treated according to a number of different protocols. Therefore, in a first part of this section, treatment strategies and results for the whole group of large-cell lymphomas in children are discussed. The second part of the section will deal with special aspects of therapy modalities in distinct subsets of LCLs in childhood.

TREATMENT STRATEGIES AND RESULTS IN LARGE-CELL LYMPHOMAS

Table 39.4 summarizes treatment protocols and results for children suffering from LCLs. In the randomized trial CCG 551 of the Childrens Cancer Group (CCG) the four-drug cytoxan, vincristine, methorexate, prednisone (COMP) therapy and the 12-drug LSA_2L_2 protocol resulted in comparable treatment outcome for patients suffering from LCLs of advance stage in contrast to patients with LBLs and SNCLs of stage III and IV [2,6] (Table 39.4). In three different therapy studies including patients of all stages of LCLs, comparable overall results were achieved with a modified LSA_2L_2 protocol probability of event-free survival (pEFS) [71% at 6 years] [7], the Adriamycin, prednisone, oncovin (APO) regimen of the Dana Farber Cancer Institute (pEFS 76%) [109] and the strategy for B-cell lymphomas of the German NHL-BFM 86 study (pEFS 75% at 7 years) [102]. In the POG 8106 study, patients with advanced-stage disease had a 2-year EFS estimate of 61% with a four-drug regimen based on high-dose methotrexate (HD-MTX), high-dose cyclophosphamide, vincristine and prednisone [8]. Similar results were reported from a POG study using the A-COP regimen, which consisted of doxorubicin, cyclophosphamide, vincristine and prednisone [10]. Bunin et al. retrospectively analyzed children treated with cytoxan, Adriamycin, vincristine, prednisone (CHOP) therapy; 9 of 12 patients with stage III disease were long-term survivors [9]. The APO, A-COP, POG 8106 and LSA_2L_2 regimens, are presented in detail in Chapters 37 and 38. The treatment regimen of LCL patients in the German study NHL-BFM 86 differed only slightly from the therapy strategy depicted in Figures 39.1 and 39.2. An exception were

Table 39.4   Treatment results in childhood large-cell lymphoma (all subtypes)

Protocol	Duration	Local radiotherapy	CNS prophylaxis	No. of patients	Stages	pEFS	Remission failure	Relapse	Reference
APO	24 months	Stage I/II, bone disease 30–50 Gy	IT MTX CRT 24 Gy	28	I–IV	76% at 6 years	1	2 CNS	109
LSA$_2$L$_2$-mod	24 months	30 Gy a$_1$	IT MTX	30	I–IV	71% at 6 years	ns	ns	7
NHL-BFM 86	2/5 months a$_2$	a$_3$	MTX 0.5 g/m^{2}a$_4$ IT triple	53a$_5$	I–IV	75% at 7 years	5 (9%)	3 local 4 other a$_6$	102
LSA$_2$L$_2$	18 months	Bulky disease	IT MTX	18	III/IV	43% at 5 years	ns	ns	6
COMP	18/6 months	20–30 Gy	IT MTX	42	III/IV	52% at 5 years	ns	ns	
POG 8106	30/54 weeks randomized	—	MTX 6g/m^2 IT triple	23	III/IV	61% at 2 years	6 (26%)	3 other a$_6$	8
A-COP	24/36 months a$_7$	21 Gy a$_1$	IT MH CRT 24 Gy	22	III/IV	67% at 4 years	4 (18%)	1 BM 2 ns	10

pEFS, Probability of event-free survival; CRT, cranial radiotherapy; IT, intrathecal; MTX, methotrexate; MH, MTX+hydrocortisone.
a$_1$, Residual tumor after induction.
a$_2$, Stages I and II – resected, 2 months (3 therapy courses); stages II – not resected, III, IV, 5 months (6 therapy courses).
a$_3$, Only in few individual cases.
a$_4$, 5 g/m^2 in stage IV patients.
a$_5$, Four patients with pleomorphic T-cell lymphoma were treated according to regimen non-B (Chapter 38) with 24 months duration.
a$_6$, New extramedullary sites other than the primary, and other than CNS.
a$_7$, Stage III, 24 months; stage IV, 36 months.

four patients with pleomorphic T-cell lymphoma who were treated according to the regimen for LBL (see Chapter 38).

Table 39.5 compares the number and the cumulative doses of the drugs used in the abovementioned protocols. Although almost all of them included steroids, cyclophosphamide and vincristine, the size of individual doses, the number of doses and the cumulative doses of these drugs differed considerably. Doxorubicin was given up to a total cumulative dose of 500 mg/m^2 in the APO, A-COP and LSA$_2$L$_2$ regimens, whereas doxorubicin was not a part of the POG 8106 regimen and was given at a much lower cumulative dose in the NHL-BFM 86 protocol. In the latter two regimens, methotrexate (MTX) was used at medium (0.5 g/m^2) or high dose (>1 g/m^2), but was given at low dose during the maintenance components of the APO, A-COP and LSA$_2$L$_2$ protocols.

An epipodophyllotoxin was included exclusively in the BFM regimen. Since treatment results were comparable in these five studies, protocols including medium- or high-dose MTX ± epipodophyllotoxin ± low cumulative dose doxorubicin in addition to cyclophosphamide, vincristine and steroids seem to be as effective as protocols which included relatively high cumulative doses of anthracyclines, and thus carry a considerable risk of late cardiac disease [110].

Stratification of treatment intensity

In the CCG study 551 and the BFM 86 study, treatment intensity was stratified according to stage. In the CCG 551 trial, patients with localized disease were randomized either to receive 6 months or 18 months therapy duration. In the NHL-BFM 86 study, patients with stage I and stage II-R (completely

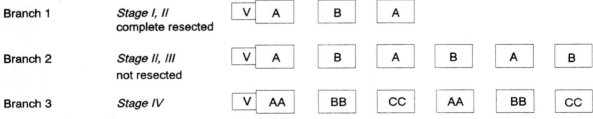

Figure 39.1   Treatment strategy for Ki-1 ALCL in studies NHL-BFM 83, NHL-BFM 86 and NHL-BFM 90. Therapy intensity was stratified into three therapy branches according to stage (modified St Jude staging system). Reproduced by permission of WB Saunders [27].

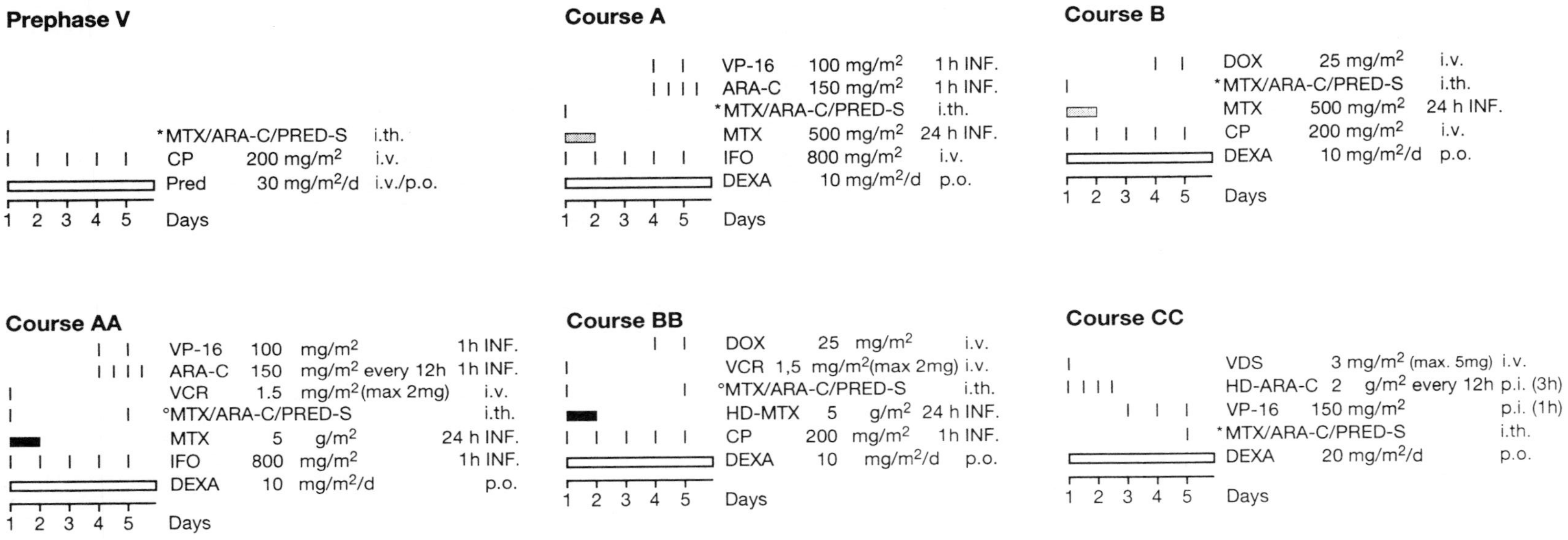

Prephase V

*MTX/ARA-C/PRED-S		i.th.
CP	200 mg/m²	i.v.
Pred	30 mg/m²/d	i.v./p.o.

Days 1 2 3 4 5

Course A

VP-16	100 mg/m²	1 h INF.
ARA-C	150 mg/m²	1 h INF.
*MTX/ARA-C/PRED-S		i.th.
MTX	500 mg/m²	24 h INF.
IFO	800 mg/m²	i.v.
DEXA	10 mg/m²/d	p.o.

Days 1 2 3 4 5

Course B

DOX	25 mg/m²	i.v.
*MTX/ARA-C/PRED-S		i.th.
MTX	500 mg/m²	24 h INF.
CP	200 mg/m²	i.v.
DEXA	10 mg/m²/d	p.o.

Days 1 2 3 4 5

Course AA

VP-16	100 mg/m²	1 h INF.
ARA-C	150 mg/m² every 12h	1 h INF.
VCR	1.5 mg/m²(max 2mg)	i.v.
°MTX/ARA-C/PRED-S		i.th.
MTX	5 g/m²	24 h INF.
IFO	800 mg/m²	1 h INF.
DEXA	10 mg/m²/d	p.o.

Days 1 2 3 4 5

Course BB

DOX	25 mg/m²	i.v.
VCR	1,5 mg/m²(max 2mg)	i.v.
°MTX/ARA-C/PRED-S		i.th.
HD-MTX	5 g/m²	24 h INF.
CP	200 mg/m²	1 h INF.
DEXA	10 mg/m²/d	p.o.

Days 1 2 3 4 5

Course CC

VDS	3 mg/m² (max. 5mg)	i.v.
HD-ARA-C	2 g/m² every 12h	p.i. (3h)
VP-16	150 mg/m²	p.i. (1h)
*MTX/ARA-C/PRED-S		i.th.
DEXA	20 mg/m²/d	p.o.

Days 1 2 3 4 5

° i.th. doses in courses AA,BB :

	MTX	ARA-C	PRED-S
<1 Y.:	3	8	2 mg
>=1 and <2 Y.:	4	10	3 mg
>=2 and <3 Y.:	5	13	4 mg
>=3 Y.:	6	15	5 mg

* i.th. doses in courses V,A,B,CC :

	MTX	ARA-C	PRED-S
<1 Y.:	6	16	4 mg
>=1 and <2 Y.:	8	20	6 mg
>=2 and <3 Y.:	10	26	8 mg
>=3 Y.:	12	30	10 mg

Figure 39.2 Prephase V and therapy courses V, A, B, AA, BB, CC in study NHL-BFM 90. MTX, Methotrexate; ARA-C, cytosine arabinoside; PRED-S, prednisolone; Pred, prednisone; CP, cyclophosphamide; VP-16, etoposide; IFO, ifosfamide; DOX, doxorubicin; VCR, vincristine; VDS, vindesine; HD, high dose; i.v., intravenously; Inf, infusion; i.th., intrathecally; p.o., orally; h, hour. In study NHL-BFM 86, teniposide was given instead of etoposide. In study NHL-BFM 83 cyclophosphamide (200 mg/m²) was given in stead of ifosfamide in course A, teniposide (165 mg/m²) and Ara-C (300 mg/m²) were given in one dose at day 5 in course A, and doxorubicin (50 mg/m²) was given in one dose at day 5 in course B. I.th. therapy consisted of MTX only. Reproduced by permission of WB Saunders [27].

Table 39.5 Number of drugs and cumulative doses of current protocols

Protocol	Prednisone (g/m²)	Dexamethasone (g/m²)	CP (mg/m²)	Ifosamide (mg/m²)	VCR (mg/m²)	Doxorubicin (mg/m²)	MTX (g/m²)	ARA-C (mg/m²)	VM26 (mg/m²)	Other	Reference
APO	20	—	—	—	71	450	a₁	—	—	a₂	109
LSA₂L₂	1.8	—	>1.2 a₃	—	>8 a₃	500/350 a₄	a₁	100×16	—	a₅	7
NHL-BFM 86 a₆	0.15	0.15	2	8	—	50	0.5×3	150×8	400	—	102
	0.15	0.3	4	12	—	150	0.5×6	150×12	600	—	
	0.15	0.3	4	12	9	150	5×6	150×12	600	—	
COMP	3.3–6.6 a₃	—	6.2–18 a₃	—	23–59 a₃	—	0.3×6–18	—	—	—	6
POG 8106	1.7	—	3.6	—	15/19 a₃	—	1.5–6×8/12 a₃,₇	—	—	—	8
A-COP	1.1	—	13.6 19.4 a₈	—	54 70 a₈	480/360 a₄	a₁	—	—	a₉	10

CP, cyclophosphamide; VCR, vincristine; MTX, methotrexate; ARA-C, cytarabine; VM26, teniposide; BCNU, bis-(2-chloroethyl) nitrosourea.

a₁, Low-dose methotrexate during maintenance.
a₂, L-Asparaginase 56000 (28000 if age > 6 years) IU/m²×5; 6-mercaptopurine 225 mg/ m²/day×5 × 31 courses.
a₃, Depending on numbers of maintenance courses.
a₄, Lower dose for patients with mediastinal radiotherapy.

a₅, L-Asparaginase 6000 IU/m² × 14, additional CP, BCNU, hydroxyurea, 6-thioguanine, ARA-C during maintenance.
a₆, Stratified for stages: stages I/II – resected, three courses; stages II – not resected, and III, six courses; stage IV, six intensified courses.
a₇, 50–200 mg/kg body weight; dose/m² body surface area was calculated by dose/kg × 30.
a₈, Stage IV disease.
a₉, 6-Mercaptopurine 75 mg/m²/day × 14 days × 16 (stage IV), 24 courses during maintenance.

Table 39.6 Treatment results in childhood Ki-1 anaplastic large-cell lymphoma

Protocol	Duration (months)	Local radiotherapy	CNS prophylaxis	No. of patients*	Outcome†	Remission failure	Relapses (site)	Reference
LSA₂L₂-mod	24	Bulky disease 20 Gy	IT MTX CRT for stage III/IV	12	pEFS 63% at 4 years	0	1 (local) 1 (other‡) 1 (CNS + other‡)	94
Milan	24	Bulky disease 30–35 Gy	—	28	71% in CCR	0	1 (CNS) 6 (ns)	103
COPAD +HDMTX+VP16 +VBL+Bleo	12–18 8 8	— — —	— MTX 3 g/m² MTX 3 g/m²	28 22 25	pEFS 52% at 5 years	6 2 4	10 (ns) 9 (ns) 5 (ns)	113,114
UKCCSG-LMB89	ns	ns	IT triple HDMTX	11	73% in CCR	3	0	115
NHL-BFM 83/86/90	2–5	—	MTX 0.5/5g/m²‡ IT triple	62	pEFS 81% at 9 years	4	3 (local + other‡) 4 (other‡)	27

* Patients of all stages included.
† Median follow-up 2.5–4 years.
‡ New extramedullary sites other than the primary and other than CNS.

CNS, Central nervous system; IT, intrathecal; MTX, methotrexate; VBL, vinblastine; Bleo, bleomycin; pEFS, probability of event-free survival; CRT, cranial radiotherapy; CCR, continuous complete remission.

resected) disease received three courses of therapy, patients of stage II-NR (not resected) and stage III received six courses, and patients of stage IV received six courses of intensified chemotherapy (Figure 39.1 and 39.2). In the APO protocol, local radiotherapy and CNS prophylaxis was stratified according to stage.

Treatment duration

These therapy regimens differed considerably in the duration of treatment. All therapy of the BFM regimen B was delivered within 2 (localized completely resected tumors) to 5 months. The duration of the POG 8106 therapy for advanced-stage disease was either 30 weeks (two maintenance cycles) or 54 weeks (six maintenance cycles), whereas in the APO, A-COP and LSA$_2$L2$_2$ protocols therapy was given over 18–24 months (Table 39.4). In all studies adverse events occurred early. Almost half of the patients who failed therapy were incomplete responders. In the complete responders, relapses were diagnosed while on treatment or shortly thereafter. In the BFM 86 trial, all relapses were observed within 8 months after diagnosis except for patients suffering from large-cell pleomorphic T-cell lymphomas. Within this small subset of patients, who were treated according to the BFM ALL-type protocol, which includes maintenance therapy for up to 24 months (see Chapter 38), relapses were observed as late as 47 months after achieving remission.

Local therapy modalities

Local therapy modalities differed in the referenced studies (Table 39.4). The APO protocol included radiation to localized disease (30–40 Gy) and bone lesions (50–54 Gy) at week 8 of therapy. No patient treated on that regimen suffered from local relapse. In the CCG 551 study radiotherapy (20–30 Gy) was given to bulky disease. The sites of relapses were not specified, however, in the reports of that trial [2,6]. No local therapy was performed in the POG study 8106 [8]. All three relapses in LCL patients in that trial occurred in extramedullary sites other than the primary. In two other POG studies in which the LSA$_2$L$_2$ or the A-COP protocols were used, radiotherapy was given to tumors which did not undergo complete resolution during chemotherapy. However, the sites of failure were not specified [7,10]. In the BFM 86 study, second-look surgery was performed in patients with incomplete resolution of tumors after two courses of chemotherapy. None of 10 patients with residual tumors which had a completely necrotic appearance by microscopic examination subsequently relapsed. Four patients with poor response during the first week of chemotherapy had bulky

viable lymphoma when the second-look operation was performed. In all three cases the disease progressed rapidly despite local radiotherapy and intensified chemotherapy.

As discussed below, the sites of failure probably differ between the subentities of LCLs in children. Hence, the potential role of local therapy modalities may also differ in subsets of LCL patients.

CNS therapy

In children suffering from LCLs the CNS is rarely involved at the time of diagnosis and rarely the site of relapse [6–8,51,102,109]. The prophylactic CNS therapy administered in various studies and the number of patients who relapsed in the CNS is given in Table 39.4. Preventive cranial irradiation (24 Gy) was included in the APO regimen and in the A-COP protocol in addition to intrathecal (IT) MTX therapy. Cranial irradiation seems, however, not to be necessary for prevention of CNS relapses. Intrathecal therapy in combination with intermediate-dose (0.5 g/m^2) or high-dose (> 1 g/m^2) methotrexate did effectively prevent CNS relapses in the POG 8106 study and the NHL-BFM 86 trial in the absence of cranial radiotherapy [8,102]. In these protocols, triple drug IT therapy (MTX, cytarabine, steroid) was used. It might be questioned, however, whether triple drug IT therapy is necessary for CNS prevention or whether MTX IT monotherapy in combination with systemic MTX may be enough. The findings of the CCG 551 trial for localized disease other than head and neck tumors suggest that IT therapy may not be necessary at all [111].

TREATMENT STRATEGIES AND RESULTS IN DISTINCT SUBSETS OF LARGE-CELL LYMPHOMAS

Ki-1 ALCL

Table 39.6 summarizes reports on the treatment and results of Ki-1 ALCL in children. Comparable overall results were achieved with quite different treatment strategies. A modified LSA$_2$L$_2$ protocol resulted in an 4-year event-free survival rate of 63% in 12 patients [94]. The protocol of the Milan Tumor Institute consisted of 2 months' induction therapy with prednisone, vincristine, cyclophosphamide, doxorubicin, HD-MTX, cytarabine, bleomycin, 6-thioguanine, and five IT MTX doses, followed by a 22-month maintenance therapy consisting of cycles of MTX/6-mercaptopurine, doxorubicin/vincristine/cyclophosphamide/prednisone and cytarabine/6-thioguanine [112]. Local radiotherapy (30–35 Gy) was applied to bulky disease during the first months of

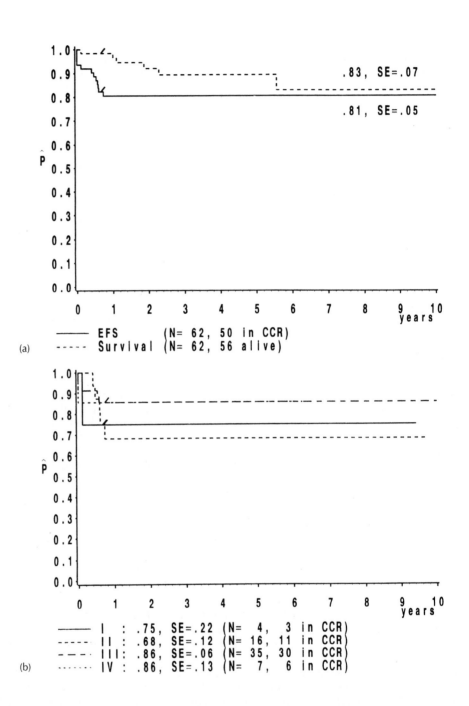

(a)
- —— EFS (N= 62, 50 in CCR)
- ----- Survival (N= 62, 56 alive)

(b)
- —— I : .75, SE=.22 (N= 4, 3 in CCR)
- ----- II : .68, SE=.12 (N= 16, 11 in CCR)
- —-— III: .86, SE=.06 (N= 35, 30 in CCR)
- ······· IV : .86, SE=.13 (N= 7, 6 in CCR)

therapy. With that regimen, 20 of 28 children suffering from Ki-1 ALCL (71%) survived event free [103]. In the NHL studies of the German BFM group patients with Ki-1 ALCL were treated according to the B-cell lymphoma regimen depicted in Figure 39.1. The treatment consisted of 5-day therapy courses, shown in Figure 39.2, which were given with short intervals in between in order to minimize tumor cell regrowth. The treatment intensity was stratified according to stage. Patients with

stage I and II completely resected disease received three courses of therapy while all others received six courses. The therapy courses for patients with stage I, II and III disease contained an intermediate dose (0.5 g/m^2) of MTX while HD-MTX 5 g/m^2 was given to patients with stage IV disease. Furthermore, stage IV patients received a third therapy element composed of high-dose cytarabine, etoposide, dexamethasone and IT therapy. Most of the patients who were defined as having stage IV disease had

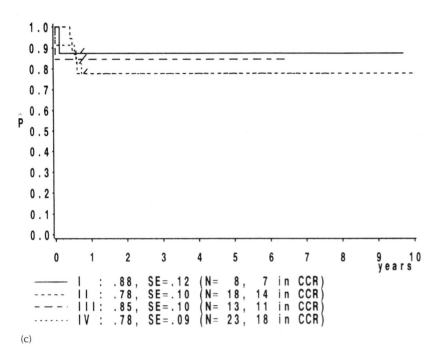

(c)

Figure 39.3 (a) Probability of duration of survival (––), and of event-free survival (-----) for 62 Ki-1 ALCL patients in studies NHL-BFM 83, NHL-BFM 86 and NHL-BFM 90 ($N = 50$ are in continuous CR, and $N = 56$ are alive). Slashes indicate the patients with shortest follow-up. SE, standard error. (b,c) The probability of duration of event-free survival according to stage. (b) Stages according to the St Jude staging system [87] with one modifcation: six patients with multifocal bone involvement without bone marrow disease were included in stage IV. (c) Stages according to the modified Ann Arbor staging system [88]. $P > 0.1$ (log-rank test) for all comparisons between stages. Reproduced by permission of WB Saunders [27].

multiple bone lesions without bone marrow disease (this was a modification of the St Jude staging system). All therapy was delivered within 2 (stage I and II-R) to 5 months. The Kaplan–Meier estimate for 9-year event-free survival in 62 patients enrolled into three consecutive BFM trials was 81% [27]. Treatment outcome according to disease stage was not significantly different (Figure 39.3).Therapy failure was characterized by early progression. Four patients did not enter remission and seven patients suffered from early relapses shortly after cessation of therapy. A similar observation was made when Ki-1 ALCL patients were treated according to the modified B-cell lymphoma protocols cyclophosphamide, oncorin, prednisone, Adriamycin (COPAD) and COPAD plus methotrexate (COPADM) of the French group (these protocols are described in Chapter 37). One-third of patients who failed therapy were nonremitters. Relapses occurred within a mean time of 8 months after achieving remission [113–115]. Interestingly, the time period during which patients are at risk for relapse in Ki-1 ALCL seems to be influenced by the form and duration of the treatment given. Patients treated according to protocols with a longer treatment duration of 24 months (LSA$_2$L$_2$ protocol and the Milan protocol) had a longer period at risk than patients treated in the BFM trials with a short therapy duration. In these long-duration protocols, relapses were observed as late as 47 months after remission [94, 103]. In this respect, Ki-1 ALCL seems to differ from SNCLs in which failure occurs early independent of the treatment strategy applied [1–6,102,107,108].

The value of involved-field radiotherapy which was included in the Milan protocol [112] and the LSA$_2$L$_2$ protocol of the Bologna group [94] is difficult to determine owing to small numbers of patients and the lack of a control group. In the German BFM-NHL studies, however, no local radiotherapy was given. In four patients with incompletely resolved tumors, second-look surgery was performed. Active residual disease was found in one patient in whom the disease subsequently progressed. Devitalized, necrotic tissue was found in only three patients who survived event free. New extramedullary sites other than the primary were the most frequent sites of failure (Tables 39.6 and 39.7). The preliminary conclusion from these observations is that local therapy modalities have little value in the treatment of Ki-1 ALCL patients.

The CNS is rarely involved in Ki-1 ALCL patients at the time of diagnosis or at relapse [27,94,103,113,114] and it is quite clear that cranial radiotherapy is not needed for the prevention of CNS relapses in Ki-1 ALCL patients without overt CNS disease at presentation. Not a single CNS relapse was observed among 137 CNS-negative patients in the French and German studies in which patients received IT therapy (MTX alone or triple therapy) in combination with intermediate dose (0.5 g/m^2) MTX or HD-MTX (3–8 g/m^2) but no cranial irradiation [27,113,114]. Owing to the small number of patients with overt CNS disease at diagnosis, no conclusions can currently be drawn as to optimal treatment in this circumstance.

Table 39.7   Site of treatment failure in childhood large-cell lymphoma

Diagosis (Kiel classification)	No. of patients	Remission failure	Relapses	Site of failure				
				Local	BM	CNS	Other†	Skin
ML, centroblastic*	35	2	0	2	—	—		
ML, immunoblastic B*	7	1	0	1	—	—		
MLBLS*	13	3	0	3	—	—		
ML, immunoblastic T*	2	0	0					
Ki-1 ALCL [27]	62	4	7	3	—	1	6	1
Pleomorphic T-cell, large cell*	6	1	3	2	—	—	2	

* Updated unpublished data of trials NHL-BFM 86 and NHL-BFM 90.
† New extramedullary sites other than the primary and other than CNS.

BM, Bone marrow; CNS, central nervous system; ML, malignant lymphoma; MLBLS, mediastinal large B-cell lymphoma with sclerosis; ALCL, anaplastic large-cell lymphoma.

Pleomorphic T-cell lymphoma of large-cell type

Since large-cell PTCL is rare in childhood, there is little existing information derived from prospectively analyzed treatment strategies. In the series of Gordon et al., 13 of the 22 children with peripheral T-cell lymphoma were encountered by the authors after relapse [34]. The nine newly diagnosed patients had a 2-year relapse-free survival rate of 61% but detailed information regarding the therapy administered are not reported. In the German study, NHL-BFM 86, three of four of the patients who were treated according to the 'ALL-type' protocol for LBLs (see Chapter 38) relapsed. Although the number of patients is small, these data do not suggest that this type of therapy represents optimal treatment for PTCL of postthymic origin. Owing to the clinical and biological relationship between large-cell PTCL and Ki-1 ALCL discussed above, one might question whether the 'B-cell lymphoma type' treatment strategy would provide better therapy for patients suffering from large-cell PTCL. Prospective trials with larger numbers of patients are needed to determine optimal treatment modalities of large-cell PTCL in childhood.

Mediastinal large B-cell lymphoma with sclerosis

No reports confined to mediastinal large B-cell lymphoma with sclerosis (MLBLS) in childhood have been published. In the German study, NHL-BFM 86, nine patients suffering from this disease were enrolled [102]. Two patients erroneously diagnosed as T-lymphoblastic lymphoma responded poorly to the ALL-type regimen for *lymphoblastic*

lymphomas. Both patients died early despite intensified chemotherapy and local radiotherapy. Seven patients with MLBLS who were treated according to the BFM B-cell lymphoma regimen without radiotherapy responded completely and survived event free. It is questionable, however, whether the different strategies employed account for this observation. The marked difference between initial good and poor responders is a frequent observation in reports dealing with adult patients suffering from this entity [61,63,116]. In these studies, progression-free survival for complete responders was reported to be 70–80%, while few patients survived if the initial response was incomplete. The proportion of complete responders, however, was higher with more intensive treatment regimen such as MACOB-B (see Chapter 42) compared to standard CHOP therapy [61,63]. Local radiotherapy was administered to some of the adult patients in all reported series. However, the value of radiation cannot be determined in view of the lack of prospective comparative studies.

Centroblastic lymphoma and immunoblastic lymphoma

In the German trial NHL-BFM 86 a similar response pattern was seen in patients suffering from centroblastic and immunoblastic lymphomas as that observed in patients with MLBLS. One patient each of 14 with centroblastic lymphoma and seven with immunoblastic lymphoma, respectively, had a poor initial response to the first two therapy courses of the B-cell therapy strategy (Figures 39.1 and 39.2) and large viable tumors were resected at second-look surgery. None of these patients could be salvaged. In contrast, none of the patients who achieved complete remission suffered from subsequent relapse.

PATTERN OF THERAPY FAILURE IN DIFFERENT SUBSETS OF LCLS

Table 39.7 summarizes the pattern of treatment failure in the different subsets of childhood LCLs as observed in BFM-NHL studies. Incomplete resolution of local disease was exclusively the site of failure in patients suffering from the B-lineage neoplasms, centroblastic, immunoblastic and MLBLS. No patient who entered remission suffered from a subsequent relapse. In contrast, in Ki-1 ALCL patients, new extramedullary sites distant from the primary were the most frequent sites of failure. Even in two of the four patients who failed to enter remission, new sites of involvement appeared after the first course of therapy whereas the primary manifestations disappeared. Similarly, two of three relapses in patients suffering from large-cell PTCL occurred at new sites. Since the majority of Ki-1 ALCL are derived from the T-cell lineage (and none of the therapy failures had a B-cell immunophenotype), the question arises whether LCLs of T-cell lineage differ from those of B-cell lineage with respect of the pattern of disease spread. Local contiguous growth seems to predominate in LCLs of B-cell lineage whereas discontiguous spread at extramedullary sites is a feature of LCLs of T-cell lineage.

ROLE OF LOCAL THERAPY MODALITIES AND MANAGEMENT OF INCOMPLETE RESPONDERS

Local therapy methods may have a different role in the treatment of different subsets of LCLs. In LCLs of T-cell lineage, local therapy modalities seems to have little value owing to the tendency for these diseases to spread to extramedullary sites. In patients with LCLs of B-cell lineage, easily performed complete resection of a localized tumor may be of advantage, providing a high chance of survival with a minimum of chemotherapy. In patients with large tumors, surgical debulking is of no value, however. In patients in whom complete remission is achieved during chemotherapy, additional involved field radiotherapy is not justified since subsequent relapse is unlikely in LCLs of B-cell lineage, and is more likely to occur at new sites in Ki-1 ALCL and PTCL.

Tumors with incomplete resolution during chemotherapy occur not infrequently in childhood NHL of all histologies. Clinical observations suggest that there are two different categories of incomplete resolution of tumors, especially in patients with LCLs of B-cell lineage (centroblastic, immunoblastic and mediastinal large B-cell lymphoma with sclerosis): an almost complete absence of shrinkage of the tumor mass, or a rapid but incomplete regression. Patients with tumors which responded rapidly but were shown at biopsy to consist of necrotic material containing infiltrates of normal lymphocytes and macrophages, had an excellent prognosis. Whether resection of such tumor remnants contributed to cure or whether the residual tumor had no implications for the course of the patient is difficult to determine. However, surgical resection may be less harmful to patients than the application of radiotherapy to tumor remnants. Tumors in which there was only slight shrinking during chemotherapy were shown to consist of viable tumor when second-look surgery was performed. From the limited experience of the BFM studies, there is little evidence that patients with a poor response to initial chemotherapy can be rescued by local therapy modalities. One patient with a large intrahepatic residual centroblastic lymphoma was observed who had long-term progression-free survival after local radiotherapy and intensified chemotherapy. In this patient, a needle biopsy had been performed, which revealed necrotic material. In six patients with persistent viable tumor, the disease progressed rapidly despite radiotherapy and intensified chemotherapy. High-dose chemotherapy and autologous hematological rescue was found to be of value for children with diffuse NHL after partial but incomplete response to firstline induction therapy [117]. Whether this approach provides effective salvage for children with poorly responding LCLs of B-cell lineage remains to be determined. The casual clinical observation of an almost absent response to conventional chemotherapy in those patients suggests highly resistant disease.

Second-look surgery is certainly less than optimal to distinguish patients at risk for subsequent progression while negative results from needle biopsies can be misleading. Imaging methods such as gallium-67 single photon emission computed tomography, MRI or immunoscintigrapy using radionuclide-labeled anti-CD30 antibodies, or monitoring of residual clonal lymphoma cells in the peripheral blood and/or bone marrow using molecular biological methods may contribute to the detection of persistent active tumor during chemotherapy as discussed in Chapters 4, 25 and 26. Prospective studies are warranted to investigate the value of such methods for monitoring treatment response in childhood LCL in order to allow for early adjustment of treatment modalities before progression of the disease takes place.

Course after relapse

Little information is available on salvage regimens

and results in children with LCLs who suffered a relapse. As mentioned above in the German BFM-NHL studies, children with centroblastic, immunoblastic and MLBLS who were unsuccessfully treated failed to enter remission, while complete responders did not suffer from relapse.

A distinct feature of Ki-1 ALCL is that patients who relapse respond well to salvage therapy. In the German BFM-NHL studies and in the series of Vecchi et al., all relapsed patients who received a salvage therapy achieved a second remission [27,94]. The course after relapse seems to be variable, however. While a rapidly fatal course with a second relapse and death shortly after autologous bone marrow transplantation (BMT) was observed, some patients are in long-term second remissions after treatment with conventional chemotherapy alone. Spontaneous regression and a long-term waxing and waning course without rescue therapy was also observed. Therefore, a uniform therapy approach for Ki-1 ALCL patients who relapse is difficult to devise. In particular, the indications as well as the type of BMT still need to be determined. In the German BFM series, autologous BMT was performed in three patients and allogeneic BMT in one after second remission had been achieved using the HD-MTX and cytarabine-containing courses depicted in Figure 39.2. Three of these four patients are long-term survivors. Anecdotal observations suggest that even after repeated relapses, long-term remissions can be achieved with salvage regimens that include BMT [118].

As observed in patients with Ki-1 ALCL, most children with peripheral T-cell lymphoma who relapsed achieved a second remission with conventional chemotherapy in the series of Gordon et al. [34]. However, without subsequent BMT, relapse-free survival in second remission was poor. BMT seems to improve the survival chance after relapse considerably. Autologous or allogeneic BMT using a thioTEPA/etoposide/total body irradiation preparative regimen resulted in an 89% 2-year relapse-free survival estimate in a prospectively analyzed series of nine patients of whom eight were transplanted after relapse [119].

Follow-up studies

Appropriate intervals between follow-up studies for LCLs includes monthly examinations in the first 6–9 months after cessation of treatment and 2-monthly assessment during the second year, after which relapse is unlikely, except for patients with PTCL. Follow-up studies should include not only examina-

tion of known sites of previous disease but also complete physical examination, especially in patients with Ki-1 ALCL and PTCL. Routine bone marrow punctures and spinal taps are not necessary, however. Monitoring of serum levels of soluble IL-2 receptor and CD30 antigen may be of value for early detection of relapses in Ki-1 ALCL patients, although IL-2 levels also increase during infections [91]. After the second year, patients should be seen every 6 months to 1 year to ascertain that no long-term side-effects have developed and to ensure that accurate records are kept of survival duration.

Summary and outlook

Various chemotherapy protocols based on quite different strategies have been proven to be efficacious for the treatment of children suffering from LCLs. In this subgroup of childhood NHL, the type of therapy strategy – ALL type versus B-cell lymphoma type – seems to have less impact on treatment outcome as compared to LBLs and SNCLs. A therapy strategy based on short-pulse therapy protocols used for B-cell lymphomas provides highly effective treatment for all subsets of LCLs, irrespective of their immunological lineage derivation. One potential advantage of the protocols being used for B-cell lymphomas is their short duration. The time pattern of therapy failure in LCLs suggests that relapse is the result of chemotherapy resistance rather than the escape of chemotherapy-sensitive cells. Prolonged therapy duration may postpone but not inhibit the clinical manifestations of relapse. Steroids, vincristine and oxazaphosphorine drugs are included in all effective therapy protocols. Anthracyclines were included in some effective protocols at high cumulative doses of more than 300 mg/m^2 but such doses are associated with considerable risk of impaired cardiac function [110]. Protocols including cytarabine, epipodophyllotoxins, and intermediate or high doses of MTX, but lower cumulative doses of anthracylines are highly effective. Cranial radiotherapy is not needed for the prevention of CNS relapse in CNS-negative patients when IT therapy in combination with at least intermediate dose systemic MTX therapy is used. The role of local therapy modalities in the treatment of LCLs in children is difficult to determine, owing to the lack of prospective comparative studies. In LCLs of T-cell lineage, local therapy methods seems to contribute little to the cure of the patients because of the tendency for discontiguous spread of the disease. LCLs of B-cell lineage may have a more locally contiguous growth pattern and complete resection of a small localized tumor may be of advantage, providing a high chance of survival with a minimum of chemotherapy. In patients with large tumors, however, debulking is of no value. The use of involved-field radiotherapy seems to be unnecessary, based on the similarly good results achieved in studies in which radiation was not used. Most tumors with a good partial but incomplete resolution during chemotherapy have been shown to consist of necrotic material and do not compromise prognosis. Surgical resection to exclude the presence of viable lymphoma may be less harmful to the patients than a policy of radiating all tumor remnants in patients. The likelihood that radiation would, in any event, not be useful is supported by its lack of utility in patients with poor initial response to chemotherapy and persistent viable tumor. High-dose chemotherapy and hematological rescue may be an option for these patients. There is evidence that patients with Ki-1 ALCL or peripheral T-cell lymphoma who relapse respond well to salvage therapy programs and long-term second remissions are possible.

New therapy options may become available in the near future, especially for the treatment of Ki-1 ALCL. 13-*cis*-Retinoic acid has induced cellular differentiation and durable remission in a case of refractory cutaneous Ki-1 lymphoma [120]. Since the Ki-1 (CD30) antigen is absent in most normal tissues [17], this antigen could be a tumor-specific target for immunotherapy in Ki-1-antigen-positive neoplasms. An anti-CD30 immunotoxin has induced responses in refractory Hodgkin's disease [121] and complete remissions in severe combined immunodeficiency mice xenografted with a chemotherapy-resistant human Ki-1 ALCL [122]. The Ki-1 molecule has been shown to be related to the nerve growth factor receptor superfamily [123] and the corresponding ligand has been cloned and found to be a member of the cytokine family with homology to tumor necrosis factor [124]. The ligand has been shown to be able to induce apoptotic cell death in Ki-1 ALCL cell lines [125]. These reagents could be of potential value in the treatment of Ki-1 ALCL.

References

1. Müller-Weihrich S, Henze G, Jobke A, et al. BFM-Studie 1975/81 zur Behandlung der Non-Hodgkin-Lymphome hoher Malignität bei Kindern und Jugendlichen. *Klin. Pädiatr.* 1982, **194**: 219–225.
2. Anderson JR, Wilson JF, Jenkin DT, et al. Childhood non-Hodgkin's lymphoma. The results of a randomized therapeutic trial comparing a 4-drug regimen (COMP) with a 10-drug regimen (LSA$_2$-L$_2$). *N. Engl. J. Med.* 1983, **308**: 559–565.
3. Müller-Weihrich S, Beck J, Henze G, et al. BFM-Studie 1981/83 zur Behandlung hochmaligner Non-Hodgkin-Lymphome bei Kindern: Ergebnisse einer nach histologisch-immunologischem Typ und Ausbreitungsstadiumstratefizierten Therapie. *Klin. Pädiatr.* 1984, **196**: 135–142.
4. Patte C, Philip T, Rodary C, et al. Improved survival rate in children with stage III and IV B-cell NHL and leukemia using multi-agent chemotherapy: Results of a study of 114 children from the French Paediatric Oncology Society. *J. Clin. Oncol.* 1986, **4**: 1219–1226.
5. Patte C, Philip T, Rodary C, et al. High survival rate in advanced-stage B-cell lymphomas and leukemias without CNS involvement with a short intensive polychemotherapy: Results from the French Pediatric Oncology Society of a randomized trial of 216 children. *J. Clin. Oncol.* 1991, **9**(1): 123–132.
6. Anderson JR, Jenkin DT, Wilson JF, et al. Long-term follow-up of patients treated with COMP or LSA$_2$-L$_2$ therapy for childhood non-Hodgkin's lymphoma: A report of CCG-551 from the Childrens Cancer Group. *J. Clin. Oncol.* 1993, **11**: 1024–1032.
7. Sullivan MP, Boyett J, Pullen J, et al. Pediatric Oncology Group experience with modified LSA$_2$-L$_2$ therapy in 107 children with non-Hodgkin's lymphoma (Burkitt's lymphoma excluded). *Cancer* 1985, **55**: 323–336.
8. Sullivan MP, Brecher M, Ramirez I, et al. High-dose cyclophosphamide – high-dose methotrexate with coordinated intrathecal therapy for advanced nonlymphoblastic lymphoma of childhood. *Am. J. Ped. Hematol. Oncol.* 1991, **13**(3): 288–295.
9. Bunin NJ, Hvizdala E, Link M, et al. Mediastinal nonlymphoblastic lymphomas in children: A clinicopathologic study. *J. Clin. Oncol.* 1986, **4**: 154–159.
10. Hvizdala EV, Berard C, Callihan T, et al. Nonlymphoblastic lymphoma in children – histology and stage-related response to therapy: A Pediatric Oncology Group Study. *J. Clin. Oncol.* 1991, **9**(7): 1189–1195.
11. Magrath IT, Janus C, Edwards BK, et al. An effective therapy for both undifferentiated (including Burkitt's) lymphomas and lymphoblastic lymphomas in children and young adults. *Blood* 1984, **63**: 1102–1111.
12. Rappaport H. Tumors of the hematopoietic system. *Atlas of Tumor Pathology,* Section III, Fasc. 8. Washington, DC: Armed Forces Institute of Pathology, 1966.
13. The Non-Hodgkin's Lymphoma Pathological Classification Project. National Cancer Institute sponsored study of classifications of non-Hodgkin's lymphomas: Summary and description of a working formulation for clinical usage. *Cancer* 1982, **49**: 2112–2135.
14. Lukes RJ, Collins RD: New approaches to the classification of the lymphomata. *Br. J. Cancer* 1975, **31** (Suppl. II): 1–28.
15. Gerard-Marchant R, Hamlin J, Lennert K, et al. Classification of non-Hodgkin's lymphomas. (Letter to the Editor). *Lancet* 1974, II: 406.
16. Lennert K, Feller AC. *Histopathology of Non-Hodgkin's Lymphomas* (based on the updated Kiel Classification). Berlin: Springer-Verlag, 1992, pp. 157–161.
17. Stein H, Mason DY, Gerdes et al. The expression of the Hodgkin's disease associated antigen Ki-1 in reactive and neoplastic lymphoid tissue: Evidence

that Reed–Sternberg cells and histiocytic malignancies are derived from activated lymphoid cells. *Blood* 1985, **66**: 848–858.

18. Schwab U, Stein H, Gerdes J, et al. Production of a monoclonal antibody specific for Hodgkin and Sternberg–Reed cells of Hodgkin's disease and a subset of normal lymphoid cells. *Nature* 1982, **299**: 65.

19. Kadin ME, Sako D, Berliner N, et al. Childhood Ki-1 lymphoma presenting with skin lesions and peripheral lymphadenopathy. *Blood* 1986, **68**: 1042–1049.

20. Agnarsson BA, Kadin ME: Ki-1 positive large cell lymphoma: A morphologic and immunologic study of 19 cases. *Am. J. Surg. Pathol.* 1988, **21**: 264–274.

21. Chott A, Kaserer K, Augustin I, et al. Ki-1-positive large cell lymphoma. A clinico-pathologic study of 41 cases. *Am. J. Surg. Pathol.* 1990, **14**: 439–448.

22. Bucsky P, Feller AC, Beck JD, et al. Zur Frage der Definition der malignen Histiozytose und des großzelligen anaplastischen (Ki-1) Lymphoms im Kindesalter. *Klin. Pädiatr.* 1989, **201**: 233–236.

23. Nakamura S, Takagi N, Kojima M, et al. Clinico-pathologic study of large cell anaplastic lymphoma (Ki-1-positive large cell lymphoma) among the Japanese. *Cancer* 1991, **68**: 118–129.

24. O'Connor NTJ, Stein H, Gatter KC, et al. Genotypic analysis of large cell lymphomas which express the Ki-1 antigen. *Histopathology* 1987, **11**: 733–740.

25. Griesser H, Tkachuk D, Reis MD, et al. Gene rearrangements and translocations in lymphoproliferative diseases. *Blood* 1989, **73**: 1402–1415.

26. Schnitzer B, Roth MS, Hyder DM, et al. Ki-1 lymphomas in children. *Cancer* 1988, **61**: 1213–1221.

27. Reiter A, Schrappe M, Tiemann M, et al. A successful treatment strategy for Ki-1 anaplastic large cell lymphoma of childhood. A prospective analysis of 62 patients enrolled in three consecutive BFM Group Studies. *J. Clin. Oncol.* 1994, **12**: 899–908.

28. Ralfkiaer E, Delsol G, O'Connor NTJ, et al. Malignant lymphomas of true histiocytic origin. A clinical, histological, immunophenotypic and genotypic study. *J. Pathol.* 1990, **160**: 9–17.

29. Fischer P, Nacheva E, Mason DY, et al. A Ki-1 (CD 30)-positive human cell line (Karpas 299) established from a high-grade non-Hodgkin's lymphoma, showing a 2;5 translocation and rearrangement of the T-cell receptor β-chain gene. *Blood* 1988, **72**(1): 234–240.

30. Rimokh R, Magaud JP, Berger F, et al. A translocation involving a specific breakpoint (q35) on chromosome 5 is characteristic of anaplastic large cell lymphoma ('Ki-1 lymphoma'). *Br. J. Haematol.* 1989, **71**: 31–36.

31. Kaneko Y, Frizzera G, Edamura S, et al. A novel translocation, t(2;5)(p23;q35), in childhood phagocytic large T-cell lymphoma mimicking malignant histiocytosis. *Blood* 1989, **73**: 806–813.

32. Le Beau MM, Bitter MA, Larson RA, et al. The t(2;5)(p23;q35): A recurring chromosomal abnormality in Ki-1-positive anaplastic large cell lymphoma. *Leukemia* 1989, **3**: 866–870.

33. Mason DY, Bastard C, Rimokh R, et al. CD30-positive large cell lymphomas ('Ki-1 lymphoma') are associated with a chromosomal translocation involving 5q35. *Br. J. Haematol.* 1990, **74**: 161–168.

34. Gordon BG, Weisenburger DD, Warkentin PI, et al. Peripheral T-cell lymphoma in childhood and adolescence. A clinicopathologic study of 22 patients. *Cancer* 1993, **71**: 257–263.

35. Ladanyi M, Parsa NZ, Offit K, et al. Clonal cytogenetic abnormalities in Hodgkin's disease. *Genes Chromosom. Cancer* 1991, **3**: 294–299.

36. Stansfeld AG, Diebold J, Kapanci Y, et al. Updated Kiel Classification for lymphomas. *Lancet* 1988, **I**: 292–293.

37. Kadin ME. Ki-1-positive anaplastic large-cell lymphoma: A clinicopathologic entity? *J. Clin. Oncol.* 1991, **9**: 533–536.

38. Chan JKC, NG CS, Hui PK, et al. Anaplastic large cell Ki-1 lymphoma. Delineation of two morphological types. *Histopathology* 1989, **15**: 11–34.

39. Penny RJ, Blaustein JC, Longtine JA, et al. Ki-1-positive large cell lymphomas, a heterogenous group of neoplasms. Morphologic, immunophenotypic, genotypic, and clinical features of 24 cases. *Cancer* 1991, **68**: 362–373.

40. Bitter MA, Franklin WA, Larson RA, et al. Morphology in Ki-1 (CD30)-positive non-Hodgkin's lymphoma is correlated with clinical features and the presence of a unique chromosomal abnormality, t(2;5) (p23;q35). *Am. J. Surg. Pathol.* 1990, **14**: 305–316.

41. Delsol G, Al Saati T, Gatter KC, et al. Coexpression of epithelial membrane antigen (EMA), Ki-1, and interleukin-2 receptor by anaplastic large cell lymphomas. Diagnostic value in so-called malignant histiocytosis. *Am. J. Pathol.* 1988, **130**: 59–70.

42. Heitger A, Gadner H, Bucsky P, et al. Das großzellige anaplastische Lymphom im Kindesalter – Klinische Erfahrungen bei einer histologisch neu definierten Entität. *Klin. Pädiatr.* 1989, **201**: 237–241.

43. Greer JP, Kinney MC, Collins RD, et al. Clinical features of 31 patients with Ki-1 anaplastic large-cell lymphoma. *J. Clin. Oncol.* 1991, **9** (Suppl. 4): 539–547.

44. Jones DB, Gerdes J, Stein H, et al. An investigation of Ki-1 positive large cell lymphoma with antibodies reactive with tissue macrophages. *Hematol. Oncol.* 1986, **4**: 315–322.

45. Carbone A, Gloghini A, De-Re V, et al. Histopathologic, immunophenotypic, and genotypic analysis of Ki-1 anaplastic large cell lymphomas that express histiocyte-associated antigens. *Cancer* 1990, **66**: 2547–2556.

46. Kamesaki H, Koya M, Miwa H, et al. Malignant histiocytosis with rearrangement of the heavy chain gene and evidence of monocyte–macrophage lineage. *Cancer* 1988, **62**: 1306–1309.

47. Carbone A, Gloghini A, Volpe R: Immunohistochemistry of Hodgkin and non-Hodgkin lymphomas with emphasis on the diagnostic significance of the BNH9 antibody reactivity with anaplastic large cell (CD30 positive) lymphomas. *Cancer* 1992, **70**: 2691–2698.

48. Kaudewitz P, Stein H, Dallenbach F, et al. Primary

and secondary cutaneous Ki-1$^+$(CD30$^+$) anaplastic large cell lymphomas: Morphologic, immunohistologic, and clinical characteristics. *Am. J. Path.* 1989, **135**: 359–367.

49. Davis TH, Morton CC, Miller-Cassman R, et al. Hodgkin's disease, lymphomatoid papulosis, and cutaneous T-cell lymphoma derived from a common T-cell clone. *N. Engl. J. Med.* 1992, **326**: 1115–1122.

50. Bucsky P, Feller AC, Reiter A, et al. Low grade malignant Non-Hodgkin's lymphomas and peripheral pleomorphic T-cell lymphomas in childhood – a BFM Study Group report. *Klin. Pädiatr.* 1990, **202**: 258–261.

51. Reiter A, Tiemann M, Ludwig WD, et al. für die BFM Studiengruppe. Therapiestudie NHL-BFM 90 zur Behandlung maligner Non-Hodgkin-Lymphoma bei Kindern und Jugendlichen. Teil 1: Klassifikation und Einteilung in strategische Therapiegruppen. *Klin. Pädiatr.* (in press).

52. Suchi T, Lennert K, Tu LY, et al. Histopathology and immunohistochemistry of peripheral T-cell lymphomas: A proposal for their classification. *J. Clin. Pathol.* 1987, **40**: 995–1015.

53. Miller JB, Variakojis D, Bitran JD, et al. Diffuse histiocytic lymphoma with sclerosis: A clinicopathologic entity with frequent occurrence of superior venacaval obstruction. *Blood* 1978, 263.

54. Miller JB, Variakojis D, Bitran JD, et al. Diffuse histiocytic lymphoma with sclerosis: A clinicopathologic entity frequently causing superior venacaval obstruction. *Cancer* 1981, **47**: 748–756.

55. Levitt LJ, Aisenberg AC, Harris NL, et al.: Primary non-Hodgkin's lymphoma of the mediastinum. *Cancer* 1982, **50**: 2486–2492.

56. Trump DL, Mann RB. Diffuse large cell and undifferentiated lymphomas with prominent mediastinal involvement. A poor prognostic subset of patients with non-Hodgkin's lymphoma. *Cancer* 1982, **50**: 277–282.

57. Perrone T, Frizzera G, Rosai J: Mediastinal diffuse large-cell lymphoma with sclerosis. *Am. J. Surg. Pathol.* 1986, **10**: 176–191.

58. Addis BJ, Isaacson PG. Large cell lymphoma of the mediastinum: A B-cell tumor of probable thymic origin. *Histopathology* 1986, **10**: 379–390.

59. Jacobson JO, Aisenberg AC, Lamarre L, et al. Mediastinal large cell lymphoma. An uncommon subset of adult lymphoma curable with combined modality therapy. *Cancer* 1988, **62**: 1893–1898.

60. Al-Sharabati M, Chittal S, Duga-Neulat I, et al. Primary anterior mediastinal B-cell lymphoma. *Cancer* 1991, **67**: 2579–2587.

61. Todeschini G, Ambrosetti A, Meneghini V, et al. Mediastinal diffuse large-cell lymphoma with sclerosis: A condition with a poor prognosis. *Am J. Clin. Oncol.* 1990, **8**: 804–808.

62. Lavabre-Bertrand T, Donadio D, Fegueux N, et al. A study of 15 cases of primary mediastinal lymphoma of B-cell type. *Cancer* 1992, **69**: 2561–2566.

63. Lazzarino M, Orlandi E, Paulli M, et al. Primary mediastinal B-cell lymphoma with sclerosis: An aggressive tumor with distinctive clinical and pathologic features. *J. Clin. Oncol.* 1993, **11**(12): 2306–2313.

64. Menestrina F, Chilosi M, Bonetti F, et al. Mediastinal large-cell lymphoma of B-type, with sclerosis: Histopathological and immunohistochemical study of eight cases. *Histopathology* 1986, **10**: 589–600.

65. Möller P, Moldenhauer G, Momburg F, et al. Mediastinal lymphoma of clear cell type is a tumor corresponding to terminal steps of B-cell differentiation. *Blood* 1987, **69**: 1087–1095.

66. Scarpa A, Bonetti F, Menestrina F, et al.: Mediastinal large-cell lymphoma with sclerosis. Genotypic analysis establishes its B nature. *Virchows Arch. A* 1987, **412**: 17–21.

67. Lamarre L, Jacobson JO, Aisenberg AC, et al. Primary large cell lymphoma of the mediastinum. A histologic and immunophenotypic study of 29 cases. *Am. J. Surg. Pathol.* 1989, **13**: 730–739.

68. Davis RE, Dorfman RF, Warnke RA. Primary large-cell lymphoma of the thymus: A diffuse B-cell neoplasm presenting as primary mediastinal lymphoma. *Hum. Pathol.* 1990, **21**: 1262–1268.

69. Franssila KO, Heiskala MK, Rapola J. Non-Hodgkin's lymphomas in childhood. A clinicopathologic and epidemiologic study in Finland. *Cancer* 1987, **59**: 1837–1846.

70. Nathwani BN, Griffith RC, Kelly DR, et al. A morphologic study of childhood lymphoma of the diffuse 'Histiocytic' type. *Cancer* 1987, **59**: 1138–1142.

71. Lee S-H, Su I-J, Chen R-L, et al. A pathologic study of childhood lymphoma in Taiwan with special reference to peripheral T-cell lymphoma and the association with Epstein–Barr viral infection. *Cancer* 1991, **68**: 1954–1962.

72. Murphy SB, Fairclough DL, Hutchison RE, et al. Non-Nodgkin's lymphomas of childhood: An analysis of the histology, staging, and response to treatment of 338 cases at a single institution. *J. Clin. Oncol.* 1989, **7**: 186–193.

73. Haaf HG, Kaatsch P, Michaelis J. Jahresbericht 1992 des Deutschen Kinderkrebs registers. *IMSD*, 1993.

74. Hutchison RE, Fairclough DL, Holt H, et al. Clinical significance of histology and immunophenotype in childhood diffuse large cell lymphoma. *Am. J. Clin. Pathol.* 1991, **95**: 787–793.

75. Anagnostopoulos I, Herbst H, Niedobitek G, et al. Demonstration of monoclonal EBV genomes in Hodgkin's disease and Ki-1 positive anaplastic large cell lymphoma by combined Southern blot and *in situ* hybridization. *Blood* 1989, **74**: 810–816.

76. Herbst H, Dallenbach F, Hummel M, et al. Epstein–Barr virus DNA and latent gene products in Ki-1 (CD30)-positive anaplastic large cell lymphomas. *Blood* 1991, **78**(10): 2666–2673.

77. Anagnostopoulos I, Hummel M, Kaudewitz P, et al. Detection of HTLV-1 proviral sequences in CD30-positive large cell cutaneous T-cell lymphomas. *Am. J. Pathol.* 1990, **137**: 1317–1322.

78. Risdall RJ, McKenna RW, Nesbit ME, et al. Virus-associated hemophagocytic syndrome. A benign histiocytic proliferation distinct from malignant histiocytosis. *Cancer* 1979, **44**: 993–1002.

79. Falini B, Pileri S, De Solas I, et al. Peripheral T-cell

lymphoma associated with hemophagocytic syndrome. *Blood* 1990, **75**: 434–444.

80. Hsu S-M, Raine L, Fanger H. Use of avidin–biotin–peroxidase complex (ABC) in immunoperoxidase techniques: A comparison between ABC and unlabeled antibody (PAP) procedures. *J Histochem. Cytochem.* 1981, **29**: 577–580.

81. Cordell JL, Falini B, Erber WN, et al. Immuno-enzymatic labeling of monoclonal antibodies using immune complexes of alkaline phosphatase and mono-clonal anti-alkaline phosphatase (APAAP) complexes. *J Histochem. Cytochem.* 1984, **32**: 219–229.

82. Schwarting R, Gerdes J, Durkop H, et al. BER-H2: A new anti-Ki-1 (CD30) monoclonal antibody directed at a formal-resistant epitope. *Blood* 1989, **74**: 1678–1689.

83. Hoane BR, Shields AF, Porter BA, et al. Detection of lymphomatous bone marrow involvement with magnetic resonance imaging. *Blood* 1991, **78**(3): 728–738.

84. Bekerman C, Port RB, Pang E, et al. Scintigraphic evaluation of childhood malignancies by 67-Ga-citrate. *Radiolgy* 1978, **127**: 719–725.

85. Parker BR: Imaging studies in the diagnosis of pediatric malignancies. In Pizzo PA, Poplack DG (eds) *Principles and Practice of Pediatric Oncology.* Philadelphia: JB Lippincott Company, 1989, pp. 127–148.

86. Falini B, Flenghi L, Fedeli L, et al. *In vivo* targeting of Hodgkin and Reed–Sternberg cells of Hodgkin's disease with monoclonal antibody Ber-H2 (CD 30): immunohistological evidence. *Br. J. Hematol.* 1992, **82**: 38–45.

87. Murphy SB: Classification, staging and end results of treatment in childhood non-Hodgkin's lymphoma: Dissimilarities from lymphomas in adults. *Semin. Oncol.* 1980, **7**(3): 332–339.

88. Lister TA, Crowther D, Sutcliffe SB, et al. Report of a committee convened to discuss the evaluation and staging of patients with Hodgkin's disease: Cotswolds meeting. *J. Clin. Oncol.* 1989, **7**: 1630–1636.

89. Magrath I, Lee YJ, Anderson T, et al. Prognostic factors in Burkitt's lymphoma: Importance of total tumor burden. *Cancer* 1980, **45**: 1507–1515.

90. Wagner DK, Kiwanuka J, Edwards BL, et al. Soluble interleukin II receptor levels in patients with undif-ferentiated and lymphoblastic lymphomas. *J. Clin. Oncol.* 1987, **5**: 1262–1274.

91. Pui CH, Ip SH, Kung P, et al. High serum interleukin-2 receptor levels are related to advanced disease and a poor outcome in childhood non-Hodgkin's lym-phoma. *Blood* 1987, **70**: 624–628.

92. Stets R, Müller-Weihrich St. Serum soluble interleukin-2 receptor levels in childhood non-Hodgkin's lym-phoma. *Med. Pediatr. Oncol.* 1992, **20**: 443.

93. Josimovic-Alasevic O, Dürkop H, Schwarting R, et al. Ki-1 (CD 30) antigen is released by Ki-1-positive tumor cells *in vitro* and *in vivo*. I. Partial characteriza-tion of soluble Ki-1 antigen and detection of the antigen in cell culture supernatants and in serum by an enzyme-linked immunosorbent assay. *Eur. J. Immunol.* 1898, **19**: 157–162.

94. Vecchi V, Burnelli R, Pileri S, et al. Anaplastic large cell lymphoma (Ki-1 +/ CD30+) in childhood. *Med. Pediatr. Oncol.* 1993, **21**: 402–410.

95. Newcom SR, Kadin ME, Ansari AA. Production of transforming growth factor-beta activity by Ki-1 positive lymphoma cells and analysis of its role in the regulation of Ki-1 positive lymphoma growth. *Am. J. Pathol.* 1988, **131**: 569–577.

96. Kadin ME, Cavaille-Coll MW, Morton CC: Tumor progression in Ki-1+ cutaneous T-cell lymphomas is related to escape from inhibition by transforming growth factor-beta. *Blood* 1990, **76** (Suppl. 1): 354a.

97. Agematsu K, Takeuchi S, Ichikawa M, et al. Spon-taneous production of interleukin-6 by Ki-1-positive large-cell anaplastic lymphoma with extensive bone destruction. *Blood* 1991, **77**(10): 2299–2301.

98. Merz H, Fliedner A, Orscheschek K, et al. Cytokine expression in T-cell lymphomas and Hodgkin's dis-ease. Its possible implication in autocrine or paracrine production as a potential basis for neoplastic growth. *Am. J. Pathol.* 1991, **139**(5): 1173–1180.

99. Merz H, Houssiau FA, Orscheschek K, et al. Inter-leukin-9 expression in human malignant lymphomas: Unique association with Hodgkin's disease and large cell anaplastic lymphoma. *Blood* 1991, **78**: 1311–1317.

100. Nishihira H, Tanaka Y, Kigasawa H, et al. Ki-1 lymphoma producing G-CSF. *Br. J. Haematol.* 1991, **80**: 556–557.

101. Arber D, Bilbao J, Bassion S: Large-cell anaplastic (Ki-1-positive) lymphoma complicated by dissemi-nated intravascular coagulation. *Arch. Pathol. Lab. Med.* 1991, **115**: 188–192.

102. Reiter A, Schrappe M, Parwaresch R, et al. Non-Hodgkin's-lymphomas of childhood and adoles-cence: Results of a therapy stratified for biological subentities and stage. A report of the BFM group. *J. Clin. Oncol.* 1995, **13**: 359–372.

103. Massimino M, Gasparini M, Rottoli L, et al. Primary anaplastic large cell non-Hodgkin lymphoma (ALC-NHL) in children. *Fifth International Conference on Malignant Lymphoma*, Lugano, 9–12 June 1993, p. 63 (abstract 85).

104. Wollner N, Burchenal JH, Lieberman PH, et al. Non-Hodgkin's lymphoma in children. A comparative study of two modalities of therapy. *Cancer* 1976, **37**: 123–134.

105. Dahl GV, Rivera G, Pui CH, et al. A novel treatment of childhood lymphoblastic non-Hodgkin's lymphoma: Early and intermittent use of teniposide plus cytarabine. *Blood* 1985, **66**: 1110.

106. Ziegler JL. Treatment results of 54 American patients with Burkitt's lymphoma: A clinicopathologic study of 30 cases. I. Clinical factors relating to prolonged survival. *Am. J. Med.* 1975, **58**: 314–321.

107. Murphy SB, Bowman WP, Abromowitch M, et al. Results of treatment of advanced-stage Burkitt's lymphoma and B-cell (SIg+) acute lymphoblastic leukemia with high-dose fractionated cyclophos-phamide and coordinated high-dose methotrexate and cytarabine. *J. Clin. Oncol.* 1986, **4**: 1732–1739.

108. Reiter A, Schrappe M, Ludwig WD, et al. Favorable outcome of B-cell acute lymphoblastic leukemia in

childhood: A report of three consecutive studies of the BFM group. *Blood* 1992, **80**: 2471–2478.

109. Weinstein HJ, Lack EE, Cassady RJ. APO therapy for malignant lymphoma of large cell 'histiocytic' type of childhood: Analysis of treatment results for 29 patients. *Blood* 1984, **64**(2): 422–426.

110. Lipshultz SE, Colan SD, Gelber RD, et al. Late cardiac effects of doxorubicin therapy for acute lymphoblastic leukemia in childhood. *N. Engl. J. Med.* 1991, **324**: 808–815.

111. Meadows AT, Sposto R, Jenkin RDT, et al. Similar efficacy of 6 and 18 months of therapy with four drugs (COMP) for localized non-Hodgkin's lymphoma of children: A report from the Childrens Cancer Study Group. *J. Clin. Oncol.* 1989, **7**: 92–99.

112. Gasparini M, Lombardi F, Gianni C, et al. Childhood non-Hodgkin's lymphoma: Prognostic relevance of clinical stages and histologic subgroups. *Am. J. Pediatr. Hematol.* 1983, **5**: 161–171.

113. Brugieres L, Caillaud JM, Patte C, et al. Malignant histiocytosis: Therapeutic results in 27 children treated with a single polychemotherapy regimen. *Med. Pediatr. Oncol.* 1989, **17**: 193–196.

114. Brugieres L, Patte C, Pacquement H, et al. Large cell anaplastic lymphoma in children: Therapeutic results in 75 patients treated with 3 consecutive polychemotherapy regimens. *Fifth International Conference on Malignant Lymphoma*, Lugano, 9–12 June 1993, p. 64 (Abstract 86).

115. Pinkerton CR, Gerrard M. Large cell anaplastic lymphoma in children. Outcome using high-grade B-ell chemotherapy. *Fifth International Conference on Malignant Lymphoma*, Lugano, 9–12 June 1993, p. 62 (Abstract 82).

116. Kirn D, Mauch P, Shaffer K, et al. Large-cell and immunoblastic lymphoma of the mediastinum: Prognostic features and treatment outcome in 57 patients. *J. Clin. Oncol.* 1993, **11**: 1336–1343.

117. Philip T, Hartmann O, Biron P, et al. High-dose therapy and autologous bone marrow transplantation in partial remission after first-line induction therapy for diffuse Non-Hodgkin's lymphoma. *J. Clin. Oncol.* 1988, **6**: 1118–1124.

118. Chakravarti V, Kamani NR, Bayever E, et al. Bone marrow transplantation for childhood Ki-1 lymphoma. *J. Clin. Oncol.* 1990, **8**: 657–660.

119. Gordon BG, Warkentin PI, Weisenburger DD, et al. Bone marrow transplantation for peripheral T-cell lymphoma in children and adolescents. *Blood* 1992, **80**(11): 2938–2942.

120. Chow JM, Cheng AL, Su IJ, et al. 13-*cis*-Retinoic acid induces cellular differentiation and durable remission in refractory cutaneous Ki-1 lymphoma. *Cancer* 1991, **67**: 2490–2494.

121. Falini B, Bolognesi A, Flenghi L, et al. Response of refractory Hodgkin's disease to monoclonal anti-CD 30 immunotoxin. *Lancet* 1992, **339**: 1195–1196.

122. Pasqualucci L, Wasik MA, Teicher B, et al. In vivo antitumor activity of Ber-H2 (CD 30)/Saporin immunotoxin against human Ki-1+ anaplastic large cell lymphoma in SCID mice. *Blood* 1993, **82**(Suppl. 1): 534a.

123. Dürkop H, Latza U, Hummel M, et al. Molecular cloning and expression of a new member of the nerve growth factor receptor family that is characteristic for Hodgkin's disease. *Cell* 1992, **68**: 421–427.

124. Smith CA, Gruss H-J, Davis T, et al. CD 30 antigen, a marker for Hodgkin's lymphoma, is a receptor whose ligand defines an emerging family of cytokines with homology to TNF. *Cell* 1993, **73**: 1349.

125. Gruss HK, Williams D, Armitage R, et al. CD 30 ligand: Molecular cloning and pathobiological role in CD30 positive malignant lymphomas. *Fifth International Conference on Malignant Lymphoma*, Lugano, 9–12 June 1993, p. 24 (Abstract 7).

CHAPTER 40

Diffuse small-cell lymphomas

SANDRA J. HORNING

Introduction

The diffuse small-cell lymphomas represent a diverse group of clinicopathologic entities that have in common a B-cell lymphoid origin, an initially indolent course, and a continuous pattern of recurring disease. Several of the subtypes discussed in this chapter were not included in the National Cancer Institute Working Formulation for Clinical Usage, a project which was intended to serve as a means for translation among existing classification schemes [1]. While the revised Kiel classification may more accurately categorize small-cell lymphomas, some expert pathologists do not feel it is entirely satisfactory [2,3]. The recent proposal for an International Consensus on the Classification of Lymphoid Neoplasms has been adopted for the subtyping of the small-cell lymphomas discussed in this chapter [4]. Table 40.1 describes these subtypes and their approximate equivalents in the Working Formulation and the Kiel classification. The diffuse small-cell lymphomas are thought to recapitulate the different compartments in the B-cell activation pathway, excluding the follicle center: small lymphocytic (SL) and lymphoplasmacytoid (LP) lymphomas arise in the interfollicular zone, the mantle cell (MC) lym-

phomas originate in the mantle zone, and the marginal zone (MZ) lymphomas arise in the marginal zone and interfollicular sinuses.

The different terminology used by leading hematopathologists and the relative rarity of newer entities such as monocytoid B-cell (MBC) lymphoma have led to a great deal of confusion for practitioners. It can still be questioned whether or not the newer diagnoses are widely recognized and reproducible among pathologists. No large-scale studies of clinical correlation exist for many of the subtypes. In addition, there is considerable overlap between the diffuse small-cell and the mucosa-associated lymphoid tissue (MALT) lymphomas, which are further discussed in Chapter 47. Extranodal small lymphocytic lymphomas have been recognized with increased frequency in recent years with the advent of monoclonal antibodies and immunophenotypic analyses. These are more completely discussed in Chapter 48.

The clinical features, prognosis, treatment and natural history of the diffuse small-cell lymphomas discussed in this chapter represent a compilation of current pathologic classification and the available clinical data. It should be appreciated that this summary represents an evolution of knowledge that is not yet complete.

Table 40.1   Nomenclature for the diffuse small-cell lymphomas

International classification	Working Formulation	Kiel classification

Small lymphocytic	Low grade
	  A. Small lymphocytic
		Low grade
		  Chronic lymphocytic leukemia, B-CLL

Lymphoplasmacytoid/
Waldenström's macroglobulinemia
	Low grade
	  A. Small lymphocytic
	     Plasmacytoid
		Low grade
		  Immunocytoma, lymphoplasmacytoid

Marginal zone*
(extranodal, nodal, splenic)
	Low grade
	  A. Small lymphocytic
		Low grade
		  Monocytoid/marginal zone
		  Immunocytoma

Mantle cell†	Intermediate grade
	  E. Diffuse small cleaved cell
		Low grade
		  Centrocytic

* Some marginal zone lymphomas may be classified in the Working Formulation as intermediate-grade, diffuse small cleaved or diffuse mixed small cleaved and large-cell lymphoma.
† Some mantle cell lymphomas may be classified as small lymphocytic lymphoma in the Working Formulation.
B-CLL, B-cell chronic lymphocytic leukemia.

Diagnosis

The descriptive histopathology and immunopathology of the diffuse small-cell lymphomas are discussed in Chapter 3. The subtypes were originally defined on the basis of their morphologic features. Subsequently, immunophenotypic profiles have been used to define their lineage and relationship to one another. Recent advances in cytogenetics and molecular biology have provided further evidence that these subtypes represent distinct pathologic entities. In practice, it is often difficult to distinguish among the indolent, B-cell lymphomas. A comparison of the salient morphologic, immunophenotypic and genetic features is provided in Table 40.2.

Small lymphocytic lymphoma is characterized by a monotonous population of small round cells, which efface the normal lymphoid architecture. Larger cells with more abundant cytoplasm, prolymphocytes and paraimmunoblasts cluster in proliferation centers or pseudofollicles, which may be present in variable number. By definition, proliferation centers are absent in MC lymphoma and thus are a valuable distinguishing feature. The small- to medium-sized lymphoid cells of MC lymphoma have an irregular contour. The pattern of MC lymphoma is usually diffuse, but a nodular variant of pure mantle zone lymphoma has been described and this can be confused with follicular small cleaved cell lymphoma. In contrast to the follicular lymphomas, MC lymphoma is characterized by the absence of large transformed cells.

The LP variant consists of small lymphocytes,

Table 40.2   Comparative pathologic features of indolent B-cell neoplasms

Category	Morphology	Immunophenotype/genotype
Small lymphocytic	Small round lymphocytes, ± proliferation centers	Faint Ig, pan-B+, CD5+, CD10–, CD23+
Lymphoplasmacytoid	Small lymphocytes with abundant basophilic cytoplasm, plasma cells	Cytoplasmic Ig, CD5–/+
Mantle cell	Small, slightly irregular lymphocytes in mantle zone, absence of large transformed cells	Strong Ig, pan-B+, CD5+, CD10–, CD23–; t(11;14)+
Follicular small cleaved cell	Small cleaved lymphocytes in nodules, presence of large transformed cells	Strong Ig, pan-B+, CD5–, CD10+; t(14;18)
Monocytoid B-cell	Small lymphocytes with abundant cytoplasm in a sinusoidal pattern	Moderate Ig, pan-B+, CD5–, CD10–, CD11c+

plasmacytoid lymphocytes (lymphocytic nuclear features with abundant basophilic cytoplasm) and plasma cells. Intranuclear inclusions (Dutcher bodies) and cytoplasmic inclusions (Russell bodies) are common. The LP variant as recently defined in the International classification, corresponds to the tissue equivalent of Waldenström's macroglobulinemia and the lymphoplasmacytic immunocytoma in the Kiel classification.

Harris and colleagues have proposed the term marginal zone lymphoma to encompass three small-cell lymphomas described in the pathologic literature: extranodal MALT lymphoma (see Chapter 47), nodal MBC lymphoma and splenic MZ lymphoma [4]. Morphologically, the MZ lymphomas are heterogeneous with features of MZ cells, MBCs, small lymphocytes and plasma cells. The capacity of marginal cells to differentiate into monocytoid B-cells or plasma cells, and to display tissue-specific homing patterns has been put forward as an explanation for the different microscopic appearances and sites of disease [5–9]. The pathologic diagnosis is made by the pattern of involvement, which may be parafollicular, interfollicular or peri-sinusoidal, as well as the cytologic features [4]. Discordant and composite MBC lymphomas are relatively common, primarily in association with other low-grade B-cell neoplasms [10–11]. Splenic MZ lymphoma is a provisional subtype of the newly proposed International classification that may overlap with splenic lymphoma with villous lymphocytes, an uncommon form of chronic B-cell leukemia characterized by small lymphocytes with short, thin cytoplasmic villi but distinct from hairy cell leukemia [12–16].

Table 40.2 describes several immunophenotypic features that assist in the differential diagnosis of the small-cell lymphomas. SL lymphomas weakly express surface immunoglobulin (Ig) and the pan-B antigens CD19, CD20 and CD22, while the expression of these markers is generally stronger in MC lymphomas [17–22]. Both express CD5, a pan-T-cell antigen that distinguishes them from follicular small cleaved cell and MZ lymphomas [17,18,23–30]. Lymphoplasmacytoid lymphomas may be CD5-negative and they have strong cytoplasmic Ig [18,31,32]. As noted in Table 40.2, SL lymphoma is usually CD23-positive while MC lymphoma is typically CD23-negative [17,20,32]. An unexplained finding of interest is the relative increase in expression of lambda light chain in MC lymphoma [3,21,27]. The immunophenotype of MZ lymphoma, CD5–, CD10–, CD11c+/–, is useful in excluding SL (CD5+), MC (CD5+) and follicular lymphomas (CD5–, CD10+, CD11c–) [17].

The application of modern immunohistochemical and genotypic techniques to cases categorized as diffuse small cleaved cell lymphoma in the Working Formulation has demonstrated that the majority represent MC lymphoma [33–35]. Rarely, small cleaved cells with the phenotype of follicular small cleaved cell lymphoma may appear in an entirely diffuse pattern. This may be noted at diagnosis or during the course of tissue sampling in patients with a prior diagnosis of follicular small cleaved cell lymphoma. It is assumed that these diffuse small cleaved cell (DSC) lymphomas represent the diffuse counterpart of follicular small cleaved lymphoma and they will not be further discussed in this chapter.

A characteristic chromosomal translocation, t(11;14) (q13;q32), has been reported in 30–80% of MC lymphomas [36–44]. The breakpoint region on chromosome 11q13 has been identified and termed *bcl-1* (B-cell leukemia/lymphoma-1); additional breakpoints have been identified near the coding region of *prad*-1, the proposed candidate *bcl-1* oncogene. *prad*-1, which is overexpressed in all cases of MC lymphoma tested to date, is homologous to the cyclin family protein designated as D1. It is hypothesized that translocations joining *bcl*-1 to the enhancer of the Ig heavy chain gene complex leads to overexpression of *prad*-1, deregulation of growth, and lymphomagenesis [45–49]. The most common cytogenetic abnormality in SL lymphoma is trisomy 12, which is present in about a third of cases [50]. Abnormalities of 13q and the t(11;14) have been reported; the latter require further study to exclude the possibility that they represent mantle cell lymphoma [37,51,52].

With the possible exception of the diffuse small cleaved cell subtype, the diffuse small-cell lymphomas do not contain the t(14;18) chromosomal translocation that is characteristic of follicular small cleaved cell lymphomas [20,34,53]. The Bcl-2 protein, however, is overexpressed in many of these lymphomas [54].

The morphologic and immunophenotypic features in many cases will not flawlessly conform to the outline in Table 40.2. For instance, many B-cell neoplasms including SL, MC, MZ and germinal center lymphomas show maturation to plasmacytoid or plasma cells. According to guidelines laid out in the International classification, these cases should be classified according to their major features. As previously noted, there is considerable overlap between the MBC and the extranodal MALT lymphomas. In establishing a diagnosis, it is important to include information about the microscopic pattern of lymph node involvement and the clinical distribution of disease as well as the morphologic and immunophenotypic features. Cytogenetic or molecular analyses may shed additional light on difficult cases.

Epidemiology

The diffuse small-cell lymphomas comprise a relatively small proportion of the non-Hodgkin's lymphomas (NHL) world-wide. As indicated in Table 40.1, most were previously included in the small lymphocytic and diffuse small cleaved cell categories of the Working Formulation, which together account for about 10% of all NHL [1]. Precise incidence figures for the subtypes are not available for the new International classification [4]. However, two recent reviews using some of the International classification categories as well as data from Europe on the incidence of centrocytic lymphoma are informative. About 20% of the NHL, in a series from Lyon, France, which included 1091 patients, were classified using current morphologic assessment as nonfollicular small B-cell lymphoma (216 cases) [55]. The two predominant subtypes, SL/LP (61 cases) and MC (52 cases), each accounted for about one-fourth of the diffuse small-cell cases, while another 20% were considered to be MALT lymphomas. There were only three MBC cases. In a retrospective assessment of 304 patients with indolent B-cell lymphoma treated on Southwest Oncology Group protocols, 56 cases of MC and 19 cases of MBC lymphoma were identified [56]. The incidence of MC lymphoma has ranged from 2.5% in the American literature (23 of 917 cases at the National Cancer Institute) to 7.7% in the European literature (87 of 1127 cases classified as centrocytic according to the Kiel nomenclature [25,57,58].

The diffuse small-cell lymphomas occur predominantly in adults aged 50 years and above [1,10,59–67]. There is a male predominance in all subtypes with the exception of MBC lymphoma, which occurs more frequently in females [10,64]. The use of different classification schemes and the relatively recent recognition of some of these entities make it difficult to recognize patterns of geographic distribution. However, it seems that MC lymphomas may be more common in southern Italy [1].

Clinical features

SMALL LYMPHOCYTIC AND LYMPHOPLASMACYTOID LYMPHOMA

The median age at diagnosis of SL reported in the literature ranges from 55 to 61 years [1,59,60,65–67]. The male to female ratio approximates 2:1

[1,59,60,66,67]. Nearly all patients have generalized adenopathy at diagnosis. The majority of patients, some 70–80%, have bone marrow involvement at presentation [1,60,65–67]. Frequent extranodal sites of involvement in addition to bone marrow include the liver and spleen [1,60,65,66]. Splenomegaly may be the presenting feature; SL represents a significant proportion of primary splenic lymphomas [68–70]. Other extranodal sites include the orbit, conjunctiva, lung and gastrointestinal tract. Cytopenias, particularly anemia and thrombocytopenia, may be due to extensive involvement of the bone marrow by lymphoma, splenomegaly, autoimmune phenomena or a combination of factors. Systemic symptoms in the form of fevers, sweats and weight loss are uncommon [1,59,60]. A subset of patients has an absolute lymphocytosis at diagnosis; an initial lymphocyte count greater than 4000/μl is usually considered to be diagnostic of chronic lymphocytic leukemia [65]. Patients are generally well at diagnosis. Less than one-third have a poor performance status, bulky tumor or an elevated serum lactic dehydrogenase (LDH) at diagnosis [55]. Table 40.3 describes the comparative clinical features of SL and the other diffuse small-cell lymphomas.

The hallmark of LP lymphoma is a monoclonal serum paraprotein of the IgM type, which is referred to as Waldenström's macroglobulinemia (WM) [65, 71–75]. Presenting features similar to SL include bone marrow involvement in nearly 100% of patients and adenopathy and splenomegaly in 20–40% [71,72]. In addition, patients with WM may manifest signs or symptoms related to the circulating paraprotein such as hyperviscosity, cryoglobulinemia or cold agglutinin anemia, or tissue deposition of IgM resulting in neuropathy, glomerular disease or amyloidosis. Anemia, monoclonal lymphocytosis and Bence Jones proteinuria occur in the majority of patients [73–75]. Neurologic, ocular or auditory impairment owing to hyperviscosity occur in about 15% of patients [71].

MANTLE CELL LYMPHOMA

It is now widely accepted that MC lymphoma is synonymous with centrocytic lymphoma as defined in the Kiel classification and intermediate lymphocytic lymphoma as described by Berard and Dorfman [2,3,76,77]. Centrocytic lymphomas were included in the Working Formulation in the category of diffuse small cleaved cell lymphomas, where they comprised the majority of cases [1]. Waldeyer's ring, bone marrow, and skin or subcutaneous sites were frequently involved by diffuse small cleaved cell lymphoma in the Working Formulation analysis [1].

Table 40.3 Clinical features of diffuse small-cell lymphoma

	Small lymphocytic	Lympho-plasmacytic	Mantle cell	Splenic villous	Monocytoid B-cell
Sex ratio (F:M)	1:2	1:2	1:3	1:1.3	2:1
Diffuse adenopathy	+	±	+	—	—
Splenomegaly	±	±	++	++	—
Bone marrow	+	+	+	+	—
Lymphocytosis	±	±	±	++	—
Gammopathy	—	+	—	+	—
Gastrointestinal	—	—	+	—	*
Histologic transformation	±	—	—	—	+
Variant form	Paraimmunoblastic		Blastic		Composite

* Mucosa-associated lymphoid tissue (MALT) lymphoma type of marginal zone lymphoma has frequent gastrointestinal involvement.
±, occasionally; +, usually; ++, nearly always.

Several clinical series, usually involving small numbers of patients, have detailed the clinical features of MC lymphoma [25,26,55,57,63,78–82]. Mantle cell lymphoma patients are typically older males who present with advanced-stage disease. There is a male predominance which ranges from 2:1 to 15:1 in reported series. Most patients present with diffuse adenopathy; only about 10% of patients have limited-stage disease. Systemic symptoms have been reported in about half. The spleen is frequently involved and may be massively enlarged. Hepatomegaly has been reported in a variable proportion of cases. The frequency of marrow involvement has varied from 54% to nearly 100%, but cytopenias are uncommon. Twenty to fifty per cent of patients have circulating tumor cells in published reports; absolute counts above 20 000/μl are uncommon. In the series reported by Berger et al., 65% of stage IV patients had multiple extranodal sites of disease [55].

A noteworthy form of gastrointestinal tract involvement, which may involve multiple areas including the stomach, duodenum, ileum, colon and rectum, has been reported in patients with MC lymphoma [83–85]. Extensive disease may take the form of multiple lymphomatous polyposis, a process that resembles familial adenomatous polyposis by endoscopy. Gastrointestinal involvement often occurs together with disseminated disease. MC lymphoma of the colon, a site which is rarely involved by other NHL subtypes, may manifest with weight loss, abdominal pain, melena or diarrhea. There is frequently a dominant mass, particularly in the ileocecal region or the stomach. It can be difficult to distinguish gastrointestinal involvement by MC from MALT lymphomas on the basis of morphology alone. Clinical features such as the widespread

nature of MC lymphoma and other pathologic features such as CD5 expression or the presence of the 11;14 translocation, both of which are present in MC lymphoma but lacking in MALT lymphomas, should be incorporated into the differential diagnostic process. Other common extranodal sites of disease include Waldeyer's ring, skin and subcutaneous tissues.

MAGINAL ZONE LYMPHOMAS

Monocytoid B-cell lymphoma is a new entity described by hematopathologists. The relatively sparse clinical data have largely been drawn from pathology consultations rather than clinical centers [10, 64,86–89]. MBC lymphomas appear to have several clinical features that distinguish them from the other indolent B-cell lymphomas. A disease of older individuals (median age 64 years), MBC is the only diffuse small-cell lymphoma with a female predominance, which is about 2:1. In contrast to the other diffuse small-cell lymphomas, lymphadenopathy is more often localized than generalized, bone marrow involvement occurs in a minority and circulating tumor cells are rare [90]. Involvement of intraparotid or paraparotid nodes and the salivary gland is common, and a significant proportion of patients have a history of autoimmune disease, particularly Sjögren's syndrome [86]. The sites of extranodal MBC lymphoma in the pathologic series have included the stomach, pharynx, tonsil, breast, thyroid, chest wall and ovary. As previously noted, the morphologic and immunogenetic features of MBC lymphoma closely resemble MALT lymphomas. The distinction between the two is made by the clinical presentation primarily in lymph nodes with or without extranodal sites or exclusively in extranodal organs.

Primary malignant lymphomas of the spleen are generally thought to arise from follicle center or mantle zone cells [91]. However, there are several reports of lymphoma involving the MZ of the white pulp of the spleen, which is a distinct, major B-cell area external to the mantle zone. In four cases of marginal zone lymphoma of the spleen reported by Schmid et al., three had involvement of the splenic hilar nodes and one had associated abdominal and intrathoracic adenopathy [5]. It is not clear how much MZ splenic lymphoma overlaps with primary splenic lymphoma with villous lymphocytes (SLVL) as reported by Catovsky and colleagues [12–16]. SLVL has been described in elderly individuals (median age 72 years) presenting with symptomatic, massive splenomegaly. Adenopathy is minimal or absent. Distinctive medium-sized lymphocytes with unevenly distributed short, thin villi are characteristic. Abnormal lymphocyte counts rarely exceed 25 000/μl. A significant proportion of patients have a circulating monoclonal paraprotein, usually IgM. Based on the paraproteinemia and the frequent plasmacytoid features, Catovsky and colleagues categorize SLVL with the lymphoplasmacytic (immunocytoma) subgroup of low-grade lymphoma [92]. SLVL can be confused with other indolent B-cell lymphomas involving the spleen [93] The distinction from hairy cell leukemia is based on the absence of the interleukin-2 receptor and the lack of tartrate acid phosphatase resistance [92,93]. In contrast to CLL and SL, MZ splenic lymphomas are CD5-negative.

Prognostic features and natural history

SMALL LYMPHOCYTIC AND LYMPHOPLASMACYTOID LYMPHOMA

SL lymphoma is an indolent disease. The median reported survivals range from 5.8 years in the Working Formulation to 10 years in a series reported from Stanford University [1,59]. As previously stated, clusters of prolymphocytes and paraimmunoblasts may impart a pseudofollicular pattern or these larger cells may be rather evenly distributed throughout nodal tissue [4,65,94]. While the presence of pseudofollicular growth centers suggests a higher-grade lesion, they appear to have no negative

effect on prognosis and they may even confer a slightly more favorable outcome [59,94]. In some cases, these larger cells may be increased in number or predominate, diffusely replacing the lymph node architecture. This histologic picture has been termed the paraimmunoblastic variant and it has been associated with an accelerated clinical course [4,60,95]. This histologic picture may be seen at diagnosis, or more commonly, in patients with a long-standing diagnosis.

A variety of clinical and histopathologic variables has been assessed for prognostic significance. Advanced stage, older age, and the presence of systemic symptoms and anemia have been associated with shortened survival. Pathologic features associated with shortened survival have included a high mitotic rate or increased expression of the Ki-67 nuclear proliferation antigen, the absence of a host T-cell infiltrate, a diffuse rather than pseudofollicular architecture, capsular invasion and an increased large-cell component [59,60,62,66,96,97].

In the analysis of Facon et al., advanced age, male sex, anemia and neutropenia were associated with shortened survival in Waldenström's macroglobulinemia [72]. In contrast, absolute IgM level, organomegaly and the percentage of neoplastic cells in the bone marrow did not confer an unfavorable prognosis. Historically, the response to chlorambucil has been considered to be the major factor predictive for survival [73]. It is notable, however, that 15–20% of deaths are attributable to causes related to neither the disease nor its treatment [72, 74]. As stated in the introduction, the proposed International classification restricts the terms lymphoplasmacytoid lymphoma or immunocytoma to the tissue counterpart of Waldenström's macroglobulinemia. In the European literature, the prognosis for lymphoplasmacytoid lymphomas is less favorable than that for small lymphocytic lymphomas. While the relatively shorter median survivals may be due to inclusion of the lymphoplasmacytoid subtype, polymorphous immunocytoma (classified as an intermediate-grade, diffuse mixed lymphoma in the Working Formulation), this does not fully explain the differences reported [57,81]. Agreement about nomenclature, the reproducibility of pathologic diagnoses and clinical correlations are required to clarify this issue.

MANTLE CELL LYMPHOMA

A profile of the natural history of the MC lymphomas has developed from the combined experience of multiple individual series [20,25–27,55–57,61–63,78,79,80–85,98]. Median survival durations range from about 3–5 years, which is significantly shorter than SL and the follicular low-grade lymphomas [99]. As noted above, pathologists have subdivided the MC lymphomas into nodular (mantle zone) and diffuse types [61,62,79]. In at least two reports, the median survival of mantle zone lymphoma was significantly prolonged, 77 and 88 months, compared with the diffuse cases in which the survival was 30 and 33 months, respectively [26,79,82]. The nodular or mantle zone pattern is thought to represent the early stages of MC lymphoma. Nodular and diffuse patterns often coexist and serial biopsies have demonstrated progression from a mantle zone to a diffuse pattern. The frequency of a nodular pattern has varied from as many as half of the cases in the Nebraska series to only one of 52 cases in the analysis of Berger et al. [55,79]. Because the architectural patterns of MC lymphoma appear to form a continuum, many pathologists find it difficult to reliably classify nodular and diffuse MC lymphoma as distinct entities.

A small proportion of mantle cell lymphomas have larger nuclei with dispersed chromatin and a high proliferation fraction [17,26]. The term 'blastic' variant has been applied because of the resemblance to lymphoblastic lymphoma. Harris and colleagues propose the term 'lymphoblastoid' variant to emphasize the resemblance to lymphoblasts rather than large transformed blasts [4]. A less favorable prognosis has been reported for MC patients with these histologic features [26]. Lennert and colleagues have described a large-cell or centrocytoid–centroblastic lymphoma, which may relate to the blastic variant of MC lymphoma [100]. A high mitotic rate, defined as >20 mitoses per high-power field, is another pathologic feature, which confers an unfavorable prognosis [82]. Expression of the Ki67 nuclear proliferation antigen correlates with mitotic rate, and higher levels of expression have been associated with a trend toward shortened survival [25,96,97].

The clinical prognostic factors identified for MC lymphoma are in agreement with those identified in other subtypes. Prognosis is determined by host factors (age, performance status) or measures of tumor burden and biologic aggressiveness (β_2 microglobulin, serum lactic dehydrogenase, number of extranodal sites, tumor bulk and hepatosplenomegaly) [55,63,77,81]. The minority of patients with limited stage disease enjoy prolonged survival, similar to the follicular low-grade lymphomas [81]. Several authors have reported that response to primary chemotherapy correlates with survival but it is notable that there was no difference in survival based upon the achievement of a very good versus poor response in one large series [81] and, similarly, no difference in survival between complete and partial responses in another study [101].

MARGINAL ZONE LYMPHOMAS

The MZ lymphomas behave in an indolent manner [10,86–90,102]. Many patients reported in the literature have never received disease-specific therapy. While it might be assumed that elderly patients with symptomatic disease have a less favorable prognosis, there is simply a paucity of clinical literature regarding these rare small-cell subtypes. In a recent analysis of 19 cases retrospectively classified by Grogan, the median survival was identical to follicular low-grade lymphoma [56].

Treatment

SMALL LYMPHOCYTIC AND LYMPHOPLASMACYTOID LYMPHOMA

The alkylating agents, cyclophosphamide and chlorambucil, have comprised the backbone of therapy for the SL/LP lymphomas. They have been used singly or in combination with prednisone and vincristine in the cyclophosphamide, vincristine and prednisone (CVP) regimen [59,67,103,104]. While responses to treatment occur regularly in the majority of patients, they are frequently less than complete and disease progression eventually occurs in nearly all patients. The median time to treatment failure ranges from less than 2 to 4 years. The use of total lymphoid irradiation or total body irradiation has not improved outcome [103]. The addition of doxorubicin in the standard CHOP (cyclophosphamide, doxorubicin, vincristine, prednisone) regimen has likewise failed to effect cures [105]. More aggressive chemotherapy such as ProMACE–MOPP (prednisone, methotrexate, doxorubicin, cyclophosphamide, etoposide, mustard, vincristine, procarbazine), used at the National Cancer Institute, or ACVB (doxorubicin, cyclophosphamide, vindesine, bleomycin), as described in the LNH-84 protocol, has also failed to provide a plateau on the disease-free survival curve [55,106]. To date there are no mature or large series detailing the efficacy of myeloablative therapy in small lymphocytic or lymphoplasmacytoid lymphoma. Plasma exchange transfusions should be considered for patients with Waldenström's macroglobulinemia who have clinical features of cryoglobulinemia, hyperviscosity or peripheral neuropathy. Chemotherapy for sustained control should follow.

More recently, the purine analogs fludarabine and 2-chloro-deoxyadenosine (2-CDA) have been assessed in SL lymphoma and Waldenström's macroglobulinemia in both previously treated and newly diagnosed patients [107–113]. Fludarabine has been administered in a dose of 25 mg/m^2 daily for 5 consecutive days every 4 weeks and 2-CDA has been given as a continuous infusion of 0.1mg/kg/day for 7 days in one or multiple cycles every 28 days. Response rates above 75%, including some complete remissions, have been reported in Waldenström's macroglobulinemia for both agents in previously untreated patients. Based on limited numbers of previously treated patients, an overall response rate from 33% to 44% has been reported in SL [107,109]. Serious infectious complications, perhaps owing to prolonged suppression of CD4+ lymphocyte populations, have been reported with the purine analogs and provide a caveat to the use of these drugs [114–116]. Repeated courses of nucleoside analogs have also been associated with severe bone marrow aplasia [117]. Clinical trials of combination therapy with purine analogs are in progress. Their precise role in the treatment of SL/LP lymphoma remains to be determined.

Prolonged freedom from relapse and probable cure of limited-stage disease has been reported with the use of radiotherapy. In the Stanford series, the 10-year freedom from relapse was 67% for 12 stage I–II patients treated with irradiation alone [59]. Owing to the absence of identified curative therapy, selected patients with indolent, stage III–IV disease have been followed without initial treatment [59,118,119]. These patients have enjoyed excellent early survival, 93% at 4 years [59]. The median time to the institution of therapy reported in these patients has ranged from 6 to 10 years [118,119]. The National Cancer Institute has conducted a clinical trial in which patients are randomized to receive immediate treatment with ProMACE–MOPP and low-dose total lymphoid irradiation or deferred therapy [106]. There is no survival advantage to aggressive therapy in this trial to date.

MANTLE CELL LYMPHOMA

The treatment most frequently reported for MC lymphoma is based on alkylating agents, either in the form of chlorambucil as a single drug or the combination of cyclophosphamide with vincristine and prednisone [20,25,26,55,81,82,98]. The rate of complete response has usually been low, less than 50%. The time to treatment failure or disease progression is generally less than 2 years. There is no evidence of a plateau (cure), on the disease-free survival curve. In contrast to the intermediate- and high-grade B-cell lymphomas, the addition of doxorubicin in combination with alkylating agents has

failed to improve prognosis as determined in a randomized trial by Meusers et al. [101]. Similarly, there is no evidence of a cured population in the experience of the Southwest Oncology Group using the CHOP regimen [56]. Table 40.4 describes seven clinical reports of MC lymphoma. Although treatment approaches have varied, median survivals are rather consistent, ranging from 40 to 62 months. The 22 cases of pure mantle zone reported by Duggan et al. provide an exception; the median survival of 88 months is similar to the follicular low-grade lymphomas.

Radiotherapy has been used for patients with limited-stage disease [81]. Richards et al. reported no deaths among seven stage I–IIE MC lymphoma patients in their series. However, the very small numbers of patients so treated and the lack of long-term follow-up make it impossible to comment on the curative potential of this approach.

Because of the initially indolent course of some MC lymphomas, they have been included in the NCI clinical trial in which patients are randomized to receive no initial therapy or immediate treatment with aggressive chemoradiotherapy [106]. Individual patients with MC in this trial have been observed for periods of up to 13 years without significant tumor progression [25]. Because of the absence of curative therapy, a small number of patients has received myeloablative therapy with stem cell rescue [120]. The results with this approach are too preliminary to be analyzed. The purine analogs, fludarabine and 2-CDA, are under study in the MC lymphomas [55]. Again, small numbers and lack of follow-up do not allow definitive conclusions. At this time, there is no known optimal therapy for MC lymphomas. Whenever possible, patients should be entered into randomized controlled trials evaluating new therapeutic approaches. However, because many patients are elderly and have pre-existing medical conditions, a conservative approach of deferred therapy may be appropriate for carefully selected, asymptomatic patients. Splenectomy has proved to be a palliative procedure in selected cases [121].

MARGINAL ZONE LYMPHOMAS

Results of treatment of MZ lymphoma are largely anecdotal. Most information is available from registry data [10, 86–88]. Since a significant proportion of patients have limited-stage disease, radiotherapy may be an attractive modality in selected cases. As mentioned above, many patients with MZ lymphoma, a disease of the elderly, have been managed with no initial treatment [10,88]. In a series of 76 cases studied by Sheibani et al., 22 patients received

Table 40.4 Clinical studies in mantle cell lymphoma

Series	Reference	N	Therapy	Median survival (months)	Comment
Swerdlow	63	18	Chlorambucil, Combination CT	45	
Richards	81	52	Chlorambucil, CVP	40	Advanced age, abnormal liver function tests prognostic
Perry	98	19	Combination CT	47	Data exclude cases with proliferation centers
Bookman	25	23	CVP, watchful waiting, P-M/MOPP	62	Complete remissions uncommon, including P-M/MOPP
Berger	55	52	Varied	52	Prognostic factors included age, LDH, β_2-microglobulin, performance status, splenomegaly, number of extranodal sites
Meusers	101	91	COP versus CHOP	32 / 37	Adriamycin did not improve prognosis in a randomized trial
Duggan	82	22	Combination CT	88	Mantle zone cases only

CT, Chemotherapy; CVP, COP, cyclophosphamide, vincristine, prednisone; P-M/MOPP, prednisone, methotrexate, Adriamycin, cyclophosphamide, etoposide, mustard, vincristine, procarbazine; CHOP, cyclophosphamide, Adriamycin, vincristine, prednisone.

some form of chemotherapy, two had radiotherapy and ten had both. The remaining 42 patients were managed with surgery alone. Of the 52 patients for whom follow-up data were available, 35 were alive and disease free, five died from lymphoma, three died from other causes and nine were alive with disease [87]. The primary management of splenic presentations has often been splenectomy. In the Southwest Oncology Group analysis of 19 cases treated with CHOP chemotherapy, patients had a continuously relapsing pattern and a median survival similar to the follicular lymphomas [56].

Relapse

SMALL LYMPHOCYTIC AND LYMPHOPLASMACYTOID LYMPHOMA

Progression of SL lymphoma is marked by increasing adenopathy, organomegaly and cytopenias. A subgroup, about 20%, of SL lymphoma patients evolve into a leukemic phase [59,60,65–67]. During the course of disease, SL lymphoma may progress to a malignancy of higher grade, a diffuse large-cell lymphoma. This phenomenon in chronic lymphocytic leukemia (CLL) is known as Richter's syndrome, where transformation is heralded by rapidly enlarging lymph nodes, systemic symptoms, elevated LDH

and extranodal involvement [122–124]. Large-cell lymphomas of the same or different clonal origin have been reported [125–129]. Richter's syndrome, which has been reported to occur in 1–10% of CLL, has an accelerated course with median survivals of less than 1 year. However, patients who respond may enjoy prolonged survival [122].

Several cases of coexistent SL lymphoma or CLL and Hodgkin's disease have been reported [129–131]. In these cases, the Reed–Sternberg cells demonstrated cytochemical and biologic properties typical of Hodgkin's disease. With limited follow-up, some of these patients went on to develop disseminated Hodgkin's disease. It is of interest in one report that 12 of 13 of these rare cases contained the Epstein–Barr virus [131].

Prolymphocytic transformation of SL lymphoma has been reported only rarely [60,132], although some cases may have been reported as the paraimmunoblastic variant [95]. In these cases, prolymphocytes similar to those in the pseudofollicular proliferation centers are admixed with the small cells typical of SL lymphoma. The clinical behavior of prolymphocytic transformation appears to be intermediate between typical SL lymphoma and the transformed tissue counterpart of classic Richter's syndrome.

MANTLE CELL LYMPHOMA

As stated earlier, most patients with MC lymphoma have a response to therapy but this is frequently less

small B-cell lymphomas: A heterogeneous group of patients with distinct clinical features and outcome. *Blood* 1994, **83**: 2829–2835.

56. Fisher RI, Dahlberg S, Grogan TM. A clinical analysis of new indolent lymphoma entities in the Revised European American Lymphoma (REAL) Classification. *Proc. Am. Soc. Clin. Oncol.* 1994, **12**: 379 (1287A).

57. Brittinger G, Bartels H, Common H, et al. Clinical and prognostic relevance of the Kiel classification of non-Hodgkin lymphomas results of a prospective multicenter study by the Kiel Lymphoma Study Group. *Hematol. Oncol.* 1984, **2**: 269–306.

58. Jaffe ES, Bookman MA, Longo DL. Lymphocytic lymphoma of intermediate differentiation – mantle zone lymphoma: A distinct subtype of B-cell lymphoma. *Hum. Pathol.* 1987, **18**: 877–880.

59. Morrison WH, Hoppe RT, Weiss LM, et al. Small lymphocytic lymphoma. *J. Clin. Oncol.* 1989, **7**: 598–606.

60. Ben Ezra J, Burke JS, Swartz WG, et al. Small lymphocytic lymphoma: A clinicopathologic analysis of 268 cases. *Blood* 1989, **73**: 579–587.

61. Weisenburger DD, Kim H, Rappaport H. Mantle-zone lymphoma: A follicular variant of intermediate lymphocytic lymphoma. *Cancer* 1982, **49**: 1429–1438.

62. Weisenburger DD, Nathwani BN, Diamond LW, et al. Malignant lymphoma, intermediate lymphocytic type: A clinicopathologic study of 42 cases. *Cancer* 1981, **48**: 1415–1425.

63. Swerdlow SH, Habeshaw JH, Dhalial HS, et al. Centrocytic lymphoma: A distinct clinicopathological and immunologic entity. A multiparameter study of 18 cases at diagnosis and relapse. *Am. J. Path.* 1983, **113**: 181–197.

64. Shin SS, Sheibani K. Monocytoid B-cell lymphoma. *Am. J. Clin. Pathol.* 1993, **99**: 421–425.

65. Pangalis GA, Nathwani BN, Rappaport H. Malignant lymphoma, well differentiated type: Its relationship with chronic lymphocytic leukemia and macroblogulinemia of Waldenstrom. *Cancer* 1977, **39**: 999–1010.

66. Evans HL, Butler JJ, Youness EL. Malignant lymphoma, small lymphocytic type: A clinicopathologic study of 84 cases with suggested criteria for intermediate lymphocytic lymphoma. *Cancer* 1978, **41**: 1440–1455.

67. Icli F, Ezdinili EZ, Costello W, et al. Diffuse well-differentiated lymphocytic lymphoma (DLWD): Response and survival. *Cancer* 1978, **42**: 1936–1942.

68. Spier CM, Kjeldsberg CR, Eyre HJ, et al. Malignant lymphoma with primary presentation in the spleen. A study of 20 patients. *Arch. Pathol. Lab. Med.* 1985, **109**: 1076–1080.

69. Narang S, Wolf BC, Neiman RS. Malignant lymphoma presenting with prominent splenomegaly. A clinicopathologic study with special reference to intermediate cell lymphoma. *Cancer* 1985, **55**: 1948–1957.

70. Kraemer BB, Osborne BM, Butler JJ. Primary splenic presentation of malignant lymphoma and related disorders. A study of 49 cases. *Cancer* 1984, **54**: 1606–1619.

71. Dimopoulos MA, Alexanian R. Waldenstrom's macroglobulinemia. *Blood* **83**: 1452–1459.

72. Facon T, Brouillard M, Duhamel A, et al. Prognostic factors in Waldenstrom's macroglobulinemia: A report of 167 cases. *J. Clin. Oncol.* 1993, **11**: 1553–1558.

73. MacKenzie MR, Fudenberg HH. Macroglobulinemia: An analysis of 40 patients. *Blood* 1972, **39**: 874–889.

74. Krajny M, Pruzanski W. Waldenstrom's macroglobulinemia: Review of 45 cases. *Can. Med. Assoc. J.* 1976, **114**: 899–906.

75. Kyle RA, Garton JP. The spectrum of IgM monoclonal gammopathy in 430 cases. *Mayo Clin. Proc.* 1987, **62**: 719–731.

76. Banks PM, Chan J, Cleary ML, et al. Mantle cell lymphoma. A proposal for unification of morphologic, immunologic, and molecular data [see comments]. *Am. J. Surg. Pathol.* 1992, **16**: 637–640.

77. Berard CW, Dorfman RF. Histopathology of malignant lymphomas. *Clin. Haematol.* 1974, **3**: 39–75.

78. Shivdasani RA, Hess JL, Skarin AT, Pinkus GS. Intermediate lymphocytic lymphoma: Clinical and pathologic features of a recently characterized subtype of non-Hodgkin's lymphoma. *J. Clin. Oncol.* 1993, **11**: 802–811.

79. Weisenburger DD, Duggan MJ, Perry DA, et al. Non-Hodgkin's lymphomas of mantle zone origin. *Pathol. Annu.* 1991, **1**: 139–158.

80. Carbone A, Poletti A, Manconi R, et al. Intermediate lymphocytic lymphoma encompassing diffuse and mantle zone pattern variants. A distinct entity among low-grade lymphomas? *Eur. J. Cancer Clin. Oncol.* 1989, **25**: 113–121.

81. Richards MA, Hall PA, Gregory WM, et al. Lymphoplasmacytoid and small cell centrocytic non-Hodgkin's lymphoma – a retrospective analysis from St Bartholomew's Hospital 1972–1986. *Hematol. Oncol.* 1989, **7**: 19–35.

82. Duggan MJ, Weisenburger DD, Ye YL, et al. Mantle zone lymphoma. A clinicopathologic study of 22 cases. *Cancer* 1990, **66**: 522–529.

83. Isaacson PG, MacLennan KA, Subbuswamy SG. Multiple lymphomatous polyposis of the gastrointestinal tract. *Histopathology* 1984, **8**: 641–656.

84. Triozzi PL, Borowitz MJ, Gockerman JP. Gastrointestinal involvement and multiple lymphomatous polyposis in mantle-zone lymphoma. *J. Clin. Oncol.* 1986, **4**: 866–873.

85. O'Briain DS, Kennedy MJ, Daly PA, et al. Multiple lymphomatous polyposis of the gastrointestinal tract. A clinicopathologically distinctive form of non-Hodgkin's lymphoma of B-cell centrocytic type. *Am. J. Surg. Pathol.* 1989, **13**: 691–699.

86. Shin SS, Sheibani K, Fishleder A, et al. Monocytoid B-cell lymphoma in patients with Sjogren's syndrome: A clinicopathologic study of 13 patients. *Hum. Pathol.* 1991, **22**: 422–430.

87. Sheibani K, Sohn CC, Burke JS, et al. Monocytoid B-cell lymphoma. A novel B-cell neoplasm. *Am. J. Pathol.* 1986, **124**: 310–318.

88. Sheibani K, Burke JS, Swartz WG, et al. Monocytoid B-cell lymphoma. Clinicopathologic study of 21 cases of a unique type of low-grade lymphoma.

Cancer 1988, **62**: 1531–1538.

89. Traweek ST, Sheibani K, Winberg CD, et al. Monocytoid B-cell lymphoma: Its evolution and relationship to other low-grade B-cell neoplasms. *Blood* 1989, **73**: 573–578.

90. Traweek ST, Sheibani K. Monocytoid B-cell lymphoma. The biologic and clinical implications of peripheral blood involvement. *Am. J. Clin. Pathol.* 1992, **97**: 591–598.

91. Burke JS. Splenic lymphoid hyperplasias versus lymphomas/leukemias. A diagnostic guide. *Am. J. Clin. Pathol.* 1993, **99**: 486–493.

92. Matutes E, Morilla R, Owusu AK, et al. The immunophenotype of splenic lymphoma with villous lymphocytes and its relevance to the differential diagnosis with other B-cell disorders. *Blood* 1994, **83**: 1558–1562.

93. Melo JV, Hegde U, Parreira A, et al. Splenic B-cell lymphoma with circulating villous lymphocytes: Differential diagnosis of B-cell leukemias with large spleens. *J. Clin. Pathol.* 1987, **40**: 642–651.

94. Dick FR, Maca RD. The lymph node in chronic lymphocytic leukemia. *Cancer* 1978, **41**: 283–292.

95. Pugh WC, Manning JT, Butler JJ. Paraimmunoblastic variant of small lymphocytic lymphoma/leukemia. *Am. J. Surg. Pathol.* 1988, **12**: 907–917.

96. Medeiros LJ, Picker LJ, Gelb AB, et al. Numbers of host 'helper' T-cells and proliferating cells predict survival in diffuse small-cell lymphomas. *J. Clin. Oncol.* 1989, **7**: 1009–1017.

97. Leith CP, Spier CM, Grogan TM, et al. Diffuse small cleaved-cell lymphoma: A heterogeneous disease with distinct immunobiologic subsets. *J. Clin. Oncol.* 1992, **10**: 1259–1265.

98. Perry DA, Bast MA, Armitage JO, et al. Diffuse intermediate lymphocytic lymphoma. A clinicopathologic study and comparison with small lymphocytic lymphoma and diffuse small cleaved cell lymphoma. *Cancer* 1990, **66**: 1995–2000.

99. Horning SJ. Natural history of and therapy for the indolent non-Hodgkin's lymphomas. *Semin. Oncol.* 1993, **20**: 75–88.

100. Ott M, Ott G, Kuse R, et al. The anaplastic variant of centrocytic lymphoma is marked by frequent rearrangement of the Bcl-1 gene and high proliferative indices. *Histopathology* 1994, **24**: 329–334.

101. Meusers P, Engelhard M, Bartels H, et al. Multicentre randomized therapeutic trial for advanced centrocytic lymphoma: Anthracycline does not improve the prognosis. *Hematol. Oncol.* 1989, **7**: 365–380.

102. Cogliatti SB, Lennert K, Hansmann ML, et al. Monocytoid B-cell lymphoma: Clinical and prognostic features of 21 patients. *J. Clin. Pathol.* 1990, **43**: 619–625.

103. Hoppe RT, Kushlan P, Kaplan HS, et al. The treatment of advanced stage favorable histology non-Hodgkin's lymphoma: A preliminary report of a randomized trial comparing single agent chemotherapy, combination chemotherapy, and whole body irradiation. *Blood* 1981, **58**: 592–598.

104. Rosenberg SA. Karnofsky memorial lecture. The low-grade non-Hodgkin's lymphomas: Challenges and opportunities. *J. Clin. Oncol.* 1985, **3**: 299–310.

105. Dana BW, Dahlberg S, Nathwani BN, et al. Long-term follow-up of patients with low-grade malignant lymphomas treated with doxorubicin-based chemotherapy or chemoimmunotherapy. *J. Clin. Oncol.* 1993, **11**: 644–651.

106. Young RC, Longo DL, Glatstein E, et al. The treatment of indolent lymphomas: Watchful waiting v. aggressive combined modality treatment. *Semin. Hematol.* 1988, **25**: 11–16.

107. Redman JR, Cabanillas F, Velasquez WS, et al. Phase II trial of fludarabine phosphate in lymphoma: An effective new agent in low-grade lymphoma. *J. Clin. Oncol.* 1992, **10**: 790–794.

108. Kay AC, Saven A, Carrera CJ, et al. 2-Chlorodeoxyadenosine treatment of low-grade lymphomas. *J. Clin. Oncol.* 1992, **10**: 371–377.

109. Hochster HS, Kim KM, Green MD, et al. Activity of fludarabine in previously treated non-Hodgkin's low-grade lymphoma: Results of an Eastern Cooperative Oncology Group study. *J. Clin. Oncol.* 1992, **10**: 28–32.

110. Pigaditou A, Rohatiner AZ, Whelan JS et al. Fludarabine in low-grade lymphoma. *Semin. Oncol.* 1993, **20** (5 Suppl. 7): 24–27.

111. Zinzani PL, Lauria F, Rondelli D, et al. Fludarabine: An active agent in the treatment of previous-treated and untreated low-grade non-Hodgkin's lymphoma. *Ann. Oncol.* 1993, **4**: 575–578.

112. Dimopoulos MA, Kantarjian H, Estey E, et al. Treatment of Waldenstrom macroglobulinemia with 2-chlorodeoxyadenosine. *Ann. Intern. Med.* 1993, **118**: 195–198.

113. Dimopoulos MA, O'Brien S, Kantarjian H, et al. Fludarabine therapy in Waldenstrom's macroglobulinemia. *Am. J. Med.* 1993, **95**: 49–52.

114. Betticher DC, Fey MF, von RA, et al. High incidence of infections after 2-chlorodeoxyadenosine (2-CDA) therapy in patients with malignant lymphomas and chronic and acute leukemias. *Ann. Oncol.* 1994, **5**: 57–64.

115. Keating MJ. Immunosuppression with purine analogues – the flip side of the gold coin [editorial]. *Ann. Oncol.* 1993, **4**: 347–348.

116. Hoffman M, Tallman MS, Hakimian D, et al. 2-Chlorodeoxyadenosine is an active salvage therapy in advanced indolent non-Hodgkin's lymphoma. *J. Clin. Oncol.* 1994, **12**: 788–792.

117. Beutler E, Koziol JA, McMillan R, et al. Marrow suppression produced by repeated doses of cladribine. *Acta Haematol.* 1994, **91**: 10–15.

118. Portlock CS, Rosenberg SA. No initial therapy for stage III and IV non-Hodgkin's lymphomas of favorable histologic types. *Ann. Intern. Med.* 1979, **90**: 10–13.

119. Horning SJ, Rosenberg SA. The natural history of initially untreated low-grade non-Hodgkin's lymphomas. *N. Engl. J. Med.* 1984, **311**: 1471–1475.

120. Vose JM, Weisenburger DD, Anderson JR, et al. Mantle cell lymphoma (MCL) has a poorer prognosis than follicular non-Hodgkin's lymphoma; however, high-dose therapy and autologous stem cell transplantation may overcome treatment resistance in MCL. *Blood* 1993, **82**: 135a (527A).

121. Coad JE, Matutes E, Catovsky D. Splenectomy in lymphoproliferative disorders: A report on 70 cases and review of the literature. *Leuk. Lymphoma* 1993, **10**: 245–264.

122. Robertson LE, Pugh W, O'Brien S, et al. Richter's syndrome: A report on 39 patients. *J. Clin. Oncol.* 1993, **11**: 1985–1989.

123. Harousseau JL, Flandrin G, Tricot G, et al. Malignant lymphoma supervening in chronic lymphocytic leukemia and related disorders. Richter's syndrome: A study of 25 cases. *Cancer* 1981, **48**: 1302–1308.

124. Trump DL, Mann RB, Phelps R, et al. Richter's syndrome: Diffuse histiocytic lymphoma in patients with chronic lymphocytic leukemia. A report of five cases and review of the literature. *Am. J. Med.* 1980, **68**: 539–548.

125. Chan WC, Dekmezian R. Phenotypic changes in large cell transformation of small cell lymphoid malignancies. *Cancer* 1986, **57**: 1971–1978.

126. Sheibani K, Nathwani BN, Winberg CD, et al. Small lymphocytic lymphoma. Morphologic and immunologic progression. *Am. J. Clin. Pathol.* 1985, **84**: 237–243.

127. van Dongen JJM, Hooijkaas H, Michiels JJ, et al. Richter's syndrome with different immunoglobulin light chains and different heavy chain gene rearrangements. *Blood* 1984, **64**: 571–575.

128. Sun T, Susin M, Desner M, et al. The clonal origin of two cell populations in Richter's syndrome. *Hum. Pathol.* 1990, **21**: 722–728.

129. Jaffe ES, Zarate OA, Kingma DW, et al. The interrelationship between Hodgkin's disease and non-Hodgkin's lymphomas. *Ann. Oncol.* 1994, **5**: S7–11.

130. Jaffe ES, Zarate OA, Medeiros LJ. The interrelationship of Hodgkin's disease and non-Hodgkin's lymphomas – lessons learned from composite and sequential malignancies. *Semin. Diagn. Pathol.* 1992, **9**: 297–303.

131. Momose H, Jaffe ES, Shin SS, et al. Chronic lymphocytic leukemia/small lymphocytic lymphoma with Reed–Sternberg-like cells and possible transformation to Hodgkin's disease. Mediation by Epstein–Barr virus. *Am. J. Surg. Pathol.* 1992, **16**: 859–867.

132. Traweek ST, Esteban JM, Rappaport H. Prolymphocytic transformation of a small lymphocytic lymphoma: Cell cycle and ploidy analysis. *Lab. Invest.* 1990, **62**: 101a.

CHAPTER 41

Follicular lymphoma

AMA ROHATINER AND T. ANDREW LISTER

Introduction

The biological and clinical enigma of follicular lymphoma centers around the paradox that, although this is an illness that responds to both chemotherapy and irradiation, for the majority of patients it remains demonstrably incurable. Thus, almost always, death occurs as a consequence of the disease, regardless of whether transformation to high-grade histology has occurred.

Some progress has been made: 50 years ago, when the only available treatment was radiotherapy, the median survival was 5 years [1]; now it is between 9 and 10 years (Figure 41.1) [2–5]. Therefore, within the context of malignant disease as a whole, follicular lymphoma has been variously described as 'indolent' and even 'benign' (surely, a misnomer), but for the younger person, a life expectancy of 10 years can hardly be considered acceptable.

This frustrating situation has encouraged various investigators over the years to try to improve the initial treatment. Stronger drugs, different drugs, more drugs, exposure to the same drugs for longer, the combination of radiotherapy and chemotherapy and biological therapies have all been tried. Most of these strategies have prolonged duration of remission but none to date has convincingly improved survival. Attempts have certainly been made to develop potentially curative therapy for follicular lymphoma. Whilst some would argue that this is naive, unrealistic and, in the light of previous failed attempts, impossible, such a nihilistic attitude is probably unjustified in the light of recent work, which has led to a much clearer understanding of the pathophysiology of the disease at the cytogenetic and molecular level. Much attention has focused on the molecular biology of follicular lymphoma, the t(14;18) translocation having been described in the majority of cases [6–9]. The development of the polymerase chain reaction (PCR) [10] has provided a technique that is increasingly being used to assess the potential 'curability' of the new treatments available; the difficulty is knowing what the presence of residual t(14;18)-containing cells in the blood or bone marrow actually signifies. Inherently, one feels that the objective of a treatment should be to remove all potentially 'malignant' cells completely and permanently. However, whether this is actually the case in follicular lymphoma is far from clear (vide infra).

The main emphasis of this chapter will be the management of the patient with follicular lymphoma. A critical review of the different available treatment options will be presented. Detailed descriptive pathology and molecular biology are reviewed elsewhere in this book. They will, however, be alluded to briefly at this point, for completeness and in order to put the illness into perspective.

HISTOPATHOLOGY

Follicular lymphoma is often considered to be the

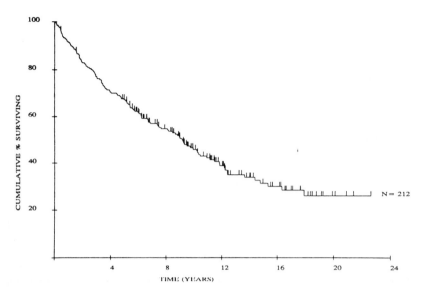

Figure 41.1 Survival of patients with follicular lymphoma treated at St Bartholomew's Hospital.

prototype of the low-grade B-cell lymphomas [11]. Histologically, it is characterized by the presence of follicular aggregates within the lymph node, not dissimilar from normal lymphoid follicles, the lymphoma cells themselves being superficially similar to the cells found within the normal germinal center [12]. The follicles can clearly be seen at low power and, indeed, the criteria for classifying follicular lymphomas depend on the presence of such follicles [13–15], which tend to be uniform in size and lack well-defined mantle zones.

There has been much debate and controversy about the subclassification of follicular lymphomas; in the Kiel classification [16], all are described as centrocytic/centroblastic without the identification of subgroups. In contrast, the Working Formulation [11] distinguishes three subtypes. Tumors composed predominantly of small cleaved cells, and those containing more equal proportions of small cleaved and large cells, fall into the 'low-grade' category (as B and C), whereas those made up of predominantly large cells are classified as being of 'intermediate grade' (D). In the recently proposed 'revised European–American (REAL) classification' [17], the nomenclature has been changed to 'follicular lymphoma, grade I, II or III'. In some clinical studies, patients with follicular large-cell lymphoma have been found to have a better prognosis and some have considered these tumors to be potentially curable [18–20] but this has also been disputed and has yet to be demonstrated [21]. Some of the discrepancy may be due to the use of different criteria for defining 'follicular' large-cell lymphoma.

In the bone marrow, the pattern of infiltration is typically paratrabecular, with small cleaved lym-phocytes (centrocytic cells) predominating, irrespective of the subtype. Even when a peripheral blood smear does not overtly contain lymphoma cells, their presence can often be demonstrated using molecular techniques (see Chapters 4 and 14).

Immunologically, follicular lymphomas represent a proliferation of mature B-cells which express B-cell markers such as CD19, CD20 and CD22, together with surface immunoglobulin (Ig) [22–24]. Most express IgM but some, IgG or IgA heavy chain. The CD10 antigen is also frequently present on the cell surface but, unlike the low-grade B-cell diffuse lymphomas, CD5 is not [22,23].

CYTOGENETICS

The t(14;18) translocation was first described by Fukuhara and Rowley in 1978 [6] and the breakpoints subsequently localized by Yunis et al. [7]. The translocation has been found in the majority of patients with follicular lymphoma [8,9] but it is also present in patients with high-grade lymphoma, some of whom have evidence of transformation from a cellular origin as follicular lymphoma [25,26].

There are interesting epidemiological differences in the incidence of t(14;18)-associated lymphomas throughout the world; they appear to be much more frequent in Europe, the United States and Australia, as compared to Japan [27,28], although the lower frequency in the latter country may be the result of a lower overall incidence of follicular lymphoma. There are also patients with follicular lymphoma who do not have the t(14;18) translocation at all [29] and those in whom the translocation at 14q32 occurs with other chromosomes [30].

There is controversy as to whether these cytogenetic changes confer a favorable or adverse prognosis. With regard to the prognostic significance of t(14;18) *per se*, its presence or absence does not appear to influence survival [31–33]. Some studies suggest that the persistence of some detectable normal metaphases in a biopsy specimen has favorable prognostic value [31] but this has also been disputed [32,33]. However, additional abnormalities of chromosome 17 have consistently been found to be associated with a poor prognosis [31,32,34].

MOLECULAR BIOLOGY

It has been demonstrated that follicular lymphomas characteristically have a rearrangement of the Ig heavy chain and light chain genes [35,36] and, as mentioned above, most are associated with the chromosomal translocation t(14;18)(q32;q21) [8,9]. A combination of cytogenetic analysis and molecular techniques has shown the t(14;18) translocation to be present in up to 95% of patients [7,37]. The molecular changes associated with the translocation can be summarized as follows: the translocation results in juxtaposition of the *bcl*-2 gene on chromosome 18 to the joining region of the Ig heavy chain gene, which is on chromosome 14. The effect of this is thought to be deregulation of the *bcl*-2 gene by the enhancer region of the Ig heavy chain gene, resulting in increased production of *bcl*-2 protein, a mitochondrial membrane protein (also present in other internal cell membranes) that inhibits 'programmed cell death', or apoptosis [38]. This can be demonstrated using monoclonal antibodies against the *bcl*-2 protein. Overexpression of *bcl*-2 in turn results in prolongation of cell survival, leading to accumulation of follicular B-cells and creating circumstances in which a further genetic event may occur. Since the 14;18 translocation has been detected by PCR in the lymphocytes of normal individuals, even children, it is apparently not sufficient to give rise to clinical follicular lymphoma. Presumably, additional genetic changes in a t(14;18)-bearing cell lead to the clinical manifestations of the illness.

Natural history

Follicular lymphoma is first alluded to in the literature in 1901 by Becker [39]. In 1925, Brill et al. described its pathology in the *Journal of the American Medical Association*, referring to a 'generalised giant lymph follicle hyperplasia of lymph nodes and spleen' [40]. Subsequently, in 1938, Symmers wrote about an illness, which was characterized pathologically by 'giant follicular lymphadenopathy', and sometimes involved the spleen [41]. A series of patients was described, some of whom had been treated by radiotherapy. Not only is this a detailed account of the pathology, it is also the first description of the course of the illness and its potential evolution.

It is salutory to remember that despite the development of several different treatment modalities, more than 50 years later, the natural history has not really been altered by therapy. In the original description, as indeed now, patients usually presented with generalized lymph node enlargement, with or without enlargement of the spleen and the diagnosis was made on the basis of a lymph node biopsy. Symmers went on to describe response to therapy in terms of regression of lymphadenopathy following local radiotherapy; characteristically, the responses were usually incomplete. He further described the typical behavior of the illness with inevitable and repeated recurrences, the histology often remaining unchanged, until the disease became resistant to radiation therapy. Some patients developed what was described as 'sarcomatous change', with dire consequences. In a third group, abnormal cells would be found in the peripheral blood and, occasionally, an illness similar to Hodgkin's disease would develop. The first three patterns of evolution remain unchanged to this day, the last seen only extremely rarely, and perhaps coincidentally. The obvious major difference is that with modern chemotherapy and improvements in supportive care, the median survival has doubled, but the inexorable pattern of recurrence, culminating in death owing to the illness, has not changed. Thus, the great majority of patients who develop follicular lymphoma die of progressive disease, usually with transformation to high-grade histology. In a recent analysis from St Bartholomew's Hospital, only 8 out of 116 patients died from causes unrelated to lymphoma.

Management

INVESTIGATION

As mentioned above, the majority of people with follicular lymphoma present with enlargement of one or more lymph nodes; they may otherwise be perfectly well. Alternatively, they may have B symptoms (weight loss, fevers and sweats at night), although the latter are seen less frequently than in Hodgkin's disease. A lymph node biopsy is mandatory in order to establish the diagnosis. When there are no accessible peripheral lymph nodes, the use of tru-cut needle biopsies has made an appreciable difference to the clinical management of such patients, laparotomy and thoracotomy being only very rarely necessary [42].

The illness may also present with symptoms of bone marrow involvement. Frequently, the bone marrow aspirate does not show any abnormality and a trephine biopsy (or indeed bilateral biopsies) is required to confirm infiltration. Involvement of the peripheral blood is not unusual, particularly in the small cleaved cell subtype [43,44], typical cells being easy to identify in the peripheral blood.

The diagnosis having been established, the next step is to define the extent of disease. Computed tomography (CT) scanning is now routine in most centers and provides a baseline. Traditionally, staging criteria have been based on the Ann Arbor classification [45,46]. The majority of patients with follicular lymphoma will have advanced disease at presentation, bone marrow infiltration being most frequently the basis upon which the person is deemed to have stage IV disease [4]. Beyond CT scanning and a bone marrow aspirate and trephine biopsy, together with measurement of the full blood count, electrolytes, urea, uric acid and liver function tests, and outside the parameters imposed by specific clinical trials, other tests are really not essential. However, with the development of prognostic indices (*vide infra* – see Chapter 35), measurement of β_2-microglobulin and lactate dehydrogenase (LDH) levels may also be useful.

EXPLANATION

The diagnosis having been established, it is then incumbent upon the doctor to explain to the patient and to the family, its implications, the possible treatment options and the likely life expectancy. Follicular lymphoma is not an easy subject to discuss: the explanation has to encompass the concept of a malignancy and the virtual inevitability of death as a consequence of the illness (unless the person is older, in which case death from an unrelated cause may supervene). The perception of the general public is that cancer implies certain death, sooner rather than later. It can therefore be difficult for a patient to understand that he or she might be quite well for a prolonged period, with treatment being required only from time to time. It can be even more difficult to accept that treatment may not necessarily be required at all initially and that such a lack of intervention does not shorten survival.

Several new approaches are being tested, including myeloablative therapy with autologous bone marrow transplantation and it should be made clear that they can be applied sequentially, if indicated or desired, during the course of the illness.

TREATMENT

No initial therapy

Follicular lymphoma is unusual amongst malignancies in that some patients with disseminated lymphoma do not appear to require any treatment at the time of presentation. Furthermore, it has been demonstrated that such deferral of treatment does not result in shorter survival [47]. Conversely, the administration of intensive therapy from the outset does not appear to afford any survival advantage [48]. This is not, however, true for the minority of patients who present with localized disease who can and should be treated with curative intent from the outset (see Chapter 30).

It is possible to argue that, since no curative treatment is currently available and chemotherapy is toxic, unpleasant and likely to interfere with a patient's normal life, treatment should only be started when there is a good reason for doing so. The philosophy developed at Stanford University is that treatment should be initiated when one or more of the following occurs: the development of systemic symptoms, painful lymph node enlargement, compromise of a vital organ such as the bone marrow or clear evidence of progressive disease. Sometimes, treatment will also have to be initiated if the patient finds it unacceptable to delay.

However, it is possible to question the basic premise upon which this approach is based. It could well be that the patients who remain well for several years and require 'no initial therapy' may be the very patients who could be cured, if an effective treatment were to be found and given to them at the outset when they had only minimal disease. Nevertheless, in the context of accepting the former approach and not treating everyone immediately, it is possible to observe two phenomena characteristic of follicular lymphoma: spontaneous regression and transformation to high-grade histology. Occasionally, a person will come to the clinic and previously easily palpable lymph nodes will have diminished in size. In the original group of patients followed at Stanford University without initial treatment, such spontaneous regressions were seen in 19 of 83 patients [47]. This number, and indeed the proportion of patients considered not to need treatment at the time of presentation, are both much higher than those seen at St Bartholomew's Hospital, London, over a 25-year period [5]. Thus, patient selection and referral patterns are important considerations.

There are a number of important points to be made in the context of transformation to diffuse histology. This may occur early in the course of the illness, after several recurrences, 9–10 years after diagnosis, or never [49–54] and the frequency with which it occurs is the same, irrespective of whether treatment is started at the time of diagnosis, or later [51]. Patients may also present with centroblastic (diffuse large-cell) lymphoma but with evidence of a residual follicular pattern, suggesting that the tumor arose from follicular lymphoma. Alternatively, there may be discordance between a peripheral lymph node, which shows follicular histology and, for example, an abdominal mass, which on biopsy reveals centroblastic lymphoma. It is also not unusual to find patients with centroblastic lymphoma in large tumor masses and concurrent, paratrabecular infiltration typical of follicular lymphoma in the bone marrow. Survival after transformation has occurred is generally very poor, often less than one year [5,50–54] (Figure 41.2). However, in one series (from Stanford), it was found that provided complete remission could be achieved, the survival of such patients was relatively good [55].

The concept of 'no initial therapy', (also sometimes called 'watch and wait policy' or 'watchful waiting') has been widely adopted. More recently, O'Brien et al. have confirmed that a strategy of no initial treatment does not shorten survival [56] and this has also been demonstrated in the much-quoted randomized study from the National Cancer Institute in which intensive chemotherapy (ProMACE–MOPP) (see Chapter 42) and total lymphoid irradiation were compared to a policy of 'watchful waiting' [48]. Follow-up of the patients originally ran-

domized continues but thus far there is no discernible difference in survival. There is, of necessity, a certain selection bias in this study, since only patients able to be observed without treatment were selected for randomization in the first place. Also, the group randomised to 'watchful waiting' was 'allowed' palliative radiotherapy in the interim.

Initial therapy

Localized disease

Radiotherapy
Whilst 80–90% of patients present with disseminated lymphoma, a small proportion will be found to have limited disease, which is potentially curable with radiation therapy. Clearly, the treatment of such patients should not be deferred. Radiotherapy at doses between 30 and 50 Gy results in at least half of the patients being free of disease at 10 years [5,57–65] (Table 41.1). The results for patients with stage I disease are in general better than for those with stage II [57]. Some centers use involved-field irradiation, some a more extensive field or total lymphoid irradiation. At St Bartholomew's Hospital, only patients with stage I disease are now treated with radiotherapy but, elsewhere, total nodal irradiation for patients with stage II follicular lymphoma has been used with very good results (83% disease-free survival) at 5 years [58].

Chemotherapy with or without radiotherapy
An alternative philosophy has been to use combination chemotherapy or the latter with radiotherapy. A randomized study compared the combination of

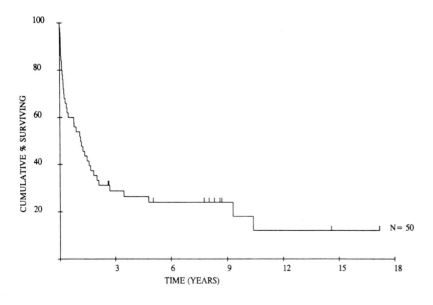

Figure 41.2 Survival from transformation at any point.

Table 41.1   Radiotherapy with or without chemotherapy for stage I and II follicular lymphoma

Reference	Treatment	No. of patients	Disease-free survival
57	IF	28	88% at 10 years
	EF		61% at 10 years
5	IF	22	83% at 10 years
	TLI		
58	IF	29	83% at 10 years
	EF		
59	IF	252	53% at 10 years
60	IF		
	EF	124	54% at 10 years
	TLI		
61	EF	24	70% at 10 years
62	IF		67%
	IF + CVP		92%
	EF	55	39%
	TLI + CVP		
63	IF		67%
	IF + CHOP or	76	64%
	IF + COP-Bleo		
64	IF or	26	54% at 5 years
	IF + CVP		
139	IF	54	48% at 10 years
	EF		

IF, Involved field; EF, extended field; TLI, total lymphoid irradiation; CVP/COP, cyclophosphamide + vincristine + prednisolone; CHOP, cyclophosphamide + Adriamycin + vincristine + prednisolone; Bleo, bleomycin.

cyclophosphamide, vincristine and prednisolone (CVP) and radiotherapy with radiotherapy alone, and no difference was demonstrated [64]. However, when the doxorubicin-containing treatment cytoxan, Adriamycin, vincristine, prednisone (CHOP) was used in a similar comparison at MD Anderson Cancer Center, there was a significant difference in recurrence-free survival at 5 years, namely 64% for combined modality therapy as compared to 37% for radiation therapy alone [63]. The situation is therefore not clear.

Advanced disease

Chemotherapy

With the development of alkylating agents, it became clear that such relatively innocuous treatment (at least in terms of lack of overt clinical toxicity at the dosage used) resulted in meaningful responses in more than 50% of patients, usually within 6 weeks of starting. An obvious advantage is that chlorambucil

Table 41.2   Alkylating agent treatment

Reference	Treatment	No. of patients	Complete remission (%)	Median survival (years)
69	Cyclophosphamide	13	46	2.5
83	Cyclophosphamide or chlorambucil	17	64	>4
248	Cyclophosphamide or chlorambucil	37	65	11
70	Chlorambucil	31	13	>4
68	Cyclophosphamide	26	42	>5
249	Predimustine	106	63	3.5

can be given orally, and this remains the bulwark of conventional treatment at most centers (Table 41.2). At St Bartholomew's Hospital, it is given as 10 mg daily for 6 weeks, followed by a 2-week interval, followed by three 14-day cycles, each separated by 14-day intervals [5]. With such relatively simple treatment, 'clinical remission' (no palpable disease) will be achieved in 75% of patients and the median duration of such a first remission will be approximately 18 months [5]. In some centers, chlorambucil is given at a lower daily dose for longer.

Whilst chlorambucil is effective (both as initial therapy and at recurrence) the responses, although clinically valuable, are often incomplete and hardly ever more than temporary. Historically, initial studies with single-agent chemotherapy have been succeeded by drug combinations and follicular lymphoma is no exception. Comparison of a combination of cyclophosphamide, vincristine and prednisolone with cyclophosphamide alone [66] was originally made in a relatively small number of patients. The demonstration that the response rate was higher with the combination led to this treatment, albeit in higher doses than used originally, becoming CVP [67]. A series of randomized studies followed [68–71] (Table 41.3). All confirmed a higher complete response rate than that seen with chlorambucil, but unfortunately, no advantage could be demonstrated in terms of survival. CVP is, however, still widely used, despite the fact that there is no demonstrable advantage in comparison with the much simpler single agent, chlorambucil.

The median duration of remission with CVP ranged between 1.5 and 3 years. Various derivative regimens were subsequently tested in an attempt to improve on these results. Regimens without an anthracycline were usually variations on a theme of COPP, which included the same drugs used in CVP with the addition of procarbazine [72–75] (Table 41.4). An alternative approach has been to use bis-(2-chloroethyl) nitrosourea (BCNU) [76].

Following the relative success of Adriamycin in the form of CHOP for intermediate- and high-grade lymphoma, the regimen was then applied to follicular lymphoma. Although the initial comparison between CHOP and CVP showed no significant difference in complete remission rate [77] and the conclusion of a very recent analysis of the outcome of patients receiving Adriamycin-containing regimens in open studies was that there is no advantage to adding Adriamycin [78], many people with follicular lymphoma are in fact treated with CHOP in the first instance (Table 41.5). The addition of bleomycin has also not made any appreciable difference to response rate, disease-free survival or survival [79–81].

Radiation therapy

The observation that lymph node recurrences were relatively unusual within an irradiated field [82] led to the evaluation of total lymphoid irradiation as treatment for follicular lymphoma and, subsequently, the combination of the latter treatment with chemotherapy. However, once more, no improvement in survival could be demonstrated [83]. Low-dose whole-body irradiation has also been tested and significant responses have been seen, although such treatment is very myelosuppressive, thrombocytopenia, in particular, being a problem [83–86]. A number of centers have also tried a combination of chemotherapy and radiotherapy, the latter usually in the form of total lymphoid irradiation or low-dose total body irradiation (TBI). The only subgroup that seems to have benefitted are patients with stage III disease: in a study from the MD Anderson Cancer Center [87], durable remissions were achieved with

Table 41.3   Treatment with CVP

Reference	No. of patients	Complete remission (%)	Median survival
68	32	41	>2 years
83	17	88	>5 years
67	75	57	N/ST
48	29	65	>5 years
250	31	65	>5 years
73	49	67	6 years 11 months
77	74	48	4 years
88	162	56	5 years 4 months
69	28	68	>5 years
70	35	37	>4 years
251	40	67	4 years

CVP, Cyclophosphamide, vincristine and prednisolone; N/ST, not stated.

In contrast, two studies in which IFN has been combined with an alkylating agent have not shown any advantage for the combination: a preliminary analysis of a study currently in progress in the United Kingdom shows no difference in response rate between patients receiving chlorambucil alone, or chlorambucil in combination with IFN [108]. Similarly, an intergroup study (Cancer and Leukemia Group B + ECOG) in the United States compared very similar treatment comprising cyclophosphamide alone, with the combination of IFN and cyclophosphamide. Once more, no advantage was demonstrated for the addition of IFN in terms of response rate, remission duration or survival, and the toxicity of the combination was significantly greater [109].

One of the difficulties in interpreting these results is that the French/Belgian study [107] had a maintenance phase, in that both IFN and the relatively intensive combination chemotherapy were given as remission induction therapy, followed by 12 months' treatment in which the chemotherapy was given less frequently. While it is difficult to separate the influence of maintenance treatment from that of the initial therapy, even patients on the maintenance arm were randomized to receive or not to receive IFN.

Interferon given as maintenance therapy (Table 41.8)   Other studies have specifically addressed the question of continuing IFN beyond the remission induction and/or consolidation stage. In the British study mentioned above [108], patients in whom a complete or 'good partial response' has been achieved in the initial part of the study are subsequently randomized for a second time to receive either no further treatment (which would be regarded as conventional management), or maintenance IFN for up to 1 year. Currently, with a median follow-up of 4.5 years, there is a remission duration advantage in favor of the group receiving maintenance IFN ($P=0.03$) but no difference in survival. These results are reminiscent of those of a European Organization for Research and Treatment of Cancer (EORTC) study in which 'CVP' was given as initial therapy, with or without 'iceberg radiotherapy' to large nodal masses. Patients were then allocated to receive no further therapy or maintenance IFN. An interim analysis shows better progression-free survival ($P=0.02$) in the IFN-treated group but no difference in survival [110].

A study from the MD Anderson Cancer Center, Houston, also shows a remission duration advantage for patients in whom complete remission was achieved with the comination of CHOP given with bleomycin, followed by IFN as maintenance therapy. Comparison with a historical control group treated with the same chemotherapy alone [111] showed duration of remission to be significantly longer in the group receiving IFN. A study is currently in progress (Southwest Oncology Group: SWOG) in which the initial treatment, ProMACE–MOPP and total lymphoid irradiation is followed by randomization to no further therapy or maintenance IFN.

The discrepancies between the various studies may to some extent be due to the fact that the selection criteria were different. Some of the studies included patients who had low-grade lymphoma but not necessarily only follicular lymphoma. The ECOG study, for example, has not been analyzed separately for patients with follicular lymphoma. In some, e.g., the GELF study, only patients considered to be in a 'poor' prognostic category were included. It is perhaps not a coincidence that the two studies with the 'best' results are those in which IFN was combined with relatively intensive, Adriamycin-containing regimens. These reservations notwithstanding, IFN is unquestionably active in follicular lymphoma but when given alone it is less effective than alkylating agents.

Several questions remain: how best should it be incorporated into current treatment programmes? Future trials will no doubt address this. There is also the pragmatic problem that IFN must be given by injection and, furthermore, is certainly not entirely

Table 41.8   Results of treatment with 'maintenance' interferon

Reference	Initial therapy	'Maintenance' IFN (dose $\times 10^6$ units + schedule)	Outcome
108	CB/CB + Hur α	3 × 3/week for up to 1 year (versus NFT)	↑ duration of remission
110	CVP ± RT	3 × 3/week for 1 year (versus NFT)	↑ progression-free survival
107	CHVP ± Hur α	5 × 3/week + CHVP for 1 year (versus CHVP alone)	↑ duration of remission ↑ survival

CB, Chlorambucil; CVP, cyclophosphamide, vincristine, prednisolone; CHVP, cyclophosphamide, Adriamycin, teniposide (VM-26), prednisolone; RT, radiotherapy; Hur α, human recombinant interferon; IFN, interferon; ↑, increased.

devoid of side-effects. Patients (perhaps especially British ones) are, in general, uncomplaining; whilst at the doses used they may not specifically complain of fatigue, many do notice a change for the better when treatment with IFN is completed. A further question is that of dose. The standard dose is an entirely empirical one: $3–5 \times 10^6$ units, subcutaneously, thrice weekly, has been given almost without question, whereas in fact it evolved from the dose originally used in the Scandinavian osteogenic sarcoma study [112] at a time when IFN was in very short supply. Higher doses have been used in chronic myeloid leukemia but have caused more side-effects [113–115]. Lower doses have not been investigated and may well be just as effective. Finally, the mechanism of action of IFN in follicular lymphoma remains unexplained.

Prognostic factors

Whilst prognostic factor analysis and the development of prognostic indices have long been in favor for intermediate- and high-grade lymphoma, it is only relatively recently that such indices have been applied to follicular lymphoma. Since complete remission is less frequently achieved in follicular lymphoma, 'progression-free survival' and survival are probably more useful end-points for prognostic factor analyses than achievement and duration of complete remission.

LOCALIZED DISEASE

A series of studies from the Princess Margaret Hospital, Toronto, has identified age, stage and B symptoms to be independent prognostic factors for patients treated with radiotherapy [59,116]. The size of the lymph node mass has also been shown to be important, the cutoff being 5 cm [59,116]. Using the Princess Margaret Hospital prognostic index, three groups can be defined: the best category comprises younger patients (less than 70 years old) with stage I or II nodal disease with a maximum diameter of less than 5 cm; the disease-free survival at 10 years is excellent at 75%. Patients with extensive stage II disease, >5 cm in diameter have a survival inferior to that of the first group (58% at 10 years with a disease-free survival of 45%). The prognosis of the third group i.e., older patients (>70 years old), irrespective of any other considerations, is very poor. Age is thus a much stronger prognostic factor than all the other parameters, such older patients having a disease-free and overall survival of <28% at 10 years [116].

ADVANCED DISEASE

Histological features

Within the three categories of the Working Formulation, patients with 'nodular mixed' histology have sometimes been found to have a significantly shorter survival [117], whereas in a report from the National Cancer Institute, this histological subtype was associated with longer duration of remission following combination chemotherapy [72]. It has also been reported to be associated with longer initial remissions when patients were treated with an Adriamycin-containing regimen [118]. However, it is widely agreed that the definition and reproducibility of these three categories is difficult, and somewhat subjective [14,15]. Thus, at St Bartholomew's Hospital, the choice of treatment is not based on the percentage of large cells in the original biopsy.

There are also conflicting reports as to the significance of high mitotic activity. One series [119] showed a mitotic index >2 to be associated with poor survival, but two other studies have not confirmed this [120,121]. The significance of other indices of cell proliferation is also unclear; shorter survival has been found to be consequent upon the finding of a high percentage of cells in S phase and high expression of the nuclear proliferation antigen Ki-67 [122–124]. Other histopathological features have also been said to have prognostic significance, e.g., the degree of 'follicularity' [125–128], absence of fibrosis between the follicles [125] and the degree of T-helper cell infiltration in the lymph node [129,130].

Cytogenetics

As mentioned above, the prognostic significance of the t(14;18) translocation remains controversial but most studies, at least in the context of conventional therapy, have not found any correlation of the presence of this translocation with either response to therapy or survival [31,131]. The development of other cytogenetic changes is, however, associated with a poor prognosis [132].

Clinical features

It is generally agreed that older age is associated with a worse prognosis [133–138], whilst women seem to have a better prognosis for no obvious reason [88,137,138]. Stage clearly correlates with survival [5,20,88,135–140], as shown in Figure 41.3 for patients treated at St Bartholomew's Hospital. The majority of patients have bone marrow involvement but infiltration of other organs seems to confer a worse prognosis [138,140,141]. The presence of B symptoms is also an adverse prognostic factor [135–137,142], as is poor performance status [88].

The concept of 'tumor burden' has been put forward as a very important prognostic factor by the French/Belgian group. In several centers, a 'high tumor burden' has been variously defined in terms of the size of lymph node masses, the number of extranodal sites involved, the degree of splenomegaly and hepatomegaly, and the presence of circulating lymphoma cells [88,135–140,142].

Hematological and biochemical parameters

Anemia has been found to have a poor prognosis in some series [5,137,142]. A high LDH level (as in large-cell lymphoma) correlates very well with both a lower response rate and shorter survival [20,88,138, 140,142] as does a high level of β_2-microglobulin. [143].

Treatment parameters

In patients with advanced disease, a very important prognostic factor for survival is response to the initial therapy [5]. However, there has been much debate as to the significance of the degree of response. A retrospective analysis from St Bartholomew's Hospital did not show any difference in survival between patients in whom a complete or 'good partial' remission had been achieved ('good partial' response being defined as no palpable disease, with minimal residual paratrabecular infiltration in the marrow and/or equivocal lymphadenopathy

on a CT scan) [5]. However, in other studies, the completeness of response has been found to discriminate in terms of long-term survival [20,140].

Prognostic indices

The development and application of prognostic indices to follicular lymphoma is fraught with problems in comparison with the generally agreed principles upon which prognostic indices for large-cell lymphoma have been based. Part of the difficulty lies in the inclusion or exclusion of specific subgroups, for example, patients with follicular large-cell lymphoma have often been excluded. Also, studies vary in terms of the entry criteria. Nonetheless, valid and reproducible prognostic indices have been proposed. Leonard et al. [137] have described an index based on age, sex, stage, hemoglobin level and performance status, which separates patients into three subgroups. Romaguera et al. [138] have, in turn, developed an index based on sex, number of extranodal sites and the size of involved lymph nodes. Two other prognostic indices originally developed for use in patients with intermediate- and high-grade lymphoma are also valid for follicular lymphoma: the LNH 84 index [144], for example, has been applied to patients with follicular lymphoma treated in Lyon [145]. Those with localized disease, less than two extranodal sites, a normal LDH level and no 'bulky' lymph nodes (less than 10 cm in diameter) have the best survival. In contrast, those with disseminated disease, 'bulky' lymph nodes, more than one extranodal site or any of these parameters, together with a high LDH level, have the worst survival, with a third intermediate group falling between these two extremes (Figure 41.4).

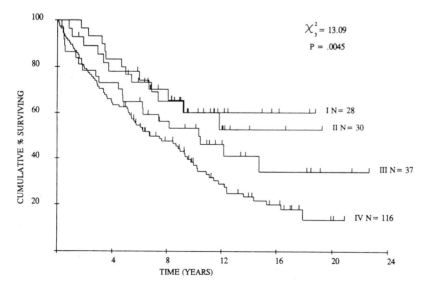

Figure 41.3 Survival of patients with follicular lymphoma treated at St Bartholomews's Hospital according to stage.

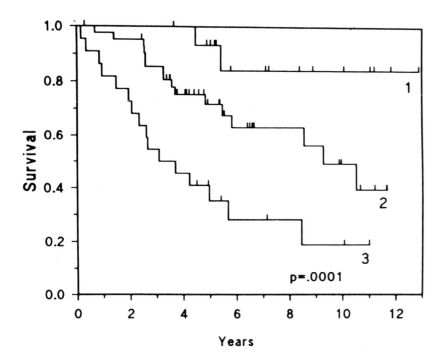

Figure 41.4 Survival for patients with follicular lymphoma treated in Lyon according to the LNH 84 Index.

More recently, the International Index for large-cell lymphoma [146] has also been applied to patients with follicular lymphoma treated in Lyon and, once more, distinct subgroups can be defined using only age, stage, LDH level and performance status [145].

Thus, at least retrospectively, these quite simple parameters can discriminate between patients with clearly different prognoses. Prospective studies will be needed to evaluate their true clinical value.

Recurrence

The virtual inevitability of recurrence in this illness makes the question of choice of treatment for recurrence an important one.

CONVENTIONAL TREATMENT

Patients in whom chlorambucil was effective at presentation are very likely to respond to it again at first, second and even third recurrence [5]. Simple to give and relatively free of toxicity, it is a good option for younger and older people alike. If however, after, for example, 6 weeks treatment there has clearly been no response, it is appropriate, at that point, to change to a more intensive regimen such as CHOP with the expectation that at least 50% of patients will respond. Patients who are asymptomatic at recur-

rence, other than the finding of one or several enlarged lymph nodes, may not need any specific treatment at that time.

SURVIVAL FROM RECURRENCE

The likelihood of response to further treatment at recurrence correlates with response to the initial therapy [5,147]. In a recent analysis from St Bartholomew's Hospital, the median survival following recurrence was 4.5 years [148]. Overall, the response rate at first recurrence was 78%, with the median duration of second remission being 13 months. Survival from first recurrence was found to correlate with only two factors on multivariate analysis: age at the time of recurrence and the number of prior treatments [148]. The latter is in fact a measure of responsiveness to treatment in that patients 'requiring' several different treatments are those in whom there is difficulty in achieving first remission. Survival after second recurrence depended on age and the 'quality' of the second remission; a greater proportion of patients in whom a second complete (as compared to a partial) remission was achieved, were alive at 10 years (53% versus 28%) [148]. Age thus appears to be overwhelmingly important, but the difficulty in precisely assessing the prognostic significance of any parameter (and age in particular), is that the proportion of patients with a specific characteristic will to some extent reflect referral patterns.

NEW APPROACHES

A number of new treatments have been evaluated and warrant mentioning separately:

1. Purine analogs:
   (a) fludarabine;
   (b) 2-chlorodeoxyadenosine (2-CDA);
   (c) deoxycoformycin;
2. Biological therapy:
   (a) interleukin-2 (IL-2);
   (b) monoclonal antibody alone;
   (c) monoclonal antibody–ricin conjugates;
   (d) radiolabeled monoclonal antibodies.
3. Myeloablative therapy with autologous bone marrow transplantation or peripheral blood progenitor cell support.

Purine analogs

Purine analogs are not in themselves new; this group of drugs includes 6-mercaptopurine, 5-fluorouracil and cytosine arabinoside. However, there has been a resurgence of interest in their use with the development of two drugs that are quite similar in structure, fludarabine and 2-CDA and the adenosine deaminase inhibitor, 2'-deoxycoformycin (DCF). All three were originally used in chronic lymphocytic leukemia (CLL) and have more recently been shown to have activity in follicular lymphoma.

Fludarabine

Fludarabine (9-β-D-arabinosyl-2-fluoro-adenine monophosphate) (Table 41.9) is an interesting drug in that it is devoid of the side-effects generally associated with cancer chemotherapy. This makes it attractive from the point of view of the patient. The main practical disadvantage is that in 1997 at least, it has to be given over a 5-day period, intravenously, which is

clearly unsatisfactory for patients traveling long distances for treatment. Its development has an interesting history: it is a fluorinated derivative of adenine arabinoside (ara-A), a drug of limited potential because it is rapidly deaminated in the bloodstream by adenosine deaminase. The 2'-fluoro derivative is relatively resistant to deamination but was in turn found to be virtually insoluble. Fludarabine was finally developed as the 5'-monophosphate form, which was both resistant to deamination and could be formulated in aqueous solution. Preclinical studies revealed activity against L1210 leukemia and P388 leukemia [149], and activity was also found against lymphoma and breast cancer in a human tumor cloning system [150].

The drug is thought to have two mechanisms of action: first, the triphosphate inhibits DNA synthesis and other enzymes including ribonuclease reductase, DNA polymerase-α, DNA primase and DNA ligase-1 [151]; but it is also cytotoxic to non-proliferating cells [152], possibly through the induction of apoptosis [153].

The dose and schedule conventionally used were first described by investigators at the MD Anderson Cancer Center, Houston, i.e., 25mg/m^2 as a bolus injection, daily for 5 days, repeated every 3–4 weeks [154–157]. This dose and schedule were adopted following prohibitive central nervous system toxicity seen when fludarabine was given at higher doses in the original phase I studies [158,159]. The dose-limiting toxicity at the currently used dose is myelosuppression, with neutropenia and infection frequently necessitating admission to hospital. A side-effect specific to fludarabine is immunosuppression, which has resulted in an increased risk of opportunistic infection [160].

The published studies to date have generally reported results in patients with recurrent or refractory disease (Table 41.9), and response rates have ranged from 38% to 55% [161–167]. It is likely that

Table 41.9 Results of treatment with fludarabine in patients with recurrent/resistant follicular lymphoma

Reference	Dose (mg/m^2/day) and schedule	Response rate
164	20: loading dose 30: × 2 days continuous infusion	8/26 (1 CR, 7 PR)
154	18 × 5, every 4 weeks	11/28 (4 CR, 7 PR)
166	25 × 5, every 3–4 weeks	19/28 (4 CR, 13 PR)
163	25 × 5, every 3–4 weeks	11/23 (5 CR, 6 PR)
165	25 × 5, every 3–4 weeks	5/11
161	25 × 5, every 4 weeks	12/38* (5 CR, 7 PR)
167	25 × 5, every 4 weeks	8/13*

* 'Low-grade lymphoma', not reported separately for follicular lymphoma.
CR, Complete remission; PR, partial remission.

higher rates would be achieved in newly diagnosed patients. At St Bartholomew's Hospital, the drug has also been found to be useful in a specific situation [165], namely, in patients in whom CHOP had failed to eradicate infiltration from the bone marrow. The exact role of fludarabine in the treatment of follicular lymphomas remains to be clarified but more information on this exciting new compound should be obtained from ongoing studies.

2-Chlorodeoxyadenosine

There are relatively few data for 2-CDA in follicular lymphoma, although the drug has some activity. In the series reported by Kay et al. [168], 17 patients out of 40 who had received a median of three different prior chemotherapy regimens responded (eight complete response and nine partial response); a later study reported by Hickish et al. [169] has confirmed activity. Further studies are awaited.

2'-Deoxycoformycin (pentostatin)

As with 2-CDA, there are few data on low-grade lymphoma. Patients with various subtypes of lymphoma were included in an Eastern Cooperative Oncology Group study; 2 out of 12 patients with low-grade histology had a partial response [170], and in a Cancer and Leukemia Group B (CALGB) study, two out of four patients with follicular lymphoma entered complete remission [171].

Biological therapy

Interleukin-2

IL-2 has been shown to have some activity in patients with follicular lymphoma when given alone, or in conjuction with lymphokine-activated killer (LAK) cells. A total of 39 patients with follicular lymphoma have been reported to date and 12 responses seen, three of them complete [172]. All of the latter patients were treated in the context of having developed recurrent lymphoma and some were considered to have resistant disease.

The mechanism of action for IL-2 +/– LAK cells is unclear; however, IL-2 is known to activate both natural killer cells and cytotoxic T-cells. In addition, when patients are treated with IL-2, a number of other cytokines are released into the circulation by activated lymphocytes and macrophages, including interleukin-6 (IL-6), interferon-γ (IFNγ), tumor necrosis factor and granulocyte–macrophage colony-stimulating factor (GM-CSF), [173]. LAK cell activity is certainly inducible from peripheral blood lymphocytes of patients with non-Hodgkin's lymphoma [174] and such cells can lyse autologous lymphoma cells *in vitro* [175]. It has also been suggested that, in addition to an indirect, immunologically mediated mechanism, there may be a direct anti-tumor effect in low-grade lymphoma, since many of the lymphoma cells have high expression of IL-2 receptors on the cell surface [176].

The main clinical problem in the early IL-2 studies was its virtually prohibitive toxicity, in particular, capillary leak syndrome and hypotension necessitating admission to the intensive care unit [177]. More recently, the drug has been given at a lower dose by continuous intravenous infusion and, although this has helped considerably, patients still complain of feeling tired and generally unwell.

In terms of responsiveness, there is a suggestion, based on a small number of observations, that patients with follicular lymphoma may be more responsive than those with other subtypes of lymphoma [178] and it may well be that the use of IL-2 in an adjuvant setting, as is currently being evaluated in patients with acute leukemia, will prove to be more effective'.

Monoclonal antibody-based treatment

Since follicular lymphoma represents a clonal proliferation of B-cells, it is, in theory anyway, an ideal target for the use of treatment based on the administration of monoclonal antibodies directed against tumor-specific B-lymphocyte antigens.

Monoclonal antibodies alone

Monoclonal antibodies were originally used in the hope that such highly specific treatment would be effective against tumor cells that were resistant to conventional chemotherapy and a number of patients with follicular lymphoma have in fact received such treatment. Unconjugated antibodies have resulted in some degree of response in patients with follicular lymphoma, either as a decrease in the number of circulating lymphoma cells, or as tangible but incomplete regression of lymphadenopathy [179–190]. The main clinical problems have been non-specific toxicity, i.e., fever, rashes, rigors and hypotension, but the usefulness of the treatment has also been limited by other factors. The majority of the antibodies used have limited inherent cytoxicity. There is also the risk of the development of human antimouse antibodies in some patients, which precludes the administration of repeated cycles of treatment. A possible way of bypassing the latter has been the construction of 'humanized' or chimeric antibodies to reduce immunogenicity.

The CAMPATH-I group of antibodies are directed against a ubiquitous B-cell antigen (CD52) expressed on both normal B-cells and on most B-cell malignancies [179]. Initially, the IgM and IgG$_2$B antibodies, CAMPATH-IM and CAMPATH-IG respectively,

Table 41.10 Myeloablative therapy with autologous hematopoietic progenitor cell support

Reference	No. of patients and situation	Treatment	*In vitro* treatment	Source of progenitor cells	Outcome (no. free of disease)
226	51 in 2nd CR or >2nd remission	CY + TBI	Initially: anti-CD20 + C', then anti-CD10 anti-CD20 + C', anti-B5	Aut. BM	32 patients for 3 months–5 years
225	64 in 2nd or >2nd remission	CY + TBI	Anti-CD20 + C'	Aut. BM	
232	46 following recurrence	CY + TBI (40 patients) or CT alone	None	Aut. BM: 6 Per. blood: 40	26 patients for 3 months–4 years and 8 months
247		CY + TBI or CT alone		Per. blood	
231	26 variable		12/26 patients + mafosphamide	Aut. BM or per. blood	20 patients for 6 months–4 years and 8 months
235	66 in 1st remission	CY + TBI	Anti-CD10 Anti-CD20 + C' Anti-B5	Aut. BM	53 patients for 3 months–2 years and 2 months
234	9 in 1st remission		Mafosphamide	Aut. BM	8 patients for 15–43 months

CY, Cyclophosphamide; TBI, total body irradiation; CT, chemotherapy; Aut., autologous; BM, bone marrow; C', complement; Per., peripheral.

row transplantation (ABMT) in patients with recurrent intermediate- and high-grade lymphoma [213–224], a similar approach has been explored in younger patients with follicular lymphoma. The total number of patients treated is still relatively small and the follow-up time relatively short, in comparison to natural history of follicular lymphoma. Most patients have been treated with cyclophosphamide and TBI, although 'drug-only' regimens have also been used (Table 41.10). In view of the propensity of follicular lymphoma to involve the bone marrow, at two centers, the Dana–Farber Cancer Institute in Boston and St Bartholomew's Hospital, London the view has been taken that *in vitro* 'purging' of the marrow should be performed, since it can at least reduce the number of clonogenic tumor cells present in the reinfused marrow preparation, even if tumor cells cannot be completely eliminated [225,226].

The results from St Bartholomew's Hospital can be summarized as follows [225]: at present, with a median follow-up of 3.5 years, one-third of patients have developed recurrent lymphoma. Freedom from recurrence does not currently correlate with the length of time the patient had had the illness prior to transplant, the presence or absence of residual disease at any site at the time of treatment, or the specific remission in which the treatment is given (second versus third or beyond). However, a comparison with an age-matched, remission-matched historical control group treated at St Bartholomew's Hospital prior to the introduction of this treatment shows a significant advantage in favor of myeloablative therapy ($P=0.001$) for patients treated in second remission (Figure 41.5). Currently, there is no difference in survival, either because there will not be such a difference or because the follow-up is still too short. When these results were analyzed jointly with the results from the DFCI, they were found to be identical [227].

At the present time, as mentioned above, there are no data to suggest that this treatment is better given earlier rather than later. The only problem with deferring the treatment is that at each recurrence the proportion of patients responding will be approximately 75% [5]; therefore the denominator will decrease each time. In practical terms this means that some patients in whom a second complete or nearly complete remission was achieved will not enter a third remission, either because of transformation or because of chemotherapy resistance.

The question whether reinfusion of lymphoma cells contributes significantly to recurrence remains contentious. Data from the DFCI suggests that 'PCR negativity' for the t(14;18) is the most important prognostic factor for freedom from recurrence [228]. In contrast, at St Bartholomew's Hospital, using only

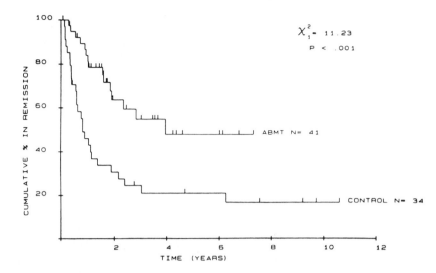

$$\chi^2_1 = 11.23$$
$$P < .001$$

Figure 41.5 Duration of remission for patients treated at St Bartholomew's Hospital receiving cyclophosphamide, total body irradiation and autologous bone marrow transplantation in second remission, compared to a historical control group receiving chlorambucil or cyclophosphamide, vincristine, prednisone.

one monoclonal antibody (anti-CD-20, as compared to three in Boston), such PCR negativity is almost never achieved [229], and yet the clinical results are the same [227].

Furthermore, the results in patients in whom the marrow has not been treated *in vitro* are also very similar to those in whom purging was performed. Schouten et al., on behalf of the European Bone Marrow Transplant Group Registry, has reported the outcome in 80 patients with low-grade lymphoma treated at centers throughout Europe [230]. With a median follow-up of 2 years' progression-free survival was 52%, irrespective of whether a TBI-containing or drug-only regimen was used. Three other studies have reported results for myeloablative therapy with untreated autologous stem cells: Colombat et al. described 26 patients in whom the myeloablative therapy was supported either by autologous bone marrow or autologous peripheral blood progenitor cells. The event-free survival was 67% at a median follow-up of between 2 and 3 years [231]. The greatest experience with peripheral blood cells is from Omaha, Nebraska; Bierman et al. have reported an actuarial 4-year event-free survival of 46% for patients with follicular lymphoma receiving myeloablative therapy supported by peripheral blood progenitor cells [232]. Very recently, high-dose therapy with peripheral blood progenitor cell support has been reported for 30 patients with follicular lymphoma treated in Heidelberg. The treatment comprised high-dose ara-C and mitoxantrone, followed by granulocyte colony-stimulating factor (G-CSF). Although the follow-up time is very short, such that the success of the approach cannot be assessed yet, it is clear that, in the majority of patients, the peripheral blood progenitor cell (PBPC) collection contained PCR-detectable lymphoma cells. However, in 6 out of 22 such patients, bone marrow

samples became PCR-negative between 3 and 16 months after reinfusion of PBPC [233].

It is frequently believed by patients and physicians alike that no further treatment is possible after any sort of transplant procedure. This is clearly not the case. Not only is further treatment possible but advisable if the person is symptomatic. There is, however, sometimes a problem with 'fragility' of the blood count; even chlorambucil alone in this situation may lead to a precipitous fall. Another fallacy is that death follows shortly after a recurrence post-transplantation. Again, this is not necessarily the case. In patients with follicular lymphoma receiving cyclophosphamide + TBI + ABMT at St Bartholomew's Hospital, 30 of 81 have developed recurrent lymphoma and 13 have subsequently died, in some of whom transformation to high-grade histology occurred. In four patients, the recurrence was asymptomatic and was detected on annual surveillance investigations.

High-dose therapy with stem cell rescue in first remission
Myeloablative therapy is now being tested as a consolidation of first remission. Nine patients have been reported by Fouillard et al. [234]; the treatment was given as consolidation of first remission, and eight of the nine patients were well and free of disease at the time of publication. A larger number of patients have been treated in first remission in Boston [235]; 53 of the 66 patients had been in unmaintained first remission for between 3 and 26 months at the time that the report was published. A study is currently in progress in Europe comparing continuous CHOP treatment with CHOP therapy followed by consolidation, consisting of myeloablative therapy and ABMT.

Myeloablative therapy and ABMT have also been

investigated after transformation to high-grade histology. A report from the DFCI described 18 such patients; the event-free survival at 4 years was only 23%, as compared to 53% for patients in whom there was no evidence of transformation [216]. Similarly, the results reported by Schouten et al., in patients in whom transformation had occurred, are considerably inferior to those achieved when similar myeloablative treatment was used prior to transformation [236].

The problem with all of these data is that longer follow-up is required before any conclusion about the potential for cure can be made. It is clear that, while some patients appear to be doing well, there is already a significant recurrence rate. Attempts to improve this treatment as a whole might include changing the myeloablative regimen, changing from autologous marrow to peripheral blood progenitor cells and, possibly, using immunological therapy, such as IFN or IL-2, afterwards.

A problem, which has only recently come to light, is that, although the early treatment-related mortality is less than 5% after myeloablative therapy, the overall figure will be higher, since a few patients [227,237] have developed myelodysplasia and, rarely, acute myelogenous leukemia. This is clearly a cause for major concern. It is impossible to know whether this relates to both previous therapy and myeloablation, or whether it is caused exclusively by the latter. The incidence is, however, considerably higher than that seen over a 25-year period at St Bartholomew's Hospital in patients with follicular lymphoma receiving conventional treatment.

While these data are preliminary and it remains possible that this intensive treatment approach, like so many before it, will eventually be demonstrated to simply prolong remission duration but not survival for the younger patient with follicular lymphoma who has already had one recurrence, it is probably, currently, the best treatment option.

Detection of lymphoma at the molecular level

In the majority of patients with follicular lymphoma, the t(14;18) translocation is present in the clonal population of cells [6–9]. Recently, much attention has been focused on the use of PCR analysis to detect residual t(14;18)-containing cells in the peripheral blood and bone marrow of patients who have completed treatment.

It has been demonstrated that, after therapy, patients initially presenting with advanced-stage disease have cells containing the *bcl*-2 rearrangement in the peripheral blood, despite the fact that by all other criteria they are considered to be in complete remission [238]. Circulating translocation-positive cells have also been shown to persist in patients who have been in remission for protracted periods of time. Price et al. found persistent cells, by PCR, in patients presenting with stage III and stage IV disease but not in those presenting with localized disease; all had been in remission for more than 10 years [239]. Furthermore, sequence analysis demonstrated that the circulating cells belonged to the original *bcl*-2 clone. In a recent study, peripheral blood from 21 patients in long-term remission after radiotherapy for stage I or II follicular lymphoma was also found to be positive for the presence of t(14;18) [240]. A further study has confirmed these findings, with 9 out of 12 patients who presented with stage I and II follicular lymphoma being found to be PCR-positive, either at diagnosis or after treatment [241]. In yet another study, untreated, early and advanced-stage patients with follicular lymphoma were examined. Bone marrow and peripheral blood samples from 28 newly diagnosed patients were assessed by morphology, PCR analysis, immunophenotyping and cytogenetic analysis. On the basis of morphology alone, bone marrow infiltration was detected in 11 of 28 patients. PCR analysis alone detected lymphoma cells in the bone marrow in 17 of the 24 assessable patients but, interestingly, morphologic examination revealed lymphoma in three bone marrow samples that were negative by PCR [242]. A study from Switzerland has demonstrated concordance with respect to the ability to detect t(14;18) between peripheral blood and bone marrow in 55 of 56 patients [243]. However, the presence or absence of t(14;18)-positive cells in the circulation has been shown to have no correlation with clinical remission status or remission duration in patients receiving conventional therapy for stage III or IV disease [244].

There has been much interest in trying to establish whether myeloablative therapy in patients with follicular lymphoma can eradicate minimal residual disease. One difficulty in exploring this issue is the presence of tumor cells in the reinfused autologous bone marrow. Gribben et al., analyzing bone marrow samples before and after *in vitro* 'purging' treatment, have reported that PCR negativity of the reinfused marrow is the single most important prognostic factor for disease-free survival [228]. More recently, the same group have examined sequential bone marrow samples from patients deemed to be in complete remission after the myeloablative therapy. Again, disease-free survival was longer in patients with no PCR detectable lymphoma cells in the marrow [245].

The use of PBPCs as opposed to autologous marrow raises the same questions about such PBPC collections. A small series from Australia suggests that tumor cell contamination of PBPC collections is not uncommon [246] and other studies have shown that progenitor cells collected from peripheral blood from patients in whom the marrow was morphologically uninvolved at the time of collection are positive by PCR analysis [233, 247].

The clinical significance and prognostic implications of such residual cells detected by PCR and evaluation of the risk of further recurrence will require prospective long-term studies.

Acknowledgment

We are most grateful to Chris Sykes for typing this manuscript.

References

1. Gall EA, Mallory TB. Malignant lymphoma: A clinico-pathological survey of 618 cases. *Am. J. Pathol.* 1942, **18**: 381–429.
2. Jones SE, Fuks Z, Bull M, et al. Non-Hodgkin's lymphoma IV. Clinicopathologic correlation in 405 cases. *Cancer* 1973, **31**: 806–823.
3. Anderson T, De Vita V, Simon R, et al. Malignant lymphoma II: Prognostic factors and response to treatment of 473 patients at the National Cancer Institute. *Cancer*, 1982, **50**: 2708–2721.
4. Brittinger G, Bartels H, Common H, et al. Clinical and prognostic relevance of the Kiel Classification of non-Hodgkin's lymphomas: Results of a prospective multicentre study by the Kiel lymphoma study group. *Haematol. Oncol.* 1984, **2**: 269–306.
5. Gallagher CJ, Gregory WM, Jones AE, et al. Follicular lymphoma: Prognostic factors for response and survival. *J. Clin. Oncol.* 1986, **4**: 1470–1480.
6. Fukuhara S, Rowley JD. Chromosome 14 translocations in non-Burkitt lymphomas. *Int. J. Cancer* 1978, **22**: 14–21.
7. Yunis JJ, Oken MM, Kaplan ME, et al. Distinctive chromosomal abnormalities in histologic subtypes of non-Hodgkin's lymphoma. *N. Engl. J. Med.* 1982, **307**: 1231–1236.
8. Fifth International Workshop on Chromosomes in Leukemia–Lymphoma. Correlation of chromosome abnormalities with histologic and immunologic characteristics in non-Hodgkin's lymphoma and adult T-cell leukemia–lymphoma. *Blood* 1987, **70**: 1554–1564.
9. Weiss LM, Warnke RA, Skear J, et al. Molecular analysis of the t(14;18) chromosomal translocation in malignant lymphomas. *N. Engl. J. Med.* 1987, **317**: 1185–1189.
10. Crescenzi M, Seto M, Herzig GP, et al. Thermostable DNA polymerase chain amplification of t(14;18) chromosome break point and detection of minimal residual disease. *Proc. Natl Acad. Sci. USA* 1988, **85**: 4869–4873.
11. Non-Hodgkin's Lymphoma Pathologic Classification Project. National Cancer Institute sponsored study of classifications of non-Hodgkin's lymphomas: Summary and description of a Working Formulation for clinical usage. *Cancer* 1982, **49**: 2112–2135.
12. Lukes RJ, Collins RD. Immunologic characterization of human malignant lymphomas. *Cancer* 1974, **34**: 1488–1503.
13. Mann RB, Berard CW. Criteria for the cytologic subclassification of follicular lymphomas: A proposed alternative method. *Hematol. Oncol.* 1983, **1**: 187–192.
14. Metter GE, Nathwani BN, Burke JS, et al. Morphological subclassification of follicular lymphoma: Variability of diagnoses among hematopathologists, a collaborative study between the repository center and pathology panel for lymphoma clinical studies. *J. Clin. Oncol.* 1985, **3**: 25–38.
15. Nathwani BN, Metter GE, Miller TP, et al. What should be the morphologic criteria for the subdivision of follicular lymphomas? *Blood* 1986, **68**: 837–845.
16. Gerard-Marchant R, Hamlin I, Lennert K, et al. Classification of non-Hodgkin's lymphomas. *Lancet* 1974, **2**: 406–408.
17. Harris NL, Jaffe ES, Stein H, et al. A revised European–American classification of lymphoid neoplasms. A proposal from the International Lymphoma Study Group. *Blood* 1994, **84**: 1361–1392.
18. Osborne CK, Norton L, Young RC, et al. Nodular histiocytic lymphoma: An aggressive nodular lymphoma with potential for prolonged disease-free survival. *Blood* 1980, **56**: 98–103.
19. Glick JH, McFadden E, Costello W, et al. Nodular histiocytic lymphoma: Factors influencing prognosis and implications for aggressive chemotherapy. *Cancer* 1982, **49**: 840–845.
20. Kantarjian HM, McLaughlin P, Fuller LM, et al. Follicular large cell lymphoma: Analysis and prognostic factors in 62 patients. *J. Clin. Oncol.* 1984, **2**: 811–819.
21. Anderson JR, Vose JM, Bierman PJ, et al. Clinical features and prognosis of follicular large-cell lymphoma: A report from the Nebraska Lymphoma Study Group. *J. Clin. Oncol.* 1993, **11**: 218–224.
22. Jaffe ES. The role of immunophenotypic markers in the classification of non-Hodgkin's lymphomas. *Semin. Oncol.* 1990, **17**: 11–19.
23. Picker LJ, Weiss LM, Medeiros LJ, et al. Immunophenotypic criteria for the diagnosis of non-Hodgkin's lymphoma. *Am. J. Pathol.* 1987, **128**: 181–201.
24. Harris NL, Nadler LM, Bhan AK. Immunohistologic characterization of two malignant lymphomas of germinal center type (centroblastic/centrocytic and centrocytic) with monoclonal antibodies: Follicular and diffuse lymphomas of small-cleaved-cell type are

related but distinct entities. *Am. J. Pathol.* 1984, **117**: 262–272.

25. Levine EG, Arthur DC, Frizzera G, et al. There are differences in cytogenetic abnormalities among histologic subtypes of the non-Hodgkin's lymphomas. *Blood* 1985, **66**: 1414–1422.

26. Richardson ME, Chen Q, Filippa DA, et al. Intermediate- to high-grade histology of lymphomas carrying t(14;18) is associated with additional nonrandom chromosome changes. *Blood* 1987, **70**: 444–447.

27. Konishi H, Sakurai M, Nakao H, et al. Chromosome abnormalities in malignant lymphoma in patients from Kurashiki: Histological and immunophenotypic correlations. *Cancer Res.* 1990, **50**: 2698–2703.

28. Maseki N, Kaneko Y, Sakurai M, et al. Chromosome abnormalities in malignant lymphoma in patients from Saitama. *Cancer Res.* 1987, **47**: 6767–6775.

29. Wlodarska I, Mecucci C, Vandenberghe E, et al. dup(12)(q13→qter) in two t(14;18)-negative follicular B-non-Hodgkin's lymphomas. *Genes Chromosom. Cancer* 1992, **4**: 302–308.

30. Ladanyi M, Offit K, Parsa NZ, et al. Follicular lymphoma with t(8;14)(q24;q32): A distinct clinical and molecular subset of t(8;14)-bearing lymphomas. *Blood* 1992, **79**: 2124–2130.

31. Levine EG, Arthur DC, Frizzera G, et al. Cytogenetic abnormalities predict clinical outcome in non-Hodgkin's lymphoma. *Ann. Intern. Med.* 1988, **108**: 14–20.

32. Schouten HC, Sanger WG, Weistenburger DD, et al. Chromosomal abnormalities in untreated patients with non-Hodgkin's lymphoma: Associations with histology, clinical characteristics, and treatment outcome. *Blood* 1990, **75**: 1841–1847.

33. Offit K, Wong G, Filippa DA, et al. Cytogenetic analysis of 434 consecutively ascertained specimens of non-Hodgkin's lymphoma: Clinical correlations. *Blood* 1991, **77**: 1508–1515.

34. Cabanillas F, Pathak S, Grant G, et al. Refractoriness to chemotherapy and poor survival related to abnormalities of chromosomes 17 and 7 in lymphoma. *Am. J. Med.* 1989, **87**: 167–172.

35. Aisenberg AC, Wilkes BM, Jacobson JO, et al. Immunoglobulin gene rearrangements in adult non-Hodgkin's lymphoma. *Am. J. Med.* 1987, **82**: 738–744.

36. Williams ME, Innes DJ Jr, Borowitz MJ, et al. Immunoglobulin and T-cell receptor gene rearrangements in human lymphoma and leukemia. *Blood* 1987, **69**: 79–86.

37. Tsujimoto Y, Cossman J, Jaffe E, et al. Involvement of the *bcl*-2 gene in human follicular lymphoma. *Science* 1985, **288**: 1440–1443.

38. Hockenberry D, Nunez G, Milliman C, et al. Bcl-2 is an inner mitochondrial membrane protein that blocks programmed cell death. *Nature* 1990, **348**: 334–336.

39. Becker E. Rein Betrag zur Lehr von den Lymphomen. *Deutsch. Med. Wochenssch.* 1901, **27**: 726.

40. Brill NE, Baehr G, Rosenthal N. Generalised giant lymph follicle hyperplasia of lymph nodes and spleen: A hitherto undescribed type. *JAMA* 1925, **84**: 668.

41. Symmers D. Giant follicular lymphadenopathy with or without splenomegaly. *Arch. Path.* 1938, **26**: 603–647.

42. Whelan JS, Reznek RH, Daniell SJN, et al. Computed tomography (CT) and ultrasound (US) guided core biopsy in the management of non-Hodgkin's lymphoma. *Br. J. Cancer* 1991, **63**: 460–462.

43. Schnitzer B, Loesel LS, Reed RE. Lymphosarcoma cell leukemia: A clinicopathologic study. *Cancer* 1970, **26**: 1082–1096.

44. Melo JV, Robinson DSF, de Oliveira MP, et al. Morphology and immunology of circulating cells in leukemic phase of follicular lymphoma. *J. Clin. Pathol.* 1988, **41**: 951–959.

45. Carbone PP, Kaplan HS, Musshoff K, et al. Report of the committee on Hodgkin's disease staging classification. *Cancer Res.* 1971, **31**: 1860–1861.

46. Rosenberg SA, Boiron M, De Vita V, et al. Report of the committee on Hodgkin's disease staging procedures. *Cancer Res.* 1971, **31**: 1862–1863.

47. Horning SJ, Rosenberg SA. The natural history of initially untreated low-grade non-Hodgkin's lymphomas. *N. Engl. J. Med.* 1984, **311**: 1471–1475.

48. Young RC, Longo DL, Glatstein E, et al. The treatment of indolent lymphomas: Watchful waiting v aggressive combined modality treatment. *Semin. Hematol.* 1988, **25**(Suppl.): 11–16.

49. Acker B, Hoppe RT, Colby TV, et al. Histologic conversion in the non-Hodgkin's lymphomas. *J. Clin. Oncol.* 1983, **1**: 11–16.

50. Ersboll J, Schultz HB, Pedersen-Bjergaard J, et al. Follicular low-grade non-Hodgkin's lymphoma: Long-term outcome with or without tumor progression. *Eur. J. Haematol.* 1989, **42**: 155–163.

51. Hubbard SM, Chabner BA, DeVita VJ Jr, et al. Histologic progression in non-Hodgkin's lymphoma. *Blood* 1982, **59**: 258–264.

52. Armitage JO, Dick FR, Corder MP. Diffuse histiocytic lymphoma after histologic conversation: A poor prognostic variant. *Cancer Treat. Rep.* 1981, **65**: 413–418.

53. Ostrow SS, Diggs CH, Sutherland JC, et al. Nodular poorly differentiated lymphocytic lymphoma: Changes in histology and survival. *Cancer Treat. Rep.* 1981, **65**: 929–933.

54. Cullen MH, Lister TA, Brearley RL, et al. Histological transformation of non-Hodgkin's lymphoma. A prospective study. *Cancer* 1979, **44**: 645–651.

55. Yuen AR, Horning SJ. Long term survival after histologic transformation of low-grade lymphoma. *Proc. Am. Soc. Clin. Oncol.* 1993, **12**: 365 (abstract 1236).

56. O'Brien ME, Easterbrook P, Powell J, et al. The natural history of low-grade non-Hodgkin's lymphoma and the impact of a no initial treatment policy on survival. *Quart. J. Med.* 1991, **80**: 651–660.

57. Chen MG, Prosnitz LR, Gonzales-Serva A, et al. Results of radiotherapy in control of stage I and II non-Hodgkin's lymphoma. *Cancer* 1979, **43**: 1245–1254.

58. Gomez GA, Barlos M, Krishnamsetty RM, et al. Treatment of early – stage I and II – nodular poorly differentiated lymphocytic lymphoma. *Am. J. Clin. Oncol.* 1986, **9**: 40–44.

59. Gospodarowicz MG, Bush RS, Brown TC, et al. Prognostic factors in nodular lymphomas: A multivariate analysis based on the Princess Margaret Hospital experience. *Int. J. Radiat. Oncol. Biol. Phys.* 1984, **10**: 489–497.

60. Paryani SB, Hoppe RT, Cox RS. Analysis of non-Hodgkin's lymphomas with nodular and favorable histologies, stages I and II. *Cancer* 1983, **52**: 2300–2307.

61. Reddy S, Saxema VS, Pelletiere EV, Hendrickson FR. Stage I and II non-Hodgkin's lymphomas: long term results of radiation therapy. *Int. J. Radiat. Oncol. Biol. Phys.* 1989, **16**: 687–692.

62. Carde P, Burgers JMV, Van Glabbeke M, et al. Combined radiotherapy-chemotherapy for early stages in non-Hodgkin's lymphoma: The EORTC controlled lymphoma trial. *Radiother. Oncol.* 1984, **2**: 301–312.

63. McLaughlin P, Fuller LM, Velasquez WS, et al. Stage I–II follicular lymphoma: Treatment results of 76 patients. *Cancer* 1986, **58**: 1596–1602.

64. Monfardini S, Banfi A, Bonadonna G, et al. Improved five-year survival after combined radiotherapy–chemotherapy for stage I and II non-Hodgkin's lymphoma. *Int. J. Radiat. Oncol. Biol. Phys.* 1980, **6**: 125–134.

65. Richards MA, Gregory WM, Hall PA, et al. Management of localised non-Hodgkin's lymphoma: The experience at St Bartholomew's Hospital 1972–1985. *Haematol. Oncol.* 1989, **7**: 1–35.

66. Hoogstraten B, Owens AH, Lenhard RE, et al. Combination chemotherapy in lymphosarcoma and reticulum cell sarcoma. *Blood* 1969, **33**: 370–377.

67. Bagley CM, De Vita VT, Berrard CW, et al. Advanced lymphosarcoma: Intensive cyclical combination chemotherapy with cyclophosphamide, vincristine and prednisolone. *Ann. Intern. Med.* 1972, **76**: 227–234.

68. Portlock CS, Rosenberg SA, Glatstein E, et al. Treatment of advanced non-Hodgkin's lymphomas with favorable histology: Preliminary results of a prospective trial. *Blood* 1976, **47**: 747–756.

69. Kennedy BJ, Bloomfield CD, Kiang DT, et al. Combination versus successive single agent chemotherapy in lymphocytic lymphoma. *Cancer* 1978, **41**: 23–28.

70. Lister TA, Cullen MH, Beard MEJ, et al. Comparison of combined and single agent chemotherapy in non-Hodgkin's lymphoma of favorable histological subtype. *Br. Med. J.* 1978, **1**: 533–537.

71. Ezdinli E, Anderson J, Melvin F, et al. Moderate versus aggressive chemotherapy of nodular poorly differentiated lymphoma. *J. Clin. Oncol.* 1985, **3**: 769–775.

72. Longo DL, Young RC, Hubbard SM, et al. Prolonged initial remission in patients with nodular mixed lymphomas. *Ann. Intern. Med.* 1984, **100**: 651–656.

73. Anderson T, Bender RA, Fisher RI, et al. Combination chemotherapy in non-Hodgkin's lymphoma: Results of long-term follow-up. *Cancer Treat. Rep.* 1977, **61**: 1057–1066.

74. Bitran JC, Golomb HM, Ultmann JE, et al. Non-Hodgkin's lymphoma, poorly differentiated and mixed-cell types: Results of sequential staging procedures, response to therapy and survey of 100 patients. *Cancer* 1978, **42**: 88–95.

75. Glick JH, Barnes JM, Ezdinli EZ, et al. Nodular mixed lymphoma: Results of a randomized trial failing to confirm prolonged disease-free survival with COPP chemotherapy. *Blood* 1981, **58**: 920–925.

76. Oken MM, Costello WG, Johnson GJ, et al. The influence of histologic subtype on toxicity and response to chemotherapy in non-Hodgkin's lymphoma. *Cancer* 1983, **51**: 1581–1586.

77. Jones SE, Grozea PN, Metz EN, et al. Superiority of Adriamycin-containing combination chemotherapy in the treatment of diffuse lymphoma. A Southwest Oncology Group Study. *Cancer* 1979, **43**: 417–425.

78. Dana BW, Dahlberg S, Nathwani BN, et al. Long-term follow-up of patients with low-grade malignant lymphomas treated with doxorubicin-based chemotherapy or chemoimmunotherapy. *J. Clin. Oncol.* 1993, **11**: 644–651.

79. Anderson KC, Skarin AT, Rosenthal DS, et al. Combination chemotherapy for advanced non-Hodgkin's lymphomas other than diffuse histiocytic or undifferentiated histologies. *Cancer Treat. Rep.* 1984, **68**: 1343–1350.

80. Peterson BA, Anderson JR, Frizzera G, et al. Nodular mixed lymphoma: A comparative trial of cyclophosphamide and cyclophosphamide, Adriamycin, vincristine, prednisone and bleomycin. *Blood* 1985, **66**: 216a (abstr. 749).

81. Rodriguez V, Cabanillas F, Burgess MA, et al. Combination chemotherapy ('CHOP-Bleo') in advanced non-Hodgkin's lymphoma. *Blood* 1977, **49**: 325–333.

82. Fuks Z, Kaplan HS. Recurrence rates following radiation therapy of nodular and diffuse malignant lymphomas. *Radiology* 1973, **108**: 675–684.

83. Hoppe RT, Kushlan P, Kaplan HS, et al. The treatment of advanced stage favorable histology non-Hodgkin's lymphoma: A preliminary report of a randomized trial comparing single agent chemotherapy, combination chemotherapy, and whole body irradiation. *Blood* 1981, **58**: 592–598.

84. Mendenhall NP, Noyes WD, Million RR. Total body irradiation for stage II–IV non-Hodgkin's lymphoma: Ten-year follow-up. *J. Clin. Oncol.* 1989, **7**: 67–74.

85. Lybeert MLM, Meerwaldt JH, Deneve W. Long-term results of low dose total body irradiation for advanced non-Hodgkin lymphoma. *Int. J. Radiat. Oncol. Biol. Phys.* 1987, **13**: 1167–1172.

86. Chaffey JT, Hellman S, Rosenthal DS, et al. Total body irradiation in the treament of lymphocytic lymphoma. *Cancer Treat. Rep.* 1977, **61**: 1149–1152.

87. McLaughlin P, Fuller LM, Velasquez WS, et al. Stage III follicular lymphoma: Durable remissions with combined chemotherapy-radiotherapy regimen. *J. Clin. Oncol.* 1987, **5**: 867–874.

88. Steward WP, Crowther D, Mcwilliam LJ, et al. Maintenance chlorambucil after CVP in the management of advanced stage, low-grade histologic type non-Hodgkin's lymphoma: A randomized prospective study with an assessment of prognostic factors. *Cancer* 1988, **61**: 441–447.

89. Ezdinli EZ, Harrington DP, Kucuk O, et al. The effect of intensive intermittent maintenance therapy in ad-

vanced low-grade non-Hodgkin's lymphoma. *Cancer* 1987, **60**: 156–160.

90. Gresser I, Brouty-Boye D, Thomas M-T, et al. Interferon and cell division. I. Inhibition of the multiplication of mouse leukemia L1210 cells in vitro by an interferon preparation. *Proc. Natl. Acad. Sci. USA* 1970, **66**: 1052–1058.

91. Gresser I, Maury C, Tovey MG. Interferon and murine leukemia VII. Therapeutic effect of interferon preparations after diagnosis of lymphoma in AKR mice. *Int. J. Cancer* 1976, **7**: 647–651.

92. Gutterman JU, Blumenschein GR, Alexanian R. Leukocyte interferon-induced tumor regression in human metastatic breast cancer, multiple myeloma and malignant lymphoma. *Ann. Intern. Med.* 1980, **93**: 399–406.

93. Horning SJ, Merigan TC, Krown SE. Human interferon alpha in malignant lymphoma and Hodgkin's disease. *Cancer* 1985, **56**: 1305–1310.

94. Louie AC, Gallagher JC, Sikora K, et al. Follow up observations on the effect of human leukocyte interferon in non-Hodgkin's lymphoma. *Blood* 1981, **58**: 712–718.

95. Quesada JR, Hawkins M, Horning S, et al. Collaborative Phase I–II study of recombinant DNA-produced leukocyte Interferon (Clone A) in metastatic breast cancer, malignant lymphoma and multiple myeloma. *Am. J. Med.* 1984, **77**: 427–432.

96. O'Connell MJ, Colgan JP, Oken MM, et al. Clinical trial of recombinant leukocyte A interferon as initial therapy for favorable histology non-Hodgkin's lymphomas and chronic lymphocytic leukemia. *J. Clin. Oncol.* 1986, **4**: 128–136.

97. Wagstaff J, Loynds P, Crowther D. A phase II study of human recombinant DNA-a2 interferon in patients with low-grade non-Hodgkin's lymphoma. *Cancer Chemother. Pharmacol.* 1986, **18**: 54–58.

98. Leavitt J, Ratanathathorn V, Ozer H, et al. Alfa-2b Interferon in the treatment of Hodgkin's disease and non-Hodgkin's lymphoma. *Semin. Oncol.* 1987, **14** (2 Suppl. 2):18–23.

99. Foon KA, Roth MS, Bunn PA. Interferon therapy of non-Hodgkin's lymphoma. *Cancer* 1987, **59**: 601–604.

100. Gresser I, Maury C, Tovey M. Efficacy of combined interferon cyclophosphamide therapy after diagnosis of lymphoma in AKR mice. *Eur. J. Cancer* 1978, **14**: 97–99.

101. Chirigos MA, Pearson JW. Cure of murine leukemia with drugs and interferon treatment. *J. Natl Cancer Inst.* 1973, **51**: 1367–1368.

102. Balkwill FR, Moodie EM. Positive interactions between human interferon and cyclophosphamide or Adriamycin in a human tumor model system. *Cancer Res.* 1984, **44**: 904–908.

103. Rohatiner AZS, Richards MA, Barnett MJ, et al. Chlorambucil and interferon for low-grade non-Hodgkin's lymphoma. *Br. J. Cancer* 1987, **55**: 225–226.

104. Chisesi T, Capnist G, Vespignani M, et al. Interferon alfa-2b and chlorambucil in the treatment of non-Hodgkin's lymphoma. *J. Invest. New Drugs* 1987, **5**: 35–40.

105. Smalley RV, Andersen JW, Hawkins MJ, et al. Interferon alpha combined with cytotoxic chemotherapy for patients with non-Hodgkin's lymphoma. *N. Engl. J. Med.* 1992, **327**: 1336–1341.

106. Andersen JW, Smalley RV. Interferon alfa plus chemotherapy for non-Hodgkin's lymphoma five-year follow-up. *N. Engl. J. Med.* 1993, **329**: 1821–1822.

107. Solal-Celigny P, Lepage E, Brousse N, et al. Recombinant interferon alfa-2b combined with a regimen containing doxorubicin in patients with advanced follicular lymphoma. *N. Engl. J. Med.* 1993, **329**: 1608–1614.

108. Price CGA, Rohatiner AZS, Steward W, et al. Interferon-a2b in the treatment of follicular lymphoma. Preliminary results of a trial in progress. *Ann. Oncol.* 1991, **2**: 141–146.

109. Peterson BA, Petrioni G, Oken MM. Cyclophosphamide vs Cyclophosphamide + Interferon-a-2b in follicular low-grade lymphomas: A preliminary report of an inter-group trial (CALGB 8691 and EST 7486). *Proc. Am. Soc. Clin. Oncol.* 1993, **12**: 1240 (abstract).

110. Hagenbeek A, Carde P, Somers R, et al. Maintenance of remission with human recombinant alpha-2 interferon (Roferon-A) in patients with stages III and IV follicular malignant non-Hodgkin's lymphoma. Results from a prospective, randomised phase III clinical trial in 331 patients. *Blood* 1992, **80** (Suppl. 1): abstract 288.

111. McLaughlin P, Cabanillas F, Hagemeister FB, et al. CHOP-Bleo plus Interferon for stage-IV low-grade lymphoma. *Ann. Oncol.* 1993, **4**: 205–211.

112. Strander H, Adamson U, Aparisi T, et al. Adjuvant interferon treatment of human osteosarcoma. *Recent Result Cancer Res.* 1979, **68**: 40–44.

113. Talpaz M, Kantarijian HM, McCredie KB, et al. Clinical investigation of human alpha interferon in chronic myelogenous leukemia. *Blood* 1987, **69**: 1280–1288.

114. Alimena G, Morra E, Lazzarino M, et al. Interferon alpha-2b as therapy for Ph'-positive chronic myelogenous leukemia: A study of 82 patients treated with intermittent or daily administration. *Blood* 1988, **72**: 642–647.

115. The Italian Cooperative Study Group on Chronic Myeloid Leukemia. Interferon Alfa-2a as compared with conventional chemotherapy for the treatment of chronic myeloid leukemia. *N. Engl. J. Med.* 1994, **330**: 820–825.

116. Sutcliffe SB, Gospodarowicz MK, Bush RS, et al. Dose of radiation therapy in localized non-Hodgkin's lymphoma. *Radiother. Oncol.* 1985, **4**: 211–223.

117. Simon R, Durrlemen S, Hoppe RT, et al. The Non-Hodgkin Lymphoma Pathologic Classification Project: Long-term follow-up of 1153 patients with non-Hodgkin lymphomas. *Ann. Intern. Med.* 1988, **109**: 939–945.

118. Peterson BA, Anderson JR, Frizzera G, et al. Combination chemotherapy prolongs survival in follicular mixed lymphoma (FML). *Proc. Am. Soc. Clin. Oncol.* 1990, **9**: 259 (abstract 1004).

119. Ackerman M, Brandt L, Johnson A, et al. Mitotic activity in non-Hodgkin's lymphoma. Relation to the

Kiel classification and to prognosis. *Br. J. Cancer* 1987, **55**: 219–223.

120. Bastion Y, Berger F, Bryon PA, et al. Follicular lymphomas: Assessment of prognostic factors in 127 patients followed for 10 years. *Ann. Oncol.* 1991 (Suppl. 2) **2**: 123–129.

121. Ellison DJ, Nathwani BN, Metter GE, et al. Mitotic counts in follicular lymphomas. *Hum. Pathol.* 1987, **18**: 502–505.

122. Macartney JC, Camplejohn RS, Morris R, et al. DNA flow cytometry of follicular non-Hodgkin's lymphoma. *J. Clin. Pathol.* 1991, **44**: 215–218.

123. Rehn S, Glimelius B, Strang P, et al. Prognostic significance of flow cytometry studies in B-cell non-Hodgkin lymphoma. *Hematol. Oncol.* 1990, **8**: 1–12.

124. Holte H, de Lange Davies C, Beiske K, et al. Ki67 and 4F2 antigen expression as well as DNA synthesis predict survival at relapse/tumor progression in low-grade B-cell lymphoma. *Int. J. Cancer* 1989, **44**: 975–980.

125. Warnke RA, Kim H, Fuks Z, et al. The coexistence of nodular and diffuse patterns in nodular non-Hodgkin's lymphomas: Significance and clinicopathologic correlation. *Cancer* 1977, **40**: 1229–1233.

126. Rappaport H, Winter WJ, Hicks EB. Follicular lymphoma: A re-evaluation of its position in the scheme of malignant lymphoma, based on a survey of 253 cases. *Cancer* 1956, **9**: 792–821.

127. Ezdinli EZ, Costello WG, Kucuk O, et al. Effect of the degree of nodularity on the survival of patients with nodular lymphomas. *J. Clin. Oncol.* 1987, **5**: 413–418.

128. Hu E, Weiss LM, Hoppe RT, et al. Follicular and diffuse mixed small-cleaved and large-cell lymphoma – A clinico-pathologic study. *J. Clin. Oncol.* 1985, **3**: 1183–1187.

129. Gelb AB, Davis R, Mo S, et al. Prognostic significance of host 'helper' T-cells and proliferating cells in diffuse small lymphocytic lymphomas: Results of a tree-structured survival analysis. *Lab. Invest.* 1992, **66**: 454 (abstract).

130. Medeiros LJ, Picker LJ, Gelb AB, et al. Numbers of host 'helper' T-cells and proliferating cells predict survival in diffuse small-cell lymphomas. *J. Clin. Oncol.* 1989, **7**: 1009–1017.

131. Pezzella F, Jones M, Ralfkiaer E, et al. Evaluation of bcl-2 protein expression and 14;18 translocation as prognostic markers in follicular lymphoma. *Br. J. Cancer* 1992, **65**: 87–89.

132. Yunis JJ, Frizzera G, Oken MM, et al. Multiple recurrent genomic defects in follicular lymphoma: A possible model for cancer. *N. Engl. J. Med.* 1987, **316**: 79–84.

133. Rudders RA, Kaddis M, DeLellis RA, et al. Nodular non-Hodgkin's lymphoma: Factors influencing prognosis and indications for aggressive treatment. *Cancer* 1979, **43**: 1643–1651.

134. Soubeyran P, Eghbali H, Bonichon F, et al. Low-grade follicular lymphomas: Analysis of prognosis in a series of 281 patients. *Eur. J. Cancer* 1991, **27**: 1606–1613.

135. Gospodarowicz MK, Bush RS, Brown TC, et al. Prognostic factors in nodular lymphomas: A multi-variate analysis based on the Princess Margaret Hospital experience. *Int. J. Radiat. Oncol. Biol. Phys.* 1984, **10**: 489–497.

136. Lepage E, Sebban D, Gisselbrecht C, et al. Treatment of low-grade non-Hodgkin's lymphomas: Assessment of Doxorubicin in a controlled trial. *Hematol. Oncol.* 1990, **8**: 31–39.

137. Leonard RCF, Hayward RL, Prescott RJ, et al. The identification of discrete prognostic groups in low-grade non-Hodgkin's lymphoma. *Ann. Oncol.* 1991, **2**: 655–662.

138. Romaguera JE, McLaughlin P, North L, et al. Multivariate analysis of prgnostic factors in stage IV follicular low-grade lymphoma: A risk model. *J. Clin. Oncol.* 1991, **9**: 762–769.

139. Lawrence TS, Urba WJ, Steinberg SM, et al. Retrospective analysis of stage I and II indolent lymphomas at the National Cancer Institute. *Int. J. Radiat. Oncol. Biol. Phys.* 1988, **14**: 417–424.

140. Portlock CS, Fischer D, Cadman E, et al. High-pulse chlorambucil in advanced, low-grade non-Hodgkin's lymphomas. *Cancer Treat. Rep.* 1987, **71**: 1029–1031.

141. Bennett JM, Cain KC, Glick JH, at el. The significance of bone marrow involvement in non-Hodgkin's lymphoma: The Eastern Cooperative Oncology Group experience. *J. Clin. Oncol.* 1986, **4**: 1462–1469.

142. Spinolo JA, Cabanillas F, Dixon DO, et al. Therapy of relapsed or refractory low-grade follicular lymphomas: Factors associated with complete remission, survival and time to treatment failure. *Ann. Oncol.* 1992, **3**: 227–232.

143. Litam P, Swan F, Cabanillas F, et al. Prognostic value of serum $\beta2$ microglobulin in low-grade lymphoma. *Ann. Intern. Med.* 1991, **114**: 855–860.

144. Coiffier B, Gisselbrecht C, Vose JM, et al. Prognostic factors in aggressive malignant lymphomas. Description and validation of a prognostic index that could identify patients requiring a more intensive chemotherapy. *J. Clin. Oncol.* 1991, **9**: 211–219.

145. Coiffier B, Bastion Y, Berger F, et al. Prognostic factors in follicular lymphomas. *Semin. Oncol.* 1993, **20** (Suppl. 5):89–95.

146. Shipp MA, Harrington D, Anderson J, et al. Development of a predictive model for aggressive lymphoma: The international NHL prognostic factors project. *N. Engl. J. Med.* 1993, **329**: 987–994.

147. Weisdorf DJ, Andersen JW, Glick JH, et al. Survival after relapse of low-grade non-Hodgkin's lymphoma: Implications for marrow transplantation. *J. Clin. Oncol.* 1992, **10**: 942–947.

148. Johnson PWM, Rohatiner AZS, Whelan JS, et al. Patterns of survival in patients with recurrent follicular lymphoma: A 20 year study from a single center. *J. Clin. Oncol.* 1995, **13**: 140–147.

149. Chun HG, Leyland-Jones B, Cheson BD. Fludarabine phosphate: A synthetic purine antimetabolite with significant activity against lymphoid malignancies. *J. Clin. Oncol.* 1991, **9**: 175–188.

150. Lathan B, Diehl V, Clark GM, et al. Cytotoxic activity of 9-β-D-arabinofuranosyl-2-fluoroadenine 5-monophosphate (fludarabine, NSC 312887) in a

human tumor cloning system. *Eur. J. Cancer Clin. Oncol.* 1988, **24**: 1891–1895.

151. Yang S-W, Huang P, Plunkett W, et al. Dual mode of inhibition of purified DNA ligase 1 from human cells by 9-β-D-arabinofuranosyl-2-fluoroadenine triphosphate. *J. Biol. Chem.* 1992, **267**: 2345–2349.

152. Plunkett W, Gandhi V. Cellular metabolism of nucleotide analogues in CLL: Implications for drug development. In Cheson BD (ed.) *Chronic Lymphocytic Leukemia: Scientific Advances and Clinical Developments.* New York: Marcel Dekker, 1993, pp. 197–219.

153. Robertson L, Chubb S, Hittelman WN, et al. Programmed death (apoptosis) in chronic lymphocytic leukemia cells after fludarabine and chlorodeoxyadenosine. *Blood* 1991, **78**: 173a (abstract 682).

154. Hochster HS, Kim KM, Green MD, et al. Activity of fludarabine in previously treated non-Hodgkin's lowgrade lymphoma: Results of an Eastern Co-operative Oncology Group study. *J. Clin. Oncol.* 1992, **10**: 28–32.

155. Danhauser L, Plunkett W, Keating M, et al. 9-β-D-Arabinofuranosyl-2-fluoroadenine 5'-monophosphate pharmacokinetics in plasma and tumor cells of patients with relapsed leukemia and lymphoma. *Cancer Chemother. Pharmacol.* 1986, **18**: 145–152.

156. Hutton JJ, Von Hoff DD, Kuhn J, et al. Phase I clinical investigation of 9-β-D-arabinofuranosyl-2-fluoroadenine 5'-monophosphate (NSC 312887), a new purine antimetabolite. *Cancer Res.* 1984, **44**: 4183–4186.

157. Hersh MR, Kuhn JG, Phillips JL, et al. Pharmacokinetic study of fludarabine phosphate (NSC 312887). *Cancer Chemother. Pharmacol.* 1986, **17**: 277–280.

158. Warrell RP Jr, Berman E. Phase I and II study of fludarabine phosphate in leukemia: Therapeutic efficacy with delayed central nervous system toxicity. *J. Clin. Oncol.* 1986, **4**: 74–79.

159. Chun HG, Davies B, Hoth D, et al. The first marine compound entering clinical trials as an antineoplastic agent. *Invest. New Drugs* 1986, **4**: 279–284.

160. Schilling PJ, Vadhan-Raj S. Concurrent cytomegalovirus and pneumocystis pneumonia after fludarabine therapy for chronic lymphocytic leukemia. *N. Engl. J. Med.* 1990, **323**: 833–834 (letter).

161. Hiddeman W, Unterhalt M, Pott C, et al. Fludarabine single-agent therapy for relapsed low-grade non-Hodgkin's lymphomas – a phase II study of the German low-grade non-Hodgkin's Lymphoma Study Group. *Semin. Oncol.* 1993, **20** (Suppl. 7): 28–31.

162. Hochster H, Cassileth P. Fludarabine phosphate therapy of non-Hodgkin's lymphoma. *Semin. Oncol.* 1990, **17**: 63–65.

163. Whelan JS, Davis CL, Rule S, et al. Fludarabine phosphate for the treatment of low grade lymphoid malignancy. *Br. J. Cancer* 1991, **64**: 120–123.

164. Leiby JM, Snider KM, Kraut EH, et al. Phase II trial of 9-β-D-arabinofuranosyl-2-fluoroadenine 5'-monophosphate in non-Hodgkin's lymphoma: Prospective comparison of response with deoxycytidine kinase activity. *Cancer Res.* 1987, **47**: 2719–2722.

165. Pigaditou A, Rohatiner AZS, Whelan JS, et al. Fludarabine in low-grade lymphoma. *Semin. Oncol.* 1993, **20** (Suppl. 7): 24–27.

166. Redman JR, Cabanillas F, Velasquez WS, et al. Phase II trial of fludarabine phosphate in lymphoma: An effective new agent in low-grade lymphoma. *J. Clin. Oncol.* 1992, **10**: 790–794.

167. Zinzani PL, Lauria F, Rondelli D, et al. Fludarabine – an active agent in the treatment of previously treated and untreated low-grade non-Hodgkin's lymphoma. *Ann. Oncol.* 1993, **4**: 575–578.

168. Kay AC, Saven A, Carrera CJ, et al. 2-Chlorodeoxyadenosine treatment of low-grade lymphomas. *J. Clin. Oncol.* 1992, **10**: 371–377.

169. Hickish T, Serafinowski P, Cunningham D, et al. 2'-Chlorodeoxyadenosine: Evaluation of a novel predominantly lymphocyte selective agent in lymphoid malignancies. *Br. J. Cancer* 1993, **6**: 139–143.

170. Cummings FJ, Kim K, Neiman RS, et al. Phase II trial of pentostatin in refractory lymphomas and cutaneous T-cell disease. *J. Clin. Oncol.* 1991, **9**: 565–571.

171. Duggan BD, Anderson JR, Dillman R, et al. 2'Deoxycoformycin (pentostatin) for refractory non-Hodgkin's lymphoma: A CALGB Phase II study. *Med. Pediatr. Oncol.* 1990, **18**: 203–206.

172. Benyunes MC, Fefer A. Interleukin-2 in the treatment of hematologic malignancies. In Atkins MB, Mier JW (eds) *Therapeutic Applications of Interleukin-2.* New York: Marcel Dekker, 1993, pp. 163–175.

173. Boldt DH, Ellis TM. Biologic effects of interleukin-2 administration on the immune system. In Atkins MB, Mier JW (eds) *Therapeutic Applications of Interleukin-2.* New York: Marcel Dekker, 1993, pp. 73–91.

174. Zamkoff KW, Watman NP, Duggan DB, et al. Inducible lymphokine-activated killer (LAK) cell activity in the peripheral blood of patients with relapsed/refractory non-Hodgkin's lymphoma (NHL). *Hematol. Oncol.* 1990, **8**: 97–104.

175. Oshimi K, Oshimi Y, Akutsu M, et al. Cytotoxicity of interleukin 2-activated lymphocytes for leukemia and lymphoma cells. *Blood* 1986, **68**: 938–948.

176. Korsmeyer SJ, Greene WC, Cossman J, et al. Rearrangement and expression of immunoglobulin genes and expression of Tac antigen in leukemia and lymphoma. *Proc. Natl Acad. Sci. USA* 1983, **80**: 4522–4526.

177. Margolin K. The clinical toxicities of high-dose interleukin-2. In Atkins MB, Mier JW (eds) *Therapeutic Applications of Interleukin-2.* New York: Marcel Dekker, 1993, pp. 331–362.

178. Weber JS, Yang JC, Topalian SL, et al. The use of interleukin-2 and lymphokine-activated killer cells for the treatment of patients with non-Hodgkin's lymphoma. *J. Clin. Oncol.* 1992, **10**: 33–40.

179. Dyer MJS, Hale G, Hayhoe FGJ, et al. Effects of CAM-PATH-1 antibodies in vivo in patients with lymphoid malignancies: Influence of antibody isotype. *Blood* 1989, **73**: 1431–1439.

180. Grossbard ML, Press OW, Appelbaum FR, et al. Monoclonal antibody-based therapies of leukemia and lymphoma. *Blood* 1992, **80**: 863–878.

181. Nadler LM, Stashenko P, Hardy R, et al. Serotherapy of a patient with a monoclonal antibody directed against a human lymphoma-associated antigen. *Cancer Res.* 1980, **40**: 3147–3154.

182. Press OW, Appelbaum F, Ledbetter JA, et al. Monoclonal antibody IF5(anti-CD20) serotherapy of human B-cell lymphomas. *Blood* 1987, **69**: 584–591.

183. Hu E, Epstein AL, Naeve GS, et al. A phase 1a clinical trial of LYM-1 monoclonal antibody serotherapy in patients with refractory B-cell malignancies. *Hematol. Oncol.* 1989, **7**: 155–166.

184. Scheinberg DA, Straus DJ, Yeh SD, et al. A phase I toxicity, pharmacology, and dosimetry trial of monoclonal antibody OKB7 in patients with non-Hodgkin's lymphoma: Effects of tumor burden and antigen expression. *J. Clin. Oncol.* 1990, **8**: 792–803.

185. Hale G, Dyer MJS, Clark MR, et al. Remission induction in non-Hodgkin lymphoma with reshaped human monoclonal antibody CAMPATH-1H. *Lancet* 1988, **2**: 1394–1399.

186. Clendeninn NJ, Nethersell ABW, Scott JE, et al. Phase I/II traiLS of CAMPATH-IH, a humanized anti-lymphocyte monoclonal antibody (MoAb), in non-Hodgkin's lymphoma (NHL) and chronic lymphocytic leukemia (CLL). *Blood* 1992, **80** (Suppl.): 158a (abstract).

187. Rankin EM, Hekman A, Somers R, et al. Treatment of two patients with B-cell lymphoma with monoclonal anti-idiotype antibodies. *Blood* 1985, **65**: 1373–1381.

188. Meeker TC, Lowder J, Maloney DG, et al. A clinical trial of anti-idiotype therapy for B-cell malignancy. *Blood* 1985, **65**: 1349–1363.

189. Brown SL, Miller RA, Horning SJ, et al. Treatment of B-cell lymphomas with anti-idiotype antibodies alone and in combination with alpha interferon. *Blood* 1989, **73**: 651–661.

190. Maloney DG, Brown S, Czerwinski D, et al. Monoclonal anti-idiotype antibody therapy of B-cell lymphoma: The addition of a short course of chemotherapy does not interfere with the antitumor effect nor prevent the emergence of idiotype-negative variant cells. *Blood* 1992, **80**: 1502–1510.

191. Swisher EM, Shawler DL, Collins HA, et al. Expression of shared idiotypes in chronic lymphocytic leukemia and small lymphocytic lymphoma. *Blood* 1991, **77**: 1977–1982.

192. Basham TY, Kaminski MS, Kitamura K, et al. Synergistic antitumor effect of interferon and anti-idiotype monoclonal antibody in murine lymphoma. *J. Immunol.* 1986, **137**: 3019–3024.

193. Kwak LW, Campbell MJ, Czerwinski DK, et al. Induction of immune responses in patients with B-cell lymphoma against the surface-immunoglobulin idiotype expressed by their tumors. *N. Engl. J. Med.* 1992, **327**: 1209–1215.

194. Tao M-H, Levy R. Idiotype/granulocyte-macrophage-colony-stimulating factor fusion protein as a vaccine for B-cell lymphoma. *Nature* 1993, **362**: 755–758.

195. Amlot PL, Stone MJ, Cunningham D, et al. A Phase I study of an anti-CD22-deglycosylated ricin A chain immunotoxin in the treatment of B-cell lymphomas resistant to conventional therapy. *Blood* 1993, **82**: 2624–2633.

196. Vitetta ES, Stone M, Amlot P, et al. Phase I immunotoxin trial in patients with B-cell lymphoma. *Cancer Res.* 1991, **51**: 4052–4058.

197. Grossbard ML, Freedman AS, Ritz J, et al. Serotherapy of B-cell neoplasms with anti-B4 blocked ricin: A phase I trial of daily bolus infusion. *Blood* 1992, **79**: 576–585.

198. Grossbard ML, Lambert JM, Goldmacher VS, et al. Anti-B4 blocked ricin: A phase I trial of 7-day continous infusion in patients with B-cell neoplasms. *J. Clin. Oncol.* 1993, **11**: 726–737.

199. Grossbard ML, Gribben JG, Freedman AS, et al. Adjuvant therapy with anti-B4 blocked ricin (anti-B4-BR) following autologous bone marrow transplantation (ABMT) for B-cell non-Hodgkin's lymphoma (NHL): Phase I/II Trials. *Blood* 1992, **80** (Suppl. 1): abstract 623.

200. Parker BA, Vassos AB, Halpern SE, et al. Radioimmunotherapy of human B-cell lymphoma with ^{90}Y-conjugated anti-idiotype monoclonal antibody. *Cancer Res.* 1990, **50** (Suppl.): 1022s–1028s.

201. Kaminski MS, Fig LM, Zasadny KR, et al. Imaging, dosimetry, and radioimmunotherapy with iodine-131-labeled anti-CD37 antibody in B-cell lymphoma. *J. Clin. Oncol.* 1992, **10**: 1696–1711.

202. Goldenberg DM, Horowitz JA, Sharkey RM, et al. Targeting, dosimetry, and radioimmunotherapy of B-cell lymphomas with iodine-131-labeled LL2 monoclonal antibody. *J. Clin. Oncol.* 1991, **9**: 548–564.

203. Press OW, Eary JF, Badger CC, et al. Treatment of refractory non-Hodgkin's lymphoma with radiolabeled MB-1 (anti-CD37) antibody. *J. Clin. Oncol.* 1989, **7**: 1027–1038.

204. DeNardo SJ, DeNardo GL, O'Grady LF, et al. Treatment of B-cell malignancies with ^{131}I Lym-1 monoclonal antibodies. *Int. J. Cancer* 1988, **42** (Suppl. 3): 96–101.

205. DeNardo GL, DeNardo SJ, O'Grady LF, et al. Fractionated radioimmunotherapy of B-cell malignancies with ^{131}I-Lym-1. *Cancer Res.* 1990, **50** (Suppl.): 1014s–1016s.

206. Press O, Eary J, Badger C, et al. Radiolabeled antibody (RAb) therapy of relapsed B-cell lymphomas. *Proc. Am. Soc. Clin. Oncol.* 1992, **11**: 318 (absract).

207. DeNardo SJ, DeNardo GL, O'Grady LF, et al. Pilot study of radioimmunotherapy of B-cell lymphoma and leukemia using ^{131}I Lym-1 monoclonal antibody. *Antibody Immunoconj. Radiopharm.* 1988, **1**: 17–33.

208. Kaminski MS, Zasadny KR, Moon S, et al. Radioimmunotherapy (RIT) of refractory B-cell lymphoma with 131-I-anti B1 (anti-CD20) antibody: Promising early results using non-marrow ablative radiation doses. *Blood* 1992, **80** (Suppl.): 43a (absract).

209. Czuczman MS, Straus DJ, Divgi CR, et al. A phase I dose escalation trial of ^{131}I-labeled monoclonal antibody OKB7 in patients with non-Hodgkin's lymphoma. *Blood* 1990, **76** (Suppl.): 345a (absract).

210. Kaminski MS, Zasadny KR, Francis IR et al. Radioimmunotherapy of B-cell lymphoma with 131I anti-B1 (anti-CD20) antibody. *N. Engl. J. Med.* 1993, **329**: 459–465.

211. Press OW, Eary JF, Frederick R et al. Radiolabeled-antibody therapy of B-cell lymphoma with autologous bone marrow support. *N. Engl. J. Med.* 1993, **329**: 1219–1224.

212. Lundberg J, Hansen R, Chitambar C, et al. Allogeneic

more aggressive chemotherapy regimens in the treatment of early-stage disease. Investigators at the National Cancer Institute (NCI) employed four cycles of ProMACE/MOPP (see Table 42.3) using 75% dosage of the myelotoxic drugs followed by IFRT in the treatment of 49 patients with stage I and IE disease [8]. Forty-seven patients entered a CR and with a median follow-up of 4 years, 94% of the patients are alive. This limited experience demonstrates that this is a very successful treatment approach for patients with very early stage disease, although aggressive therapy such as this is probably unnecessary.

Whether there is a need for RT in addition to 'full' course chemotherapy is being addressed in a study being conducted by the Eastern Cooperative Oncology Group (ECOG). Patients are randomized to receive eight cycles of CHOP alone or the same chemotherapy followed by IFRT. The data from Connors et al. and from the NCI would suggest that RT adds to chemotherapy by allowing fewer cycles of chemotherapy to be given with equivalent results, by reducing the toxicity of chemotherapy and by allowing the use of less chemotherapy, which is of particular importance in the treatment of the elderly, although the long-term toxicity of this approach is unknown. Moreover, it is also possible that a smaller number of cycles, even without radiation therapy, would provide as effective therapy for these patients. This possibility has not been addressed.

The best approach to the management of a patient with early-stage disease remains to be defined and therefore, if possible, patients should be encouraged to participate in a clinical trial. If this is not possible, the currently available data would suggest that either eight cycles of CHOP or three cycles of CHOP followed by RT to an involved field given at tumoricidal doses is a reasonable approach to treatment.

ADVANCED DISEASE (II BULKY, III, IV)

Investigators at the NCI were among the first to demonstrate that some patients with advanced-stage disease are curable. Using combination chemotherapy regimens (C-MOPP, a regimen based on the successful four-drug regimen used at the NCI for the treatment of Hodgkin's disease in which cyclophosphamide was used in place of mustine, and BACOP, which included bleomycin, Adriamycin, cyclophosphamide, vincristine and prednisone), they were able to achieve complete remission in 45% of treated patients with approximately 75–80% of these being durable remissions [9,10]. In these early studies relapses beyond two years posttherapy were rare and therefore a disease-free survival of 2 years was tantamount to cure. Based on these observations,

subsequent trials were focused on achieving higher rates with the assumption being that this would translate into increased numbers of patients cured of their disease.

The CHOP regimen was one of the first combination therapy programs to utilize the drug Adriamycin. This regimen was employed in serial studies in the SWOG and it remains the gold standard against which newer treatments must be compared [11,12]. Utilizing the CHOP regimen, an increased percentage of patients did achieve CR. Unfortunately, this did not translate into increased cure rates. Relapses and deaths were not limited to the first 2 years after treatment and, in fact, relapses were seen as long as 6 and 7 years after the completion of therapy.

Recognizing the need to improve on the results achieved with the CHOP regimen, new and more complex regimens were developed in the 1980s. These regimens are frequently referred to as second- and third-generation regimens to distinguish them from the earlier regimens such as CHOP. The newer regimens continued to employ the most active anti-lymphoma drugs, cyclophosphamide and Adriamycin, but in addition, other drugs with less single-agent activity against lymphoma, such as methotrexate, cytarabine and bleomycin, were introduced into the treatment regimens. Initial single institution phase II results were very promising, suggesting that the number of patients cured of their disease might be double that achieved with the CHOP regimen. Two examples of second-generation regimens are M-BACOD (see Table 42.3) which was developed and piloted at the Dana–Farber Cancer Center, and the ProMACE/MOPP regimen, which was developed and piloted at the NCI [13,14]. Unique to M-BACOD was the use of high-dose methotrexate given during the period of myelosuppression induced by the standard drugs, cytoxan and doxorubin, which were given at the beginning of the chemotherapy cycle. Patients participating in the M-BACOD study were relatively young with a median age of 48. It is important to note that patients entered on study included those with early-stage (I, IE, II, IIE) as well as those with advanced-stage (III, IV) disease. The initial results were excellent with a reported CR rate of 72% and a projected 5-year survival of 65%. Unfortunately, with longer follow-up, the 3-year survival declined to 54%.

ProMACE/MOPP also included high-dose methotrexate and, in addition, etoposide along with standard lymphoma drugs. In the pilot study, 74 patients with stage II, III and IV diffuse mixed, diffuse large-cell and undifferentiated lymphoma were treated. A CR was achieved in 74% of patients and the projected 4-year survival was 65%. In a recent update of this series, now with 9 years of follow-up, however, the long-term survival has decreased to 50% [15]. It should be noted that the median age of patients treated in this study was 44 years as compared to a median age of 55 years for patients treated on previous CHOP studies. Furthermore this NCI study included patients with stage II disease, whereas prior studies from the NCI of first-generation regimens included only patients with stage III and IV disease.

In an attempt to improve on the results seen with the second-generation regimens, several single institutions piloted and reported results with third-generation regimens. These third-generation regimens include MACOP-B (see Table 42.3), which is an intensive 12-week treatment program employing conventional drugs given on a weekly basis, m-BACOD in which two doses of moderate dose methotrexate are substituted for the high-dose methotrexate (MTX) of M-BACOD, and ProMACE/CytaBOM (see Table 42.3), in which cytarabine and bleomycin are added to the ProMACE drugs [16–18]. As with the second-generation regimens, early results were very promising with third-generation regimens, in which CR rates ranging from 68% to 86% and projected survival rates of 58–69% were observed.

The SWOG conducted comfirmatory phase II trials of these three third-generation regimens [19–21]. Unfortunately, results were considerably worse compared to the initial single insitution results. CR rates ranging from 49% to 65% were observed and survival projections ranged from 50% to 61%. In fact, the results were very similar to those which had been obtained with CHOP. These results are not surprising because, as noted above, the single institution studies included more younger patients with less advanced disease compared to the SWOG trials. While these results implied that third-generation regimens may have no advantage over CHOP, an accurate assessment of their relative value could not be made without randomized trials. Such studies were conducted, since the increased cost and toxicity of the third-generation regimens is acceptable only if they are associated with significant improvements in outcome. Initially, CHOP was compared to one of the newer chemotherapy regimens. ECOG compared CHOP to m-BACOD and found no difference between the two arms with regard to outcome but more toxicity was seen on the m-BACOD arm [22]. The Australian and New Zealand Lymphoma Group conducted a randomized trial comparing CHOP to MACOP-B. Similar results were obtained on both treatment arms but again CHOP was found to be less toxic than the newer regimen [23]. These data have been confirmed and extended by a large clinical trial conducted in the USA. The results of this study, a phase III, randomized comparison of CHOP versus m-BACOD versus ProMACE/CytaBOM versus MACOP-B (Intergroup trial 0067) have recently been published [24].

In this study, 1138 previously untreated patients with bulky stage II, stage III and stage IV disease, and diffuse mixed-cell, follicular large-cell, diffuse large-cell, immunoblastic and small noncleaved cell lymphomas, were randomized between 1986 and 1991 to one of four treatment arms. Each of the regimens was administered exactly as had been described in the prior phase II studies. A total of 239 patients were deemed ineligible, primarily as a result of central pathology review. The reported results were those for the 899 eligible patients. As a whole, the group of treated patients had very poor prognostic characteristics. The median age of the patients was 56 years and 25% of patients were over the age of 64. Bulky disease was present in 40% of cases and the LDH was elevated in 46%. The four treatment arms were well balanced for these and all other patient characteristics. At the time of publication of the results, the median follow-up was 49 months with a maximum follow-up of 84 months.

No differences among the four treatment arms were seen with respect to the complete response rate or the overall response rate. Because assessment of CR is sometimes difficult, owing to persistent abnormalities on CT scan after treatment, the time to failure, which is a measure of time to progression, relapse or death from any cause was also analyzed in order to provide a more accurate estimate of the fraction of patients who were cured by the initial treatment. Forty-three per cent of all eligible patients were estimated to be alive without disease at 3 years. By treatment arm, 43% on the CHOP and m-BACOD arms, 44% on the ProMACE-CytaBOM arm and 40% on the MACOP-B arm were projected to be alive without disease at 3 years. The projected overall survival at 3 years for all eligible patients was 52%: 49% on MACOP-B, 51% on m-BACOD, 53% on ProMACE-CytaBOM and 55% on CHOP.

The toxicities observed in the phase III study were similar to those seen in the initial phase II studies. Severe toxicities were predominantly infectious occurring during granulocytopenia. Fatal toxicities were seen in 1% of CHOP-treated patients, 5% of M-BACOD, 3% of ProMACE-CytaBom and 6% of MACOP-B-treated patients.

Although all four regimens were therapeutically equivalent in the entire patient group, it remains possible that one or more subsets of patients might have a better outcome when treated with one of the third-generation regimens rather than CHOP. With this in mind, patients were divided into risk groups, using the International NHL Prognostic Factors Projects Predictive Model described above. There were no observed differences in time to treatment failure or overall survival with low, low-intermediate, high-intermediate or high-risk groups when analyzed according to treatment arm. The possibility that other patient subsets, e.g., defined by cytogenetic or molecular abnormalities, might have a better prognosis with one or other of these drug combinations remains to be determined.

Hence, based on the available data, CHOP remains the standard treatment for patients with advanced-stage aggressive lymphoma. With a projected disease-free survival of 43%, it is obvious that CHOP is not ideal and there is clearly a need for better therapies. For this reason, we strongly advocate the inclusion of as many patients as possible in clinical trials.

Salvage therapy

As is obvious from the results of the Intergroup trial, there are large numbers of patients with advanced-stage intermediate- and high-grade lymphoma who are either refractory to initial therapy or who relapse after an initial response to first-line therapy. Effective salvage therapy is needed for these patients. If they are candidates for bone marrow transplant (usually autologous), this should be considered because this approach offers an extended disease-free survival in 20–25% of patients [25–27]. Patients who have had a good response to initial therapy and those who have relapsed disease which is sensitive to conventional dose salvage therapy are the subsets of patients most likely to benefit from this procedure [28,29].

Because of advanced age, bone marrow involvement, poor performance status and other medical problems, many patients will not be candidates for atologous bone marrow transplantation (ABMT). These patients are usually offered conventional dose salvage therapy. Many salvage regimens have been reported to have activity in relapsed disease, but comparison of salvage regimens is difficult, if not impossible, since many regimens have been used in only small numbers of patients, and selection criteria and patient characteristics have varied widely.

The DHAP (dexamethasone, high-dose cytarabine and cisplatin) regimen, however, which is one of the more commonly used drug combinations, has been used as salvage therapy in approximately 300 patients [30,31]. Results from several series employing this regimen have consistently shown response rates greater than 50% with complete responses in 15–30%. DHAP is commonly used prior to ABMT to 'debulk' the lymphoma and the response to this regimen is frequently used to determine if relapsed disease is 'sensitive' or resistant. As noted above, patients with sensitive relapse are more likely to benefit from ABMT than patients with relapsed disease which is resistant to salvage therapy.

Other approaches to salvage therapy have been explored. Monoclonal antibody therapy has been used and two recent reports have suggested some promise for this approach [32,33]. Cytokine therapy with interleukin-2 has shown minimal activity; perhaps newer cytokines will have greater activity [34]. Finally, approaches aimed at reversing the drug resistance present at the time of relapse (and presumably accounting for the relapse) are being explored [35].

Patient follow-up

Patients with diffuse aggressive lymphoma require follow-up for the remainder of their lives. The period of greatest risk of relapse is during the 24 months following completion of therapy. Approximately one month after completion of therapy patients should undergo a restaging evaluation. This involves the repetition of all tests which were abnormal prior to the initiation of therapy. Patients who have achieved a CR should be examined at 1-month intervals during the first year and 2-month intervals during the second year following completion of therapy. Following a 2-year disease-free interval, patients should be evaluated every 3 months.

References

1. The Non-Hodgkin's Lymphoma Pathologic Classification Project. National Cancer Institute sponsored study of classifications off non-Hodgkin's lymphomas: Summary and description of a working formulation for clinical usage. *Cancer* 1982, **49**: 2112–2135.
2. The International Non-Hodgkin's Lymphoma Prognostic Factors Project. A predictive model for aggressive non-Hodgkin's lymphoma. *N. Engl. J. Med.* 1993, **329**: 987–994.
3. Hall PA, Richards MA, Gregory WM, et al. The prognostic value of Ki67 immunostaining in non-Hodgkin's lymphoma. *J. Pathol.* 1988, **154**: 223–235.
4. Horst E, Meijer CJLM, Radaszkiewicz T, et al. Adhesion molecules in the prognosis of diffuse large cell lymphoma: Expression of a lymphocyte homing receptor (CD44), LFA-1 (CD 11a/18), and ICAM-1 (CD54). *Leukemia* 1990, **4**: 595–599.
5. Schouten HC, Sanger WG, Weisenburger DD, et al. Chromosomal abnormalities in untreated patients with non-Hodgkin's lymphoma: Associations with histology, clinical characteristics and treatment outcome. *Blood* 1990, **75**: 1841–1847.
6. Jones SE, Miller TP, Connors JMJ. Long term follow-up and analysis for prognostic factors for patients with

limited stage diffuse large cell lymphoma treated with initial chemotherapy with or without adjuvant radiotherapy. *Clin. Oncol.* 1989, **7**: 1186–1191.

7. Connors JM, Klimo P, Fairey RN, et al. Brief chemotherapy and involved field radiation therapy for limited-stage histologically aggressive lymphoma. *Ann. Intern. Med.* 1987, **107**: 25–30.

8. Longo DL, Glatstein E, Duffey PL, et al. Treatment of localized aggressive lymphomas with combination chemotherapy followed by involved-field radiation therapy. *J. Clin. Oncol.* 1989, **7**: 1295–1302 .

9. DeVita VT, Canellos GP, Chabner B, et al. Advanced diffuse histiocytic lymphoma, a potentially curable disease. *Lancet* 1975, **1**: 248–250.

10. Schein PS, DeVita VT, Hubbard S, et al. Bleomycin, adriamycin, cyclophosphamide, vincristine, and prednisone (BACOP) combination chemotherapy in the treatment of advanced diffuse histiocytic lymphoma. *Ann. Intern. Med.* 1976, **85**: 417–422.

11. Jones SE, Grozea PN, Metz EN, et al. Superiority of adriamycin-containing combination chemotherapy in the treatment of diffuse lymphoma: A Southwest Oncology Group Study. *Cancer* 1979, **43**: 417–425.

12. Jones SE, Grozea PN, Miller TP, et al. Chemotherapy with cyclophosphamide, doxorubicin, vincristine and prednisone alone or with levamisole or with levamisole plus BCT for malignant lymphoma: A Southwest Oncology Group study. *J. Clin. Oncol.* 1985, **3**: 1318–1324.

13. Skarin AT, Canellos GP, Rosentha, DS, et al. Improved prognosis of diffuse histiocytic and undifferentiated lymphoma by use of high dose methotrexate alternating with standard agents (M-BACOD). *J. Clin. Oncol.* 1983, **1**: 91–98.

14. Fisher, R., DeVita VT, Hubbard SM, et al. Diffuse aggressive lymphomas: Increased survival after alternating flexible sequences of ProMACE and MOPP chemotherapy. *Ann. Intern. Med.* 1983, **98**: 304–309.

15. Long DL, DeVita VT, Duffey PL. Superiority of ProMACE-CytaBOM over ProMACE-MOPP in the treatment of advanced diffuse aggressive lymphoma: Results of a prospective randomized trial. *J. Clin. Oncol.* 1991, **9**: 25–38.

16. Connors JM, Klimo P. MACOP-B chemotherapy for malignant lymphomas and related conditions: 1987 update and additional observations. *Semin. Hematol.* 1933, **25**: 41–46.

17. Shipp MA, Harrington DP, Klatt MM, et al. Identification of major prognostic subgroups of patients with large cell lymphoma treated with m-BACOD or M-BACOD. *Ann. Intern. Med.* 1986, **104**: 757–765.

18. Longo DL, DeVita V T, Duffey PL, et al. Superiority of ProMACE-CytaBOM over ProMACE-MOPP in the treatment of advanced diffuse aggressive lymphoma: Results of a prospective randomized trial. *J. Clin. Oncol.* 1991, **9**: 25–38.

19. Miller TP, Dahlberg S, Weick JK, et al. Unfavorable histologies of non-Hodgkin's lymphoma treated with ProMACE-CytaBOM: A group wide Southwest Oncology Group Study. *J.·Clin. Oncol.* 1990, **8**: 1951–1958.

20. Dana BW, Dahlberg S, Miller TP, et al. m-BACOD treatment for intermediate and high-grade lymphomas: A Southwest Oncology Group study. *J. Clin. Oncol.* 1990, **8**: 1155–1162.

21. Weick JK, Dahlberg S, Fisher RI, et al. Combination chemotherapy for intermediate-grade and high-grade non-Hodgkin's lymphoma with MACOP-B: A Southwest Oncology Group Study. *J. Clin. Oncol.* 1991, **9**: 748–753.

22. Gordon LI, Harrington D, Anderson J, et al. Comparison of a second generation combination chemotherapeutic regimen (m-BACOD) with a standard regimen (CHOP) for advanced diffuse non-Hodgkin's lymphoma. *N. Engl. J. Med.* 327: 1342–1349.

23. Cooper IA, Wolf MM, Robertson TI, et al. Randomized comparison of MACOP-B and CHOP in patients with intermediate grade non-Hodgkin's lymphoma. *J. Clin. Oncol.* 1994, **12**: 769–778.

24. Fisher RI, Gaynor ER, Dahlberg S, et al. Comparison of standard regimen (CHOP) with three intensive chemotherapy regimens for advanced non-Hodgkin's lymphoma. *N. Engl. J. Med.* 1993, **328**: 1002–1006.

25. Carey PJ, Proctor SJ, Taylor P, et al. Superiority of second over first generation chemotherapy in a randomized trial for stage III–IV intermediate and high-grade non-Hodgkin's lymphoma (NHL): The 1980–1985 EORTC trial. *Blood* 1991, **77**: 1593–1598.

26. Philip T, Chauvin F, Armitage J, et al. Parma international protocol – pilot study of DHAP followed by involved field radiotherapy and BEAC with autologous bone marrow transplantation. *Blood* 1991, **77**: 1587–1592.

27. Armitage JO. Bone marrow transplantation in the treatment of patients with lymphoma. *Blood* 1989, **73**: 1749–1758.

28. Gribben JG, Goldstone AH, Linch DC, et al. Effectiveness of high-dose combination chemotherapy and autologous bone marrow transplantation for patients with non-Hodgkin's lymphomas who are still responsive to conventional dose therapy. *J. Clin. Oncol.* 1989, **7**: 1621–1629.

29. Brandwein JM, Callum J, Sutcliffe SB, et al. Analysis of factors affecting hematopoietic recovery after autologous bone marrow transplantation for lymphoma. *Bone Marrow Transplant.* 1990, **6**: 291–294.

30. Press OW, Livingston R, Mortimer J, et al. Treatment of relapsed non-Hodgkin's lymphomas with dexamethasone, high-dose cytarabine and cisplatin before marrow transplantation. *J. Clin. Oncol.* 1991, **9**: 423–431.

31. Velasquez WS, Cabanillas F, Salvadore P, et al. Effective salvage therapy for lymphoma with cisplatin in combination with high dose ara-C and dexamethasone. *Blood* 1988, **71**: 117–122.

32. Kaminski MS, Zasadny KR, Francis IR, et al. Radioimmunotherapy of B-cell lymphoma with [131I] anti-B1 (Anti CD-20) antibody. *N. Engl. J. Med.* 1993, **329**: 459–465.

33. Press OW, Eary JF, Appelbaum FR, et al. Radiolabeled antibody therapy of B-cell lymphoma with autologous bone marrow support. *N. Engl. J. Med.* 1993, **329**: 1219–1224.

34. Bernstein ZP, Vaickus L, Friedman N, et al. Interleukin-2 lymphokine-activated killer cell therapy of non-Hodgkin's lymphoma and Hodgkin's disease. *J. Immunother.* 1991, **10**: 141–146.

35. Dalton WS, Grogan TM, Meltzer PSJ. Drug resistance in multiple myeloma and non-Hodgkin's lymphoma: Detection of P-glycoprotein and potential circumvention by addition of verapamil to chemotherapy. *Clin. Oncol.* 1989, **7**: 415–424.

CHAPTER 43

Cutaneous T-cell lymphomas

YOUN H. KIM AND RICHARD T. HOPPE

Introduction

Cutaneous T-cell lymphomas (CTCL) collectively describe non-Hodgkin's, T-cell lymphomas that have primary cutaneous involvement. Mycosis fungoides and its clinical variant, Sézary syndrome, constitute major subsets of CTCL. With advances in surface antigen characterization, using immunologic and molecular probes, CD30 (Ki-1) lymphomas have emerged as a distinct subset of CTCL with its own spectrum of clinical and histologic heterogeneity.

Mycosis fungoides and Sézary syndrome

Mycosis fungoides (MF) is distinguished from other non-Hodgkin's lymphomas (NHL) by its unique clinical and histopathologic features [1,2]. MF typically presents as an indolent cutaneous eruption with erythematous scaly patches or plaques. The diagnosis of MF is often preceded by a 'premycotic' period which may range from several months to several years or longer. Patients in this 'premycotic' phase frequently have nonspecific scaly skin erup-

tions and nondiagnostic skin biopsies. The histologic hallmark of MF is the 'Pautrier microabscesses', which are clusters of tumor cells in the epidermis.

Sézary syndrome (SS) is a clinical variant of MF, which usually presents without the indolent phase and is characterized by generalized erythroderma, lymphadenopathy and circulating neoplastic T-cells, i.e., Sézary cells, in the peripheral blood. Patients may present initially with all components of SS or may present with only one component, e.g., generalized erythroderma, and, subsequently, progress to develop other clinical features of SS. With progression of the disease, SS patients may develop infiltrating tumors of the skin and extracutaneous sites.

EPIDEMIOLOGY

Although MF and SS are uncommon forms of NHL, they are the most common lymphoma with primary involvement of the skin. The annual incidence in the United States is estimated at 0.29 cases per 100 000 [3], which suggests approximately 500–600 new cases each year. MF and SS are diseases of older adults with the median age at diagnosis between 55 and 60 years. Both occur in individuals of less than 30 years, although essentially never in children [4]. There is 2:1 male predominance and Blacks have a two-fold greater risk for developing MF/SS than whites.

The etiology of MF and SS remains undetermined. Various studies and case reports have suggested an association with genetic factors, environmental exposure or an infectious etiology. A few studies have demonstrated histocomaptibility antigen associations with MF and SS, specifically, Aw31, Aw32, B8, Bw38 and DR5 [5,6]. Chromosomal abnormalities have been identified in tumor cells, mostly deletions and translocations in chromosome 1 or 6 [7]. The significance of these immunogenetic findings and chromosomal abnormalities is unclear.

Chronic antigenic stimulation has been proposed by some investigators as an etiological factor [8,9]. Prolonged exposure to contact allergens, for example, has been postulated as affecting the host immune response in some way such that the development of MF and SS is more likely. A subsequent case-controlled study did not, however, support this hypothesis since MF patients do not appear to have an altered immune response to skin allergens [10]. Toxic environmental exposures, such as industrial chemicals, pesticides and herbicides, have been implicated as potential oncogenic factors [11–13]. However, well-designed, case-controlled studies have failed to support this possibility.

A search for a viral etiology of MF and SS has been pursued for many years [14–18], with a particular focus on human T-lymphotrophic virus-1 (HTLV-1), a virus that was initially isolated from a patient erroneously believed to have SS. However, extensive testing of patient blood and tissues for HTLV-1 have not provided clear evidence for the involvement of this virus in the pathogenesis of MF and SS.

CLINICAL FEATURES

MF is characterized by heterogeneous cutaneous manifestations [1,2]. The initial cutaneous presentation of MF can be as patches, plaques, tumors or generalized erythroderma. A patient may present with more than one morphologic type of skin disease or the disease may evolve from one morphologic type to another in the course of time. The most common initial presentation is with patch and plaque disease. Patches or plaques in MF are often localized, typically in a 'bathing trunk' distribution, although any area of the body can be involved. However, the skin involvement can be much more extensive and sometimes progress to tumors or generalized erythroderma involving essentially the entire skin surface. In the more generalized presentations, the palms and soles are frequently involved, nails may be dystrophic and scalp involvement can result in alopecia. Pruritus is the most common symptom in these patients and may prompt a visit to the dermatologist. Patches and plaques often resemble the lesions of psoriasis and eczematous dermatitis, leading to delay in establishing the correct diagnosis.

Less frequently, the initial skin manifestation of MF are tumor-like (the so-called *d'emblée* presentation) or consist of generalized erythroderma. Extensive involvement of the face with indurated plaques or tumors can result in 'leonine facies' reminiscent of the facies observed in patients with lepromatous leprosy. Rarely, patients present with a solitary cutaneous lesion, either as a scaly indurated plaque or a nodular lesion [19].

The extent of extracutaneous disease tends to correlate with the extent and type of skin involvement, which, in MF, is subdivided into four T (tumor)-stages [1,2]. Extracutaneous manifestations are extremely rare in patients with stage T1 disease, infrequent in patients with T2 disease (8%), and most likely in patients with T3 (30%) or T4 (42%) disease [1]. Patients who present with limited cutaneous involvement (T1) only, may never progress to more advanced T-stages, especially when appropriate treatment is administered. Although MF may be a systemic disease from the outset, the clinical behavior is such that extracutaneous involvement is usually preceded by progression of skin involvement. Any visceral sites can be involved with MF, although many detected only at autopsy. The most common sites of involvement detected premortem include the lungs, gastrointestinal tract, liver and central nervous system. Involvement of the oral cavity may occur when the disease is advanced and is associated with a poor prognosis [20].

STAGING

The standard clinical staging system for MF is based on the TNMB classification and is based on the extent and type of skin involvement (T-stage), the presence of lymph node (N-stage) or visceral disease (M-stage), and the detection of abnormal (Sézary) cells in the peripheral blood (B-stage) [21]. Tables 43.1 and 43.2 summarize the TNMB classification and the overall clinical staging systems. Accurate staging is important because therapeutic approaches in MF are largely based on the clinical stage of the disease.

In general, the initial evaluation of newly diagnosed patients with MF includes a comprehensive physical examination, a chemistry panel and complete blood count with examination for circulating Sézary (malignant) cells, and a chest X-ray. If the patient has palpable lymphadenopathy, a lymph node biopsy or aspiration should be performed to determine the N-stage. Patients with extensive skin involvement may often have dermatopathic or re-

Table 43.1 TNMB classification for mycosis fungoides

T (Skin)
  T1   Limited patch/plaque (< 10% of total skin surface)
  T2   Generalized patch/plaque (≥10% of total skin surface)
  T3   Tumors
  T4   Generalized erythroderma

N (Nodes)
  N0   Lymph nodes clinically uninvolved
  N1   Lymph nodes enlarged, histologically uninvolved (includes 'reactive' and 'dermatopathic' nodes)
  N2   Lymph nodes clinically uninvolved, histologically involved
  N3   Lymph nodes enlarged and histologically involved

M (Viscera)
  M0   No visceral involvement
  M1   Visceral involvement

B (Blood)
  B0   No circulating atypical (Sézary) cells (< 5%)
  B1   Circulating atypical (Sézary) cells (≥ 5%)

active lymphadenopathy (N1), rather than involvement of the node by lymphoma (N2 and 3) [22,23].

Suspected sites of visceral involvement must be confirmed by appropriate imaging studies and histologic evaluation when possible. Routine imaging studies in patients with early stages of MF is unproductive [24]. Significant bone marrow involvement with an infiltrative histologic pattern is extremely rare in patients with limited skin disease [25] and is most often present in patients who meet the clinical criteria for Sézary syndrome. Significant bone marrow disease is usually reflected by the presence of readily detectable Sézary cells in the peripheral blood. Therefore, bone marrow biopsy is not routinely employed as part of the initial staging procedure for MF patients.

Table 43.2 Clinical staging system for mycosis fungoides

Clinical stages	TNM classification*		
IA	T1	N0	M0
IB	T2	N0	M0
IIA	T1–2	N1	M0
IIB	T3	N0–1	M0
IIIA	T4	N0	M0
IIIB	T4	N1	M0
IVA	T1–4	N2–3	M0
IVB	T1–4	N0–3	M1

* The 'B' classification does not alter clinical stage.

DIAGNOSIS AND PROGNOSTIC INDICATORS

MF is a disease with heterogeneous manifestations and a correspondingly broad prognosis. Over the last 20 years, there have been significant advances in the identification of clinical, peripheral blood and tissue evidence of the presence of MF that may aid early diagnosis and help to determine the prognosis. The identification of prognostic factors, whether clinical, histopathological or molecular, is not only important for defining the clinical stage of each patient but it is also critical to the valid interpretation of therapeutic trials and the selection of appropriate treatment modalities.

Clinical and histologic parameters of predictive value

Previous studies directed towards the identification of prognostic indicators in MF have consistently shown that the skin (T) stage is the single most important determinant of survival duration [1,3,22, 26–28]. Patients with limited skin involvement (T1) have an excellent prognosis, whereas, patients with tumor-stage (T3) or erythrodermic MF (T4) have a poor prognosis. Patients with lymph node (N2, N3) or visceral involvement (M1), or Sézary syndrome also have a poor prognosis. Median survival data from Stanford [1] demonstrated that the majority of patients with T1 disease never progress to subsequent stages and that most died from causes unrelated to MF. The median survival of patients with generalized patches and plaques (stage T2) was 10.7 years (129 months), that of tumor stage (T3) was 3.3 years (39 months) and that of erythrodermic stage (T4) was 3.7 years (45 months).

A multicenter study of 152 consecutive patients with MF and SS at all stages led to the proposal that patients should be divided into three distinct prognostic groups designated as 'good-risk', 'intermediate-risk' and 'poor-risk' as determined by clinical and histologic analysis of skin, lymph nodes, blood and visceral sites [22]. Adverse prognostic features identified by univariate analysis included: one or more cutaneous tumors or generalized erythroderma, adenopathy, blood smear involvement with Sézary cells, lymph node effacement, eosinophilia and visceral involvement. Multivariate analysis showed that the presence of visceral disease and the type of skin involvement remain as important independent prognostic factors. Various other studies [26], including the series reported by the multicenter MF Cooperative Group [27], have demonstrated that the extent and type of skin involvement, T-stage, and the number and sites of palpable lymph nodes are significant prognostic indicators in MF and SS. A recent study evaluating the potential predictive value of the histologic patterns of lymph node disease revealed that the cell morphology of the involved lymph node correlated with survival, analogous to observations in other NHL [29].

Although all these previous studies support the T-stage as the single most important prognostic parameter, even within a single T-stage the survival profile may be very heterogeneous. For example, in a recent study of 106 T4 patients managed at Stanford, various clinical parameters, including patient's age at presentation, sex and race, duration of symptoms before diagnosis, lymph node and peripheral blood involvement, and the type of their first significant treatment, were evaluated as potential correlates of survival. In a multivariate analysis, patient's age at presentation (<65 versus ≥ 65), overall clinical stage (III versus IV) and peripheral blood involvement (B0 versus B1) were found to be statistically significant, independent prognostic factors. The median survival of the most favorable prognostic group (age < 65 years, overall stage = III, B-stage = 0) was 10.2 years (122 months) and that of the worst prognostic group (age ≥ 65, overall stage = IV, B-stage = 1) was 1.1 years (13 months). These results demonstrate that within the erythrodermic (T4) patient group, a number of subsets, with variable survival expections exist. It is important to take account of these prognostic factors when analyzing survival and/or treatment efficacy data in erythrodermic MF and SS patients.

The single most important diagnostic tool in MF/SS is still considered to be histology. The criteria for establishing a histologic diagnosis vary, however, among pathologists, which poses dilemmas for the clinician and may lead to difficulties in interpreting the results of clinical trials. All agree that neoplastic cells must be present in the epidermis (epidermotropism or Pautrier microabscesses) to make a definitive diagnosis of MF. Attempts to use histologic parameters such as the absence or loss of epidermotropism [30], the percentage of blastic cells [31], the mitotic index or the thickness of tumor cell infiltrate [28], as markers of predictive value have not been successful when T-stage is also considered, since these parameters do not appear to predict prognosis independently of T-stage.

Cytokine, immunohistochemical and molecular markers

Cytokines

An abnormal cytokine profile, either in tissue or peripheral blood, has been implicated in the patho-genesis or pathophysiology of MF and SS [32–35]. Whether these abnormalities are of pathogenetic significance or are secondary to the disease is unclear. Soluble interleukin-2 receptors (sIL-2R) have received particular attention and serum sIL-2R levels have been measured in MF and SS, peripheral T-cell lymphomas, inflammatory skin diseases and benign erythrodermas [33,36,37]. These studies have shown that serum sIL-2R values are significantly higher in SS than in other malignant or inflammatory T-cell diseases, and that the serum levels correlate with stage, clinical course and hematologic parameters such as the Sézary cell count.

Recently it has also been demonstrated that the peripheral blood mononuclear cells from SS patients express higher levels of interleukin-4 (IL-4) and lower levels of IL-2 and interferon-γ (IFNγ) upon phytohemagglutinin (PHA) stimulation compared with those of normal controls. This cytokine profile is similar to that of murine T-helper 2 (T_{H2}) cells [35] and may be a marker of advanced CTCL. The low level of expression of IFNγ has led to the suggestion that IFNγ may be a useful therapeutic modality. Upregulated expression of IL-4 and IL-5 has also been implicated in hypereosinophilia, while elevated immunoglobulin E (IgE) has been observed in some SS patients [38]. Most patients with significant eosinophilia had circulating Sézary cells and tended to have more advanced skin disease [22].

Adhesion molecules (integrins)

The role of adhesion molecules has been studied in detail in MF and SS, because of the unique epidermotropism that characterizes the histopathology of this subtype of CTCL [39–44]. Epidermotropism indicates the ability of the tumor cells to infiltrate the epidermis and is demonstrated by the presence of these cells in the epidermis. In many studies, the expression of intercellular adhesion molecule 1 (ICAM-1) on keratinocytes in areas of epidermotropism but not ouside these areas has been reported. Consistent with this finding are descriptions of downregulation of ICAM-1 expression on keratinocytes associated with lack of epidermotropism [40]. Other investigators have implicated $\alpha3\beta1$ integrin [very late antigen-3 (VLA-3)] expression by Sézary cells as relevant to their ability to infiltrate the epidermis [43]. Using a monoclonal antibody against $\alpha3$, they reported that increased $\alpha3$ expression (indicative of VLA-3 expression) correlated with increased epidermotropism, whereas the lack of epidermotropism and increased extracutaneous involvement were correlated with a loss of $\alpha3$ expression.

More recently, a group of adhesion molecules

labeled as 'cutaneous lymphocyte antigen' (CLA) has been described on lymphocytes. CLA appears to be involved in the skin-selective homing ability of this subset of peripheral lymphocytes [45,46]. Increased expression of both CLA on pathogenic T-cells and its ligand, E-selectin (endothelial cells), have been demonstrated in the tissue and peripheral blood of various inflammatory diseases and malignant T-cell lymphomas, including MF and SS [47]. A number of studies have shown high levels of expression of CLA on the malignant cells of MF, particularly in patients with erythroderma (T4) [44].

T-Cell antigen markers (immunophenotyping)

With the development of monoclonal antibodies against specific surface epitopes on T-cells, immunohistochemical staining for T-cell antigens has become an integral, although not an essential, tool in the diagnosis, assessment of prognosis and management of MF. Most often, immunophenotyping provides supportive or confirmatory evidence for the histological diagnosis, which remains the primary diagnostic tool. In the majority of cases, the tumor cells in MF and SS exhibit a CD4 (helper/inducer) phenotype, but in more than two-thirds of cases, there is a loss of Leu-8 and CD7 antigen expression. Pan-T-cell antigens, CD2, CD3, CD5, are usually present; the loss of the expression of one or more of these antigens has been associated with aggressive disease or disease progression [1]. Other markers of T-cell activation, such as CD25 (Tac) antigen, are variably expressed, and therefore cannot be used as a diagnostic or a reliable prognostic marker. Ki-67, an antigen expressed by actively proliferating cells, is also variably expressed, being most often positive in patients with more advanced disease. Tumor cells in MF/SS occasionally transform into an anaplastic large-cell lymphoma expressing the Ki-1 (CD30) antigen – a situation which is associated with a poor prognosis [48–50].

In small number of cases of MF and SS, CD8 (cytotoxic/suppressor)-positive tumor cells may predominate and CD4 is not expressed. In such cases the expression of CD2 and CD7 has been reported to be of prognostic significance, a CD2–, CD7+ phenotype being associated with a more rapid progression of disease and lack of response to therapy, and a CD2+, CD7– phenotype with a more favorable outcome [51]. In contrast to CD8+ expression by tumor cells, the presence of large numbers of tumor-infiltrating lymphocytes expressing CD8, presumably reflecting a significant host response, has been associated with a more favorable prognosis [52].

The results of immunohistochemical studies must be interpreted with caution. Occasionally, benign inflammatory skin diseases may show a lack of CD5, CD7 or Leu-8 antigens. It is important to note that there can be discordant expression of antigens between intraepidermal and intradermal T-cells in MF and SS [53]. This discordance, which is defined by the characteristic lack of CD5 or CD7 antigens in the epidermal but not in the intradermal T-cells, has only been observed in biopsies from patients with MF/SS and not in biopsies of benign inflammatory lesions. Significant differences in antigen expression have also been observed in biopsies obtained from different lesions in the same patient.

Molecular methods and markers

Advances in molecular biology techniques and their application to studies of T-cell receptor (TCR) gene rearrangement have permitted the investigation of the clonality and degree of differentiation of MF/SS cells in tissues and peripheral blood [54–57]. Traditionally, Southern blot analysis (SBA) has been the most widely used technique for the assessment of TCR gene rearrangements. Newer techniques based on polymerase chain reaction (PCR) amplification have significantly increased the sensitivity of detecting clonality in the early stages of MF/SS. The assessment of TCR gene rearrangement can be a useful adjunctive tool in establishing a diagnosis when routine histologic and immunohistologic studies are equivocal [1,58–60]. Monoclonality is characteristic of MF/SS and potentially malignant dermatoses, such as lymphomatoid papulosis and cutaneous lymphoid hyperplasia, whereas polyclonality is typically associated with benign inflammatory dermatoses. However, monoclonality is not diagnostic of neoplasia – clonal TCR rearrangements have been observed in benign dermatoses, such as pityriasis lichenoides et varioliformis acuta.

SBA analysis of peripheral blood mononuclear cells in MF patients have revealed that clonal TCR β-gene rearrangements in the peripheral blood are uncommon in patients with nonerythrodermic (T1, T2, T3) disease [61], but are more prevalent in erythrodermic MF and present in most cases of SS [62,63]. Approximately a third of patients with histologically proven lymph node involvement have clonal rearrangements detectable in peripheral blood cells. Such patients usually have a rapidly fatal course.

The presence of clonal TCR gene rearrangements in lymph nodes of MF patients has also been correlated with histologic findings and prognosis [64]. TCR gene rearrangements are absent in histologically uninvolved lymph nodes, present in half of the dermatopathic lymph nodes, in which there are clusters of atypical cells, and found in the majority of lymph nodes effaced by lymphoma. The presence of TCR rearrangements also correlates with the presence of palpable lymphadenopathy and is associated with a shorter survival.

TREATMENT APPROACHES

There are multiple therapeutic options for MF and SS. Selection of a specific treatment plan is based on the clinical stage of the disease, the assessment of prognostic factors, the accessibility of different treatment approaches, the patient's age and other social and medical problems, and the cost–benefit ratio. The most important factor in designing a treatment plan is the clinical stage of the patient (Figure 43.1). For patients with T1 and T2 disease without extracutaneous involvement, the treatment plan will usually be limited to topical therapeutic measures, whereas patients with any extracutaneous disease should receive some form of systemic therapy as part of their regimen. There is no evidence that early aggressive systemic therapy is preferable to conservative therapy in the management of limited disease. Despite decades of experience in the treatment of MF and SS, well-designed, prospective, controlled clinical studies comparing the efficacy of various therapies, whether traditional, newer or investigative, is lacking.

Nonspecific, symptomatic treatment of MF and SS patients is an integral component of the overall therapeutic regimen. Pruritus and xerosis, either as a result of the disease or therapy, can be severe in these patients, and thus supportive measures such as aggressive emolliation, topical steroids, and oral antipruritics should be utilized as necessary.

Traditional therapies

Despite advances in treatment methods in MF and SS, the traditional therapies are still used as the primary therapeutic modality in the majority of patients with stage I and II disease, although in some patients these may be subsequently supplemented with other treatment approaches.

Phototherapy

Phototherapy involves using ultraviolet (UV) radiation in the form of UVA or UVB wavelengths, which can be used alone, together or with psoralen, a photosensitizing agent. The long-wave UVA has the advantage over UVB in its greater depth of penetration into the dermal infiltrates of MF. For early limited diseases, UVB alone [65] or home UV phototherapy (UVA+UVB) [66] has been shown to be effective.

Psoralen with UVA (PUVA), also referred to as photochemotherapy, is clearly the most commonly used form of phototherapy for MF and SS patients. PUVA therapy was initially developed for treatment of psoriasis and is widely used in dermatology for various dermatoses. PUVA is indicated as primary therapy in minimally infiltrated patch and plaque-type MF and erythrodermic MF without evidence of extracutaneous disease. It is also given as palliative therapy in patients with advanced disease, often in combination with other treatment. The efficacy of PUVA in MF has been demonstrated by many investigators [1,2,67–69].

Initially, PUVA treatments are given 2–3 times per week, with a minimum of 48 hours between treatments to monitor the delayed erythema reaction (the reaction observed with UVB or UVA without psoralen is more immediate). The initial dose of UVA and the rate at which the dose is increased is dependent upon the skin type and additional factors that are relevant to photosensitivity. Erythrodermic patients tend to require very low starting doses with very small dose increments. After a maximal steady-state response has been achieved, the frequency of PUVA treatments is decreased to a maintenance level. Refractory lesions can be supplemented with local measures such as radiation therapy or topical chemotherapy.

In a long-term follow-up study of 82 patients treated with PUVA therapy, with a mean follow-up period of 45 months, complete response was observed in 88% of patients with limited plaque (T1) disease and 52% with generalized plaque (T2) disease [68]. A smaller number of their patients with erythrodermic (T4) MF had excellent responses but most relapsed when the treatments were decreased to a maintenance level. Patients with tumor stage T3 disease in this study had only partial responses. In a 10-year follow-up study of 29 patients at Stanford treated with PUVA [67], an overall complete response rate of 59% was observed in plaque-type (*n*=16) and erythrodermic MF (*n*=13) patients. The three nonresponders had SS. Complete response was observed in 54% of erythrodermic MF, none of which had SS, and in 63% of patients with plaque disease. Despite continued maintenance therapy, most patients in both groups relapsed after a mean disease-free interval of 10.7 months in early-stage disease and 22.2 months in advanced disease (stages III and IV).

Psoralens intercalate between pyrimidines within DNA and, upon UVA irradiation, form photoadducts and DNA cross-links [70]. This process results in direct cytotoxic and antiproliferative effects, as well as possibly immunomodulatory effects, through either a direct effect on T-cells or an indirect effect by modulating cytokine production [71]. The optimal

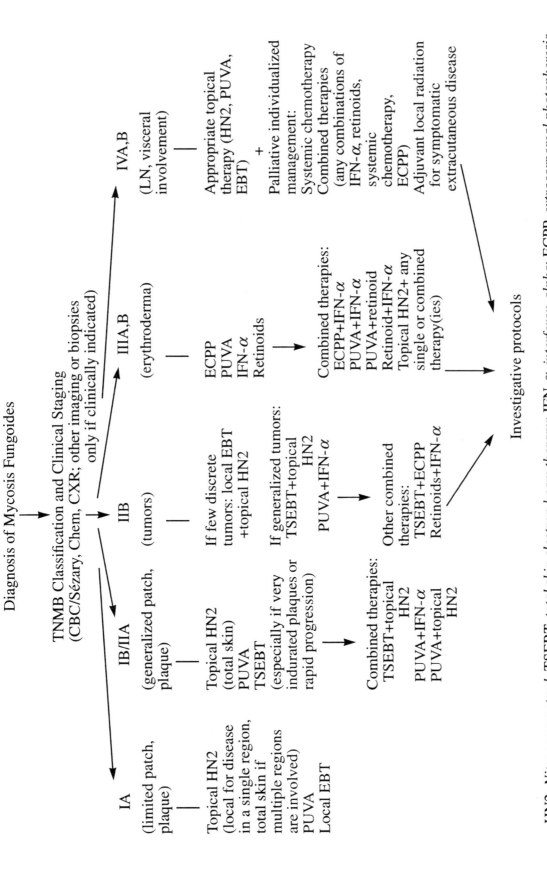

Figure 43.1 Management of patients with mycosis fungoides.

HN2, *Nitrogen mustard*; TSEBT, *total skin electron beam therapy*; IFN-α, *interferon-alpha*; ECPP, *extracorporeal photopheresis*.

patients treated with TSEBT who have previously received prolonged or multiple sequential treatments with other topical therapies, such as PUVA and topical HN2 [88].

Megavoltage photon irradiation
Megavoltage photon irradiation can provide effective palliative therapy for extracutaneous involvement, especially lymph nodes, brain, oropharynx and localized visceral involvement [1]. With disease progression, nodal involvement may become symptomatic, resulting in edema and pain, especially of the extremities. Total doses similar to those for cutaneous disease, i.e., up to 3000 cGy, are necessary to control disease successfully at these sites.

Systemic chemotherapy

In contrast to other types of NHL, conventional systemic chemotherapy is usually not very effective for the treatment of MF and SS. Most of the systemic chemotherapeutic agents that are used for NHL have been used in MF and SS, either as single agents or as combination regimens, with variable rates of complete remission (0–57%) [1]. Patients who achieve a complete response rarely have long-term disease-free survival with systemic chemotherapy alone. In most cases, the median duration of response is less than 1 year. The most commonly utilized single agents are methotrexate and chlorambucil. Frequently used combination regimens include cyclophosphamide, vincristine and prednisone (CVP), or CVP combined with other agents such as VP-16, adriamycin or methotrexate. A study by investigators at the National Cancer Institute demonstrated that early aggressive therapy with combination chemotherapy and TSEBT did not result in a more favorable survival outcome compared with a group of patients managed more conservatively, with sequential topical regimens followed by systemic treatment after failure of topical therapies [99].

Because of the lack of a sustained effect with systemic chemotherapy, this approach is limited to patients with refractory, progressive disease or for palliation of extracutaneous disease [1,69], used often in conjunction with other forms of topical therapy, especially palliative radiation therapy.

Newer therapies

The efficacy of many of the newer, emerging therapies for CTCL has not been definitively established, and, although their use as primary therapy may be justified in some circumstances, it is important to balance carefully their potential benefit versus their cost, toxicity and convenience of administration.

Extracorporeal photopheresis

Also known as extracorporeal or 'systemic' photochemotherapy, extracorporeal photopheresis (ECPP) is considered by some investigators to be the treatment of choice for erythrodermic (T4) MF and SS [69,100, 101]. Since its introduction in the mid-1980s [102], the efficacy of ECPP has been demonstrated mostly in erythrodermic (T4) MF and SS patients [101,103, 104] and its effectiveness in T1, T2 and T3 disease remains undetermined. The largest study of patients with erythrodermic MF/SS [101] revealed that the majority (83%) experienced some level of response to ECPP. The complete response rate was lower (20%), but 41% of patients experienced at least 50% improvement in their skin disease. The best responders were those erythrodermic (T4) patients with disease limited to the skin and a lower CD4/CD8 ratio in the peripheral blood at the start of therapy. Patients with advanced disease, with large numbers of circulating Sézary cells or extensive extracutaneous disease infrequently had a significant response.

ECPP is a method of delivering PUVA systemically by utilizing an extracorporeal technique [100]. The patient is given a photoactivating drug (8-methoxypsoralen), the white blood cells are collected (leukapheresis) and irradiated with UVA, and then the irradiated cells are returned to the patient. The ECPP instrument performs the leukapheresis and delivers the UVA treatment. A standard complete ECPP regimen for CTCL consists of 2 consecutive days of therapy, each consisting of six cycles of leukapheresis. During these six cycles, a total of 240 ml of buffy coat lymphocytes are photoirradiated. The 2-day ECPP treatment is usually repeated at 4-week intervals, the frequency of administration being adjusted according to clinical response. After maximal, stable response has been achieved, the frequency of treatments is gradually decreased then stopped completely, unless the disease relapses or flares during the weaning process or when maintenance therapy is given. Maintenance therapy is given every 4–6 weeks; a repeat attempt at weaning can be done at a later time. If complete response is not achieved or flares are not controlled with ECPP alone, adjunctive therapy can be used, such as interferon or topical therapies. A minimum of 4–6 treatments should be given before ECPP is considered a failure.

The mechanism of action of ECPP remains unclear. It is strongly believed by some investigators that there is a dual effect: a direct cytotoxic or antiproliferative effect on the neoplastic cells and an 'immune-enhancing' effect on immunocompetent lymphocytes against the neoplastic cells [101,105, 106]. The 'immune-enhancing' effect is presumed to occur as a result of the induction of suppressor/

cytotoxic T-cells with specificity against the malignant clone of T-cells and/or via modulation of cytokine production [71,107].

One of the greatest advantages of ECPP is that the adverse effects are minimal [100]. Some patients may experience nausea, mostly as the result of the ingested psoralen, and some experience a transient low-grade fever or slight malaise after treatment. As with the conventional PUVA, photoprotection should be used for up to 24 hours after administration of psoralen. However, in contrast to conventional PUVA, the skin surface is not irradiated as part of treatment; therefore, the risk of secondary cutaneous tumors is not a significant issue.

Interferon-α

Among the interferons, interferon-α (IFNα) has the most profound antitumor effect against MF/SS. Recombinant IFNα is commercially available for intramuscular or subcutaneous administration. A detailed description of its mechanisms of action and associated adverse effects has been provided in other chapters. IFNα therapy has generally been used for the palliation of refractory or advanced disease, and is often combined with other topical or systemic therapies. More recently, IFNα has been shown in several small clinical trials to be effective as a primary therapeutic agent for MF and SS [108–111]. The reported overall response rates range between 53% and 74%, with complete response rates of 21% and 35%. Larger studies will be needed before IFNα can be considered part of the standard repertoire.

Currently, administration of IFNα for MF and SS is initiated usually at a low dose of 3–5 million units (MU) given daily or three times a week, and is gradually increased, depending on the clinical response and the severity of adverse effects [108,110]. In earlier studies, high doses (50 MU/m^2) of IFNα were used but this was associated with considerable toxicity, necessitating dose reductions [112,113]. Subsequent clinical trials using an intermittent high-dose regimen have demonstrated reponses in patients with refractory advanced MF and SS, and fewer side-effects than the previous high-dose regimen [114]; however, further studies are necessary to establish efficacy of this regimen as primary therapy. Intralesional administration of IFNα has also been reported to result in complete or partial clearing of skin lesions [115,116].

Retinoids

Retinoids are vitamin A analogs that have been used for many years for various cutaneous disorders other than CTCL. More recently, the retinoids have been shown to be beneficial in the management of MF and SS – overall response rates of approximately 45% with 20% complete response rates have been reported [117,118]. Retinoids, like IFNα, have been mostly used in patients with refractory or advanced disease, usually as an adjuvant to other topical or systemic therapy. The systemic retinoids are administered orally and are commercially available as isotretinoin (13-*cis*-retinoic acid, Accutane) or etretinate (Tegison). Newer retinoids with potentially higher potency but without increased toxicity are presently undergoing clinical trial to determine their efficacy and safety [119,120].

All retinoids have multiple biological effects that vary according to the biological system and the drug concentration [121–125]. They have been shown to promote differentiation and inhibit proliferation, to inhibit keratinization, to decrease sebum production and to modulate immunologic function.

The initiation doses for isotretinoin is 1 mg/kg/day and for etretinate 0.5–1.0 mg/kg/day, which can be adjusted according to the level of clinical response and the severity of adverse effects [69]. In most cases, the disease relapses after discontinuation of retinoid therapy.

The toxicity profile of different forms of retinoids are similar and many of these adverse effects are dose-dependent [69,123,126]. Most commonly, patients experience photosensitivity and dryness of the skin and mucous membranes. Other adverse effects include myalgia, arthralgia and fatigue, and less commonly, headaches, which on rare occasions are due to pseudotumor cerebri. The well-known teratogenic effects of retinoids must be carefully addressed in female patients of childbearing age. Because of its potential hepatotoxic and hyperlipidemic effects, liver function and serum lipid levels (triglycerides/cholesterol) should be monitored in each patient during treatment. Potential long-term cumulative dose toxicity of retinoids include the development of bony changes such as hyperostosis.

Monoclonal antibody therapy

Advances in immunologic methods and the characterization of the cell surface antigens of neoplastic cells in MF and SS have allowed the development of specific antigen-targeted monoclonal antibody therapies. Both murine and chimeric (murine/human) monoclonal antibodies have been evaluated for efficacy and safety as primary therapy for early and advanced disease MF and SS.

Initially, murine monoclonal antibodies raised against mature human T-cell surface antigens were used for MF and SS patients [127–129]. The development of human antimouse immunoglobulin antibodies (HAMA) during treatment and modulation of target antigen expression limited the efficacy of the murine antibody therapies. Radiolabeled antibodies have been utilized in order to enhance antitumor effects [130]. Subsequently, chimeric (murine/human) anti-CD4 monoclonal antibodies have been tested in clinical trials designed to reduce the risk of HAMA development as well as providing treatment which, while affecting the neoplastic cells, should have a more limited effect on T-cell subsets than the previously used pan-T-cell monoclonal antibodies [131]. However, although the overall clinical response rates were high, they were generally modest and short-lived (median duration of 2 weeks).

The toxicities of monoclonal antibody therapy are generally mild and include low-grade fevers, malaise, pruritus, urticaria and occasional dyspnea [1,69]. With radiolabeled antibodies, myelosuppression may be observed [130].

Other investigational therapies

Recombinant toxins
As an alternative therapeutic approach in the treatment of CTCL, recombinant fusion toxins have been developed. This involves the use of growth factor–cytotoxin fusion proteins designed specifically to kill defined neoplastic cell populations [132]. The first example of this approach is the interleukin-2 (IL-2)–diphtheria toxin fusion protein. This fusion protein is cytotoxic only to cells expressing high-affinity IL-2 receptors. Once bound to such cells, the fusion protein is internalized by endocytosis, which is followed by inhibition of protein synthesis and eventual cell death. A phase I clinical trial [133] using the IL-2–diphtheria toxin fusion protein has demonstrated significant clinical response with minimal toxicity in a group of patients with refractory disease, showing potential benefit in the management of CTCL.

Purine analogs
The three major purine analogs, fludarabine monophosphate (FAMP), 2-chlorodeoxyadenosine (2-CDA) and 2-deoxycoformycin (pentostatin), have been studied to evaluate their efficacy and toxicity in MF and SS [134]. In a clinical trial using FAMP [135], the investigators observed an overall response rate of 19%, with only 1 out of 31 patients achieving complete response. The major toxicity observed was bone marrow suppression. Pulmonary fibrosis, thought to be secondary to FAMP, was encountered in one patient. Only 12 patients with refractory advanced disease have been studied with 2-CDA [136]. The overall response rate was 33%, with two patients achieving complete response. The potentially life-

threatening bone marrow toxicity observed with 2-CDA was much more severe than that with FAMP.

Pentostatin, an inhibitor of adenosine deaminase, has been shown to be beneficial not only for CTCL [137,138], but also for other NHL and hairy cell leukemia [139]. The overall response rate in MF may be as high as 50% [138].

Phosphocholines
Topical application of hexadecylphosphocholine has been shown to be beneficial in a recent study of 12 patients with MF [140]. Phosphocholines inhibit tumor cell growth directly by inhibition of protein kinase C and induction of cellular differentiation. They may also have immunoregulatory properties via stimulation of cytokine release, activation of monocytes and the enhancement of peptide expression in the context of class II MHC. The overall response rate to hexadecylphosphocholine was 50%, with a complete response rate of 17%. Similar response rates were observed for cutaneous B-cell lymphoma patients that were included in these studies.

Bone marrow transplantation
Although autologous bone marrow transplantation (ABMT) has been recognized as a potentially curative therapy for certain subsets of NHL, its efficacy in CTCL has not been established. In a study of six MF patients with advanced, extracutaneous disease, ABMT was successfully performed and managed without life-threatening infections [141]. Five of the six patients had complete clinical responses, although three of these responses lasted less than 100 days. Further studies need to be performed to determine the benefit of ABMT in light of its high cost and potential life-threatening complications.

COMBINED MODALITY THERAPIES

As demonstrated in the previous sections, single modality therapy for MF and SS may not be sufficient to achieve a good or sustained clinical response. Therefore, therapeutic approaches combining two or more modalities, especially those that have complementary mechanisms of action, can be particularly beneficial in the management of MF and SS. In most cases, a combined modality approach is utilized for patients with refractory or advanced diseases, especially with extracutaneous involvement. The more commonly utilized combination therapies will be described in this section.

PUVA + INFα
The clinical efficacy of combined PUVA and IFNα

has been demonstrated in MF and SS [68,142–144]. In these studies, the initial PUVA treatment was three times per week, and IFNα was administered intramuscularly three times per week starting at low doses and gradually being increased to intermediate doses as tolerated. The studies included patients in clinical stages IB–IVB, and an overall response rate of approximately 90%, with more than 60% achieving a complete response, has been observed. In a small series of five patients who were unresponsive to PUVA alone, a complete response rate of 100% was observed when these patients were treated with combined PUVA + IFNα [144].

Etretinate + IFNα

IFNα combined with etretinate has been reported to produce an overall response rate of 42–77% in patients at stages I–IVB, with a complete response rate of 15–54% [145–147]. Patients with SS did not respond as well as those with non-Sézary stage IV disease.

ECPP + IFNα

The combination of ECPP and IFNα dramatically cleared the skin, lymph node and peripheral blood involvement of a patient with rapidly deteriorating SS, who remained in remission after 22 months of follow-up [148]. However, it is unclear whether this combined therapy is more effective than treatment with INFα alone.

Pentostatin + IFNα

A phase II clinical study has been performed to assess the efficacy and toxicity of alternating administration of pentostatin (deoxycoformycin) and IFNα in patients with refractory or advanced MF and SS [149]. Pentostatin was administered intravenously at 4 mg/m^2 on days 1–3, and IFNα was given intramuscularly at 10 MU/m^2 on day 22 and 50 MU/m^2 on days 23–26. The overall response rate was 41% with 5% of patients achieving complete response. All nonresponders had visceral involvement.

Cutaneous Ki-1 (CD30/BER-H2)-positive lymphomas

Ki-1 (CD30) lymphomas are emerging as a distinct subgroup of cutaneous T-cell lymphomas [50]. In 1982, Schwab et al. described the Ki-1 antigen, which is expressed on the surface of Hodgkin's disease and Reed–Sternberg cells, and a subset of normal lymphoid cells [150]. More recently, the

Ki-1 (CD30/Ber-H2) antigen has been found to be present on highly activated B- and T-cells, and on the atypical lymphocytes of lymphomatoid papulosis [151–153]. Lymphomatoid papulosis (LyP) is a benign lymphoproliferative process characterized by skin infiltrates of activated and atypical T-cells expressing the Ki-1 antigen. LyP can be present alone, presenting with erythematous papules or plaques that spontaneously resolve, or it can present in association with other malignant lymphoid processes such as Hodgkin's disease, MF and Ki-1-positive lymphomas.

There is a spectrum of clinical and histologic presentations of Ki-1 (CD30) lymphomas. Most Ki-1 (CD30) lymphomas are histologically anaplastic large-cell lymphomas, but there are subsets of nonanaplastic Ki-1 lymphomas such as immunoblastic and pleomorphic lymphomas. Although the morphologic distinction between anaplastic and nonanaplastic lymphomas is not sharp, neither do the clinical and prognostic characteristics of these two morphologic subsets differ greatly. Therefore, subclassification according to these morphologic features appears not to be necessary at this time [154,155]. Ki-1 (CD30)-positive lymphoma can present as a primary cutaneous process or may occur as a result of transformation of other lymphoproliferative conditions such as MF or LyP (Table 43.3). Also, Ki-1 (CD30) lymphoma can present as a primary noncutaneous large-cell lymphomas [48]. In this chapter, we shall focus on primary cutaneous Ki-1 (CD30)-positive large-cell lymphomas.

PRIMARY CUTANEOUS Ki-1 (CD30) LARGE-CELL LYMPHOMA

Clinical presentation

Primary cutaneous Ki-1(CD30) large-cell lymphoma (LCL) usually occurs in adults although it has been reported in children [156,157]. The most common clinical presentation is as solitary or localized cutaneous nodules, noduloplaques, or tumors resembling skin lesions of lymphocytoma cutis (cutaneous lymphoid hyperplasia) or those observed in primary cutaneous B-cell lymphomas [158–160]. Occasionally, the skin lesions consist of multiple smaller papules or large ulcerating tumors, and are usually confined to a single anatomical region [161]. The skin lesions of primary cutaneous Ki-1 (CD30)-positive LCLs tend to progress without treatment, although they can undergo partial or complete spontaneous regression [154]. Extracutaneous involvement occurs in a minority of patients and is usually confined to the regional peripheral lymph nodes.

Table 43.3 Cutaneous Ki-1 (CD30) large-cell lymphomas

	Primary cutaneous Ki-1 (CD30) LCL	Secondary cutaneous Ki-1 (CD30) LCL
Pre-existing lymphoproliferative disease	None	MF/SS, LyP, primary noncutaneous Ki-1 LCL
Extent of skin involvement	Usually regional	More generalized
Extracutaneous involvement	Uncommon	Common
Prognosis	Favorable	Unfavorable*
Treatment	Usually local or topical therapy	Often systemic therapy ± local or topical adjunctive modality

* Secondary Ki-1 LCL arising in LyP may have a more favorable prognosis.
LCL, Large-cell lymphomas; MMF/SS, mycosis fungoides/Sézary syndrome; LyP, lymphamatoid papulosis.

In the rare presentation in which there are multiple, generalized skin lesions, there is a higher risk of a more extensive systemic involvement. In addition to a thorough physical examination, screening blood work and a chest X-ray, additional staging work-up is recommended, including abdominal and pelvic computed tomograpy (CT) and bone marrow biopsy, to look for the presence of extracutaneous disease. However, the extent of a staging evaluation should be tailored to individual patient circumstance, especially in cases where systemic chemotherapy or any other aggressive treatment will not be tolerated. In general, patients with primary cutaneous Ki-1 (CD30)-positive large-cell lymphoma (LCL) have a favorable prognosis compared with those with primary cutaneous Ki-1 (CD30)-negative LCL, with 4-year survival rates of 90% and <25%, respectively [50,154,160].

Diagnosis

The diagnosis of primary cutaneous Ki-1 (CD30)-positive LCL is established when patients with the clinical features described above have histologic and immunohistologic features characteristic of this disease. Unlike MF and SS, the skin biopsy typically does not show epidermotropism and thus the large Ki-1 (CD30)-positive tumor cells are found densely infiltrating the dermis, forming large clusters or nodules [48]. In most of the cases, the tumor cells have the morphologic features of large anaplastic cells with abundant cytoplasm. However, in some cases, the cells are more pleomorphic or immunoblastic in appearance [50,160,162]. Most of the primary cutaneous Ki-1 (CD30)-positive LCLs are T-cell in origin, although, extremely rarely, they can be of B-cell origin [154,160]. As in MF and SS, the Ki-1 (CD30)-positive T-cells also express CD4 antigen, but do not express the CD2, CD3 and CD5 antigens that would be present on normal CD4 lymphocytes.

They also tend to express other activation antigens such as CD25, T9 and HLA-DR, and cutaneous lymphocyte-associated antigen (HECA-452) [163]. In general, these Ki-1 (CD30)-positive cells do not express the leukocyte common antigen (LCA), CD15 (Leu-M1) or epithelial membrane antigen (EMA) [164], a potential source of confusion with nonlymphoid tumors if LCA were used as a primary means of distinction.

Some cases of LyP can be confused with primary cutaneous Ki-1 (CD30)-positive LCL because of the occasional overlap of histologic features. Occasionally, the classical, self-healing skin lesion characteristic of LyP may have histologic features similar to Ki-1 (CD30)-positive LCL [165]. In other cases, a patient may present with skin lesions clinically consistent with Ki-1 (CD30)-positive LCL, but the histologic findings may be more characteristic of LyP type A [154,166]. These overlap cases may lead to a delay in diagnosis and therapy. Because of the similarities or overlapping features between LyP type A and Ki-1 (CD30)-positive LCL, attempts have been made to describe these entities as a spectrum of Ki-1 (CD30)-positive lymphoproliferative disorders [50]. 'Regressing atypical histiocytosis', which is similar, with respect to its tendency to spontaneously regress, to LyP, but histologically, immunophenotypically and genotypically resembles Ki-1 (CD30)-positive LCL [161,167], has been included in this spectrum as primary cutaneous Ki-1 (CD30)-positive LCL with overlapping clinical features of LyP.

Primary noncutaneous Ki-1 (CD30)-positive LCL occurs more commonly in children and adolescents, and is associated with an unfavorable prognosis [154,156–158,166]. Cytogenetic studies have revealed a 2;5(p23;q35) chromosomal translocation in many cases of the primary noncutaneous type in contrast to the lack of association of this translocation in the primary cutaneous disease [162,168].

SECONDARY CUTANEOUS Ki-1 (CD30)-POSITIVE LARGE-CELL LYMPHOMAS

The secondary cutaneous Ki-1 (CD30)-positive LCLs are anaplastic LCLs that arise in patients with pre-existent MF/SS [48,49,169], LyP [170,171] or primary noncutaneous Ki-1 (CD30)-positive LCL. These secondary forms of Ki-1 (CD30)-positive LCLs must be distinguished from the primary cutaneous Ki-1 (CD30)-positive LCLs because of the difference in prognosis, which, in most patients with secondary cutaneous Ki-1 (CD30)-positive LCLs arising from pre-existent lymphomas, has been poor [48]. However, recent reports have indicated that patients whose secondary cutaneous Ki-1 (CD30)-positive LCL evolving from LyP have a very favorable prognosis except for those who have extracutaneous involvement at the time of evolution [171].

MANAGEMENT OF CUTANEOUS Ki-1 (CD30)-POSITIVE LARGE-CELL LYMPHOMAS

The management of cutaneous Ki-1 (CD30)-positive LCLs differs for primary and secondary forms [50]. After diagnosis of cutaneous Ki-1 (CD30)-positive LCLs, appropriate staging studies should be performed to identify any concurrent extracutaneous disease. The initial therapy largely depends on the extent of the cutaneous involvement and presence of extracutaneous disease. Patients with localized skin involvement without extracutaneous disease are treated with local measures such as radiation therapy or surgical excision. The additional benefit of local radiation therapy after surgical excision or spontaneous resolution of a solitary lesion is undetermined. For localized primary cutaneous Ki-1 (CD30)-positive LCLs, recent studies have shown that systemic chemotherapy as initial treatment does not result in higher cure or clinical response rate, longer remission or lower risk of relapse as compared with local radiation therapy or surgical excision [154]. Systemic chemotherapy is indicated in patients who have extracutaneous involvement or who have extensive cutaneous disease and are at high risk for extracutaneous involvement. Refractory localized skin disease can be treated with supplemental radiation therapy. Oral etoposide has been demonstrated to be a safe and effective therapy for Ki-1 (CD30)-positive LCLs [172].

References

1. Hoppe R, Wood G, Abel E. Mycosis fungoides and the Sézary syndrome: pathology, staging, and treatment. *Curr. Probl. Cancer* 1990, **14**: 295–371.
2. Kuzel T, Roenigk H Jr, Rosen S. Mycosis fungoides and the Sézary syndrome: A review of pathogenesis, diagnosis, and therapy. *J. Clin. Oncol.* 1991, **9**: 1298–1313.
3. Weinstock M, Horm J. Mycosis fungoides in the United States – increasing incidence and descriptive epidemiology. *JAMA* 1988, **260**: 42–46.
4. Burns M, Ellis C, Cooper K. Mycosis fungoides-type cutaneous T-cell lymphoma arising before 30 years of age. Immunophenotypic, immunogenotypic and clinicopathologic analysis of nine cases. *J. Am. Acad. Dermatol.* 1992, **27**: 974–978.
5. Safai B, Myskowski P, Dupont B, et al. Association of HLA-DR5 with mycosis fungoides. *J. Invest. Dermatol.* 1983, **80**: 395–397.
6. Rosen S, Radvany R, Roenigk HJ, et al. Human leukocyte antigens in cutaneous T-cell lymphoma. *J. Am. Acad. Dermatol.* 1985, **12**: 531–534.
7. Johnson G, Dewald G, Strand W, et al. Chromosomal studies in 17 patients with the Sézary syndrome. *Cancer* 1985, **55**: 2426–2433.
8. Tan R, Butterworth C, McLaughlin H, et al. Mycosis fungoides – a disease of antigen persistence. *Br. J. Dermatol.* 1974, **91**: 607–616.
9. Rowden G, Lewis M. Langerhans cells: Involvement in the pathogenesis of mycosis fungoides. *Br. J. Dermatol.* 1976, **95**: 665–672.
10. Whittemore A, Holly E, Lee I, et al. Mycosis fungoides in relation to environmental exposures and immune response: A case-control study. *J. Natl Cancer Inst.* 1989, **81**: 1560–1567.
11. Fischman A, Bunn PJ, Guccion J, et al. Exposure to chemicals, physical agents, and biologic agents in mycosis fungoides and the Sézary syndrome. *Cancer Treat. Rep.* 1979, **63**: 591–596.
12. Cohen S, Kurt S, Braverman I, et al. Mycosis fungoides: Clinicopathologic relationships, survival and therapy in 59 patients with observations on occupation as a new prognostic factor. *Cancer* 1980, **46**: 2654–2666.
13. Tuyp E, Burgoyne A, Aitchison T, et al. A case-control study of possible causative factors in mycosis fungoides. *Arch. Dermatol.* 1987, **123**: 196–200.
14. Wantzin G, Thomsen K, Nissen N, et al. Occurrence of human T-cell lymphotrophic virus (type I) antibodies in cutaneous T-cell lymphoma. *J. Am. Acad. Dermatol.* 1986, **15**: 598–602.
15. Poiesz B. Detection and isolation of type C retrovirus particles from fresh and cultured lymphocytes of a patient with cutaneous T-cell lymphoma. *Proc. Natl Acad. Sci. USA* 1980, **77**: 7415–7419.
16. Ranki A, Niemi K, Nieminen P, et al. Antibodies against retroviral core proteins in relation to disease outcome in patients with mycosis fungoides. *Arch. Dermatol. Res.* 1990, **282**: 532–538.
17. Hall W, Liu C, Schneewind O, et al. Deleted HTLV-I

provirus in blood and cutaneous lesions of patients with mycosis fungoides. *Science* 1991, **253**: 317–320.

18. Whittaker S, Ng Y, Rustin M, et al. HTLV-1-associated cutaneous disease: A clinocopathological and molecular study of patients from the U.K. *Br. J. Dermatol.* 1993, **128**: 483–492.

19. Oliver G, Winkelmann R. Unilesional mycosis fungoides: A distinct entity. *J. Am. Acad. Dermatol.* 1989, **20**: 63–70.

20. Sirois D, Miller A, Harwick R, et al. Oral manifestations of cutaneous T-cell lymphoma. A report of eight cases. *Oral. Surg. Med. Pathol.* 1993, **75**: 700–705.

21. Bunn P, Lamberg S. Report of the committee on staging and classification of cutaneous T-cell lymphomas. *Cancer Treat. Rep.* 1979, **63**: 725–728.

22. Sausville E, Eddy J, Makuch R, et al. Histopathologic staging at initial diagnosis of mycosis fungoides and the Sézary Syndrome: Definition of three distinctive prognostic groups. *Ann. Intern. Med.* 1988, **109**: 372–382.

23. Vonderheid E, Diamond L, Lai S, et al. Lymph node histopathologic findings in cutaneous T-cell lymphoma. A prognostic classification system based on morphologic assessment. *Am. J. Clin. Pathol.* 1992, **97**: 121–129.

24. Kulin P, Marglin S, Shuman W, et al. Diagnostic imaging in the initial staging of mycosis fungoides and Sézary syndrome. *Arch. Dermatol.* 1990, **126**: 914–918.

25. Salhany K, Greer J, Cousar J, et al. Marrow involvement in cutaneous T-cell lymphoma. A clinicopathologic study of 60 cases. *Am. J. Clin. Path.* 1989, **92**: 747–754.

26. Green S, Byar D, Lamberg S. Prognostic variables in mycosis fungoides. *Cancer* 1981, **47**: 2671–2677.

27. Lamberg S, Green S, Byar D, et al. Clinical staging for cutaneous T-cell lymphoma. *Ann. Intern. Med.* 1984, **100**: 187–192.

28. Marti R, Estrach T, Reverter J, et al. Prognostic clinicopathologic factors in cutaneous T-cell lymphoma. *Arch. Dermatol.* 1991, **127**: 1511–1516.

29. Vonderheid E, Diamond L, van Vloten W, et al. Lymph node classification systems in cutaneous T-cell lymphoma. Evidence for the utility of the Working Formulation of Non-Hodgkin's lymphoma for clinical usage. *Cancer* 1994, **73**: 207–218.

30. Yamamura T, Aozasa K, Sano S. The cutaneous lymphomas with convoluted nucleus. *J. Am. Acad. Dermatol.* 1984, **10**: 796–803.

31. Vonderheid E, Tan D, Johnson W, et al. Prognostic significance of cytomorphology in the cutaneous T-cell lymphomas. *Cancer* 1981, **47**: 119–125.

32. Rook A, Vowels B, Jaworsky C, et al. The immunopathogenesis os cutaneous T-cell lymphoma. Abnormal cytokine production by Sézary T-cells [editorial]. *Arch. Dermatol.* 1993, **129**: 486–489.

33. Bernengo M, Fierro M, Novelli M, et al. Soluble interleukin-2 recptor in Sézary syndrome: Its origin and clinical application. *Br. J. Dermatol.* 1993, **128**: 124–129.

34. Dalloul A, Laroche L, Bagot M, et al. Interleukin-7 is a growth factor for Sézary lymphoma cells. *J. Clin. Invest.* 1992, **90**: 1054–1060.

35. Vowels B, Cassin M, Vonderheid E, et al. Aberrant cytokine production by Sézary syndrome patients: Cytokine secretion pattern resembles murine Th2 cells. *J. Invest. Dermatol.* 1992, **99**: 90–94.

36. Gilmore S, Benson E, Kelly J. Serum interleukin-2 receptor levels and cutaneous T-cell lymphoma. *Austral. J. Dermatol.* 1991, **32**: 101–105.

37. Zachariae C, Larsen C, Kaltoft K, et al. Soluble IL2 receptor serum levels and epidermal cytokines in mycosis fungoides and related disorders. *Acta Derm. Venereol.* 1991, **71**: 465–470.

38. Borish L, Dishuck J, Cox L, et al. Sézary syndrome with elevated serum IgE and hpereosinophilia: Role of dysregulated cytokine production. *J. Allergy Clin. Immunol.* 1993, **92**: 123–131.

39. Shioara T, Moriya N, Gotoh C, et al. Differential expression of lymphocyte function-associated antigen 1 (LFA-1) on epidermotropic and non-epidermotropic T-cell clones. *J. Invest. Dermatol.* 1989, **93**: 804–808.

40. Nickoloff B, Griffiths C, Baadsgaard O, et al. Markedly diminished epidermal keratinocyte expression of intercellular adhesion molecule-1 (ICAM-1) in Sézary syndrome. *JAMA* 1989, **261**: 2217–2221.

41. Ralfkiaer E, Thomsen K, Vejlsgaard G. Expression of a cell adhesion protein (VLA beta) in normal and diseased skin. *Br. J. Dermatol.* 1991, **124**: 527–532.

42. Sterry W, Mielke V, Konter U, et al. Role of beta 1-integrins in epidermotropism of malignant T-cells. *Am. J. Pathol.* 1992, **141**: 855–860.

43. Savoia P, Novelli M, Fierro M, et al. Expression and role of integrin receptors in Sézary syndrome. *J. Invest. Dermatol.* 1992, **99**: 151–159.

44. Heald P, Yan S, Edelson R, et al. Skin-selective lymphocyte homing mechanisms int the pathogenesis of leukemic cutaneous T-cell lymphoma. *J. Invest. Dermatol.* 1993, **101**: 222–226.

45. Picker L, Kishimoto T, Smith C, et al. ELAM-1 is an adhesion molecule for skin-homing T-cells. *Nature* 1991, **349**: 796–799.

46. Berg E, Yoshino T, Rott L, et al. The cutaneous lymphocyte antigen is a skin lymphocyte homing receptor for the vascular lectin endothelial cell-leukocyte adhesion molecule 1. *J. Exp. Med.* 1991, **174**: 1461–1466.

47. Borowitz M, Weidner A, Olsen E, et al. Abnormalities of circulating T-cell subpopulations in patients with cutaneous T-cell lymphoma: Cutaneous lymphocyte-associated antigen expression on T-cells correlates with extent of disease. *Leukemia* 1993, **7**: 859–863.

48. Kaudewitz P, Stein H, Dallenbach F: Primary and secondary cutaneous Ki-1+ (CD 30+) anaplastic large cell lymphomas. *Am. J. Pathol.* 1989, **135**: 359–367.

49. Wood G, Bahler D, Hoppe R, et al. Transformation of mycosis fungoides: T-Cell receptor beta-gene analysis demonstrates a common clonal origin for plaque-type mycosis fungoides and CD30+ large cell lymphoma. *J. Invest. Dermatol.* 1993, **101**: 296–300.

50. Willemze R, Beljaards R. Spectrum of primary cutaneous CD30 (Ki-1)-positive lymphoproliferative disorders. *J. Am. Acad. Dermatol.* 1993, **28**: 973–980.

51. Agnarsson B, Vonderheid E, Kadin M. Cutaneous T-cell lymphoma with suppressor/cytotoxic (CD8) phenotype: Identification of rapidly progressive and chronic

subtypes. *J. Am. Acad. Dermatol.* 1990, **22**: 569–577.

52. Hoppe R, Madeiros L, Warnke R, et al. CD8+ tumor infiltrating lymphocytes influence the long term survival of patients with mycosis fungoides. *J. Am. Acad. Dermatol.* 1995, **32**: 448–453.

53. Michie S, Abel E, Hoppe R, et al. Discordant expression of antigens between intraepidermal and intradermal T-cells in mycosis fungoides. *Am. J. Pathol.* 1990, **137**: 1447–1451.

54. Weiss L, Hu E, Wood G, et al. Clonal rearrangement of the T-cell receptor gene in mycosis fungoides and dermatopathic lymphadenopathy. *N. Engl. J. Med.* 1985, **313**: 539–544.

55. Wood G, Weiss L, Warnke R, et al. The immuno-pathology of cutaneous lymphomas: Immunopheno-typic and immunogenotypic characteristics. *Semin. Dermatol.* 1986, **5**: 334–345.

56. Wood G. Recent advances in the molecular biology of cutaneous lymphomas and related disorders. *Semin. Dermatol.* 1991, **10**: 172–177.

57. Lessin S, Rook A, Rovera G. Molecular diagnosis of cutaneous T-cell lymphoma: Polymerase chain reaction amplification of T-cell antigen receptor beta-chain gene rearrangements. *J. Invest. Dermatol.* 1991, **96**: 299–302.

58. Zelickson B, Peters M, Muller S, et al. T-cell receptor gene rearrangement analysis: Cutaneous T-cell lymphoma, peripheral T-cell lymphoma, and premalignant and benign cutaneous lymphoproliferative disorders. *J. Am. Acad. Dermatol.* 1991, **25**: 787–796.

59. Terhune M, Cooper K. Gene rearrangements and T-cell lymphomas. *Arch. Dermatol.* 1993, **129**: 1484–1490.

60. Weinberg J, Rook A, Lessin S. Molecular diagnosis of lymphocytic infiltrates of the skin. *Arch. Dermatol.* 1993, **129**: 1491–1500.

61. Bakels V, Van Oostveen J, Gordijn R, et al. Frequency and prognostic significance of clonal T-cell receptor beta-gene rearrangements in the peripheral blood of patients with mycosis fungoides. *Arch. Dermatol.* 1992, **128**: 1602–1607.

62. Weiss L, Wood G, Hu E, et al. Detection of clonal T-cell receptor gene rearrangement in the peripheral blood of patients with mycosis fungoides/Sézary syndrome. *J. Invest. Dermatol.* 1989, **92**: 601–604.

63. Bakels V, Van Oostveen J, Gordijn R, et al. Diagnostic value of T-cell receptor beta gene rearrangement analysis on peripheral blood lymphocytes of patients with erythroderma. *J. Invest. Dermatol.* 1991, **97**: 782–786.

64. Lynch J, Linoilla I, Sausville E, et al. Prognostic implications of evaluation for lymph node involvement by T-cell antigen receptor gene rearrangement in mycosis fungoides. *Blood* 1992, **79**: 3293–3299.

65. Ramsay D, Lish K, Yalowitz C, et al. Ultraviolet-B phototherapy for early-stage cutaneous T-cell lymphoma. *Arch. Dermatol.* 1992, **128**: 931–933.

66. Resnik K, Vonderheid E. Home UV phototherapy of early mycosis fungoides: Long-term follow-up observations in thirty-one patients. *J. Am. Acad. Dermatol.* 1993, **29**: 73–77.

67. Abel E, Sendagorta E, Hoppe R, et al. PUVA treatment of erythrodermic and plaque-type mycosis fungoides: Ten-year follow-up study. *Arch. Dermatol.* 1987, **123**: 897–901.

68. Roenigk HJ, Kuzel T, Skoutelis A, et al. Photo-chemotherapy alone or combined with interferon alpha-2a in the treatment of cutneous T-cell lymphoma. *J. Invest. Dermatol.* 1990, **95**: 198S–205S.

69. Holloway K, Flowers F, Ramos-Caro F. Therapeutic alternatives in cutaneous T-cell lymphoma. *J. Am. Acad. Dermatol.* 1992, **27**: 367–378.

70. Edelson R. Light-activated drugs. *Sci. Am.* 1988, **259**: 68–75.

71. Edelson R. Photopheresis: A clinically relevant immunobiologic response modifier. *Ann. N. York Acad. Sci.* 1991, **636**: 154–164.

72. Group BP. British photodermatology group guidelines for PUVA. *Br. J. Dermatol.* 1994, **130**: 246–255.

73. Abel E. *Clinical and Histologic Changes in PUVA-related Skin.* Boston: GK Hall Medical Publishers, 1984.

74. Gupta A, Anderson T. Psoralen photochemotherapy. *J. Am. Acad. Dermatol.* 1987, **17**: 703–734.

75. Farber E, Epstein J, Nall L, et al. Current status of oral PUVA therapy for psoriasis: Eye protection revisions. *J. Am. Acad. Dermatol.* 1982, **6**: 851–855.

76. Stern R, Laird N, Melski J, et al. Cutaneous squamous cell carcinoma in patients treated with PUVA. *N. Engl. J. Med.* 1984, **310**: 1156–1161.

77. Stern R, Abel E, Wintroub B, et al. Genital tumors among men with psoriasis exposed to psoralens and ultraviolet A radiation (PUVA) and ultraviolet B radiation. *N. Engl. J. Med.* 1990, **322**: 1093–1097.

78. Rhodes A, Harrist T, Momtaz T-K. The PUVA-induced pigmented macule: A lentiginous proliferation of large, sometimes cytologically atypical, melano-cytes. *J. Am. Acad. Dermatol.* 1983, **9**: 47–58.

79. Ramsay D, Halperin P, Zeleniuch-Jacquotte A. Topical mechlorethamine therapy for mycosis fungoides. *J. Am. Acad. Dermatol.* 1988, **19**: 684–691.

80. Vonderheid E, Tan E, Kantor A, et al. Long-term efficacy, curative potential, and carcinogenicity of topical mechlorethamine chemotherapy in cutaneous T-cell lymphoma. *J. Am. Acad. Dermatol.* 1989, **20**: 416–428.

81. VanScott E, Kalmanson J. Complete remissions of mycosis fungoides lymphoma induced by topical nitrogen mustard (HN2). Control of delayed hypersensitivity to HN2 by desensitization and by induction of specific immunologic tolerance. *Cancer* 1973, **32**: 18–30.

82. Price N, Hoppe R, Deneau D. Ointment-based mechloethamine treatment for mycosis fungoides. *Cancer* 1983, **52**: 2214–2219.

83. Taylor J, Halprin K, Levine V, et al. Mechlorethamine hydrochloride solution and ointment. *Arch. Dermatol.* 1980, **116**: 783–785.

84. Hoppe R, Abel E, Deneau D, et al. Mycosis fungoides: Management with topical nitrogen mustard. *J. Clin. Oncol.* 1987, **5**: 1796–1803.

85. Vonderheid E. Topical mechlorethamine chemotherapy. Considerations on its use in mycosis fungoides. *Int. J. Dermatol.* 1984, **23**: 180–186.

86. Waldorf D, Haynes H, VanScott E. Cutaneous hypersensitivity and desensitization to mechlorethamine in

patients with mycosis fungoides lymphomas. *Ann. Intern. Med.* 1967, **67**: 282–290.

87. Constantine V, Fuks Z, Farber E. Mechlorethamine desensitization in therapy for mycosis fungoides. Topical desensitization to mechlorethamine (nitrogen mustard) contact hypersensitivity. *Arch. Dermatol.* 1975, **111**: 484–488.

88. Abel E, Sendagorta E, Hoppe R. Cutaneous malignancies and metastatic squamous cell carcinoma following topical therapy for mycosis fungoides. *J. Am. Acad. Dermatol.* 1986, **14**: 1029–1038.

89. Smoller B, Marcus R. Risk of secondary cutaneous malignancies in patients with long-standing mycosis fungoides. *J. Am. Acad. Dermatol.* 1994, **30**: 201–204.

90. Zackheim H, Epstein E, Crain W. Topical carmustine (BCNU) for cutaneous T-cell lymphoma: A 15-year experience in 143 patients. *J. Am. Acad. Dermatol.* 1990. 22: 802–810.

91. Hoppe R, Fuks Z, Bagshaw M. Radiation therapy in the management of cutaneous T-cell lymphoma. *Cancer Treat. Rep.* 1979, **63**: 625–632.

92. Karzmark C, Loevinger R, Steele R, et al. A technique for large-field, superficial electron therapy. *Radiology* 1960, **74**: 633–644.

93. Nisce L, Safai B, Kim J. Effectiveness of once weekly total skin electron beam therapy in mycosis fungoides and Sézary syndrome. *Cancer* 1981, **47**: 870–876.

94. Hamminga B, Noordijk E, van Vloten W. Treatment of mycosis fungoides. Total-skin electron-beam irradiation vs topical mechlorethamine therapy. *Arch. Dermatol.* 1982, **118**: 150–153.

95. van Vloten W, DeVroome H, Noordijk E. Total skin electron beam irradiation for cutaneous T-cell lymphoma (mycosis fungoides). *Br. J. Dermatol.* 1985, **112**: 697–702.

96. Lo T, Salzman F, Moschella S, et al. Whole body surface electron irradiation in the treatment of mycosis fungoides. An evaluation of 200 patients. *Radiology* 1979, **130**: 453–457.

97. Tadros A, Tepperman B, Hryniuk W, et al. Total skin electron irradiation for mycosis fungoides: Failure analysis and prognostic factors. *Int. J. Radiat. Oncol. Biol. Phys.* 1983, **9**: 1279–1287.

98. Price N, Hoppe R, Constantine V, et al. The treatment of mycosis fungoides: Adjuvant topical mechlorethamine after electron beam therapy. *Cancer* 1977, **40**: 2851–2853.

99. Kaye F, Bunn P, Steinberg S, et al. A randomized trial comparing combination electron-beam radiation and chemotherapy with topical therapy in the initial treatment of mycosis fungoides. *N. Engl. J. Med.* 1989, **321**: 1784–1790.

100. Edelson R, Heald P, Perez M, et al. Photopheresis update. *Prog. Dermatol.* 1991, **25**: 1–6.

101. Heald P, Rook A, Perez M, et al. Treatment of erythodermic cutaneous T-cell lymphoma with extracorporeal photochemotherapy. *J. Am. Acad. Dermatol.* 1992, **27**: 427–433.

102. Edelson R, Berger C, Gasparro F, et al. Treatment of cutaneous T-cell lymphoma by extracorporeal photochemotherapy. *N. Engl. J. Med.* 1987, **316**: 297–303.

103. Wieselthier J, Koh H. Sézary syndrome: diagnosis,

prognosis, and critical review of treatment options. *J. Am. Acad. Dermatol.* 1990, **22**: 381–401.

104. Armus S, Keyes B, Cahill C, et al. Photopheresis for the treatment of cutaneous T-cell lymphoma. *J. Am. Acad. Dermatol.* 1990, **23**: 898–902.

105. Marks D, Rockman S, Oziemski M, et al. Mechanisms of lymphocytotoxicity induced by extracorporeal photochemotherapy for cutaneous T-cell lymphoma. *J. Clin. Invest.* 1990, **86**: 2080–2085.

106. Peterseim J, Kuster W, Gebauer H, et al. Cytogenetic effects during extracorporeal photopheresis: Treatment of two patients with cutaneous T-cell lymphoma. *Arch. Dermatol. Res.* 1991, **28**: 81–85.

107. Vowels B, Cassin M, Boufal M, et al. Extracorporeal photochemotherapy induces the production of tumor necrosis factor-alfa by monocytes: Implications for the treatment of cutaneous T-cell lymphoma and systemic sclerosis. *J. Invest. Dermatol.* 1992, **98**: 686–692.

108. Vagna M, Papa G, Defazio D, et al. Interferon alpha-2a in cutaneous T-cell lymphoma. *Eur. J. Haematol.* 1990, **52**(Suppl.): 32–35.

109. Papa G, Tura S, Mandelli F, et al. Is interferon alpha in cutaneous T-cell lymphoma a treatment of choice? *Br. J. Dermatol.* 1991, **79**(Suppl.): 48–51.

110. Olsen E, Rosen S, Vollmer R, et al. Interferon alfa-2a in the treatment of cutaneous T-cell lymphoma. *J. Am. Acad. Dermatol.* 1989, **20**: 395–407.

111. Hagberg H, Juhlin L, Scheynius A, et al. Low dosage alpha-interferon treatment in patients with advanced cutaneous T-cell lymphoma. *Eur. J. Haematol.* 1988, **40**: 31–34.

112. Bunn P, Foon K, Ihde D, et al. Recombinant leukocyte A interferon: An active agent in advanced cutaneous T-cell lymphomas. *Ann. Intern. Med.* 1984, **101**: 484–487.

113. Bunn P, Ihde D, Foon K. The role of recombinant interferon alfa-2a in the therapy of cutaneous T-cell lymphomas. *Cancer* 1986, **57**: 1689–1695.

114. Kohn E, Steis R, Sausville E, et al. Phase II trial of intermittent high-dose recombinant interferon alfa-2a in mycosis fungoides and the Sézary syndrome. *J. Clin. Oncol.* 1990, **8**: 155–160.

115. Wolff J, Zitelli J, Rabin B, et al. Intralesional interferon in the treatment of early mycosis fungoides. *J. Am. Acad. Dermatol.* 1985, **13**: 604–612.

116. Vonderheid E, Thompson R, Smiles K, et al. Recombinant interferon alfa-2b in plaque-phase mycosis fungoides. *Arch. Dermatol.* 1987, **123**: 757–763.

117. Kessler J, Jones S, Levine N, et al. Isotretinoin and cutaneous helper T-cell lymphoma (mycosis fungoides). *Arch. Dermatol.* 1987, **123**: 201–204.

118. Claudy A, Rouchouse B, Boucheron S, et al. Treatment of cutaneous lymphoma with etretinate. *Br. J. Dermatol.* 1983, **109**: 49–56.

119. Tousignant J, Raymond G, Light M. Treatment of cutaneous T-cell lymphoma with the arotinoid Ro 13–6298. *J. Am. Acad. Dermatol.* 1987, **16**: 167–171.

120. Hoting E, Meissner K. Arotinoid-ethylester effectiveness in refractory cutaneous T-cell lymphoma. *Cancer* 1988, **62**: 1044–1048.

121. Dennert G, Lotan R. Effects of retinoic acid on the immune system. Stimulation of T killer cell induction.

Eur. J. Immunol. 1978, **8**: 23–29.

122. Lotan R. Effects of vitamin A and its analogs (retinoids) on normal and neoplastic cells. *Biochem. Biophys. Acta* 1980, **605**: 33–91.

123. Dicken C. Reinoids: A review. *J. Am. Acad. Dermatol.* 1984, **11**: 541–552.

124. DiGiovanna J. Retinoids for the future: Oncology. *J. Am. Acad. Dermatol.* 1992, **27**: S34-S37.

125. Smack D, Korge B, James W. Keratins and keratinization. *J. Am. Acad. Dermatol.* 1994, **30**: 85–102.

126. Saurat J. Side effects of systemic retinoids and their clinical management. *J. Am. Acad. Dermatol.* 1992, **27**: 29–S33.

127. Miller R, Levy R. Response of cutaneous T-cell lymphoma to therapy with hybridoma monoclonal antibody. *Lancet* 1981, **2**: 226–230.

128. Miller R, Oseroff A, Stratte P, et al. Monoclonal antibody therapeutic trials in seven patients with T-cell lymphoma. *Blood* 1983, **62**: 988–995.

129. Dillman R, Shawler D, Dillman J, et al. Therapy of chronic lymphocytic leukemia and cutaneous T-cell lymphoma with T101 monoclonal antibody. *J. Clin. Oncol.* 1984, **2**: 881–891.

130. Rosen S, Zimmer M, Goldman-Leikin R, et al. Radioimmunodetection and radioimmunotherapy of cutaneous T-cell lymphomas using an ^{131}I-labeled monoclonal antibody: An Illinois Cancer Council Study. *J. Clin. Oncol.* 1987, **5**: 562–573.

131. Knox S, Levy R, Hodgkinson S, et al. Observations on the effect of chimeric anti-CD4 monoclonal antibody in patients with mycosis fungoides. *Blood* 1991, **77**: 20–30.

132. Williams D, Snider C, Strom T, et al. Structure/function analysis of interleukin-2-toxin (DAB486IL-2): Fragment B sequences required for the delivery of fragment A to the cytosol of target cells. *J. Biol. Chem.* 1990, **265**: 11885–11889.

133. Hesketh P, Caguioa P, Koh H, et al. Clinical activity of a cytotoxic fusion protein in the treatment of cutaneous T-cell lymphoma. *J. Clin. Oncol.* 1993, **11**: 1682–1690.

134. Saven A, Piro L. The newer purine analogs. Significant therapeutic advance in the management of lymphoid malignancies. *Cancer* 1993, **72**: 3470–3483.

135. Von Hoff D, Dahlberg S, Hartstock R, et al. Activity of fludarabine monophosphate in patients with advanced mycosis fungoides: A Southwest Oncology Group study. *J. Natl Cancer Inst.* 1990, **82**: 1353–1355.

136. Kuzel T, Samuelson E, Roenigk H, et al. Phase II trial of 2-chlorodeoxyadenosine (2-CDA) for the treatment of mycosis fungoides or the Sézary syndrome. *Proc. Annu. Meet. Am. Soc. Clin. Oncol.* 1992, **11**: 1089A.

137. Dang-Vu A, Olsen E, Vollmer R, et al. Treatment of cutaneous T-cell lymphoma with 2-deoxycoformycin (pentostatin). *J. Am. Acad. Dermatol.* 1988, **19**: 692–698.

138. Cummings F, Kim K, Neiman R, et al. Phase II trial of pentostatin in refractory lymphomas and cutaneous T-cell disease. *J. Clin. Oncol.* 1991, **9**: 565–571.

139. Brogden R, Sorkin E. Pentostatin. A review of its pharmacodynamic and pharmacokinetic properties, and therapeutic potential in lymphoproliferative disorders. *Drugs* 1993, **46**: 652–677.

140. Dummer R, Krasovec M, Roger J, et al. Topical administration of hexadecylphosphocholine in patients with cutaneous lymphomas: Results of a phase I/II study. *J. Am. Acad. Dermatol.* 1993, **29**: 963–970.

141. Bigler R, Crilley P, Micaily B, et al. Autologous bone marrow transplantation for advanced stage mycosis fungoides. *Bone Marrow Transplant.* 1991, **7**: 133–137.

142. Kuzel T, Gilyon K, Springer E, et al. Interferon alfa-2a combined with phototherapy in the treatment of cutaneous T-cell lymphoma. *J. Natl Cancer Inst.* 1990, **82**: 203–207.

143. Kuzel T, Roenigk HJ, Samuelson E, et al. Therapy of mycosis fungoides with interferon alfa-2a combined with phototherapy: phase I and II trial long-term follow-up. *Proc. Annu. Meet. Am. Soc. Clin. Oncol.* 1991, **10**: 939A.

144. Mostow E, Neckel S, Oberhelman L, et al. Complete remissions in psoralen and UV-A (PUVA)-refractory mycosis fungoides-type cutaneous T-cell lymphoma with combined interferon alfa and PUVA. *Arch. Dermatol.* 1993, **129**: 747–752.

145. Dreno B. Roferon-A (interferon alpha 2a) combined with Tegason (etretinate) for treatment of cutaneous T-cell lymphomas. *Stem Cells* 1993, **11**: 269–275.

146. Dreno B, Claudy A, Meynadier J, et al. The treatment of 45 patients with cutaneous T-cell lymphoma with low doses of interferon alpha 2a and etretinate. *Br. J. Dermatol.* 1991, **125**: 456–459.

147. Altomare G, Capella G, Pigatto P, et al. Intramuscular low dose alpha-2b interferon and etretinate for treatment of mycosis fungoides. *Int. J. Dermatol.* 1993, **32**: 138–141.

148. Rook A, Prystowsky M, Cassin M, et al. Combined therapy for Sézary syndrome with extracorporeal photochemotherapy and low-dose interferon alfa therapy. *Arch. Dermatol.* 1991, **127**: 1535–1540.

149. Foss F, Ihde D, Breneman D, et al. Phase II study of pentostatin and intermittent high-dose recombinant interferon alfa-2a in advanced mycosis fungoides/Sézary syndrome. *J. Clin. Oncol.* 1992, **10**: 1907–1913.

150. Schwab U, Stein H, Gerdes J, et al. Production of a monoclonal antibody specific for Hodgkin and Sternberg–Reed cells of Hodgkin's disease and a subset of normal lymphoid cells. *Nature* 1982, **299**: 65–67.

151. Stein H, Mason D, Gerdes J, et al. The expression of Hodgkin's disease-associated antigen Ki-1 in reactive and neoplastic lymphoid tissue: Evidence that Reed–Sternberg cells and histiocytic malignancies are derived from activated lymphoid tissue. *Blood* 1985, **66**: 848–858.

152. Kadin M, Nasu K, Sako D, et al. Lymphomatoid papulosis: A cutaneous proliferation of activated helper T-cells expressing Hodgkin's disease-associated antigens. *Am. J. Pathol.* 1985, **119**: 315–325.

153. Kaudewitz P, Stein H, Burg G, et al. Atypical cells in lymphomatoid papulosis express the Hodgkin cell-associated antigen Ki-1. *J. Invest. Dermatol.* 1986, **86**: 350–354.

154. Beljaards R, Kaudewitz P, Berti E, et al. Primary cutaneous large cell lymphomas: definition of a new type of cutaneous lymphoma with a favorable prognosis: A European multicenter study on 47 patients. *Cancer* 1993, **71**: 2097–2104.

155. Gianotti R, Alessi E, Caicchini S, et al. Primary cutaneous pleomorphic T-cell lymphoma expressing CD30 antigen. *Am. J. Dermatopathol.* 1991, **13**: 503–508.

156. Kadin M, Sako D, Berliner N, et al. Childhood Ki-1 lymphoma presenting with skin lesions and peripheral lymphadenopathy. *Blood* 1986, **68**: 1042–1049.

157. Vecchi V, Burnelli R, Pileri S, et al. Anaplastic large cell lymphoma (Ki-1/CD30+) in childhood. *Med. Ped. Oncol.* 1993, **21**: 402–410.

158. Chott A, Kaserer K, Augustin I, et al. Ki-1 positive large cell lymphoma: A clinicopathologic study of 41 cases. *Am. J. Surg. Pathol.* 1990, **14**: 439–448.

159. Greer J, Kinney M, Collins R, et al. Clinical features of 31 patients with Ki-1 anaplastic large cell lymphoma. *J. Clin. Oncol.* 1991, **9**: 539–547.

160. Beljaards R, Meijer C, Scheffer E, et al. Prognostic significance of CD 30 (Ki-1/Ber-H2) expression in primary cutaneous large-cell lymphomas of T-cell origin: A clinicopathologic and immunohistochemical study in 20 patients. *Am. J. Pathol.* 1989, **135**: 1169–1178.

161. Camisa C, Helm T, Sexton C, et al. Ki-1-positive anaplastic large-cell lymphoma can mimic benign dermatoses. *J. Am. Acad. Dermatol.* 1993, **29**: 696–700.

162. Kinney M, Collins R, Greer J, et al. A small-cell-predominant variant of primary Ki-1 (CD30)+ T-cell lymphoma. *Am. J. Surg. Pathol.* 1993, **17**: 859–868.

163. Noorduyn A, Beljaards R, Pals S, et al. Differential expression of the HECA-452 antigen (cutaneous lymphocyte associated antigen, CLA) in cutaneous and non-cutaneous T-cell lymphomas. *Histopathology* 1992, **21**: 59–64.

164. Beljaards R, Meijer C, Scheffer E. Differential diagnosis of cutaneous large cell lymphomas using monoclonal antibodies in paraffin-embedded skin biopsies. *Am. J. Dermatopathol.* 1991, **13**: 342–349.

165. Kadin M. The spectrum of Ki-1+ cutaneous lymphomas. *Curr. Probl. Dermatol.* 1990, **19**: 132–143.

166. Chan J, Ng C, Hui P, et al. Anaplastic large cell Ki-1 lymphoma: delineation of two morphologic cases. *Histopathology* 1989, **15**: 11–34.

167. Motley R, Jasani B, Ford A, et al. Regressing atypical histiocytosis, a regressing cutaneous phase of Ki-1-positive anaplastic large cell lymphoma. *Cancer* 1992, **70**: 476–483.

168. Bitter M, Franklin W, Larson R. Morphology in Ki-1 (CD30) positive non-Hodgkin's lymphomas is correlated with clinical features and the presence of a unique chromosomal abnormality. *Am. J. Surg. Pathol.* 1990, **14**: 305–316.

169. Banerjee S, Heald J, Harris M. Twelve cases of Ki-1 positive anaplastic large cell lymphoma of the skin. *J. Clin. Pathol.* 1991, **44**: 119–125.

170. Harrington D, Braddock S, Blocher K, et al. Lymphomatoid papulosis and progression to T-cell lymphoma: An immunophenotypic and genotypic analysis. *J. Am. Acad. Dermatol.* 1989, **21**: 951–957.

171. Beljaards R, Willemze R. The prognosis of patients with lymphomatoid papulosis associated with other types of malignancies. *Br. J. Dermatol.* 1992, **126**: 596–602.

172. Rijlaarsdam J, Huygens P, Beljaards R, et al. Oral etoposide in the treatment of cutaneous large cell lymphomas. *Br. J. Dermatol.* 1992, **127**: 524–528.

CHAPTER 44

Other peripheral T-cell lymphomas

ALAIN DELMER AND ROBERT A. ZITTOUN

Introduction

Among T-cell non-Hodgkin's lymphomas, lymphoblastic lymphoma and mycosis fungoides have long been recognized as fundamentally different clinicopathological entities, which have distinct natural histories and organ and tissue tropisms, and which require very different therapeutic approaches. More recently the underlying reason for this difference has been identified: lymphoblastic lymphoma is derived from thymic, i.e., precursor T-cells, and mycosis fungoides from postthymic T-cells. The advances in basic immunology that led to the identification of major divisions in the lineage of non-Hodgkin's lymphomas stemmed from the recognition, in the early 1970s, of the basic subdivision of the immune system into B- and T-cell lineages. The first descriptions of T-cell lymphomas were published at the end of this decade [1–6] and the subsequent expansion in the number of entities identified as neoplastic counterparts of postthymic T-cells has led to the designation of this group of lymphomas as peripheral T-cell lymphomas (PTCLs). Two major advances led to the recognition that many lymphomas are of T-cell origin: the development of monoclonal antibodies against T-cell antigens, which permitted immunophenotyping on cryostat sections [7,8]; and progress in molecular biology,

which has permitted rearrangements in the T-cell receptor genes (TCR) to be identified [8–11]. PTCLs encompass a wide spectrum of clinicopathologic entities that demonstrate marked clinical, morphological and immunological diversity. They can be broadly classified into cutaneous T-cell lymphomas, i.e., those which have a particular predilection for the skin (classically mycosis fungoides and Sézary syndrome) and the remainder, many of which were formerly classified as diffuse mixed-cell lymphomas. Some entities such as the angioimmunoblastic lymphadenopathy with dysproteinemia (AILD) or angiocentric immunoproliferative lesions (AIL), the malignant condition of which has been repeatedly debated, have also fallen within the scope of PTCLs. In this chapter, we discuss the PTCLs other than mycosis fungoides and Sézary syndrome, which are described in Chapter 43.

PTCLs represent approximately 10–20% of all NHLs in Western countries, but they account for up to 50% of NHLs in Asia, half of which are related to the type C retrovirus, human T-cell lymphotropic virus (HTLV-1), which is endemic in some districts of Japan and the Caribbean. HTLV-1-related adult T-cell leukemia–lymphoma (ATLL) has rather monomorphic clinical and immunopathological characteristics, and is consistently associated with a poor outcome. In contrast, PTCLs not related to HTLV-1 infection exhibit numerous features which will be reviewed in this chapter.

Whether or not T-cell phenotype as a whole has prognostic relevance is still controversial. Ongoing prospective trials on properly phenotyped non-Hodgkin's lymphoma (NHL) cohorts will certainly address this issue, at least for the high-grade PTCLs, but no specific therapeutic recommendation may be presently given for most subtypes of PTCLs. It seems probable that the broad range of entities that fall within this category will lead, as in the case for B-cell lymphomas, to the necessity for a number of therapeutic approaches, dictated by the nature of the individual entity rather than by simply its origin from the T-cell lineage.

Recently, the possible role of Epstein–Barr virus (EBV) in the pathogenesis of PTCLs has emerged from the recognition of EBV genome and its latent gene products in the tumor cells of a significant percentage of cases. Otherwise, it is likely that the differential release of various cytokines by the tumor cells and/or the accompanying reactive B- and T-cells is responsible for the diversity of clinical and histomorphological characteristics of PTCLs. Little detailed information is available yet, but numerous investigations of cytokine production and response are in progress.

Epidemiology

HTLV-1-RELATED T-CELL LYMPHOMAS

The overall incidence of NHLs in Asia (Japan, China) is lower than in Western countries. It has been estimated, on average, at 3.5 and 2.0 per 100 000 of the population per annum in males and females respectively [12]. PTCLs account for 40–50% of NHLs in these countries, but they represent 75% of NHLs in the Kyushu district of Japan, the region in which HTLV-1 infection was first identified as being associated with an increased risk of ATLL [13]. Since estimates of the incidence of PTCLs in Asia are quite similar to those of Western countries (see below), it would appear that the higher frequency of T-cell lymphomas in Asia is mainly a consequence of a deficit in B-cell lymphomas.

An epidemiologic survey of HTLV-1 infection has shown a highly geographic restriction. The main endemic areas have been identified as the southern islands of Japan, the Caribbean and French-speaking West Africa, but areas of lower seroprevalence have been identified in South America, West Africa and the Philippines [14]. Epidemiologic studies have demonstrated the role of breast feeding, blood transfusion and semen in the transmission of HTLV-1 infection.

The annual incidence of ATLL among HTLV-1 carriers has been estimated at 2.0 and 0.5 per 1000 in males and in females, respectively, and the cumulative risk for ATLL in HTLV-1 carriers during a 70-year life span is 1–5% [12]. The age distribution of ATLL is unimodal with a male to female ratio of 1.3 and a median age at diagnosis of 50–55 years [15]. Therefore, assuming, as appears to be the case, that most patients are infected during infancy, the latency before the development of ATLL is long, often extending over several decades.

PTCL IN WESTERN COUNTRIES

The overall incidence of PTCLs in Western countries is probably about 2–4 per 100 000 per year in males and roughly half this in females, based on USA (White) incidence rates of 20 and 12, respectively, and frequencies of 10–20% of all NHLs [16–18], although large-scale epidemiologic surveys that have specifically addressed this issue are not available. In the German Kiel Registry, the overall frequency of T-cell phenotype was 17.1%, and T-cell lymphomas accounted for 8.9% and 8.2% of the low-grade and high-grade categories, respectively [19]. In one series [20], PTCLs represented up to 30% of 361 cases of intermediate- and high-grade NHL. However, as it was stated by the authors, this unusually high incidence of PTCLs was probably biased by the fact that these cases were selected from a larger series because of adequate phenotypic analysis and that the phenotyped cases were those for which morphological examination was conflicting.

In nonendemic areas, some T-cell proliferations containing HTLV-1-specific sequences integrated into DNA have occasionally been described even though serologic analysis for HTLV-1 antibodies was negative. However, in one study, HTLV-1-specific polymerase sequences were systematically assessed by the polymerase chain reaction (PCR) in a series of 27 HTLV-1-seronegative patients with PTCL and four seropositive control patients. None of the PTCL samples were PCR positive, demonstrating, in this study, full concordance with serologic analysis [21].

The median age at presentation in patients with PTCL is usually 55–60 years. However, PTCL may occur in younger adults or in children, mainly within the subset of anaplastic large-cell lymphoma (ALCL) [22]. A preceding disorder of the immune system is occasionally present. In one series [23], 36 out of 134 patients had an underlying condition, including autoimmune diseases (arthritis, Grave's disease, sarcoidosis), ataxia telangiectasia (one case), lymphoma of unspecified type (11 cases), and lymphoproliferative disorders (15 cases), such as AILD, atypical dermatitis and lymphomatoid papulosis. In recent years the latter conditions have been reclassified as lymphomas from the beginning, rather than conditions upon which lymphoma may be superimposed, although they may have an indolent phase prior to transformation into a more aggressive and overtly malignant condition. Thus, what has been considered an 'underlying condition' in earlier series may actually be the initial manifestations of lymphoma. The development of small intestinal large-cell lymphoma of T-lineage is a rare but well-documented complication of celiac disease [24].

Although the majority of lymphoproliferations arising in the context of acquired immune deficiency are of B-cell origin, some PTCLs have occasionally been reported either in organ transplant recipients [25–26] or in human immunodeficiency virus (HIV)-infected patients [27–30]. In one case of CD4+, CD25+ T-cell lymphoma in an HIV-1 patient, a pathogenetic role for HIV-1 was strongly suggested by its monoclonal integration in the tumor genome and the production of HIV p24 antigen by the tumor cells [28]. However, additional cases of this kind have not been reported. As has been regularly observed for B-cell NHLs, EBV has also been detected in some PTCL cases occurring either posttransplant [26] or in patients with HIV infection [30], suggesting that EBV may contribute to the pathogenesis of these lymphomas.

Diagnosis

MORPHOLOGICAL CLASSIFICATIONS

There is no universally accepted, satisfactory scheme for the histological subclassification of PTCLs that encompasses the morphologic diversity of PTCLs. Several proposals have been made [31], including that from Suchi et al. [32] subsequently incorporated into the updated Kiel classification [33], which is widely used in Europe. In this classification, PTCLs are divided, mainly on the basis of tumor cell size, into low-grade and high-grade categories (Table 44.1). The former includes leukemic proliferations of postthymic lymphocytes (T-cell chronic lymphocytic leukemia, T-cell prolymphocytic leukemia [34], leukemia of large granular lymphocytes [35]), cutaneous T-cell lymphomas (mycosis fungoides and Sézary syndrome), lymphoepithelioid T-cell lymphoma (Lennert's lymphoma), T-zone lymphoma, AILD-type lymphoma and pleomorphic, small-cell type. The high-grade category includes pleomorphic, medium- and large-cell subtypes, immunoblastic lymphoma of T-cell type and anaplastic large-cell lymphoma. The prognostic value of such a separation is questionable in view of the rather poor outcome of the so-called low-grade PTCLs [36–38]. Some cases, as well as angiocentric immunoproliferative lesions (angiocentric lymphomas), do not fit this scheme and must, therefore, be considered 'unclassified'.

More recently, Stein et al. [39] have proposed that

Table 44.1 Classification of peripheral T-cell lymphomas (PTCLs) (Suchi et al. [32] and Stansfeld et al. [33]) and distribution of PTCLs within this classification

Classification	Chott et al. [120]	Hôtel-Dieu [193]
Low-grade	37	12
T-cell chronic lymphocytic leukemia and T-prolymphocytic leukemia	3	
Small cerebriform cell (mycosis fungoides, Sézary syndrome)	—*	—*
Lymphoepithelioid (Lennert's lymphoma)	4	2
AILD-type lymphoma	22	10
T-Zone	6	—
Pleomorphic, small cell	2	—
High-grade	38	35
Pleomorphic, medium and large cell	24	24
Immunoblastic	1	3
Anaplastic large cell	13	8
Unclassified, low- and high-grade		

* Epidermotropic T-cell lymphomas excluded.

AILD, Angioimmunoblastic lymphadenopathy with dysproteinemia.

Table 44.4 Expression of α/β and γ/δ T-cell receptors in PTCLs (from Gaulard et al. [66])

		T-cell subset antigen expression				CD56	TCR Gene
	n (%)	CD4+CD8–	CD4–CD8+	CD4+CD8+	CD4–CD8–	expression	rearrangements
'Common' $\alpha\beta$-TCR type* CD3+, βF1+, TCRδ-1–	39 (69%)	31	2	2	2	1/15	β-chain 16/18
TCR-$\gamma\delta$ type*† CD3+, βF1–, TCRδ-1+	6 (10%)	0	0	0	4	4/6	δ-chain 5/5 (β-chain 2/5)
'TCR silent' type CD3+ or CD3–, βF1–, TCRδ-1–	12 (21%)	8	0	1	3	3/11	β-chain 8/10

* For each category, CD4 expression could not be evaluated in two cases.
† Five cases corresponded to T$\gamma\delta$ lymphomas with hepatosplenic presentation while the other was a lethal midline granuloma.
βF1 and TCRδ-1 monoclonal antibodies recognize the β-chain of TCRα/β and an invariant epitope of the δ-chain of TCRγ/δ, respectively.
TCR, T-cell receptor.

represent a type of T-cell lymphoma that probably arises from the small subset of normal T-γ/δ lymphocytes. These lymphomas frequently present with hepatosplenomegaly [67] and the tumor cells also express CD56 (a natural killer marker) in most cases (four out of six). In Gaulard's third group (12 cases), the tumor cells were TCRα/β and TCRγ/δ-negative and they variably expressed the CD3 molecule. A nonproductive rearrangement of the TCRβ-chain gene was observed in eight of ten of these cases. Thus, immunogenotypic studies are not only a helpful tool for the diagnosis of PTCLs, but they may also provide insights into the pathogenesis and classification of these disorders.

CYTOGENETICS

Several numerical and structural karyotypic changes have been reported in T-cell neoplasias. However, most studies have been performed in T-cell chronic lymphocytic leukemia or T-lymphoblastic leukemia/lymphoma, and the data on cytogenetic abnormalities in PTCLs are relatively few, except for ATLL. A variety of nonrandom translocations involving the TCR sites (TCRα and TCRγ, TCRβ and TCRγ on chromosomes 14q11, 7q34, and 7p15, respectively) have been described in PTCLs but none of these is common [68–71]. In PTCLs, no single chromosomal region has been found to be consistently implicated. The most frequent structural abnormalities involve chromosomes 1, 2, 4, 6, 14 and 17, although noticeable variations exist from one study to another [68,71,72]. The most common numerical aberrations are trisomies 3 and 5, gain of an X chromosome [71], along with trisomy 21, or deletion of an X or Y chromosome in ATLL [72]. Karyotypic changes may represent the only marker of clonality [73–76].

Indeed, the first evidence for the clonal nature of AILD was provided by the finding of trisomy 3 or 5 [73,74]. Schlelgelberger et al. [71] have recently reported that the chromosomal abnormalities observed among the various types of PTCL are distinct and parallel the Kiel classification. High-grade PTCLs are frequently associated with triploid and tetraploid clones, as well as complex abnormalities. The only chromosome aberration that appears, at present, to be restricted to a specific type of high-grade PTCL is the t(2;5)(p23;q35) translocation observed in large-cell anaplastic lymphoma of T- and null phenotype [77,78]. This translocation has recently been cloned and involves the nucleophosmin (NPM) gene on chromosome 5q35 and a new kinase (ALK for anaplastic large-cell kinase) gene on chromosome 2p13 [79].

EBV DETECTION IN PTCL

The role of EBV in the pathogenesis of African Burkitt's lymphoma, B-cell posttransplant immunoproliferative disorders and nasopharyngeal carcinoma is generally accepted, although the molecular pathways involved remain to be elucidated [80]. The possible implication of EBV in the pathogenesis of PTCLs has also been investigated recently [81]. The overall frequency of EBV detection in tumor tissue from patients with PTCL is higher than in B-cell lymphomas but there are significant variations in EBV association among PTCL subtypes [82]. EBV is detected in most cases of angiocentric immunoproliferative lesions (nasal T-cell lymphoma, lethal midline granuloma, lymphomatoid granulomatosis) [83–87], a significant number of ALCL [88] and AILD-type lymphoma [89,90], while in other subtypes it is detected in approximately 10–20% of cases, regardless of whether the patients originate from Asia [91] or Europe [92] (Table 44.5). The EBV genome has been shown to be monoclonally integrated into the tumor DNA [83,91]. Moreover, RNA *in situ* hybridization with EBER (EBV-encoded RNA)-1 and -2 probes, combined with morphology or immunostaining with T-cell antibodies has demonstrated that the latently infected cells were tumor T-

Table 44.5   EBV Detection in PTCLs

Reference	No. of patients	Histologic subtype	Methods	No. positive (%)	Comments
Harabuchi et al. [83]	5	Lethal midline granuloma (LMG)	SB DNA ISH	5 (100%)	EBNA2 and LMP1 positive in all cases
Kanavaros et al. [86]	7	Nasal T-cell lymphoma	RNA ISH* DNA ISH	7 (100%)	LMP1 positive in all cases EBV detected in tumor cells whatever the site (nose, lymph node, skin)
Borisch et al. [87]	12	Nasal T-cell lymphoma: 6 other nasopharyngeal lymphomas: 6	PCR RNA ISH*	Nasal T-cell 6/6 (100%) Other 3/6 (50%)	EBV subtype 2 in 3/6 nasal T-cell lymphomas In the other T-cell lymphomas arising in nasopharyngeal region, EBV-positive cells were bystander cells
Katzenstein et al. [84]	29	Lymphomatoid granulomatosis	PCR	21 (72%)	
Herbst et al. [88]	47	ALCL (Including 26 T-ALCL)	PCR RNA ISH* Immunostaining†	15 (32%)	EBV detected in 5/18 (28%) T-ALCL by PCR LMP1 and EBNA2 were positive in 2/18 (11%) and in none of T-ALCL, respectively In most cases, EBV-positive cells were tumor cells
Su et al. [91]	50	Not specified for the entire cohort	SB DNA ISH	10 (20%)	EBV clonotypically integrated into DNA from tumor tissue Positive cases included AILD-type: 4, pleomorphic type: 4, immunoblastic type: 1 and angiocentric lymphoma: 1
Hamilton-Dutoit et al. [82]	187	High-grade B-NHL: 105 PTCL: 82	Immunostaining† DNA ISH	B-Cell 4/105 (4%) PTCL 8/82 (10%)	EBV detected in 7/48 (15%) pleomorphic type PTCL (EBNA2 positive in two of them) and none of 19 T-ALCL
Korbjuhn et al. [92]	81	Pleomorphic type	PCR RNA ISH*	38 (47%)	EBV found in the tumor cells of 30/38 PCR-positive cases, while mainly found in the bystanders cells in the other cases LMP1 positive in 18/81 (22%)
DeBruin et al. [93]	40	Pleomorphic type: 25 T-ALCL:15 (All extranodal)	PCR RNA ISH*	17/34 (50%) by PCR 7/40 (18%) by ISH	By ISH, EBV was detected in the tumor cells of nasal T-cell lymphomas (5/5) and lung lymphomas (2/6) only, but not in GI tract (n=12) and cutaneous (n=17) lymphomas
Weiss et al. [90]	23	AILD: 6 AILD-type: 17	PCR RNA ISH*	22/23 (96%)	When RNA ISH was coupled with immunostaining, most EBV-positive cells were CD20+ B-cells (3/3)

SB, Southern blot; ISH, *in situ* hybridization; PCR, polymerase chain reaction; EBNA2, Epstein–Barr virus nuclear antigen-2; LMP1, latent membrane protein-1; ALCL, anaplastic large-cell lymphoma; AILD, angioimmunoblastic lymphadenopathy with dysproteinemia; B-NHL, B-cell non-Hodgkin's lymphoma; GI, gastrointestinal.

* With EBER (Epstein–Barr virus encoded RNAs) probes.
† For the study of LMP1 and EBNA2 expression.

cells [83,88,92], although bystander reactive B-cells might also be positive in some cases [92]. Conversely, in a study referring to 23 cases of AILD-like PTCLs, most of the EBV-positive cells have been shown to express the B-lineage antigen CD20, whereas a minority of them were stained for the T-lineage-associated antigen CD43 [90]. In a study of extranodal T-cell lymphomas with similar morphology but originating from a variety of sites, the detection of EBV appeared to be site restricted, i.e., tumors arising in nasal cavities and the lung were normally positive, while cutaneous and gastrointestinal tract lymphomas were usually negative [93]. Moreover, EBV detection was not associated with angiocentricity in these cases. Although EBV-associated PTCL has been reported occasionally in immunocompromised patients [26,30], patients whose tumor samples showed latent EBV infection, did not have overt immune deficiency.

The latent membrane protein 1 (LMP-1) of known ability to transform cells *in vitro* [80], and EBNA-2 have been detected by immunostaining in a low percentage of PTCL cases, with the exception of nasal T-cell lymphomas, where they are consistently expressed [82,83,86,87,92]. The ZEBRA protein that triggers viral replication is nearly always undetectable [88]. How and when EBV infects the tumor T-cells that do not express the recognized EBV receptor CD21, and to what extent EBV contributes to the pathogenesis of PTCLs are still unsolved issues. One possibility is that EBV infects immature normal cells and tumors arise in their progeny cells [80].

Whatever the site from which the lymphoma arises, EBV-associated PTCLs may present special clinical features, such as the development of a hemophagocytic syndrome [94].

CYTOKINES EXPRESSION IN PTCLS

The histomorphological diversity of PTCLs, in which there is frequent admixture of nonneoplastic B- and T-cells and neoplastic T-cells, hyperplasia of venules in AILD-type lymphoma, variable content of epithelioid cells in Lennert's lymphoma or of macrophages, with or without erythrophagocytosis, in ALCL, is probably due to the release of various cytokines by the tumor cells. Some clinical or laboratory features may also be explained in this way. The putative role of cytokines, or at least their production by tumor cells, may be investigated in a number of ways including tumor cell culture and characterization of the biological activities of supernatants, mRNA analysis by Northern blot and *in situ* hybridization, immunostaining with antibodies directed to cytokines, and use of the PCR. The results of

such studies must be interpreted cautiously, since *in vitro* culture may not reflect *in vivo* conditions, while overexpression of a given cytokine at the mRNA level does not mean necessarily that the protein is overexpressed, since regulation may be posttranslational [95].

Omishi et al. [96] have studied 18 PTCL cases by Northern blot analysis and immunochemistry with a panel of monoclonal antibodies directed against several cytokines. They found overexpression of interleukin-4 (IL-4) in seven cases, all of which were associated with serum hyperglobulinemia, and overexpression of interferon-γ (IFNγ) in seven cases characterized by a high content of epithelioid cells on tissue sections (Table 44.6). High expression of interleukin-6 (IL-6) mRNA has been detected in the tumor tissue from some patients with ALCL [97], including one who presented with extensive bone destruction [98]. Other cytokines have also been implicated in the pathogenesis of ALCL and the finding of interleukin-9 (IL9) expression in ALCL (2/6) and also in Hodgkin's disease (6/13) has suggested that IL-9 may play a role in the pathogenesis of both these disorders, probably acting as an autocrine growth factor [99]. This finding also raises a question about the relationship between these two diseases. The role of interleukins in causing hypereosinophilia and/or high eosinophil content of tissue sections often observed in PTCLs has been supported by demonstration of IL-5 in supernatants from tumor cells cultured *in vitro*, and by the overexpression of IL-5 mRNA [100,101]. However, owing to the complexity of the cytokine network, histological features of this kind may not be the result of the expression of only one cytokine, as illustrated in two cases of PTCL where hypereosinophilia was probably related to the combined secretion of IL-5, IL-3 and granulocyte–macrophage colony-stimulating factor (GM-CSF) [102]. Moreover, in AILD-type PTCL, hypergammaglobulinemia has been associated not only with IL-4 but also IL-6 overexpression [103]. It is noteworthy that there is a strong heterogeneity in cytokine expression even among lymphoma types that are morphologically homogeneous [96,97,103]. This topic is dealt with further in Chapter 9.

Clinical characteristics

PTCLs usually express even more clinical diversity than B-cell NHLs and there is a close, but not absolute, relationship between some unusual clinical features and certain histological features, genotype, phenotype and the presence of HTLV-1 infection. A

Table 44.6 Expression of cytokines in PTCLs

Reference	No. of patients	Histologic subtype	Investigated cytokine(s)	Methods	Results and correlations with pathological or clinical features
Ohnishi et al. [96]	18	AILD-type: 3 TZL: 3, LeL: 1 Pleomorphic type: 9 Other: 2	IL-1, IL-2, IL-3, IL-4, IL-6, IFNγ, TNFα, G-CSF, GM-CSF	Immuno-chemistry	IL-4 expressed in 7/18 cases, all of them associated with hypergammaglobulinemia IFNγ expressed in 7/18 cases characterized by a marked content of histiocytes or epitheliod cells IL-1, IL-2, IL-6 and G-CSF never detected IL-3 detected in 1/15 cases, TNFα in 1/16 and GM-CSF in 2/17
Merz et al. [97]	14	AILD-type: 4 LeL: 1 Pleomorphic type: 6 T-ALCL: 3	IL-2, IL-3, IL-4 IL-5, IL-6 IFNγ, GM-CSF	Northern blot RNA ISH	IFNγ expressed in 7/12 cases IL-6 expressed in 4/13 cases (T-ALCL in three cases) GM-CSF detected in 1/13 cases, IL-3 in 1/8 and IL-4 in 1/14 No established correlation with pathological or clinical features
Merz et al. [99]	14	AILD-type: 4 LeL: 1 Pleomorphic type: 6 T-ALCL: 3	IL-9	Northern blot RNA ISH	IL-9 expressed in two cases, both of ALCL subtype (in the same study, IL-9 message was detected in 6/13 cases of Hodgkin's disease)
Agematsu et al. [98]	1	T-ALCL	IL-6	Northern blot cell culture	Detection of a large amount of IL-6 in culture supernatant Extensive osteolytic bone lesions at presentation
Samoszuk et al. [101]	3	Large-cell immunoblastic	IL-5	RT-PCR	Detection of IL-5 transcripts in the three cases, all characterized by a significant infiltration of tissues by eosinophils and eosinophilia
Fermand et al. [102]	2	Pleomorphic: 1 Unclassified cutaneous nonepidermotropic: 1	IL-5, IL-3 GM-CSF	Cell culture RT-PCR	Both patients with leukemic manifestations and hypereosinophilia Culture supernatants stimulated the growth of eosinophil colonies GM-CSF, IL-3 and IL-5 transcripts detected in one case, GM-CSF transcripts only in the other case
Hsu et al. [103]	4	AILD-type	IL-1β, TNFα IL-4, IL-6	Immuno-chemistry	IL-6 strongly expressed in 1/4 cases with a significant plasma cell tissue infiltration and serum hypergammaglobulinemia IL-4 weakly positive in a minority of cells from the same case TNFα and IL-1β not detected in any cases

ISH, *In situ* hybridization; RT-PCR, reverse transcriptase–polymerase chain reaction; IL, interleukin; IFNγ, interferon-γ; TNFα, tumor necrosis factor-α; G-CSF, granulocyte colony-stimulating factor; GM-CSF, granulocyte–macrophage colony-stimulating factor; AILD, angioimmunoblastic lymphadenopathy with dysproteinemia; TZL, T-zone lymphoma; LeL, lymphoepithelioid lymphoma; ALCL, anaplastic large-cell lymphoma.

combination of these characteristics has permitted the definition of several clinicopathological entities.

HTLV-1-RELATED ADULT T-CELL LYMPHOMA–LEUKEMIA

Following the first description of ATLL in Japan as a unique entity with a fulminant course [104], and the subsequent reports of identical cases in the Caribbean and the USA [105–108] coupled to the recognition of HTLV-1 as an etiological factor of the disease [13], the Japanese Lymphoma Study Group has conducted several nationwide surveys of the epidemiologic and clinical aspects of ATLL, and has identified less aggressive forms of ATLL, referred to as chronic and smoldering ATLL. Although the distinction between these different ATLL subtypes remains difficult in many instances, criteria that would help the early identification of each of them have recently been proposed [109].

Acute ATLL

The clinical presentation of acute ATLL is quite similar regardless of whether it occurs in an HTLV-1 endemic or nonendemic region. Patients are usually critically ill with poor performance status, severe systemic symptoms and disseminated disease. However, because of the immune deficiency associated with ATLL, fever may be also related to infection. Infectious complications have been detected at diagnosis in up to 27% of patients in the Japanese experience. These were either bacterial (frequently pneumonia), fungal or viral, or even due to *Strongyloides stercoralis* infestation [109]. Superficial lymphadenopathy is present in most cases, and hepatomegaly and/or splenomegaly in 30–50% of cases. Mediastinal involvement is infrequent. Skin and lung lesions are observed in 40% and 20% of patients, respectively. Skin lesions are variable, including small papules, plaques, tumors or erythroderma, with epidermotropism. Pautrier's microabscesses as found in cutaneous T-cell lymphoma mycosis fungoides/Sézary syndrome are observed in two-thirds of cases in histologic sections [110]. Central nervous system (CNS) disorders are present in many patients and may be related to either lymphomatous leptomeningitis or metabolic disturbances, such as hypercalcemia.

Leukemic manifestations are unique to acute ATLL, unlike the lymphoma type, which is defined by the lack of leukemic manifestation, i.e., no lymphocytosis (lymphocyte count $< 4 \times 10^9/l$) and 1% or less abnormal circulating T-lymphocytes [109]. Although patients with the lymphoma type usually display a better general condition and less extranodal disease at diagnosis, their overall survival rate does not differ significantly from that of patients with the acute type [111]. In acute type ATLL, leukocytosis is in excess of $30 \times 10^9/l$ in 35% of cases, with polynucleosis and lymphocytosis composed of atypical lymphoid cells and ATLL cells. Marked anemia (hemoglobin level < 10 g/dl) and thrombocytopenia (platelet count $< 100 \times 10^9/l$) are observed in 10 and 20% of patients, respectively. ATLL cells, which have been designed 'flower cells' in the Japanese literature, are very distinctive (Figure 44.1). They are pleomorphic, small to large in size with a high nucleus/cytoplasm ratio, deeply indented irregular nuclei and basophilic cytoplasm without granules. They consistently express a helper/inducer CD4+ phenotype, along with activation markers CD25 and HLA-DR, but do not express the CD7 antigen. However, despite their helper/inducer phenotype, ATLL cells have been shown to have no enhancing effect or even a suppressive effect on pokeweed mitogen (PWM)-driven immunoglobulin (Ig) synthesis in B-lymphocytes, probably by activating normal CD8+ suppressor cells rather than acting themselves as suppressor cells [112]. A suppressor/cytotoxic CD8+ phenotype has been occasionally reported in ATLL, but these cases did not differ from CD4+ ATLL with regard to clinical presentation and outcome. Bone marrow is frequently involved but, as previously noticed in Sézary syndrome, there is no absolute correlation between the presence of leukemic manifestations and bone marrow infiltration.

Hypercalcemia is a very common feature of ATLL, occurring in approximately 50% of cases at presentation, although it has been initially reported at an even higher frequency in cases originating from the USA [105]. It has been related to increased osteoclastic bone resorption, but the mechanisms

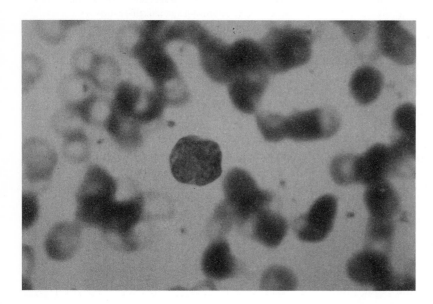

Figure 44.1 A 'flower' cell of ATLL.

that lead to hypercalcemia appear complex, implicating the production of either parathyroid hormone-related protein (PTHrP) or calcitriol (1,25-dihydroxy-vitamin D_3), or the local release of OAF (osteoclast-activating factor)-like substance [113]. Extensive lytic bone lesions with pathological fractures resembling those observed in myeloma or metastatic solid tumors have not been reported.

Other relevant laboratory features, observed in 30% of patients or more, include a highly elevated LDH level (≥ 3 N), increased uric acid, hyperbilirubinemia and hypoalbuminemia.

Histopathological examination of lymph nodes, if done, most often reveals pleomorphic, medium-sized lymphoma cells, although pleomorphic small-cell type, pleomorphic predominantly large-cell type or even immunoblastic type may also be observed.

The outcome of treatment is usually very poor, with low response rates to chemotherapy, rapid relapse in the few responders whatever the chemotherapy regimen used and short median survival. Patients mostly die from hypercalcemia or opportunistic infections.

Chronic and smoldering ATLL

Smoldering and chronic types of ATLL have a smaller tumor mass, a less aggressive course and a longer survival than acute ATLL. Median age at diagnosis is in the same range as acute ATLL.

The chronic type is also distinguished from the acute type by the absence of extranodal disease, other than skin or lung lesions, normal calcemia, and normal or moderately elevated LDH level (< 2 N). Lymphocytosis is present with a variable proportion of abnormal T-cells and a few ATLL flower cells may occasionally be observed.

The smoldering type is similar to the chronic type, but patients should have no organomegaly and a normal lymphocyte count ($< 4 \times 10^9$/l) with more than 5% abnormal T-cells in peripheral blood. Hypergammaglobulinemia is frequently observed.

A defect in cellular immunity results in a high frequency of opportunistic infectious episodes in these diseases. Both smoldering and chronic types can often progress to acute ATLL after a more or less prolonged course. The sudden flare-up of the disease with development of features characteristic of acute ATLL has been referred to as a 'crisis type' (compare blast crisis in chronic myeloid leukemia) [114]. Because chemotherapy is not curative, and may in fact worsen the immune defect, immediate therapy has not been recommended so far for either the chronic or smoldering forms of ATLL.

GENERAL CHARACTERISTICS OF PTCLs NOT RELATED TO HTLV-1

Descriptions of the clinical features of PTCLs must be interpreted cautiously. The first reports on PTCLs included small numbers of patients collected because of a particular clinical or laboratory feature, such as lung involvement [3] or hypergammaglobulinemia [5], and as such did not reflect the real frequency of these manifestations in PTCLs. In addition, numerous studies, especially those devoted to angiocentric lymphomas or AILD-type T-cell lymphoma, have focused on the histopathological, immunophenotypic and genotypic aspects that have allowed the insertion of these entities into the spectrum of PTCLs, but clinical characteristics have not been detailed. Finally, most studies have analyzed patient series that include the whole range of pathological subtypes such that the characterization of individual subtypes is difficult.

Clinical aspects

When compared to B-cell lymphomas, PTCLs usually present with more advanced disease, more extranodal disease, a higher frequency of systemic symptoms and spleen involvement, but a lower incidence of bulky disease and gastrointestinal (GI) tract involvement [23,44–47,115–120].

Lymphadenopathy is present in 80% of cases and is the most common presenting symptom. In some instances, lymphadenopathy – and also skin lesions – may wax and wane for several weeks or months before diagnosis, as classically described in B-cell low-grade NHLs. Mediastinal and abdominal lymphadenopathy are reported in 15–30% and 60% of cases, respectively, and bulky masses in excess of 10 cm in diameter are less frequent than in B-cell NHLs. However, mediastinal involvement may sometimes be as bulky and compressive of mediastinal structures as encountered in T-lymphoblastic lymphoma [45,46]. Splenic involvement is common and some PTCLs may present with predominant splenomegaly ('primary lymphoma of the spleen') [45,46,49,67]. Tonsil involvement has been reported more specifically in lymphoepithelioid lymphoma [36].

The main extranodal sites are liver, bone marrow, skin, lung and pleura, and the CNS, the incidence of each being variable in different series (Table 44.7). The occurrence of CNS involvement is rather low, both at presentation and during the course of the disease, suggesting that the mature T-cell malignancies exhibit less neurotropism than thymic or prethymic stage-derived neoplasms. The expression of CD56 on tumor cells, which has been shown to react with antibodies against neural cell adhesion molecule (NCAM), has been associated with

with the exception of one study [136]. In addition, there is usually a deficit of one or more pan-T-antigens, while double immunostaining has shown that most proliferating cells were either CD4+ or CD8+ [137].

Characteristic chromosomal changes include trisomies 3 or 5 and an additional X chromosome [71,73,74]. A clonal rearrangement of the TCR β-chain gene has been shown in most cases [11,36,59, 60,62,138,139], although in some instances TCRβ rearrangement has been associated with a clonal rearrangement of the Ig heavy chain gene (Table 44.8). Sometimes it has not been possible to demonstrate clonality. This has led Frizzera et al. [140] to define three levels or subtypes of AILD-type lymphoma: the reactive, benign or 'true' AILD with polyclonal proliferation, normal cytogenetics and a germline configuration of DNA (or, at least, no evidence, within the level of sensitivity of the tests employed, of monoclonal disease); malignant or

AILD-type T-cell lymphoma with a detectable clonal rearrangement of TCR genes and chromosomal abnormalities; and an intermediate state called AILD dysplasia. Similarly, Nakamura and Suchi [36] have distinguished three groups of AILD lymphomas according to the degree of nuclear atypia, the number of clear cells and the number of immunoblast-like cells present in the biopsy. This distinction, based on morphological criteria alone, has been supported by the observation that increasing rate of detectable TCR β-chain gene rearrangement is associated with increasing numbers of recognizable tumor cell features. Although Nakamura's study has shown a correlation, with borderline statistical significance, between the histologic appearance and survival, the clinical usefulness of such stratifications among patients with AILD/AILD-type lymphomas remains doubtful.

The presenting manifestations of well-characterized AILD-type lymphoma do not differ from

Table 44.9 Main clinical and laboratory characteristics at presentation and outcome of patients with AILD-type lymphoma

	Watanabe et al. [136]	Archimbaud et al. [141]	Tobinai et al. [139]	Nakamura et al. [36]	Siegert et al. [37]
No. of patients (M:F ratio)	21 (5.7:1)	30 (1:1)	36 (6.2:1)	56 (3.2:1)	39 (1.6:1)
Median age (years)(range)	$\simeq$ 60 (35–80)	58 (33–82)	58 (36–80)	59 (40–90)	59 (25–82)
Clinical features					
B symptoms	10 (48%)	13 (43%)	31 (86%)	—	29 (74%)
Drug allergy	—	6 (20%)	8 (22%)	—	—
Generalized adenopathy	21 (100%)	30 (100%)	34 (94%)	52 (93%)	—
Splenomegaly	7 (33%)	16 (53%)	25 (69%)	38 (68%)‡	—
Hepatomegaly	7 (33%)	13 (43%)	26 (72%)	—	—
Skin rash	10 (48%)	10 (33%)	21 (58%)	25 (44%)	—
Bone marrow involved	—	11/20 (55%)	—	7 (35%)	—
Ann Arbor stage					
I	—		—	1 (2%)	1 (2%)
II	—	5 (17%)*	—	3 (5%)	3 (8%)
III	—		—	29 (52%)	18 (46%)
IV	—	25 (83%)†	—	23 (41%)	17 (44%)
Laboratory features					
Eosinophilia	9 (43%)	11 (37%)	—	—	—
Elevated LDH level	12 (57%)	6/12 (50%)	—	—	—
Hypergammaglobulinemia	16 (76%)	18 (60%)	30 (83%)	—	—
Positive antiglobulin test	3/17 (18%)	12/27 (44%)	14 (45%)	—	—
Median overall survival (months)	14	24	18	11–14	15

* Stages I and II combined.
† Stages III and IV combined.
‡ Including spleen and liver enlargement.
AILD, Angioimmunoblastic lymphadenopathy with dysproteinemia; LDH, lactate dehydrogenase.

those described in the first reports on AILD [36,37, 136,139,141] (Table 44.9). The median age of patients at the time of presentation is about 60 years with a male to female ratio of 3 to 6:1. Advanced disease (stages III and IV), generalized lymph node swelling and hypergammaglobulinemia are almost constant features, while hepatosplenomegaly and skin rash are observed in half the patients. However, the frequency of autoimmune phenomena is not provided in the most recent studies, which have focused on diagnostic criteria and outcome. The median overall survival time is short, ranking from 14 to 30 months [36,37,139,140]. Infection is the direct cause of death in the majority of cases, supervening mainly in patients who have achieved only partial remission or whose disease is progressing [37]. Most of the lymphomas that have been previously reported to complicate the evolution of AILD must now be viewed, in light of the current understanding of AILD, as the result of histologic progression from a low-grade AILD-type T-cell lymphoma towards a large T-cell lymphoma [36]. Nevertheless, the occurrence of high-grade B-cell lymphoma has also been reported in rare patients with AILD-type PTCL. Since the malignant T-cells of AILD-type lymphoma are believed to release cytokines, yet to be identified, which are responsible for the polyclonal B-cell hyperplasia consistently observed on lymph node sections, it is likely that the onset of B-cell lymphoma results from genetic changes occurring in the hyperplastic B-cell population.

Angiocentric lymphomas

The unifying term of angiocentric immunoproliferative lesions (AIL) was first proposed by Jaffe [142] to include lymphomatoid granulomatosis and lethal midline granuloma (also referred to as polymorphic reticulosis, midline malignant reticulosis or malignant centrofacial granuloma), diseases that were initially reported as separate entities based on their predominant sites of involvement.

Lymphomatoid granulomatosis

Lymphomatoid granulomatosis (LG) has been described as a systemic disease predominantly involving the lungs, but also numerous extranodal sites such as skin, CNS, kidneys, nasopharynx, skeletal muscles or peripheral nerves [143]. LG predominantly affects males with a male to female ratio of approximately 3:1. Initial pulmonary symptoms are cough, dyspnea or chest pain, often present for weeks or months prior to diagnosis. Hemoptysis is uncommon. Occasionally, the disease is discovered on routine chest X-ray in asymptomatic patients [144]. The most frequent extrapulmonary manifestations at presentation (observed in 20–50% of cases) are B symptoms, skin lesions, cranial or peripheral nerve motor involvement leading to weakness or sensory deficits [144,145]. Superficial lymphadenopathy is observed in less than 10% of patients. The most common chest radiographic finding is that of multiple bilateral nodules from 1 to 5 cm in diameter, but pulmonary consolidation or diffuse bilateral reticulonodular infiltrates can be seen [144] (Figure 44.2). The frequency of hilar or mediastinal adenopathy and pleural effusion have been variously reported from 0% to 30% of cases [144,146]. The skin lesions usually consist of purplish nodules involving the trunk, upper or lower limbs and/or the face, which spontaneously undergo central necrosis and sometimes ulceration. Skin lesions may be the primary manifestation (the so-called angiocentric T-cell lymphoma of skin [147]). When the disease presents as isolated pulmonary lesions without extrapulmonary organ involvement, the diagnosis must usually be established from material obtained by open lung biopsy.

Although variable and apparently unpredictable from the presenting symptoms [144], the prognosis of LG is usually poor, reported mortality rates ranging from 50% to 85%. The median overall survival is short – 14 months in the largest series in the literature [145]. However, some patients may experience a protracted clinical course despite multiple recurrences after treatment or, occasionally, even in the absence of treatment [144]. The evolution towards overt malignant lymphoma has been reported to occur in 12% to 47% of cases [145,146].

Midline lethal granuloma

Midline lethal granuloma (MLG) encompasses an uncommon group of disorders characterized by a progressive necrotizing and destructive process, with or without a gross tumor mass, and involving the upper airways. The most common sites of disease are the nasal fossae, nasal septum, nasopharynx, palate, and adjacent soft tissue or bone structures. The median age is about 50 years with a strong male predominance, and most of the reported cases originate from Asia. The patients often present with a history of long-standing sinusitis with purulent and foul-smelling nasal discharge. Other complaints related to the anatomical extension of the disease include nasal obstruction, sore throat, cheek and orbital swelling or dysphagia. The outcome is usually very poor with, if not already present at diagnosis, rapid dissemination to cervical lymph nodes, liver, spleen, lungs, skin and bone marrow [83,148,149].

LG and MLG display similar histopathological features, consisting of granulomatous lesions with a

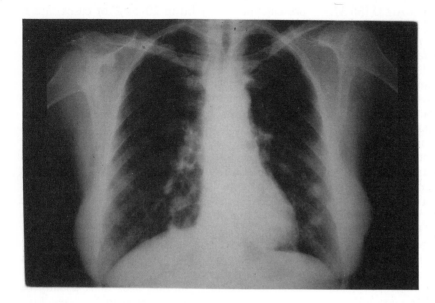

Figure 44.2 Chest X-ray showing multiple pulmonary nodules in a patient with lymphomatoid granulomatosis.

characteristic angiocentric and angioinvasive pattern with infiltration of vessel walls, extensive necrosis and a polymorphous cell infiltrate. Phenotypic analysis has shown that atypical cells express T- but not B-cell-associated markers, and often fail to express pan-T-differentiation antigens as do most mature T-cell neoplasms [86,87,149]. Nasal T-cell lymphomas, particularly, may express only CD2, or CD2 and CD7 lacking other pan-T-lineage markers [86]. Studies of TCR gene rearrangements are scarce and have yielded contradictory results. Although a TCR β-chain gene rearrangement has been observed in a few cases [63,64], most studies have not demonstrated TCR β-, γ- or δ-chain gene rearrangements [86,150]. In addition, in nasal T-cell lymphomas, tumor cells consistently express the natural killer (NK)-related CD56 antigen, but usually not other NK markers, such as CD16 and CD57 [86]. This is consistent with the finding that CD56 expression in T-cell lymphomas is associated with a particular pattern of extranodal involvement [57,58].

Lipford et al. [151] have proposed dividing AILs (as has been done for AILD lymphomas) into three histological categories (from grade I lesions, with a benign appearance to grade III lesions, or overt angiocentric lymphoma). These grades appeared to correlate with clinical aggressiveness and outcome. However, the clinical usefulness of such a distinction is unclear, and it remains uncertain whether all AILs are neoplastic or whether the natural history is one of progression from a preneoplastic to an overt neoplastic process. Such a distinction may be semantic rather than biologically meaningful – presumably there must be a preneoplastic phase at some point, even though evolution to a true neoplastic process may not be definable by morphology.

Additional evidence that AILs are clonal processes, as well as progress in the understanding of the pathogenesis of AILs, have been provided by the demonstration that in most cases clonally integrated EBV genomes can be demonstrated in tumor cells [83–86]. Moreover, the higher than expected frequency of EBV subtype 2 detection in AILs has raised the hypothesis that patients may have occult immune deficiency [87]. AIL has also been described occasionally in patients with either acquired immune deficiency syndrome [29] or HTLV-1 infection [152].

Although AILs/angiocentric lymphomas have a striking propensity for involving the upper respiratory tract, it must be remembered that they account for a minor proportion only of lymphomas arising in the nose or nasopharynx, at least in Western countries [153].

Lymphomatoid papulosis

Lymphomatoid papulosis (LP) is a clinically benign cutaneous disorder characterized by a chronic course in which there is repeated occurrence of self-healing papulonodular lesions, mostly on the forearms, that resolve spontaneously with scarring [154] (Figure 44.3). However, in contrast to the benign clinical course of LP, its histology, consisting of large, atypical clear cells resembling Reed–Sternberg cells or the cells of anaplastic large-cell lymphoma, is suggestive of a malignancy. These large cells usually express the phenotypic profile of activated helper CD4+ T-cells with loss of one or more pan-T-markers, and expression of CD30 and CD15. A clonal rearrangement of the TCR β- and/or γ-chain genes has been found in most studied cases [64,65]. Interestingly, at least two different T-cell clones were

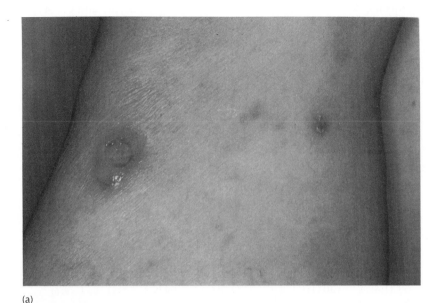

(a)

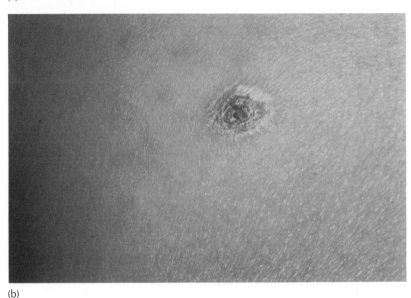

(b)

Figure 44.3 Lymphomatoid papulosis: (a) hemorrhagic and ulcerated skin lesion; (b) the same lesion after healing.

identified in one patient with multiple concomitant lesions [64], while in another patient the same TCR β-chain gene rearrangement pattern was observed in two separate lesions taken 11 months apart [65].

These studies have provided evidence that LP represents a clonal T-cell proliferation and may explain why a significant proportion of patients (about 10–20%) eventually develop malignant lymphoma, most commonly mycosis fungoides but also large-cell type (frequently anaplastic). Case-control epidemiologic studies have shown that patients with LP have a significantly increased frequency of prior or coexisting lymphoproliferative disorders such as Hodgkin's disease, lymphoma of the skin or mycosis fungoides [155]. This pathological association is unlikely to be fortuitous, especially since the same clonal TCR gene rearrangement has been found in samples obtained from each disease phase in a patient who successively developed Hodgkin's disease, LP and mycosis fungoides [156].

Anaplastic large-cell lymphoma

ALCL is now widely (but not universally) accepted as a subgroup of NHL. Its morphological features, which include partial lymph node infiltration, a tendency of the large neoplastic cells to form cohesive sheets and involvement of lymph node sinuses, have led in the past to it being misdiagnosed as malignant histiocytosis, metastatic anaplastic carcinoma, or in some cases Hodgkin's disease. ALCL cells characteristically express the CD30 antigen (recognized by the Ki-1 and BerH2 monoclonal antibodies on frozen and paraffin-embedded sections, respectively) [157], which has been shown to belong to the nerve growth factor (NGF)/tumor necrosis factor (TNF) receptor superfamily [56]. The typical phenotype of tumor cells is CD30+, CD45+, CD15–, EMA+, keratin– and lysozyme– with frequent expression of the activation markers CD25

and CD71 [158]. Immunophenotypic and genotypic studies have shown that most ALCLs (50–70%) are of T-cell origin, whereas a B-cell phenotype is observed in 15–30% of cases, and in 10–20% of cases the cell lineage could not be determined ('null' phenotype) [159–166] (Table 44.10). In some instances, T-cell low-grade malignancies such as mycosis fungoides, lymphomatoid papulosis or AILD-type lymphoma (and also low-grade B-cell lymphomas) may evolve into ALCL (secondary ALCL).

Primary ALCL more commonly occurs in children and young adults. Peripheral lymphadenopathy

Table 44.10 Main clinical characteristics, phenotype and outcome in patients with anaplastic large-cell lymphoma (ALCL)

	Chott et al. [159]	Greer et al. [160]	Nakamura et al. [162]	Shulman et al. [163]	Pileri et al.¶ [166]	Reiter et al. [165]
No. of patients (M:F ratio)	41 (1.3:1)	31 (1.4:1)	30 (1:1.3)	31 (1.4:1)	69 (2.1–1.5:1)	62 (1.9:1)
Median age (years)(range)	50 (5–91)	35 (4mo-78)	28‡ (2–80)	44 (16–86)	27–34 (15–59)	9.7 (0.8–17.6)
Phenotype						
T	28 (68%)	24 (77%)	24 (80%)	13/27 (48%)	40 (58%)	32/52 (62%)
B	4 (10%)	4 (13%)	0	8/27 (30%)	19 (27%)	3/52 (6%)
Null	9 (22%)	3 (10%)	6 (20%)	6/27 (22%)	9 (13%)ll	15/52 (29%)b
B symptoms	24 (59%)	13 (42%)	7 (23%)	6 (19%)	36 (52%)	26 (42%)
Peripheral lymphadenopathy	23 (56%)	26 (84%)	22 (73%)	—	—	46 (74%)
Mediastinal mass	2 (5%)	5 (16%)	2 (7%)	—	52 (75%)a	18 (29%)
Extranodal disease, any	10 (24%)	13 (42%)	—	20 (65%)	—	37 (60%)d
Skin	4 (10%)	7 (23%)	9 (30%)§	10 (32%)	—	9 (14%)
Bone	3 (7%)	2 (6%)	0	—	—	13 (21%)
Bone marrow	7/23 (30%)	1/30 (3%)	4 (13%)	2/26 (8%)	4 (6%)	0
Lung	2 (5%)	2 (6%)	0	—	5/28 (18%)c	4 (6%)
Soft tissue	2 (5%)	—	—	—	—	13 (21%)
Ann Arbor Stage						
I	14 (37%)	6 (19%)	—	5 (16%)	0	8 (13%)
II	7 (18%)	8 (26%)	—	4 (13%)	38 (55%)	18 (29%)
III	6 (16%)	8 (26%)	—	6 (19%)	17 (25%)	13 (21%)
IV	11 (29%)	9 (29%)	—	15 (52%)	14 (20%)	23 (37%)
CR rate	6/25 (24%)	21/23 (91%)	—	25/31 (85%)	38/69 (55%)	58/62 (93%)
Median OS (months)	13	Not reached	Not reached	Not reached	Not reached	Not reached
Survival % (years)	—	73% (2)*	52% (5)	≃ 70% (4)	66–68% (4)	83% (9)
DFS.FFP % (years)	—	39% (2)†	—	—	68–79% (4)	81% (9)

* Stages I–II: 75%; stages III–IV: 48%.
† Stages I–II: 62%; stages III–IV: 20%.
‡ Mean.
§ Primary cutaneous lymphoma in five cases.
¶ Series divided into two groups: ALCL, common-type (CT)(n=41, left number when applicable) and ALCL, Hodgkin-related (HR)(n=28, right number when applicable).
ll One patient with hybrid phenotype.
a 24/41 (58%) in ALCL-CT and 28/28 (100%) in ALCL-HR.
b Two patients with 'histiocytic' phenotype.
c Contiguous lung involvement in patients with ALCL-HR.
d Only extranodal disease in six cases (10%).
OS, Overall survival; DFS, disease-free survival; FFP, freedom from progression; CTR, complete remission; ≃, approximately (deduced from figures).

is the most common presenting site, occurring in 80% of cases (Table 44.10). A mediastinal mass is rather infrequent. Extranodal disease is very common, ranging in published series from 25% to 65% of cases [159–163]. Skin is the most frequent site of extranodal involvement and sometimes, particularly in children, the only site of disease [167,168]. Bone marrow involvement is rarely found.

The t(2;5)(p23;q35) translocation has been found in up to 70% of cases of T-type ALCL and therefore represents the cytogenetic abnormality, which is the most consistently associated with a specific subtype of T-cell lymphoma [78].

Although the first reports described an overall poor prognosis of patients with ALCL, more recent studies have reported a good response to chemotherapy and prolonged survival, even after relapse [163–166] (Table 44.10).

Small intestine PTCLs

Compared to B-cell NHLs, primary or secondary gastrointestinal (GI) tract involvement is rare in T-cell lymphomas. However, PTCLs may arise primarily in the small intestine, either as a complication of a documented enteropathy, such as celiac disease or a more or less well-defined small bowel inflammatory disease (dermatitis herpetiformis, Crohn's disease, nonspecific jejunoileitis), or it may arise as *de novo* GI tract disease. In the former group designated as enteropathy-associated T-cell lymphoma (EATCL), tumor cells apparently derive from gut mucosa intraepithelial T-lymphocytes and express the MLA antigen (recognized by diverse monoclonal antibodies such as HML-1) [169]. EATCLs are mainly defined by the presence of villous atrophy adjacent to and distant from the lymphoma site, and a high density of intraepithelial lymphocytes. They may also occur in patients without a previous history of malabsorption [170]. Presenting symptoms are not specific and include weight loss, abdominal pain, and acute abdomen as a result of perforation and/or obstruction. In most cases, the disease is confined to the abdomen, with preferential involvement of the jejunum, either with or without involvement of mesenteric lymph nodes. Histologically, the appearance is usually that of high-grade PTCL, either pleomorphic medium and large-cell type, or immunoblastic type. Pleomorphic small-cell or anaplastic large-cell types may also be encountered. Besides the histopathologic features and presence of malabsorption, EATCL differs from non-EATCL by the multifocal pattern of small intestine involvement, the high frequency of local relapses and the overall poorer prognosis.

Interestingly, Wright et al. have reported a patient with malabsorption, jejunitis and intense intraepithel-ial lymphocytosis in whom the immunophenotypic, genotypic (rearrangement of TCR β- and γ-chain genes) and cytogenetic abnormalities (deletion of chromosomes Y and 9) of lymphoid cells led to the hypothesis that adult-onset celiac disease might be a form of low-grade lymphoma [76].

$T\gamma/\delta$ PTCL

Phenotypic and genotypic studies in PTCLs have allowed the definition of distinct patterns of TCR expression [66]. The uncommon $T\gamma/\delta$ phenotype (CD3+, CD2+, other pan-T-antigens–, TCR$\alpha\beta$–, TCR$\gamma\delta$+, CD56+) has been associated with peculiar clinical and pathological features [67,171]. Patients present with predominant hepatomegaly and/or splenomegaly but usually have no lymphadenopathy. Tumor cells are monomorphic and medium sized with a sinusal/sinusoidal pattern of infiltration in the spleen, the liver and bone marrow. Although the number of reported cases is few, this PTCL subtype appears to be an aggressive one, eventually progressing to a blast-like terminal phase [172]. The $T\gamma/\delta$ phenotype is not restricted to hepatosplenic presentation, however, and has also been reported in nasal T-cell lymphoma [66,86].

Cutaneous large-cell T-lymphomas

The skin is frequently involved in patients with PTCLs and primary skin involvement in subtypes other than mycosis fungoides (MF) or lymphomatoid papulosis has been described [173,174]. Such lymphomas are usually high grade, according to the current histopathological classifications, and of either large-cell, pleomorphic, immunoblastic or anaplastic large-cell type. Some are unclassifiable. They accounted for 27% of cases in an unselected, retrospective study of 52 patients with non-MF cutaneous lymphoma [174] and in this series usually presented as a single, red to violaceous nodule or tumor, or alternatively as multiple lesions confined to a circumscribed area of skin. Although these lymphomas were designated primary cutaneous lymphoma because skin involvement was the presenting manifestation, many patients were shown to have disseminated disease after a staging work-up. The diagnosis of T-cell lineage was based on the usual immunopathological criteria, and the expected loss of one or more pan-T-antigens was observed in most cases. This phenotypic anomaly has also been observed in cutaneous pseudo T-cell lymphomas, which must therefore be differentiated from genuine T-cell lymphomas on the basis of clinical and morphological characteristics [175]. Interestingly, whatever the pathologic subtype, the expression of CD30 antigen on tumor cells has been associated with localized disease and a significantly better outcome [168,173].

Hemophagocytic syndrome and PTCL

Hemophagocytic syndrome (HS) has been recently observed to be an associated feature of some PTCLs, mainly in oriental populations. The main clinical and biological manifestations of HS include pronounced systemic manifestations, high fever, jaundice, marked hepatosplenomegaly, profound pancytopenia, abnormal liver function tests, blood coagulation disorders with prolonged prothrombin and partial activated thromboplastin times, hypofibrinogenemia and hypertriglyceridemia [94,176]. The diagnosis of HS is based on the finding of benign-looking hemophagocytizing histiocytes in bone marrow. The proliferation of phagocytizing histiocytes is also observed on tissue sections from the spleen or lymph nodes, and may overwhelm the lymphomatous component [176]. HS may occur at any time in the patient's clinical course, either at initial presentation, accompanying relapse or even during apparent complete remission [94]. In this circumstance, the prognosis is very poor with a median survival of less than 2 months from the onset of HS, despite treatment with high-dose steroids or chemotherapy [94]. The pathogenesis of HS remains poorly understood. Histiocyte activation is likely to result from the release by tumor T-cells of cytokines, such as IFNγ, tumor necrosis factor (TNF) or IL-1. The preferential, but not exclusive occurrence of HS in angiocentric lymphomas, which are frequently associated with EBV infection, along with the previous reports of EBV-related virus-associated hemophagocytic syndrome (VAHS) without obvious evidence of lymphoma, suggest a predominant role for EBV in the triggering of HS.

Other low-grade PTCLs

Among nodal low-grade PTCLs, lymphoepithelioid type (Lennert's lymphoma) has appeared to display some clinical features that differ from those of other PTCLs, outlined above. Lymphoepithelioid lymphoma (LeL) is characterized by its high content of epithelioid cells and an exclusive helper/inducer CD4+ phenotype [43]. Patients present predominantly with peripheral nodal disease, usually involving cervical areas. Thoracic or deep abdominal lymphadenopathy and hepatosplenomegaly are rather infrequent at initial presentation [36,177]. Nevertheless, some patients presenting with predominant splenomegaly have been reported [45]. Extranodal disease and bone marrow involvement are rare. Tonsil involvement has been reported in 8% [177] to 35% [36] of cases. Overall prognosis is rather poor, with a reported median survival ranging from 16 to 32 months [36,177].

T-zone lymphoma has appeared to take an intermediate position between AILD-type lymphoma and LeL with regard to the respective frequency of organ involvement at presentation [36]. Although the number of patients for whom survival data are available is low, T-zone lymphoma and LeL seem to have a similar outcome.

Prognostic factors

PROGNOSTIC FACTORS IN ATLL

The very poor prognosis of patients with HTLV-1-related ATL has been stressed since the first reports of the disease [104]. Indeed, the presence of serum anti-HTLV-1 antibodies is the most adverse prognostic parameter of T-cell lymphomas in Asia [178]. However, the presenting manifestations and outcome are variable among patients with ATLL and, although median survival in most series is less than a year, 'smoldering' and chronic types of the disease have been identified [109]. In one Japanese series of 854 patients, which included all subtypes of ATLL diagnosed between 1983 and 1987, the overall median survival was 10 months, and the projected 2- and 4-year survival rates were 28% and 12%, respectively [179]. In this series, five parameters were shown by multivariate analysis to be strongly correlated with a short survival. These were age over 40 years, a poor performance status, a high number of involved sites, a high serum lactate dehydrogenase (LDH) level and hypercalcemia. The presence of leukemic manifestations, previously reported as an unfavorable feature [178], was not correlated with survival in this study. Recently, based largely on these results, criteria for distinguishing ATLL subtypes at the onset of the disease, have been proposed. One important difference between patients who have a chronic course and those with an acute course is the percentage of Ki-67-positive circulating lymphoid cells, which is significantly lower in patients with chronic ATLL than in acute ATLL. This parameter appears to be a better correlate of the length of survival than even the serum LDH level [180].

PTCLs NOT RELATED TO HTLV-1

Early reports suggested that PTCLs were an unfavorable subset of NHLs in which both low response rates to chemotherapy and short survival could be expected [3,47,117]. However, subsequent studies aimed at comparing the outcome of T- and B-cell lymphomas have yielded contradictory results. A particularly controversial issue is whether or not the separation of PTCLs into low- and high-grade categories on the basis of morphological features has prognostic significance, and whether or not a T-cell phenotype *per se* is associated with a poorer outcome. The discrepancies among published series in this respect may be explained by the usually small number of PTCL patients included in each series, the frequent admixture of several morphological subtypes owing to the lack of a widely accepted subclassification system for T-cell lymphomas, and the heterogeneity of primary treatment within a given series.

The reported median overall survival in low-grade PTCLs is consistently less than 30 months in either AILD-type lymphoma [36,37,139,141] or lymphoepithelioid lymphoma [36,38,177]. This poor outcome is quite unexpected for so-called low-grade lymphoid malignancies, and compares unfavorably with that of B-cell low-grade lymphomas. Most of the patients reported in these series were treated with either prednisone, a single alkylating agent or CVP (cyclophosphamide, vincristine, prednisone), and it has been suggested that the use of a more aggressive, anthracycline-containing regimen, might lead to a better outcome [37,177]. In some studies survival difference between small-cell, diffuse small- and large-cell, and diffuse large-cell subtypes of T-cell lymphomas were not observed [23,44], although other reports have yielded the opposite results [36,45]. This suggests that morphology is not a good predictor of prognosis in the T-cell lymphomas.

The prognostic relevance of immunophenotype (T versus B) has been addressed in several studies, the main results of which are summarized in Table 44.11. Whereas several studies failed to show statistically significant differences among T-cell and B-cell lymphomas with respect to complete remission (CR) rates, relapse rates or overall survival [6,17,18,118,181], a T-cell phenotype was associated with a significantly shorter duration of freedom from relapse (FFR) in two studies [16,20]. The largest of them originated from a French group (GELA), and included more than 350 patients with intermediate- or high-grade NHL according to the Working Formulation, among which one-third were of T-cell origin [20]. All of these patients received the same intensive treatment. The CR rate (75%) was similar in both T- and B-cell groups, but the relapse rate was significantly higher in patients with T-cell lymphomas (43% for T-cell lymphomas versus 23% for B-cell lymphomas). However, this did not result in a significant difference in overall survival between the two groups, probably because patients with PTCL survived for longer periods of time after relapse than B-cell lymphoma patients. In this study, a multivariate analysis showed that the T-cell phenotype was the only prognostic variable that predicted FFR duration. Within the T-cell group itself, the well-identified adverse prognostic factors such as poor performance status, advanced stage, numerous extranodal sites, bulky disease and elevated LDH level, were significantly correlated with the likelihood of a shorter overall survival.

Although the expression of a helper/inducer CD4+ CD8− phenotype by the tumor cells has been associated with a better outcome in some studies [44], T-cell subset antigen expression has not been demonstrated to be a prognostic indicator in most reports. A low

Table 44.11 Prognostic significance of T-cell phenotype

	Lippman et al. [16]		Armitage et al. [17]		Cheng et al. [181]		Coiffier et al. [20]		Kwak et al. [18]	
Phenotype	T	B	T	B	T	B	T	B	T	B
No. of patients	20	83	19	91	34	36	108	253	21	77
CR rate (%)	50	62	53	74	62	67	72	71	95	84
Median OS (months)	18	35	—	—	≃ 15	≃ 15	42	50	—	—
Median FFP/DFS (months)	*10.8*	*42.7*	—	—	—	—	*34*	*not reached*	—	—
% Survival	—	NS —	41	50†	—	NS —	—	NS —	79	52§
% FFP	*0*	*55**	70	75†	—	NS —	≃ 45	≃ 75‡	54	38§

* At 2 years.
† At 3 years.
‡ At 4 years.
§ At 5 years.

OS, Overall survival; DFS, disease-free survival; CR, complete remission; FFP, freedom from progression; ≃, approximately (deduced from figures); NS, not significant.
Only the differences between values in italics are statistically significant.

proliferative activity, with less than 10% of cells being in the S+G$_2$M phases of the cell cycle, as assessed by flow cytometry, has been associated with a favorable prognosis [182].

Treatment

ATLL

In acute ATLL, conventional chemotherapy has resulted in very low CR rates, ranging from 20% with cyclophosphamide, doxorubicin, vincristine and prednisone (CHOP)-like regimen, vincristine, endoxan (cyclophosphamide), prednisone and Adriamycin (VEPA) or VEPA and methotrexate (VEPA-M), to 42% with more aggressive alternating regimens [111]. The reported CR rates in the lymphoma subtype were slightly higher, but patients still exhibited a poor outcome with a median survival time of 8 months and a projected 3-year survival rate of 15% [111]. This resistance to chemotherapy may be explained, in part, by the frequent expression of the multidrug resistance gene (mdr-1) product, P-glycoprotein, on the tumor cell surface, either at diagnosis or shortly after exposure to cytostatic agents [183]. In view of these poor results, several alternative treatment approaches have been explored. For example, several phase II trials of deoxycoformycin have been conducted in Japan. In the largest one, in which 31 patients were enrolled, the overall response rate was 32%, including two CRs [111]. In refractory or relapsed patients, treatment with IFNβ and IFNγ has led to transient responses [184]. Treatment with an anti-CD25 monoclonal antibody has been administered safely in 19 patients, among whom seven achieved remissions (including two CRs) that lasted from 9 weeks to more than 3 years [185]. The most impressive results have been achieved with a treatment combining the antiviral drug, zidovudine (1000 mg/day), and IFNα (6 x 10^6 IU/day) [186]. A major response, including five CRs, was observed in seven out of ten patients with either previously untreated ($n = 5$) or refractory ($n = 5$) ATLL. The longest follow-up in this series was 3 years. Although the number of patients was small and the results have not yet been confirmed, this approach is promising and might profitably be explored earlier in the course of the disease – perhaps initially in chronic or smoldering types.

PTCLs NOT ASSOCIATED WITH HTLV-1

Since the prognostic value of immunophenotype remains controversial, no specific recommendation for the treatment of T-cell lymphomas has been made. However, it does appear that patients with the so-called low-grade PTCLs might benefit from an anthracycline-based multidrug regimen rather than palliative treatment, when their general condition makes it feasible. This applies particularly to AILD-type lymphomas, where prednisone alone is unlikely to induce a durable CR, except in a minority of patients, and where secondary chemotherapy might be associated with increased toxicity in patients whose general condition and immune defects have worsened during steroid therapy [37]. Treatment with low-dose IFNα (3 × 10^6 IU/day) has been reported to induce CR or partial response in two-thirds of patients with AILD-type lymphoma who have either refractory disease or contraindications to chemotherapy [187]. Cyclosporin A has also been shown to be effective in such patients [188].

In the absence of data indicating that T- and B-cell lymphomas in intermediate- and high-grade categories of the Working Formulation require different therapy, most oncologists still use the same induction therapy for both groups. However, since the T-cell phenotype has been associated with a significantly shorter FFP duration, at least in some studies, some have added intensification or maintenance treatment. The preliminary results observed with maintenance therapy similar to that used in acute lymphocytic leukemia in patients who achieved CR with a lymphoma regimen, suggest that this approach is at least worthy of further study [119]. Another approach for which few data currently exist is high-dose therapy with hematopoietic stem cell support performed in first CR. While this has yet to be demonstrated as useful in patients with high-risk B-cell lymphoma, this does not exclude the possibility of a beneficial effect in patients with PTCL. However, the outcome of patients with recurrent NHL appears to be similar after high-dose therapy and autologous bone marrow transplantation, regardless of whether the lymphoma was of T- or B-cell origin [189].

INFα has well established activity in cutaneous T-cell lymphomas and may be of value in relapsing PTCL [190]. Recently, 13-*cis*-retinoic acid (RA) was shown to have activity in T-cell lymphomas, both *in vitro*, on T-lymphoma cell lines, and *in vivo* [191,192]. Administered at the dose of 1 mg/kg/day, 13-*cis*-RA induced CR or partial response in six out of 12 patients with PTCL, whereas none of the six patients with B-cell lymphoma responded [192]. If these results are confirmed, 13-*cis*-RA might offer a nontoxic alternative therapy for relapsing or elderly patients with PTCL.

References

1. Lennert K, Mohri N. Malignant lymphoma, lymphocytic, T-zone type (T-zone lymphoma). In Lennert K (ed.) *Malignant Lymphomas Other than Hodgkin's Disease.* Berlin: Springer Verlag, 1978, pp. 196–209.
2. Pinkus GS, Said JW, Hargreaves H. Malignant lymphoma, T-cell type: A distinct morphologic variant with large multilobated nuclei, with a report of four cases. *Am. J. Clin. Pathol.* 1979, **72**: 540–550.
3. Waldron JA, Leech JH, Glick AD, et al. Malignant lymphoma of peripheral T-lymphocyte origin. Immuno-ologic, pathologic, and clinical features in six patients. *Cancer* 1977, **40**: 1604–1617.
4. Palutke M, Tabaczka P, Weise RW, et al. T-Cell lymphomas of large cell type. A variety of malignant lymphomas: 'Histiocytic' and mixed lymphocytic-'histiocytic'. *Cancer* 1980, **46**: 87–101.
5. Watanabe S, Shimosato Y, Shimoyama M, et al. Adult T-cell lymphoma with hypergammaglobuline-mia. *Cancer* 1980, **46**: 2472–2483.
6. Levine AM, Taylor CR, Schneider DR, et al. Immunoblastic sarcoma of T-cell versus B-cell origin: I. clinical features. *Blood* 1981, **58**: 52–61.
7. Picker LJ, Weiss LM, Medeiros LJ, et al. Immunophenotypic criteria for the diagnosis of non-Hodgkin's lymphoma. *Am. J. Pathol.* 1987, **128**: 181–201.
8. Knowles DM. Immunophenotypic and antigen receptor gene rearrangement analysis in T-cell neoplasia. *Am. J. Pathol.* 1989, **134**: 761–785.
9. Knowles DM, Pelicci PG, Dalla-Favera R. T-Cell receptor beta chain gene rearrangements: Genetic markers of T-cell lineage and clonality. *Hum. Pathol.* 1986, **17**: 546–551.
10. Cossman J, Uppenkamp M, Sundeen J, et al. Molecular genetics and the diagnosis of lymphoma. *Arch. Pathol. Lab. Med.* 1988, **112**: 117–127.
11. Griesser H, Feller AC, Minden M, et al. Rearrangement of β-chain of the T-cell antigen receptor and immunoglobulin genes in lymphoproliferative disorders. J. Clin. Invest. 1986, **78**: 1179–1184.
12. Tajima K. Malignant lymphomas in Japan: Epidemiological analysis of adult T-cell leukemia/lymphoma (ATL). *Cancer Metastasis Rev.* 1988, **7**: 223–241.
13. Gallo RC, Kalyanaraman VS, Sarngadharan MG, et al. Association of the human type C retrovirus with a subset of adult T-cell cancers. *Cancer Res.* 1983, **43**: 3892–3899.
14. Mueller N. The epidemiology of HTLV-I infection. *Cancer Causes Control* 1991, **2**: 37–52.
15. Shimoyama M. Peripheral T-cell lymphoma in Japan: recent progress. *Ann. Oncol.* 1991, **2** (Suppl. 2): 157–162.
16. Lippman SM, Miller TP, Spier CM, et al. The prognostic significance of the immunophenotype in diffuse large-cell lymphoma: A comparative study of the T-cell and B-cell phenotype. *Blood* 1988, **72**: 436–441.
17. Armitage JO, Vose JM, Linder J, et al. Clinical significance of immunophenotype in diffuse aggressive non-Hodgkin's lymphoma. *J. Clin. Oncol.* 1989, **7**: 1783–1790.
18. Kwak LW, Wilson M, Weiss LM, et al. Similar outcome of treatment of B-cell and T-cell diffuse large-cell lymphomas: The Stanford experience. *J. Clin. Oncol.* 1991, **9**: 1426–1431.
19. Lennert K, Feller AC (eds). *Histopathology of Non-Hodgkin's Lymphomas (Based on the Updated Kiel Classification).* Berlin: Springer Verlag, 1992.
20. Coiffier B, Brousse N, Peuchmaur M, et al. Peripheral T-cell lymphomas have a worse prognosis than B-cell lymphomas: A prospective study of 361 immunophenotyped patients treated with the LNH 84 regimen. *Ann. Oncol.* 1990, **1**: 45–50.
21. Henni T, Divine M, Gaulard P, et al. Polymerase chain reaction (PCR) amplification demonstrates the absence of human T-cell lymphotropic virus (HTLV)-I specific pol sequences in peripheral T-cell lymphomas. *J. Clin. Immunol.* 1990, **10**: 282–286.
22. Kadin ME. Ki-1/CD30+ (anaplastic) large-cell lymphoma: Maturation of a clinicopathologic entity with prospects of effective therapy. *J. Clin. Oncol.* 1994, **12**: 884–887.
23. Armitage JO, Greer JP, Levine AM, et al. Peripheral T-cell lymphoma. *Cancer* 1989, **63**: 158–163.
24. Swinson CM, Slavin G, Coles EC, et al. Coeliac disease and malignancy. *Lancet* 1983, **i**: 111–115.
25. Garvin J, Self S, Sahovic EA, et al. The occurrence of a peripheral T-cell lymphoma in a chronically immunosuppressed renal transplant patient. *Am. J. Surg. Pathol.* 1988, **12**: 64–70.
26. Waller EK, Ziemianska M, Bangs CD, et al. Characterization of posttransplant lymphomas that express T-cell-associated markers: Immunophenotypes, molecular genetics, cytogenetics, and heterotransplantation in severe combined immunodeficient mice. *Blood* 1993, **82**: 247–261.
27. Nasr SA, Brynes RK, Garrison CP, et al. Peripheral T-cell lymphoma in a patient with acquired immune deficiency syndrome. *Cancer* 1988, **61**: 947–951.
28. Herndier BG, Shiramizu BT, Jewett NE, et al. Acquired immunodeficiency syndrome-associated T-cell lymphoma: Evidence for Human Immunodeficiency Virus type 1-associated T-cell transformation. *Blood* 1992, **79**: 1768–1774.
29. Gold JE, Ghali V, Gold S, et al. Angiocentric immunoproliferative lesion/T-cell non Hodgkin's lymphoma and the acquired immune deficiency syndrome: A case report and review of the literature. *Cancer* 1990, **66**: 2407–2413.
30. Thomas JA, Cotter F, Hanby AM, et al. Epstein–Barr virus-related oral T-cell lymphoma associated with human immunodeficiency immunosuppression. *Blood* 1993, **81**: 3350–3356.
31. Winberg CD. Peripheral T-cell lymphoma: Morphologic and immunologic observations. *Am. J. Clin. Pathol.* 1993, **99**: 426–435.
32. Suchi T, Lennert K, Tu LY, et al. Histopathology and immunohistochemistry of peripheral T-cell lymphomas: A proposal for their classification. *J. Clin. Pathol.* 1987, **40**: 995–1015.
33. Stansfeld AG, Diebold J, Kapanci Y, et al. Updated

Kiel classification for lymphomas. *Lancet* 1988, **i**: 292–293.

34. Matutes E, Brito-Babapulle V, Swansbury J, et al. Clinical and laboratory features of 78 cases of T-prolymphocytic leukemia. *Blood* 1991, **78**: 3269–3274.

35. Loughran TP Jr. Clonal diseases of large granular lymphocytes. *Blood* 1993, **82**: 1–14.

36. Nakamura S, Suchi T. A clinicopathologic study of node-based, low-grade, peripheral T-cell lymphoma. Angioimmunoblastic lymphoma, T-zone lymphoma, and lymphoepithelioid lymphoma. *Cancer* 1991, **67**: 2565–2578.

37. Siegert W, Agthe A, Griesser H, et al. Treatment of angioimmunoblastic lymphadenopathy (AILD)-type T-cell lymphoma using prednisone with or without the COPBLAM/IMVP-16 regimen. *Ann. Intern. Med.* 1992, **117**: 364–370.

38. Siegert W, Nerl C, Engelhard M, et al. Peripheral T-cell non-Hodgkin's lymphomas of low malignancy: Prospective study of 25 patients with pleomorphic small cell lymphoma, lymphoepithelioid cell (Lennert's) lymphoma and T-zone lymphoma. *Br. J. Haematol.* 1994, **87**: 529–534.

39. Stein H, Dienemann D, Dallenbach F, et al. Peripheral T-cell lymphomas. *Ann. Oncol.* 1991, **2** (Suppl. 2): 163–169.

40. Cerf-Bensussan N, Jarry A, Brousse N, et al. A monoclonal antibody (HML-1) defining a novel membrane molecule present on human intestinal lymphocytes. *Eur. J. Immunol.* 1987, **17**: 1279–1285.

41. Winberg CD, Sheibani K, Krance R, et al. Peripheral T-cell lymphoma: Immunologic and cell-kinetic observations associated with morphological progression. *Blood* 1985, **66**: 980–989.

42. Horschowski N, Sainty D, Sebahoun G et al. Histological evolution of peripheral T-cell lymphomas: Study of six cases. *Pathol. Biol.* 1991, **39**: 692–696.

43. Patsouris E, Noel H, Lennert K. Histological and immunohistological findings in lymphoepithelioid cell lymphoma (Lennert's lymphoma). *Am. J. Surg. Pathol.* 1988, **12**: 341–350.

44. Coiffier B, Berger F, Bryon PA, et al. T-Cell lymphomas: Immunologic, histologic, clinical and therapeutic analysis of 63 cases. *J. Clin. Oncol.* 1988, **6**: 1584–1589.

45. Pinkus GS, O'Hara CJ, Said JW. Peripheral/post-thymic T-cell lymphomas: A spectrum of disease. Clinical, pathologic, and immunologic features of 78 cases. *Cancer* 1990, **65**: 971–998.

46. Delmer A, Caulet S, Bryard F, et al. Peripheral T-cell lymphomas. Clinical, morphological and evolutive features in 22 cases. *Presse Med.* 1990, **19**: 851–855.

47. Brisbane JU, Berman LD, Neiman RS. Peripheral T-cell lymphoma: A clinicopathologic study of nine cases. *Am. J. Clin. Pathol.* 1983, **79**: 285–293.

48. Mirchandani I, Palutke M, Tabaczka P, et al. B-Cell lymphomas morphologically resembling T-cell lymphomas. *Cancer* 1985, **56**: 1578–1583.

49. Stroup RM, Burke JS, Sheibani K, et al. Splenic involvement by aggressive malignant lymphomas of B-cell and T-cell types. *Cancer* 1992, **69**: 413–420.

50. Winberg CD, Sheibani K, Burke JS, et al. T-Cell-rich lymphoproliferative disorders: Morphologic and immunologic differential diagnoses. *Cancer* 1988, **62**: 1539–1555.

51. Rodriguez J, Pugh WC, Cabanillas F. T-Cell rich B-cell lymphoma. *Blood* 1993, **82**: 1586–1589.

52. Picker LJ, Brenner MB, Weiss LM, et al. Discordant expression of CD3 and T-cell receptor beta-chain antigens in T-lineage lymphoma. *Am. J. Pathol.* 1987, **129**: 434–444.

53. Henni T, Gaulard P, Divine M, et al. Comparison of genetic probe with immunophenotype analysis in lymphoproliferative disorders: A study of 87 cases. *Blood* 1988, **72**: 1937–1943.

54. Weiss LM, Crabtree GS, Rouse SV, et al. Morphologic and immunologic characterization of 50 peripheral T-cell lymphomas. *Am. J. Pathol.* 1985, **118**: 316–324.

55. Borowitz MJ, Reichert TA, Brynes RK, et al. The phenotypic diversity of peripheral T-cell lymphomas: The Southeastern Cancer Study Group experience. *Hum. Pathol.* 1986, **17**: 567–574.

56. Diehl V, Bohlen H, Wolf J. CD30: Cytokine-receptor, differentiation marker or a target molecule for specific immune response? *Ann. Oncol.* 1994, **5**: 300–302.

57. Kern WF, Spier CM, Hanneman EH, et al. Neural cell adhesion molecule-positive peripheral T-cell lymphoma: A rare variant with a propensity for unusual sites of involvement. *Blood* 1992, **79**: 2432–2437.

58. Wong KF, Chan JKC, Ng CS, et al. CD56 (NKH1)-positive hematolymphoid malignancies: An aggressive neoplasm featuring frequent cutaneous/mucosal involvement, cytoplasmic azurophilic granules and angiocentricity. *Hum. Pathol.* 1992, **23**: 798–804.

59. O'Connor NTJ, Crick A, Wainscoat JS, et al. Evidence for a monoclonal T-lymphocyte proliferation in angioimmunoblastic lymphadenopathy. *J. Clin. Pathol.* 1986, **39**: 1229–1232.

60. Weiss LM, Strickler JG, Dorfman RF, et al. Clonal T-cell populations in angioimmunoblastic lymphadenopathy and angioimmunoblastic lymphadenopathy-like lymphoma. *Am. J. Pathol.* 1986, **122**: 392–397.

61. Feller AC, Griesser H, Schilling CV, et al. Clonal gene rearrangement patterns correlate with immunophenotype and clinical parameters in patients with angioimmunoblastic lymphadenopathy. *Am. J. Pathol.* 1988, **133**: 549–556.

62. Takagi N, Nakamura S, Ueda R, et al. A phenotypic and genotypic study of three node-based, low-grade peripheral T-cell lymphomas: Angioimmunoblastic lymphoma, T-zone lymphoma, and lymphoepithelioid lymphoma. *Cancer* 1992, **69**: 2571–2582.

63. Gaulard P, Henni T, Marolleau JP, et al. Lethal midline granuloma (polymorphic reticulosis) and lymphomatoid granulomatosis. Evidence for a monoclonal T-cell lymphoproliferative disorder. *Cancer* 1988, **62**: 705–710.

64. Weiss LM, Wood GS, Trela M, et al. Clonal T-cell populations in lymphomatoid granulomatosis. Evidence of a lymphoproliferative origin for a clinically benign disease. *N. Engl. J. Med.* 1986, **315**: 475–479.

65. Kadin ME, Vonderheid EC, Sako D, et al. Clonal composition of T-cells in lymphomatoid papulosis. *Am. J. Pathol.* 1987, **126**: 13–17.

66. Gaulard P, Bourquelot P, Kanavaros P, et al. Expression of the alpha/beta and gamma/delta T-cell receptors in 57 cases of peripheral T-cell lymphomas. Identification of a subset of $\gamma\delta$ T-cell lymphomas. *Am. J. Pathol.* 1990, **137**: 617–628.

67. Farcet JP, Gaulard P, Marolleau JP, et al. Hepatosplenic T-cell lymphoma: Sinusal/sinusoidal localization of malignant cells expressing the T-cell receptor $\gamma\delta$. *Blood* 1990, **75**: 2213–2219.

68. Sanger WG, Weisenburger DD, Armitage JO, et al. Cytogenetic abnormalities in noncutaneous peripheral T-cell lymphoma. *Cancer Genet. Cytogenet.* 1986, **23**: 53–59.

69. Cosimi MF, Casagranda I, Ghiazza G, et al. Rearrangements on chromosome 7 and 14 with breakpoints at 7q35 and 14q11 in angioimmunoblastic lymphadenopathy and IBL-like T-cell lymphoma. *Pathologica* 1990, **82**: 391–397.

70. Berger R. Chromosomal abnormalities in T-cell malignant lymphoma. *Bull. Cancer* 1991, **78**: 283–290.

71. Schlegelberger B, Himmler A, Gödde E, et al. Cytogenetic findings in peripheral T-cell lymphomas as a basis for distinguishing low-grade and high-grade lymphomas. *Blood* 1994, **83**: 505–511.

72. Kamada N, Sakurai M, Miyamoto K, et al. Chromosome abnormalities in adult T-cell leukemia/lymphoma: A Karyotype Review Committee report. *Cancer Res.* 1992, **52**: 1481–1493.

73. Kaneko Y, Maseki N, Sakurai M, et al. Characteristic karyotypic pattern in T-cell lymphoproliferative disorders with reactive 'angioimmunoblastic lymphadenopathy with dysproteinemia-type' features. *Blood* 1988, **72**: 413–421.

74. Schlegelberger B, Nolle I, Feller AC, et al. Angioimmunoblastic lymphadenopathy with trisomy 3: the cells of the malignant clone are T-cells. *Hematol. Pathol.* 1990, **4**: 179–183.

75. Donner LR, Dobin S, Harrington D, et al. Angiocentric immunoproliferative lesion (lymphomatoid granulomatosis). A cytogenetic, immunophenotypic, and genotypic study. *Cancer* 1990, **65**: 249–254.

76. Wright DH, Jones DB, Clark H, et al. Is adult-onset coeliac disease due to a low-grade lymphoma of intraepithelial T lymphocytes? *Lancet* 1991, i:1373–1374.

77. Kaneko Y, Frizzera G, Edamura S, et al. A novel translocation, t(2;5)(p23;q35), in childhood phagocytic large T-cell lymphoma mimicking malignant histiocytosis. *Blood* 1989, **73**: 806–813.

78. Mason DY, Bastard C, Rimokh R, et al. CD30-positive large cell lymphomas ('Ki-1 lymphoma') are associated with a chromosomal translocation involving 5q35. *Br. J. Haematol.* 1990, **74**: 161–168.

79. Morris SW, Kirstein MN, Valentine MB, et al. Fusion of a kinase gene, ALK, to a nucleolar protein gene, NPM, in non-Hodgkin's lymphoma. *Science* 1994, **263**: 1281–1284.

80. Cohen JI. Molecular biology of Epstein–Barr virus and its mechanims of B-cell transformation. In Straus (moderator). *Epstein–Barr Virus Infections: Biology, Pathogenesis, and Management. Ann. Intern. Med.* 1993, **118**: 45–58.

81. Jones JF, Shurim S, Abramowsky C, et al. T-Cell lymphomas containing Epstein–Barr viral DNA in patients with chronic Epstein–Barr infections. *N. Engl. J. Med.* 1988, **318**: 733–741.

82. Hamilton-Dutoit SJ, Pallesen G. A survey of Epstein–Barr virus gene expression in sporadic non-Hodgkin's lymphomas: Detection of Epstein–Barr virus in a subset of peripheral T-cell lymphomas. *Am. J. Pathol.* 1992, **140**: 1315–1325.

83. Harabuchi Y, Yamanaka N, Kataura A, et al. Epstein–Barr virus in nasal T-cell lymphomas in patients with lethal midline granuloma. *Lancet* 1990, i: 128–130.

84. Katzenstein AA, Peiper S. Detection of Epstein–Barr virus genomes in lymphomatoid granulomatosis: Analysis of 29 cases by the polymerase chain reaction technique. *Mod. Pathol.* 1990, **3**: 435–441.

85. Peiper SC. Angiocentric lymphoproliferative disorders of the respiratory system: Incrimination of Epstein–Barr virus in pathogenesis. *Blood* 1993, **82**: 687–690.

86. Kanavaros P, Lescs MC, Brière J, et al. Nasal T-cell lymphoma: A clinicopathologic entity associated with peculiar phenotype and with Epstein–Barr virus. *Blood* 1993, **81**: 2688–2695.

87. Borisch B, Hennig I, Laeng RH, et al. Association of the subtype 2 of the Epstein–Barr virus with T-cell non-Hodgkin's lymphoma of the midline granuloma type. *Blood* 1993, **82**: 858–864.

88. Herbst H, Dallenbach F, Hummel M, et al. Epstein–Barr virus DNA and latent gene products in Ki-1 (CD30)-positive anaplastic large cell lymphomas. *Blood* 1991, **78**, 2666–2673.

89. Knecht H, Sahli R, Shaw P, et al. Detection of Epstein–Barr virus DNA by polymerase chain reaction in lymph node biopsies from patients with angioimmunoblastic lymphadenopathy. *Br. J. Haematol.* 1990, **75**: 610–614.

90. Weiss LM, Jaffe ES, Liu XF, et al. Detection and localization of Epstein–Barr viral genomes in angioimmunoblastic lymphadenopathy and angioimmunoblastic lymphadenopathy-like lymphoma. *Blood* 1992, **79**: 1789–1795.

91. Su IJ, Hsieh HC, Lin KH, et al. Aggressive peripheral T-cell lymphomas containing Epstein–Barr viral DNA: A clinicopathologic and molecular analysis. *Blood* 1991, **77**: 799–808.

92. Korbjuhn P, Anagnostopoulos I, Hummel M, et al. Frequent latent Epstein–Barr virus infection of neoplastic T-cells and bystander B-cells in human immunodeficiency virus-negative European peripheral pleomorphic T-cell lymphomas. *Blood* 1993, **82**: 217–223.

93. de Bruin PC, Jiwa M, Oudejans JJ, et al. Presence of Epstein–Barr virus in extranodal T-cell lymphomas: Differences in relation to site. *Blood* 1994, **83**: 1612–1618.

94. Yao M, Cheng AL, Su IJ, et al. Clinicopathological spectrum of haemophagocytic syndrome in Epstein–

Barr virus-associated peripheral T-cell lymphoma. *Br. J. Haematol.* 1994, **87**: 535–543.

95. Hsu SM, Waldron JW, Hsu PL, et al. Cytokines in malignant lymphomas: review and prospective evaluation. *Hum. Pathol.* 1993, **24**: 1040–1057.

96. Ohnishi K, Ichikawa A, Kagami Y, et al. Interleukin 4 and γ-interferon may play a role in the histopathogenesis of peripheral T-cell lymphoma. *Cancer Res.* 1990, **50**: 8028–8033.

97. Merz H, Fliedner A, Orscheschek K, et al. Cytokine expression in T-cell lymphomas and Hodgkin's disease. Its possible implication in autocrine or paracrine production as a potential basis for neoplastic growth. *Am. J. Pathol.* 1991, **139**: 1173–1180.

98. Agematsu K, Takeuchi S, Ichikawa M, et al. Spontaneous production of interleukin-6 by Ki-1 positive large-cell anaplastic lymphoma with extensive bone destruction. *Blood* 1991, **77**: 2299–2301.

99. Merz H, Houssiau FA, Orscheschek K, et al. Interleukin-9 expression in human malignant lymphomas: Unique association with Hodgkin's disease and large cell anaplastic lymphoma. *Blood* 1991, **78**: 1311–1317.

100. Matsuzaki M, Shimamotop Y, Enokihara H, et al. High Eo-CSF activity in T-cell non-Hodgkin's lymphoma with eosinophilia. *Clin. Lab. Haemat.* 1992, **14**: 251–255.

101. Samoszuk M, Ramzi E, Cooper DL. Interleukin-5 mRNA in three T-cell lymphomas with eosinophilia. *Am. J. Hematol.* 1993, **42**: 402–404.

102. Fermand JP, Mitjavila MT, Le Couedic JP, et al. Role of granulocyte–macrophage colony-stimulating factor, interleukin-3 and interleukin-5 in the eosinophilia associated with T-cell lymphoma. *Br. J. Haematol.* 1993, **83**: 359–364.

103. Hsu SM, Waldron JA, Fink L, et al. Pathogenic significance of interleukin-6 in angioimmunoblastic lymphadenopathy-type T-cell lymphoma. *Hum. Pathol.* 1993, **24**: 126–131.

104. Uchiyama T, Yodoi J, Sagawa K, et al. Adult-T-cell leukemia: Clinical and hematologic features of 16 cases. *Blood* 1977, **50**: 481–492.

105. Bunn PA, Schechter GP, Jaffe E, et al. Clinical course of retrovirus-associated adult T-cell lymphoma in the United States. *N. Engl. J. Med.* 1983, **309**: 257–264.

106. Catovsky D, Greaves MF, Rose M, et al. Adult T-cell lymphoma-leukemia in blacks from the West Indies. *Lancet* 1983, **i**: 639–643.

107. Gibbs WN, Lofters WS, Campbell M, et al. Non-Hodgkin's lymphoma in Jamaica and its relation to adult T-cell leukemia–lymphoma. *Ann. Intern. Med.* 1987, **106**: 361–368.

108. Ratner L, Poiesz BJ. Leukemias associated with human T-cell lymphotropic virus type I in a non-endemic region. *Medicine* 1988, **67**: 401–422.

109. Shimoyama M. Diagnostic criteria and classification of clinical subtypes of adult T-cell leukemia-lymphoma. A report from the Lymphoma Study Group (1984–1987). *Br. J. Haematol.* 1991, **79**: 428–437.

110. Jaffe ES, Cossman J, Blattner WA, et al. The pathologic spectrum of adult T-cell leukemia/lymphoma in the United States. Human T-cell leukemia/lymphoma virus-associated lymphoid malignancies. *Am. J. Surg.*

Pathol. 1984, **4**: 263–275.

111. Shimoyama M. Treatment of patients with adult T-cell leukemia-lymphoma: An overview. In Takatsuki K, Hinuma Y, Yoshida M (eds). *Advances in Adult T-Cell Leukemia and HTLV-1 Research. Gann. Monogr. Cancer Res.* 1992, **39**: 43–56.

112. Morimoto C, Matsuyama T, Oshige C, et al. Functional and phenotypic studies of Japanese adult T-cell leukemia cells. *J. Clin. Invest.* 1985, **75**: 836–843.

113. Seymour JF, Gagel RF. Calcitriol: The major humoral mediator of hypercalcemia in Hodgkin's disease and non-Hodgkin's lymphomas. *Blood* 1993, **82**: 1383–1394.

114. Kawano F, Yamaguchi K, Nishimura H, et al. Variation in the clinical courses of adult T-cell leukemia. *Cancer* 1985, **55**: 851–856.

115. Greer JP, York JC, Cousar JB, et al. Peripheral T-cell lymphoma: A clinicopathologic study of 42 cases. *J. Clin. Oncol.* 1984, **2**: 788–798.

116. Weisenburger DD, Astorino RN, Glassy FJ, et al. Peripheral T-cell lymphoma. A clinicopathologic study of a morphologically diverse entity. *Cancer* 1985, **56**: 2061–2068.

117. Grogan TM, Fielder K, Rangel C, et al. Peripheral T-cell lymphoma: Aggressive disease with heterogenous immunotypes. *Am. J. Clin. Pathol.* 1985, **83**: 279–288.

118. Horning SJ, Weiss LM, Crabtree GS, et al. Clinical and phenotypic diversity of T-cell lymphomas. *Blood* 1986, **67**: 1578–1582.

119. Liang R, Todd D, Chan TK, et al. Peripheral T-cell lymphoma. *J. Clin. Oncol.* 1987, **5**: 750–755.

120. Chott A, Augustin I, Wrba F, et al. Peripheral T-cell lymphomas: A clinicopathologic study of 75 cases. *Hum. Pathol.* 1990, **21**: 1117–1125.

121. Hanson CA, Brunning RD, Gajl-Peczalska K, et al. Bone marrow manifestations of peripheral T-cell lymphoma. A study of 30 cases. *Am. J. Clin. Pathol.* 1986, **86**: 449–460.

122. Caulet S, Delmer A, Audouin J, et al. Histopathological study of bone marrow biopsies in thirty cases of T-cell lymphoma with clinical, biological and survival correlations. *Hematol. Oncol.* 1990, **8**: 155–168.

123. Gaulard P, Kanavaros P, Farcet JP, et al. Bone marrow histologic and immunohistochemical findings in peripheral T-cell lymphoma: A study of 38 cases. *Hum. Pathol.* 1991, **22**: 331–338.

124. Gherardi R, Gaulard P, Prost C, et al. T-Cell lymphoma revealed by a peripheral neuropathy. A report of two cases with an immunohistologic study on lymph nodes and nerve biopsies. *Cancer* 1986, **58**: 2710–2716.

125. Gaulard P, Zafrani ES, Mavier P, et al. Peripheral T-cell lymphoma presenting as predominant liver disease: A report of three cases. *Hepatology* 1986, **6**: 864–868.

126. O'Shea JJ, Jaffe ES, Lane HC, et al. Peripheral T-cell lymphoma presenting as hypereosinophilia with vasculitis. Clinical, pathologic and immunologic features. *Am. J. Med.* 1987, **82**: 539–545.

127. Diez-Martin JL, Lust JA, Witzig TE, et al. Unusual presentation of extranodal peripheral T-cell lymphomas with multiple paraneoplastic features. *Cancer*

1991, **68**: 834–841.

128. Marsh WL, Stevenson DR, Long HJ. Primary leptomeningeal presentation of T-cell lymphoma. Report of a patient and review of the literature. *Cancer* 1983, **51**: 1125–1131.

129. Schnitzer B, Smid D, Lloyd R. Primary T-cell lymphoma of the adrenal glands with adrenal insufficiency. *Hum. Pathol.* 1986, **17**: 634–636.

130. Delmer A, Audouin J, Rio B, et al. Peripheral T-cell lymphoma presenting as hypereosinophilia with vasculitis. *Am. J. Med.* 1988, **84**: 565–566.

131. Frizzera G, Moran EM, Rappaport H. Angio-immunoblastic lymphadenopathy with dysproteinemia. *Lancet* 1974, **i**: 1070–7073.

132. Lukes RJ, Tindle BH. Immunoblastic lymphadenopathy: A hyperimmune entity resembling Hodgkin's disease. *N. Engl. J. Med.* 1975, **292**: 1–8.

133. Knecht H. Angioimmunoblastic lymphadenopathy: Ten years' experience and state of current knowledge. *Semin. Hematol.* 1989, **26**: 208–215.

134. Pangalis GA, Moran EM, Nathwani BN, et al. Angioimmunoblastic lymphadenopathy. Long-term follow-up study. *Cancer* 1983, **52**: 318–321.

135. Nathwani BN, Rappaport H, Moran EM, et al. Malignant lymphoma arising in angioimmunoblastic lymphadenopathy. *Cancer* 1978, **41**: 578–606.

136. Watanabe S, Sato Y, Shimoyama M, et al. Immunoblastic lymphadenopathy, angioimmunoblastic lymphadenopathy, and IBL-like T-cell lymphoma. *Cancer* 1986, **58**: 2224–2232.

137. Namikawa R, Suchi T, Ueda R, et al. Phenotyping of proliferating lymphocytes in angioimmunoblastic lymphadenopathy and related lesions by the double immunoenzymatic staining technique. *Am. J. Pathol.* 1987, **127**: 279–287.

138. Lipford EH, Smith HR, Pittaluga S, et al. Clonality of angioimmunoblastic lymphadenopathy and implications for its evolution to malignant lymphoma. *J. Clin. Invest.* 1987, **79**: 637–642.

139. Tobinai K, Minato K, Ohtsu T, et al. Clinicopathologic, immunophenotypic, and immunogenotypic analyses of immunoblastic lymphadenopathy-like T-cell lymphoma. *Blood* 1988, **72**: 1000–1006.

140. Frizzera G, Kaneko Y, Sakurai M. Angioimmunoblastic lymphadenopathy and related disorders: A retrospective look in search of definitions. *Leukemia* 1989, **3**: 1–5.

141. Archimbaud E, Coiffier B, Bryon PA, et al. Prognostic factors in angioimmunoblastic lymphadenopathy. *Cancer* 1987, **59**: 208–212.

142. Jaffe ES. Pathologic and clinical spectrum of postthymic T-cell malignancies. *Cancer Invest.* 1984, **2**: 413–424.

143. Liebow AA, Carrington CRB, Friedman PJ. Lymphomatoid granulomatosis. *Hum. Pathol.* 1972, **3**: 457–558.

144. Koss MN, Hochholzer L, Langloss JM, et al. Lymphomatoid granulomatosis: A clinicopathologic study of 42 patients. *Pathology* 1986, **18**: 283–288.

145. Kazenstein AA, Carrington CB, Liebow AA. Lymphomatoid granulomatosis: A clinicopathologic study of 152 cases. *Cancer* 1979, **43**: 360–373.

146. Fauci AS, Haynes BF, Costa J, et al. Lymphomatoid granulomatosis, prospective trial and therapeutic experience over years. *N. Engl. J. Med.* 1982, **306**: 68–74.

147. Chan JKC, Ng CS, Ngan KC, et al. Angiocentric T-cell lymphoma of the skin. An aggressive lymphoma distinct from mycosis fungoides. *Am. J. Surg. Pathol.* 1988, **12**: 861–876.

148. Ishii Y, Yamanaka N, Ogama K, et al. Nasal T-cell lymphoma as a type of so-called 'lethal midline granuloma'. *Cancer* 1982, **50**: 2336–2344.

149. Chan JKC, Ng CS, Lau WH, et al. Most nasal/nasopharyngeal lymphomas are peripheral T-cell neoplasms. *Am. J. Surg. Pathol.* 1987, **11**: 418–429.

150. Medeiros LJ, Peiper SC, Elwood L, et al. Angiocentric immunoproliferative lesions: A molecular analysis of eight cases. *Hum. Pathol.* 1991, **22**: 1150–1157.

151. Lipford EH, Margolick JB, Longo DL, et al. Angiocentric immunoproliferative lesions: A clinicopathologic spectrum of post thymic T-cell proliferations. *Blood* 1988, **72**: 1674–1681.

152. Shimokawa I, Ushijima N, Moriuchi R, et al. A case of angiocentric immunoproliferative lesions (angiocentric lymphoma) associated with human T-cell lymphotropic virus type 1. *Hum. Pathol.* 1993, **24**: 921–923.

153. Weiss LM, Arber DA, Strickler JG. Nasal T-cell lymphoma. *Ann. Oncol.* 1994, **5**(Suppl. 1): S39-S42.

154. Sanchez NP, Pittelkow MR, Muller SH, et al. The clinicopathologic spectrum of lymphomatoid papulosis: Study of 31 cases. *J. Am. Acad. Dermatol.* 1983, **8**: 81–94.

155. Wang HH, Lach L, Kadin ME. Epidemiology of lymphomatoid papulosis. *Cancer* 1992, **70**: 2951–2957.

156. Davis TH, Morton CC, Miller-Cassman R, et al. Hodgkin's disease, lymphomatoid papulosis, and cutaneous T-cell lymphoma derived from a common T-cell clone. *N. Engl. J. Med.* 1992, **326**: 1115–1122.

157. Stein H, Mason DY, Gerdes J, et al. The expression of the Hodgkin's disease associated antigen Ki-1 in reactive and neoplastic tissue: Evidence that Reed–Sternberg cells and histiocytic malignancies are derived from activated lymphoid cells. *Blood* 1985, **66**: 848–858.

158. Kadin ME. Primary Ki-1-positive anaplastic large-cell lymphoma: A distinct clinicopathologic entity. *Ann. Oncol.* 1994, **5**(Suppl. 1): S25-S30.

159. Chott A, Kaserer K, Augustin I, et al. Ki-1-positive large cell lymphoma: A clinicopathologic study of 41 cases. *Am. J. Surg. Pathol.* 1990, **14**: 439–448.

160. Greer JP, Kinney MC, Collins RD, et al. Clinical features of 31 Ki-1 anaplastic large-cell lymphomas. *J. Clin. Oncol.* 1991, **9**: 539–547.

161. Penny RJ, Blaustein JC, Longtine JA, et al. Ki-1-positive large cell lymphomas, a heterogenous group of neoplasms. Morphologic, immunophenotypic, genotypic, and clinical features of 24 cases. *Cancer* 1991, **68**: 362–373.

162. Nakamura S, Takagi MC, Kojima M, et al. Clinicopathologic study of large-cell anaplastic lymphoma (Ki-1-positive large-cell lymphoma) among the Japanese. *Cancer* 1991, **68**: 118–129.

163. Shulman LN, Frisard B, Antin JH, et al. Primary Ki-1 anaplastic large-cell lymphoma in adults: Clinical characteristics and therapeutic outcome. *J. Clin. Oncol.* 1993, **11**: 937–942.

164. Sandlund JT, Pui CH, Santana VM, et al. Clinical features and treatment outcome for children with CD30+ large-cell non-Hodgkin's lymphoma. *J. Clin. Oncol.* 1994, **12**: 895–898.

165. Reiter A, Schrappe M, Tiemann M, et al. Successful treatment strategy for Ki-1 anaplastic large-cell lymphoma of childhood: A prospective analysis of 62 patients enrolled in three consecutive Berlin–Frankfurt–Munster Group studies. *J. Clin. Oncol.* 1994, **12**: 899–908.

166. Pileri S, Bocchia M, Baroni CD, et al. Anaplastic large cell lymphoma (CD30+/Ki-1+): Results of a prospective clinico-pathological study of 69 cases. *Br. J. Haematol.* 1994, **86**: 513–523.

167. Kadin ME, Sako D, Berliner N, et al. Childhood Ki-1 lymphoma presenting with skin lesions and peripheral lymphadenopathy. *Blood* 1986, **68**: 1042–1049.

168. Beljaards RC, Meijer CJLM, Scheller, E et al. Primary cutaneous CD30-positive large cell lymphoma: Definition of a new type of cutaneous lymphoma with a favorable prognosis. *Cancer* 1993, **71**: 2097–2104.

169. Spencer J, Cerf-Bensussan N, Jarry A, et al. Enteropathy-associated T-cell lymphoma (malignant histiocytosis of the intestine) is recognized by a monoclonal antibody (HML-1) that defines a membrane molecule on human mucosal lymphocytes. *Am. J. Pathol.* 1988, **132**: 1–5.

170. Chott A, Dragosics B, Radaszkiewicz T. Peripheral T-cell of the intestine. *Am. J. Pathol.* 1992, **141**: 1361–1371.

171. Lin MT, Shen MC, Su IJ, et al. Peripheral T γ/δ lymphoma presenting with idiopathic thrombocytopenic purpura-like picture. *Br. J. Haematol.* 1991, **78**: 280–282.

172. Mastovich S, Ratech H, Ware RE, et al. Hepatosplenic T-cell lymphoma: An unusual case of a γ/δ T-cell lymphoma with a blast-like terminal transformation. *Hum. Pathol.* 1994, **25**: 102–108.

173. Beljaards RC, Meijer CJLM, Scheller E, et al. Prognostic significance of CD30 (Ki-1/Ber-H2) expression in primary cutaneous large-cell lymphomas of T-cell origin. A clinicopathologic and immunohistochemical study in 20 patients. *Am. J. Pathol.* 1989, **135**: 1169–1178.

174. Joly P, Charlotte F, Leibowitch M, et al. Cutaneous lymphomas other than mycosis fungoides: Follow up study of 52 patients. *J. Clin. Oncol.* 1991, **9**: 1994–2001.

175. Rijlaarsdam JU, Scheffer E, Meijer CJLM, et al. Cutaneous pseudo-T-cell lymphomas. A clinicopathologic study of 20 patients. *Cancer* 1992, **69**: 717–724.

176. Falini A, Pileri S, DeSolas I, et al. Peripheral T-cell lymphoma associated with hemophagocytic syndrome. *Blood* 1990, **75**: 434–444.

177. Patsouris E, Engelhard M, Zwingers Th, et al. Lymphoepithelioid cell lymphoma (Lennert's lymphoma): Clinical features derived from analysis of 108 cases. *Br. J. Haematol.* 1993, **84**: 346–348.

178. Shimoyama M, Ota K, Kikuchi M, et al. Chemotherapeutic results and prognostic factors of patients with advanced non-Hodgkin's lymphoma treated with VEPA or VEPA-M. *J. Clin. Oncol.* 1988, **5**: 128–141.

179. Shimoyama M, Takatsuki K, Araki K, et al. for the Lymphoma Study Group (1984–1987). Major prognostic factors of patients with adult T-cell leukemialymphoma: A cooperative study. *Leuk. Res.* 1991, **15**: 81–90.

180. Yamada Y, Murata K, Kamihira S, et al. Prognostic significance of the proportion of Ki-67-positive cells in adult T-cell leukemia. *Cancer* 1991, **67**: 2605–2609.

181. Cheng AL, Chen YC, Wang CH, et al. Direct comparisons of peripheral T-cell lymphoma with diffuse B-cell lymphoma of comparable histological grades – Should peripheral T-cell lymphoma be considered separately? *J. Clin. Oncol.* 1989, **7**: 725–731.

182. Grierson HL, Wooldridge TN, Purtilo DT, et al. Low proliferative activity is associated with a favorable prognosis in peripheral T-cell lymphoma. *Cancer Res.* 1990, **50**: 4845–4848.

183. Kuwazuru Y, Hanada S, Furukawa T, et al. Expression of P-glycoprotein in adult T-cell leukemia cells. *Blood* 1990, **76**: 2065–2071.

184. Tamura K, Makino S, Araki Y, et al. Recombinant interferon beta and gamma in the treatment of adult T-cell leukemia. *Cancer* 1987, **59**: 1059–1062.

185. Waldmannn TA, White JD, Goldman CK, et al. The interleukin-2 receptor: A target for monoclonal antibody treatment of Human T-cell Lymphotropic Virus I-induced adult T-cell leukemia. *Blood* 1993, **82**: 1701–1712.

186. Gill PS, Masood R, Cai J, et al. Novel (antiviral) therapy for adult T-cell leukemia secondary to HTLV-I infection. *Blood* 1992, **80**(Suppl. 1): 74a.

187. Siegert W, Nerl C, Meuthen I, et al. Recombinant human interferon-α in the treatment of angioimmunoblastic lymphadenopathy: Results in 12 patients. *Leukemia* 1991, **5**: 892–895.

188. Murayama T, Imoto S, Takahashi T, et al. Successful treatment of angioimmunoblastic lymphadenopathy with dysproteinemia with cyclosporin A. *Cancer* 1992, **69**: 2567–2570.

189. Vose JM, Peterson C, Bierman PJ, et al. Comparison of high-dose therapy and autologous bone marrow transplantation for T-cell and B-cell non-Hodgkin's lymphomas. *Blood* 1990, **76**: 424–431.

190. Gisselbrecht C, Coiffier B, Simon M, et al. IFN therapy in peripheral T-cell lymphoma (PTCL). *Third International Conference in Malignant Lymphoma,* Lugano, Switzerland, June 10–13, 1987 (abstract).

191. Su IJ, Cheng AL, Tsai TF, et al. Retinoic acid-induced apoptosis and regression of a refractory Epstein–Barr virus-containing T-cell lymphoma expressing multidrug-resistance phenotype. *Br. J. Haematol.* 1993, **85**: 826–828.

192. Cheng AL, Su IJ, Chen CC, et al. Use of retinoic acids in the treatment of peripheral T-cell lymphoma: A pilot study. *J. Clin. Oncol.* 1994, **12**: 1185–1192.

193. Hôtel-Dieu 1993 (Table 44.1).

CHAPTER 45

Lymphoproliferative disorders in immunocompromised individuals

IAN T. MAGRATH, AZIZA T. SHAD AND JOHN T. SANDLUND

Introduction

The lymphoproliferative disorders (LPD) that occur in association with congenital, iatrogenically induced and acquired immunodeficiencies are a morphologically heterogenous group of lymphoid proliferations that are predominantly of B-cell immunophenotype and may be polyclonal or monoclonal [1–12]. In this context, the term LPD, as used here, ranges from polyclonal entities that would not express malignant behavior in a normal host, and indeed, would probably be rapidly eliminated, to presumptively fully transformed monoclonal neoplasms that would behave as an aggressive neoplasm even in an immunocompetent individual. It is perhaps only the latter that warrant use of the term 'malignant lymphoma' although this term has been employed in cases of LPD that have a more aggressive, atypical appearance. There seems little doubt that LPD results, in most patients, directly from the underlying T-cell immunodeficiency, which permits the survival of cells, particularly Epstein–Barr virus (EBV)-infected B-cells, which would normally be eliminated by cytotoxic T-cells. This initial expansion of B-cells is usually polyclonal, but the increased proliferation and life span of these cells increases the likelihood that genetic changes may occur, such that one of the clones may develop into a true monoclonal malignancy [1,13]. While the majority of LPDs are probably not truly neoplastic by this above definition, when lymphoid proliferation is entirely unchecked, the usual criteria of a neoplastic process (e.g., monoclonality, genetically aberrant) are, in any event, irrelevant to outcome – even the EBV-driven B-cell proliferation of infectious mononucleosis can result in the death of an immunosuppressed individual. In less severely immunosuppressed patients, in whom immunoregulation is still partially effective, the evolution from polyclonality (which may be subclinical) to monoclonality may have occurred by the time the patient presents with LPD. This does not necessarily signify the presence of genetic changes that result in the deregulation of oncogenes, but could equally represent clonal selection related to the varying degrees to which different clones survives in various microenvironments or are recognized or killed by T-cells (clonal selection of EBV-transformed B-cells also occurs *in vitro*, in the absence of T-cells). It is perhaps this clonal selection that makes widespread monoclonal processes somewhat more difficult to eradicate simply by withdrawal of immunosuppression than polyclonal processes, but there is no *a priori* reason to believe that it will be a significant factor in determining the response to therapeutic agents, a presumption that appears to be borne out by observation. Inherited defects in DNA repair are sometimes associated with immunodeficiency, e.g., in Bloom's syndrome and ataxia telangiectasia (AT), and may, in these conditions, be the predominant factor in the predisposition to lymphoma development [4,8,9,11]. In these circumstances, the neoplasms that emerge usually contain similar genetic lesions to those present in lymphomas arising in the general population.

With the rapidly growing numbers of individuals undergoing organ transplantations each year (most of whom are maintained on immunosuppressive therapy for life), the more widespread use of immunosuppressive drugs, such as methotrexate, for autoimmune disorders, and the increasing number of patients receiving T-cell depleted, mismatched bone marrow transplantations, coupled to the current human immunodeficiency virus (HIV) epidemic, the patient population at risk for the development of LPD continues to increase. These patients require different treatment strategies from those used in the non-Hodgkin's lymphomas arising in the general population and, moreover, because of the underlying disease or previous allograft, patients at high risk for the development of LPD are readily identified such that preventive measures represent a potentially important component of the interventional strategy.

In this chapter, we shall discuss the epidemiology, pathogenesis, clinical manifestations and treatment of LPD associated with pre-existing immunodeficiency. Since HIV-associated LPD and the epidemiology and pathogenesis of LPD arising in patients with inherited immunodeficiencies has been discussed in other chapters, only brief reference to these topics will be made here. The major emphasis will be on LPD in allograft recipients, although similar treatment principles apply to LPD in immunosuppressed individuals regardless of the cause of the immunosuppression.

Epidemiology and pathogenesis

CONGENITAL IMMUNODEFICIENCIES

Lymphoproliferative disorders are potentially fatal complications of primary immunodeficiencies. It has been estimated that patients with congenital immunodeficiencies are 100–10 000 times more likely to develop cancer, and that 25% of them will develop a tumor, in particular a lymphoid neoplasm, some time during their life [4,5]. A recent report from the Immunodeficiency Cancer Registry (ICR) indicated that NHL constitutes more than 50% of all reported tumors in patients with immune deficiencies [5]. The largest number of cases of lymphoma in the ICR were reported in patients with AT (69 out of 160), followed by Wiskott–Aldrich syndrome (59 out of 78), common variable immunodeficiency (55 out of 120) and severe combined immunodeficiency (SCID) (31 out of 42). Nearly half the patients were diagnosed before reaching 10 years of age, and there was a slight preponderance of males (which reflects the large proportion of X-linked disorders such as Wiskott–Aldrich syndrome and SCID). Other inherited immunodeficiencies associated with LPDs include predominantly antibody deficiency syndromes, such as hyperimmunoglobulin (Ig) M (IgM) syndrome, X-linked agammaglobulinemia, IgA and IgG subclass deficiencies, Bloom's syndrome (characterized by chromosomal instability and increased susceptibility of cultured fibroblasts to γ-irradiation [14]), and phagocytic defect diseases such as the Chediak–Higashi syndrome. Although LPDs in patients with congenital immunodeficiencies are usually EBV associated, and of the B-cell type, a T-cell phenotype may occasionally be seen.

At least three major biological factors, either alone, or in conjunction with each other, are thought to be involved in the pathogenesis of LPD in this population of patients. These are: (1) EBV virus; (2) imbalanced production of cytokines secondary to host defects in immunoregulation; and (3) genetic defects resulting in ineffective or aberrant rearrangement of immunoglobulin and T-cell receptor genes during lymphopoiesis [13]. The first two of these factors are relevant to B-cell proliferation: EBV can drive B-cell proliferation through its latent genes, while predominance of 'TH2' cytokines, such as interleukins-4 and -6 (IL-4 and IL-6), activates the B-cell or humoral compartment of the immune system. Inherited defects in enzymes involved in DNA recombination and repair, in addition to affecting immunocompetence through impairment of lymphocyte differentiation, also increase the likelihood that genetic abnormalities will occur, some of which may influence lymphocyte growth and differentiation. The relative importance of these factors differs in different immunodeficiency syndromes and has been discussed further in Chapter 19.

IATROGENICALLY INDUCED IMMUNODEFICIENCIES

Organ transplant recipients

Immunosupressed organ transplant recipients have an increased risk of developing cancer [3,4]. Prevention of rejection requires long-term immunosuppression, which places recipients at an increased risk of both infections and posttransplant LPDs (PT-LPDs). The relative risk of developing a PT-LPD in such a setting is approximately 25–49 times greater than that expected in the general population [15,16]. The occurrence rate varies according to the organ transplanted, the age of the patient, the number of transplants a patient has had, and the type and dose of immunosuppressive therapy administered. The incidence appears to be highest in heart (1.8–9.8%) and combined heart–lung (4.6–9.4%) transplants [17–19], followed by renal transplants (1–3%) [20], liver transplants (2%) [15], and bone marrow transplants (especially when HLA mismatched and T-cell depleted) (1–2%) [21,22]. Individuals receiving cyclosporin A [23] and monoclonal antibody OKT3 [24] are amongst those at highest risk of developing an LPD. Hodgkin's disease is rare in the transplanted patient.

PT-LPDs account for 11% of second neoplasms in patients receiving regimens containing azathioprine or cyclophosphamide, compared to 16% in patients receiving cyclosporin A-based regimens. The time to development of the LPD is also shorter in the cyclosporin A group (32% occur within 4 months of transplant) as compared to 11% in the azothiaprine/cyclophosphamide group. The addition of OKT3 to the immunosuppressive regimen following cardiac transplantation has been reported to increase the incidence of PT-LPD nine-fold; the risk increases sharply after cumulative doses greater than 75 mg [24].

PT-LPDs in children differ from those in adults, both in frequency and presentation, being approximately six times higher in children than in adults (19% compared with 2.7%), and more likely to present with a picture resembling fulminating acute infectious monocucleosis [25]. In contrast to PT-LPD in adults, improved monitoring of cyclosporin A levels has not led to a decrease in PT-LPD in children. This is probably because many children have not been previously exposed to EBV and thus are more likely to develop a primary EBV infection. In Nalesnik's series of PT-LPD, for example, 94% of children and 42% of adults developed primary EBV infection [18]. Because of the lack of immunological memory, the proliferation of EBV-infected B-cells will be much less readily controlled [26]. An increased incidence of both EBV infections and PT-LPDs has been observed in children following the use of the immunosuppressant FK-506. In a series of 51 children treated with FK-506 following liver transplantation [25], the incidence of PT-LPD was much higher in the group given FK-506 (13.7%) than in the cyclosporin A group (2.2%). In children under the age of 5 years the difference was even greater (18.9% compared to 2.9%). The likeliest interpretation of these data is that the higher incidence of fulminant EBV infections and PT-LPDs observed in association with FK-506 is the result of more severe immunosuppression resulting from its use, compared to cyclosporin A.

PT-LPDs (after solid organ and post-bone marrow transplantation) are most commonly of B-cell origin and are nearly always associated with EBV, although cases in which EBV has not been detected even by sensitive hybridization techniques have been reported [26]. A few cases of T-cell PT-LPDs have been described [26–28]. The reason for their paucity is unknown, but may relate to the tendency for immunosuppressive drugs and some acquired forms of immunosuppression (e.g., HIV infection) to create an imbalance in T-cell helper (T_H) populations that favors a T_{H2}, i.e., B-cell promoting, pattern, and reduces the size of T-cell populations.

Bone marrow transplant recipients

Allogeneic bone marrow transplantation (BMT) differs from solid organ transplantation in that the patient receives a new immune system from an HLA-matched (or partially matched) donor, following ablation of his/her own immune system with radiation and chemotherapy. The temporary immunosuppression caused by marrow ablation (and therefore elimination of all precursor cells of the immune system as well as those of the hematopoietic system) recovers as mature lymphocytes and macrophages are generated from the donated bone marrow, but full recovery is delayed by the use of immunosuppressive therapy (cyclosporin A, methotrexate, prednisone) designed to prevent rejection of the graft and graft-versus-host disease (GVHD) [29]. Full immune constitution following a BMT, even without the added impediment of immunosuppressive therapy, takes from 6 months to 2 years [30]. Factors that contribute to the development of LPDs in this group of patients include acute or chronic GVHD (which results in lymphocyte activation), and prolonged immunosuppression, which, as in organ transplant recipients, impairs the regulation of the outgrowth of EBV-containing B-cells. Interestingly, the incidence of LPD in patients undergoing standard matched BMT is low. For example, only six cases were observed in a series of 1000 patients undergoing HLA-matched transplants at the Fred Hutchinson Cancer Center in Seattle [31]. However, with the increasing numbers of T-cell depleted, HLA-mismatched transplants being carried out today, there has been a significant rise in the EBV-associated LPDs, with actuarial risks of 6–12% being reported [32]. The addition of antithymocyte globulin in the early posttransplant period has been reported to increase this risk to 8% [22]. The LPDs arising in this setting are of donor cell origin (host lymphocytes having been ablated), contain EBV, and are usually observed in the first 6 months after bone marrow allografting, the period during which there is profound deficiency of T-cell function consequent upon the prior immunoablative cytoreduction. This can only be relieved by the emergence of functional donor T-cells [29,32–34].

Immunosuppressed patients not receiving an allograft

Another group of patients at risk for developing an LPD are those who are immunosuppressed secondary to the use of dose-intensive chemotherapy regimens for neoplasia, e.g., patients with leukemias. Only eight such patients have been reported so far, all of whom developed an EBV-positive LPD while on maintenance therapy [9]. LPDs have also been described in patients on immunosuppressive therapy (azothioprine, cyclophosphamide, methotrexate, and chlorambucil) for the treatment of various types of autoimmune disorders, including rheumatoid arthritis [35]. In this group, the relative risk of developing an LPD has been reported to be 11 times greater than in the general population. EBV association is rare, and has only been confirmed in one case [36].

Pathogenesis

Many authors have hypothesized that the development of PT-LPDs is a multistep process, which is related to EBV infection in the vast majority of patients [37,38]. Immunosuppressive therapy is believed to lead to reactivation of latent EBV infection in organ allograft recipients, as demonstrated in a prospective study involving 88 allograft recipients, where a four-fold increase in antibody titers to viral capsid antigen (VCA) occurred within 3 weeks of transplantation in 38% of individuals [39]. Primary infection with EBV may also occur in seronegative

patients (almost exclusively children), and in bone marrow transplant recipients in whom host EBV-containing cells are ablated by the preparative regimen. The successful control of EBV infection in an immunocompetent host ultimately depends on the establishment of an EBV-specific, major histocompatibility complex (MHC)-restricted, cytotoxic T-cell response, which is able to control latently infected B-cells. These T-cells react against EBV latent antigens, including EBV nuclear antigens (EBNAs) 1–6 and the latent membrane proteins (see Chapter 12). Humoral responses, antibody-dependent cellular toxicity, natural killer cell activity and endogenous interferons play a smaller role [1]. Two aspects of defective T-cell function are relevant to the outgrowth of PT-LPD. Firstly, impairment of the EBV-specific cytotoxic T-cell response is a crucial element in pathogenesis. This is supported by the mixed pattern of expression of EBV latent genes seen in many LPDs (even within the same LPD) [39a]. EBNA-2 and latent membrane protein (LMP)-1, for example, are not infrequently expressed in both PT-LPD and HIV-associated lymphomas [39b,39c], whereas EBNA-2 gene is expressed, if at all, only in a small minority of cells in EBV-associated neoplasms in normal hosts. It is reasonable to believe that LPDs that express EBNA-2 and other immunogenic latent genes would be eliminated in a normal host by the cytotoxic T-cell response.

In addition to cytotoxic T-cells, however, subsets of helper T-cells are also likely to be relevant, since T helper cells regulate many B-cell functions, either directly (e.g., by the expression of CD40 ligand, which binds to the corresponding receptor on B-cells) or indirectly, through the mediation of cytokines. IL-4, for example, is a B-cell growth factor, one pathway it utilizes being the induction of shedding of CD23, another B-cell surface molecule which, in its soluble form, acts as a B-cell growth factor [40]. IL-4 also directs B-cells to switch to the synthesis of IgE. Interferon-γ (IFNγ) and interferon-α (IFNα) inhibit these effects of IL-4 [41]. It is the balance of these cytokines that regulates the size of the B-cell population. B-Cell proliferation and function is favored by the T_{H2} subset of helper T-cells, i.e., cells which produce, when activated, IL-4, IL-5, IL-6, IL-9, IL-10 and IL-13, while T_{H1} cells, which produce IL-2, IFNγ and tumor necrosis factor-β (TNFβ), tend to suppress B-cell growth [42]. Recently, Mathur et al. measured serum levels of IL-4, IFNα and IgE in eight patients with recently diagnosed PT-LPD [43]. They compared the findings in these patients with those in healthy recipients of organ transplants (i.e., without LPD) receiving immunosuppressive therapy and normal EBV-seropositive controls. Levels of serum IL-4 were significantly elevated in both patients with LPD and healthy immunosuppressed organ transplant recipients, compared to normal individuals. Patients with PT-LPD, however, demonstrated a combination of significantly lower levels of serum IFNα and significantly higher levels of serum IgE, than either healthy EBV-seropositive individuals or healthy recipients of organ transplants receiving immunosuppressive therapy. These findings suggest that patients at risk to develop LPD have an imbalance between T_{H1} and T_{H2} responses, favoring T_{H2}-cells at the expense of T_{H1}-cells, and resulting in expansion of the B-cell compartment and rather poor cytotoxic T-cell responses, including T-cells specifically reactive against EBV. Other factors, such as the presence of foreign antigens introduced by the allograft, may also contribute to the immunological imbalance, perhaps because T-cells are activated by the foreign antigens; aberrations in the T-cell response may occur because of the drug-induced immunosuppression.

Whatever the precise mechanism, the net result is the expansion of multiple clones of EBV-containing B-cells, which tend to become fewer in number over time. This may relate to the elimination or control of clones which are more readily recognized by the residual T-cell response, or perhaps simply to competition among the clones for available growth factors, including antigens already encountered and sequestered in follicular center cells. The net result is that the number of proliferating clones decreases with time, the process becoming oligoclonal and finally monoclonal. This does not mean, however, that monoclonal lesions emerge later after transplant than polyclonal lesions. In fact, the time from transplant to diagnosis is similar in both in cyclosporin A-treated patients [18]. Clonal evolution can only occur when sufficient control is exerted over the B-cell clones to prevent rapid demise from overwhelming proliferation (as occurs, for example, in patients who encounter EBV for the first time or in bone marrow transplant recipients in whom all previous immunity against EBV is lost as a consequence of the myeloablative therapy). Thus, clonal evolution is likely to be influenced by the degree of immunosuppression. While the process of clonal selection is going on, it favors the development of genetic lesions. Some may be subtle (i.e., not recognized), but still able to contribute to the emergence of a single clone, while others may be identical to those associated with specific B-cell neoplasms that arise in the normal population. The latter suggests that there is also deregulation of B-cell ontogeny, since for reasons discussed elsewhere in this volume, chromosomal translocations, which are usually present in true malignant lymphomas, are more likely to occur in precursor cells.

A report by Knowles et al. [15] supports this paradigm as demonstrated in their recent study of 28 B-cell PT-LPDs (from 22 patients). These investigators conducted a detailed molecular analysis of LPDs, looking for rearrangements and/or mutations in selected proto-oncogenes (*bcl*-1, *bcl*-2, c-*myc*, H-, K- and N-*ras*) and p53. They made correlations with the morphological characteristics, presence of EBV infection and clonality (based on analysis of heavy and light chain rearrangements, and analysis of EBV terminal repeat sequences). They described three distinct clinicopathological categories of B-cell LPD, which are likely to be stages in a continuous spectrum: polyclonal (plasmacytic) hyperplasia; a monoclonal, although polymorphic process without oncogene or tumor suppressor gene abnormalities; and essentially monomorphic tumors possessing oncogene or p53 abnormalities (Table 45.1). These same investigators also demonstrated that separate PT-LPDs occurring synchronously in a single organ or patient may be histologically similiar, yet clonally distinct with respect to IgH gene rearrangements, oncogene alterations and EBV association, supporting the notion that clonal evolution occurs continuously from the underlying polyclonal process and that different clones may emerge at different sites [44]. Based on this observation, it would seem that a representative biopsy of only one of the several PT-LPD lesions in a given patient may not accurately reflect the clonality or pathological nature of the patient's disease. Moreover, true genetic transformation could be present at one site but not at another.

Table 45.1 Classification of posttransplant lymphoproliferative disorders (PT-LPDs)*

1. Plasmacytic hyperplasia
   Commonly arise in the oropharynx or lymph nodes
   Nearly always polyclonal
   Usually contain multiple clones of EBV
   No oncogene and tumor suppressor gene alterations

2. Polymorphic B-cell hyperplasia and polymorphic B-cell lymphoma
   Can involve lymph nodes or extranodal sites
   Nearly always monoclonal
   Usually contain a single clone of EBV
   No oncogene or tumor suppressor gene alterations

3. Immunoblastic lymphoma or multiple myeloma
   Present with widely disseminated disease
   Always monoclonal
   Contain a single clone of EBV
   Contain alterations of one or more oncogenes or tumor suppressor genes (N-*ras*, p53, c-*myc*)

EBV, Epstein–Barr virus.
* Based on Knowles et al. [15].

This could have an impact upon the choice of therapy.

It is important to note that the term 'monoclonal' is not synonymous with neoplasia and, moreover, it simply indicates that a single clone is sufficiently represented in the cell population studied to be detected by the assay used. In the case of a Southern blot for immunoglobulin gene analysis, a single clone is detected if it constitutes 5–10% of the cell population. When EBV terminal repeat analysis is performed, considerable less representation of a single clone within the population (certainly less than 1%) is required, because multiple genomes are present in each cell. Thus, many LPDs referred to as 'monoclonal' may actually consist of multiple, even very large numbers of clones, one of which is sufficiently represented to be detected by the assay used. The extent to which this is true will depend upon the rapidity with which a single clone replaces all other clones in the initial polyclonal population. Occasionally, as occurs in Wiscott–Aldrich syndrome, for example, the outgrowth of a single clone may occur *de novo*; such clones sometimes persist for some time (usually measured in months) before regressing and are clearly not malignant even though such a clone could theoretically undergo malignant transformation. True neoplasia is, of course, also monoclonal but when neoplastic cells are interspersed among nonneoplastic yet expanded B-cell populations, the presence of the monoclonal neoplastic population could be missed unless molecular analysis capable of detecting it is performed. This situation has been described in patients with HIV-associated lymphomas in whom monoclonality at the c-*myc* locus but polyclonality at the immunoglobulin locus has been described in the same lymph node sample [45].

ACQUIRED IMMUNE DEFICIENCIES

With the advent of the acquired immunodeficiency syndrome (AIDS), there has been a sharp increase in the incidence of HIV-associated lymphomas. The risk of acquiring an HIV-associated LPD has been estimated to be approximately 30% after 3 years of treatment for HIV infection [46] and it has been calculated that between 8% and 27% of all non-Hodgkin's lymphomas (NHL) in the USA may be related to HIV infection [47]. The majority of HIV-associated lymphomas are of the B-cell type, and usually fall into the category of diffuse large-cell (immunoblastic) lymphoma or small noncleaved cell lymphoma (SNCC). Immunoblastic lymphomas tend to occur in patients with severe immunosuppression, are usually EBV-associated (80%), uncommonly possess c-*myc*/immunoglobulin translocations, and

their incidence increases with age. SNCL occur predominantly in patients in the first two decades of life, are more frequently the AIDS-defining illness (i.e., they often occur in patients who are not yet grossly immunosuppressed), are usually associated with a c-*myc*/immunoglobulin translocation, and are less often EBV-associated (35–40%) than immunoblastic lymphomas. Lymphomas involving the central nervous system are almost always immunoblastic lymphomas and are uniformly associated with EBV [48]. The HIV-associated LPDs are discussed in detail in Chapter 20.

Histopathology

The histological appearance of B-cell LPD in patients with underlying immunodeficiency syndromes is heterogeneous, but these disorders can be broadly classified as polymorphic or monomorphic. The relative proportions of polymorphic to monomorphic LPDs vary in different immunodeficiency syndromes and, particularly in the PT-LPDs, different lesions in the same patient may exhibit varying degrees of polymorphism. Individual cells have an appearance ranging from activated lymphocytes, through immunoblasts with varying degrees of plasmacytoid differentiation, to mature plasma cells. Most of these same cell types can be seen in EBV-transformed lymphoblastoid cell lines (although terminal differentiation to plasma cells is rare *in vitro*), which is consistent with the notion that the origin of a large number of the LPDs arising in immunodeficient patients represent B-cells transformed by EBV and that the observed polymorphism is primarily a manifestation of variability in the degree of differentiation of these activated B-cells. Occasionally, cell types resembling germinal center cells are seen, but these are likely to be left over from the underlying normal germinal centers, for LPD commonly effaces the normal nodal architecture. Some patients, particularly those with HIV infection or with AT, have diseases that are indistinguishable from NHL occurring in the general population. Patients with PT-LPD, however, are more likely to have polymorphic processes that differ markedly, histologically, from NHL occurring in the absence of underlying immunosuppression. Frizzera et al. divided these cases into polymorphic hyperplasia and polymorphic lymphoma [37,38], based on histological evidence suggesting a more or less aggressive process; in addition to disruption of the normal nodal architecture, invasion of blood vessels, nerves and normal tissue, PT-LPDs have varying degrees of cytological atypia and necrosis. However, the underlying implication that polymorphic hyperplasia is benign and polymorphic lymphoma malignant has been questioned. Intermediate forms between Frizzera's hyperplasia and lymphoma are observed, while different patterns may be evident in biopsies from separate sites. Moroever, similar features may be seen in the lymph nodes of normal patients with infectious mononucleosis, so that these seemingly aggressive characteristics do not signify that the process is irreversible or that genetic changes relevant to true lymphoid neoplasia are present.

The fraction of PT-LPDs that have a monomorphic appearance is usually referred to as immunoblastic lymphoma, although occasionally an appearance indistinguishable from multiple myeloma is seen. Typical monomorphic lymphomas of large noncleaved cell type, Burkitt's lymphoma and Burkitt-like lymphomas do occur, but are relatively uncommon in PT-LPD, accounting, for example, for only some 14% of the series of Nalesnik and colleagues [18]. In contrast, in HIV-related lymphomas, polymorphic forms are uncommon and the majority of cases can be classified either as SNCC or immunoblastic lymphoma. In AIDS, as in PT-LPD, occasional cases are indistinguishable from multiple myeloma, although these tumors, which may be seen in young adults, are usually EBV-associated [48a] and may even contain *myc*/immunoglobulin translocations.

Recently, Knowles, Frizzera and others proposed a new classification of PT-LPDs. They distinguished three major categories (Table 45.1). The first, plasmacytic hyperplasia, includes lesions in which the underlying architecture of the lymph node is retained, but germinal centers tend to be hypoplastic and the interfollicular area is infiltrated with plasmacytoid lymphocytes and plasma cells, with rare immunoblasts. This morphological category is polyclonal and is likely to have been included in the polymorphic category described by Nalesnik et al. [18]. In the series by Knowles et al. [15], in contrast to that of Nalesnik et al., all cases of PT-LPD occurring in the tonsils and adenoids belonged to this category. The second category of Knowles et al. encompasses Frizzera's polymorphic hyperplasia and polymorphic lymphoma categories, but in spite of the apparent morphological differences between these two, they appeared on the basis of a molecular analysis to be a homogeneous group, characterized by monoclonality but without structural changes in oncogenes or tumor suppressor genes. While in earlier studies polymorphic lesions had been shown to be either polyclonal or monoclonal, this may have been a result of the inclusion of Knowles plasmacytic hyperplasia in this category. The second category may have a parallel in the EBV 'immortalized' cells that grow *in vitro* as cell lines. The cells

vary with respect to their degree of plasmacytic differentiation and they rapidly become monoclonal *in vitro*, but do not normally develop chromosomal changes characteristic of particular neoplasms. Finally, Knowles et al. identified a category of 'true' neoplasia, characterized by an appearance of immunoblastic lymphoma or multiple myeloma, in association with structural changes in oncogenes or p53. All tumors in this category were also monoclonal.

The borderland between neoplasia and nonneoplastic lymphoproliferation, i.e., a lymphoproliferative process that would progress in an individual without pre-existing immunodeficiency versus lymphoproliferation that would be readily controlled in a normal individual, is extremely difficult, if not impossible to define on the basis of morphology alone. The expression of highly immunogenic EBNAs, such as EBNA-2, in tumors that are morhologically similar to immunoblastic lymphoma supports this notion. Moreover, whether or not the process would result in the death of an immunocompetent individual is irrelevant to the outcome in the immunosuppressed individual. What matters to the clinician is the extent to which any given morphological classification provides information regarding the therapy to which the patient is most likely to respond. At present, morphology is not very useful in this regard – nor is clonality when considered alone. In the meantime, it would be reasonable to confine the term 'lymphoma' to monoclonal lesions that are histologically identical to malignant lymphomas that can occur in the normal population, or to lesions in which a genetic defect that has been observed in lymphomas in the general population is detectable. It should be borne in mind, however, as already mentioned, that truly neoplastic cells (i.e., possessing genetic changes associated with a specific lymphoma) may, at least early in the evolution of the neoplasm, account for only a fraction of the cells in a given lesion.

Clinical characteristics

The clinical manifestations of LPDs are also quite variable. The presentation may range from localized indolent nodal or extranodal disease to a fulminant, rapidly progressive syndrome with high-grade fever, massive lymphadenopathy and splenomegaly [1,49, 50]. The central nervous system (CNS) is frequently involved. Allograft recipients chronically receiving immunosuppressive drugs, particularly older patients who received an organ graft some years before, more commonly present with slow-growing extranodal masses, which are often localized, while individuals with congenital immunodeficiency and BMT recipients more often present with aggressive, disseminated disease, in the case of BMT recipients, shortly after (within months) of the transplant [1].

Patients with LPD may present with a syndrome that closely resembles infectious monocumeosis, including fever, lymphadenopathy, splenomegaly tonsillitis and pharyngitis. In children particularly, pharyngeal adenopathy may cause acute, life-threatening airway obstruction. Gastrointestinal symptoms are frequently encountered, owing to masses of lymphoid tissue within or adjacent to bowel, and LPD may cause bowel obstruction or perforation. A third common type of presentation is with organ dysfunction, particularly, lung, liver and kidney, while CNS symptoms may herald CNS involvement. Systemic symptoms including fever, malaise and weight loss may occur with any of these presentations [49,50]. The relative frequency of involvement of various sites is shown in Table 45.2.

It has been suggested that the organ distribution of LPD lesions is determined partly by the allograft itself, and partly by the type and intensity of the immunosuppressive regimen. CNS involvement, for example, appears to be most frequent (40%) in patients on immunosuppressive regimens that do not contain cyclosporin A [51], while the lungs have been reported to be involved in almost 60–80% of heart–lung transplant recipients, and only 30% of kidney, liver or bone marrow recipients. Certain organs appear to be involved more often in particular groups of patients. For example, the liver is a frequent site of involvement in BMT recipients (50%), the lungs in heart (54%) or BMT (38%) recipients, the CNS in renal transplant patients (24%), and the kidneys in BMT (41%) or liver transplants recipients (33%).

In Leblond's series [49], the interval between transplantation and a diagnosis of LPD ranged from 60 days to 4140 days, with a mean of 771 days and a median of 210 days. It was shorter in heart and lung recipients (60–1980 days with a median of 150 days) than in kidney recipients (180–4140 days, with a median of 420 days). Patients treated with cyclosporin A also tend to develop LPD earlier than patients treated with azathioprine [18]. Perhaps not surprisingly, the median interval to the appearance of LPD decreased as the intensity of the immunosuppressive regimen increased.

Diagnosis

The diagnosis of a LPD should be suspected in the presence of suggestive physical findings and a history of either an inherited immunodeficiency disorder or organ/bone marrow transplant. Confirmation requires biopsy of one or more involved areas and, wherever possible, additional studies, including immunophenotyping, cytogenetics, molecular analysis and examination for the presence of EBV genomes in the lymphoid cells.

There are no definitive laboratory abnormalities that are characteristic for LPD. Relevant investigations at diagnosis should include at least a peripheral blood count, renal profile, liver function tests, lactic dehydrogenase (LDH) level, and immunoglobulin electrophoresis. An elevated LDH and monoclonal immunoglobulin spikes, if present, may be useful markers to follow disease. Bilateral bone marrow aspirates and biopsies should be performed to rule out involvement, even though this is rare.

Owing to the propensity of the LPDs to involve any organ, including the CNS, radiological evaluation of the patient should include a computed tomography (CT) scan or magnetic resonance image (MRI) of the head, neck, chest and abdomen. The uptake of gallium-67 by LPDs is variable [1]. It is often worth performing this study at presentation, however, since it can be helpful in detecting occult sites of disease and following the patient.

EBV serology is frequently abnormal in patients with B-cell LPD, but serological patterns vary and, to a degree, relate to the underlying disease. Many patients have very high anti-VCA titers but lack anti-EBNA antibodies. This, however, is not a consistent finding, and some patients with X-linked lymphoproliferative (XLP) or XLP-like syndromes,

Table 45.2 Common sites of involvement in B-cell lymphoproliferative disorders

Site	% of patients
Lymph nodes	59
Liver	31
Lung	29
Kidney	25
Bone marrow	25
Small intestine	22
Spleen	21
Central nervous system	19
Large intestine	14
Tonsils	10
Adrenals	9
Skin/soft tissue	7
Blood	6
Heart	5
Salivary glands	4

Prepared with information obtained from Romagnani [42].

for example, may be unable to mount a humoral response to EBV. For the detection of EBV genomes, *in situ* hybridization, in which an EBV-specific probe is reacted with viral DNA present in tissue sections (Figure 45.1), is probably the most reliable method available today, and the presence of EBV in a pathologically consistent lesion is strongly suggestive of a diagnosis of LPD. EBV clonality can also be detected by Southern blot (or polymerase chain reaction, but the sensitivity of this assay may be misleading, since EBV-containing normal lymphocytes may be detectable in an otherwise EBV-negative pathological lesion), and if terminal repeat region probes are used, the technique can also be used to assess clonality [52].

It is important to perform biopsies on as many sites of LPD as is conveniently possible in a given patient, for reasons discussed earlier.

Prevention of LPD

Improved understanding of the causes of LPD in patients with inherited and acquired immunodeficiency disorders should lead to the development of strategies for preventing its development. In patients with inherited disorders, the most obvious preventative measure is reversal of the immunodeficiency itself by performing a bone marrow transplantation – an approach which is, of course, primarily undertaken to treat the underlying disease. While this approach can be highly successful, it is disease-dependent, since the increased risk of neoplasia in some inherited immunodeficiency syndromes, as already mentioned, is not simply related to immunodeficiency, but may sometimes be the result of chromosomal fragility or defective DNA repair, e.g., in Bloom's syndrome and AT. In fact, immunological reconstitution provides the possibility of determining whether the immunosuppression is the primary cause of the predisposition to LPD, or whether associated chromosomal fragility or defects in DNA repair are paramount. In children with SCID and Wiskott–Aldrich syndrome, full immunological reconstitution appears to prevent LPD. In one series of 48 SCID patients, for example, no LPD occurred over a period of more than 20 years of follow-up [53]. In a small number of patients with these diseases in whom reconstitution was partial, however, the increased risk of LPD persisted [54]. In contrast, relief of immunosuppression in AT by transplantation does not appear to prevent LPD, suggesting that the markedly increased tendency of such patients to develop chromosomal translocations is the primary cause of their predisposition to LPD [55]. In the XLP syndrome, boys are unable to control primary EBV infection and many die from fulminating infectious mononucleosis, but allogeneic BMT has led to successful immunological reconstitution and prevention of LPD even in patients suffering acutely from infectious mononucleosis [56]. An alternative approach that has met with some success in preventing EBV infection and its potentially devestating consequences in the XLP syndrome is the use of intravenous immunoglobulin containing neutralizing antibodies against EBV [57].

In the acquired immunodeficiency disorders, complete reversal of immunosuppression is frequently not possible. HIV-associated LPD, for example, is not prevented by the partial improvement in immune function occasioned by antiretroviral therapy, while in patients iatrogenically immunosuppressed to permit allografting, the discontinuation of all immunosuppressive drugs will result in graft rejection. Reduction of the risk of PT-LPD, however, can be accomplished by careful choice of the immunosuppressive regimen, and/or by addressing the specific issue of immunological responsiveness to EBV-infected cells. In this context, the all-embracing term 'immunosuppression' belies the qualitative and quantitative differences that result from different drug regimens, and it is not surprising that different drug regimens are associated with differences in the risk of developing LPD. The increased risk associated with the use of anti-CD3 monoclonal antibodies and FK-506 have already been alluded to, but risk is also a function of dose. The risk of developing LPD appeared to increase, for example, when cyclosporin A was first introduced into the immunosuppressive regimens of organ transplant recipients. From 4% to 10% of patients developed LPD in early studies [58–60], but in subsequent studies, in which lower doses of the drug were used as the sole immunosuppressive agent, less than 1% of patients developed LPD [61,62].

The increased incidence of LPD in patients who

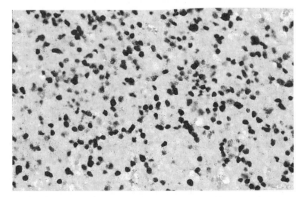

Figure 45.1 Demonstration of EBV association in an LPD by *in situ* hybridization with an EBER (a small, EBV-coded RNA molecule) probe.

receive T-cell-depleted allografts [21,63–65] also has implications for prevention, for this finding suggests that EBV-specific cytotoxic T-cells present in whole bone marrow preparations prevent outgrowth of LPD. The findings also imply that in patients undergoing allografting it ought to be possible to preserve or replenish those elements of the immune system relevant to the development of LPD (e.g., immunological memory for EBV-coded antigens) while maintaining sufficient immunosuppression to prevent graft rejection. BMT is, of course, a special case, since the patient becomes a chimera in whom the hematopoietic and immune systems are of donor origin – as will be all LPDs that evolve, assuming that chimerism is complete. In this circumstance, immunocompetent donor cells can be administered, without fear of rejection, to the transplant recipient to compensate for the absence of immunological memory in the newly developing immune system. In addition, LPD of donor origin appears to be confined to the first 6 months or so after transplantation – the period of severe immunosuppression. The infusion of whole leukocyte preparations, however, entails significant risk, particularly if given soon after the transplant, since donor T-cells can react against normal host tissues and induce GVHD [66] (T-cells that develop from the transplanted marrow will have developed in the context of host tissues such that most host-reactive cells should have been eliminated). Thus, a more attractive approach is to use EBV-specific T-cell clones. Early data from St Jude Children's Research Hospital in Memphis suggest that this approach is likely to be successful [67].The St Jude investigators showed reversal of evidence of EBV reactivation in three recipients of bone marrow allografts (namely, a marked reduction in the levels of EBV DNA detected in circulating cells), and minimal toxicity in these three and seven other patients who received infusions of EBV-specific T-cells as prophylaxis.

Another approach to the prevention of EBV-associated LPD in BMT recipients is the avoidance of EBV infection from the donor – the origin of the virus that causes EBV-associated LPD in many patients, since the preparative regimens used prior to BMT have been shown to eliminate the host B-cell population that harbours EBV [68]. The availability of donors is usually sufficiently limited that choosing an EBV-negative donor is not practical, but methods to eliminate EBV-containing cells from the donated bone marrow could be developed. Indeed, the depletion of B-cells from the bone marrow product (some of which will contain EBV in a seropositive donor) does appear to reduce markedly the increased risk of development of LPD in patients who receive T-cell-depleted bone marrows [21,69], although whether infused EBV-infected B-cells give

rise to LPD directly in such patients, or whether activation of EBV replication and infection of other B-cells, including newly developed B-cells (from the grafted marrow), is required for an LPD to develop is not known. The risk of EBV infection subsequent to transplantation can be reduced by eliminating leukocytes from blood products administered to the patient by the use of leukocyte filters (EBV-seronegative donors are likely to be very few) and limiting exposure to the saliva of seropositive individuals (90% of the population), the other potential source of EBV infection of the BMT recipient.

While there is good evidence for activation of the EBV replicative cycle in immusuppressed individuals [39,39c], the role this plays in the development of LPD is unknown. If EBV replication is a necessary component of the development of LPD, e.g., because the B-cells that normally harbor EBV genomes are incapable of developing into proliferating cells, such that only virus release and infection of other, transformation susceptible cells, can result in LPD, it might be expected that acyclovir or ganciclovir, both of which inhibit EBV replication, would reduce the incidence of LPD (acyclovir, or ganciclovir, is now used almost routinely in patients undergoing BMT or organ transplants in order to prevent cytomegalovirus disease, but also appear to reduce the risk of infection or reactivation of other herpesviruses [70]). Interestingly, in SCID mice inoculated with human lymphocytes from seropositive donors, the administration of acyclovir did not prevent or delay outgrowth of LPD, although ganciclovir did delay outgrowth of LPD when lymphocytes from seronegative donors were used in conjunction with active infection with EBV [71]. In spite of these results, retrospective comparison of the incidence of EBV-associated LPD in the recipients of T-cell-depleted bone marrow allografts who received or did not receive acyclovir has suggested that this drug may prevent LPD: Trigg et al. reported that LPD developed in 6 out of 25 patients who did not receive acyclovir but in none of 40 patients who received it [65]. In this context, the demonstration by Rooney et al. [67] that EBV reactivation, a potential marker of increased risk for the development of EBV-associated disease, can be measured by quantification of circulating EBV, could prove to be of value in identifying high-risk patients in whom preventative strategies can be explored. Similarly, since patients with EBV-associated LPD have been shown to have significantly lower levels of serum IFNα and higher levels of IL-4 than normal seropositive individuals or posttransplant patients who do not have LPD [43], i.e., a predominantly T_{H2} cytokine profile, it may be possible to identify patients at high risk to develop LPD by measurement of serum IFNα

and/or IL-4 (or other cytokines, or immunoglobulin E). The ability to identify patients at high risk for the development of EBV-associated LPD would permit more more efficient testing of preventative strategies, such as the adminstration of acyclovir, ganciclovir, IFNα or IFNγ, or the use, in allogeneic BMT recipients, of specifically immune donor T-cells.

Treatment

The selection of an optimal treatment approach for an immunosuppressed patient with a lymphoproliferative disorder is not always straightforward, and is made more difficult by the relatively small size of published series and the diversity of approaches that have been employed, coupled to variability in histological categorization and the investigations performed. In making a sound decision, both the type of lymphoproliferative disorder and the underlying immunodeficiency syndrome must be taken into consideration. Some of the lymphoproliferative lesions that arise in patients after allografting exist at the borderland of neoplasia and may regress following withdrawal of iatrogenic immunosuppression, while others fulfill all criteria of malignant neoplasia and may progress in spite of intensive chemotherapy. It is particularly important to recognize that immunosuppressed patients tolerate chemotherapy poorly, largely because of the increased risk of opportunistic infections. Patients with LPD after BMT appear to have a worse prognosis (until recently, the majority of patients died [32,33]) than patients who develop LPD after organ transplantation, in whom 40–50% of patients survive [26,72]. Such differences may relate to the degree of immunosuppression (and the possibility of discontinuing or reducing the dose of immunosuppressive drugs in organ transplant recipients), tolerance to chemotherapy used in the treatment of the LPD, the type of therapy administered or the type of lymphoproliferative syndrome. In general, patients with monoclonal disease and those who present late have a worse prognosis than those who present early with polyclonal disease [18,49], but in the absence of lymphoma-specific genetic derrangements, such as a c-*myc*/immunoglobulin translocation, chemotherapy is not necessarily the treatment of choice for all patients with monoclonal disease. Regression of monoclonal lesions following reduction of the dose of immunosuppressive drugs is well documented [72], as is response to IFNα. Other factors, particularly the extent of disease and rapidity of progression, should be taken into consideration, while in specific diseases the severity of tissue damage associated with some treatment modalities is

considerably enhanced. For example, patients with AT are particularly radiosensitive and may develop severe local toxicity even when low doses of radiation are administered; they may also develop greater toxicity with radiomimetic drugs such as bleomycin, and appear to be at increased risk for the development of hemorrhagic cystitis in association with the administration of oxazaphosphorines [73,74]. The latter is readily prevented by administration of mesna.

A treatment algorithm for LPD is shown in Table 45.3. The main therapeutic approaches currently in use include withdrawal of immunosupression, IFNα (often with intravenous gammaglobulin), anti-B-cell monoclonal antibodies, immunotherapy with T-cells

Table 45.3 Treatment of B-cell lymphoproliferative disease in immunosuppressed patients

---

Inherited immunodeficiency syndromes

Polyclonal or monoclonal with no genetic abnormalities

Localized
  Radiation/surgery (low dose in AT)

Generalized
  Interferon-α
  Anti-B-cell monoclonal antibodies
  Chemotherapy if no response, rapidly progressive or recurrent

Monoclonal with a specific genetic abnormality
  Chemotherapy

Post-organ transplant

Polyclonal or monoclonal with no genetic abnormalities
  Reduce dose of immunosuppressive drugs if possible

Localized
  Radiation/surgery

Generalized
  Interferon-α
  Anti-B-cell monoclonal antibodies
  Chemotherapy if no response, rapidly progressive or recurrent

Monoclonal with a specific genetic abnormality
  Chemotherapy

Post-bone marrow transplant

  Donor leukocyte infusions, preferably EBV-specific
  Interferon-α
  Anti-B-cell monoclonal antibodies
  Chemotherapy if no response or recurrence

Monoclonal with a specific genetic abnormality
  Chemotherapy

AT, Ataxia telangiectasia; EBV, Epstein–Barr virus.

and cytotoxic drugs. The mere documentation of monoclonality is not an indication for cytotoxic chemotherapy, but chemotherapy should be considered as first-line treatment in patients in whom the disease is monoclonal and contains non-random genetic lesions, and it should be strongly considered in patients in whom there is widespread disease undergoing rapid progression. Chemotherapy is also indicated in patients with progressive disease in whom other approaches to therapy have failed. A combination of chemotherapy and IFNα may be considered in some circumstances.

WITHDRAWAL OF IMMUNOSUPPRESSION

Withdrawal or reduction of immunosuppressive drugs in patients with LPD after organ transplantation or with autoimmune disease can lead to regression even in patients with monoclonal LPD, if localized, but this approach is rarely successful in patients with widespread LPD, whether polyclonal or monoclonal [18,38,75,75a]. It appears that complete removal of immunosuppressive drugs is not essential for regression to occur. Nalesnik et al., for example, have suggested that posttransplant LPD always results from overimmunosuppression – which does not necessarily relate to the dosage of immunosuppressive drugs [72] – and that as much as a 50% reduction in cyclosporin A dosage can frequently be accomplished with only a small risk of organ rejection. Evidence of regression often occurs within days and is unlikely to occur if there has been no reduction in size within a period of two weeks – or, of course, if there is disease progression. In the presence of genetic abnormalities in oncogenes, or a p53 mutation, the likelihood of regression upon reduction of immunosuppression is small [15].

INTERFERON-α

If withdrawal of immunosuppression fails, or is not possible, IFNα, with or without intravenous immunoglobulin, should be considered. The available data suggest that clonality does not appear to influence the likelihood of success of IFNα [76], but perhaps other parameters, such as the level of serum IFNα, may prove to be predictors of response. IFNα can inhibit the effects of IL-4 on B-cells, including CD23 expression and production of soluble CD23, cell growth and immunoglobulin class switching [77]. Since IFNγ has similar effects, it would be of interest to study the effect of this cytokine (or a combination if IFNα and IFNγ) on LPD.

B-CELL MONOCLONAL ANTIBODIES

Murine anti-B-cell monoclonal antibodies specific for B-cell membrane antigens, including CD21, CD24 and CD23, have been shown to prevent the growth in SCID mice of B-cell lines obtained from patients with lymphoproliferative disease [78]. Anti-CD24 and anti-CD21 antibodies also inhibited the growth of the LPD in the patients from whom the cell lines were derived. In a larger series of patients with LPD following bone marrow (14) or organ transplants (12), these same antibodies, administered daily for 10 days, induced complete remission in 16 patients with oligoclonal LPD, but not in 7 patients with monoclonal LPD. Two patients who had oligoclonal proliferation as well as CNS involvement achieved systemic but not CNS remission, and died from progression of their CNS disease [34]. Stephan et al. reported the direct injection of monoclonal antibodies into the cerebrospinal fluid (via an Ommaya reservoir) in a patient with CNS LPD with excellent results [79].

In a more recent report, Leblond et al. treated ten patients with post-organ transplant LPD with anti-CD21 and anti-CD24 antibodies for 10 days after failure of reduction of immunosuppressive therapy to halt disease progression [49]. Eight patients, three of whom had monoclonal disease, achieved a sustained complete remission within 2 weeks to 3 months. One of these patients subsequently developed a second malignancy and died. Two patients with CNS disease received intraventricular monoclonal antibodies and one achieved a partial response, while the other had no response.

ANTIVIRAL (EBV) STRATEGIES

Acyclovir has been used in patients with EBV-associated LPD as well as patients suffering from XLP with fulminant infectious mononucleosis, but no clear benefits have been demonstrated in spite of some reports of regression, particularly in young patients with an infectious mononucleosis-like syndrome occurring in the first 9 months of immunosuppression. In these cases simultaneous reduction of immunosuppression may have been the element that led to regression [50,75,80–82]. The lack of a clear benefit of acyclovir is not surprising, since its action is to inhibit virion replication; there is no reason to suppose it would have a significant effect on the growth of LPD cells which contain EBV in a latent state – indeed, viral replication leads to cell death, so that inhibition of the lytic cycle is actually undesirable, although only a small percentage, at most, of LPD cells are likely to be producing virus at any point in time. Acyclovir has been shown to be ineffective in older patients who present years after the transplantation with a localized EBV-associated tumor mass [82]. However, while ineffective in the treatment of established LPD, acyclovir may have a role in prevention, as discussed above.

Infusions of donor T-cells have been successful in patients with monomorphic EBV-associated LPD after T-cell-depleted allogeneic BMT. Papadopoulos treated five patients with 10^6 CD3-positive cells per kilogram of body weight – a dose approximately ten times lower than that provided by an unmodified (i.e., without T-cell depletion) bone marrow allograft, but some ten times higher than that administered in a T-cell-depleted allograft [22]. All five achieved a complete remission. Two patients subsequently died of progressive pulmonary failure; in both cases, the onset of pulmonary dysfunction was associated with the development of LPD at other sites. Three patients were alive and free of disease at 10,16 and 16 months at the time of publication; all three developed mild chronic GVHD (two had also had acute, grade II GVHD of the skin [22]). To avoid GVHD, Rooney et al. used *in vitro* cultured, EBV-specific cytotoxic T-cell lines derived from cells obtained from donor peripheral blood on the day of marrow harvest [67]. T-Cells were stimulated by irradiated autologous EBV-transformed B-cells and cultured in the presence of IL-2. In a patient with LPD diagnosed as immunoblastic lymphoma that developed 3 months after BMT, a complete response was observed after four infusions of EBV-specific cytotoxic T-cells [60]. Of additional interest in this case was the observation that both EBNA-2 and LMP-1 were expressed in this tumor. Both antigens are capable of exciting an immune response in an immunocompetent individual, and their expression is likely to have been responsible for the regression observed after administration of the cytotoxic lymphocytes. This lymphoma, in other words, despite its morphological appearance, would not have developed in an immunocompetent individual.

ROLE OF LOCAL THERAPY

Perhaps surprisingly, a fraction of patients who develop LPD post-organ transplant appear to have localized disease – usually in the head and neck, gastrointestinal tract, or in a solid organ - quite frequently the grafted organ. This could be a consequence of antigenic stimulation of host lymphocytes by the grafted organ, although there is no evidence to support this hypothesis. Why involvement of the grafted organ occurs particularly in patients who receive heart–lung transplants is not known [19]. Allograft involvement occurs in some 15–30% of kidney transplant recipients, and in a smaller fraction of heart transplants [16,18,83]. LPD arising from donor cells in organ transplant recipients is much less common than is the case in BMT recipients, but does occasionally occur [84,85], raising the possibility that donor lymphocytes present in the graft may be protected from host immunosurveillance. In any event, if the LPD is confined to the grafted organ, suggesting that this environment is particularly favorable, removal of the organ (usally only feasible if it is a kidney) or local radiation therapy may be effective. Local therapy is usually performed in concert with a reduction of immunosuppression and is particularly indicated when there is a local mass effect, e.g., airway or intestinal obstruction, or bowel perforation.

While the use of local radiation is attractive in immunosuppressed patients who have localized disease, since such patients will tolerate chemotherapy poorly, in patients with disseminated disease in whom chemotherapy is planned, the addition of radiation therapy is not recommended, since it is likely to add to toxicity and there is no evidence that it will increase efficacy.

CHEMOTHERAPY

The treatment of LPD with chemotherapy has, in general, been disappointing. Perhaps the major reason for this has been the empirical application of the drug regimens used in patients who develop diffuse large B-cell lymphomas *de novo* for patients with LPD. This approach has led, not surprisingly, to a high incidence of serious toxicity, at least in part accounting for the poor survival rates obtained. For example, three toxic deaths occurred among five patients with posttransplant lymphomas treated initially with chemotherapy by Leblond et al. [49]. Similar experiences have been reported by others [18,75,86,87]. In addition, since the pathogenesis of LPD is different from that of *de novo* lymphoma, there is no reason to believe that standard regimens represent the best approach. There is, perhaps, good reason to return to basics, and ask the questions 'which patients with LPD should be treated with chemotherapy?' and 'what chemotherapy should be used?'. At the present time, there are no definitive answers to these questions, but the present state of our knowledge does permit the application of reasonable guidelines to the first question, while the answer to the second will only come from empirical clinical trials, the conduct of which will require collaboration among transplant surgeons and oncologists.

Which patients should be treated with chemotherapy?

Chemotherapy cannot be undertaken lightly in immunosuppressed patients. Consideration should, therefore, be first given to treatment approaches which do not entail chemotherapy. In transplant recipients the dosage of immunosuppressive therapy should be reduced as much as possible, but patients with widespread disease are unlikely to respond to this approach. When disease is localized, surgery and/or radiation should also be considered. Patients in whom a reduction of immunosupression fails are candidates for IFNα or anti-B-cell antibody therapy. In allogeneic BMT recipients, infusion of donor T-cells is rapidly becoming the treatment of choice. Patients in whom these approaches have failed, or patients in whom the LPD is associated with characteristic genetic abnormality, are candidates for chemotherapy.

What chemotherapy should be used?

Since patients with underlying immunosuppression tolerate chemotherapy poorly, there seems little point in continuing to use standard, multidrug regimens, e.g., cytoxan, Adriamycin, vincristine, prednisone (CHOP) or similar combinations, which in general have produced survival rates of less than 20% [55,75,86,87]. It seems more reasonable to examine the efficacy of regimens that are minimally myelosuppressive and immunosuppressive. Our approach in children with LPD associated with immunosuppression at the National Cancer Institute (NCI), Bethesda, has been to explore the efficacy of two simple drug regimens – one that includes only cyclophosphamide and high-dose methotrexate, and another which contains ifosfamide and high-dose cytosine arabinoside (Ara-C) (Figure 45.2). Cyclophosphamide and high-dose methotrexate alone have been shown to be reasonably effective in patients with Burkitt's lymphoma [88]. Each of the drugs in these regimens is given at full dosage, and myelosuppression is minimized by using granulocyte colony-stimulating factor. Only three cycles of therapy are given, since prolonged therapy is unlikely to be tolerated, and in any event is not known to be advantageous. Prophylactic acyclovir, pneumocystis prophylaxis, and in HIV-positive patients for whom the regimens are also used, antiretroviral therapy are administered during and after chemotherapy. In the small number of patients (8) with either HIV-associated or transplant-associated LPD refractory to IFNα, the cyclophosphamide/methotrexate regimen has been well tolerated and good responses have been seen. The second regimen, ifosfamide and Ara-C, has so far been reserved for patients who relapse, but has also been shown to be active and tolerable, although too few patients have been treated with either regimen to date to provide an accurate estimate of efficacy. Ultimately, the possibility of incorporating both drug combinations into an alternating regimen is an attractive one. They have both been well tolerated, even by heavily immunosuppressed patients.

Patients with AT, who generally have heightened susceptibility to radiation and chemotherapy are a special case. Their predisposition to the development of LPD appears to be reflected by on an increased tendency of antigen receptor genes to undergo hybrid rearrangement, e.g., for T-cell receptor (TCR)-β to recombine with TCRγ, or TCRα with the immunoglobulin heavy chain locus, or, at least, for such rearrangements to persist [89–91]. The majority of lymphoid proliferations that arise in such patients contain genetic abnormalities, such as chromosomal translocations, and they appear to be true neoplasms with the same histological spectrum present in lymphomas occurring in the general population. Whether they possess the full quota of genetic abnormalities present in neoplasms arising in the general population is not known, but it remains possible that neoplastic growth on a background of immunosuppression may occur with fewer genetic lesions. If this were so, it could have an important impact on outcome on the response to chemotherapy. Lymphomas arising in AT patients might also be more chemosensitive because, as a consequence of the inherited defect, they are more susceptible to DNA-damaging agents. Patients with AT and Bloom's syndrome do not tolerate radiation, even relatively low doses, and it is clearly best avoided. At present, it would appear logical to treat lymphomas arising in patients with AT and Bloom's syndrome with simple regimens such as the one described above.

TREATMENT OF PATIENTS WITH ISOLATED CNS DISEASE

The treatment of patients with lymphoproliferative disease confined to the CNS on a background of immunosuppression is controversial. Approaches include radiation therapy, the infusion of monoclonal antibodies into the ventricular system via an Ommaya reservoir, and chemotherapy, emphasizing high-dose methotrexate (and/or Ara-C) and intrathecal drugs. The first two approaches have met with mixed success, although only a very small number of patients have, to date, been treated with intraventricular monoclonal antibodies. Chemotherapy alone is largely untried, although a pilot study of the treatment of primary CNS lymphoma in nonimmunosup-

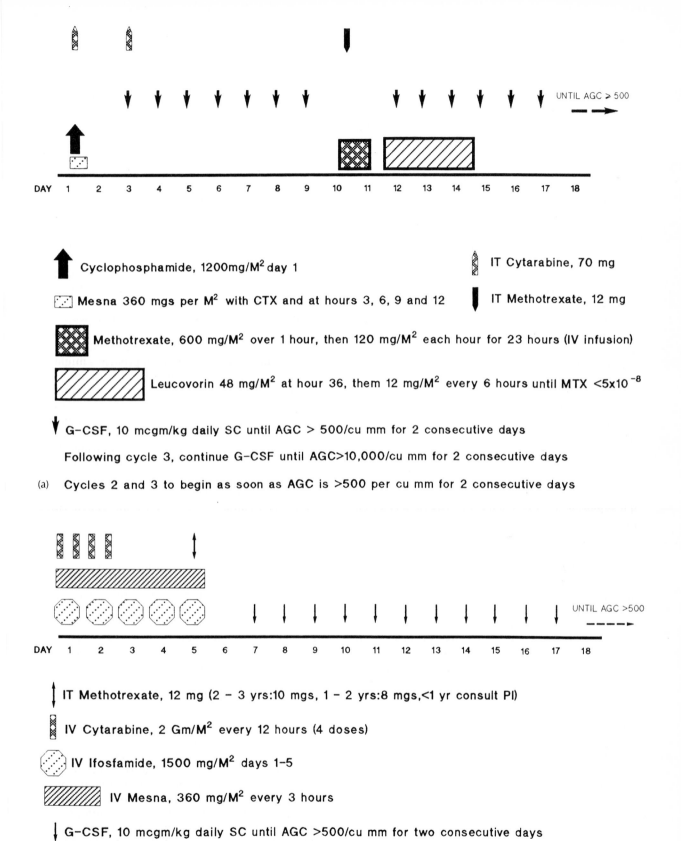

Figure 45.2 Schema of the NCI experimental chemotherapy protocol for patients with LPD. (a) Therapy for newly diagnosed patients. (b) Therapy for relapsed patients.

Interestingly, patients with primary CNS (P-CNS) lymphoma seem to have the poorest prognosis of all, with median survival of approximately 2.5 months, despite therapeutic intervention [9]. These individuals have evidence of profound HIV-associated immunodeficiency, with a history of AIDS prior to the lymphoma in 73%, and median CD4 cells of approximately 30/μl [9].

Primary central nervous system lymphoma

Lymphoma isolated to the CNS was first described in association with AIDS in 1983 [60] and was considered an AIDS-defining diagnosis from the outset of the epidemic. HIV-infected patients with P-CNS lymphoma do very poorly and are often diagnosed only at the time of autopsy, after the occurrence of multiple prior AIDS-defining illnesses [24,61,62]. The true prevalence and incidence of the condition, then, is largely unknown. Characteristics of CNS lymphoma in AIDS are provided in Table 46.1.

Interestingly, AIDS-related P-CNS lymphoma is universally associated with the EBV. Thus, as demonstrated by MacMahon and colleagues in a group of 21 such cases [48], all expressed the EBV early region protein (EBER), indicative of latent infection, while 45% expressed the latent membrane protein of EBV (LMP-1), which has transforming and oncogenic properties [63]. In contrast, only one of 14 (7%) cases of *de novo* P-CNS lymphoma expressed these EBV-related proteins. Likewise,

Meeker et al. [64] have also demonstrated uniform presence of EBV genome in five cases of AIDS-related P-CNS lymphoma. These studies raise the distinct possibility that the etiology of large-cell primary CNS lymphoma in AIDS may involve ongoing B-cell proliferation induced by EBV, in a site (brain) relatively protected by mechanisms of normal immune surveillance.

The vast majority of patients with P-CNS lymphoma are diagnosed with immunoblastic or large-cell lymphomas, similar to the case in patients with *de novo* P-CNS lymphomatous disease [9,29,48,65]. However, approximately 25% of patients with AIDS-related P-CNS lymphoma have the small noncleaved pathologic type, which is distinctly uncommon in patients with *de novo* disease, occurring in less than 5% [62,66].

Patients with P-CNS lymphoma present with mass lesions in the brain. These lesions are usually quite large (3–4 cm); approximately half are multifocal, although the lesions are fewer in number than one would normally expect to see in cerebral toxoplasmosis; 1–3 large masses are commonly found [67,68]. Ring enhancement may be seen, similar to the lesions of toxoplasmosis but distinct from patients with *de novo* P-CNS lymphoma, in whom ring enhancement is not expected [66]. Magnetic resonance imaging (MRI scan) may be more sensitive than the CAT scan in identifying primary CNS lymphoma, or in distinguishing it from other pathologic processes [68]. Results of lumbar puncture may be helpful, if not clinically contraindicated, in confirming the pathologic diagnosis. The cerebrospinal fluid (CSF) contains malignant cells in approximately 25% of patients with AIDS-related P-CNS lymphoma [61, 66]. In the absence of diagnostic material from the

Table 46.1 Characteristics of central nervous system (CNS) involvement in AIDS lymphoma

	Systemic AIDS lymphoma with CNS involvement	Primary CNS lymphoma
Sites of involvement	Leptomeningeal (cerebrospinal fluid)	Mass lesions within brain, at any site
Pathologic type	Immunoblastic, large-cell diffuse, or small noncleaved	Immunoblastic or large cell, diffuse
Evidence of EBV infection	100% (CSF)	100% (tumor tissue)
History of AIDS prior to lymphoma	37%	73%
Median CD4 cells at diagnosis of NHL	187/μl	30/μl
Median survival	Approximately 6 months	2–3 months

EBV, Epstein–Barr virus; NHL, non-Hodgkin's lymphoma; CSF, cerebrospinal fluid.

CSF, definitive diagnosis may only be made by actual brain biopsy [69]. Unfortunately, many such patients are never taken to biopsy, owing to the unjustified fear of potential contagion to operating room personnel [70] or in the belief that treatment would be ineffective [69]. These attitudes have impeded progress in the understanding and treatment of P-CNS lymphoma.

P-CNS lymphoma may involve any site within the brain, similar to the case in P-CNS lymphoma unrelated to AIDS [66,71]. Autopsy series have demonstrated that these lymphomas are universally multicentric [62]. More common sites of involvement *ante mortem* include the cerebrum, cerebellum and brainstem [62]. Approximately 75% of the tumors are located adjacent to ventricular surfaces or cortical convexities, indicating the propensity to spread along CSF pathways [66].

Symptoms of P-CNS lymphoma include focal neurologic deficits, such as paresis or cranial nerve palsies. Seizures occur in approximately 25% [66], and headaches are also common. Interestingly, altered mental status may be the only presenting complaint, and may be quite subtle in nature, such as change in personality or behavior. Confusion, lethargy, and/or memory loss may also be seen [61,62]. Mental status changes have been reported in approximately 50% of patients with AIDS-related P-CNS lymphoma compared with 35% of those with *de novo* disease [66].

Patients with P-CNS lymphoma have far-advanced immunodeficiency, related to long-standing underlying HIV infection [9]. They are usually quite frail, and may have multiple pathologic processes occurring simultaneously in the brain and elsewhere.

The optimal therapy for patients with AIDS-related P-CNS lymphoma remains undefined at the present time. In *de novo* P-CNS lymphoma, complete remission is expected in approximately 90% after use of whole-brain radiotherapy; disease-free survival is relatively short, however, and the median survival is only approximately 18 months [65,66]. Recently, use of systemic chemotherapy prior to the institution of cranial radiation has been tested, in an attempt to improve long-term outcome; early results are quite promising, with median survival in the range of 4 years [72]. While potentially efficacious, however, the use of systemic chemotherapy in patients with AIDS-related P-CNS lymphoma poses the additional threat of chemotherapy-induced immunodeficiency.

The use of cranial radiation in patients with AIDS-related P-CNS lymphoma has resulted in complete remission in approximately 20–50% of patients [73–76]. Median survival, however, has been only in the range of 2–3 months, with death often due to opportunistic infections. If left untreated, median survival is approximately 1–3 months, with death due to lymphoma, or to other opportunistic conditions [77]. Of importance, however, is the fact that radiation therapy is associated with significant improvement in the quality of survival in approximately 75% of treated individuals, indicating a definite role for such intervention, even if used solely for palliation of disease [75].

Recently, national protocols have been activated, which seek to explore the role of short courses of systemic chemotherapy, followed by whole-brain radiation in patients with AIDS-related P-CNS lymphoma. Results of these studies are awaited with great interest, especially considering the fact that the incidence of these lymphomas is expected to increase significantly as survival is prolonged in HIV disease.

Treatment

The optimal therapy for AIDS-related lymphoma remains to be defined. However, advances have been made over the past decade, which have resulted in higher rates of complete remission, longer survival times and greater ease in the administration of chemotherapy, with fewer toxicities. These are summarized in Table 46.2.

At the outset of the AIDS epidemic in the early 1980s, it was common practice to employ very dose-intensive regimens in patients with intermediate- or high-grade lymphoma, in the belief that multidrug resistance might be avoided, with greater likelihood of response [78]. Building upon the CHOP regimen [79], additional combinations were thus designed, including M-BACOD [80], ProMACE-CytoBOM [81,82], MACOP-B [83] and others, which appeared to be associated with higher response rates, from 60% with CHOP, to over 80% with MACOP-B. While initially promising, however, a subsequent large, prospective national trial has recently demonstrated no real difference in complete remission rates or rates of long-term disease-free survival when the CHOP regimen was compared to MACOP-B, ProMACE-CytaBOM or M-BACOD (see Chapter 42) [84].

In the early 1980s, since patients with AIDS-related lymphoma were known to have extensive, extranodal disease of high-grade pathologic type, it seemed reasonable to employ very dose-intensive regimens, similar to the trials being explored in *de novo* lymphoma. Unfortunately, these regimens were associated with low rates of response and high rates of opportunistic infection. Thus, the COMP regimen was associated with a 28% complete remission rate

Table 46.2   Selected therapeutic results: AIDS-related lymphoma

Regimen	No. of patients	Patients included	CR (%)	Opportunistic infections (%)	References
NOVEL: High-dose Ara-C, methotrexate and other agents	9	All	33	78	87
COMET A	38	All	58	NS	27
Low-dose m-BACOD	35	All	51	20	57
Low-dose m-BACOD + Zalcitabine	25	All	56 (equivalent in poor-risk patients)	11	90
CHOP with delayed GM-CSF	24	All	60–70	NS	89
Infusional cyclophosphamide, hydroxyldaunamycin, etoposide	21	All	62	14 episodes	94
Oral CCNU, etoposide cyclophosphamide, procarbazine	18	All	39	11	92
LNH-84	141	Good risk	63	NS	96
Low-dose chemotherapy with azidothymidine (AZT)	37	Poor risk	14	43	91

CR, Complete remission rate; GM-CSF, granulocyte–macrophage colony-stimulating factor.

(CR) in 19 patients with AIDS-related small non-cleaved lymphoma [85], while ProMACE-MOPP resulted in a 20% CR rate in 15 patients [86]. A novel regimen, containing high-dose cytosine arabinoside, high-dose methotrexate, high-dose cyclophosphamide and other agents resulted in a CR rate of only 33%, while 78% of patients developed opportunistic infections, from which they died [87]. A similar regimen, cyclophosphamide, vincristine, methotrexate, etoposide, cytosine arabinoside (termed COMET-A), yielded complete remission in 58% of a group of 38 patients, although the median duration of survival was only 5.2 months, which was statistically shorter than that achieved with other less intensive 'standard' regimens [27].

With these data in mind, the national AIDS Clinical Trials Group (ACTG), sponsored by the National Institutes of Allergy and Infectious Disease (NIAID) in the USA embarked upon a trial of a low-dose modification of the M-BACOD regimen. A CR of approximately 50% was achieved in 35 evaluable patients, with durable remissions in 75% and median survival of 18 months in this group [57]. With routine use of prophylactic intrathecal cytosine arabinoside, no case of isolated CNS relapse was encountered. Opportunistic infections developed in 20%, consisting of PCP in all, despite the use of

prophylaxis for this organism. Interestly, although low dosages of chemotherapy were employed and the total treatment time was shortened (four cycles), absolute granulocyte counts (AGC) less than 1000/mm^3 occurred in 60%, while 20% had AGC nadir counts of less than 500/mm^3. No differences in response rate or survival were seen in patients with various pathologic subtypes of disease, although those with prior AIDS, low CD4 counts or bone marrow involvement fared less well [57].

ADDITION OF HEMATOPOIETIC GROWTH FACTORS

In an attempt to improve both response rates and toxicity profile, Walsh et al. conducted a phase I/II trial of the low-dose m-BACOD regimen together with granulocyte–macrophage colony stimulating factor (GM-CSF) [88]. Sequential dose escalations of the m-BACOD could safely be administered when given together with GM-CSF, with acceptable toxicity. Although *in vitro* data had suggested that GM-CSF might increase HIV replication, this was not observed, at least, when measured by serial HIV p24 antigen levels [88].

Kaplan et al. studied the use of CHOP chemotherapy, either with or without GM-CSF, beginning either 24 h after completion of chemotherapy or more 'delayed', and given from days 4–13 post-chemotherapy [89]. Later institution of GM-CSF was associated with a statistically higher mean nadir of absolute neutrophil count, fewer days in hospital, and fewer chemotherapy cycles complicated by neutropenia and fever [89]. Serum HIV p24 antigen levels fell after the first week of chemotherapy in the GM-CSF-treated subjects, with a transient increase in p24 antigen at week 3, which was not observed in patients treated with CHOP alone. The clinical significance of this finding could not be determined.

ADDITION OF ANTIRETROVIRAL AGENTS

The low-dose m-BACOD regimen was recently modified by Levine et al. by the addition of ddC (Zalcitabine) for antiretroviral therapy and given to 28 patients [90]. Because of the known neurotoxicity of ddC, vincristine was initially withheld, and then added and escalated in successive cohorts of patients. Interestingly, only minimal (grade 1 and 2) neurotoxicity was documented, in two patients who had not received vincristine. Bone marrow toxicity was also relatively mild, with 15% of patients experiencing nadir granulocyte counts less than 500/mm^3. Only four patients required the use of hematopoietic growth factors (granulocyte colony-stimulating factor; G-CSF). Opportunistic infections occurred in 11%. The CR was 56% and was durable in 75% of these. Median survival of complete responders has not been reached but is in excess of 18 months. Interestingly, CR was equivalent in patients with poor prognostic indicators of disease, including history of a AIDS (CR=60%); CD4 cells less than 200/mm^3 (CR=53%) and bone marrow involvement [90].

The concomitant use of zidovudine (AZT) with chemotherapy has been more problematic, owing to the combined bone marrow suppressive effects. Tirelli et al. employed low-dose chemotherapy (cyclophosphamide, doxorubicin, teniposide, prednisone, vincristine; and bleomycin) with zidovudine (500 mg/day by mouth) in 37 patients with poor-prognosis AIDS lymphoma [91]. Of 21 (57%) patients who actually received any zidovudine, only 12 (32%) were able to complete a full course of combined chemo- and antiretroviral therapy. Opportunistic infections occurred in 43% of those receiving zidovudine and in 31% of those who did not. The complete remission rate was only 14%, and median survival for the group was 3.5 months.

ALTERNATIVE ROUTES OF CHEMOTHERAPY ADMINISTRATION

An oral regimen for treatment of AIDS-related lymphoma was recently employed by Remick et al. in 18 patients [92]. The median CD4 cell count was 73/μl and 27% had a history of AIDS-defining opportunistic infections. Of note was the fact that no patient had small noncleaved (Burkitt or non-Burkitt) lymphoma; ten had diffuse large-cell disease, seven had immunoblastic lymphoma and one had diffuse mixed lymphoma. The regimen employed consisted of 1-(2-chloroethyl)-3-cyclohexyl-1-nitrosourea (CCNU) (100 mg/m^2 day 1), etoposide (200 mg/m^2, days 1–3), cyclophosphamide (100 mg/m^2, days 22–31) and procarbazine (100 mg/m^2, days 22–31). A complete remission rate of 39% was achieved. Median duration of CR was 7 months and median survival of complete responders was 15 months. Grade 3 or 4 neutropenia occurred in 64% of cycles, while opportunistic infections developed in 11%. Therapy-related deaths occurred in 11% and treatment was stopped secondary to toxicity in 40%. Only one patient completed all five cycles of therapy as planned [92].

Infusional chemotherapy was employed by Sparano et al., consisting of a 4-day continuous infusion of cyclophosphamide (750 mg/m^2), doxorubicin (50 mg/m^2) and etoposide (240 mg/m^2), each dose representing the full dosage over four days. This was repeated every 28 days six times. Twelve patients were initially reported [93] with a recent update including a total of 21 subjects [94]. Complete remission was achieved in 62% with median survival of 18 months. Severe neutropenia (<500/μl) occurred in 38% of cycles; dose reduction for toxicity was required in 47% of cycles, and for 79% of patients who received at least two cycles. Fourteen episodes of opportunistic infections occurred and resulted in death in one patient with disseminated aspergillosis [94].

USE OF DOSE-INTENSIVE REGIMENS

Various regimens of dose-intensive chemotherapy have been employed over the past several years, primarily in patients with good prognosis disease. Bermudez used the MACOP-B regimen in 12 patients, half of whom had intermediate-grade lymphoma. A complete remission rate of 67% was achieved with median survival of 7 months. Five of the eight complete responders had Karnofsky performance scores of 100% with no history of prior AIDS [95].

Gisselbrecht et al. tested the intensive LNH-84 regimen in 141 patients with good prognosis AIDS lymphoma, as evidenced by excellent performance status, no history of prior opportunistic infections and relatively high CD4 cells at study entry (median = 227/mm³). A complete response rate of 63% was seen with median survival of 9 months [96]. Drug dosages were given as planned in 80% of patients, although 70% experienced treatment delays secondary to bone marrow suppression, which reduced the relative dose intensity actually administered. Independent factors predicting shorter survival included CD4 cells less than 100/mm³, performance status of 3 or 4, immunoblastic pathologic type and history of prior AIDS (present in 9%). In the absence of all such factors, the median survival was 2 years [96].

It is evident from these data that patients with 'good prognosis' AIDS-related lymphoma may be able to tolerate various dose-intensive regimens of combination chemotherapy. However, the real issue has been whether dose-intensive regimens actually confer an advantage in terms of response or survival. In order to address this issue, a large, prospective randomized trial has recently been completed, through the AIDS Clinical Trials Group (ACTG) of the National Institutes of Allergy and Infectious Disease [97]. A total of 192 patients were stratified by prognostic characteristics, and then randomized to receive either low-dose m-BACOD [57], or standard dose M-BACOD with GM-CSF [88]. Complete remission rates were equivalent, at approximately 50%. Median time to recurrence following complete response was 106 weeks for standard dose therapy (P = ns). Grade 3 or higher chemotherapy toxicity occurred in 66 of 94 (70%) patients assigned to standard dose therapy and in 50 of 98 (51%) patients assigned to low dose treatment (P = 0.008). These results were similar in patients with good prognostic, or poor prognostic disease. It is thus apparent from this large, randomized trial that low dose chemotherapy is associated with significantly less toxicity, and similar response rates and survival time when compared to standard dose therapy with adjunctive colony stimulating factor support [97].

USE OF BIOLOGIC AGENTS

Preliminary data have recently been published regarding use of various biologic agents in patients with AIDS lymphoma. With the understanding that IL-6 may function as a growth factor in these lymphomas, Emillie et al. employed a monoclonal antibody against IL-6 in ten patients. Stabilization of disease was seen in four, with disappearance of systemic B symptoms. However, no patient experienced a tumor response [98].

An immunotoxicin, B4-blocked ricin, directed against a B-cell antigen, has been given to nine patients with refractory or relapsed AIDS lymphoma

by Levine et al. [99]. This immunotoxin was generated by conjugating the potent toxin, ricin, to a mouse-derived IgG1 monoclonal antibody directed against the CD19 antigen on normal and malignant B-lymphocytes [100]. In this dose-escalating, phase I trial, no significant toxicity has been encountered, at doses of 5, 10 and 20 μg/kg, given by continuous infusion over 28 days. Responses have been seen in 22%, including the complete regression of a large rectal mass in one and partial remission of hepatic disease in a second individual. Human antimouse (HAMA) and human antiricin antibodies (HARA) developed in three individuals [99].

With evidence of efficacy in patients with refractory disease, Scadden et al. have now employed B4-blocked ricin, given by continuous infusion over 7 days, together with the low-dose m-BACOD regimen, in a phase I/II study [101]. The maximally tolerated dose of B4-blocked ricin appears to be 20 μg/kg in this setting. The monoclonal antibody was administered during cycles three and four, in those patients achieving complete or partial remission after two cycles of m-BACOD alone. In 18 evaluable patients to date, a CR rate of 67% was achieved after m-BACOD. The efficacy of B4-blocked ricin could not be assessed in this study, although toxicity appears to be acceptable. Four patients developed either HAMA and/or HARA responses. This trial is still in progress and further data are awaited [101].

Interleukin-2 has also undergone preliminary testing, based upon preclinical data in the severe combined immunodeficient (SCID)-human mouse model in which IL-2 prevents the development of EBV-associated lymphoproliferative disease [102].

SPONTANEOUS REGRESSION OF AIDS LYMPHOMA

While extremely rare, several patients with AIDS-related high-grade lymphoma have been reported in whom spontaneous regression of malignant disease occurred [103,104]. In one patient, an 11 × 7 cm lymphomatous mass in the neck spontaneously disappeared, although recurrence in the testes occurred 14 months later [103]. Another patient with isolated pulmonary involvement experienced significant regression of tumor after use of zidovudine [13].

References

1. Peters BS, Beck EJ, Coleman DG, et al. Changing disease patterns in patients with AIDS in a referral center in the United Kingdom: the changing face of AIDS. *Br. Med. J.* 1991, **302**: 203–207.

2. Levine AM. HIV related lymphoma: The epidemic shifts (Editorial). *J. Natl Cancer Inst.* 1991, **83**: 662–663.
3. Ross R, Dworsky R, Paganini-Hill A, et al. Non-Hodgkin's lymphomas in never married men in Los Angeles. *Br. J. Cancer* 1985, **52**: 785.
4. Centers for Disease Control. Revision of the case definition of acquired immunodeficiency syndrome for national reporting – United States. *Ann. Intern. Med.* 1985, **103**: 402.
5. Gail MH, Pluda JM, Rabkin CS et al. Projections of the incidence of non-Hodgkin's lymphoma related to acquired immunodeficiency syndrome. *J. Natl Cancer Inst.* 1991, **83**: 695–701.
6. Beral V, Peterman T, Berkelman R, et al. AIDS-associated non-Hodgkin lymphoma. *Lancet* 1991, **337**: 805–809.
7. d'Arminio Monforte A, Vago L, Mainini F. Primitive cerebral lymphoma and systemic lymphomas in 637 autopsies from AIDS cases. *VIIIth International Conference on AIDS*, Amsterdam, 1992.
8. Roithmann S, Tourani JM, Andrieu JM. AIDS-associated non-Hodgkin's lymphoma. *Lancet* 1991, **338**: 884–885.
9. Levine AM, Sullivan-Halley J, Pike MC, et al. HIV-related lymphoma: Prognostic factors predictive of survival. *Cancer* 1991, **68**: 2466–2472.
10. Biggar RJ, Rabkin CS. The epidemiology of acquired immunodeficiency syndrome-related lymphomas. *Curr. Opin. Oncol.* 1992, **4**: 883–893.
11. Casabona J, Melbye M, Biggar RJ. Kaposi's sarcoma and non-Hodgkin's lymphoma in European AIDS cases. No excess risk of Kaposi's sarcoma in Mediterranean countries. *Int. J. Cancer* 1991, **47**: 49–53.
12. Moore RD, Kessler H, Richman DD, et al. Non-Hodgkin's lymphoma in patients with advanced HIV infection treated with Zidovudine. *JAMA* 1991, **265**: 2208–2211.
13. Baselga J, Krown SE, Telzak EE, et al. AIDS-related pulmonary NHL regressing after zidovudine therapy. *Cancer* 1993, **71**: 2332–2334.
14. Pluda JM, Venzon DJ, Tosato G, et al. Parameters affecting the development of non-Hodgkin's lymphoma in patients with severe human immunodeficiency virus infection receiving antiretroviral therapy. *J. Clin. Oncol.* 1993, **11**: 1099–1107.
15. Pluda JM, Yarchoan R, Jaffe ES, et al. Development of non-Hodgkin's lymphoma in a cohort of patients with severe human immunodeficiency virus (HIV) infection on long-term antiretroviral therapy. *Ann. Intern. Med.* 1990, **113**: 276.
16. Levine AM, Bernstein L, Sullivan-Halley, J, et al. Role of zidovudine anti-retroviral therapy in one pathogenesis of AIDS-related lymphoma. *Blood* 1995, **86**: 4612–4616.
17. Monfardini S, Vaccher E, Tirelli U. AIDS associated non-Hodgkin's lymphoma in Italy: Intravenous drug users versus homosexual men. *Ann. Oncol.* 1990, **1**: 208–211.
18. Ragni MV, Belle SH, Jaffe RA, et al. Acquired immunodeficiency syndrome-associated non-Hodgkin's lymphomas and other malignancies in patients with hemophila. *Blood* 1993, **81**: 1889–1897.
19. NCI Non-Hodgkin's Lymphoma Classification Project Writing Committee: Classification of Non-Hodgkin's lymphomas: Reproducibility of major classification systems. *Cancer* 1985, **55**: 91–95.
20. Carbone A, Tirelli U, Vaccher E, et al. A clinicopathologic study of lymphoid neoplasias associated with human immunodeficiency virus infection in Italy. *Cancer* 1991, **68**: 842–852.
21. Ziegler JL, Beckstead JA, Volberding PA et al. Non-Hodgkin's lymphoma in 90 homosexual men: Relation to generalized lymphadenopathy and the acquired immunodeficiency syndrome. *N. Engl. J. Med.* 1984, **311**: 565–570.
22. Levine AM, Gill PS, Meyer PR, et al. Retrovirus and malignant lymphoma in homosexual men. *JAMA* 1985, **254**: 1921–1925.
23. Knowles DM, Chamulak GA, Subar M, et al. Lymphoid neoplasia associated with the acquired immunodeficiency syndrome (AIDS): The New York University experience. *Ann. Intern. Med.* 1988, **108**: 744–753.
24. Lowenthal DA, Straus DJ, Campbell SW, et al. AIDS-related lymphoid neoplasia: The Memorial Hospital experience. *Cancer* 1988, **61**: 2325–2337.
25. Ioachim HL, Dorsett B, Cronin W, et al. Acquired immunodeficiency syndrome associated lymphomas: Clinical, pathological, immunologic and viral characteristics of 111 cases. *Hum. Path.* 1991, **22**: 659–673.
26. Levine AM. Acquired Immunodeficiency Syndrome-related lymphoma (Review). *Blood* 1992, **80**: 8–20.
27. Kaplan LD, Abrams DI, Feigal E, et al. AIDS-associated non-Hodgkin's lymphoma in San Francisco. *JAMA* 1989, **261**: 719–724.
28. Lukes RJ, Parker JW, Taylor CR, et al. Immunologic approach to non-Hodgkin's lymphomas and related leukemias. Analysis of the results of multiparameter studies of 425 cases. *Semin. Hematol.* 1978, **15**: 322–351.
29. Raphael M, Gentilhomme O, Tulliez M, et al. Histopathologic features of high-grade non-Hodgkin's lymphomas in acquired immunodeficiency syndrome. The French study group of pathology for human immunodeficiency virus-associated tumors. *Arch. Pathol. Lab. Med.* 1991, **115**: 15–20.
30. Stansfeld AG, Diebold J, Kapanci Y, et al. Updated Kiel classification for lymphomas. *Lancet* 1988, **i**: 292–293.
31. Hui PK, Feller AC, Lennert K. High grade non-Hodgkin's lymphoma of B-cell type I. *Histopathology* 1988, **12**: 127–143.
32. Horning SJ, Rosenbery SA. The natural history of initially untreated low-grade non-Hodgkin's lymphomas. *N. Engl. J. Med.* 1984, **311**: 1471.
33. Konrad RJ, Kricka LJ, Goodman DBP, et al. Brief report: Myeloma-associated paraprotein directed against the HIV-1 p24 antigen in an HIV-1 seropositive patient. *N. Engl. J. Med.* 1993, **328**: 1817–1819.
34. Ciobanu N, Andreef M, Safai B, et al. Lymphoblastic neoplasia in a homosexual patient with Kaposi's sarcoma. *Ann. Intern. Med.* 1983, **98**: 151.
35. Presant CA, Gala K, Wiseman C, et al. Human immunodeficiency virus associated T-cell lymphoblastic lymphoma in AIDS. *Cancer* 1987, **60**: 1459.

36. Janier M, Katlama C, Flageul B, et al. The Pseudo-Sezary syndrome with CD8 phenotype in a patient with the acquired immunodeficiency syndrome (AIDS). *Ann. Intern. Med.* 1989, **110**: 738.

37. Goldstein J, Becker N, DelRowe J, et al. Cutaneous T-cell lymphoma in a patient infected with HIV, type 1. *Cancer* 1990, **66**: 1130.

38. Crane GA, Variakojis D, Rosen ST, et al. Cutaneous T-cell lymphoma in patients with human immuno-deficiency virus infection. *Arch. Dermatol.* 1991, **127**: 989.

39. Sternlieb J, Mintzer D, Kwa D, Gluckman S. Peripheral T-cell lymphoma in a patient with the acquired immunodeficiency syndrome. *Am. J. Med.* 1988, **85**: 445.

40. Baurmann H, Miclea JM, Ferchal F, et al. Adult T-cell leukemia associated with HTLV-I and simultaneous infection by HIV type 2 and human herpes-virus 6 in an African woman: A clinical, virologic and familial serologic study. *Am. J. Med.* 1988, **85**: 853.

41. Shibata D, Brynes R, Rabinowitz A, et al. HTLV-1 associated adult T-cell leukemia lymphoma in a patient infected with HIV-1. *Ann. Intern. Med.* 1989, **111**: 871–875.

42. Thomas JA, Cotter F, Hanby AM, et al. Epstein–Barr virus-related oral T-cell lymphoma associated with human immunodeficiency virus immunosuppression. *Blood* 1993, **81**: 3350–3356.

43. Gonzalez-Clemente JM, Ribera JM, Campo E, et al. Ki-1 positive anaplastic large cell lymphoma of T-cell origin in an HIV infected patient. *AIDS* 1991, **5**: 751–755.

44. Carbone A, Tirelli U, Gloghini A, et al. Human immunodeficiency virus-associated systemic lymphomas may be subdivided into two main groups according to Epstein–Barr viral latent gene expression. *J. Clin. Oncol.* 1993, **11**: 1674–1681.

45. Chadburn A, Cesarman E, Jagirdar J, et al. CD30 (Ki-1) positive anaplastic large cell lymphomas in individuals infected with the HIV. *Cancer* 1993, **72**: 3078–3090.

46. Anagnostopoulos I, Herbst H, Niedobitek G, et al. Demonstration of monoclonal EBV genomes in Hodgkin's disease and Ki-1 positive anaplastic large cell lymphoma by combined Southern blot and in situ hybridization. *Blood* 1989, **74**: 810–816.

47. Herbst H, Dallenbach F, Hummel M, et al. Epstein Barr virus DNA and latent gene products in Ki-1 (CD30) positive anaplastic large cell lymphomas. *Blood* 1991, **78**: 2666–2673.

48. MacMahon EME, Glass JD, Hayward, SD, et al. Epstein Barr virus in AIDS-related primary central nervous system lymphoma. *Lancet* 1991, **338**: 969–974.

49. Jones SE, Fuks Z, Bellm M, et al. Non-Hodgkin's lymphoma: IV. Clinico-pathologic correlation of 405 cases. *Cancer* 1973, **31**: 806–823.

50. Armenakas NA, Schevchuk MM, Brodherson M, et al. AIDS presenting as primary testicular lymphoma. *Urology* 1992, **40**: 162–164.

51. Holladay AO, Siegel RJ, Schwartz DA. Cardiac malignant lymphoma in acquired immune deficiency syndrome. *Cancer* 1992, **70**: 2203–2207.

52. Gill PS, Chandraratna P, Meyer PR, et al. Malignant lymphoma: Cardiac involvement at initial presentation. *J. Clin. Oncol.* 1987, **5**: 216–224.

53. Podzamczer D, Ricat I, Bolao F, et al. Gallium-67 scan for distinguishing follicular hyperplasia from other AIDS associated diseases in lymph nodes. *AIDS* 1990, **4**: 683.

54. Hill M, Cunningham D, MacVicar D, et al. Role of magnetic resonance imaging in predicting relapse in residual masses after treatment of lymphoma. *J. Clin. Oncol.* 1993, **11**: 2273–2278.

55. Radin DR, Esplin J, Levine AM, et al. AIDS-related non-Hodgkin's lymphoma: Abdominal CT findings in 112 patients. *Am. J. Roentgenol.* 1993, **160**: 1133–1139.

56. Sider L, Weiss AJ, Smith MD, et al. Varied appearance of AIDS-related lymphoma in the chest. *Radiology* 1989, **171**: 629–632.

57. Levine AM, Wernz JC, Kaplan L, et al. Low dose chemotherapy with central nervous system prophylaxis and azidothymidine maintenance in AIDS-related lymphoma: A prospective multi-institutional trial. *JAMA* 1991, **266**: 84–88.

58. Shipp MA, for The International Non-Hodgkin's Lymphoma Prognostic Factors Project. A predictive model for aggressive non-Hodgkin's lymphoma. *N. Engl. J. Med.* 1993, **329**: 987–994.

59. Silverman BA, Rubinstein A. Serum lactate dehydrogenase levels in adults and children with acquired immunodeficiency deficiency syndrome (AIDS) and AIDS-related complex: Possible indicator of B-cell lymphoproliferation and disease activity. *Am. J. Med.* 1985, **78**: 728–736.

60. Snider WD, Simpson DM, Aronyk KE, Nielsen SL. Primary lymphoma of the nervous system associated with acquired immune-deficiency syndrome. *N. Engl. J. Med.* 1983, **308**: 45.

61. Gill PS, Levine AM, Meyer PR, et al. Primary central nervous system lymphoma in homosexual men: Clinical, immunologic and pathologic features. *Am. J. Med.* 1985, **78**: 742–748.

62. So YT, Beckstead JH, Davis RL: Primary central nervous system lymphoma in acquired immune deficiency syndrome: A clinical and pathological study. *Ann. Neurol.* 1986, **20**: 566–572.

63. Wang D, Liebowitz D, Kieff E: An EBV membrane protein expressed in immortalized lymphocytes transforms established rodent cells. *Cell* 1985, **43**: 831–840.

64. Meeker TC, Shiramizu B, Kaplan L, et al. Evidence for molecular subtypes of HIV-associated lymphoma: Division into peripheral monoclonal, polyclonal and central nervous system lymphoma. *AIDS* 1991, **5**: 669.

65. De Angelis LM, Yahalom J, Rosenblum M, et al. Primary CNS lymphoma: Managing patients with spontaneous and AIDS-related disease. *Oncology* 1987, **1**: 52.

66. Fine HA, Mayer RJ. Primary central nervous system lymphoma (Review). *Ann. Intern. Med.* 1993, **119**: 1093–1104.

67. Gill PS, Graham RA, Boswell W, et al. A comparison

of imaging, clinical and pathologic aspects of space occupying lesions within the brain in patients with acquired immunodeficiency syndrome. *Am. J. Physiol. Imaging* 1986, **1**: 134–141.

68. Ciricillo SF, Rosenblum ML. Use of CT and MR imaging to distinguish intracranial lesions and to define the need for biopsy in AIDS patients. *J. Neurosurg.* 1990, **73**: 720.

69. Galetto G, Levine AM. AIDS-related primary central nervous system lymphoma. *JAMA* 1993, **269**: 92–93.

70. Corn BW, Trock BD. Impact of medical speciality on the approach to AIDS patients with intracranial mass lesions. *Proc. Am. Soc. Clin. Oncol.* 1992, **11**: 44.

71. Shibata S. Sites of origin of primary intracerebral malignant lymphoma. *Neurosurgery* 1989, **25**: 14–19.

72. DeAngelis LM, Yahalom J, Heinemann MH, et al. Primary CNS lymphoma: Combined treated with chemotherapy and radiotherapy. *Neurology* 1990, **40**: 80–86.

73. Formenti SC, Gill PS, Lean E, et al. Primary central nervous system lymphoma in AIDS: Results of radiation therapy. *Cancer* 1989, **63**: 1101–1107.

74. Goldstein JD, Dickson DW, Moser FG, et al. Primary central nervous system lymphoma in acquired immunodeficiency syndrome: A clinical and pathologic study with results of treatment with radiation. *Cancer* 1991, **67**: 2756–2765.

75. Baumgartner JE, Rachlin JR, Beckstead JH, et al. Primary central nervous system lymphomas: Natural history and response to radiation therapy in 55 patients with acquired immunodeficiency syndrome. *J. Neurosurg.* 1990, **73**: 206–211.

76. Nisce LZ, Kaufmann T, Metroka C. Radiation therapy in patients with AIDS-related central nervous system lymphomas. *JAMA* 1992, **267**: 192–193.

77. Bishburg E, Eng RHK, Slim J, et al. Brain lesions in patients with acquired immunodeficiency syndrome. *Arch. Intern. Med.* 1989, **149**: 941–943.

78. Goldie JH, Coldman AJ, Gudauskas GA. Rationale for the use of alternating non-cross resistant chemotherapy. *Cancer Treat. Rep.* 1982, **66**: 439–449.

79. McKelvey EM, Gottlieb JA, Wilson HE, et al. Hydroxyldaunomycin (Adriamycin) combination chemotherapy in malignant lymphoma. *Cancer* 1976, **38**: 1484.

80. Skarin AT, Canellos GP, Rosenthal DS, et al. Improved prognosis of diffuse histiocytic and undifferentiated lymphoma by use of high dose methotrexate alternating with standard agents (M-BACOD). *J. Clin. Oncol.* 1983, **1**: 91–98.

81. Fisher RI, DeVita VT Jr, Hubbard SM, et al. Diffuse aggressive lymphomas: Increased survival after alternating flexible sequence of ProMACE and MOPP chemotherapy. *Ann. Intern. Med.* 1983, **98**: 304.

82. Fisher RI, DeVita VT, Hubbard SM, et al. Randomized trial of ProMACE-MOPP versus ProMACE-CytaBOM in previously untreated, advanced stage, diffuse aggressive lymphomas. *Proc. Am. Soc. Clin. Oncol.* 1984, **3**: 242.

83. Klimo P, Connors JM. MACOP-B chemotherapy for the treatment of diffuse large cell lymphoma. *Ann. Intern. Med.* 1985, **102**: 596.

84. Fisher RI, Gaynor E, Dahlberg S, et al. Comparison of a standard regimen (CHOP) with three intensive chemotherapy regimens for advanced non-Hodgkin's lymphoma. *N. Engl. J. Med.* 1993, **328**: 1002–1006.

85. Odajnyk C, Subar M, Dugan M, et al. Clinical features and correlates with immunopathology and molecular biology of a large group of patients with AIDS associated small non-cleaved lymphoma (SNCL). *Blood* 1986, **68**: 1331a.

86. Dugan M, Subar M, Odajnyk C, et al. Intensive multiagent chemotherapy for AIDS related diffuse large cell lymphoma. *Blood* 1986, **68**: 124a.

87. Gill PS, Levine AM, Krailo M, et al. AIDS-related malignant lymphoma: Results of prospective treatment trials. *J. Clin. Oncol.* 1987, **5**: 1322–1328.

88. Walsh C, Wernz J, Levine AM, et al. Phase I study of m-BACOD and granulocyte macrophage colony stimulating factor (GM-CSF) in HIV associated non-Hodgkin's lymphoma. *J. AIDS* 1993, **6**: 265–271.

89. Kaplan LD, Kahn JO, Crowe S, et al. Clinical and virologic effects of recombinant human granulocyte-macrophage colony-stimulating factor in patients receiving chemotherapy for human immunodeficiency virus-associated non-Hodgkin's lymphoma: Results of a randomized trial. *J. Clin. Oncol.* 1991, **9**: 929.

90. Levine AM, Tulpule A, Espina B, et al. Low dose methotrexate, bleomycin, adriamycin, cyclophosphamide, oncovin and dexamemasone with Zalcitabine in patients with AIDS-related lymphoma: Effect on HIV and serum interleukin-6 levels over time. *Cancer* 1996, **78**: 517–526.

91. Tirelli U, Errante D, Okssenhendler E, et al. Prospective study with combined low-dose chemotherapy and zidovudine in 37 patients with poor prognosis AIDS-related non-Hodgkin's lymphoma. *Ann. Oncol.* 1992, **3**: 843–847.

92. Remick SC, McSharry JJ, Walt BC, et al. Novel oral combination chemotherapy in the treatment of intermediate-grade and high-grade AIDS-related non-Hodgkin's lymphoma. *J. Clin. Oncol.* 1993, **11**: 1691–1702.

93. Sparano JA, Wiernik PH, Strack M, et al. Infusional cyclophosphamide, doxorubicin, etoposide in human immunodeficiency virus and human T-cell leukemia virus type 1-related non-Hodgkin's lymphoma: A highly active regimen. *Blood* 1993, **81**: 2810–2815.

94. Sparano JA, Wiernik PH, Dutcher JP, et al. Infusion cyclophosphamide, doxorubicin, and etoposide in HIV-related non-Hodgkin's lymphoma: A follow up report of a highly active regimen. *Blood* 1993, **82**: 386a.

95. Bermudez M, Grant KM, Rodvien R, et al. Non-Hodgkin's lymphoma in a population with or at risk for acquired immunodeficiency syndrome: Indications for intensive chemotherapy. *Am. J. Med.* 1989, **86**: 71.

96. Gisselbrecht C, Oksenhendler E, Tirelli U, et al, for the French Italian Cooperative Group: Human immunodeficiency virus-related lymphoma treatment with intensive combination chemotherapy. *Am. J. Med.* 1993, **95**: 188–196.

97. Kaplan L, Straus D, Testa M, Levine AM. Randomized trial of standard dose M-BACOD with GM-CSF versus reduced dose m-BACOD for systemic HIV associated lymphoma: ACTG 142. *Proc. ASCO* 1995, **14**: 288.

98. Emillie D, Marfaing A, Merrien D, et al. Treatment of AIDS-lymphomas with an anti-IL-6 monoclonal antibody. *Blood* 1993, **82**: 387a.

99. Levine AM. Personal communication.

100. Investigator's brochure. *Anti-B4 Blocked Ricin.* Boston, MA: ImmunoGen, 1990.

101. Scadden DT, Doweiko J, Schenkein D, et al. A phase I/II trial of combined immunoconjugate and chemotherapy for AIDS-related lymphoma. *Blood* 1993, **82**: 386a.

102. Baiocchi RA, Caligiuri MA. Low dose IL-2 prevents the development of Epstein–Barr virus associated lymphoproliferative disorder in the SCID-human mouse. *Blood* 1993, **82**: 385a.

103. Daniels D, Lowdell CP, Glaser MG. The spontaneous regression of lymphoma in AIDS. *Clin. Oncol.* 1992, **4**: 196–197.

104. Karnad AB, Jaffar A, Lands RH. Spontaneous regression of acquired immune deficiency syndrome related, high-grade, extranodal non-Hodgkin's lymphoma. *Cancer* 1992, **69**: 1856–1857.

CHAPTER 47

Treatment of malignant neoplasms of the mucosa-associated lymphoid tissues

PHILIP A. SALEM AND DENNIE V. JONES

Introduction

Neoplasms arising from the mucosa-associated lymphoid tissues (MALTs) make up a large portion of the extranodal non-Hodgkin's lymphomas and are relatively common lymphomas whose incidence varies by geographic location. While these neoplasms often arise in the mucosa of the lung, pharynx and small intestine, areas well endowed with MALT, they frequently occur in the stomach, salivary glands, thyroid and other regions, which are normally devoid of lymphoid tissues. MALT-lymphomas as a group tend to remain localized for a prolonged period and, during this time, are amenable to regional treatment strategies. When they disseminate, they usually metastasize to another site within the organ of origin or to another MALT-containing organ.

Within the gastrointestinal tract the precursor cells which eventually populate the gut as immunoglobulin A (IgA)-secreting plasmacytes originate from immature B-lymphocytes of the Peyer's patches and appendix, where specific T-cells induce IgA-specific isotype switching [1–5]. It is while they are within the Peyer's patches that these precursor cells encounter antigens from the lumen of the gut. From there, they migrate first to the mesenteric lymph nodes, where they undergo expansion, and then to the thoracic duct, where they become large lymphocytes. These cells make up one-tenth of the thoracic duct cell population and, although they are in a stage of active DNA synthesis, they have a limited proliferative capacity. They home specifically and exclusively toward the lamina propria of the gut, where they differentiate into IgA-producing plasmacytes [2,6]. The small lymphocytes, which constitute the remainder of the thoracic duct lymphocyte population, retain the capacity to proliferate, and appear to circulate continuously in the peripheral lymphoid tissues, the thoracic duct and the bloodstream. In contrast to the large lymphocytes, these small lymphocytes lodge in any site, not necessarily the gut, as long as specific antigen is present, and then divide and differentiate into IgA-secreting plasma cells [5].

This ability to migrate is the result of the expression of a complex array of specific glycoproteins, including the lymphocyte homing receptors and other cell adhesion molecules that recognize complementary molecules in target sites [6–14]. Pals et al. have suggested that the expression of lymphocyte homing receptors may explain the pattern of dissemination of disease in a variety of non-Hodgkin's lymphomas [14], and it is thus conceivable that a similar mechanism may be involved in the metastatic pattern of MALT lymphomas.

MALT lymphomas often follow a protracted clinical course, although lesions involving large areas of mucosal surfaces may be associated with considerable morbidity. Other non-Hodgkin's lymphomas may metastasize to the mucosal lining of the aerodigestive tract, but because they do not originate from MALTs, their biologic behavior is similar to that of lymphomas arising at other lymphoid sites in the body. It is believed that MALT lymphomas develop after a prolonged, sometimes inappropriate, stimulation of the immune system. In some instances, this stimulation is the result of an autoimmune phenomenon, but in others it is secondary to a chronic, minimally invasive mucosal infection. Neoplasms which possibly have an infectious etiology appear to have a prolonged premalignant phase that is usually reversible with readily available antibiotics. By virtue of their ability to eradicate infection, these antibiotics eliminate, or markedly reduce, the source of the chronic antigenic stimulation and, consequently, reverse the process which may ultimately evolve into neoplasia. Four types of MALT lymphomas will be considered in this chapter: immunoproliferative small intestinal disease, low-grade gastric B-cell lymphoma, monocytoid B-cell lymphoma and enteropathy-associated T-cell lymphoma. To be complete, there is evidence to support a MALT origin for Burkitt's lymphoma; however, the clinical and biological behavior of this disease is radically different from all other MALT-derived neoplasms and therefore it will be discussed elsewhere in this book.

Immunoproliferative small intestinal disease

Immunoproliferative small intestinal disease (IPSID) usually starts as a benign-appearing, diffuse small bowel mucosal infiltration of lymphocytes and/or plasma cells, and if left untreated, it evolves into large-cell immunoblastic lymphoma, which was initially called Mediterranean lymphoma. The term 'Mediterranean lymphoma' has been recently discarded as the disease has been shown to be endemic outside of the Mediterranean basin. Furthermore, lymphoma does not necessarily develop in all patients with IPSID [15–26]. Most of the cases described have been Arabs and non-European Jews, but the disease has also been noted in Iranians and South African Blacks. Very few cases of IPSID have been reported from the industrialized nations but most of these have been in immigrants from regions where the disease is endemic.

In contrast to other non-Hodgkin's lymphomas that afflict patients regardless of their socioeconomic status, most patients with IPSID are from the lower socioeconomic strata. Also, in contrast to non-IPSID lymphomas, IPSID occurs exclusively between the ages of 15 and 40 years, while non-IPSID lymphomas may occur at any age, with a peak incidence in the sixth decade.

There is no established etiology for IPSID at present. Virtually all those afflicted by this disease come from communities in which poor hygiene and chronic malnutrition are prevalent [25–29]. Improvements in living conditions in some areas where this disease is endemic have been associated with a corresponding decrease in the incidence of IPSID [25]. These regions are also characterized by a high prevalence of intestinal parasitoses and infectious enteritis, and bowel flora are known to stimulate the proliferation of intestinal IgA-producing lymphocytes, the presumed normal counterparts of the aberrant cells of IPSID. However, no infectious agent or dietary factor has been identified that predisposes a patient to the development of IPSID. Interestingly, biopsy specimens from the intestines of apparently healthy individuals living in these same endemic regions demonstrate an increase in the number of lymphocytes and plasma cells in the lamina propria, a reflection of the more florid infiltration that occurs in IPSID [30].

It is conceivable that the immunosuppression which is frequently associated with the malnutrition often seen among the poorer populations of developing nations may play a permissive role in the genesis of this disease [31,32]. Severe malnutrition is associated with multiple immune deficits, including T-cell depletion, decrease in lymphocyte differentiation, decrease in levels of several of the complement components and a reduction in the function of phagocytic cells. Specific defects in the mucosal immune system are also observed, including atrophy of the gut-associated lymphoid follicles, decreased numbers of mucosal T-cells and IgA-positive B-cells, decreased levels of secretory IgA and a reduction in specific antibody responses. Vitamin A deficiency is associated with reduced lymphocyte mucosal homing [31,32]. Immunodeficiency is, in turn, associated with the development of non-Hodgkin's lymphoma predominantly of the diffuse large-cell and immunoblastic subtypes. It is of note that a clinical syndrome that resembles IPSID has been described in some victims of AIDS [33].

The natural course of IPSID appears to include a potentially reversible premalignant phase that if untreated degenerates into a malignant lymphoma [34–38]. After the initial insult to the alimentary canal, which probably consists of prolonged antigenic stimulation, cellular proliferation within the Peyer's patches and mesenteric lymph nodes occurs. This proliferation will eventually lead to changes in the anatomy and function of the intestine, and permit bacterial overgrowth, which then provides further antigenic stimulation. This is subsequently followed, in most cases, by the appearance of an aberrant α heavy chain (IgA)-producing clone (α heavy chain disease, αHCD), where the neoplastic cells produce an abnormal α heavy chain paraprotein that may be found in the serum and/or intestinal fluid. Some cases of nonsecretory αHCD in which the paraprotein is only found within the cell have also been reported [39–41].

To date, there have been no large therapeutic trials in this disease, and most authors have reported observations based on only one or a few patients. Studies with larger numbers of patients have employed retrospective data in most instances and used multiple treatment regimens, making it difficult to derive specific treatment recommendations. Furthermore, many authors have not reported the clinical stage of their patients, and most of those who had, have used the Galian staging system [41,42] (Table 47.1). In this system, IPSID is divided into stages A, B and C: in stage A, plasmacytes infiltrate the small intestinal mucosa, and mesenteric lymph nodes and dystrophic changes are rare; stage B is characterized

by increasing dysplasia in both the intestine and lymph nodes; in stage C, an immunoblastic lymphoma is found within the intestinal wall, mesenteric lymph nodes or other nodal or extranodal sites. Another system, the Salem system [35] (Table 47.2), is more accurate in reflecting the anatomical extent of the disease. However, survival data for a large population of patients, evaluated by either of these staging systems, have not yet been reported.

In Galian stage A disease, which corresponds to Salem stage O disease, sustained clinical and pathologic remissions may be obtained with a prolonged (six months or more) trial of antibiotics (Table 47.3). Most investigators have used tetracycline, although metronidazole, with or without ampicillin, appears to be an effective alternative [43–55].

The major problem in the interpretation of data relating to the role of antibiotics in the prelymphomatous phase of IPSID is the lack of adequate staging. Most patients were not staged by laparotomy and, therefore, it is conceivable that some of them had lymphoma in the mesenteric lymph nodes, although the histological expression of the disease in the small bowel mucosa appeared benign. In spite of this, the data are strongly suggestive that more than half of the patients considered to have early and prelymphomatous IPSID achieve a complete or a partial response with antibiotics alone. These responses are durable and may last for decades, and indeed some of these patients may well be cured. This suggests that infection is at least partially responsible for the biological and anatomical changes that eventually lead to IPSID lymphoma, and more importantly, that eradication of infection would reverse these changes and lead to cure. This observation constitutes the first milestone in the story of chemoprevention of cancer in man. Of great interest was the observation by Ramot that a patient with an established IPSID lymphoma (confirmed histologically by three pathologists) had definite

Table 47.1 Galian staging system [42]

Stage	Small intestine	Lymph nodes
A	Lymphoplasmacytic or plasmacytic infiltration of lamina propria; variable villous atrophy	Plasmacytic infiltration; nodal architecture generally preserved
B	Atypical lymphoplasmacytes or plasmacytes with immunoblast-like cells with extension to at least submucosa; subtotal or total villous atrophy	Atypical plasmacytic infiltrate with immunoblast-like cells; subtotal or total effacement of nodal architecture
C	Frankly malignant invasion through entire intestinal wall	Malignant effacement of entire lymph node

Table 47.2 Salem staging system [35]

Stage	Definition
0	Diffuse benign-appearing mucosal cellular infiltrate, (+) α heavy chain protein and no evidence of lymphoma by staging laparotomy
I	Malignant lymphoma in either the intestine (Ii) or in the mesenteric lymph nodes (In), but not in both
II	Malignant lymphoma in both intestine and mesenteric lymph nodes
III	Involvement of retroperitoneal or extra-abdominal lymph nodes
IV	Involvement of noncontiguous extranodal tissues

regression of disease on antibiotics alone. This was indeed a historical observation, because never before had an established lymphoma been shown to respond to antibiotics. This suggests that even in advanced malignancy, eradication of infection may still reverse (at least partially) the carcinogenic process. Unfortunately, no other patients with established IPSID lymphoma have been treated with antibiotics alone and thus it is not possible to determine to what extent antibiotics may be useful in the treatment of the advanced lymphomatous phase.

In the lymphomatous phase of IPSID, single-agent cytotoxic chemotherapy [46,51,52], such as chlorambucil or cyclophosphamide, has been used, but with limited success [56–61] (Table 47.4). Steroids are often used in drug combinations but appear to have limited activity.

Table 47.3 Results of antibiotic therapy for prelymphomatous phase – immunoproliferative small intestinal disease

Author	No. of patients	Treatment* Antibiotic/dose	Duration (months)	Response† CR	PR	Duration (years)
Gilinsky	11	MNA/antihelmenthics	Unknown	7	3	Mean, 9.6
Banisadre	7	TCN, 500 mg/day	9–30	Unknown		Unknown
Ben-Ayed	6	MNA and AMP TCN	7–24	2		3.5
Malik	6	TCN + folic acid	Unknown	1		Unknown
Russell	5	TCN, 1.0 g/day	1	Improvement		Unknown
Price	5	TCN	Unknown	3		0.5, 0.5, 2.5
Salem	3	TCN, 2 g/day	12	2		14, 15
Lewin	3	Antibiotics Antiparasitics	Unknown	2		4, 5
Bowie	3	TCN	9	1		10
Manousos	2	TCN, 2 g/day TCN/MNA	3 Unknown	1‡ Pd§		6
Rambaud	2	Colimycin/rifampin (1) minocycline/MNA (1)	Unknown 2	1¶		
Ramot	1	TCN	Unknown			
Matuchansky	1	TCN, 2 g/day		1		1
O'Keefe	1	TCN, 250 g/day	12	1		1
Chaqui	1	Antibiotics	Unknown	1		2

* TCN, tetracycline; MNA, metronidazole; AMP, ampicillin.
† CR, Complete response: asymptomatic, absence of α heavy chains, no histologic evidence of disease; PR, partial response: asymptomatic, decrease in α heavy chains, histologic evidence of disease persists but is improved, with a decrease in the infiltrate and with a partial restoration of villi; MR, minor response: improvement in symptoms, persistence of α heavy chains, no change in histologic picture; PD, progressive disease.
‡ This patient subsequently received radiotherapy and chemotherapy, and had a CR of 3.75+ years.
§ This patient received weekly cyclophosphamide and continued TCN, and had a CR after 3 months. The patient remained free of disease after 3.5 years.
¶ One patient had a CR after chemotherapy.

Table 47.4 Results of single-agent chemotherapy in lymphomatous phase – immunoproliferative small intestinal disease

| Author | No. of patients | Treatment* | | | Response† | |
		Agent	Steroids	Antibiotics	Level	Duration (months)
Al-Bahrani	13	CTX	+	TCN	13 CR/PR	9–59
Ramot	11	MUS	+	Achromycin	Short response	Unknown
Doe	3	LPAM or CTX	+	Broad spectrum	3 CR	6+ to 18+
Tabbane	3	Chlor	–	Antibiotics	PD	
Malik	2	LPAM	+		2 CR	Unknown
Rambaud	1	LPAM	+		MR	
Manousos	1	CTX	+	TCN/MNA	CR	40

* LPAM, Melphalan; CTX, cyclophosphamide; Chlor, chlorambucil; Pred, prednisone; TCN, tetracycline; MNA, metronidazole; VCR, vincristine; MUS, mustargen (mechlorethamine).
† CR, Complete response; PR, partial response; PD, progressive disease.

Much of the recent literature has examined the application of combination chemotherapy regimens (Table 47.5). However, these reports suffer from major problems: (1) they fail to document the rate and duration of response to a particular regimen; (2) they are anecdotal in nature; (3) they are retrospective; (4) they use different drug regimens and treatment modalities; and (5) they deal with small numbers of patients [45,50,62–64].

Many of the larger trials have incorporated abdominal radiotherapy for some patients, but it is difficult to determine from these reports what contribution radiotherapy may have made [43,44,48, 58,65,66] (Table 47.6). The published experience of

Table 47.5 Results of combination chemotherapy for lymphomatous phase – immunoproliferative small intestinal disease

| Author | No. of patients | Treatment* | | Response† | | |
		Chemotherapy	Steroid	CR	PR	Duration (months)
Gilinsky	17	CHOP or MUS + CTX + VCR + Chlor or XRT + VP16 + DOX or XRT + Pred	—	7 – 'Good' 5 – 'Temporary'		Mean survival 20.1
Ben-Ayed	14	CHVP # based	+	9		20–55
Lewin	9	MUS + CTX + VCR + Chlor or Sequential single agents	—	Unknown		Mean survival 32
Salem	6	CHOP	—	2	1	14–24
Rambaud	2	CHOP	+	1		12–24
Bowie	1	COMP	+		1	72
Matuchansky	1	M-BACOP	+	1		12
Rogers	1	COMP	+		1	12

* M-BACOP, Methotrexate, bleomycin, doxorubicin, cyclosphosphamide, vincristine, prednisone; Pred, prednisone; COMP, cyclophosphamide, vincristine, methotrexate, prednisone; XRT, radiotherapy; CHOP, cyclphosphamide, doxorubicin, vincristine, prednisone; CHVP, cyclophosphamide, doxorubicin, teniposide, prednisone; MUS, mustargen; CTX, cyclophosphamide; VCR, vincristine; Chlor, chlorambucil; VP16, etoposide; DOX, doxorubicin.
† CR, Complete response; PR, partial response.

Table 47.6 Results of combination chemotherapy and radiation therapy in lymphomatous phase – immunoproliferative small intestinal disease

		Treatment*		Response†		
Author	No. of patients	Regimen*	No. of patients receiving radiotherapy	CR	PR	Duration/mean survival (months)
Asselah	120	CHOP	+/–		Unknown	
Al-Bahrani	82	CTX or 'more aggressive conventional chemotherapy'	+/–	5 year survival 22.7		
Banisadre	43	CVP	43	4	Unknown	
Gilinsky	17	VP16 + DOX or Pred	5 8		Unknown	20
Lewin	13	MUS + CTR + VCR + Pred or sequential single agents	9		Unknown	Unknown
Price	5	Unknown	5	4		Unknown

* CHOP, Cyclophosphamide, doxorubicin, vincristine, prednisone; Pred, prednisone; MUS, mustargen; CTX, cyclophosphamide; VCR, vincristine; VP16, etoposide; DOX, doxorubicin; CVP, cyclophosphamide, vincristine, prednisone.
† CR, Complete response; PR, partial response.

the treatment of IPSID with radiotherapy alone (or with steroids) has been anecdotal. Novis et al. [67,68] reported two patients who received 3 Gy of external-beam radiotherapy to the abdomen plus corticosteroids. One of them achieved a CR and remained in CR for greater than 12 years. Lewin et al. [49] treated nine patients with a combination of radiotherapy and chemotherapy, consisting of either sequential single agents or a combination of cyclophosphamide, nitrogen mustard, vincristine and prednisone. Four patients received radiotherapy alone. There was no mention of response rate or duration of response in this report though an improved survival rate was noted in those patients who received more than 2.75 Gy, as compared to those who received less than 2 Gy. To date, there have been no reports of large trials of patients treated with radiotherapy alone to determine the exact role of radiotherapy in the treatment of this disease, if any.

It is clear from this literature that immunoblastic lymphoma of IPSID is sensitive to chemotherapy and that at least 50% of patients treated achieve a complete response. Because of the varied nature of the treatment strategies reported, it is difficult to advocate one particular regimen, although combination anthracycline-based therapy appears to be superior at this time. Rambaud and Halphen [69] have advocated an aggressive approach, suggesting that as the overwhelming majority of these patients are young, those who are rapidly rendered free of disease should be considered candidates for high-dose

chemotherapy with bone marrow transplantation. However, there are no data to support the use of dose-intensive chemotherapy with marrow support in this population, and with the marginal nutritional status of the patients at the outset of therapy and their overall poor performance status, it is unlikely that these patients could tolerate such therapy.

Surgery plays little role in the treatment of this disease other than in diagnosis, staging and the treatment of rare abdominal catastrophes. Some researchers advocate resection of areas of bulky transmural disease prior to the initiation of antineoplastic therapy in order to avoid a potential catastrophe, but such lesions are uncommon in IPSID [24]. Additionally, as this disease involves virtually the entire small bowel, resection for cure is impossible. A small series of four patients with gastric αHCD was reported by Tungekar [17]. Two patients were treated with subtotal gastrectomy and two with total gastrectomy. One patient who had a total gastrectomy received in addition, radiotherapy and cyclophosphamide, vincristine and prednisone (CVP); and one of the two patients with subtotal gastrectomy was given CVP chemotherapy. Three of the four were alive and in complete remission after 10–30 months of follow-up. The follow-up of the fourth patient, in whom a distinction between lymphoma and gastritis could not be made on the basis of biopsy specimens, although α heavy chain proteins were present, was not reported.

In summary, all patients suspected of having

IPSID should have their disease evaluated by staging laparotomy unless surgery is contraindicated. While many patients are examined by upper endoscopy, the absence of lymphoma on multiple peroral intestinal biopsies does not rule out the presence of lymphoma in the mesenteric lymph nodes. Stool studies should be obtained for ova, parasites and other fecal pathogens, and specific infections should be treated if found. Careful attention should be paid to both fluid and nutritional status, and intravenous fluids and hyperalimentation should be used as necessary. Therapy of patients with Galian stage A (Salem stage O) may begin with antibiotics alone, such as tetracycline or metronidazole and ampicillin for at least 6 months. If at least a partial response is not achieved within 6 months, then the possibility of an underlying lymphoma should be ruled out and antineoplastic agents should be considered. While there is no chemotherapeutic regimen of choice, the present data suggest that anthracycline-containing regimens offer the highest response rates and the best survival advantages and regimens like CHOP, although potentially more toxic in this population of patients with severe malnutrition, should be used.

Low-grade B-cell gastric lymphoma

Primary lymphomas of the stomach account for less than 10% of all gastric malignancies but recent studies have suggested that the incidence of this neoplasm is increasing [70,71]. The stomach is the single most common primary site of extranodal lymphomas in the West [72–74] and is often involved upon dissemination of primary nodal lymphomas [75]. A variety of histologic subtypes of primary gastric lymphomas have been reported but most of these behave much the same as their nodal counterparts. However, low-grade B-cell gastric lymphoma (LBGL) of the stomach is histologically similar to MALT-derived lymphomas from other sites, and it accounts for 41–67% of the cases diagnosed [76–78].

While this disease has a follicular appearance, unlike nodal or gastrointestinal primary follicular lymphomas, there is no evidence of an underlying t(14;18) translocation or *bcl*-2 gene expression [79,80]. However, LBGL may be similar to IPSID in that an infectious etiology has been suspected, and recent evidence has strongly implicated a role for *Helicobacter pylori* in its development [81–86]. *H. pylori* colonization in the gastric mucosa is relatively common, and 50–60% of normal asymptomatic people may be found to harbor this organism. However, the rate of *H. pylori* infection in patients with gastric LBGL is much higher (92%) [81] and comparable with that seen in patients with gastric ulceration (97%) [87], and gastric adenocarcinoma (80%) [88]. Some investigators have suggested that a possible association between *H. pylori* infection and gastric LBGL exists. Wotherspoon et al. [81] reported the presence of *H. pylori* in the gastric mucosa of 92% of 110 patients with LBGL. Parsonnet et al. [89] found *H. pylori* in 91% (10 of 11) of patients with gastric lymphoma, as compared to 64% of a control group. Finally, Doglioni et al. [90] compared *H. pylori* prevalence rates from the Veneto region of northern Italy with those of several geographic locations within the United Kingdom. The Veneto region had an incidence of gastric lymphoma more than 13-fold higher than that of the chosen geographical locations within the United Kingdom (Llanelli District, Wales; Salisbury District, Wiltshire; and the Gloucester District, Gloucestershire), and more than three times the incidence of gastric carcinoma. This higher incidence of gastric lymphomas and carcinomas was associated with a higher incidence of *H. pylori* infection (87% versus 50–60%). Other authors have noted that lymphoid follicles are absent in the stomach mucosa of healthy individuals and in patients with reflux gastritis, but they are found in 54–100% of patients with *H. pylori*-related gastritis [91,92].

It is unknown how *H. pylori* causes gastric mucosal damage. One interesting finding is that not only does *H. pylori* elicit both a local and systemic antibody response, but it also shares several antigens with gastric epithelial cells. In a recent study, Negrini et al. [93] demonstrated that nearly 90% of patients who are seropositive for *H. pylori* also have autoantibodies directed against the mucosa of the body and antrum of the stomach. Additionally, these autoantibodies are fairly specific for gastric mucosa, as they are only weakly reactive with human salivary ducts, renal tubules and endometrial tissues. This suggests that the damage to the mucosa and the accumulation of lymphoid cells are, at least in part, autoimmune phenomena [94]. It also explains the emergence of LBGLs in the salivary and thyroid glands in the setting of Sjögren's syndrome and Hashimoto's thyroiditis, respectively [95–100]. Further evidence along these lines is that, when cells from patients with gastric LBGL are coincubated with *H. pylori*, there is stimulation of the release of interleukin-2 and tumor-derived immunoglobulin, upregulation of interleukin-2 receptor expression, and stimulation of growth of both the neoplastic cells and nonneoplastic T-cells [82]. These responses are reduced when the T-cells are removed from the culture. These findings are specific for gastric

LBGL, as there is no response to *H. pylori* with either cells from high-grade gastric lymphomas, or LBGLs from other sites [94].

An additional finding possibly explaining *H. pylori*-related mucosal damage is that of Crabtree et al. [87], who described the presence of a 120 kD protein elaborated by some strains of *H. pylori* and associated with epithelial damage and inflammatory changes in the mucosa [86]. It is unknown whether this protein is related to a 128–130 kD cytotoxin that is found in *H. pylori* culture-broth supernatants.

The association of gastric MALT-lymphoma with *H. pylori* has led to interesting speculation that this neoplasm may be treated in its earliest phase of development by antibiotics in a manner akin to that of IPSID. In fact, several lines of evidence support this hypothesis. For example, Genta et al. [92] demonstrated that eradication of *H. pylori* with triple combination therapy (metronidazole, tetracycline hydrochloride and bismuth subsalicylate) was associated with a decrease in the number of gastric lymphoid follicles, although the follicles were not completely eliminated in any patient over the span of the 1-year period of observation (two patients were observed for 20 and 21 months). Wotherspoon et al. [84] noted complete histologic and molecular remissions upon completion of therapy in five of six patients with gastric LBGL who were treated either with ampicillin and omeprazole, or with ampicillin, metronidazole and tripotassium dicitrobismuthate (Table 47.7). All patients had monoclonal DNA rearrangements as demonstrated by polymerase chain reaction or Southern blot analysis prior to the initiation of therapy. Similarly, Stolte and Eidt [91] reported that 12 of 12 patients with gastric MALT lymphoma and *H. pylori* experienced objective tumor regression after a 2-week course of ampicillin and omeprazole. These authors carefully pointed out that they were unsure of the depth of invasion of the lesions, as neither a full-thickness biopsy at laparotomy nor an endoscopic echosonography were performed. All patients treated lacked gross masses and had only the endoscopic appearance of 'gastritis'. However, disease in all patients was histologically consistent with malignant lymphoma and monoclonality was demonstrated in all by the application of the polymerase chain reaction. Based on the treatment experience of IPSID, a 2-week course of antibiotics may be too short to produce a complete remission in these patients.

There are a variety of reports on the therapy of gastric lymphoma, but many of these involve non-MALT histologies and utilize different therapeutic strategies. However, because of the tendency to remain localized until very late in the course of the disease, these lesions often lend themselves to a regional approach, such as radiotherapy or radical surgical resection with curative intent. Patients may thus experience a prolonged disease-free interval, although local relapse may occur if a portion of the organ of origin remains in place, or in distant MALT-related sites. One possible explanation for local relapse after a prolonged disease-free interval, as put forth by Wotherspoon et al., is that in at least some cases of gastric LBGL, the disease may be multifocal, despite the appearance of one dominant lesion, with some of the lymphomatous deposits at some distance from the predominant tumor [101]. Alternatively, if relevant pathogenetic factors are not eliminated, the possibility must be considered that late relapse sometimes represents the development of a new neoplastic clone.

As with most of the histologic subtypes of gastric lymphoma, an optimal therapeutic regimen has yet to be devised. Chemotherapy has been used and a variety of regimens have been administered, often with results consistent with responses seen in other low-grade lymphomas. A complete or near-complete response is achieved in more than half of the patients, followed by relapse in some of the patients, sometimes years after the initial treatment. The most commonly employed regimens are: COP (cyclophosphamide, vincristine and prednisone) and CHOP (COP with Adriamycin), or a variant. Unfortunately, most reports of large series of gastric lymphoma are retrospective, use multiple regimens, and omit response rates by histology and chemotherapeutic regimen, thus making it difficult, at best, to deter-

Table 47.7   Results of antibiotic therapy for gastric low-grade B-cell lymphoma

Author	No. of patients	Agent*	Response†	
			Level	Duration/survival interval
Wotherspoon	6	AMP + MNA + BIS (5)	5 CR	Unknown
		AMP + OMEP (1)	1 Regression	
Stolte	12	AMOX + OMEP	12 Regressions	Unknown

* AMOX, Amoxicillin; OMEP, omeprazole; AMP, ampicillin; MNA, metronidazole; BIS, tripotassium dicitrobismuthate.
† CR, Complete response.

mine the optimal regimen. In one interesting study, 14 of 16 patients with gastric MALT-LBGL received monotherapy with cyclophosphamide. Of the remaining two patients, one had rapidly progressing disease at initial presentation and received CHOP with radiotherapy to the gastric bed, and the other had undergone a partial gastrectomy and received radiotherapy prior to referral to the authors' institutions [96]. All patients had follow-up for at least 1 year, and the median follow-up was 4.5 years. Of the patients treated with monotherapy, eight experienced a complete remission, and one had a partial remission, giving a total response rate of 56%. However, all 16 patients remained alive at last follow-up, with only two lost to follow-up. It is of note that those patients who relapsed remained sensitive to rechallenge with cyclophosphamide. No evidence of a myelodysplastic syndrome was noted, despite the use of daily therapy for a year or more. While interesting, these data await confirmation by other investigators.

In general, however, there are several major difficulties in evaluating the published series of patients with gastric lymphoma. Most large trials include patients whose disease reflects a number of histologic subtypes that may have different biologic behaviors, even when all patients are treated alike, but in reporting their results, most authors do not adequately analyze treatment and response data by histology. While some authors have identified MALT lesions in their series, they have not analyzed these patients separately. Furthermore, when chemotherapy was used, multiple treatment regimens have been utilized. In the large series of 307 cases reported by Radaszkiewicz et al. [77], where 125 patients were noted to have MALT lesions, 37% of patients received radiotherapy and/or chemotherapy, but no mention is made of any of the chemotherapy agents used. They only stated that multiple regimens were used. In their evaluation of 56 patients with gastric lymphoma, Castrillo et al. [95] do not recommend any particular chemotherapy combination. They suggest that patients with low-grade histologic lesions should be treated with resection, whereas those with high-grade lesions should receive multi-agent chemotherapy. Swaroop et al. [102] used 'chemotherapy and radiotherapy only' in 30 patients and noted a 'good complete response rate'. Pinotti et al. [71] treated 119 patients having gastric lymphoma, of whom 28 had a surgical resection followed by adjuvant chemotherapy or radiation therapy, and 20 had chemotherapy or radiation without resection. Single-agent chlorambucil or CVP was used for low-grade lesions, whereas CHOP was used for high-grade lesions. A 5-year survival rate of 89% was noted in those patients who had undergone resection, compared to a 33% survival rate in those who had no resection. However, it was impossible to determine which patients had MALT neoplasms and how such patients had responded. Cogliatti et al. [78] reported the results of treatment of 145 patients, of whom 71 had a low-grade B-cell lymphoma. Although a variety of combination chemotherapeutic regimens were used in 43 patients (33 of them also received radiotherapy), a 5-year survival rate for patients with low-grade B-cell lymphoma was 91%, compared to 76% for the group as a whole. Again, the specific treatment regimens and the results of therapy in patients with LBGL exclusively were not mentioned.

Many investigators still recommend a radical gastrectomy as essential for maximal disease control and report increased 5- and 10-year survival rates in patients who undergo a complete resection [77,103–105]. Some, such as Ichiyoshi et al. [105], even recommend radical resection including the extraperigastric nodes along the celiac, common hepatic and splenic arteries followed by adjuvant chemotherapy, without specifying a chemotherapeutic regimen. Not all authors are in agreement with this approach and, instead, some advocate radiotherapy to the tumor bed followed by systemic chemotherapy [106,107]. Not only were these researchers able to document comparable disease-free survival rates but also they provided further evidence that surgical resection may provide no additional benefit [107,108]. Authors who support the use of surgical resection also cite the elimination of potential complications such as bleeding or perforation which may occur with the use of either chemotherapy or radiotherapy should the tumor remain in its primary site as an additional benefit, though these appear to be relatively uncommon complications [98,106].

Recognizing the propensity for these malignancies to recur, postoperative adjuvant therapy has been advocated. Except for one report by Shiu et al. [109] that noted a doubling of patient's survival rate using adjuvant radiotherapy, there is no evidence that such an approach is beneficial and some authors have even noted a decrease in survival rate in patients treated with adjuvant radiotherapy. As noted by Walker [104], the 5-year survival rate in patients who received adjuvant radiotherapy was 71.5%, compared to 82.4% in those treated with resection alone. A lack of beneficial effect is not unexpected, as both surgery and radiotherapy are purely local modalities. In one small study (Ben-Shaher et al.) the necessity of gastric resection was specifically addressed [110]. Eleven patients with limited disease were treated. Of the five who underwent surgical resection, two patients had postoperative radiotherapy and another had postoperative chemotherapy for disease-positive surgical margins. Of the six patients whose disease was not approached surgically, three were treated with radiotherapy alone, two with a combination of radiotherapy and chemotherapy, and one with chemotherapy alone. Ten of the 11 patients achieved and remained in a complete response of 2–44 months' duration, with a median follow-up of 24 months. While these data are interesting, the number of treated patients is very small, making a statistical comparison impossible. Also, the chemotherapeutic regimens and the radiotherapeutic treatments were not described in detail.

In conclusion, the optimal treatment of LBGL of MALT origin remains to be determined. All patients with this disease should be adequately staged and the depth of invasion of the gastric wall by lymphoma should be evaluated. Patients with early disease and lymphoma confined to the mucosa and submucosa should be studied for *H. pylori* colonization. In the presence of *H. pylori* infection, these patients should be treated with antibiotics for an adequate period of time necessary to eradicate the infection. The duration of antibiotic therapy is not known; however, extrapolation from experience in the treatment of immunoproliferative small intestinal disease leads us to believe that this duration should be prolonged. Patients who achieve a complete remission on antibiotic therapy alone should be observed only and followed every few months. Upon relapse, these patients may be treated as other patients with MALT-LBGL. Patients with more advanced disease should probably be treated with the combination of chemotherapy plus surgery or chemotherapy plus radiation therapy. It is unclear at the moment as to whether surgical resection offers any additional benefits to radiation therapy (or vice versa). However, patients who are candidates for surgical resection should, for the moment at least, undergo surgery, while patients who have advanced disease or where surgery is contraindicated should receive radiation therapy. Irrespective of whether patients are scheduled to receive radiation therapy or surgery, it is advisable to begin with systemic chemotherapy (using CHOP or a CHOP-based regimen). Initial chemotherapy will demonstrate whether the disease is sensitive to chemotherapy and would permit chemotherapy to be pursued until a complete remission were achieved in patients with tumors shown to be sensitive to this treatment. In patients who achieve a complete remission, surgery or radiotherapy may be used. Of course, surgery then has the added advantage of documenting whether there is residual disease in the stomach or not.

Monocytoid B-cell lymphoma

An entity which is closely related to MALT-LBGL is monocytoid B-cell lymphoma. The nonneoplastic monocytoid B-cell, which was initially labeled as an immature sinus histiocyte, and which is also known as a parafollicular B-lymphocyte, is found in the intrasinusoidal and paracortical regions of reactive lymph nodes. These cells are commonly found in AIDS-related adenopathy and toxoplasmosis. Such cells may also be observed in other inflammatory lymphadenopathies, as well as in Hodgkin's disease and other non-Hodgkin's lymphomas [111–120]. Monocytoid B-cell lymphoma was recognized relatively recently, with Sheibani et al. documenting the first cases in 1986 [115]. It is thought that monocytoid B-cell lymphoma is very closely related to LBGL. To date, most reports consist of small groups of patients.

The underlying etiology of monocytoid B-cell lymphoma remains to be determined. In common with MALT lymphomas and in distinct contrast to follicular lymphomas, *bcl*-2 oncogene rearrangement in this disease is rare [121,122]. However, the presence of monocytoid B-cells in HIV-associated lymphadenopathy, and the association of monocytoid B-cells (and the subsequent lymphoma) in patients with a variety of autoimmune diseases, suggest that a disturbance of the normal immune regulation may play a role in the development of this disease.

The natural history of monocytoid B-cell lymphoma is similar to that of other low-grade MALT lymphomas and is characterized by a prolonged clinical course, high rates of complete remission induction, late relapses and good long-term survival rates. The majority of patients present for evaluation of peripheral lymphadenopathy and approximately one-third of patients complain of B symptoms. As might be expected, patients with greater tumor bulk and those presenting with a higher stage of disease fare relatively poorly.

The treatment of this disease has been extremely heterogeneous (Table 47.8), and a variety of combination chemotherapy regimens, such as COP, CHOP, ABVD (doxorubicin, bleomycin, vincristine and dacarbazine), KNOSPE (chlorambucil and prednisone) and m-BACOD (methotrexate, bleomycin, doxorubicin, cyclophosphamide, vincristine and dexamethasone) have been used with initial success, although disease in at least half of the patients eventually relapses [120,123,124]. Cogliatti et al. [124] reported 15 complete and three partial responses in 21 patients treated with a variety of regimens and multimodal strategies, although half the patients had disease that relapsed at a mean of 20 months. Shin et al. [125] obtained a complete response in 12 of 13 cases of monocytoid B-cell lymphoma associated

Table 47.8 Results of treatment for monocytoid B-cell lymphoma

Author	No. of patients	Agent*	Response†		
			CR	PR	Duration/survival (years)
Cogliatti	18	COP + CHOP + ABVD + KNOSPE	15	3	28.2
Aozasa	6	Unknown 5		24.3	
Banerjee	1	DICE + VAPEC-B	1		22 3

* COP, Cyclophosphamide, vincristine, prednisone; CHOP, cyclophosphamide, doxorubicin, vincristine, prednisone; DICE, doxorubicin, ifosfamide, cyclophosphamide, etoposide; ABVD, doxorubicin, bleomycin, vinblastine, dacarbazine; VAPEC-B, doxorubicin, cyclophosphamide, etoposide, vincristine, bleomycin, prednisone; KNOSPE, chlorombucil, prednisone.
† CR, Complete response; PR, partial response.

with Sjögrens' syndrome. Shin and Sheibani [121] reported that, of 100 patients in their registry, 65 had adequate follow-up data and that only five of these had died of disease. Forty-five had received chemotherapy and/or radiotherapy, but the specifics were not discussed. To date, while most reports state that patients have responded favorably to chemotherapy and/or radiotherapy, there was no documentation of the chemotherapeutic agents used, or treatment details of radiotherapy. No prospective trials have been conducted to determine the optimal treatment strategy. Until such information is at hand, this malignancy should be approached as any other low-grade MALT lymphoma.

Enteropathy-associated T-cell lymphoma

The vast majority of MALT-related malignancies are of B-cell origin. Peripheral T-cell lymphomas, while frequently presenting in extranodal sites such as the skin, as in cutaneous T-cell lymphoma and Sézary syndrome, rarely involve MALT-associated tissues at presentation. One exception to this is enteropathy-associated T-cell lymphoma (EATCL).

First described in 1962, EATCL was initially termed malignant histiocytosis of the intestine [126]. However, the malignant cell was later shown to be of lymphocytic, not monocytic, lineage [127,128]. EATCL usually develops in patients with long-standing celiac disease and/or dermatitis herpetiformis. It occurs in 7–12% of such patients [129,130]. As patients with celiac disease have a 50–100-fold greater risk of developing lymphoma, some authors have suggested that this disease may, in fact, be a premalignant phase [130]. Occasionally, a patient will present with EATCL, and will subsequently develop mild or asymptomatic celiac sprue.

Small intestinal lymphoma arising in celiac disease occurs more commonly in Europe, particularly among the Irish, but it is relatively uncommon in North America. This suggests that there may be a genetic predisposition to EATCL. There is ample evidence to postulate a role for genetic factors in the etiology of celiac sprue, such as a higher incidence in the relatives of affected patients, and an association with the HLA-A1, HLA-B8, HLA-DR3, HLA-DR5/DR7 and HLA-DQw2 histocompatibility antigens [129,131]. However, not all patients with celiac sprue express these antigens and, conversely, not all patients with these antigens are affected by sprue. Recently, several reports have surfaced that implicate the Epstein–Barr virus (EBV) in the etiology of EATCL [132,133]. Although EBV has been associated with the development of malignancy, such as Burkitt's lymphoma, nasopharyngeal carcinoma and, infrequently, the Reed–Sternberg cells of Hodgkin's disease [134], until recently it was thought that EBV-associated T-cell lymphomas were rare [135]. Using Southern blot hybridization, Pan et al. [133] observed that only one of 30 patients with nodal T-cell lymphomas but four (36%) of 11 patients with EATCL had EBV DNA within the tumor cells. Likewise, Borisch et al. [132] used amplification by the polymerase chain reaction to detect EBV DNA in the neoplastic cells of a patient who had received a prior renal transplant and had developed EATCL. It is unclear, at present, whether such an association is causative or coincidental.

The malignant cells of EATCL appear to be derived from the intraepithelial lymphocytes [136, 137]. Although the function of these cells remains speculative at present, the cells are cytolytic upon stimulation. EATCL is usually a high-grade malignancy associated with a rapidly progressive course and a poor clinical outcome. Most patients present with exacerbation of their symptoms, such as a worsening of the malabsorption syndrome and a loss of responsiveness to a gluten-restricted diet. Approximately a quarter of the patients present with an intestinal perforation [138,139]. The treatment of this disease is difficult at best. There is no evidence that a gluten-free diet will prevent the development of EATCL; in fact, in one study it was noted that such a diet was associated with an increased risk of developing a small bowel lymphoma [140]. Once a lymphoma has developed, patients often experience a worsening of what may have been a marginal nutritional status at the outset [138,139]. EBV may play a role in the etiology of a small subset of patients with EATCL but antiviral therapy for EBV infection is ineffective [141]. Curative surgical resection is precluded by the large area of gut involvement, although the lymphoma tends to be localized in the jejunum and surgery should be reserved for the emergency therapy of abdominal catastrophes. A variety of combination chemotherapy regimens have been used. Chott et al. [142] noted that, of 27 T-cell lymphomas of the intestines, 14 were EATCL. Multiple modalities were used in this series: 14 (of the original 27) patients received chemotherapy (the regimens were not specified) and the median survival for the entire group was 4 months. Mead et al. [143] treated nine patients (five following attempted resection) with four different chemotherapy regimens and observed responses in five. Grogan et al. [144] treated eight patients with M-BACOD. Compared to nine patients with B-cell gastrointestinal lymphoma who were similarly treated, patients with EATCL has a poorer response rate (38% versus 100%), a worse 2-year disease-free survival rate (13% versus 100%), and an inferior overall median survival interval (12 months, range of 3–45 months, versus 49+ months, range of 15–90+ months). In general, responses were usually brief and therapy was poorly tolerated owing to the malnourished state of most of these patients. To date, there has been no carefully controlled study of a particular regimen in a significant population of patients with EATCL.

Conclusions

The MALT lymphomas represent a distinct subset of non-Hodgkin's lymphomas, and present a unique research opportunity to understand the genesis of lymphomas and the relationship between infection and cancer. While these lymphomas tend to have a prolonged clinical course similar to that of low-grade

nodal lymphomas, it is clear that they are biologically different from their nodal counterparts. Most of these diseases are associated with an indolent phase that appears to arise from an inappropriate or excessive prolonged stimulation of the mucosal immune system, and which is associated with considerable morbidity. In this indolent phase, early changes often appear to be benign but with time, and if left untreated, malignant lymphoma emerges. Clear examples of this slow transition from benign to malignant disease include: Sjögren's syndrome and salivary gland lymphoma, Hashimoto's thyroiditis and thyroid lymphoma, celiac sprue and EATCL, the prelymphomatous phase of IPSID and IPSID lymphoma. Most interesting, is the potential causative link between infection and the development of malignant lymphoma, as in IPSID, gastric MALT lymphoma, Burkitt's lymphoma and perhaps a small subset of patients with EATCL. The observation that antibiotics may reverse the prelymphomatous phase of IPSID and possibly the early phase of established gastric MALT lymphomas is of considerable importance, and opens the door wide for future research to delineate the nature of the relationship between infection and cancer. Also, the reversibility of IPSID by antibiotics constitutes the first milestone of chemoprevention of cancer in man. MALT lymphomas constitute an important cancer model and future efforts should be directed towards studies of the basic mechanisms underlying the pathogenesis of these diseases.

References

1. Tseng J. Migration and differentiation of IgA precursor cells in the gut-associated lymphoid tissue. In Husband AJ (ed.) *Migration and Homing of Lymphoid Cells*, Vol. II. Boca Raton: CRC Press, Inc. 1988, pp. 77–97.
2. Phillips-Quagliata JM, Roux ME, Arny M, et al. Migration and regulation of B-cells in the mucosal immune system. *Ann. N. York Acad. Sci.* 1983, **409**: 194–203.
3. Cebra JJ, Kamat R, Gearhart P, et al. The secretory IgA system of the gut. In *Immunology of the Gut*. CIBA Foundation Symposium 46. Amsterdam: Elsevier/Excerpta Medica/North Holland, 1977, pp. 5–22.
4. Husband AJ, Monie JH, Gowans JL. The natural history of the cells producing IgA in the gut. In *Immunology of the Gut*. CIBA Foundation Symposium 46. Amsterdam: Elsevier/Excerpta Medica/North Holland, 1977, pp. 29–42.
5. Kawanishi H, Strober W. Regulatory T-cells in murine Peyer's patches directing IgA-specific isotype switching. *Ann. N. York Acad. Sci.* 1983, **409**: 243–256.

6. McWilliams M, Phillips-Quagliata JM, Lamm ME. Mesenteric lymph node B lymphoblasts which home to the small intestine are precommitted to IgA synthesis. *J. Exp. Med.* 1977, **145**: 866–875.

7. Gallatin WM, St John TP, Siegelman M, et al. Lymphocyte homing receptors. *Cell* 1986, **44**: 673–680.

8. Jalkanen S, Reichert RA, Gallatin WM, et al. Homing receptors and the control of lymphocyte migration. *Immunol. Rev.* 1986, **91**: 39–60.

9. Woodruff JJ, Clarke LM, Chin YH. Specific cell adhesion mechanisms determining migration pathways of recirculating lymphocytes. *Annu. Rev. Immunol.* 1987, **5**: 201–222.

10. Holzmann B, Weissman IL. Peyer's patch-specific lymphocyte homing receptors consist of a VLA-4-like α chain with either of two integrin β chains, one of which is novel. *EMBO J.* 1989, **8**: 1735–1741.

11. Holzmann B, McIntyre BW, Weissman IL. Identification of a murine Peyer's patch-specific lymphocyte homing receptor as an integrin molecule with an α chain homologous to human VLA-4α. *Cell* 1989, **56**: 37–46.

12. Sher BT, Bargatze R, Holzmann B, et al. Homing receptors and metastasis. *Adv. Cancer Res.* 1988, **51**: 361–390.

13. Jalkanen S, Wu N, Bargatze RF, et al. Human lymphocyte and lymphoma homing receptors. *Annu. Rev. Med.* 1987, **38**: 467–476.

14. Pals ST, Horst E, Ossekoppele GJ, et al. Expression of lymphocyte homing receptors as a mechanism of dissemination in non-Hodgkin's lymphoma. *Blood* 1989, **73**: 885–888.

15. Al-Mondhiry H. Primary lymphomas of the small intestine: East–west contrast. *Am. J. Hematol.* 1986, **22**: 89–105.

16. Cohen JH, Gonzalvo A, Krook J, et al. New presentation of alpha heavy chain disease: North American polypoid gastrointestinal lymphoma. Clinical and cellular studies. *Cancer* 1978, **41**: 1161–1168.

17. Tungekar MF, Omar YT, Behbehani K. Gastric alpha heavy chain disease. *Oncology* 1987, **44**: 360–366.

18. Guardia J, Mirada A, Moragas A, et al. Alpha chain disease of the stomach. *Hepatogastroenterology* 1980, **27**: 238–239.

19. Azar HA. Cancer in Lebanon and the Middle East. *Cancer* 1962, **15**: 66–78.

20. Seligmann M, Danon F, Hurez D, et al. Alpha-chain disease: A new immunoglobulin abnormality. *Science* 1968, **162**: 1396–1397.

21. Seijffers MJ, Levy M, Hermann G. Intractable watery diarrhea, hypokalemia, and malabsorption in a patient with Mediterranean type of abdominal lymphoma. *Gastroenterology* 1968, **55**: 118–124.

22. World Health Organization. Alpha chain disease and related small intestinal lymphoma: A memorandum. *Bull. WHO* 1976, **54**: 615–624.

23. Ramot B, Shahin N, Bubis JJ. Malabsorbtion syndrome in lymphoma of the small intestine. *Isr. J. Med. Sci.* 1965, **1**: 221–226.

24. Khojasteh A, Haghshenass M, Haghighi P. Current concepts immunoproliferative small intestinal disease: A third-world lesion. *N. Engl. J. Med.* 1983, **308**: 1401–1405.

25. Rizk W, Shamseddine N, Taleb N. Epidemiology of GI NHL in Lebanon and the Middle East. *Fifth International Conference on Malignant Lymphoma,* June 1993, Lugano, Switzerland, p. 93 (abstract).

26. Salem PA, Nassar VH, Shahid MJ, et al. 'Mediterranean abdominal lymphoma', or immunoproliferative small intestinal disease. Part I: Clinical aspects. *Cancer* 1977, **40**: 2941–2947.

27. Haghighi P, Nasr K. Primary upper small intestinal lymphoma (so-called Mediterranean lymphoma). *Pathol. Annu.* 1973, **8**: 231–255.

28. Rambaud JC. Small intestinal lymphomas and alpha-chain disease. *Clin. Gastroenterol.* 1983, **12**: 743–766 (abstract).

29. Doe WF. Alpha chain disease: Clinicopathological features and relationship to so-called Mediterranean lymphoma. *Br. J. Cancer* 1975, **31** (Suppl. 2): 350–355.

30. Asselah F, Slavin G, Sowter G, et al. Immunoproliferative small intestinal disease in Algerians. I. Light microscopic and immunochemical studies. *Cancer* 1983, **52**: 227–237.

31. Chandra RK. Mucosal immune responses in malnutrition. *Ann. N. York Acad. Sci.* 1983, **409**: 345–351.

32. Chandra RK. Nutrition, immunity and infection: Present knowledge and future directions. *Lancet* 1983, **1**: 688–691.

33. Pape JW, Liautaud B, Thomas F, et al. Characteristics of the acquired immunodeficiency syndrome (AIDS) in Haiti. *N. Engl. J. Med.* 1983, **309**: 945–950.

34. Seligmann M, Rambaud JC. Alpha-chain disease: A possible model for the pathogenesis of human lymphomas. In Twomey JJ, Good RA (eds) *The Immunopathology of Lymphoreticular Neoplasms.* New York: Plenum Medical Books, 1978, pp. 425–447.

35. Salem P, El-Hashimi L, Anaissie E, et al. Primary small intestinal lymphoma in adults. A comparative study of IPSID versus non-IPSID in the Middle East. *Cancer* 1987, **59**: 1670–1676.

36. Rambaud JC, Matuchansky C. Alpha chain disease: Pathogenesis and relation to Mediterranean lymphoma. *Lancet* 1973, **1**: 1430–1432.

37. Crow J, Asselah F. Immunoproliferative small intestinal disease in Algerians. II. Ultrastructural studies in alpha-chain disease. *Cancer* 1984, **54**: 1908–1913.

38. Nasr K, Haghighi P, Bakhshandeh K, et al. Primary upper small intestinal lymphoma: A report of 40 cases from Iran. *Am. J. Digest. Dis.* 1970, **21**: 213–223.

39. Matuchansky C, Cogne M, Lemaire M, et al. Nonsecretory α-chain disease with immunoproliferative small intestinal disease. *N. Engl. J. Med.* 1989, **320**: 1534–1539.

40. Cogne M, Preud'homme JL. Gene deletions force nonsecretory α-chain disease plasma cells to produce membrane-form α-chain only. *J. Immunol.* 1990, **145**: 2455–2458.

41. Cammoun M, Jaafoura H, Tabbane F, et al. Immunoproliferative small intestinal disease without alpha-

109. Shiu MH, Karas M, Nisce L, et al. Management of primary gastric lymphoma. *Ann. Surg.* 1982, **195**: 196–202.

110. Ben-Shahar M, Ben-Arie Y, Epelbaum R, et al. MALT lymphoma of the stomach: Is surgical resection necessary? *Fifth International Conference on Malignant Lymphoma*, June 1993, Lugano, Switzerland (abstract).

111. Miettinen M. Histological differential diagnosis between lymph node toxoplasmosis and other benign lymph node hyperplasias. *Histopathology* 1981, **5**: 205–216.

112. Sheibani K, Fritz RM, Winberg CD, et al. 'Monocytoid' cells in reactive follicular hyperplasia with and without multifocal histiocytic reactions: An immunohistochemical study of 21 cases including suspected cases of toxoplasmic lymphadenitis. *Am. J. Clin. Pathol.* 1984, **81**: 453–458.

113. Chambers TJ, Stansfeld AG. Histiocytosis and histiocytic neoplams. In Stansfeld AG (ed.) *Lymph Node Biopsy Interpretation.* Edinburgh: Churchill Livingstone, 1985, pp. 345–379.

114. Nizze H, Cogliatti SB, von Schilling C, et al. Monocytoid B-cell lymphoma: Morphological variants and relationship to low-grade B-cell lymphoma of the mucosa-associated lymphoid tissue. *Histopathology* 1991, **18**: 403–414.

115. Sheibani K, Sohn CC, Burke JS, et al. Monocytoid B-cell lymphoma: A novel B-cell neoplasm. *Am. J. Pathol.* 1986, **124**: 310–318.

116. Harris NL. Low-grade B-cell lymphoma of mucosa-associated lymphoid tissue and monocytoid B-cell lymphoma: Related entities that are distinct from other low-grade B-cell lymphomas. *Arch. Pathol. Lab. Med.* 1993, **117**: 771–775.

117. Ortiz-Hidalgo C, Wright DH. The morphological spectrum of monocytoid B-cell lymphoma and its relationship to lymphomas of mucosal-associated lymphoid tissue. *Histopathology* 1992, **21**: 555–561.

118. Spencer J, Finn T, Pulford KAF, et al. The human gut contains a novel population of B lymphocytes which resemble marginal zone cells. *Clin. Exp. Immunol.* 1985, **62**: 607–612.

119. Piris M, Rivas C, Morente M, et al. Monocytoid B-cell lymphoma, a tumor related to the marginal zone. *Histopathology* 1988, **12**: 383–392.

120. Traweek ST, Sheibani K, Winberg CD, et al. Monocytoid B-cell lymphoma: Its evolution and relationship to other low-grade B-cell neoplasms. *Blood* 1989, **73**: 573–578.

121. Shin SS, Sheibani K. Monocytoid B-cell lymphoma. *Am. J. Clin. Pathol.* 1993, **99**: 421–425.

122. Sheibani K, Ben-Ezra J. Molecular biology of monocytoid B-cell lymphoma: Absence of HTLV-I, HTLV-II, and HIV genome and rearranged *bcl*-2 genes in neoplastic monocytoid B-cells. *Lab. Invest.* 1990, **62**: 92A (abstract).

123. Banerjee SS, Harris M, Eyden BP, et al. Monocytoid B-cell lymphoma. *J. Clin. Pathol.* 1991, **44**: 39–44.

124. Cogliatti SB, Lennert K, Hansmann M-L, et al. Monocytoid B-cell lymphoma: Clinical and prognostic features of 21 patients. *J. Clin. Pathol.* 1990, **43**: 619–625.

125. Shin SS, Sheibani K, Fishleder A, et al. Monocytoid B-cell lymphoma in patients with Sjögren's syndrome: A clinicopathologic study of 13 patients. *Hum. Pathol.* 1991, **22**: 422–430.

126. Gough KR, Read AE, Naish JM. Intestinal reticulosis as a complication of idiopathic steatorrhoea. *Gut* 1962, **3**: 232–239.

127. Isaacson PG, O'Connor NT, Spencer J, et al. Malignant histiocytosis of the intestine: A T-cell lymphoma. *Lancet* 1985, **2**: 688–691.

128. Selby WS, Gallagher ND. Malignancy in a 19-year experience oestinal. In Sleisenger MH, Fordtran JS (eds) *Gastrointestinal Disease*, 5th edn. Philadelphia: W. B. Saunders, 1993, pp. 1078–1095.

129. Trier JS. Celiac sprue. In Sleisenger MH, Fordtran JS (eds) *Gastrointestinal Disease*, 5th edn. Philadelphia: W. B. Saunders, 1993, pp. 1078–1095.

130. Moroz C, Marcus, H, Zahavi I, et al. Is coeliac disease a premalignant state? *Lancet* 1988, **2**: 903–904.

131. Freeman HJ, Weinstein WM, Shnitka TK, et al. Primary abdominal lymphoma: Presenting manifestation of celiac sprue or complicating dermatitis herpetiformis. *Am. J. Med.* 1977, **63**: 585–594.

132. Borisch B, Hennig I, Horber F, et al. Enteropathy-associated T-cell lymphoma in a renal transplant patient with evidence of Epstein–Barr virus involvement. *Virchows Arch. A [Pathol. Anat. Histopathol.]* 1992, **421**: 443–447.

133. Pan L, Diss TC, Peng H, et al. Epstein–Barr virus (EBV) in enteropathy-associated T-cell lymphoma (EATL). *J. Pathol.* 1993, **170**: 137–143.

134. Coates PJ, Slavin G, d'Ardenne AJ. Epstein–Barr virus localises to Reed–Sternberg cells in a minority of Hodgkin's disease tissues. *J. Pathol.* 1991, **163**: 172A (abstract).

135. Jones JF, Shurin S, Abramowsky C, et al. T-cell lymphomas containing Epstein–Barr viral DNA in patients with chronic Epstein–Barr virus infections. *N. Engl. J. Med.* 1988, **318**: 733–741.

136. Salter DM, Krajewski AS. Histogenesis of malignant histiocytosis of the intestine. *Gastroenterology* 1987, **92**: 2050.

137. Stein H, Dienemann D, Sperling M, et al. Identification of a T-cell lymphoma category derived from intestinal mucosa-associated T-cells. *Lancet* 1988, **2**: 1053–1054.

138. Domizio P, Owen RA, Shepherd NA, et al. Primary lymphoma of the small intestine. A clinicopathological study of 119 cases. *Am. J. Surg Pathol.* 1993, **17**: 429–442.

139. Cooper BT, Read AE. Coeliac disease and lymphoma. *Q. J. Med.* 1987, **63**: 269–274.

140. Holmes GKT, Prior P, Lane MR, et al. Malignancy in coeliac disease: Effect of a gluten free diet. *Gut* 1989, **30**: 333–338.

141. Straus SE, Cohen JI, Tosato G, Meier J. Epstein–Barr virus infections: Biology, pathogenesis, and management. *Ann. Intern. Med.* 1993, **118**: 45–58.

142. Chott A, Dragosics B, Radaszkiewicz T. Peripheral T-cell lymphomas of the intestine. *Am. J. Pathol.* 1992, **141**: 1361–1371.

143. Mead GM, Whitehouse JM, Thompson J, et al. Clinical features and management of malignant

histiocytosis of the intestine. *Cancer* 1987, **60**: 2791–2796.

144. Grogan L, Devaney D, Corbally N, et al. Enteropathy-associated T-cell lymphoma with multiple skip lesions identified a distinct clinicopathological subset of primary small bowel lymphoma with poor prognosis. *Fifth International Conference on Malignant Lymphoma*, June 1993, Lugano, Switzerland, p. 138 (abstract).

CHAPTER 48

Extranodal lymphomas

FRANCO CAVALLI

Introduction

Although lymphomas are usually considered as tumors of the lymph nodes, a substantial percentage of non-Hodgkin's lymphomas (NHLs) arise from other lymphoid tissue, such as tonsil or Peyer's patches, and also from sites such as the stomach, which normally contain no lymphoid tissue. These lymphomas are referred to as primary extranodal lymphomas.

The relative incidence of extranodal lymphoma varies considerably in different series but, conservatively estimated, at least a quarter of all NHLs are probably of extranodal origin [1]. Despite the relative prominence of extranodal lymphomas, the literature on their incidence, and on the majority of specific types and sites, is sparse and often contradictory. This is primarily because these tumors, numerous when considered together, are distributed so widely throughout the body that it is difficult to assemble an adequate series based on any given site. Hence, for the most part, it is necessary to resort to data from literature reviews or series assembled largely by selective referral.

In this light, data collected prospectively from population-based registries have an advantage, since they are not biased by referral policy [2]. A major disadvantage of these data sources, however, is the lack, in general, of common treatment protocols. This has been partially eliminated in data collected recently which predominantly consist of patients treated on the basis of a consensus reached before the registry was started [2,3].

Another problem with establishing the prevalence and incidence of extranodal lymphomas concerns their definition, in the presence of both nodal and extranodal disease. The following definition has recently been applied [3]: lymphomas are considered extranodal when after routine staging procedures there is either no or only 'minor' nodal involvement along with a clinically 'dominant' extranodal component. Minor nodal or dominant extranodal components were respectively defined as < 25% or > 75% of the total tumor volume [3]. Another methodological problem relates to the debate about whether tonsils and Waldeyer's ring should be considered as nodal or extranodal sites. Recent immunohistological and clinical data strongly suggest that primary tonsilar and Waldeyer's ring lymphomas should be considered to be of nodal origin [2–6].

RISING INCIDENCE

In view of the methodological problems discussed so far, it is not surprising that there are large differences in incidence among countries: USA 24% [1], Israel 36% [7], Denmark 37% [3], Holland 41% [2] and Italy 48% [8]. Little is known about the incidence in developing countries where methodological problems are even greater; there have, however, been frequent allusions to a higher incidence of extranodal than nodal lymphomas in less developed countries [9].

In Western countries, the more realistic data are probably those derived from population-based registries, according to which it has been estimated that 35–40% of all lymphomas are of extranodal origin [2–3].

It has recently been demonstrated that NHLs are rapidly increasing in incidence – an increase which, at least in the USA in the last 20 years, has been exceeded only by lung cancer in women and malignant melanoma [10]. This emerging epidemic of NHL has recently been reviewed and discussed [9–11]. From the US data it appears that between 1974 and 1988 increases in incidence were proportionately greater for the extranodal forms [11]; incidence rates increased by 1.7–2.5% per year for nodal cases compared to 3.0–6.9% for extranodal cases. The extranodal sites with the greatest rise in incidence were the stomach, intestines and skin, with increases of 49%, 56% and 67%, respectively [11]. However, the largest proportionate increases occurred in the brain and other areas of the nervous system (244%), and in the eye (140%). Similar data have been reported for Denmark, where recent data show an annual increase of 4–5% in newly diagnosed NHL [12]. The corresponding rate of increase in the USA is 3.3% per year [9]. Analogous to the US data, the main contribution of the Danish results to the overall increase in incidence derived from lymphomas with diffuse histology and those with extranodal localization. It is of interest that, as in the USA [9], in Denmark there appears to be a nonrandom geographic variation in the increase, suggesting a significant impact of environmental factors. Another report from Denmark confirmed the fact that among extranodal lymphomas, central nervous system (CNS) lymphomas are those with the most rapidly rising incidence [13].

PATIENT CHARACTERISTICS: NODAL VERSUS EXTRANODAL LYMPHOMAS

Older series reporting detailed characteristics of patients suffering from extranodal lymphomas are of limited value because of the recent refinements in staging and diagnostic procedure as well as the changing nomenclature of histological classification [1]. More recent data, especially those derived from population-based registries, are more consistent with respect to definitions.

In three recent series [2–3,14] the distributions by age and sex of nodal and extranodal NHLs were very similar; the only exception occurred in a series [3] in which patients with nodal NHL tended to be younger ($P = 0.05$). In all three series there were two important and consistently statistically significant differences: extranodal cases were more frequently

localized (45–50% were stage IE or III1E) and were less frequently of low-grade histology (12–20% of all extranodal NHLs). In this context it must be noted that for extranodal lymphomas the Ann Arbor staging classification is often modified according to Musshoff [15], whereby modified stage III1E corresponds to confluent loco-regional lymph nodes only. Patients with localized extranodal lymphomas more often present with diffuse large-cell and high-grade histologies [2,14]. Generally, patients with extranodal lymphomas tend less often to present with B symptoms than do patients suffering from lymphomas arising in the lymph nodes [3]. The degree of concurrent nodal involvement has been adequately evaluated in only one recent series [3] in which multivariate analysis showed that about one-third of 463 patients with extranodal NHLs had minor nodal involvement along with a clinically dominant extranodal component; the presence of this simultaneous nodal component did not influence survival [3].

TREATMENT OUTCOME

As shown in Table 48.1, the survival rates for various specific sites of localized extranodal lymphoma vary widely – from a 5-year actuarial rate of > 75% for skin, orbit, thyroid and gastrointestinal lymphoma to < 50% for testis, bone and brain lymphomas. This pronounced heterogeneity of outcome of the various primary extranodal presentations is one of the main justifications for a detailed consideration of the different sites of origin of these lymphomas and particularly of localized disease.

Whether extranodal lymphomas have an overall survival similar to that of nodal cases as a whole remains a matter of controversy. In two recent reports there was no difference [2,14], while in a third [3], although after a 7-year observation period the overall survival for extranodal NHLs was 46% versus 49% for nodal cases ($P = 0.05$), a recent reanalysis of these data (Figure 48.1) showed, in more than 2500 patients, a highly significant survival

Table 48.1 Localized extranodal lymphoma: 5-year survival [14]

Skin	92%	Waldeyer's	72%
Gastrointestinal	77%	Breast	63%
Soft tissue	77%	Genitourinary*	52%
Orbit	76%	Bone	47%
Gastrointestinal	76%	Lung	44%
Gynecological	75%	Brain	24%

Data from Princess Margaret Hospital, Toronto (1967–1988).
* Including testes.

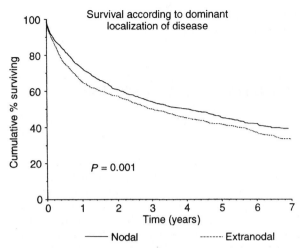

Figure 48.1 Seven-year survival of nodal (*N* = 1690) versus extranodal (*N* = 1103) NHL cases from the Danish LYFO registry (data from 1/24/94).

difference in favor of nodal cases ($P = 0.001$). However, considering the many variables which influence site-specific outcome in extranodal lymphomas, it is questionable whether such an overall difference has clinical relevance. Such analyses might be more meaningful if patients were grouped according to grade of malignancy [2]. When this was done in a recent series, striking differences in survival and relapse-free survival between nodal and extranodal lymphomas were observed [2], since localized low-grade malignancy and disseminated intermediate-grade NHL fared significantly better when extranodal than when nodal. However, patients with disseminated, high-grade extranodal NHL clearly had the worst prognosis. These results suggest that the differences in distribution of stages cannot be solely responsible for the differences observed within grades of malignancy in these analyses.

SITES OF INVOLVEMENT

Table 48.2 summarizes the localization of site-specific primary extranodal lymphomas in 236 patients from a Dutch population-based registry [2]. Similar frequencies have been reported in other series from the Western hemisphere. Overall, gastro-intestinal localizations, which, in most series, account for about one-third of all cases, represent the most common form of extranodal lymphoma. If tonsils and Waldeyer's ring are considered extranodal, ear, nose and throat localizations are the second most frequent site of involvement, averaging about one-fifth of all cases. Extranodal lymphomas can arise in almost all organs: from Table 48.2 it is apparent that

Table 48.2 Localization of site-specific primary extranodal lymphoma (*N* = 236)

Localization	Total	Localization	Total
Gastrointestinal (GI)	86	Others	101
Stomach	54	Bone marrow only	33
Colon	14	Brain, spinal cord, etc.	15
Small intestine	13	Lung	9
Multiple GI sites	3	Bone	6
Rectum	2	Connective tissue	5
		Breast	5
ENT	49	Orbit	5
Tonsil*	25	Skin (other than mycosis fungoides)	4
Waldeyer's ring*	11	Testis	4
Tongue	5	Thyroid gland	4
Parotid	3	Pleura	2
Nose, sinus	3	Kidney	2
Floor of mouth	1	Multiple organs	2
Buccal mucosa	1	Gall bladder	1
		Ovary	1
		Prostate	1
		Lacrimal gland	1
		Conjunctiva	1

* Generally considered as nodal lymphomas.
Data from population-based tumor registry, Northern Holland [2].

bone marrow only (about 15%) and brain (about 10%) are two of the organs most often involved. As previously stated (see Table 48.1), the primary organ of origin greatly influences the outcome. There are, however, other differences related to primary localization. Testis and thyroid lymphomas are seen almost exclusively in patients >50 years, while there is a significantly higher incidence of hepatic and intestinal lymphomas at younger ages. Salivary gland and thyroid lymphomas are significantly more common in females, while intestinal and pulmonary lymphomas are more often found in males [3]. NHLs of the stomach, salivary glands and thyroid are more frequently localized, whereas extranodal lymphomas of the lungs, liver, bones and testes are mostly widespread [2,3]. With respect to histological classification, low-grade histology is most frequent in cases involving salivary glands or bone marrow. Intermediate-grade histology, particularly of the centrocytic type (mantle cell), is more common in gastric and intestinal lymphomas, while high-grade histology is predominant in NHLs of the CNS, testes, bones, liver, lungs and, to some extent, the stomach [2,3]. It must be noted that in certain localizations (e.g., orbit, head and neck, intestine) the distribution of the histologic subtypes is very similar to that reported within the International Working Formulation.

Certain extranodal sites have characteristic patterns of either B- or of T-cell disease. Cutaneous lymphoma clearly comprises a wide range of lymphomas of T-cell origin, even though a small subset of B-cell cutaneous lymphomas has recently been described [16]. Little is known about the pattern of B- or T-cell disease in extranodal lymphomas in certain geographic areas such as the Far East, where T-cell lymphomas are generally much more prevalent than in the Western hemisphere. However, a high incidence of B-cell lymphomas in the oral cavity (in contrast to lymphomas in the Waldeyer's ring) was recently reported from Japan [17] while T- or natural killer (NK) cell lymphomas are quite common in South East Asia and some parts of Latin America.

METHODOLOGICAL CONCLUSION

The differences in presentation, clinical stage, histology and survival strongly suggest that primary nodal and extranodal NHL are distinct entities [2,3]. However, the site of involvement represents the most important discriminatory factor among extranodal lymphomas; this is partly the result of differences in natural history, but mainly to differences in management strategy which arise from organ-specific problems (e.g., brain, stomach, thyroid, eye, etc.). Given this heterogeneity, the various primary extranodal presentations will be examined separately.

Primary gastrointestinal lymphoma

The gastrointestinal (GI) tract is the most frequently involved extranodal localization in NHL [1,14]. In hospital- and population-based series published thus far, GI-NHL accounts for 4–20% (on average 12–13%) of all NHLs and 30–40% of all extranodal cases [18,19]. In the Western world, the most common locations are stomach (approximately 50–60%), small intestine (approximately 30%) and large intestine (approximately 10%). Localized esophageal lymphoma is extremely rare. In the small intestine, ileal (ileocecal) presentations are the most common (approximately 60%), followed by jejunal (approximately 30%) and duodenal sites (approximately 10%). Colorectal lymphomas most commonly occur in the cecum. These proportions can differ geographically, with small intestinal lymphomas being more common than gastric lymphomas in the Middle East. This special type of extranodal lymphoma (immunoproliferative small intestinal disease; IPSID) is discussed in detail elsewhere in this volume.

NHL represents 3–10% of all gastric neoplasias [20], and is thus the most common malignancy of the stomach after adenocarcinoma. NHL accounts for about one-fifth of all intestinal cancers [21], but for less than 1% of all large bowel malignancies [18]. It has been suggested that the incidence of gastric and intestinal lymphoma may have increased over the last two decades [11]. Whether this is the result of an actual increase or of more efficient case registration is as yet unclear. Recent data from a Danish population-based registry involving almost 2500 NHL cases collected over a 9-year period (1983–1991) did not demonstrate an increase in the incidence of gastric or intestinal lymphomas [18]. A recent analysis performed in demographically comparable communities of the UK and Italy [22] revealed a much higher incidence of gastric NHL in northeastern Italy than in the corresponding UK communities (13.2×10^5/year versus 1×10^5/year), suggesting the existence of geographic variations in the incidence of gastric NHL [22]. Infection by *Helicobacter pylori* has been cited as an environmental factor of possible etiologic relevance in those cases of gastric NHL deriving from the so-called mucosa-associated lymphoid tissue (MALT) [23]. (MALT lymphomas are extensively discussed in Chapters 21 and 47 of this book.) There is less epidemiological information on intestinal NHLs available than on gastric NHLs. Patients with celiac disease have a 200-fold increased risk of developing intestinal lymphoma, the so-called enteropathy-associated T-cell lymphoma (EATCL) and some authors even favor the hypothesis that adult-onset celiac disease is itself a form of low-grade lymphoma [24].

DIAGNOSIS, CLASSIFICATION AND STAGING

Presenting symptoms are generally the result of the local lesion (pain, obstruction, hemorrhage). Fever and night sweats are uncommon and, if they do occur, are more often associated with a T-cell phenotype and/or intestinal localization [18]. Weight loss, however, is common, although this is more often a consequence of the localization of the primary lymphoma rather than a constitutional symptom of the disease.

Radiological appearances are often suggestive of the presence of a GI-NHL. Within the stomach, lymphoma is most common at the pyloric antrum, followed by the body, and then the cardia. Computed tomography (CT) is useful for evaluating the regional node size and might also reveal wall thickening. The intraluminal component is, however, not readily imaged [14]. In the past, surgery was regarded as an essential component of the diagnostic work-up on the grounds that it provided large biopsy specimens for diagnosis. Its current role as a treatment option, mainly for gastric lymphomas, will be dealt with later. From a purely diagnostic viewpoint, however, improved endoscopy and imaging techniques are sufficiently advanced that its role, at least in gastric lymphomas, must be questioned [25]. In fact, sufficient material for diagnosis is currently obtained in more than 90% of cases by endoscopic biopsy, although this approach does not permit a distinction to be made between stages I and II (as defined by Musshoff) [15], a distinction that may, in fact, have no therapeutic relevance. Furthermore, the introduction of endoscopic ultrasonography has helped to assess the degree of involvement of the stomach wall and to identify patients at high risk of bleeding and/or perforation [26].

It is not always possible to establish whether lymphomas are of gastric origin. Recently [19,27], cases in which the stomach is most probably the site of origin have generally been accepted as primary gastric lymphomas, irrespective of the extent of dissemination within the abdominal cavity.

GI tract lymphomas comprise a number of distinct clinico-pathological entities which have been variously defined according to the histological classification in vogue at the time; in the Working Formulation, most are of intermediate- or high-grade malignancy, with low-grade lymphomas representing only 15–20% [18,19]. Intestinal lesions more often tend to be high grade than do gastric lymphomas [18,27]. In view of the current lack of consensus concerning classification and staging of GI-NHL, a workshop was recently organized at the Fifth International Conference on Malignant Lymphoma in Lugano (June 1993) to consider the problems of evaluating patients with GI tract lymphoma [27]. The attendees concurred that there is a compelling need for a new classification for primary GI tract lymphomas because of their unique histology, special features and origin in mucosal tissue. Adoption was recommended of the classification presented in Table 48.3, which follows the principles of the Kiel classification and is based on the proposal of Isaacson et al. [28], with revision of the name of centrocytic lymphoma in accord with Banks et al. [29].

The applicability of the Ann Arbor staging system to GI tract lymphoma has often been questioned. In view of the features specific to the latter, an alternative staging system was proposed by Blackledge et al. [30]. Moreover, the modifications proposed by Musshoff [15] have been of value in identifying subsets of patients with different prognoses. At the Lugano workshop, a revised version of the Blackledge staging system was recommended for future general use [27] (Table 48.4).

Regardless of treatment modality, several prognostic factors have been shown to be associated with a poor prognosis, namely, stage > I, involvement of para-aortic versus regional lymph nodes, large tumor size, penetration of the serosa and intestinal as

Table 48.3 Histological classification of gastrointestinal non-Hodgkin's lymphomas [27]

B-cell

Lymphomas of mucosa-associated lymphoid tissue (MALT)
    Low-grade B-cell lymphoma of MALT
    High-grade B-cell lymphoma of MALT, with or without evidence of a low-grade component
    Mediterranean lymphoma (immunoproliferative, small intestinal disease), low grade, mixed or high grade
Malignant lymphoma, centrocytic (mantle cell)
Burkitt's-like lymphoma
Other types of low- or high-grade lymphoma corresponding to peripheral lymph node equivalents

T-Cell

Enteropathy-associated T-cell lymphoma (EATL)
Other types not associated with enteropathy

Table 48.4 Staging system for gastrointestinal non-Hodgkin's lymphomas [27]

Stage I	Tumor confined to gastrointestinal tract without serosal penetration:
	    Single primary site
	    Multiple, noncontiguous lesions

Stage II	Tumor extending into abdomen from primary site – nodal involvement
	    II_1 Local (gastric/mesenteric)
	    II_2 Distant (para-aortic/para-caval)

Stage II_E	Penetration of serosa to involve adjacent 'structures' (enumerate actual site of involvement, e.g., stage IIE (pancreas), stage IIE (large intestine), stage IIE (postabdominal wall) Perforation/peritonitis
Stage IV	Disseminated extranodal involvement or a gastrointestinal tract lesion with supradiaphragmatic nodal involvement

opposed to gastric origin [1]. With regard to histological subtype, low-grade MALT lymphomas have a relatively good prognosis, while those of mantle cell type and EATCL have proven to have a very poor prognosis [27,31,32].

TREATMENT

It is now clear that combination chemotherapy is the treatment of choice for patients with advanced local involvement (stage II2) or with multiple node involvement (stage IIE with residual disease) or disseminated disease. In a recent prospective study including more than 700 patients with aggressive lymphomas, about 15% of the 91 patients were believed to have primary gastrointestinal lymphoma [33]. In that study, no difference in therapy outcome was observed between patients with an advanced aggressive lymphoma and the subset in which the lymphoma was deemed to have arisen in the GI.

Advanced GI-NHLs thus appear to behave in the same manner as other advanced lymphomas, with comparable histology and prognostic index [34]. The outcome of patients who present with more advanced disease in the abdomen is characterized by a long-term success rate of approximately 40% [34]. These results are indirectly supported by data (to be discussed later) derived from series in which patients with more localized GI-NHLs were treated with chemotherapy alone.

Analogous to events in other chemosensitive neoplasms (e.g., testicular tumors), the effectiveness of combination chemotherapy in advanced cases of GI-NHL has engendered a reconsideration of the

role of primary surgery in less advanced cases, where surgery has, historically, been the initial procedure of choice. This is particularly true for gastric lymphomas. For primary intestinal lymphoma, however, there are as yet no studies which clearly demonstrate that surgery is unnecessary [25].

Even though there is a dearth of randomized studies comparing surgery alone with the addition of adjuvant chemotherapy, combined modality treatment is nowadays considered the procedure of choice for patients with primary intestinal lymphoma [14, 25,34]. In the large series of the Milan Cancer Centre [34], it is noteworthy that, with such an approach, primary gastric and intestinal lymphomas appear to have similar outcomes if they are comparable with respect to histology and prognostic index; in the past, the prognosis for intestinal lymphomas was considered to be generally worse [18,25].

Much more controversial nowadays is the situation with cases of gastric lymphoma in which there is limited involvement. Traditionally, surgery has played a major role in the treatment of localized gastric lymphoma by simultaneously solving diagnostic and therapeutic problems. Since endoscopy and CT scan have become generally available, the necessity of surgery for biopsy and staging has, as previously stated, almost entirely disappeared [25–27]. The possible advantage of debulking as well as the lessening of the risk of bleeding perforation were other reasons for advocating surgery as a primary treatment. The role of debulking has never been properly defined in this situation. Moreover, the presence of a bulky mass is sometimes itself an obstacle to surgical intervention. The risk of bleeding perforation during chemotherapy or radiotherapy has been generally overestimated, as was well demonstrated by recent series [33,35,36]. Surgery, moreover, does not necessarily prevent these complications, as episodes of bleeding or perforation have also been reported after surgery. Nevertheless, the risk does exist and can be estimated at about 5%. On the other hand, surgical resection of the stomach has an intrinsic mortality (about 8–10%) – comparable, if not superior, to the risk of bleeding. Finally, postsurgical complications can delay subsequent chemo- or radiotherapy and can also adversely affect the performance status.

In view of these facts, new approaches have been advocated. Taal et al. [26] recently published a retrospective study of 119 patients with localized gastric NHLs treated with either radiotherapy alone (after clinical staging) or with surgery followed by adjuvant radiotherapy. The survivals at 5 years were 70% and 37%, respectively, for patients with stage I and II disease, with no difference between the results for patients receiving radiotherapy alone, or radiotherapy after surgical resection. The study was not randomized but no obvious bias in the selection of the treatment procedure was detected. They therefore propose that radiotherapy is the treatment of choice for nonbulky lesions in stage I or II disease. For larger tumors, results are less satisfactory and these authors advocate the addition of combination chemotherapy. It is also possible that improved results in patients with stage I and II disease would be achieved by including chemotherapy in the treatment regimen. It has been suggested by the results of at least three series [33,35,36] that chemotherapy, sometimes combined with radiotherapy [36], is as effective as surgery and that gastrectomy was thus redundant. In another study [37], 106 cases of localized gastric lymphoma reported to a population-based Danish registry were analyzed. Of these, 67 had surgical resection, 51 chemotherapy and 55 radiotherapy, or combinations thereof. None of the treatment modalities showed any relative superiority with respect to survival ($P = 0.13$); the overall 5-year survival was 67%. By Cox regression analysis the pretherapeutic presence of fever or lactate dehydrogenase (LDH) elevation had a far more significant influence on survival than did any of the treatments or treatment combinations. Of note is the fact that, in these series, surgical resection was associated with a significantly higher risk of late complications than was radiotherapy.

However, confirmation of these results, with comparability of patient populations, is required and essential, since the cure fraction with surgery with or without adjuvant chemotherapy is high, with 70–75% of stage I patients and 40–50% of stage II patients still alive at 5 years [38]. As in other chemosensitive tumors, it is nevertheless possible that, in future, surgery will be resorted to as a potential approach to salvage should complete remission not be achieved.

The therapeutic approach in cases presenting with a gastric lymphoma of MALT origin [28] remains controversial. Furthermore, it is not yet clear whether high-grade MALT lymphoma should be treated differently from low-grade MALT lymphomas [38]. In at least some centers, a 'wait-and-see' attitude has been advocated for low-grade MALT gastric lymphoma, while others still suggest surgical intervention [34]. Recently, however, antibiotic therapy alone was suggested [39]. Experience with this new and distinct entity is still insufficient, and larger and prospectively registered series are needed to clarify the situation.

Primary lymphoma of the genitourinary tract

Genitourinary lymphomas are rare, constituting < 5% of all extranodal NHLs [12]. Testicular lymphomas comprise the vast majority of genitourinary lymphomas, with all other sites being very rare. More common, however, is a secondary involvement of genitourinary sites in advanced lymphoma.

PRIMARY TESTICULAR LYMPHOMA

The literature regarding the natural history of testicular lymphoma is extensive and rather homogeneous [14,40–47], although data derived from population-based studies are rare [40–42]. Primary testicular lymphoma represents 1–2% of all NHLs, which corresponds to an annual incidence rate of about $0.25/10^5$ males. A much higher incidence of subclinical testicular involvement is to be expected based on data from autopsy studies [48]. Primary testicular lymphoma is predominantly a disease of older men, with the highest prevalence in the seventh to the ninth decades. Eighty-five per cent are older than 60 years and lymphoma is the most common testicular tumor in that age group [40,48,49]. Testicular lymphoma is also the most common bilateral testicular tumor [45,46]. In a population-based study [40], synchronous bilaterality was present in more than 5% of the cases, while metachronous involvement was less common (< 3%). In other series, bilaterality occurred at an average of 19% [47,49].

The usual presentation is a painless testicular swelling and definitive diagnosis is almost always obtained by high inguinal orchiectomy. In contrast to the presentation of most cases of nonlymphomatous testicular cancer, primary lymphomas commonly involve the spermatic cord, and epididymis and vascular invasion is frequent. Histologically, almost all cases are diffuse (2/3 diffuse centroblastic) and well over 90% are of intermediate or high-grade malignancy. In a recent series 11% were of T- and 89% of B-immunophenotype [40].

A detailed staging evaluation is necessary, since, in addition to the contralateral testis, the disease has a high propensity for involving para-aortic and mediastinal nodes, liver and spleen, bone marrow, lung, CNS and skin. Autopsy studies have revealed noncontiguous lung involvement in 86% of lethal cases, suggesting micrometastatic dissemination by the hematogeneous route [50].

The literature reports a uniformly poor prognosis

Histologically, the vast majority of lymphomas are of diffuse large-cell type [13,14], while in AIDS-related lymphomas there is a prevalence of high-grade histologies [72]. No follicular lymphomas have thus far been reported to present as PCNSL, while there are anecdotal cases of T-cell origin [13]. Extensive necrosis can sometimes render histological subclassification very difficult [13]. Cerebrospinal fluid (CSF) studies commonly show abnormalities, including elevated protein levels and increased cell counts, but cytology is positive only in about one-fifth of the cases [13,78]. The use of immunopheno-typing can, however, reveal the presence of a monoclonal lymphatic population in the cerebro-spinal fluid, even in the presence of negative cytology [80]. An ophthalmologic examination with a slit lamp is mandatory, since at least one-fifth of the patients will already have ocular involvement at the time of diagnosis [13,78]. In non-AIDS patients systemic involvement outside the CNS is almost never present at diagnosis and therefore extensive staging is not required.

Historically, whole-brain radiation with no less than 40 Gy has been the treatment of choice. Despite this dosage, which is curative in most localized non-Hodgkin's lymphomas at other sites, in PCSNL the local recurrence rate is approximately 90%, although in less than 10% will there be systemic progression. Moreover, higher doses have not improved local control rates [14]. A significant proportion of patients will recur in the nonirradiated neuraxis. This fact, together with frequent meningeal involvement, would favor the use of craniospinal radiation. Nowadays, however, intrathecal chemotherapy in combination with whole-brain irradiation is more often used [78,81].

With the use of radical irradiation alone for unselected patients with non-HIV-associated PCNSL, the 5-year survival rate is 5–10% with a median survival between 9 and 24 months [13,14]. A few, selected series have recently reported improved outcome with the use of a combined modality approach (radiotherapy, intrathecal and systemic chemotherapy) with median survivals on the order of 20–30 months [78,81–83]. These results, although suggestive, are preliminary and there are no larger nonselected series or randomized trials in progress, so that the impact of combined modality therapy on survival remains to be defined.

SPECIAL PRESENTATIONS

Primary leptomeningeal lymphoma

In rare instances, malignant lymphoma presents as a localized leptomeningeal·disease in the absence of parenchymal brain involvement [84]. Diagnosis is commonly made by positive CSF cytology. Treatment has generally focused on intrathecal chemotherapy, with craniospinal or regional neuraxis irradiation. The prognosis is poor, similar to that of primary parenchymal brain lymphoma.

OCULAR LYMPHOMA

Ocular lymphomas are restricted to the globe, usually the vitreous, retina and chorioid. In contrast to orbital lymphoma, ocular lymphoma is commonly associated with PCNSL. About 20% of patients with PCNSL have initial ocular involvement [13,14,85], while 60–100% (depending on the length of follow-up) of patients who initially present with ocular lymphoma develop cerebral lymphoma [85]. The eye is a direct extension of the brain, and PCNSL and ocular lymphoma may represent different aspects of a single disease. At presentation, 20–40% of patients with PCNSL have multifocal disease, and almost all patients have multiple sites of tumor at autopsy [13,14,85]. Thus, ocular lymphoma represents another site of multifocal CNS lymphoma, although it is very rare – only 150 well-documented cases have been reported to date [85].

Ocular lymphoma is one cause of chronic vitreitis or uveitis. In most patients the cause is not identified, and corticosteroids produce a prompt and durable remission. Primary or secondary resistance to steroid treatment is a common clinical feature of ocular lymphoma and therefore this diagnosis should be considered in patients with steroid-resistant chronic uveitis. Treatment with ocular and whole-brain radiotherapy and chemotherapy, including high-dose Ara-C, can contribute to a lengthy remission with improved vision and neurologic function [85]. Ocular radiotherapy should include both eyes even when only unilateral disease is apparent. In fact, most patients will develop bilateral involvement [14,85]. Unfortunately, despite treatment, eventual ocular or CNS relapse is the rule and the prognosis, therefore, remains poor.

Primary extradural lymphoma

Spinal cord compression is a well-recognized presentation of lymphoma and accounts for approximately 1% of all localized NHLs [1,14]. While the lesion is commonly imaged by myelography, the diagnosis is generally arrived at on the basis of tissue biopsy at the time of decompressive surgery. The most common histology is diffuse large-cell lymphoma. CSF studies are, in most cases, initially negative; however, data on recurrences in the CSF or other extradural sites are discordant [14,83]. When treated with radiotherapy alone, about two-thirds of patients with primary extradural lymphoma will recur [14]. Nowadays, after surgery patients are treated with a combined modality comprising radiotherapy, intrathecal and systemic chemotherapy. Combined modality treatment will yield a 10-year survival approaching 90%. This favorable outcome, the high rate of local control with radiotherapy and the propensity for systemic progression (in the absence of combination chemotherapy) demonstrate that the natural history of primary extradural lymphoma is very different from that of PCSNL, and similar to that of other non-CNS extranodal lymphomas.

Head and neck lymphoma

The head and neck region is the second most frequent site of localized extranodal presentation of NHL. Ranking by site of tumor presentation reveals tonsil to be the most common, followed by nasopharynx, oral cavity, salivary glands, paranasal sinuses and base of the tongue (Table 48.5). At the end of this section we will also discuss thyroid and orbital lymphomas, even though they are not usually included with head and neck lymphomas. As stated earlier, there is controversy as to whether tonsils and Waldeyer's ring should, in general, be considered as nodal or extranodal sites, but recent immunohistological and clinical data strongly suggest that primary tonsilar and Waldeyer's ring lymphomas should be considered to be of nodal origin [2,6,14]. Therefore, we will not discuss the latter localizations in detail here, since their treatment is logically based on data obtained from the therapy of lymphomas of nodal origin. However, indications for local radiotherapy might be more stringent for these lymphomas than for nodal lymphomas in general [86,87]. Nevertheless, more than 50% of patients with stage I malignant lymphoma of Waldeyer's ring treated with radiotherapy alone will recur [88].

Table 48.5 Stages I and Ii head and neck lymphoma presenting at extranodal sites: the experience at Princess Margaret Hospital 1967–1988 (from Sutcliffe and Gospodarowicz [14]

Waldeyer's ring		Non-Waldeyer's ring	
Tonsil	35.0%	Oral cavity	16.0%
Nasopharynx	17.5%	Salivary glands	9.6%
Base of tongue	5.2%	Paranasal sinuses	8.0%
Larynx and hypopharynx	1.3%	Nasal cavity	2.2%

The signs and symptoms of NHL arising in an extranodal site are similar to those of a head and neck squamous cancer, and only by biopsy can the distinction be made. Long-term results in patients presenting with extranodal lymphomas in the head and neck area vary greatly, depending not only on histology, but also on sites of presentation. From a series of 156 patients with head and neck lymphomas, the 5-year survival according to site was as follows: salivary gland (61%), oral cavity (57%), tonsil (49%), base of tongue (47%), nasopharynx (36%) and paranasal sinuses (12%) [87].

One problem related to most sites in the head and neck area is the precise definition of disease bulk. Recent advances in imaging, particularly CT and MRI, have greatly facilitated the definition of disease extent, even though documentation of precise margins remains difficult for some localizations (e.g., paranasal sinus) [89–91].

An important aspect of the natural history of primary head and neck lymphoma is its relationship to GI tract involvement, either concurrent with diagnosis or at subsequent relapse [86]. Therefore, GI tract investigation should be included in the required staging procedures in patients with apparently localized head and neck presentations. The GI tract is clearly also the most frequent extranodal site of disease progression [86, 92–94]. This is particularly true for lymphomas originating in the tonsil [86,92–95].

LYMPHOMA OF THE ORAL CAVITY (INCLUDING SALIVARY GLANDS)

There are only very limited data on the overall distribution of sites within the oral cavity for lymphomas [96,97]. Among 70 cases of primary extranodal NHLs of the oral region, where localization was the palate in 21 patients, the gingiva in 17, the parotid gland in 13, the tongue in eight, the cheek in seven, the florae of mouth in three and the lip in one [97]. It might be argued that this series from Japan may not be representative of Western countries. However, from a second Japanese series we know that the immunophenotypic distribution of oral lymphomas in Japan is similar to that seen in the Western world [17]. The vast majority of lymphomas in the oral cavity are of intermediate- and high-grade malignancy, with follicular lymphomas representing only 15–20% of case, although it must be remembered that follicular lymphoma is uncommon in Japan [96,97]. However, at least in Japan, almost 20% of the cases appear to be true histiocytic lymphoma [97]. This latter finding will be considered later in the discussion of nasal lymphomas.

There are few therapeutic principles that apply specifically to primary localization in the palate and gingiva, but mutilating surgery should be avoided and a combination of chemo- and radiotherapy administered, depending on the histologic subtype [96].

More knowledge has been accumulated concerning primary lymphomas of salivary glands, the vast majority of which are located in the parotid [98–100]. Primary lymphomas of the salivary gland account for 5–6% of all salivary gland tumors [98,99] and somewhat less than 5% of lymphomas from all sites [1,14]. Several studies of large numbers of patients undergoing parotidectomy have reported an incidence rate of 1–4% for lymphoma [99,101].

It is generally believed that the majority of lymphomas presenting in the parotid gland actually arise in the lymph nodes associated with the gland, despite classification as extranodal lymphomas [102]. The gland parenchyma is often secondarily involved, making determination of the actual origin of lymphoma presenting in this region almost impossible [99,102]. However, treatment of these patients is not affected by the tissue of origin, and thus this issue is of little clinical relevance. Whether some (and how many) of these lymphoma are of MALT origin remains to be determined [99]. The average age at diagnosis is more than 60 years and there is a predominance of females, corresponding to the well-described preponderance of women in patients with Sjögren's syndrome, which predisposes to salivary gland lymphoma [99,103].

Sjögren's syndrome is characterized by lymphocytic infiltration of salivary and lachrymal glands, hypergammaglobulinemia and high levels of circulating autoantibodies, including rheumatoid factor and antinuclear antibodies. Patients with this autoimmune disease have a risk of developing NHLs more than 40 times greater than that of a matched, nonsicca population [103]. The steps involved in the transition from autoimmunity to B-cell neoplasia are not well understood. Before developing frank lymphoma, these patients often have recurrent swellings of the salivary gland, which exhibit a 'prelymphoma' lesion on biopsy [104]. Recent studies have shown that oligoclonal rearrangements of the immunoglobulin genes and, in some instances, translocations of the proto-oncogene, *bcl*-2, precede the development of a frank lymphoma [104].

About half of patients with salivary gland lymphoma will have low-grade histology, while stage I disease is reported in about 40% of cases [99]. Survival statistics for parotid lymphoma vary greatly from series to series, with a reported long-term survival of 50–75% [100,101,105]. Overall, the survival rates quoted for most series are higher than for most other localizations of extranodal lymphoma. Several studies have, however, reported a worse prognosis in patients with Sjögren's syndrome and NHL [99,106].

Another association which has been reported in a few times [100,107] is that of NHL with a benign tumor of the parotid gland, the papillary lymphomatous cystadenoma (Warthin's tumor). The role of surgery in its treatment is limited to excisional biopsy, while further therapy has to be tailored to stage, and (particularly) to histologic subtype [99].

LYMPHOMA OF PARANASAL SINUSES

Lymphoma of the paranasal sinuses accounts for 2–7% of extranodal lymphomas [14,108]; about 200 cases have so far been reported in the literature [108,109]. The relative rarity of this neoplasm has precluded focused clinical trials, and its inclusion in the literature with other lymphomas of the head and neck has obscured its definition as a clinical entity with a distinct natural history and response to therapy. Recent reports have, in fact, emphasized the tendency of these lymphomas to present with bulky localized disease, to relapse in noncontiguous nodal and extranodal sites after radiation therapy, and to spread frequently to the central nervous system [87,109–115].

The local bulkiness of the disease at the time of diagnosis may be related to the origin of the lymphoma in a sinus and its growth into potentially clinically silent sites such as the parapharyngeal space or infratemporal fossa [14]. In addition, because lymph node involvement is uncommon, most patients present only after locally advanced disease has caused pain, nasal obstruction or facial distortion. Thus, the tumor node metastasis (TNM) staging system may reflect the extent of disease more accurately than the Ann Arbor staging system [108]. In most series, the majority of patients with paranasal sinus lymphoma present with T3 or T4 disease [87,108,116]. The biologic behavior of paranasal sinus lymphomas may also be more aggressive than that of other extranodal lymphomas of the head and neck because the vast majority present with intermediate- or high-grade lymphoma [108,109,116,117]. Moreover, in contrast to thyroid gland and Waldeyer's ring lymphomas, for instance, none of the paranasal sinus lymphomas seem to originate in gut-associated lymphoid tissue (GALT, a subtype of MALT). In addition, no predilection for GI-tract relapse has been observed for paranasal sinus lymphomas. These lymphomas are characterized by a prolonged localized growth phase and a comparatively low rate of distant relapse, some of which occur in other GALT sites [28,118,119]. Gospodarowicz et al. [112] have recently shown that survival with GALT lymphomas is superior to that of other extranodal lymphomas, irrespective of stage and histology.

In the past, treatment results in patients with paranasal sinus lymphoma have been dismal, with a 5-year survival of only 12–15% [87]. In patients treated with radiation therapy alone, systemic recurrence has generally been within the first year after therapy, despite excellent local control [108]. Moreover, several series indicate that patients are at high risk for leptomeningeal relapse [108,109,111,117]. Recently, therefore, a combined approach including systemic chemotherapy, involved-field radiation therapy and CNS prophylaxis has been advocated [108,109]. In one series in which radiotherapy usually preceded chemotherapy, 14 patients were treated; 11 achieved a complete response and eight have relapsed, while the median survival of the entire group is 24 months. The authors conclude that, although combined modality therapy with CNS prophylaxis has improved outcome, prognosis remains poor and these patients would be considered for experimental consolidation therapy such as autologous bone marrow transplantation (ABMT) [109]. In the most recent series of four patients [108], all responded and none have relapsed after more than 2 years. In this case, chemotherapy preceded radiotherapy and this sequence may be more optimal in view of the aggressive biologic behavior of this lymphoma. While these results await confirmation, it should be borne in mind that treatment for paranasal sinus lymphoma remains difficult and long-term results uncertain, even with more modern approaches.

NASAL LYMPHOMA

Nasal lymphomas represent a controversial subset of malignant lymphomas, owing in part to the difficulty of recognizing them, both clinically and pathologically. Clinically, nasal lymphomas are part of the clinical spectrum of lethal midline granuloma or midfacial necrotizing lesions [114,120]. Pathologically, a mixed infiltrate is often found, which is difficult to distinguish from reactive processes. The incidence of nasal lymphoma is difficult to ascertain, given the problems with diagnosis, the tendency to group these uncommon lymphomas with those arising in adjacent structures such as the sinuses and nasopharynx, and the varying incidence among different populations. In Western populations, nasal lymphomas account for about 1% of all NHLs [117,121]. In this latter series, B-cell lymphomas predominate, although other series have reported a preponderance of T-cell phenotype [122, 123].

Nasal lymphomas are much more prevalent in Asian countries where they represent the second largest group of extranodal lymphomas after GI lesions [124,125], and most of them have a T-cell phenotype [120,124,125].

In the Working Formulation most cases of nasal lymphoma would fit into intermediate- or high-grade lymphoma. Some investigators have used the term 'angiocentric immunoproliferative lesion' to describe these lymphomas [126]. In contrast, nasal lymphomas of B-cell phenotype are more monomorphous and do not demonstrate angiocentricity [120].

Nasal T-cell lymphomas characteristically demonstrate a highly unusual phenotype [120] with a restricted pattern of pan-T-antigens, an absence of T-cell receptor antigen gene rearrangements and in the majority of cases, expression of the NK cell antigen CD56, which would suggest a NK cell derivation for this neoplasm. Moreover, recent data strongly suggest that EBV may play an important role in the pathogenesis of this disease [120,123].

Thus, although nasal T-cell lymphoma appears to be a distinctive type of neoplasm, NHLs with similar characteristics have on rare occasions been identified at other sites. Most commonly, these reports have described similar findings at other locations in the respiratory tract, including the nasopharynx, the nasal sinuses, the oropharynx, the larynx and the lung [119,122,126,127]. Treatment, as reported in the literature has been inconsistent, with some groups using localized radiotherapy alone, and others, multiagent chemotherapy with or without additional radiation therapy [120]. Although reports on long-term results are sparse and inconclusive [120], about one-half of the patients succumb to the disease.

PRIMARY ORBITAL LYMPHOMA

Lymphoma of extraocular orbital space is considerably more common than intraocular lymphoma (lymphoma of the eye) and the two types of presentation should be clearly distinguished because of their different natural histories [14].

Primary orbital lymphomas, those involving the anterior compartment of the orbital cavity: the eye lids, lachrymal gland and conjunctiva, and those in the posterior or retrobulbar compartment, account for about 2% of all lymphomas. Traditional histopathological classification has proven complex; presently, however, it seems that most low-grade cases could be considered to be of MALT origin [128–130]. Only a minority of orbital lymphomas are intermediate- or high-grade, while most of them have a low-grade histology. This might be reflected in the 60–75% 10-year survival rates reported for most series [14,131–134].

Radiation therapy has been the common form of treatment for primary orbital lymphoma and high local control rates can be achieved with moderate-dose radiation (25–35 Gy). At this dosage, visual complications are limited, but doses above 35 Gy result in an increased risk of complications [131]. About 1/3 to 1/4 of the patients will progress after local radiotherapy – in either the contralateral orbit, or with systemic disease. It appears that retrobulbar involvement carries a higher risk of disease failure than anterior compartment disease [133]. So far there are few data indicating that combined modality therapy should be applied, although this should be considered in the few patients showing an aggressive histology subtype. In most instances, however, primary orbital lymphoma should still be treated with low-dose radiotherapy only [131].

THYROID LYMPHOMA

Primary NHL of the thyroid is uncommon, accounting for only 5% of thyroid neoplasms and less than 2% of extranodal lymphomas [1]. The majority of patients have an intermediate- or high-grade lymphoma [135], which clinically is often reflected by a rapidly enlarging neck mass accompanied by compression of surrounding structures such as the larynx or the esophagus. Elderly women are most often affected, perhaps because of the tendency of this neoplasm to occur against a background of Hashimoto's thyroiditis [136]. The prevalence of aggressive histologies is somewhat surprising, since thyroid lymphomas have been thought to be grouped with the MALT lymphomas [130,137].

The optimal treatment of thyroid lymphoma is controversial. Surgery was used extensively in older studies, but since the introduction of thyroid biopsy and fine-needle aspiration, surgery has ceased to play a major role and debulking surgery should, in any case, be discouraged [138]. Two-hundred and one patients with stage IE and IIE thyroid lymphoma were recently analyzed in detail in an evaluation of the relative merits of radiotherapy and chemotherapy. Distant and overall relapse rates were significantly lower in the group that received combined modality treatment than in those given radiotherapy alone. Local relapse was also less but the difference was not statistically significant. It is important to note that in thyroid lymphoma distant relapses occur twice as often as local failure. In only a small number of patients with disease confined to the neck and in whom the mediastium was included in the treatment port were the results with radiation alone superior to those of combined modality treatment [135]. The authors of this review concluded that more than 30% of thyroid lymphomas with clinically localized disease relapse at a distant site and that the addition of chemotherapy to radiation significantly lowers distant and overall recurrence, and should therefore be regarded as the treatment of choice in most patients. How the two modalities should be combined remains to be determined. In a recent report, patients with thyroid lymphoma and a tumor mass less than 10 cm were treated with 6–9 weeks of chemotherapy and involved-field radiation therapy, and only two of 23 relapsed [139].

The success of chemotherapy alone in both systemic and localized extranodal lymphomas [140] raises the question of the role of radiation. The propensity for patients with thyroid lymphoma to have bulky local disease, however, might be an adverse risk factor for local control with chemotherapy alone. In two recent series a 25% rate of recurrence was in fact reported in patients treated only with chemotherapy [7,13]. It would therefore seem that radiation therapy still has a role to play in the local control of thyroid lymphoma, although this may depend upon the chemotherapy employed.

Primary lymphoma of bone

Non-Hodgkin's lymphoma involving bone is relatively common in patients with advanced disease, but constitutes less than 5% of localized extranodal presentations [1,14,141,142]. The most common sites of presentation are the femur and long bones, followed by the ileum and scapula. Pain is the usual symptom and radiological findings comprise a lytic and, less commonly, a sclerotic or mixed lesion [14]. The vast majority of the cases are of B-cell phenotype and belong to the intermediate- to high-grade category [141–146]. Only a few cases of low-grade histology have been described and these usually have plasmacytoid features [146]. No follicular lymphomas seem, thus far, to have been reported [147]. The median age of patients with primary lymphoma of bone is 55 years [141], but about 3% of all lymphomas in children are localized to bone [143]. In the latter instance, the most prevalent histology is lymphoblastic lymphoma.

Most patients present with stage IE lesions, with about one-fifth having involved regional lymph nodes (stage IIE) at diagnosis. Historically, radiotherapy alone has resulted in an overall 5-year survival rate of 40–50% [14,141–143]. Most series do not show an advantage for doses in excess of 40 Gy [14,141,147]. Risk factors for loco-regional relapse include large tumor bulk and the use of limited radiation fields restricted to gross disease [14].

The use of a combined modality approach has recently been advocated [14,141,142,144,148,149]. In one report [141] survival was significantly better for patients treated by both chemotherapy and radiation therapy (88% at 5 years) than for those who received radiotherapy alone (40% at 5 years), although the study was not randomized. In one recent report dealing with children, all patients were treated with chemotherapy alone [143]. The authors of that study feel that the addition of radiotherapy to modern, intense combination chemotherapy is superfluous, especially in view of its potential for producing serious long-term effects. In another recent series, radiation therapy is advocated only as adjuvant treatment following initial chemotherapy [142]. At least in adults, however, long-term follow-up has revealed only modest morbidity related to radiation fields [14,141]. The situation might, however, be different for children: in a series of 11 children treated with an Adriamycin-containing regimen concomitant with radiation therapy (median tumor dose 50 Gy), the overall 8-year actuarial survival was 83%. While no relapses were seen, two patients developed second bone tumors in the radiation field [149].

In conclusion, while improved long-term results have been obtained with modern approaches, the exact role of radiation therapy versus cytotoxic agents as well as of combined modality treatment in primary lymphoma of bone remains to be established.

Primary extranodal lymphoma – other sites

PRIMARY LYMPHOMA OF THE BREAST

Primary lymphoma of the breast comprises approximately 2% of all localized extranodal lymphomas [1,2], and less than 0.5% of breast tumors [150]. Review of the literature shows two distinct clinicopathologic groups [151,152]; one, which affects young women, is frequently bilateral, is often associated with pregnancy, and is generally a high-grade malignancy lymphoma [151,152]. The second group affects older women, has clinical features identical to those of carcinoma of the breast and is generally of B-cell phenotype [151]; this is also true for Japanese women [152]. In this second group, most cases have an intermediate-grade histology, with large-cell lymphoma being the most common type [14,151–153].

However, a few cases of low-grade lymphomas have been described [152,153] – some breast lymphomas of MALT origin have been reported in the Western world [60,130,151,154], but none in Japan [152]. This could also be a matter of definition, since the criteria for defining lymphomas of MALT origin have recently been expanded [130].

Patients present with a breast mass, frequently rather large, with or without ipsilateral adenopathy. Lymphomatous involvement of the breast is generally represented on the mammogram as a circumscribed mass without tumor calcifications [155,156]. Its appearance, however, is generally nonspecific, and an accurate diagnosis, consisting of fine-needle aspiration cytology or biopsy, is required. Historically, radiotherapy to the breast and the regional lymph nodes has been employed following surgery. With doses of 35–40 Gy, local control is achieved in 4/5 of patients and overall survival rates of 40–60% at 10 years are reported [14,150,157]. Despite good local control, systemic failure occurs in at least half of the patients. Prognostic factors for disease progression include large tumor bulk and nodal involvement. Adjuvant combination chemotherapy has recently been used [158–161]. Long-term results with combination chemotherapy added to radiation are still sparse and therefore the relative merits of this modality cannot yet be assessed. It would, however, seem reasonable to routinely use chemotherapy, at least in patients with bulky disease, nodal involvement, and an intermediate- or high-grade histology.

PRIMARY LYMPHOMA OF THE LUNG

While the lung is frequently involved by disseminated lymphoma, isolated pulmonary lymphoma is rare, accounting for less than 1% of all extranodal localized disease [14].

Three categories of primary pulmonary lymphoma can be distinguished. In rare instances, large-cell lymphoma can present primarily in the lung [14]; a second variant is represented by T-cell lymphoma presenting as an angiocentric process within the framework of the so-called lethal midline granuloma [120,162,163] while the most common variant, lymphocytic or lymphoplasmacytoid lymphoma, has often been considered to be a pseudotumor [60,164]. A long, indolent natural history is characteristic of these low-grade primary lung lesions, for which the concept of BALT (bronchus-associated lymphoid tissue) lymphoma, as a part of the MALT lesions, has been developed [28,118,119,165]. These lesions should be treated as localized, low-grade lymphomas [14].

PRIMARY LYMPHOMA OF THE LIVER

Primary lymphoma of the liver and of the gall bladder has been only reported infrequently [60,166, 167]. Its presentation may mimic various liver diseases, since single or multiple masses as well as a diffuse infiltration of the liver have been described [168]. Both T- and B-cell lymphomas have been reported, with the majority of cases having diffuse large-cell histologies [168]. Partial hepatectomy for solitary lesions has been described [168], but given the commonly observed extensive intrahaepatic disease, the addition of chemotherapy seems warranted.

PRIMARY LYMPHOMA OF THE ESOPHAGUS

Although lymphoma may involve any part of the GI tract, either primarily or secondarily, esophageal involvement is exceedingly rare [169]; only a few cases have been reported in the literature. Diagnosis is generally made by biopsy, since roentgenographic studies and endoscopic findings are not specific [169]. No precise therapeutic rules have been established, but combined radio- and chemotherapy seems advisable [169].

PRIMARY CARDIAC LYMPHOMA

Primary malignant lymphomas of the heart are extremely rare [170]. In a series of more than 500 primary tumors and cysts of the heart, only seven were primary lymphomas [171]. These tumors present with a variety of clinical manifestations and are rarely diagnosed *ante mortem*.

References

1. Freeman C, Berg JW and Cutler SJ. Occurrence and prognosis of extranodal lymphomas. *Cancer* 1972, **29**: 253–260.
2. Otter R, Gerrits WBJ, Sandt MM, et al. Primary extranodal and nodal non-Hodgkin's lymphoma: A survey of a population-based registry. *Eur. J. Cancer Clin. Oncol.* 1989, **25**: 1203–1210.
3. D'Amore F, Christensen BE, Brincker H, et al. Clinico-pathological features and prognostic factors in extranodal non-Hodgkin's lymphomas. *Eur. J. Cancer* 1991, **27**: 1201–1208.
4. Chan JKC, Ng CS, Lo STH. Immunohistological characterization of malignant lymphomas of the Waldeyer's ring other than the nasopharynx. *Histo-*

pathology 1987, **15**: 885–899.
5. EORTC Lymphoma Cooperative Group. Protocol No. 20855. Brussels, EORTC, 1985.
6. EORTC Lymphoma Cooperative Group. Protocol No. 20856, Brussels, EORTC, 1985.
7. Modan B, Shane M, Goldman B, et al. Nodal and extranodal malignant lymphomas in Israel: An epidemiological study. *Br. Haematol. J.* 1969, **16**: 53–59.
8. Banfi A, Bonadonna G, Carnevali G, et al. Preferential sites of involvement and spread in malignant lymphomas. *Eur. J. Cancer* 1968, **4**: 319–324.
9. Weisenburger DD. Epidemiology of non-Hodgkin's lymphoma: Recent findings regarding an emerging epidemic. *Ann. Oncol.* 1994, **5** (Suppl. 1): S19-S24.
10. Levine Ph, Hoover RN. The emerging epidemic of non-Hodgkin's lymphoma: Current knowledge regarding aetiologic factors. *Cancer Res.* 1992, **42** (Suppl.): S5425–S5474.
11. Devesa SS, Fears T. Non-Hodgkin's lymphoma time trends: United States and international data. *Cancer Res.* 1992, **52** (Suppl.): S5432-S5440.
12. D'Amore F, Mortensen LS, and Storm H. Rising incidence and non-random geographic distribution of non-Hodgkin's lymphoma in western Denmark. *Ann. Oncol.* (submitted).
13. Krogh-Jensen M, D'Amore F, Jensen JMK, et al. Incidence, clinico-pathological features and outcome of primary central nervous system lymphomas. Population-based data from a Danish lymphoma registry. *Ann. Oncol.* 1995, **5**: 349–354.
14. Sutcliffe SB, Gospodarowicz MK. Clinical features and management of localized extranodal lymphomas. In Keating A, Armitage J, Burnet A, et al. (eds) *Haematological Oncology*, Vol. 2. Cambridge: Cambridge University Press, 1992, pp. 189–223.
15. Musshoff K. Klinische Stadieneinteilung der Nicht-Hodgkin Lymphome. *Strahlentherapie* 1977, **153**: 218–221.
16. Wood GS, Ngan BY, Tung R, et al. Clonal rearrangements of immunoglobulin genes in progression to B-cell lymphoma in cutaneous lymphoid hyperplasia. *Am. J. Pathol.* 1989, **135**: 13–19.
17. Takahasihi H, Fujita S, Okabe A, et al. Immunophenotypic analysis of extranodal non-Hodgkin's lymphomas in the oral cavity. *Pathol. Res. Pract.* 1993, **189**: 300–311.
18. D'Amore F, Brincker H, Grønbæk K, et al. Non-Hodgkin's lymphoma of the gastrointestinal tract: A population-based analysis of incidence, geographic distribution, clinico-pathologic presentation features and prognosis. *J. Clin. Oncol.* 1994, **12**: 1673–1684.
19. Herrmann R, Panahon AM, Barcos M, et al. Gastrointestinal involvement in non-Hodgkin's lymphoma. *Cancer* 1980, **46**: 215–222.
20. Hockey MS, Powell J, Crocker J, et al. Primary gastric lymphoma. *Br. J. Surg.* 1987, **74**: 483–487.
21. Williamson RCN, Welch CE, Malt RA. Adenocarcinoma and lymphoma of the small intestine: Distribution and aetiologic association. *Ann. Surg.* 1983, **197**: 172–178.
22. Doglioni C, Wotherspoon AC, Moschini A, et al.

High incidence of primary gastric lymphoma in northeastern Italy. *Lancet* 1992, **339**: 834–835.

23. Wotherspoon AC, Ortiz-Hidalgo C, Falzon MR, et al. *Helicobacter pylori*-associated gastritis and primary B-cell gastric lymphoma. *Lancet* 1991, **338**: 1175–1176.

24. Wright DH, Jones DB, Clark H, et al. Is adult-onset coeliac disease due to a low-grade lymphoma of intraepithelial T lymphocytes? *Lancet* 1991, **337**: 1373–1374.

25. Rossi A, Rohatiner AZS, Lister TA. Primary gastrointestinal non-Hodgkin's lymphoma: Still an unresolved question? *Ann. Oncol.* 1993, **4**: 802–803.

26. Taal BG, Burgers JMB, Van Heerde P, et al. The clinical spectrum and treatment of primary non-Hodgkin's lymphomas of the stomach. *Ann. Oncol.* 1993, **4**: 839–846.

27. Rohatiner AZS. Report on a workshop convened to discuss the pathological and staging classification of gastrointestinal tract lymphoma. *Ann. Oncol.* 1994, **5**:397–400.

28. Isaacson P, Spencer G, Wright DH. Classifying primary gut lymphomas. *Lancet* 1988, **2**: 1148–1149.

29. Banks PM, et al. Mantle cell lymphoma; a proposal for unification of morphologic, immunologic and molecular data. *Am. J. Surg. Path.* 1992, **16**: 637–640.

30. Blackledge G, Bush H, Dodge OG, et al. A study of gastrointestinal lymphoma. *Clin. Oncol.* 1979, **5**: 209–219.

31. Domizio P, Owen RA, Shepherd NA, et al. Primary lymphoma of the small intestine: A clinical pathological study of 119 cases. *Am. J. Surg. Path.* 1993, **17**: 429–442.

32. Morton JE, Leyland MJ, Vaughan, et al. Primary gastrointestinal non-Hodgkin's lymphoma: A review of 175 British national lymphoma investigation cases. *Br. J. Cancer* 1993, **67**: 776–782.

33. Salles G, Herbrecht R, Tilly H, et al. Aggressive primary gastrointestinal lymphomas: Review of 91 patients treated with the LNH-83 regimen. A study of the GELA. *Am. J. Med.* 1991, **90**: 77–84.

34. Tondini C, Giardini R, Buzzetti F, et al. Combined modality treatment for primary gastrointestinal non-Hodgkin's lymphoma: The Milan Cancer Institute experience. *Ann. Oncol.* 1993, **4**: 831–837.

35. Gobbi PG, Dionigi P, Barbieri F, et al. The role of surgery in the multimodal treatment of primary gastric non-Hodgkin's lymphomas. A report of 76 cases and review of the literature. *Cancer* 1990, **65**: 2528–2536.

36. Maor MH, Velasquez WS, Fuller LM, et al. Stomach conservation in stages I_E and II_E gastric non-Hodgkin's lymphoma. *J. Clin. Oncol.* 1990, **8**: 266–271.

37. Brinker H and D'Amore F. Treatment strategies in localized gastric non-Hodgkin's lymphomas: 'To cut or not to cut'. *Eur. J. Cancer* (in press).

38. Rossi A, Lister TA. Primary gastric non-Hodgkin's lymphoma: A therapeutic challenge. *Eur. J. Cancer* 1993, **29A**: 1924–1926.

39. Wotherspoon AC, Doglioni C, Disst C, et al. Regression of low-grade B-cell gastric lymphoma of MALT type following eradication of helicobacter pylori. *Lancet* 1993, **342**: 575–577.

40. Møller MB, D'Amore F, Christensen BE. Testicular lymphoma: A population-based study of incidence, clinico-pathological correlations and prognosis. *Eur. J. Cancer* 1994, **30A**: 1760–1764.

41. Otter R, Willemze R. Extranodal non-Hodgkin's lymphoma. *Neth. J. Med.* 1988, **33**: 49–51.

42. Duncan PR, Checa F, Gowing NFC, et al. Extranodal non-Hodgkin's lymphoma presenting in the testicle. *Cancer* 1980, **45**: 1578–1584.

43. Liang R, Chiu E, Loke SL. An analysis of 12 cases of non-Hodgkin's lymphomas involving the testis. *Ann. Oncol.* 1990, **1**: 383.

44. Tepperman BS, Gospodarowicz MK, Bush RS, et al. Non-Hodgkin lymphoma of the testis. *Radiology* 1982, **142**: 203–208.

45. Kiely JM, Massey BD, Harrison EG, et al. Lymphoma of the testis. *Cancer* 1970, **26**: 847–852.

46. Bach DW, Weissbach L, Hartlapp JH. Bilateral testicular tumor. *J. Urol.* 1983, **129**: 989–991.

47. Turner RR, Colby TV, MacKintosh FR. Testicular lymphomas: A clinico-pathologic study of 35 cases. *Cancer* 1981, **48**: 2095–2102.

48. Givler RL. Testicular involvement in leukemia and lymphoma. *Cancer* 1969, **23**(6): 1290–1295.

49. Doll DC, Weiss RB. Malignant lymphoma of the testis. *Am. J. Med.* 1986, **81**: 515–524.

50. Paladugu RR, Bearman RM, Rappaport H. Malignant lymphoma with primary manifestation in the gonad: A clinico-pathologic study of 38 patients. *Cancer* 1980, **45**: 561–567.

51. Roche H, Rus E, Pons A, et al. Stage IE non-Hodgkin's lymphoma of the testis: A need for a brief aggressive chemotherapy. *J. Urol.* 1989, **141**: 554–556.

52. Connors JM, Klimo P, Voss N, et al. Testicular lymphoma: Improved outcome with early brief chemotherapy. *J. Clin. Oncol.* 1988, **6**: 776–781.

53. Dobkin SF, Brem AS, Caldamone AA. Primary renal lymphoma. *J. Urol* 1991, **146**: 1588–1590.

54. Parveen T, Navarro-Roman L, Medeiros J, et al. Low-grade B-cell lymphoma of MALT arising in the kidney. *Arch. Pathol. Lab. Med.* 1993, **117**: 780–783.

55. Richmond J, Sherman RS, Diamond HD, et al. Renal lesion associated with malignant lymphoma. *Am. J. Med.* 1962, **32**: 184–207.

56. Kandel LB, Mc Cullough DL, Herrison LH. Primary renal lymphoma presenting with perirenal masses. *Br. J. Radiol.* 1988, **61**: 1077–1078.

57. Aign AB, Philips M. Primary malignant lymphoma of the urinary bladder. *Urology* 1986, **28**: 235–237.

58. Bostwick TG, Mann RB. Malignant lymphomas involving the prostate. *Cancer* 1985, **56**: 2932–2938.

59. Simson RH, Bridger JE, Anthoni PP, et al. Malignant lymphoma of the lower urinary tract. *Br. J. Urol.* 1990, **65**: 254–260.

60. Pelstring RJ, Essll JH, Kurtin BJ, et al. Diversity of organ site involvement among malignant lymphomas of mucosa-associated tissues. *Am. J. Clin. Pathol.* 1991, **96**: 738–745.

61. Paladugu RR, Bearman RN, Rappaport H. Malignant lymphoma with primary manifestation in the gonad: A clinico-pathologic study of 38 patients. *Cancer* 1980, **45**: 561–571.

62. Woodruff JD, Castillord RD, Novak ER. Lymphoma of the ovary. A study of 35 cases from the Ovarian Tumor Registry of the American Gynaecological Society. *Am. J. Obstet. Gynaecol.* 1963, **85**: 912–918.

63. Young RH, Harris NL, Scully RE. Lymphoma-like lesions of the lower female genital tract: A report of 16 cases. *Int. J. Gynaecol. Pathol.* 1985, **4**: 289–299.

64. Harris NL, Scully RE. Malignant lymphoma and granulocytic sarcoma of the uterus and vagina. A clinico-pathological analysis of 27 cases. *Cancer* 1984, **53**: 2530–2545.

65. Litam JB, Cabanillas F, Smith TL, et al. Central nervous system relapse in malignant lymphomas: Risk factors and implication for prophylaxis. *Blood* 1979, **54**: 1249–1257.

66. Levitt LJ, Dawson DM, Rosenthal DS, et al. CNS involvement in the non-Hodgkin's lymphomas. *Cancer* 1980, **45**: 545–552.

67. Cavalli F, Bernier J. Non-Hodgkin's lymphoma in adults. In Peckham M, Veronesi U, Pinedo H (eds) *Textbook of Oncology: Malignant Lymphoma in Adults.* Oxford: Oxford University Press, 1995, pp. 1768–1787.

68. Spaun E, Midholm S, Pedersen NT, et al. Primary malignant lymphoma of the central nervous system. *Surg. Neurol.* 1985, **24**: 646–650.

69. Hochberg FH, Miller DC. Primary central nervous system lymphoma. *J. Neurosurg.* 1988, **68**: 835–853.

70. Hobson DE, Anderson BA, Carr I, et al. Primary non-Hodgkin's lymphoma of the central nervous system: Mannitoba experience and review of literature. *Can. J. Neurol. Sci.* 1986, **13**: 55–61.

71. Pluda JM, Yarchoan R, Jaffe ES, et al. Development of non-Hodgkin lymphoma in a cohort of patients with severe human immuodeficiency virus (HIV) infection on long-term antiretroviral therapy. *Ann. Intern. Med.* 1990, **113**: 276–282.

72. Karp JE, Broder S. Acquired immunodeficiency syndrome and non-Hodgkin's lymphomas. *Cancer Res.* 1991, **51**: 4743–4756.

73. Frizzera G, Roasi J, Dehner L, et al. Lymphoreticular disorders in primary immunodeficiences: New findings based on an up-to-date histologic classification of 35 cases. *Cancer* 1980, **46**: 692–699.

74. De Angelis LM. Primary central nervous system lymphoma as a secondary malignancy. *Cancer* 1991, **67**: 1431–1435.

75. Davenport RD, O'Donnell LR, Schnitzer B, et al. Non-Hodgkin's lymphoma of the brain after Hodgkin's disease. *Cancer* 1991, **67**: 440–443.

76. Sherman ME, Erozan YS, Mann RB, et al. Stereotactic brain biopsy in the diagnosis of malignant lymphoma. *Am. J. Clin. Pathol.* 1991, **95**: 878–883.

77. Spillane JA, Kendall BE, Moseley IF. Cerebral lymphoma: Clinical radiological correlation. *J. Neurol. Neurosurg. Psychiat.* 1982, **45**: 199–208.

78. De Angelis LM, Yahalom J, Thaler HT, et al. Combined modality therapy for primary CNS lymphoma. *J. Clin. Oncol.* 1992, **10**: 635–643.

79. O'Neill BP, Illig JJ. Primary central nervous system lymphoma. *Mayo Clin. Proc.* 1989, **64**: 1005–1020.

80. Kranz BR, Thierfelder S, Gerl A, et al. Cerebrospinal fluid immunocytology in primary central nervous system lymphoma. *Lancet* 1992, **340**: 727.

81. Shibamoto Y, Tsutsui K, Dodo Y, et al. Intracranial lymphoma treated by high-dose radiotherapy and systemic Vincristine/Doxorubicin/Cyclophosphamide/Prednisolone chemotherapy. *Cancer* 1990, **65**: 1907–1912.

82. Pollack IF, Lunsford LD, Flickinger JC, et al. Prognostic factors in the diagnosis and treatment of primary central nervous system lymphoma. *Cancer* 1989, **63**: 939–947.

83. Mackintosh FR, Colby TV, Podolsky WY, et al. Central nervous system involvement in non-Hodgkin's lymphoma: An analysis of 105 cases. *Cancer* 1992, **49**: 586–595.

84. Lachance TH, O'Neill BP, MacDonald DR, et al. Primary leptomeningeal lymphoma: Report of 9 cases, diagnosis with immunocytochemical analysis and review of the literature. *Neurology* 1991, **41**: 95–100.

85. Peterson K, Gordon KV, Heinemann MH, De Angelis LM. The clinical spectrum of ocular lymphoma. *Cancer* 1993, **72**: 843–849.

86. Banfi A, Bonadonna G, Ricci SB, et al. Malignant lymphoma of Waldeyer's ring: Natural history and survival after radiotherapy. *Br. Med. J.* 1972, **3**: 140–143.

87. Jacobs C. Lymphomas of extranodal head and neck sites. *Cancer Treat. Res. 1987,* **32**: 269–284.

88. Takagi T, Sampi K, Lida K. Stage I malignant lymphoma of Waldeyer's ring: Frequent relapse after radiation therapy. *Ann. Oncol.* 1992, **3**: 137–139.

89. De Pena CA, van Tassel P, Lee YY. Lymphoma of the head and neck. *Radiol. Clin. North Am.* 1990, **28**: 723–743.

90. Matsumoto S, Shibuya H, Tatera S, et al. Comparison of CT findings in non-Hodgkin's lymphoma and squamous cell carcinoma of the maxillary sinus. *Acta Radiol.* 1992, **33**: 523–527.

91. Han MH, Chang KH, Kim IO, et al. Non Hodgkin's lymphoma of the central skull base: MR manifestations. *J. Comput. Assist. Tomogr.* 1993, **17**: 567–571.

92. Liang R, Ngo RP, Todd D, et al. Management of stage I-II diffused aggressive non-Hodgkin's lymphomas of the Waldeyer's ring: Combined modality therapy versus radiotherapy alone. *Haematol. Oncol.* 1987, **5**: 223–230.

93. Hoppe RT, Burke IS, Glatstein E, et al. Non-Hodgkin's lymphoma, involvement of Waldeyer's ring. *Cancer* 1978, **42**: 1096–1104.

94. Wulfrank D, Speelman T, Pauwles C, et al. Extranodal non-Hodgkin's lymphoma of the head and neck. *Radiother. Oncol.* 1987, **8**: 199–207.

95. Makepeace AR, Fermont DC, Bennett MH. Non-Hodgkin's lymphoma of the tonsil. Experience of

treatment over a 27-year period. *J. Laryngol. Otol.* 1987, **101**: 1151–1158.

96. Munro A. Lymphomas of the oral cavity and oropharynx. In Stafford N, Waldron J (eds) *Management of Oral Cancer.* New York: Oxford University Press, 1989, pp. 196–200.
97. Takahashi N, Tsuda N, Tezuka F and Okabe H. Primary non-Hodgkin's lymphoma of the oral region. *J. Oral. Pathol. Med.* 1989, **18**: 84–91.
98. Takahashi H, Tsuda N, Tezuka F, et al. Non-Hodgkin's lymphoma of the major salivary gland: A morphologic and immunohistochemical study of 15 cases. *J. Oral. Pathol. Med.* 1990, **19**: 306–312.
99. Mehle ME, Kraus DH, Wood BG, et al. Lymphoma of the parotid gland. *Laryngoscope* 1993, **103**: 17–21.
100. Reiner M, Goldhirsch A, Luscieti T, et al. Association of Warthin's tumor with Sijögren's syndrome and malignant non-Hodgkin's lymphoma. *Ear Nose Throat J.* 1979, **58**: 345–349.
101. Gleeson MJ, Bennett MH, Cawson RA. Lymphomas of salivary glands. *Cancer* 1986, **58**: 699–704.
102. Batsakis JG. Primary lymphomas of the salivary glands. *Ann. Otol. Rhinol. Laryngol.* 1986, **95**: 107–108.
103. Kassan SS, Thomas TL, Moutsopoulos HM, et al. Increased risk of lymphoma in Sikka syndrome. *Ann. Intern. Med.* 1978, **89**: 888–892.
104. Pisa EK, Pisa P, Kang HI, et al. High frequency of t(14;18) translocation in salivary gland lymphomas from Sjögren's syndrome patients. *J. Exp. Med.* 1991, **174**: 1245–1250.
105. Freedman SI. Malignant lymphomas of the major salivary glands. *Arch. Otolaryngol.* 1971, **93**: 123–127.
106. Hiltprand JJ, McGuirt WF, Matthews BL. Primary malignant lymphoma of the parotid gland. Two case reports. *Otolaryngol Head Neck Surg.* 1990, **102**: 77–81.
107. Shikhani AH, Shikhani LT, Kuhajda FP, et al. Warthin's tumor-associated neoplasm: Report of two cases and review of the literature. *Ear Nose Throat J.* 1993, **72**: 264–269.
108. Cooper DL, Ginsberg SS. Brief chemotherapy, involved field radiation therapy, and central nervous system prophylaxis for paranasal sinus lymphoma. *Cancer* 1992, **69**: 2888–2893.
109. Long G, van der Pas M, Jacobs C. Combined modality treatment of non-Hodgkin's lymphomas of the paranasal sinuses. *Proc. Am. Soc. Clin. Oncol.* 1990, **9**: A1023.
110. Robbins KT, Fuller LM, Vlasak M, et al. Primary lymphomas of the nasal cavity and paranasal sinuses. *Cancer* 1985, **56**: 814–819.
111. Burton GV, Atwater S, Borowitz MJ, et al. Extranodal head and neck lymphoma: Prognosis and patterns of recurrence. *Arch. Otolaryngol. Head Neck Surg.* 1990, **116**: 69–73.
112. Gospodarowicz MK, Sutkliffe SB, Brown TC, et al. Patterns of disease in localized extranodal lymphomas. *J. Clin. Oncol.* 1987, **5**: 875–880.
113. Makepeace AR, Fermont DC, Bennett MH. Non-Hodgkin's lymphoma of the nasopharynx, paranasal sinus and palate. *Clin. Radiol.* 1989, **81**: 721–727.
114. Kondo M, Mikata A, Inuyama Y, et al. Treatment of non-Hodgkin's lymphoma in the nasal cavities: A failure analysis. *Acta Radiol. Oncol.* 1986, **25**: 91–97.
115. Sofferman RA, Cummings CW. Malignant lymphoma of paranasal sinuses. *Arch. Otolaryngol. Head Neck Surg.* 1975, **101**: 287–292.
116. Tran LM, Mark R, Fu YS, et al. Primary non-Hodgkin's lymphomas of the paranasal sinuses and nasal cavity, a report of 18 cases with stage I$_E$ disease. *Am. J. Clin. Oncol.* 1992, **15**: 222–225.
117. Frierson HF Jr, Mills SE, Innes DJ. Non-Hodgkin's lymphoma of the sinonasal region: Histologic subtypes and their clinicopathologic features. *Am. J. Clin. Oncol.* 1984, **81**: 721–727.
118. Isaacson PG, Spencer J. Malignant lymphoma of mucosa-associated lymphoid tissue. *Histopathology* 1987, **11**: 445–462.
119. Stein H, Dienemann D, Dallenbach F, et al. Peripheral T-cell lymphoma. *Ann. Oncol.* 1991, **2** (Suppl. 2): 163–169.
120. Weiss LM, Arber DA, Stickler JG. Nasal T-cell lymphoma. *Ann. Oncol.* 1994, **5** (Suppl. 1): S39-S42.
121. Fellbaum C, Hansmann ML, Lennert K. Malignant lymphomas of the nasal cavity and paranasal sinuses. *Virchows Arch. A [Pathol. Anat.]* 1989, **414**: 399–405.
122. Ratech H, Burke JS, Blayney DW, et al. A clinicopathologic study of malignant lymphomas of the nose, paranasal sinuses and hard palate, including cases of lethal midline granuloma. *Cancer* 1989, **64**: 2525–2531.
123. Kanavaros P, Lescs MC, Briere J, et al. Nasal T-cell lymphoma: A clinicopathologic entity associated with peculiar phenotype and with Epstein–Barr virus. *Blood* 1993, **81**: 2688–2695.
124. Ho FCS, Todd D, Loke SL, et al. Clinico-pathological features of malignant lymphomas in 294 Hong Kong Chinese patients: Retrospective study covering an eight-year period. *Int. J. Cancer* 1984, **34**: 143–148.
125. Ng CS, Chan JKC, Lo STH, et al. Immunophenotypic analysis of non-Hodgkin's lymphomas in Chinese: A study of 75 cases in Hong Kong. *Pathology* 1986, **18**: 419–425.
126. Aviles A, Rodriguez L, Goodsman R, et al. Angiocentric T-cell lymphoma of the nose, paranasal sinuses and hard palate. *Haematol. Oncol.* 1992, **10**: 141–147.
127. Weiss LM, Picker LJ, Grogan TM, et al. Absence of clonal beta and gamma T-cell receptor gene rearrangements in a subset of peripheral T-cell lymphomas. *Am. J. Pathol.* 1988, **130**: 436–442.
128. Harris NL, Harmon DC, Pilch BZ, et al. Immunohistologic diagnosis of orbital lymphoid infiltrates. *Am. J. Surg. Pathol.* 1984, **8**: 83–91.
129. Kanowles DM, Jakoviec FA, Halper JP. Immunologic characterization of ocular adnexal lymphoid neoplasm. *Am. J. Oftal.* 1979, **87**: 603–619.
130. Harris NL. Extranodal lymphoid infiltrates and mucosa-associated lymphoid tissue (MALT). A unifying concept. *Am. J. Surg. Pathol.* 1991, **15**: 879–884.
131. Minehan KJ, Martenson JA, Garrity JA, et al. Local

$791. The high-income economies had a GNP of more than $791. The low- and middle-income group are sometimes referred to as 'developing economies'. It should, however, be noted that incomes do not always reflect the level of development. Some high-income economies are still considered to be developing countries by their own governments or by the United Nations (UN). It may also be appropriate to consider former socialist economies of Europe (FSE), which include the European Republics of the former Soviet Union as well as formerly socialist economies of Eastern and Central Europe as a distinct group, separate from the developing countries. Thus, although there are a number of exceptions, the WB/IMF grouping, by and large, aids discussion of the subject under present consideration and makes sense from the public health point of view.

There are currently 83 countries listed as developing economies in the WB report [2]. These include, among others, China, India, Pakistan, Bangladesh, Egypt, Nigeria, Ghana, Niger, Madagascar, Indonesia, Tanzania, Iran, Mexico, Brazil, Argentina and Venzuela. The developing countries represent nearly 75.7% of the world population. They are scattered all over the globe. The WB report also divides the world into eight demographic regions including India, China, the Mid-East crescent (which includes Pakistan as well as central Asian Republics), Latin America and Sub-Saharan Africa. The developing countries comprise the bulk of these regions, exceptions being the few established market economies (e.g., Japan) and FSE.

The developing countries are a diverse group. There are profound geographic differences among them, their climates and terrain, ranging from tropical rain forests to deserts. They also have different ethnic backgrounds and vary markedly with respect to their levels of development. They share, however, a number of common features, which have a bearing on the epidemiology as well as the management of the NHL and which separate them clearly from the industrial countries.

POOR ECONOMIC CONDITIONS

The basic characteristic of developing countries is their relatively low level of economic development. Not only do they have lower GNP than the industrial nations, but the percentage of the GNP spent on health-related problems is also very low (Table 49.1).

Table 49.1 Basic health indicators

	Population structure		% of children affected by stunting	Prevalence of anemia in pregnant women	Doctors/ 1000 population 1988–1992	Hospital beds/ 1000 population 1985–1990	Health expenditure as % of GDP 1985–1990
	Under 15 years (%)	Over 60 years (%)					
Sub-Saharan Africa	46	5	39	41	0.12	1.4	4.5
India	37	7	27	88	0.41	0.7	6.0
China	27	9	8	25	1.37	2.6	3.5
Latin America and Caribbean	36	7	5	35	1.25	2.7	4.0
Mid East	41	6	—	—	1.04	2.9	4.1
Demographically developing group	36	7	46	49	0.78	2.0	4.7
Formerly socialist and established market economies	20	18	4	4	3.09	9.3	8.7

Data source: World Development Report [2].

This is reflected in the relative lack of doctors and paramedical staff. Similarly, relatively few hospital beds are available.

DIFFERENT DISEASE BURDEN

The disease pattern in developing countries differs greatly from that of the developed economies (Table 49.2). Communicable diseases are far more common such that a very large proportion of the available health resources must be devoted to their prevention and treatment. Consequently, less effort can be put into the treatment of malignant diseases, especially those in which a cure is unlikely (which presently includes NHL). However, many of the parasitic diseases, such as malaria, helminthic and diarrheal diseases, may have a possible role in the pathogenesis of NHL as will be discussed subsequently. Acquired immunodeficiency syndrome (AIDS) is a rapidly growing menace in the developing countries, especially in Africa. It is disrupting the social and economic fabric, and may also rapidly change the incidence of NHL in these areas.

POPULATION STRUCTURE

In many of the developing countries, there has been rapid increase in population. Characteristically, children under 15 years account for a large proportion of the total population, ranging from 27% to 46% (Table 49.1). Older people (over 60 years) are relatively few in number (5–7%). Because some types of NHL occur more frequently in a particular age group, the pattern of lymphoma observed in developing countries is likely to be different.

Since there are only a few facilities in developing countries where a malignancy such as NHL can be efficiently diagnosed and managed, and because of the large populations that are dependent upon these facilities, each center must manage very large numbers of patients. This makes their task difficult, but at the same time creates potentially advantageous opportunity to carry out research projects and provide the results of clinical trials much more rapidly than can be accomplished in smaller centers.

COLONIAL LEGACY

Many of the developing countries had been under colonial rule in the recent past; they have been ruled by European powers, predominantly England, France, Belgium and the Netherlands for 150–200 years. This has left a legacy of Western social organization even though there is a paucity of money and technology. However, in most countries, the local traditions and beliefs have remained a fairly strong influence. This has resulted in a paradoxical situation where, even in the presence of modern centers of excellence, a very large percentage of people still prefer indigenous medicine. This inevitably delays proper diagnosis and treatment.

AGRICULTURAL ECONOMIES

Another feature common to most developing countries is that their economies are based on agriculture. The bulk of the population resides in villages where the quality of life is poor. A very small proportion has access to a clean water supply, sewage disposal,

Table 49.2 Burden of disease in males by cause 1990 (hundreds of thousands of DALY lost)

Diseases	SSA	India	China	Other Asia	Latin America	ME crescent	FSE	EME	FSE and EME	DD
Communicable	1046.8	704.0	228.0	438.0	225.3	347.2	24.5	42.3	66.8	2990.9
Non-communicable	287.9	601.3	609.6	359.7	238.6	264.0	231.6	399.0	630.6	2351.0
Malignant neoplasia	22.5	65.7	113.1	41.4	25.3	26.5	49.9	99.5	249.4	294.6
Lymphoma	3.2	3.1	2.6	1.8	1.7	1.6	1.6	4.8	6.4	13.9
Leukemia	0.7	3.2	8.1	2.7	1.5	1.9	1.7	3.5	5.2	18.1
Infectious & parasitic	763.7	404.9	117.6	258.4	137.7	80.2	8.0	18.2	26.3	1862.5
HIV	93.7	27.1	0.0	8.0	34.1	2.6	1.4	12.4	13.7	165.5
Diarrheal	157.3	136.4	20.7	78.5	31.5	75.1	1.1	1.2	2.3	499.4
Malaria	161.0	4.8	0.1	12.9	2.2	1.3	0.0	0.0	0.0	182.3
Intestinal helminths	4.2	10.6	32.6	27.6	12.0	2.8	0.0	0.0	0.0	91.8

Data from World Development Report [2], pp. 218–19.

SSA, Sub-Saharan Africa; ME, Mid East; FSE, formerly Socialist Economies; DALY, disability-adjusted life years; EME, established market economies; DD, demographically developing group.

health care and educational facilities. Most people are unemployed or marginally employed with a low income. As a result, they suffer from numerous ailments like malnutrition, malaria, gastrointestinal diseases and tuberculosis. There is also a strong temptation to migrate to the more affluent cities, which results in urban overcrowding and deterioration of the quality of urban life.

Thus, the developing countries, which comprise a very large segment of the human population, have the common characteristics of poverty, poor nutrition, poor health facilities and a rapidly growing population consisting of a very high proportion of children. In effect, their environments are radically different and much more diverse than those of industrial countries. In this chapter we shall discuss the bearing of these characteristics on the pattern and management of the NHL.

Difficulties in studying NHL in developing countries

There are numerous difficulties in studying and interpreting data pertaining to any cancer, but perhaps especially NHL, in a developing country. Although there have been recent improvements in this regard, many of the problems still remain. There is a lack of information about the magnitude and pattern of NHL owing to a lack of reliable data, i.e., population-based information is not available. The number of population-based registries in the developing countries are few, although more registries have been established in recent years. However, even data from population registries must be interpreted with caution; census data are often inadequate and medical facilities are mostly concentrated in the large urban centers. Thus, the information derived exclusively from such centers is not necessarily representative. Patients from rural areas frequently come to the city to stay with relatives while receiving therapy, and addresses provided are not always accurate.

The paucity of resources also has an impact on medical practice. The diagnosis of NHL, for example, requires expertise as well as good laboratory facilities. Both are usually lacking. In Pakistan (population 112 million) there are less than 100 trained histopathologists and laboratory facilities are limited to a few institutions. In recent years, the diagnosis and management of NHL has markedly improved, owing to the availability of immunological markers such as monoclonal antibodies. Immunophenotyping has not only provided new

insights into the nature of various tumors but has also aided the management of these cases. Thus, immunophenotyping facilities have now moved from research laboratories to routine pathology laboratories. Although these newer techniques have been used in certain research institutions in the developing countries, their cost precludes their routine use and the mainstay of diagnosis in the developing countries will continue to be histomorphology.

The nomenclature and classification of NHL is another area where lack of agreement on standardized nomenclature – at both international and national levels – makes it extremely difficult to compare studies from different countries or sometimes from within the same country. Nomenclature is constantly changing as new classifications are introduced. The introduction of the New Working Formulation in 1982 [3] provided a significant step towards the resolution of this confusion, but newer classification schemes have since been introduced and entities not then recognized have been identified so that considerable confusion still exists, particularly in developing countries where communication within a country and with experts in other countries is considerably more difficult.

In addition to inadequacies with respect to diagnosis, there is a lack of other basic health facilities in developing countries (Table 49.1). Compared to developed economies, the number of doctors and nurses are inadequate and hospital beds are few. Specialized oncology centers and trained oncologists are even fewer. In Black Africa there are less than 75 full-time cancer specialists for a population of 285 million [4]. It has been estimated, that there is a shortage of about 3000–4000 radiotherapists and 5000–10000 radiotherapy technicians in the developing countries [4,5].

In view of the constraints and handicaps for the study of NHL in developing countries, efforts to conduct research would appear, at first sight, to be futile, especially when extensive clinical and biological information is available from the more advanced countries. However, there are numerous advantages of studying NHL in the setting that exists in the Third World. This was amply shown by the work carried out by Denis Burkitt many years ago [6] when, in a very primitive setting, he carefully documented the natural history and unique associations of the tumor that now bears his name. The studies on immunoproliferative small intestinal disease (IPSID), which has been dubbed a cancer of the Third World, provides another example of such opportunities. Unfortunately, the developing countries are in a state of flux. There are large migrations owing to war and political turmoil, and even more to population shifts from rural to urban areas in search of better economic opportunities. This has resulted in changes in life styles and living conditions, which may have begun to obscure critical associations [7]. The emergence of AIDS has further compounded this picture. Its rapid spread in the Third World, owing to lack of resources to control it, may eventually override all other variables associated with the NHL. However, carefully conducted longitudinal studies could, in the presence of the dramatic differences in life styles and the environment in the developing countries, coupled to the fluxes discussed above, provide a unique opportunity to understand the influences of the environment on the pattern of neoplasia.

Incidence of NHL in developing countries

As pointed out above, information about NHL in the developing countries does not, generally, achieve the desired standard of accuracy. This does not mean that it is of no value. Population-based data are available from a few centers but a large number of institutions in various countries have published the relative frequencies of NHL in their own hospitals – nearly all countries have hospital-based tumor registries, which provide (relative) frequency data about most tumors, including NHL. Excellent studies on special tumors such as Burkitt, IPSID and mucosa-associated lymphoid tissue (MALT) are also available. Thus, useful information does exist, although it should be interpreted with the inherent deficiencies kept in mind. One of the major handicaps is the use of nomenclature, which at times is difficult to translate into that in current usuage. For example, histiocytic and lymphocytic tumors presumably refer to large-cell and small-cell/small cleaved cell lymphomas according to the Working Formulation, but are difficult to interpret with confidence.

A very useful compilation of available information from 67 developing countries has been published by the International Agency for Research on Cancer (IARC) [8]. Although the majority of series are from hospital- or pathology-based registries serving a single center, or a region or an entire country, a number of population-based statistics are also given, although multicenter studies in which a review of all histological material has been conducted have been carried out only rarely. The quality of the data is, therefore, obviously variable. However, they do provide some information about the prevalence of NHL. It may, therefore, be important to study and analyze these data, even though suboptimal.

The classification of tumors in the IARC mono-

graph is mainly according to International Classification of Diseases (ICD) ICD-8 and ICD-9. The diagnosis of lymphomas other than Hodgkin's disease are listed under ICD-200 (lymphosarcomas) and ICD-202 (other lymphomas). Hodgkin's disease is listed under ICD-201. Burkitt's lymphoma (BL) and Kaposi's sarcoma are given as subgroups of lymphosarcoma where needed.

There are wide variations among different countries, sometimes between neighboring countries, in the incidence and frequency of NHL and, while these numbers doubtless include artefacts, it can be generally stated that NHL are amongst the ten most common tumors in the world. They are more common than Hodgkin's disease (HD) in most countries. They are particularly frequent in Northern Africa, equatorial Africa and the Middle East, extending into Iran and Pakistan. They are comparatively less frequent in the Far East and Latin America (Table 49.3). Thus, it appears that there are wide and significant variations in the frequency of lymphoma in different developing countries.

AFRICA

Africa is a large continent, which contains different climatic areas as well as diverse population and ethnic groups. The frequency of NHL is generally high, constituting, for example, 26% of all malignant tumors in Uganda. There are reasonably well-defined areas of high or low frequency within the continent. The frequency is highest in West Africa and Equatorial regions. However, as the distance from the equator increases, the prevalence of NHL, mainly as a result of a reduction in the frequency of BL, falls.

EGYPT

Malignant lymphomas and leukemia are fairly frequent tumors in Egypt comprising 12–19% of all cancers. NHL constitutes 62% of all lymphomas and HD accounts for 32%. The NHL/HD ratio is 2.5:1, but is reversed in the pediatric age group. High- and intermediate-grade lymphomas are predominant (87%), with Burkitt's comprising 32% of cases. The patients present late with a large tumor burden. Extranodal tumors account for 34% of all NHL with large-cell lymphoma being the most common tumor. The most frequent site is soft tissues, i.e., extranodal (17%), being in the gastrointestinal tract. Follicular lymphoma constitutes about 3% of the total, and *bcl*-2 rearrangement appears to be low in follicular lymphomas (28.5%) compared to 77.7% in the USA [9,10].

Table 49.3 Frequency of lymphosarcoma and other lymphomas in developing countries (males)

Country	ICD-200 and 202 (lymphosarcoma and other lymphomas)*	NHL/HD ratio	Ranking
Africa			
Algeria (Oran and Constantine)	7.9	1.2	3
Tunisia (Instuit Salah Azaiz)	9.6	3.2	4
Sudan (Sudan Cancer Registry)	9.2	2.5	2
Kenya (National Registry)	10.9	2.8	1
Uganda (West Nile)	26.1	22.2	1
Zambia (Cancer Registry Lusaka)	6.1	3.3	5
Zimbabwe (Bulawayo Cancer Registry)	1.9	1.3	10
Nigeria (Ibadan)	14.8	3.4	2
Gabon (Libreville)	9.2	21.3	2
Asia			
Turkey (National Histopathology Survey)	4.7	2.0	7
Iran (Iranian Cancer Organization)	3.4	3.3	7
Isfahan	9.7	2.0	2
Iraq (Baghdad)	7.1	1.93	5
Pakistan			
(Karachi)	3.4	1.4	10
(Rawalpindi)	6.0	0.98	4
India			
(Chandigarh)	4.9	1.5	4
(Dibrugarh)	0.9	0.6	14
(Trivandrum)	2.8	2.0	9
(Madras)	3.6	1.1	7
Burma (Rangoon)	2.2	1.4	17
Indonesia			
(Yogyakarta)	4.0	5.5	4
(Semurang)	6.3	3.0	5
Malaysia	3.4	2.0	9
Phillipines (Manila)	2.1	5.4	9
South America			
Argentina (La Plata)	1.2	0.85	17
Peru (Lima)	5.6	6.8	15
Brazil (Cancer Registry of Caera)	3.8	2.8	5
Costa Rica (National Tumor Registry)	2.6	1.7	16

Data source: Parken [8].

* Percentage of all malignant tumors.

NHL, Non-Hodgkin's lymphoma; HD, Hodgkin's disease; ICD, International Classification of Diseases.

SUDAN

The predominant tumors are lymphocytic and 'histiocytic' lymphomas, while BL is not as frequent as in other parts of Africa. This disease is more frequent in southern Sudan. It is possible that the increased frequency in the southern parts of the country is the result of its proximity to the so-called 'lymphoma belt' [11,12].

EAST AFRICA

NHL appear to have a fairly high frequency throughout East Africa [13]; HD is less common. In Kenya, lymphomas comprise 11% of all tumors [14]; BL accounts for 50% of lymphomas. Among 247 non-Burkitt tumors, lymphocytic lymphoma (28%) and 'histiocytic' types (18.6%) were particularly common. About 60% were in stage III and IV. There is geographic variation in the frequency of BL, with highland regions having lower rates than the hyperendemic malarial regions near the coastal and lake belts. BL in the lake districts and coastal belts accounts for 63% of all Burkitt's cases in East Africa. The patients from these areas present with facial tumors, while those from the highlands, who tend to be older, have abdominal presentations. In Tanzania [15], five families with multiple cases of BL have been described either occuring alone or in association with other neoplasia. It has been suggested that these familial tumors may have occurred as a result of genetic factors, but specific genetic abnormalities have yet to be described and an important influence of local environmental factors could not be excluded. In Uganda, BL is the predominant lymphoma [16,17]. A comparison of the pattern of NHL in Uganda with that in a number of other countries revealed that, except for BL, the pattern was similar.

In Zambia [18], NHL consituted 78% of all lymphoreticular neoplasms with BL accounting for 21% of cases. HD was comparatively uncommon. It appears that high-grade tumors are slightly less common than in countries located on the equator, such as Kenya and Uganda. Zimbabwe, being further away from the lymphoma belt, shows a lower frequency of BL. The pattern in Zimbabwe appears to be intermediate between those of developed and developing countries, although follicular lymphomas are infrequent [19]. In another study [20], low-grade lymphoma comprised 17% of NHL, with 87% of patients having advanced disease and extranodal spread.

SOUTH AFRICA

South Africa provides an interesting opportunity to study three distinct populations, i.e., Whites, Coloreds and Blacks. There are important variations in the occurrence of various NHL among these populations. BL has been shown to occur much less frequently than in equatorial Africa, consistent with the original descriptions of the climatically delimited geographical distribution of this tumor [21]. The number of cases of NHL is greater in Natal, where the climate is more humid and Whites are twice as often affected as Asians. Among Blacks, NHL are uncommon. This is in contrast to the situation elsewhere in Africa.

NIGERIA

Nearly a quarter of the tumors collected in two large series in Nigeria [22,23] were of lymphoreticular origin (1078 out of 4515). BL accounted for 33% of NHL cases. Interestingly, malignant lymphoma appears to have a higher incidence, even after the exclusion of BL. Another interesting feature is the much lower incidence in older age groups. In another study of 508 cases of lymphoma, 413 were NHL and 71% of the NHL were high-grade malignancies, with BL accounting for 41.5%. It was concluded from this study that, in spite of improvement in the level of socioeconomic development, the proportion of BL and its clinical characteristics have not changed in the last three decades [24].

GABON

In Gabon, a country in equatorial Africa, NHL comprised 93% of lymphoma, while HD accounted for only 7%. The highest age peak, almost exclusively as a result of BL, was in children, although the median age of all NHL patients was 44 years. Follicular lymphomas were infrequent (1.5%). BL was the most common histological category (25.4%). The high-grade tumors were the larger group, while small-cell tumors were the least common [25].

In summary, NHL in Africa appears to have a fairly high frequency. It shows significant geographic variations and its distribution is strongly associated with environmental factors. There are also considerable ethnic variations between Whites, Blacks, Colored Indian and Arab populations, as well as within Blacks. The incidence peaks at a considerably younger age as compared to the industrial countries, and the tumors are in general more aggressive.

NHL in Asia

It appears that NHL is, in general, less common in Eastern Asia and Southeast Asia than in the Middle East. This increased frequency in the Middle East extends into Pakistan and the Western regions of India. In India there are differences between the northern and southern parts of the country, a pattern reflected in Pakistan [26], where NHL is also less common in the south, where data are available mainly from immigrant populations from India. This north–south difference in Pakistan is also reflected in the mother tongue of the cases. In the Pushto-speaking population, which is mainly concentrated in the north of the country, the frequency is higher than in Urdu-speaking communities. In the Middle East the higher frequency is, to some extent, the resuult of a higher proportion of BL and intestinal lymphomas. HD, as in African countries, is less common than NHL, constituting between 7.9% (China) and 32.9% (Malaysia) of all lymphomas [27 28].

CHINA

China is a vast country with a population of over a billion people. Lymphoma is one of the ten most common tumors. In a comparative study between Guanghou and Nebraska, NHL comprised 82% of all cases of lymphoma in China, compared to 84% in Nebraska. Median age was lower (42 years compared to 63 years). Chinese patients had more agressive lymphomas than American patients [29]. Although BL is rare in Asia and the Far East, this series from China has reported a frequency of 15.6% [29]. Among 317 patients from Taiwan, 125 were typed as T-cell and 180 as B-cell – a very different T:B of BL ratio to that seen in industrial countries. In Taiwan, however, the prevalence of T-cell lymphoma is similar to that in nonendemic areas of adult T-cell leukemia/lymphoma (ATLL) in Japan [30]. In Hong Kong, 32% [31], and in Shanghai, 28% of cases were reported to be T-cell in origin [32]. Extranodal lymphomas are very common in Hong Kong, with gastrointestinal (GI) tract involvement occurring in 63% [31].

PHILIPPINES

NHL comprises 82% of cases of lymphoma in the Philippines. The vast majority are diffuse. Follicular tumors account for only 8%. The intermediate- and high-grade tumors constitute the majority. The low-grade tumors comprise 23.3% [33].

INDIA

The differences among various regions of India have already been mentioned. In one study, 68.2% of 1540 cases were NHL, while HD accounted for 31.8%. Follicular lymphomas comprised 10% of NHL. The majority of cases were high and intermediate grade with diffuse large cell accounting for 39.1%, and BL 5% [34,35].

PAKISTAN

Lymphoma was the most common tumor in males in Pakistan in one study [26,36], while in females it was one of the ten most common tumors. In children it accounted for 23.91% of cancers in males and 15.96% in females. NHL accounted for 65% of all

lymphomas. The majority of cases were diffuse. It is interesting that small-cell lymphoma had a high frequency (15.42%). The intermediate- and high-grade tumors constituted the bulk of NHL, large-cell lymphoma being the most common tumor. Among the high-grade lymphomas, immunoblastic lymphoma accounted for 7.1% and BL 6.3%.

IRAN

Lymphoma constitutes 8.7% of all malignant tumors and NHL 67.4% of all lymphomas. The peak age is 41.5. Abdominal lymphoma appears to be common [37]. In a study of childhood lymphoma in southern Iran, frequency rates were intermediate between those of South America, Africa and Asia [38].

Clinical features of NHL in the developing countries

AGE

The age of onset of NHL in children does not differ markedly among different regions of the world. Most cases occur between the ages of 3 and 11 years, the mean age being 7 years [26,38,39]. In Egypt and Pakistan, the median age of pediatric NHL is 7 years and most of the cases occur between 5 and 9 years of age [26,40,55]. BL, which is the most common tumor in children, is uncommon under the age of 3 years [41]. The age of presentation of BL has not changed in the last three decades despite improvement in socioeconomic conditions. In adults the age of onset of NHL is different in developing and developed countries. In a multi-center study of diffuse aggressive lymphoma from several centers in industrial nations, 41% of patients were over 60 years of age [42]. Similarly, in a recently reported series of 547 NHL patients from Saskatchawan, Canada, the median age was 65 years [43]. The mean age at presentation is different for each grade and within the same grade there are differences among different histological subtypes, e.g., the mean age for immunoblastic lymphomas is 51 years, compared to 30 years for the small noncleaved cell lymphomas [44]. Lymphoblastic lymphomas have a mean age of 17 years. Slightly more than half of these patients were over 65 years of age. In comparison to these data from industrial countries, a median age of 45 years was observed in 238 NHL patients from India [34]. Similar studies from other countries confirm the younger median age in developing countries – 44 years in Gabon [25], 41 years in Nigeria [45–47] and 42 years in Pakistan [26]. In another Indian study, there was a bimodal age distribution with peaks at 25 and 55 years of age [34]. Some African countries have also reported a bimodal distribution, where the first peak is seen in children up to 14 years and is almost exclusively related to BL [48]. In South Africa, interestingly, the median age at presentation is 10–15 years lower in Blacks as compared to Whites, and an intermediate pattern is seen in patients with mixed ancestry [48].

Overall, it is quite evident that the average age of patients with NHL at presentation in the developing countries is almost a decade younger than in industrial nations and this difference is clearly not solely the result of an excess of BL in the pediatric population. In contrast to the overall lower median age, Chinese and Hong Kong patients with follicular lymphomas, predominantly a disease of industrial nations, were reported to have similar clinical features and age distribution to patients in Western countries [49,50].

SEX

Wide differences exist in the sex distribution of NHL patients in different regions of the world. Developed countries have generally reported a slight male predominance [42,51]. In comparison, most of the studies from the developing countries have reported a much greater male predominance, with male to female ratios varying from 1.7:1 to 6:1. In pediatric NHL, male to female ratios vary from 2.8:1 to 4:1 [52,53]. Lymphoblastic lymphomas have an even greater male predominance, with the male to female ratio being as high as 5:1. Reasons for the marked male predominance in developing countries remain unclear, but socioeconomic and cultural factors may be partly responsible, since male members of these societies have increased access to health care facilities.

DURATION OF SYMPTOMS

Although it is generally felt that patients in the developing countries present at a relatively later stage, there are few studies in which the duration of symptoms prior to presentation has been carefully studied but some data are available. The median duration of symptoms in children was reported to be 5.4 months in a study from the Armed Forces Institute of Pathology (AFIP), Rawalpindi, Pakistan [36]. In adults, Garg et al. reported the median

duration of symptoms to be 5 months in northern Indian adults with 18% of patients having symptoms for more than 15 months prior to diagnosis [34]. These findings were based upon an analysis of 238 patients with NHL of all histologic grades. In a study from Pakistan, 65% of the patients presented within 3 months. However, a fairly significant percentage (20%) of patients in this series had symptoms for more than 9 months prior to the diagnosis [36]. The impact of the duration of symptoms prior to diagnosis on subsequent response to therapy and survival has never been properly documented in the majority of developing countries.

The mode of presentation of NHL in children is generally similar in the developing and developed worlds, but African BL has a characteristic clinical pattern. In equatorial Africa, children with BL frequently present with the distinctive feature of a massively swollen face. They have rapidly expanding masses in the jaws, more often in the maxilla, with radiologic evidence of effacement of the dental laminae durae. These facial changes are frequently associated with intra-abdominal tumors, orbital lesions and involvement of the kidneys and adrenals [48]. In Egypt, the most common site of involvement at presentation is the abdomen, followed by peripheral lymphadenopathy and mediastinal involvement [51]. More typical manifestations of equatorial African BL, such as jaw tumors, are infrequently observed in Egypt. Abdominal involvement with NHL is generally reported to involve the ileocecal region, appendix, ascending colon or some combination of these sites. In Nigeria, 68% of patients with BL present with abdominopelvic tumors [54]. In Pakistan, 43% of children with NHL present with abdominal manifestations and only a rare patient has jaw involvement [36]. In Chinese children, the most common presentation is a mass, which is mostly observed in the abdomen or neck [53].

Patients in the developing countries generally present at a relatively advanced stage in comparison with Western patients. In a study of 213 patients with pediatric NHL from Egypt, 55.4% had stage III disease and 35.68% stage IV disease [55]. In Algeria, out of 59 cases of abdominal BL, 3 patients were in stage II, 20 in stage III and 9 in stage IV [56]. An additional 17 were classed as stage 'III/IV'. In our own analysis of pediatric NHL, 74% of patients presented with stage III or IV disease. In Saudi Arabia, 46% were in stage III or IV [57].

In Western countries, histologic grade may play a major role in determining the stage of the disease at the time of presentation [41]. The majority of patients with low-grade NHL have stage III or IV disease, 54–73% with intermediate-grade adult NHL have stage III or IV disease, and about half with high-grade NHL present in an advanced stage. In comparison, more than 70% of all patients with NHL in the developing countries present with stage III and IV disease [34]. In studies from South Africa, Blacks usually have late stage and bulky disease [48].

EXTRANODAL LYMPHOMA

Differences between industrial and developing countries appear to exist with respect to the frequency and sites of extranodal lymphomas (Table 49.4). In a recently reported Danish study, 37% of patients presented with extranodal disease [58] and 30% of these involved the GI tract. Forty-four per cent were high grade, 17% intermediate grade and 27% low grade; 12% remained unclassified. Half of the patients presented with stage I and II disease, and 27% had B symptoms. In another study by Maksymiuk et al. [44] from Canada, 27% of patients presented with extranodal disease and 41% of these extranodal lymphomas were of GI tract origin. It is important to emphasize that the presence of extranodal disease may also be partly dependent upon the grade of NHL. For example, marrow involvement is observed in a higher fraction 30–70% of patients with low-grade lymphomas, than 10–30% of patients with intermediate and 12–50% of patients with high-grade NHL.

In comparison to these data from the industrial countries, most of the studies from the developing countries have reported a higher incidence of extranodal disease at presentation [31–37,60]. The frequency of primary extranodal NHL in Asia varies from 28.5% to 45% [30]. The most common site of involvement is the GI tract, followed by Waldeyer's ring. In Hong Kong [31], GI tract involvement

accounts for 63% of extranodal cases. Small intestinal involvement with NHL is frequently observed in certain parts of Asia, particularly the Middle East. A study of 417 cases of NHL in Lebanon revealed that 44% of the patients had extranodal involvement [61]. The most common extranodal site was the GI tract, which was observed in 46.5% cases, followed by Waldeyer's ring involvement in 19% of cases. Small intestinal involvement was three times more common than stomach and IPSID accounted for a large number of patients with small intestinal lymphoma. Gastric NHL is of particular interest. In contrast to a continuous decline in the incidence and mortality rates of gastric adenocarcinomas during the past several decades, the frequency of primary gastric lymphomas has increased. The stomach is the most common site of primary extranodal lymphomas in adults in industrial countries [62] but is less common in developing countries. Among other sites of involvement, testicular involvement is common (11.8%) in Pakistani patients [36]. The tumors were bilateral in most cases and occurred predominantly in an older age group. The majority were diffuse large-cell lymphomas (76.4%).

HISTOLOGICAL TYPES

Of potential importance to an understanding of pathogenesis are differences in the histologic subtypes of NHL between developed and developing countries (Table 49.5). In the USA, 33% of all patients with NHL have low-grade, 38% have intermediate-grade and 17% high-grade NHL [3]. A recent study from Canada reported a very similar frequency of low-grade lymphomas [44]. In comparison, low-grade lymphomas are less frequent in

Table 49.4 Frequency and sites of extranodal lymphomas

	Hong Kong [31]	Pakistan [36]	Egypt [9]	USA [59]
Extranodal (%)	28.5	26.81	34	24
Site				
Nose	9.2	1.18	0.32	2.2
Waldeyer's ring/oral cavity	7.9	17.36	22.33	16.8
GI tract	63.2	43.71	16.83	36.7
Stomach		10.1	9.83	
Small intestine		16.7	4.85	
Large intestine		9.58	6.15	
CNS	—	2.3	0.97	1.6
Skin	2.6	7.7	4.21	7.5
Orbit	1.3	0.59	0.32	2.5
Thyroid	3.9	—	—	—
Bone	3.9	2.3	11.0	4.7
GU tract	3.9	11.37	5.61	2.2

GI, Gastrointestinal; GU, genitourinary; CNS, central nervous system.

Table 49.5 Relative frequency of histological types of non-Hodgkin's lymphoma (%)

Type (Working Formulation)	China [29]	Pakistan [26]	Egypt [9]	India [34]	USA [3]
Low grade	12.5	19.74	9.3	12.1	33.7
Small lymphocyte	3.6	12.2	7.3	3.8	3.6
Follicular small cleaved	5.2	2.2	1.09	5.9	22.5
Follicular mixed	3.6	4.26	0.98	2.5	7.5
Intermediate grade	39.1	58.94	59.8	—	37.0
Follicular large cell	5.2	7.24	1.85	0.4	3.8
Diffuse medium	5.7	—	15.58	29.4	6.9
Diffuse mixed	15.6	1.36	—	9.2	6.7
Diffuse large cell	12.5	33.09	37.25	—	19.7
Diffuse small cleaved	—	5.2	5.12	—	—
High grade	43.2	21.3	27.4	—	17.2
Immunoblastic	12.0	7.9	11.6	—	7.9
Lymphoblastic	15.6	6.25	4.25	—	4.2
Small noncleaved (Burkitt)	15.6	7.24	6.21	5.2	5.0
Miscellaneous	5.2	—	1.7	—	—

most developing countries while intermediate- and high-grade types constitute the bulk of tumors. Follicular lymphomas are distinctly uncommon and constitute less than 10% of all cases. Some countries, such as Pakistan [36] and Zimbabwe [19], however, have an intermediate pattern between developed and developing countries. In low-grade lymphoma, small-cell tumors are infrequent except in Pakistan and Zimbabwe. This could be partly explained by the age structure of this population, for older people constitute a small minorty.

In developing countries, the intermediate-grade lymphomas, with large-cell lymphoma predominating, comprise the most common subtype. This histological category, which is known to be heterogeneous, could well differ biologically from large-cell lymphomas in Western countries but there are insufficient data at present to make any comments.

In children, no marked differences are observed, in general, in histologic subtypes between developing and developed countries with the exception of equatorial Africa. A recent study from Pakistan reported that lymphoblastic lymphoma accounted for 33% of the patients, small noncleaved lymphomas for 43% and large-cell lymphoma for 17% of patients with NHL [36]. In a number of African countries, Burkitt's lymphoma is the most common histologic subtype [25,48].

Follicular lymphoma

Follicular lymphomas are worthy of special mention, since they are uncommon in developing countries, ranging from 1.5% [25] to 13.2% [36]. In the developed countries, on the other hand, the tumor is much were frequent, comprising up to a third of all NHL. The reason for this is unclear. The follicular lymphomas are known to transform into more aggressive types [63,64] and it is possible that the reason for their low frequency may be late reporting by the patients in developing countries. Other explanations, however, are possible and this issue is worthy of further study.

There is some evidence that 14;18 translocations may be present in a lower proportion of patients. Thus, in Egypt [9], 28.5% were reported to be positive, while 80% of follicular lymphomas in the USA have 14;18 translocation. While it is possible that these tumors, which have the same morphology, may be biologically different from those in the developed countries, further investigations will be required to determine whether this is so.

IMMUNOLOGIC TYPES

In the developed countries, the vast majority of NHL are of B-cell type with only 10–20% being of T-cell origin [65,66]. Similar figures are quoted for most developing countries. In Egypt, Pakistan and Malaysia, T-cell lymphomas comprise about 20% [9,26,67]. However, in the Far East, the frequency of T-cell lymphomas is much higher. In China, Xu et al. [68] reported 28.1% T-cell and 31.6% B-cell (surprisingly, the remainder were null or histiocytic). The proportions of T-cell lymphomas from Hong Kong and Taiwan were 25% and 42.33%, respectively [31,69]. No ATLL cases were seen in Chinese and

Hong Kong series, but cases have been documented in Taiwan. The majority of peripheral T-cell lymphomas present with advanced disease, i.e., in stage III and IV. A large proportion of patients (74.5%) had extranodal involvement. The involvement of the nose and nasopharynx is common [70]. Whereas in an American series, such tumors are mostly of the B-cell type [71], in the Far East, nearly all of them are of T-cell origin [72].

This increase in the frequency of T-cell lymphomas does not necessarily signify an increased incidence of T-cell lymphomas. Indeed, in Chinese and Japanese residents of ATLL nonendemic areas, the incidence of T-cell lymphomas, corrected for age differences, is similar to that reported in the USA [70,73].

Subtypes of NHL of special relevance to developing countries

BURKITT'S LYMPHOMA

Burkitt's lymphoma is an interesting tumor for a number of reasons. Although it is dealt with in detail elsewhere in this volume, a few points will be emphasized here.

This tumor has stimulated worldwide interest since Burkitt's description in 1958 [74]. The characteristic facial involvement observed much earlier had been recorded by Cook [75], but it was Burkitt's painstaking search all over the continent that led to the plotting of the lymphoma belt on the map of Africa. His dedication and ability to collect valuable information in spite of very limited resources should encourage research workers in the developing countries, who are often dismayed by the paucity of resources and inadequate infractructure.

BL is common in Africa, where a broad band about 10° north and 10° south of equator contains most of the cases. However, at higher altitudes and in regions with averge temperatures or minimal rainfall, the prevalence is much lower. This has been related to the endemicity of malaria [76]. Outside Africa, the occurrence of BL in Papua New Guinea is well documented. However, even here the rates for the highlands are lower [77]. Intermediate rates are observed in North Africa, the Middle East and Pakistan [9,36,57]. It is also less common in India [34] and East Asia [31,78]. In China [29], higher rates have been reported. In the rest of the world,

sporadic cases have been recorded in all countries. Outside endemic areas, the proportion of adults with the disease is higher. In Pakistan, 20% of patients were adults [36] and, in the USA, more than half of all patients are adults, while 26.6% are over 30 years [78].

There appears to be a gradient in the frequency of BL among developing and industrial countries, which is probably a consequence of socioeconomic factors [79]. Even in endemic areas, changes in the clinical presentation differ in regions with differing degrees of prevalence. This may be related to changes in the age of infection by Epstein–Barr virus (EBV) or differences in the frequency of malaria.

BL provides an example of a tumor in which environmental factors prevalent in developing countries probably play a part in the pathogenesis. There is considerable evidence to support a role for malaria and it has been proposed that severe EBV infection occurring early in life in conjunction with malaria increases the pool of B-cells susceptible to a chromosomal translocation. Wright [80] has suggested that the tumor cells may express receptors which cause them to home to mucosa-associated lymphoid tissue.

ADULT T-CELL LEUKEMIA/LYMPHOMA

ATLL is endemic in Southern Japan, Jamaica, West Africa and Taiwan [50,81–83]. It occurs sporadically elsewhere [84,85]. ATLL was first diagnosed as a clinicopathological entity in Japan by Uchiyama in 1977 and was subsequently demonstrated to be associated with human T-cell leukemia/lymphoma virus-1 (HTLV-1) infection [86,87]. The clinical spectrum varies from acute disease, characterized by lymphadenopathy, hepatosplenomegaly, skin lesions, elevated white blood cell count with many multi-lobed lymphocytes, hypercalcemia, elevated lactate dehydrogenase, and rapidly fatal outcome to chronic disease, which is associated with skin lesions, mildly abnormal lymphocytosis, little or no organomegaly or lymphadenopathy, and a prolonged course. The mean age of HTLV-1-positive patients with ATLL is 41 years. ATLL constitutes the largest number of patients with NHL in Jamaica. Considerable evidence, discussed in Chapter 13, supports an etiological role for HTLV 1 in ATLL, including a high frequency of antiviral antibodies, isolation of the virus, the finding of proviral sequences in leukemic cells and a higher incidence in regions of high HTLV-1 prevalence.

IMMUNOPROLIFERATIVE SMALL INTESTINAL DISEASE

Although IPSID is rarely encountered in the developed countries, it is a prevalent, debilitating illness in developing countries. In Middle Eastern and Mediterranean countries, it constitutes one of the most frequent forms of primary small intestinal lymphoma [57], where it primarily afflicts adolescents and young adults of low socioeconomic status. Symptoms include chronic diarrhea, malabsorption syndrome, weight loss and frequent growth retardation, clubbing of fingers and toes, abdominal pain and occasionally abdominal mass. The pathologic hallmark of IPSID is extensive lymphoplasmacytic infiltration of the small intestinal mucosa, particularly the duodenum and proximal jejunum. Immunologically, the disease is characterized by monoclonal proliferation of lymphocytes with or without an excess of α-heavy chains in the body fluids. Although initially potentially reversible by treatment with antibiotics, IPSID frequently evolves into a frank small intestinal lymphoma of B-cell origin. The management of IPSID depends upon the histologic appearance and stage of disease. Patients in the earlier stages can be treated with antibiotic therapy but those with more advance stages require chemotherapy (see Chapter 47). More than 50% of patients receiving aggressive multiagent chemotherapy for stage C disease have been reported to achieve a complete response. Our own experience with IPSID is in general agreement with experiences reported by other investigators [88–91].

Potental pathogenetic factors of relevance to developing countries

Non-Hodgkin's lymphoma are tumors of the immune system which are predisposed to by underlying immune defects or stresses imposed on the immune system by environmental factors. There are a number of environmental factors which are peculiar to the developing countries and which may influence the immune system. An examination of these aspects of life style and the environment which apply predominantly to developing countries could provide insights into pathogenetic mechanisms.

THE IMMUNE SYSTEM IN MALNUTRITION AND REPEATED INFECTIONS

The immune system of individuals from developing countries is affected by a number of challenges to which members of more affluent societies are not exposed. The process starts even before the birth of a child. The expectant mothers are usually from a poor socioeconomic background and are poorly educated. They are heavily infested by parasites and suffer from repeated infections. Their diet also lacks micronutrients such as iron, zinc, calcium and folic acid [92–94]. Nearly 45% are anemic and malnourished. These women have repeated pregnancies at short intervals; as a result the fetus suffers retarded growth and organ development resulting in premature births and abortions.

Low birth weight is common in developing countries – 30% of live births in Indians as compared to only 5% in Japan and Switzerland [2]. The majority of infants are small for gestational age. They suffer from excessive mortality as they are more prone to repeated infections, especially opportunistic organisms like *Pneumocystis carinii*. Malnutrition continues postnatally as the infants are likely to be bottle fed owing to an inadequate maternal milk output. This often causes enteritis as the water used to prepare the feed is usually contaminated. In one nutritional survey in Pakistan, about 60% of children were found to be malnourished and chronic malnutrition was observed in 43% [95]. In another, larger study, only 43% of children were normal according to Western standards. The rest were either stunted (40%), or wasted (11%) or both (6%) [96]. Low birth weight, improper weaning and repeated infections were probably responsible for these findings. Malnutrition appears to affect the individual in a number of ways. The incidence of diarrheal diseases is increased and episodes of diarrhea last longer [97] resulting in further malnutrition. Fever and respiratory infections are also increased [98,99].

Malnutrition has severe effects on the immune system. There is thymic atrophy, lymphocyte depletion and impaired immunity persisting for years [100–102]. CD4+ and CD8+ cells are reduced in number, interleukin-1, interleukin-2 and interferon, and T-lymphocyte responsiveness is decreased. There may be loss of cutaneous sensitivity to tuberculosis antigens [103–105] and the homing pattern of lymphocytes may be impaired. The antibody response is less affected, although antibody affinity may be decreased. The concentration of secretory immunoglobulin A is decreased [106–109] facilitating invasion of mucosae by bacteria. This results in repeated GI and respiratory infections. In one study, GI infections caused morbidity in 56% of children during the summer [110]. Various pathogens, including *E. coli*, *Rotavirus*, *Salmonella* and *Shigella*, appear to be common causes of infantile diarrhea [111,112]. Gastrointestinal infection disrupts mucosal barriers and exposes the intestinal tract to a variety of antigens. In experimental animals such infections have been shown to impair the development of immune systems. The challenge posed by repeated infections to the immature or compromised immune system causes further imbalance in T- and B-lymphocyte subset proliferations, and further immunosuppression occurs.

The impairment of T-cell regulatory function coupled to intense antigenic stimulation is reflected in the considerable mesenteric lymph node enlargement that is observed in Pakistani children subjected to laparotomy for noninfective conditions. These lymph nodes show moderate to marked reactive hyperplasia. There is a marked, and presumably unregulated, B-cell response, which results in high levels of immunoglobulins. The levels in Pakistani children are about double those of British children [113]. This is indirect evidence that the B-cell population pool is greater in such children than in the West. Similar findings have been reported in Ghanian children [114].

PROTOZOA AND WORMS

Parasitic infestation is widespread in the developing world and constitutes a major public health problem (Table 49.1). In many cases, multiple infestations are present in the same individual. The prevalence of parasitic infestation depends on socioeconomic as well as climatic conditions. In many cases, more than one parasite is involved. A large percentage of the population has no access to adequate sanitation or a safe water supply [2].

Ascaris, *Ankylostoma* and whip worms each infest between 170 and 400 million school children each year [2]. In a Pakistani urban population, 47% of stool specimens were positive for parasites [115]. In rural areas this rate is almost certainly higher. In a study carried out in expatriate workers in the United Arab Emirates [116] an overall incidence of 23.1% was observed. *Ankylostoma* was most common in Indians (39.6%), and *Ascaris* and *Trichomonas* in Philippinos (35.6% and 40.2%). *Entamoeba histolytica* was much less frequent, being most commonly observed in Iranians (2.8%). *Giardia lamblia* was also most common in Iranians (54.2%). These rates were much lower than those reported from the home countries of these various ethnic groups, where the prevailing parasites were *Giardia*, *Schistosoma*

and *Entamoeba* [117,118]. In Yemen, 53% of stool specimens were positive for intestinal parasites [119].

It is obvious that a large proportion of Third World residents, especially children, carry a very heavy load of parasites, which affect them in a number of ways. They increase malnutrition and anemia, which, in turn, increases susceptibility to a number of other diseases. The infestations are usually chronic, as it is not in the interest of the parasites to kill their hosts. This leads to the persistent circulation of numerous foreign antigens, i.e., persistent antigenic stimulation and the formation of immune complexes. The levels of serum immunoglobulins are raised in some infections, e.g., immunoglobulin (Ig) M in trypanosomiasis and malaria, IgG in malaria and IgE in worm infestation, suggesting that some of the antigens released by the parasites can act as polyclonal antigens for lymphocytes, in addition to their provocation of specific immune responses. It has been proposed that continued polyclonal stimulation leads to depletion of antigen-reactive B-lymphocytes and ultimately immunosuppression. The release of enormous quantities of soluble antigens by the parasite can also lead to reduced host response to other antigens by the process of antigenic competition. Nonspecific immune response is a universal feature of parasitic infections and has been shown to be true both for antibody production as well as for cell-mediated responses [120].

HELICOBACTER PYLORI

H. pylori has been recently reported to be associated with low-grade B-cell lymphoma of the stomach. It has been suggested that while the stomach does not possess organized lymphoid tissue, mucosa-associated lymphoid tissue (MALT) appears in response to infection by *H. pylori* [121,122]. It has been further shown [123] that cellular proliferation in low-grade B-cell lymphoma is stimulated by the appropriate strain of *H. pylori*. *H. pylori* also activated specific T-cells with release of cytokines, such as interleukin-2 (IL-2) with resultant activation and proliferation of B-cells. The coculture of tumor cells with *H. pylori* also resulted in the release of Ig. This Ig was not reactive with the organisms, indicating that the aberrant B-cell clone was dependent on the theokine-rich microenvironment provided by the organisms (presumably via T-cells) rather than on the bacteria themselves. It was also shown that eradication of *H. pylori* is associated with regression of MALT lymphoma [124].

These findings are of great importance from a number of perspectives. *H. pylori* infection is very common in developing countries. In Vietnam, Ivory

Coast, Algeria and Peru [125,126], *H. pylori* rates are higher and seropositivity occurs earlier in life than in France and the USA [125–127]. This was shown to be related to low socioeconomic status, the consumption of uncooked vegetables [125–128] and contamination of the water supply, features which are much more prevalent in economically developing countries [129].

Viruses associated with NHL

It was in the early part of this century that Rous first documented a role for a filtrable agents in the causation of tumors. Since then, viruses have been increasingly incriminated. Many of them are ubiquitous, others are geographically more restricted. Some, like the human immunodeficiency virus (HIV), have spread widely in recent years, and several other virus infections have different epidemiology and disease patterns in developing countries.

EPSTEIN–BARR VIRUS

EBY has been associated with BL as well as a number of other lymphoid and epithelial malignancies. This virus is present in all human populations and infects perhaps 90% of the world's population. The age of acquisition of EBV, however, is much earlier in developing countries. In the West, most students reach university without having an encounter with the virus [130]. In developing countries, however, most children acquire EBV by the age of 6 years, often considerably before, and predominantly through an asymptomatic primary infection [131]. The acquisition of EBV during the early childhood may be an important factor in the pathogenesis of EBV-associated neoplasms. In a seroepidemiologic survey of Chinese, Indo-Pakistanis, Africans and Europeans having different relative risks for developing BL and nasopharyageal carcinoma [132], it was found that by the age of 2–3 years, 97% of Ugandan, 20% of Singapore Chinese and 30% of Indian children show serological evidence (presence of antibodies against the EBV capsid antigen) of previous acquisition of this virus. By the age of 10 years, 100% of Ugandans, 75% of Chinese, 85% of Indians and 65% of European children are seropositive. Apart from the acquisition of infection at an earlier age, the degree of antibody response against EBV also seems to be important. In the same survey it was also found that the initial antibody response was brisk in the case of Ugandan children, who showed very high levels of anti-EBV capsid antibodies. However, soon after, they experienced a dramatic fall in their titer. On the other hand, Indians living in Singapore had the strongest immune response to EBV capsid antigen, a high titer of antibodies persisting for many years. The early age of acquisition of EBV infection presumably depends upon cultural factors but it has been suggested that the extent of the immune response may be, at least in part, a consequence of genetic factors [133]. It has been clearly demonstrated that high titers of EBV antibodies are present 7-54 months before the development of BL and that these titers are significantly higher in children who later developed BL compared those who did not [134].

It is possible that the higher anti-EBV titers indicate an underlying defect in the immune system (e.g., impaired T-cell regulation), either genetic or possibly related to the timing of EBV infection in relationship to other infections. The ability of EBV to induce continuous B-cell lines *in vitro* is well known [135], but such cell lines do not grow as tumors when implanted subcutaneously in nude mice [136].

COFACTORS WITH EBV

Malarial infection

Malarial infection may be an important cofactor in the development of BL by still unknown complementary mechanisms, although excessive B-cell proliferation caused by the early acquisition of EBV superimposed on a background of immunosuppression resulting from chronic malarial infection is likely to be relevant [137]. Malaria may allow an increase or a qualitative change in the number or types of cells that are transformed by EBV [138].

Antimalarials

The use of antimalarial drugs, such as chloroquine, may also be relevant to the pathogenesis of BL. Chloroquine has been found to activate many viral infections, e.g., *Herpes zoster*. Furthermore, it activates the *tat* gene of HIV. As this drug is used widely in regions endemic for malaria, it may have a role in the etiology of BL [139], although any effect it may have on EBV could be counterbalanced by its effect on malaria.

Herbal medicines

The members of plant family Euphorbiaceae contain active substances in the form of diterpene esters. These esters have been found to activate EBV in cell lines containing the virus [140]. In Tanzania, Uganda and Kenya, more than 90 species of the Euphorbiaceae family are found. Many such plants are used as herbal medicines and are taken in various forms, mostly by chewing [141]. Moreover, their leaves are boiled and their decoctions are used as cough suppressants and purgatives. Their roots are also used as antihelminthics against tapeworms as well as therapy for many sexually transmitted diseases. The juice of these plants is poured over the wounds for the purpose of blood clotting. Their fresh branches are roasted and chewed as a remedy for pharyngitis and dyspepsia [142].

It has been hypothesised that the inflammatory cells around the decaying milk teeth contain B-cells, which may contain EBV genomes. These viruses may be activated under the action of diterpene esters, released on chewing Euphorbia, thus predisposing to the development of BL of the jaw [143]. There are, as yet, however, no epidemiological studies that directly connect the use of these plant extracts with an increased incidence of BL. BL is not as uncommon as was initially believed in Western children, although the incidence is markedly lower than in Equatorial Africa [143], and in up to 85% of such cases, evidence for EBV association is lacking [144].

HUMAN IMMUNODEFICENCY VIRUS

The AIDS epidemic has led to a vast increase in the number of immunocompromised persons, especially in Africa. In Sub-Saharan Africa, males and females are affected equally. In certain regions, up to 25% of the young, sexually active population (20–39 years of age) are infected with HIV [145]. About one half of all HIV-infected cases occur in Sub-Saharan Africa (estimated to be more than 6.5 million in June 1993). The worst affected segment of the society was initially female prostitutes, working predominantly in the cities and along truck routes. They acted as a core high-risk group, from whom the virus made its way into the general population [146]. In Asia, Thailand is experiencing a very serious HIV epidemic. In late 1987, only 1% of the intravenous drug addicts were found to be seropositive for anti-HIV, but now more than 40% of them are known to be affected by HIV. The problem is growing day by day in this group. The next most badly hit group was that of female prostitutes. By June 1989, 44% of prostitutes in Chiangmai province were infected with HIV, while in other provinces the prevalence of the infection was between 1% and 5% [147]. It is presumed that by the year 2000, the number of HIV-infected persons will rise to 3–5 million in Thailand [148]. Similarly, India has about 1 million individuals infected with HIV. These cases are mainly concentrated in the few large cities [149]. The impact of the AIDS epidemic on the incidence of lymphomas in developing countries has yet to be quantified.

HUMAN T-LYMPHOTROPIC VIRUS-1

The frequency of the ongoing infection with this virus varies from one area to another. In southwestern Japan, especially the islands around Okinawa, 15% of the entire population are HTLV-1 carriers. In some families, the rates of viral carriage may reach 38.5% [150]. In Jamaica, the overall prevalence is as much as 6% of the general population, while in other Caribbean islands it varies from 1% to 4% [151]. In Guam, for example, 3.71% of the tested persons were anti-HTLV-1 positive and no difference was found regarding the age, urban or rural residence, social class or quality of housing. Its presence has been noted in Taiwan, Sub-Saharan Africa, south and central America, the Solomon islands and Western Asia [152]. The virus has been found to be endemic in the Iranian province of Khorassan, New Guinea and many islands in the south Pacific Ocean [153, 154].

HTLV-1 is considered to be important in the etiology of acute T-cell leukemia (ATL) with dermal infiltration in Japan but it frequently causes solid T-cell lymphoma in the Caribbean patients. Its impact on the incidence of lymphomas in other regions has been poorly documented.

Other factors

Farmers and agricultural workers have been found to have higher risks for NHL [155,156]. There is evidence that exposure to herbicides and pesticides is relevant to this risk. In Sweden [157] a six-fold risk of lymphoma was reported in persons exposed to phenoxyacetic acid or chlorophenols. A two-fold increase was reported in Kansas in users of phenoxy herbicides [158]. An increased risk of lymphoma in dogs after use of herbicide on lawns has also been described [159].

In developing countries no efforts have been made to study this problem systematically, although concern has been expressed over the effects of pesticide on agriculture workers and others. Pesticides have penetrated the food chains to an alarming degree. In Israel, pesticide residue in dairy products was found to be up to 100 times that found in US dairy products

[160]. In India, insecticides have been shown to have contaminated milk and other foods [161,162].

At a hypothetical level, infection with retroviruses infecting farm animals could be a risk factor. A higher risk for the development of lymphoma is seen in meat inspectors and abattoir workers [155]. In the Third World, where the bulk of the population is rural and engaged in farming, these factors merit serious study, particularly since, in general, there is greater laxity with regard to the control and use of such substances and the employment of safety measures. There are also many inherent reasons why it may be difficult to enforce strict compliance of safety measures in the hot and humid climates of most developing countries [163]. Among the variety of mechanisms that can be envisaged whereby these miscellaneous factors may be relevant to lymphomagenesis are mutagenesis, viral oncogenesis and chronic antigenic stimulation [164].

CONSANGUINITY

A consanguineous marriage is often viewed with disfavor in developed countries, especially in societies of European origin. In many developing countries, however, such a marriage in often resorted to out of necessity. This provides a number of social benefits as well as support to women. It has been estimated that at least 6.5% of couples worldwide contract consanguinous marriages. The proportion in Asia and Africa is 8–10 times higher than that in Europe and America [165]. The coefficient of inbreeding, which takes into account the type of relationship and its frequency in the population, is 1.15 in the USA, 34.90 in Japan, 209.30 in India [166] and 241 in Iraq [167].

There are a number of medical conditions associated with consanguinity, including birth defects and hemoglobinopathies. However, its major effect is to increase homozyogosity and decrease heterozygosity such that the chance of a child inheriting two identical copies of a gene is increased. Consanguinity, therefore, favors the manifestation of rare recessive disorders, because the chance that a carrier of a recessive gene will marry another is increased markedly when the marriage partners are related. Further, the decrease in heterozygosity will be detrimental as it will decrease the flexibility of responses to environmental challenges in populations by affecting genetic loci (e.g., the major histocompatibility antigen loci) of the human leukocyte antigen system that are concerned with immunity to infection [168].

A number of inherited disorders associated with primary immunodeficiencies, such as Wiskott–Aldrich syndrome, ataxia telangiectasia and common variable immunodeficiency [169] are associated with a marked increase in incidence of NHL. It would be interesting to know if such syndromes are related to consanguinity.

The possible effect of consanguinity on the occurrence of lymphoma has not been examined to date. A preliminary study in Pakistan showed that nearly half of marriages of the parents of patients with lymphoma were between first or second cousins. In children with lymphoma there were twice as many consanguinous marriages among parents as nonconsanguinous marriages. High-grade lymphoma was more frequent in the consanguinous group while the opposite was true for intermediate-grade lymphomas. These are preliminary observations. It is obvious that additional studies are needed to further define the relevance of consanguinity to lymphoma development.

It appears that the immune system in the developing countries is under considerable stress. A low birth weight child who is born of an anemic and malnourished mother is already immune deficient. He or she is exposed to an environment that provides a persistent and severe antigenic challenge through repeated infections. This results in a vicious cycle, which further depresses immune responses. The situation is complicated by rampant parasitic infestation. There is proliferation of B-cells and an increased B-cell pool. This increases the likelihood of a chance mutation, which could ultimately lead to monoclonal proliferation (Figure 49.1). While the relative importance of the roles played by various factors (outlined above) remains to be elucidated, all of these factors have been incriminated in the causation of lymphoid neoplasia. Further study of their contribution to the causation of these tumors in the environment prevailing in the developing world would be worthwhile, since more definitive information could lead to the development of control and preventive measures. This might prove relevant to numerous countries, including the industrial nations.

Management

The management of NHL in developing countries poses special problems. As has been pointed out previously, developing countries possess inadequate resources, both human and financial, relevant to the proper managment of any cancer, including NHL. The treatment centers in large cities are entirely inadequate. It has been estimated that out of about 170000 cancer cases in Indonesia only about 30000 are seen by a cancer specialist [4]. Additional factors

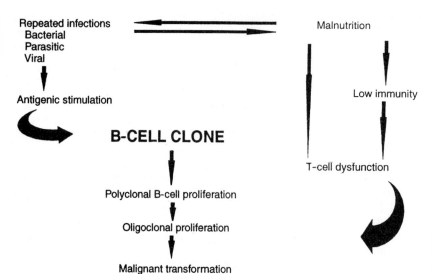

Figure 49.1 A possible mechanism for the pathogenesis of non-Hodgkin's lymphoma.

that adversely affect treatment results include late presentation, an inadequate supply of drugs, a high default rate (for treatment and follow-up) and lack of adequate facilities for supportive care [34,37,48,50, 170–172].

The cost of treatment is well beyond the means of the average patient. In Pakistan it varies from about 1000 to 10 000 US dollars, depending upon the chemotherapy regimen used. It is therefore not surprising that many patients do not receive treatment even when it is available. In a follow-up of 79 cases diagnosed at the AFIP in Pakistan in 1989–1990, it was found that 15 (19.3%) did not receive any treatment at all and only one patient from the entire group, a patient with follicular lymphoma, was alive at 1 year. Among these patients, eight were treated with radiotherapy alone, and among 48 who were prescribed CHOP therapy, nearly 50% received only 1–3 courses instead of the recommended six [26].

TRADITIONAL MEDICINE

A large number of patients opt for traditional medicine, either initially, or after receiving some conventional treatment. The reasons for this include cost of treatment, a poor ultimate prognosis and freedom from the toxicity associated with conventional medicine. The contents and nature of the medicines used in traditional medicine are generally unknown. It is reasonable to assume that in most Third World countries the desperation of these patients is frequently exploited.

In China, the study of traditional medicine has

been organized on more rational lines and a number of institutes and departments are engaged in studies on indigenous medicine. At a recent oncology conference [173], 43 papers were presented from China and Japan on the use of traditional medicine in oncology. A number of claims for the efficacy of these drugs in treatment of various cancers as well as their ameliorating effect on the side-effects of chemotherapy and radiotherapy were made. There is a need to examine such claims more closely through independent controlled studies.

CONVENTIONAL TREATMENT

In spite of these problems, good treatment results can be achieved in developing countries. Series of children with NHL reported from Egypt and Pakistan, who received appropriate chemotherapy, for example, have disease-free survival rates of 50–60% [40,51, 54,58,174–177]. Long-term survival of children with NHL in some centers in developing countries in which intensive protocols have been used have been reported to be similar to survival rates achieved in Western countries [34,54].

There have been very few series from developing countries that have reported a large number of adult patients who received adequate chemotherapy. Among existing publications, most authors comment upon the poor results obtained in adults with NHL. Results of therapy, for example, were reportedly poor in Blacks in South Africa [48]. Garg et al. reported a median survival of 16 months in patients with NHL treated in India [34]. Survival for 'diffuse histiocytic lymphoma' was reported as only 6 months in

Table 49.6 Characteristics of non-Hodgkin's lymphoma in developing countries

1. High relative frequency
2. Younger age group
3. Male predominance
4. Low frequency of follicular lymphomas
5. High incidence of extranodal tumors
6. Late presentation
7. Large tumor load
8. Lower frequency of low-grade tumors
9. Higher frequency of intermediate- and high-grade tumors

comparison to 10 months for diffuse mixed NHL. Adult patients (n=58) who received effective therapy had a median survival of 24 months. However, the follow-up in this study was very short. Almost a quarter of the deaths were the result of infection or septicemia. These results are inferior to those reported in the Western literature. In our own analysis of patients with low-grade NHL, complete remission was observed in approximately half of the patients and another quarter achieved partial remission. The cause of death was mostly disease related. In aggressive NHL, 46% achieved a complete response and 18% of patients achieved a partial remission. No difference in clinical response rate was observed in patients receiving CHOP therapy versus the new generation regimens. Most of the patients died of their disease. These results indicate that the majority of adult patients with NHL in the developing countries have a poor prognosis, even when treated with regimens similar to those used in the West.

Some of the characteristic features of NHL that, doubtless, contribute to this are shown in Table 49.6. There is a need for further study and understanding of these differences, and to do so will require the use of modern tools for the study of development of the immune system and its vulnerability to malnutrition and repeated antigenic insults. Such studies may provide clues which could help in understanding the pathogenesis of lymphoid neoplasia and may lead to the development of treatment regimens that are more appropriate for patients in developing countries, in whom both the biology of the predominant neoplasms encountered and the ability to tolerate chemotherapy and its complications may well differ markedly.

References

1. Bannock G, Bangore RE, Rees R. *The Penguin Dictionary of Economics*. Harmondsworth, Middlesex, Penguin Books, 1972.
2. World Development Report. *Investing in Health. World Development Indicators*. New York, Oxford University Press, 1993.
3. National Cancer Institute sponsored study of classifications of non-Hodgkin's lymphoma. *Cancer*, 1982, **49**: 2112–2135.
4. Racoveanu NT. Constraints and possible solutions. In *Radiotherapy in Developing Countries*. Vienna, International Atomic Energy Agency, 1987, pp. 311–402.
5. Taylor CBG. *Radiotherapy in Africa. Document IAEA/IYE/115*. Vienna, International Atomic Energy Agency, 1987.
6. Burkitt DP. *The Beginnings of the Burkitt's Lymphoma Story. Burkitt Lymphoma. A Human Cancer Model*. IARC Scientific Publication no. 60. Lyon, International Agency for Research on Cancer, 1985, pp. 11–15.
7. Williams OKO. Influence of life style on the pattern of leukaemia and lymphoma subtypes among Nigerians. *Leuk. Res.* 1985, **9**: 741.
8. Parken DM. Cancer occurrence in developing countries. IARC Scientific Publication no. 75. Lyon, International Agency for Research on Cancer, 1986.
9. El-Bolkainy MN. *Epidemiological, Immunological and Clinical Studies on Lymphoma and Leukaemia in Egypt*. Project report NC1. Cairo, Egypt, 1994.
10. Young JI, Miller JW. Incidence of malignant tumours in US Children. *J. Pediatr.* 1975, **86**: 256.
11. Ahmad MAM, Omer A, EI Hassan AM. Malignant lymphomas at the Pathology Department, University of Khartoum, Sudan. *E. African Med. J.* 1984, **61**: 627–629.
12. Yagi KI, Abdul Rehman E, Abbas KUD, et al. Burkitt's lymphoma in Sudan. *Int. J. Oral Surg.* 1984, **13**: 517–527.
13. Linsel CA. Cancer incidence in Kenya, 1957–63. *Br. J. Cancer* 1967, **21**: 20.
14. Kasili EG. Leukaemia and lymphoma in Kenya. *Leuk. Res.* 1982, **9**: 747–752.
15. Brubaker G, Levin AG, Steel CM, et al. Multiple cases of Burkitt's lymphoma and neoplasia in the North Mara District of Tanzania. *Int. J. Cancer* 1980, **26**: 165–170.
16. Serck-Hansen A. Histiocytic medullary reticulosis.In Templeton AC (ed.) *Tumours in a Tropical Country. A Survey of Uganda 1964–68*. New York, Springer Verlag, 1973, p. 292.
17. Wright DH. Lymphoreticular neoplasms. In Templetion AC (ed.) *Tumours in a Tropical Country. A Survey of Uganda, 1964–68*. New York, Springer Verlag, 1973, p. 270.
18. Naik KG, Bhagwandeen SB. Pattern of lymphomas in Zambia. *E. African Med. J.* 1977, **54**: 491.
19. Levy LM. The pattern of haematological and lymphoreticular malignancy in Zimbabwe. *Trop. Geogr. Med.* 1988, **40**: 109–114.
20. Levy LM. Low grade non Hodgkin's lymphoma in Zimbabwe. Clinical features and stage. *Oncology* 1988, **45**: 8–10.
21. Oettle AG. Cancer in Africa, especially in regions south of the Sahara. *J. Natl Cancer Inst.* 1964, **33**: 383.

22. Edington GM, Hendrickse M. Incidence and frequency of lymphoreticular tumours in Ibadan and the Western State of Nigeria. *J. Natl Cancer Inst.* 1973, **50**: 1623.

23. Edington GM, Maclean CMU. Incidence of the Burkitt's tumour in Ibadan, Western Nigeria. *Br. Med. J.* 1964, **1**: 264.

24. Okpala IE, Akong EE, Okpala UJ. Lymphomas in University College Hospital, Ibadan, Nigeria. *Cancer* 1991, **68**: 1356–1360.

25. Walter PR, Klotz F, Alfy Gattas T, et al. Malignant lymphomas in Gabon (equatorial Africa): A morphologic study of 72 cases. *Hum. Pathol.* 1991, **22**: 1040–1043.

26. Ahmad M, Khan AH, Mansoor A. *Non-Hodgkin's Lymphoma, Perspective in Pakistan.* Rawalpindi, AFIP, 1993.

27. The Nationwide Lymphoma Pathology Cooperative Group (NLPCG). A retrospective histologic study of 9009 cases of malignant lymphoma in China using NLPCG Classification. *Jap. Clin. Oncol.* 1985, **15**: 645.

28. Bosco J, Cherrian B, Lin HP, et al. Leukemia and lymphoma in Malaysia. *Leuk. Res.* 1985, **9**: 789–791.

29. Harrington DS, Ye YL, Weisenburger DD, et al. Malignant lymphoma in Nebraska and Gangzhou, China: A comparative study. *Hum. Pathol.* 1987, **18**: 924–928.

30. Shih I, Lee Y, Liang DC. Non-Hodgkin lymphoma in Asia. *Haematol. Oncol. Clin. North Am.* 1991, **5**: 983–1001.

31. Ho FC, Todd D, Loke SL, et al. Clinico-pathological features of malignant lymphomas in 294 Hong Kong Chinese patients: Retrospective study covering an eight year period. *Int. J. Cancer* 1984, **34**: 143–148.

32. Xu LZ, Tu LY, Liu YF, et al. Phenotypic expression of Non-Hodgkin's lymphoma in China. *J. Natl Cancer Inst.* 1984, **73**: 635–638.

33. Calderon B, Villalon A, Augustin B, et al. Malignant lymphoma in Manila. A clinicopathologic study at the University of the Philippines–Philippine General Hospital Medical Centre. *Jap. J. Clin. Oncol.* 1986, **16**: 21–27.

34. Garg A, Dawar R, Agarwal V, et al. Non-Hodgkin lymphoma in Northern India. *Cancer*, 1985, **56**: 972–977.

35. Kushwaha MR, Chandra D, Misra NC, et al. Leukaemias and lymphomas at Lucknow, India. *Leuk. Res.* 1985, **9**: 799–802.

36. Ahmad M, Khan AH, Mansoor A, et al. Non-Hodgkin's lymphoma clinicopathological pattern. *J. Pak. Med. Assoc.* 1992, **42**: 205–209.

37. Banisadre M, Navab F, Mojtabai A, et al. High frequency of lymphoma in Iran. *J. Cancer* 1975, **3**: 2–6.

38. Haghighi P, Mostofavi N, Dezhbaknsh F, et al. Childhood lymphoma in southern Iran. *Cancer*, 1979, **44**: 254–257.

39. Murphy SB. Classification, staging and end results of treatment of childhood non-Hodgkin's lymphoma and dissimilarities from lymphomas in adults. *Semin. Oncol.* 1980, **7**: 332–339.

40. Aziz Z, Malik IA. Clinico-pathological features and management of children with non-Hodgkin's lymphoma in Pakistan: A retrospective analysis. *Int. J. Ped. Hematol. Oncol.* (in press).

41. Magrath IT. African Burkitt's lymphoma: History, biology, clinical features, and treatment. *Am. J. Ped. Hemol. Oncol.* 1991, **13**: 222–246.

42. International Non-Hodgkin's Lymphoma Prognostic Factors Project. A Predictive model for aggressive non-Hodgkin's lymphoma. *N. Engl. J. Med.* 1993, **329**: 987–994.

43. Maksymiuk AW, Bratvold JS, Ezzat W, et al. Non-Hodgkin's lymphoma in Saskatchewan. *Cancer* 1994, **73**: 711–719.

44. Levine AM, Pavlova Z, Pockros AW, et al. Small non cleaved follicular center cell (FCC) lymphoma: Burkitt and non-Burkitt variants in the United States: I. Clinical features. *Cancer* 1983, **52**: 1073–1079.

45. Adedeji MO. The malignant lymphomas in Benin city, Nigeria. *East African Med. J.* 1989, **66**: 134–140.

46. Okpala IE, Akang EE, Okpala UJ. Lymphomas in University College Hospital, Ibadan, Nigeria. *Cancer* 1991, **68**: 1356–1360.

47. Thomas JO. Histological subtypes of non-Hodgkin's malignant lymphoma in Ibadan. *E. African Med. J.* 1992, **69**: 460–463.

48. Jacobs P. The malignant lymphomas in Africa. *Haematol. Oncol. Clinics North Am.* 1991, **5**: 953–982.

49. Liang R, Todd D, Chan TK, et al. Follicular non-Hodgkin's lymphoma in Hongkong Chinese: A retrospetive analysis. *Hematol. Oncol.* 1988, **6**: 29–37.

50. Gallagher CJ, Gregor YWM, Jones AE, et al. Follicular lymphoma: Prognostic factors for response and survival. *J. Clin. Oncol.* 1986, **4**: 1470.

51. Newell GR, Cabinillas FG, Hagemeister FJ, et al. Incidence of lymphoma in the US classified by the working formulation. *Cancer* 1987, **59**: 857–861.

52. Abdel Hadi S, El-Tannir O, Hussain MH, et al. Pediatric non-Hodgkin's lymphoma abdominal presentations: A comparative study between two treatment regimens at the National Cancer Institute, Cairo. *Hematol. Oncol.* 1991, **9**: 275–279.

53. Wang JH, Chang TK, Hsieh YL, et al. Non-Hodgkin's lymphoma in childhood: Five years survey in VGH-Taipei. *Chung-Hua-I-Hsueh Tsa Chin* 1989, **44**: 249–255.

54. Obafunwa JO, Akinsete I. Malignant lymphomas in Jos, Nigeria: A ten year study. *Central African Med. J.* 1992, **38**: 17–25.

55. Gad-EI-Mawla N, Hamza MR, Abdel-Hadi S, et al. Prolonged disease free survival in pediatric non-Hodgkin's lymphoma using fosfamide-containing combination chemotherapy. *Hematol. Oncol.* 1991, **9**: 281–286.

56. Ladjadj Y, Phillip T, Lenoir EM, et al. Abdominal type Burkitt lymphomas in Algeria. *Br. J. Cancer* 1984, **49**: 503–512.

57. Ibrahim EM, Satti MB, AL Idrissi MY, et al. Non Hodgkin's lymphoma in Saudi Arabia: Prognostic factors and an analysis of the outcome of combination chemotherapy only for both localized and advanced disease. *Eur. J. Cancer Clin. Oncol.* 1988, **24**: 391–401.

58. d'Amore F, Christensen BE, Brincker H, et al. Clinicopathological features and prognostic factors in extranodal non-Hodgkin's lymphomas. Danish LYFO study group. *Eur. J. Cancer* 1991, **27**: 1201–1208.

59. Freeman C, Berg JW, Cutler SJ. Occurrence and prognosis of extranodal lymphoma. *Cancer* 1972, **29**: 252.

60. Sarpel SG, Paydas S, Tuncer T, et al. Non Hodgkin's lymphoma in Turkey. *Cancer* 1988, **62**: 1653–1657.

61. Salem P, Anaissie E, Allan C, et al. Non Hodgkin's lymphomas in the Middle East. A study of 417 patients with emphasis on clinical features. *Cancer* 1986, **58**: 1162–1166.

62. Severson RK, Davis S. Increasing incidence of primary gastric lymphoma. *Cancer* 1990, **66**: 1283–1287.

63. Acker B, Hoppe RT, Colby TV, et al. Histology conversions in the non-Hodgkin's lymphoma. *J. Clin. Oncol.* 1983, **1**: 11–16.

64. Ersboll J, Schultz HB, Pedersen-Bjergaard J, et al. Follicular low grade non-Hodgkin's lymphoma: Long term outcome with or without tumour progression. *Eur. J. Haematol.* 1989, **42**: 155–163.

65. Jaffe ES. Pathologic and clinical spectrum of post thymic malignancies. *Cancer Invest.* 1984, **2**: 413–426.

66. Tubbs RR, Fishleder A, Weiss RA, et al. Immuno-histologic cellular phenotypes of lymphoproliferation disorders. Comprehensive evaluation of 564 cases including 257 classified by international working formulation. *Am J. Pathol.* 1983, **113**: 207–221.

67. Mancer K. The spectrum of lymphoma in Malaysia: A histological study utilizing immunophenotyping. *Malay J. Pathol.* 1990, **12**: 77–88.

68. Xu LZ, Tu LY, Lul F, et al. Phenotypic expression of non-Hodgkin's lymphoma in China. *J. Natl Cancer Inst.* 1984, **73**: 635.

69. Su IH Jen, Shih LY, Kadin ME, et al. Pathologic and immunologic characterization of malignant lymphoma in Taiwan. *Am. J. Clin. Pathol.* 1985, **84**: 715–723.

70. Ng CS, Chan JKC. Malignant lymphoma in China – what is the East West difference? *Hum. Pathol.* 1988, **19**: 614.

71. Frierson HF Jr, Innes DJ Jr, Milh SE, et al. Immuno-phenotypic analysis of sinonasal non-Hodgkin's lymphoma. *Hum. Pathol.* 1989, **20**: 636.

72. Chan JKC, Ng CS, Lan WH, et al. Most nasal/naso-pharyngeal lymphomas are peripheral T cell lymphoma. *Am. J. Surg. Pathol.* 1987, **11**: 418.

73. Ng CS, Chan JKC, Lo STH, et al. Immunophenotypic analysis of non-Hodgkin lymphoma in Chinese. A study of 75 cases in Hongkong. *Pathology* 1986, **18**: 419.

74. Burkitt DP. A sarcoma involving the jaw in African children. *Br. J. Surg.* 1958, **197**: 218–233.

75. Hutt MSR, Burkitt DP. Aetiology of Burkitt's lymphoma. *Lancet* 1973, **1**: 439.

76. Parkin DM, Sohier R, O'Conor GT. Geographic distribution of Burkitt's lymphoma. In *Burkitt's Lymphoma. A Human Cancer Model.* Lyon, IARC, 1985, pp. 155–164.

77. Wilkey IS. Malignant lymphoma in Papua New Guinea: Epidemiological aspects *J. Natl Cancer Inst.* 1973, **50**: 1703–1711.

78. Levine PH, Connelly RR, Mackay FW. Burkitt's lymphoma in USA cases reported to lymphoma registry compared with population based incidence and mortality data. In *Burkitt's Lymphoma. A Human Cancer Model.* Lyon, IARC, 1985, pp. 212–224.

79. deThé, G. Epstein–Barr virus and Burkitt's lymphoma world wide: The causal relationship. In *Burkitt's Lymphoma. A Human Cancer Model.* Lyon, IARC, 1985, pp. 165–176.

80. Wright DH. Histogenesis of Burkitt's lymphoma: A B-cell tumour of mucosa-associated lymphoid tissue. In *Burkitt's Lymphoma. A Human Cancer Model.* Lyon, IARC, 1985, pp. 37–45.

81. Takatsuki K, Uchiyama J, Sagawa K, et al. Adult T cell leukaemia in Japan. In Seno S, Takaku K, Irino S (eds) Adult T cell leukaemia in Japan. *Topics in Hematology.* Amsterdam, Excerpta Medica, 1977, pp. 73–77.

82. Gibbs WN, Lofters WS, Campbell M, et al. Non-Hodgkin's lymphoma in Jamaica and its relation to adult T-cell leukaemia lymphoma. *Ann. Intern. Med.* 1987, **106**: 361–368.

83. Catovsky D, Greaves MF, Rose M, et al. Adult T cell lymphoma–leukaemia in blacks from the West Indies. *Lancet* 1982, **1**: 639–642.

84. Blayney DW, Jaffe ES, Blattner WA, et al. The human T cell leukaemia/lymphoma virus associated with American adult T cell leukaemia/lymphoma. *Blood* 1983, **62**: 401–405.

85. Bunn PA Jr, Schecter GP, Jaffe E, et al. Clinical course of retrovirus associated adult T cell lymphoma in the United States. *N. Engl. J. Med.* 1983, **309**: 257–264.

86. Poiesz BJ, Ruscetti FW, Gazdar AF, et al. Detection and isolation of type C retrovirus particles from fresh and cultured lymphocytes of a patient with cutaneous T cell lymphoma. *Proc. Natl Acad. Sci. USA* 1980, **77**: 7415–7419.

87. Yoshida M, Miyoshi I, Hinuma Y. Isolation and characterization of retrovirus from cell lines of human adult T cell leukaemia and its implications in the disease. *Proc. Natl Acad. Sci. USA* 1982, **79**: 2031–2035.

88. Shih LY, Liaw SJ, Hsueh S, et al. Alpha chain disease: Report of a case from Taiwan. *Cancer* 1987, **59**: 545–548.

89. Seligman M, Mihaesco E, Preud'homme JL, et al. Heavy chain disease: Current findings and concepts. *Immunol. Rev.* 1979, **48**: 145.

90. Tandon HD, Vij JC, Tandon RT, et al. Alpha chain disease in India. *J. Assoc. Physicians India* 1980, **28**: 171–176.

91. Atichartakarn V, Kurathong S, Nitiyanand P, et al. Alpha chain disease in Thailand. *Southeast Asian J. Trop. Med. Public Health* 1982, **13**: 120–126.

92. Ferraz EM, Gray RH, Cunha TM. Determinants of preterm delivery and intrauterine growth retardation in northeast Brazil. *Int. J. Epidemiol.* 1990; **19**: 101–108.

93. Lima M, Figueira F, Ebrahim GJ. Malnutrition

among children of adolescent mothers in a squatter community of Recife. *Brazil. J. Trop. Pediatr.* 1990, **36**: 14–19.

94. Robyn C, Keita MS, Neuris S. Intrauterine growth retardation in Africa. In Senterre J (ed.) *Intrauterine Growth Retardation*. Nestle Nutrition Workshop Series 18. New York, Nestec Ltd Vevey/Raven Press, 1989, pp. 165–181.

95. *Micronutrient Survey of Pakistan*, Vol. I. Government of Pakistan, 1978.

96. National Nutrition Survey. *1987–87 Report*. Nutrition Division National Institute of Health, Government of Pakistan, 1988, pp. 2–3.

97. Martorell R, Yarbrough C. The energy cost of diarrheal diseases and other common diseases in children. In Chen L, Scrimshaw NS (ed) *Diarrhoea and Malnutrition. Interactions, Mechanisms and Interventions.* New York, Plenum Press, 1983, pp. 125–141.

98. Scrimshaw NS, Taylor CE, Gordon JE. *Interactions of Nutrition and Infection*. Geneva, World Health Organization, 1968.

99. Chandra RK, Newberne PM. *Nutrition, Immunity and Infection. Mechanisms of Interactions.* New York, Plenum Press, 1977.

100. Chandra RK. 1990 McCollum Award Lecture. Nutrition and immunity: Lessons from the past and new insights into the future. *Am. J. Clin. Nutr.* 1991, **53**: 1087–1101.

101. Dutz W, Kohout E, Rossipal E, Vessal K. Infantile stress, immune modulation, and disease patterns. *Pathol. Ann.* 1976, **11**: 415–454.

102. Ghavami H, Dutz W, Mohallattee M, et al. Immune disturbances after severe enteritis during the first six months of life. *Int. J. Med. Sci.* 1979, **15**: 364–368.

103. Chandra RK. Rosette-forming T lymphocytes and cell mediated immunity in malnutrition. *Br. Med. J.* 1974, **2**: 608–609.

104. Ferguson AC, Lawlor GR Jr, Neurmann CG, et al. Decreased rosette-forming lymphocytes in malnutrition and intrauterine growth retardation. *J. Pediatr.* 1974, **85**: 717–723.

105. Chandra RK. McCollum Award Lecture. Nutrition and immunity. Lessons from the past and new insights into the future. *Am. J. Clin. Nutr.* 1990, **53**: 1087–1101.

106. Chandra RK. Serum complement and immunoconglutin in malnutrition. *Arch. Dis. Child.* 1975, **50**: 225–229.

107. Chandra RK. Nutritional deficiency and susceptibility to infection. *Bull. WHO* 1979, **57**: 167–177.

108. McMurray DN, Rey H, Casazza LJ, et al. Effect of moderate malnutrition and concentrations of immunoglobulin and enzymes in tears and saliva of young Colombian children. *Am. J. Clin. Nutr.* 1977, **30**: 1944–1948.

109. Sirishinha S, Suskind R, Edelmann R, et al. Olson RE. Secretory and serum IgA in children with protein caloric malnutrition. *Pediatrics* 1975, **55**: 166–170.

110. Ghafoor A. An overview of research on communicable disease in Pakistan. *Proc. PMRC Med. Res. Congr.*, Islamabad, 1984, pp. 29–39.

111. Khan MA, Ghafoor A, Burney MI. Aetiological agents of diarrhea in infancy and childhood. *J. Pakistan Med. Assoc.* 1985, **35**: 274–279.

112. Khan MA, Ghafoor A, Burney MI. Role of toxogenic bacteria in acute infantile diarrhoea. *J. Pakistan Med. Assoc.* 1984, **34**: 266–269.

113. Hashmi JA, Siddiqui M, Sadaruddin F. Serum immunoglobulin and transferrin in pre-school children. *J. Pakistan Med. Assoc.* 1977, **27**: 386–388.

114. Neumann CG, Lawlor CG Jr, Stiehm ER, et al. Immunologic responses in malnourished children. *Am. J. Clin. Nutr.* 1975, **28**: 89–104.

115. Amjad Z, Munir MA, Ghafoor A. Intestinal parasite infections among referred patients from Rawalpindi/Islamabad. *Sci. Int.* 1990, **2**: 57–62.

116. Osama MG, Ibrahim, Benen A, et al. Prevalence of intestinal parasites among expatriate workers in ALAIN, USA. *Ann. Saud. Med.* 1993, **13**: 126–129.

117. Khan MU, Shahidullah M, Barua DK, et al. The efficacy of periodic deworming in an urban slum population for parasitic control. *Ind. J. Med. Res.* 1986, **83**: 82–88.

118. Elkins DB, Haswell-Elkins M, et al. The epidemiology and control of intestinal helminths in the Pulicat lake region of Southern India. *Trans. Roy. Soc. Trop. Med. Hyg.* 1986, **80**: 774–792.

119. Farag AH. Intestinal parasitosis in the population of Yemen Arab Republic. *Trop. Geog. Med.* 1985, **37**: 29–31.

120. Roitt I. *Essential Immunology*, 6th edn, London, Blackwell Scientific Publications, 1990, pp. 164–171.

121. Wyatt JI, Rathbone BJ. Immune response of gastric mucosa to *Campylobacter pylori*. *Scand. J. Gastroenterol.* 1988, **23**: 44–49.

122. Stole M, Eidt S. Lymphoid follicles in the antral mucosa, immune response to *Campylbacter pylori*. *J. Clin. Pathol.* 1989, **42**: 1269–1271.

123. Hussel T, Isaacson PG, Crabtree JE, et al. The response of cells from low grade B cell gastric lymphomas of mucosa associated lymphoid to *Helicobacter pylori*. *Lancet* 1993, **342**: 571–574.

124. Wotherspoon AC, Doglioni C, Diss TC, et al. Regenesis of primary low grade lymphoma of mucosa associated turn type after eradication of *Helicobacter pylori*. *Lancet* 1993, **342**: 575–577.

125. Megrand F, Brassens-Rabbe M, Denis F, et al. Seroepidemiology of lymphoblastic pylori infection in various populations. *Clin. Microbiol.* 1989, **27**: 1870–1873.

126. Klein DD, Graham DD, Gaillour A, et al. (Gastrointestinal Physiology Working Group). Water source as a risk factor for *Helicobacter pylori* infection in Peru via children. *Lancet* 1991, **337**: 1505–1506.

127. Hopkin RJ, Runnel RO, Donnerghre M, et al. Seroprevalence of *Helicobacter pylori* prevalence in seventh day adventists and other groups in Maryland: Lack of association with Def. *Arch. Int. Med.* 1990, **150**: 2347–2348.

128. Perez-Perez G, Dworkin B, Chodos J, et al. *Campylobacter pylori* antibodies in humans. *Ann. Intern. Med.* 1988, **109**: 11–17.

129. Hopkin RJ, Pablo AV, Ferreccio C, et al. Seroprevalence of *Helicobacter pylori* in Chile: Vegetables may

serve as one route of transmission. *J. Infect. Dis.* 1993, **168**: 222–226.

130. University Health Physicians and PHLS Laboratories. A joint investigation. Infectious mononucleosis and its relationship to EB virus antibody. *Br. Med. J.* 1971, **4**: 643–646.

131. Evans AS. New discoveries in infectious mononucleosis. *Mod. Med.* 1974, **47**: 113–122.

132. deThé G, Day N, Geser A, et al. Epidemiology of the Epstein–Barr virus: Preliminary analysis of an international study. In deThé, Epstein MA, Hausen H (eds) *Oncogenes and Herpesviruses II* IARC Scientific Publication no. 110: ii Vol. 2. Lyon, IARC, 1975, pp. 3–100.

133. deThé G, Ho JHC, Muir CS. Nasopharyngeal carcinoma. In Evans AS (ed.) *Viral Infections of Humans. Epidemiology and Control*, 2nd edn. New York, Plenum Press, 1984, pp. 621–652.

134. deThé G, Geser A, Day NE. Epidemiological evidence for causal relationship between Epstein–Barr virus and Burkitt's lymphoma from a Ugandan prospective study. *Nature*, 1978, **274**: 756–761.

135. Pope JH, Horne MK, Scott W. Transformation of foetal human leukocytes *in vitro* by filtrates of a human leukaemia cell line containing herpes like virus. *Int. J. Cancer* 1958, **3**: 857–866.

136. Nilsson K, Giovenella BC, Stehlin JS, et al. Tumorigenecity of human hematopoetic cell lines in athymic nude mice. *Int. J. Cancer* 1977, **19**: 337–344.

137. Lenoir GM. Role of the virus, chromosomal translocation and cellular oncogenes in the aetiology of Burkitt's lymphoma. In Epstein MA, Achong BG (eds) *The Epstein–Barr Virus.* London, William Heinemann Medical Books, 1986, pp. 184–206.

138. Miller G. *Virology, Epstein–Barr Virus.* In Field BN (ed.) New York, Raven Press, 1985, pp. 563–590.

139. Maheshwari PK, Srikantan V, Bhartiya D. Chloroquine enhanced replication of Semiliki Forest virus and encephalomyocarditis virus in mice. *J. Virol.* 1991, **65**: 992–995.

140. Zeng Y, Zhong JM, Mo YK, et al. Epstein Barr virus early antigen induction in Raji cells by Chinese medicinal herbs. *Intervirol.* 1983, **19**: 201–204.

141. Kokwaso O. Euphorbiaceae. In Kokawaro JO (ed.) *Medicinal plants of East Africa.* Nairobi, East Africa Literature Bureau, 1976, pp. 85–100.

142. Ito Y. Vegetable activators of the viral genome and the causation of Burkitt's lymphoma and nasopharyngeal carcinoma. In Epstein MA, Achong BG (eds) *The Epstein–Barr virus.* London, William Heinemann Medical Books, 1986, pp. 208–232.

143. Bouffet E, Freppaz D, Pinkerton R, et al. Burkitt's lymphoma. A model for clinical oncology. *Eur. J. Cancer* 1991, **27**: 504–509.

144. Lenoir GM, Philip T, Sohier R. Burkitt type lymphoma–EBV association and cytogenetic markers in case from various geographical locations. In Magrath IT, O'Conor GT, Ramat B (eds) *Pathogenesis of Leukaemias and Lymphomas. Environmental Influences.* New York, Raven Press, 1984, pp. 283–295.

145. Piot P, Carael M. Epidemiological and sociological aspects of HIV infection in developing countries. *Br.*

Med. J. 1988, **44**: 68–88.

146. World Health Organization Global Programme on AIDS. *The HIV/AIDS Pandemic: 1993 Overview* (WHO/GPA/CVP/EVN 93.1). Geneva, World Health Organization, 1993.

147. Siraprapasiri T, Thanpasertsuks S, Rhodklay A, et al. Risk factors for HIV among prostitutes in Chiangmai, Thailand. *AIDS* 1991, **5**: 579–582.

148. Viravaidya M. *Epidemiological Model of HIV in Thailand.* Bangkok, Population and Community Development Association, December 1990.

149. World Health Organization. *AIDS/HIV Infection in South East Asia.* Regional office for South East Asia. New Delhi, WHO, 7 November, 1992.

150. Kajiyama W, Kashiwagi S, Hiyashi J, et al. Intrafamilial clustering of anti-ATLA positive persons. *Am. J. Epidemiol.* 1986, **124**: 800–806.

151. Maqtutes E, Dalgesh AG, Weiss RA, et al. Studies in healthy HTLV-1 carriers from the Carribbean. *Int. J. Cancer* 1986, **38**: 41–45.

152. Weber T, Hunsmann S, Stevens W, et al. Human retroviruses. *Baillière's Clin. Haematol.* 1992, **5**: 273–314.

153. Sidi Y, Meytes D, Shohat B. Adult T cell lymphoma in Israeli patients of Iranian origin. *Cancer*, 1990, **65**: 590–593.

154. Kazura JW, Saxinger WC, Wenger J. Epidemiology of human T cell leukaemia virus type I infection in East Province, Papua New Guinea. *J. Infect. Dis.* 1987, **155**: 1100–1107.

155. Scherr, PA, Hutchison GB, Neiman RS. Non Hodgkin's lymphoma and occupational exposure. *Cancer Res.* 1992, **52** (Suppl.): 5503S–5509S.

156. Cantor KP. Forming and mortality from non Hodgkin's lymphoma. A case control study. *Int. J. Cancer* 1982, **29**: 239–247.

157. Hardell L, Eriksson M, Lenner P, et al. Malignant lymphoma and exposure to chemical, especially organic solvents cholorophenols and phenoxy acids: A case control study. *Br. J. Cancer* 1981, **43**: 169–176.

158. Hoar SK, Blair A, Honles FF, et al. Agricultural herbicide use and risk of lymphoma and soft tissue sarcoma. *JAMA* 1986, **256**: 1141–1147.

159. Hayer HM, Tarone RF, Cantor KO, et al. Case control study of canine malignant lymphoma positive association with dog owner use of 2-4 dichlorophenoxyacetic acid herbicide. *J. Natl Cancer Inst.* 1991, **83**: 1226–1231.

160. Westin JB. Carcinogen in Israeli milk: A study in regulatory failure. *J. Int. Health Serv.* 1993, **23**: 497–517.

161. Makery I, Bopal M. Organochlorine pesticide residue in dairy milk in and around Delhi. *J. ADAC Int.* 1993, **76**: 283–286.

162. Battu RS, Singh P, Joia BS, et al. Contamination of stored food and feed commodities from indoor use of HCH and DDT in Malaria. *Sci. Total Environment* 1989, **78**: 173–178.

163. Ong C, Jeyaratnam J, Koh D. Factors influencing the assessment and control of occupational hazards in developing countries. *Environ. Res.* 1993, **60**: 112–123.

164. Pearce N, Beth Waite P. Increasing incidence of non Hodgkin's lymphoma, occupational and environmental factors. *Cancer Res.* 1992, **52**(19 Suppl.): 54965–55005.

165. Bittles AH. *Consanguineous Marriage: Current Global Incidence and its Relevance to Demographic Research.* Population Studies Center, University of Michigan, Research report, 1990, pp. 90–186.

166. Levitan M. *Textbook of Human Genetics*, 3rd edn. New York, Oxford University Press, 1988, Vol. 10, pp. 236–252.

167. Hamamy HA, Al-Hakkak ZS. Consanguinity and reproductive health in Iraq: *Hum. Hered.* 1989, **39**: 271–275.

168. Modell B, Kuliev AM. *Social and Genetic Implications of Customary Consanguineous Marriages among British Pakistanis.* Occasional papers, second series, no. 4, Galton Institute, London, 1992, pp. 23.

169. Fillipovich AH, Mathur A, Kamat D, et al. Primary immunodeficies. Genetic risk factors for lymphoma. *Cancer Res.* 1992, **52** (Suppl.): 5465S–5467S.

170. Abinya NA, Nyabola LO. Some clinicopathologic and prognostic data in malignant lymphomas seen at Kenyatta National Hospital over a 13 years period. *E. African Med. J.* 1989, **66**: 757–763.

171. Patil PS, Elem B, Gwavana NJ, et al. The pattern of pediatric malignancy in Zambia (1980–1989): A hospital based histopathological study. *J. Trop. Med. Hyg.* 1992, **95**: 124–127.

172. Campbell OB, George AD, Shokunbi WA, et al. Problems in the management of mycosis fungoides in Nigeria. *Trop. Geogr. Med.* 1991, **43**: 317–322.

173. Tenth Asia Pacific Cancer Conference Abstacts. *Traditional Medicine in Cancer Management.* Beijing, International Academic Publishers, 1991, pp. 341–354.

174. Murphy SB, Hustu HO, Rivera G, et al. End results of treating children wih localized non-Hodgkin's lymphoma with a combined modality approach of lessened intensity. *J. Clin. Oncol.* 1983, **1**: 326–330.

175. Magrath IT, Jarus C, Edwards BK. An effective therapy for both undifferentiated (including Burkitt's) lymphomas and lymphoblastic lymphomas in children and young adults. *Blood*, 1984, **63**: 1102–1111.

176. Ziegler JL. Treatment results of 54 American patients with Burkitt's lymphoma are similar to the African experience. *N. Engl. J. Med.* 1977, **297**: 75–80.

177. Olweny CL, Katongole-Mbidde E, Otim D, et al. Long term experience with Burkitt's lymphoma in Uganda. *Int. J. Cancer* 1980, **26**: 261–266.

CHAPTER 50

Important topics for future clinical trials in non-Hodgkin's lymphomas

ALESSANDRO M. GIANNI AND GIANNI BONADONNA

Introduction

Clinical trials have always represented the most effective method of assessing the relative merits of different treatment modalities in all forms of malignant lymphomas [1]. More importantly, prospective randomized trials have provided the opportunity to test biological hypotheses that have emerged from prior clinical experience and laboratory research. Today, the non-Hodgkin's lymphomas comprise an ever-expanding world of lymphoproliferative malignancies with different morphologic and molecular characteristics [2]. The biologic diversity of these tumors has complicated the design and evaluation of controlled trials because it has introduced numerous variables, of putative prognostic significance, that must be taken into consideration.

In spite of its known limitations, the National Cancer Institute Working Formulation has been useful to clinical oncologists and hematologists in that it has clearly identified two major groups of lymphomas, namely those having an aggressive course and those with an indolent clinical course. Although both groups are somewhat heterogeneous, for each includes a number of clinicopathologic entities and patient subsets, clinicians have learned that, in general, the term 'aggressive' is associated with lymphomas that are potentially curable while the term 'indolent' includes patients with prolonged median survival, although no treatment so far administered is known to be curative. Recognition of these differences is crucial, for in deciding the most important topics for current and future clinical trials, the major reasons for the failure of prior treatments must be identified and addressed if the stumbling blocks which have prevented the achievement of better results during decades of purely empirical trials are to be overcome.

Aggressive lymphomas

DOSE INTENSITY AND DOSE SIZE

As already detailed in other sections of the book, the first generation of polychemotherapy regimens induced complete response in 45–55% and long-term survival in 30–35% of all patients with advanced lymphomas. One of the most widely used drug combinations was CHOP (cyclophosphamide, doxorubicin, vincristine and prednisone), which was, for many years, considered standard therapy. In an effort to further improve these results, a number of second- and third-generation regimens were designed. The major differences from earlier combinations were the incorporation of 6–9 different drugs (first-generation regimens generally included only four drugs), and their administration at full doses, with intervals between courses as close as possible within the limits of toxicity. To assess the dose quantitatively as a function of the time of administration, Hryniuk [3] developed a simple mathematical formula calculating the amount of drug(s) delivered per unit time (week), regardless of the schedule of administration. Using this useful parameter, termed dose intensity, Hryniuk and his coworkers, by retrospectively analyzing a large number of clinical trials, found a possible relationship between chemotherapy dose intensity and favorable outcome in a variety of malignancies, including non-Hodgkin's lymphomas. Since its initial publication, the concept of dose intensity has influenced the design of virtually all subsequent chemotherapy programs, including third-generation regimens such as MACOP-B and ProMACE-CytaBOM (see Chapter 42).

Unfortunately, when rigorously challenged within the context of prospective, randomized trials, the concept of dose intensity as a major determinant of curability has somewhat faded away, at least in the field of lymphomas. In fact, the recently updated United States National High-Priority Lymphoma Study [4] found no significant difference either in the failure-free or overall survival in over 1000 patients treated with first-generation CHOP (four drugs, dose intensity 0.26) as compared with third-generation combinations, including MACOP-B (six drugs, with a doubled dose intensity of 0.51) and ProMACE-CytaBOM (nine drugs, dose intensity 0.48). This setback led Fisher and coworkers [4] to conclude that only new, innovative approaches are likely to improve current therapeutic results significantly in lymphoma, and Ultman and co-editors to state that 'in aggressive non-Hodgkin's lymphomas the therapy of the nineties is back to where it started in 1975 [5].

This conclusion, also supported by the results of another recent study testing m-BACOD versus CHOP in advanced diffuse non-Hodgkin's lymphomas [6], was not totally unexpected. First, the approach of retrospectively analyzing treatment outcome to assess the impact of dose intensity is open to a variety of criticisms, as thoroughly discussed by Gurney [7,8]. The most important criticism is the consideration that a low delivered dose intensity may be more an effect than the cause of a poor outcome. For instance, patients with advanced disease often cannot receive the drug regimen as planned, because they present with the worst prognostic features and are too unwell to tolerate it. This major bias is very unlikely to be, and perhaps cannot be, properly dealt with in retrospective analyses. Moreover, there is an important basic explanation for the marginal, if any, impact of prospectively assessed dose intensity [4–6,] on the treatment outcome in aggressive lymphomas. Dose intensity is only one of the variables that are likely to influence therapy outcome, the others being cumulative dose, drug schedule and dose size [9]. If we assume that the most important objective of curative chemotherapy is to kill tumor cells exhibiting either intrinsic or acquired drug resistance, the leading variable should no longer be considered dose intensity, but rather dose size. This sensible principle has been clearly expressed by Coldman and Goldie [10] in an effort to mould the emerging concept of dose intensity to fit their somatic mutation theory for drug resistance [11]. According to their notable analysis [10] high-dose intensive therapy is much more effective in eliminating sensitive cells than in killing *de novo* resistant cells or preventing the acquisition of resistance after exposure to cytotoxic agents. The latter are more likely to be dealt with by larger individual doses. Thus, high dose size rather than high dose intensity is most likely to maximally influence the cure rate (as opposed to response rate) in combination chemotherapy regimens. To express this concept in a simple way, if the amount of drug given is ineffective (i.e., unable to prevent resistance and to kill *de novo* resistant cells), it will remain ineffective, no matter how frequently this dose is administered. In conclusion, even if it were unwise to deny a contributory role of dose intensity, both *in vitro* and *in vivo* experimental evidence point to dose size as the most fundamental parameter of success when chemotherapy is administered with curative intent.

The importance of dose size as a critical determinant of chemotherapy outcome has been clearly established in non-Hodgkin's lymphomas, albeit in a subset of patients. The use of high-dose therapy to salvage relapsed or refractory patients with aggressive lymphomas began in the late 1970s [12,13]; a decade later this treatment modality was shown to be able to cure a small, yet sizeable, proportion of otherwise incurable patients [14]. However, the benefit of high-dose therapy with bone marrow support emerging from these studies and from later nonrandomized studies did not clearly establish a role for this approach in the initial management of aggressive lymphomas. As a consequence, a handful of randomized studies designed to assess the relative efficacy of high-dose therapy was subsequently begun, first in Europe, with the PARMA and Groupe d'Etude des Lymphomes Aggressifs (GELA) studies [15,16], and then with other cooperative studies [17,18,19a]. The general strategy included randomization to standard therapy versus a course of myeloablative, high-dose treatment as consolidation following prior, standard-dose salvage therapy [15] or first line induction treatment [16–19a]. Only the patients who had achieved a good partial or complete response after this induction phase were considered eligible, and randomized for further standard versus high-dose consolidation. The results of these studies are conflicting, with two studies [15,16] reporting superior results from high-dose therapy, while the others found either no benefit [17,19a], or only a limited advantage from early applications of a myeloablative regimen [18]. These differences might be explained, at least in part, by the inclusion of patients with widely different histologies, by the use of high-dose progams with less than optimal antilymphoma activity [17], and by different prognostic criteria for patient selection [17]. The importance of the latter factor has been recently stressed by Vitolo et al. [19b], and by Haioun and coworkers [16]. In particular, the latter found a superior disease-free survival in the high-dose arm of their randomized trial only for patients with high-intermediate- or high-risk-lymphoma, and no difference for the low- or low-intermediate-risk subgroups. Interestingly, in the Verdonck study more than half of the patients had a low or low-intermediate risk according to the International Prognostic Index [19c].

An additional, more basic, and possibly more important explanation for the negative results reported stems from the treatment strategy utilized in virtually all studies testing the high-dose approach; the submyeloablative course was invariably delivered as a consolidation phase, i.e., at the end of several cycles of conventional drug combinations (e.g., DHAP, MACOP-B or F-MACHOP). If we assume, on the basis of the high response rate and frequent curability, that intrinsic tumor cell resistance is not a common problem in aggressive lymphomas, the same assumption cannot be held to be true for drug resistance acquired after exposure to toxic agents. The somatic mutation model of Goldie and Coldman [11] predicts an inverse relationship between dose size and development of drug resistance. Thus, when we expose malignant cells to noneradicating drug doses we might allow, and even favor, the emergence of resistant clones. The model also predicts that, in order to reduce the probability of the emergence of drug-resistant cells, the initial chemotherapy doses play a disproportionately important role as compared with late cycles. According to this model, the use of high doses as final consolidation regimen is suboptimal. We are trying to kill with high drug doses malignant lymphoma cells whose resistance has been permitted to develop, if not favored, as a consequence of exposure to standard drug doses. In conclusion, the proper application of the Goldie and Coldman model [11] is to deliver high-dose therapy at the time of diagnosis and not after multiple standard drug courses.

The induction versus consolidation approach of high-dose chemotherapy also has to face several practical difficulties. Even if not absolutely myeloablative, high-dose regimens requiring bone marrow support leave the patient with a reduced, at times indefinitely reduced, hematological reserve. Thus, such approaches are virtually incompatible with the timely administration of further myelotoxic agents. Since it is almost inconceivable that a tumor can be eradicated by a single drug course (although in very sensitive tumors, a very high drug dose might do so) some investigators have proposed tandem and even multiple sequential courses of high-dose submyeloablative therapy, each followed by bone marrow reinfusion. However, this bold approach is highly unlikely to be of practical value in the initial management of non-Hodgkin's lymphomas. The repeated exposure to the high morbidity, and even mortality, risks of multiple myeloablative regimens is least acceptable in a population of patients with finite chances of being cured with standard drug treatments.

HIGH-DOSE SEQUENTIAL THERAPY (THE MILAN EXPERIENCE)

The major challenge to the frontline application of high-dose therapy is the ability to design a regimen which can achieve a substantial increase in both dose intensity and dose size, without causing unacceptable toxicity. Ideally, such a regimen should be widely applicable outside specialized centers. In an effort to reconcile these conflicting requirements, we designed, in 1984, the scheme of chemotherapy outlined in Table 50.1 and applied it to aggressive non-Hodgkin's lymphomas with a poor prognosis. To allow immediate initiation of chemotherapy, even in patients with a poor performance status, the treatment began with a standard-dose course of APO (doxorubicin, prednisone and vincristine) chemotherapy lasting for 2–3 weeks. This was immediately followed by four courses of high-dose chemotherapy (cyclophosphamide, methotrexate, etoposide and melphalan, plus either total body irradiation or, more recently, mitoxantrone). Although developed before the publication of the Coldman and Goldie revision [10], the Milan high-dose sequential (HDS) schema conforms well to the main precepts emerging from their model, for it employs the maximal tolerable doses of several noncross-resistant agents given as early as possible after diagnosis. Moreover, the four high-dose cycles are delivered as close together as possible within the limits of hematological toxicity. Thus, HDS is also a high dose-intense regimen although dose intensity cannot be calculated according to the original formula of Hryniuk, which requires repeated administrations of the same drug(s). Initially tested in 25 patients with high-risk refractory or relapsed Hodgkin's disease, the HDS regimen proved to be highly effective and well tolerated [20]. It was even better tolerated after the introduction of growth factors, like granulocyte–macrophage colony-stimulating factor (GM-CSF) or granulocyte colony-stimulating factor (G-CSF), given with the dual

intent of accelerating hematopoietic recovery following high-dose cyclophosphamide and etoposide, and optimizing the harvest of peripheral blood progenitor cells. The reinfusion of these committed hematopoietic progenitors after the final myeloablative course of therapy resulted in the reduction of the ensuing severe pancytopenic phase to the point that hematosuppression can no longer be considered the limiting toxicity of these treatment cycles.

Having developed a high-dose approach with a very favorable therapeutic index, we conducted a randomized clinical trial in which HDS and standard-dose MACOP-B were compared in high-risk aggressive lymphomas. All 75 patients so far enrolled into the study had at least one poor prognostic factor (advanced stage, several extranodal sites of involvement or bulky disease) and completed the therapeutic program irrespective of the sensitivity of their tumor to induction treatment. The 5-year updated results of this randomized study have recently been presented [21]. After a median follow-up of 43 months, the Kaplan–Meier analysis demonstrated that HDS was definitely more effective than MACOP-B (94% versus 61% complete response rates, 93% versus 68% relapse-free survival rates, 88% versus 41% freedom from progression rates and 78% versus

Table 50.1   High-dose sequential (HDS) chemotherapy regimen in aggressive non-Hodgkin's lymphomas

Drug or procedure	Dose (mg/m^2)	Route	Approximate day of treatment
Adriamycin	50	i.v.	−45
Vincristine	1.4	i.v.	−45
Prednisone	40	p.o.	From −45 to 0
Cyclophosphamide	7000	i.v.	0
GM-CSF or G-CSF (μg/kg/day)	5	s.c. and i.v.*	1–14 (ca)
CPC harvest†			14 (ca)
Vincristine	1.4	i.v.	16
Methotrexate + leukovorin rescue	8000	i.v.	16
Etoposide	2000	i.v.	23
GM-CSF or G-CSF (μg/kg/day)	5	s.c.	26–36 (ca)
Mitoxantrone	60	i.v.	38
Melphalan	180	i.v.	39
CPC reinfusion‡			40
GM-CSF or G-CSF (μg/kg/day)	5	s.c.	41–51 (ca)
Local-regional radiotherapy (Gy)	2.5–3		60–90 (ca)

* The growth factor was administered subcutaneously from day 1 through day 10, and intravenously (continuous infusion) from day 11 until discontinuation.
† Circulating progenitor cells (CPC) were harvested through leukapheresis. Target dose was 8×10^6 CD34+ cells/kg body weight.
‡ CPC were the sole source of hematopoietic reconstitution only if the dose was $\geq 8 \times 10^6$ CD34+ cells/kg body weight.

i.v., intravenous; s.c., subcutaneous.

33% event-free survival rates, respectively). All the reported differences were statistically significant ($P < 0.05$). These data confirm beyond reasonable doubt that high-dose therapy, when delivered upfront for the treatment of a sensitive tumor, effectively prevents the emergence of resistant clones and eradicates, if present, neoplastic cells with intrinsic partial resistance.

In conclusion, the early administration of high doses of presently available drugs (made possible by the proper use of hematopoietic growth factors and peripheral blood progenitor cells) appears to be a new, promising strategy to overcome drug resistance and to increase the cure rate of aggressive lymphomas. Of course, the same results may be achievable through alternative strategies. The identification of new, more effective cytotoxic drugs or biological agents with different mechanisms of action remains a high priority, as well as the development of compounds capable of inactivating biochemical mechanisms of tumor cell resistance to presently available drugs (e.g., cyclosporin and derivates). These alternative strategies for aggressive lymphomas are central to the therapeutic approach of follicular lymphomas and will be mentioned in more detail below.

Indolent lymphomas

The indolent or low-grade lymphomas represent a heterogeneous group of B-cell lymphoproliferative disorders that reflect the functional and morphologic heterogeneity of the normal B-cell system. Their clinical hallmark is a relatively long natural history with treatment responses interspersed with multiple relapses. According to the National Cancer Institute Working Formulation, they include the following histopathologic subtypes: diffuse small lymphocytic, follicular small cleaved cell lymphoma, and follicular mixed small cleaved cell and large-cell lymphoma. Modern pathologists also include additional histologic subtypes such as diffuse intermediate lymphocytic lymphoma (mantle zone lymphoma), monocytoid B-cell lymphoma, as well as a number of T-cell lymphomas because they all share an indolent clinical course.

In contrast to the rapidly expanding insights into the biology of the lymphatic system and the pathogenesis of lymphoproliferative disorders, comparatively little progress has been achieved in the treatment of low-grade lymphomas. After decades of empirical trials, including attempts to deliver high-dose chemotherapy with autologous bone marrow transplantation, overall survival has remained essen-

tially unchanged, i.e., 7–12 years from initial diagnosis. Most important, even after aggressive forms of therapy, there is no consistently observed plateau in the survival curves, suggesting that these patients are incurable with current approaches.

The reasons for the lack of cure in indolent lymphomas, in spite of response to a variety of treatments, has not been completely elucidated. However, an important clue to the explanation may be found, at least in part, in the overexpression of the *bcl-2* oncogene or in other, similar, molecular pathogenetic mechanisms [22]. As described in detail in other sections of this book (see Chapters by Dalla Favera and Horning), the *bcl-2* oncogene becomes activated by t(14;18)(q32;q21) chromosomal translocations in the vast majority of follicular lymphomas occurring in Western countries. Furthermore, it is expressed at high levels in the absence of gene rearrangements in a high proportion of B-cell chronic lymphocytic leukemias [22]. The protein encoded by *bcl-2* contributes to neoplastic cell expansion primarily by prolonging cell survival through its ability to block apoptosis. Thus, *bcl-2* represents the first example of a new class of oncogenes that do not affect cell proliferation but increase cell survival. Deregulated *bcl-2* is also a representative of a new category of drug-resistant genes and exerts a profound influence on the relative sensitivity of neoplastic lymphoid cells to killing by a variety of growth-inhibiting compounds, which is often mediated by the apoptotic pathways. *bcl-2* does not prevent drugs from reaching molecular targets, but allows malignant cells to resume proliferation between cycles of chemotherapy [23, 24].

In spite of the abrogation of apoptotic pathways which differentiates low-grade from high-grade lymphomas and most intermediate-grade lymphomas in terms of the potential for new curative treatments, there are a number of recent lymphocytolytic compounds deserving further trials. The new nucleoside and probably some of the anthracycline analogs (e.g., idarubicin) appear more effective than the alkylating agents in providing improved palliation for indolent lymphomas. Furthermore, immunologic approaches could offer the possibility of eliminating the residual malignant cells responsible for relapses following chemotherapy-induced remissions while antisense oligonucleotides have at least the theoretical possibility of inhibiting tumor cell growth.

Nucleoside analogs

The newer nucleoside agents, i.e., deoxycoformycin (DCF), fludarabine (FDB) and 2-chlorodeoxyadenosine (2-CDA) have been shown in recent years to have significant therapeutic efficacy in lymphoid malignancies. These antimetabolites are prodrugs that must enter cells and be phosphorylated to the nucleoside phosphate before they can exert biologic activity.

Several recently published studies have demonstrated activity for fludarabine delivered as a single agent in patients with chronic lymphocytic leukemia and indolent lymphomas [25,26]. The drug is generally well tolerated at the currently used dose schedules (18–30 mg/m^2/day for 5 days every 4 weeks). Myelosuppression is the predominant toxicity and patients show a greater propensity for infection with opportunistic organisms. The overall response rate ranges from 45% to 75% and the complete remission rate from 10% to 35%, depending on whether patients were or were not previously treated. The duration of response has been long (>30 months) in most responders. At the MD Anderson Cancer Center [27], fludarabine (25 mg/m^2/day for 3 days) has been tested in combination with other drugs such as mitoxantrone (10 mg/m^2 on day 1) and dexamethasone (20 mg/day on days 1–5). In 28 patients refractory to previous treatment regimens, the complete remission rate was 32% and the partial response rate was 57%. This high response rate may be explained by the marked ability of FDB to inhibit DNA repair, such as that following damage caused by mitoxantrone, and therefore interact with other chemotherapeutic agents. Studies on *LoVo* cell lines have also revealed that FDB can increase the synergism between cytarabine and cisplatinum. Thus, combining FDB with agents that damage DNA (e.g., radiation, mitoxantrone, cisplatinum) may represent a useful strategy for combination therapy. For all these reasons, future randomized studies should test FDB-containing regimens in frontline therapy for both intermediate-grade and low-grade lymphomas with the specific aim of increasing the frequency of prolonged complete remissions. The abovementioned biologic effects should also stimulate the development of study protocols exploring the combinations of FDB plus cisplatinum with or without cytarabine, and FDB plus radiation therapy.

2-CDA is another halogenated purine analog whose clinical activity in lymphoproliferative disorders has been delineated during the past few years [28]. The most impressive results have been documented so far in the treatment of hairy cell leukemia, in which an 85–90% complete remission rate has been achieved. Substantial activity (response rate of 45–70%) has also been observed in previously treated indolent lymphomas including chronic lymphocytic leukemia. Severe and protracted pancytopenia, as well as infections owing to immunosuppression of CD4 and CD8 populations of T-cells are the most important adverse effects, especially in heavily pretreated patients [29]. Recent clinical investigations have reported that there is no consistent evidence of cross-resistance between FDB and 2-CDA [29–31] despite their similar structure. This observation should stimulate further studies in which both drugs are used in patients with indolent lymphomas in an attempt to prolong the survival of relapsing patients. Another area worthy of investigation is represented by the possibility of combining 2-CDA with other cytotoxic drugs in an attempt to increase the frequency of durable complete remission [32]. As already observed with FDB [33], the major goal will be to determine the most appropriate doses to use when used in a combination regimen, particularly in elderly patients or in patients with poor marrow reserve.

Immunotherapy

Hopes and disappointments have characterized, with impressive regularity, the history of cancer immunotherapy. However, in recent years, a few clinical studies with interferons combined with cytotoxic chemotherapy have raised the possibility that the rates of response, event-free survival and probably also overall survival may be raised in advanced follicular lymphoma [34–36]. Despite these observations, the interferon studies have provided no evidence so far that a fraction of patients can be cured. In an attempt to further improve the reported findings, new initiatives in follicular lymphomas should explore the addition of interferons to the novel nucleoside analogs, given either alone or in combination with mitoxantrone and dexamethasone.

The treatment approaches with immunotoxins and recombinant toxins – a new class of cytotoxic agents composed of monoclonal antibodies and growth factors coupled to bacterial or plant toxins – are still in an early stage of development [37–39]. Preliminary results of the current clinical trials suggest the possible clinical use of immunotoxins in leukemia and lymphoma patients. Immunotoxins can be used to kill T-cells in bone marrow without killing critical pluripotent stem cells which are ultimately responsible for lymphohematopoietic recovery. They can also be used to purge bone marrows of leukemia/lymphoma cells *ex vivo* before aggressive conditioning and autologous bone marrow transplants. In the treatment of stage III and IV malignant lymphomas it remains to be demonstrated that immunotoxins are potent enough to eliminate all tumor cells. However, since immunotoxins disrupt protein synthesis by a different mechanism than conventional therapies, it may be worth testing them in sequential combinations with DNA-targeting drugs or radiation. The major strength of this new kind of treatment may be the elimination of residual tumor cells after conventional treatment(s), thus reducing the number of relapses.

Antisense oligonucleotides

The first demonstration than an antisense RNA molecule, i.e., a ribonucleotide molecule complementary to a messenger RNA (mRNA), is capable of blocking translation was provided in 1963 by Singeret al. [40] using a cell-free system. In fact, they showed that the addition of polyadenylic acid to a cell-free extract was able to prevent the translation of polyuridilic acid completely and thus the *in vitro* synthesis of the polypeptide polyphenylalanine. The modern phase of antisense approach started in 1984, following the report by Pestka and coworkers [41], who used antisense RNA to block the translation of specific mRNAs in living cells. We now know that the use of exogenously supplied oligonucleotides is effective in blocking viral replication, protein synthesis and cell proliferation, and that their effect occurs not only in cells in culture, but also when administered to living animals [42]. These latter studies opened the way to the potential use of antisense oligonucleotides as chemotherapeutic agents [43].

The major appeal of an antisense strategy is its potential specificity against tumor cells. In an ever-increasing number of human tumors, mRNA molecules unique to the transformed cells that result from DNA rearrangements or mutations taking place during oncogenesis have been identified. Blocking of these tumor-specific mRNAs with antisense oligonucleotides should fulfill, at least in principle, the Ehrlich's dream for a magic bullet. In the case of non-Hodgkin's lymphomas, several target sequences have been identified that might be exploited for an antisense-mediated selective control of lymphoma cell growth. Overexpression or altered expression of the *bcl*-2, c-*myc*, *bcl*-6 and Epstein–Barr virus viral genes in lymphoma cells of different histological types are all possible targets for antisense strategies. It has to be acknowledged, nonetheless, that this approach is still at an early phase of development,

and that major advances must be made before antisense molecules could be considered a practical approach to cancer therapy, including the therapy of lymphomas.

Conclusions

The failure to cure about half of advanced aggressive lymphomas will probably find a partial solution, at least in suitable patients, from high-dose chemotherapy plus hematopoietic progenitor cell support. The 5-year results of our own prospective randomized trial which has utilized high-dose sequential treatment as initial therapy [21] will stimulate similar initiatives. They should be aimed at confirming that dose size is indeed the critical variable that is needed to overcome the present plateau in the cure rate in high-grade lymphomas. Future trials will be necessary to refine certain important aspects of treatments, including the deletion of total body irradiation, the use of more than one hematopoietic growth factor and the possible use of monoclonal antibodies to kill residual tumor cells.

On the opposite front, i.e., that of low-grade lymphomas, it appears less likely that new initiatives will achieve cure. In fact it is disappointing that the application of modern therapy, including myeloablative treatment and stem cell rescue, has failed to eradicate an apparently sensitive disease. The presence of *bcl*-2, which plays an important role in the natural history of low-grade lymphomas, probably also represents a significant obstacle to therapeutic progress aimed at cure. Thus, in our opinion, treatment research should be aimed at improved palliation. Within this strategy, the new structurally related nucleoside analogs have shown striking activity and warrant further investigation. Clinical trials should be designed to examine these drugs in combination with other agents, including interferon, in an attempt to improve the familiar pattern of continuous relapse. The results of future studies will require careful interpretation, with attention to patient selection factors, dose, schedule and toxicity in elderly patients. Immunotherapy approaches other than interferon should be further explored with the ultimate goal of exploring the feasibility of broad application in phase II studies.

References

1. Bonadonna G. Modern treatment of malignant lymphomas: A multidisciplinary approach? *Ann. Oncol.* 1994, **5** (Suppl. 2): S5–S16.

2. Magrath I. Molecular basis of lymphoma genesis. *Cancer Res.* 1992, 5529S–5540S.

3. Hryniuk WM. Average relative dose intensity and the impact on design on clinical trials. *Semin. Oncol.* 1987, **14**: 65–74.

4. Fisher RI, Gaynor ER, Dahlberg S, et al. A phase III comparison of CHOP vs m-BACOD vs ProMACE-CytaBOM vs MACOP-B in patients with intermediate- or high-grade non-Hodgkin's lymphoma: Results of SWOG-8516 (Intergroup 0067), the National High-Priority Lymphoma Study. *Ann. Oncol.* 1994, **5** (Suppl. 2): S91–S95.

5. Stupp R, Samuels BL, Ultmann JE. Management of lymphoma in the 1990s. *Ann. Oncol.* 1994, **5** (Suppl. 2): S1–S3.

6. Gordon LI, Harrington D, Andersen J, et al. Comparison of a second-generation combination chemotherapeutic regimen (m-BACOD) with a standard regimen (CHOP) for advanced diffuse non-Hodgkin's lymphoma. *N. Engl. J. Med.* 1992, **327**: 1342–1349.

7. Gurney H, Dodwell D, Thatcher N, et al. Escalating drug delivery in cancer chemotherapy: A review of concepts and practice – Part 1. *Ann. Oncol.* 1993, **4**: 23–24.

8. Gurney H, Dodwell D, Thatcher N, et al. Escalating drug delivery in cancer chemotherapy: A review of concepts and practice – Part 2. *Ann. Oncol.* 1993, **4**: 103–115.

9. De Vita VT. Principles of chemotherapy. In De Vita VT, Hellman S, Rosenberg SA (eds) *Cancer: Principles and Practice of Oncology*, 4th edn. Philadelphia: JB Lippincott Co, 1993, pp. 276–292.

10. Coldman AJ, Goldie JH. Impact of dose-intense chemotherapy on the development of permanent drug resistance. *Semin. Oncol.* 1987, **14** (Suppl. 4): 29–33.

11. Goldie JH and Coldman AJ. A mathematic model for relating the drug sensitivity of tumors to their spontaneous mutation rate. *Cancer Treat. Rep.* 1979, **63**: 1727–1733.

12. Appelbaum FR, Herzig GP, Ziegler JL et al. Successful engraftment of cryopreserved autologous bone marrow in patients with malignant lymphoma. *Blood* 1978, **52**: 85–92.

13. Kaizer H, Leventhal B, Wharam ND. Cryopreserved autologous bone marrow transplantation in the treatment of selected paediatric malignancies. A preliminary report. *Transplant. Proc.* 1979, 1: 208–211.

14. Desch CE, Lasala MR, Smith TJ et al. The optimal timing of autologous bone marrow transplantation in Hodgkin's disease patients after a chemotherapy relapse. *J. Clin. Oncol.* 1992, **10**: 200–209.

15. Philip T, Guglielmi C, Hagenbeek A, et al. Autologous bone marrow transplantation as compared with salvage chemotherapy in relapses of chemotherapy-sensitive non-Hodgkin's lymphoma. *N. Engl. J. Med.* 1995, **333**: 1540–1545.

16. Haioun C, Lepage E, Gisselbrecht Ch, et al. Autologous bone marrow transplantation versus sequential chemotherapy for aggressive non-Hodgkin's lymphoma in first complete remission. *Blood* 1995, **86** (Suppl. 1): 457 (Abstract 1816).

17. Verdonck LF, Wim LJ, van Putten MSc, et al. Comparison of CHOP chemotherapy with autologous bone marrow transplantation for slowly responding patients with aggressive non-Hodgkin's lymphoma. *N. Engl. J. Med.* 1995, **332**: 1045–1051.

18. Martelli M, Vignetti M, Zinzani PL, et al. High-dose chemotherapy followed by autologous bone marrow transplantation versus dexamethasone, cisplatin, and cytarabine in aggressive non-Hodgkin's lymphoma with partial response to front-line chemotherapy: A prospective randomized Italian multicenter study. *J. Clin. Oncol.* 1996, **14**: 534–542.

19a. Gisselbrecht C, Lepage E, Morel P, et al. Short and intensified treatment with autologous stem cell transplantation versus ACBV regimen in poor prognosis aggresive lymphoma. Prognostic factors of induction failure. *Ann. Oncol.* 1996, **7** (Suppl. 3): 18 (Abstract 56).

19b. Vitolo U, Cortellazzo S, Liberati AM, et al. Intensified and high dose chemotherapy with granulocyte colony-stimulating factor and autologous stem cell transplantation support as first line therapy in high risk large cell lymphoma. *J. Clin. Oncol.* 1996 (in press).

19c. The International Non-Hodgkin's Lymphoma Prognostic Factors Project. A predictive model for aggressive non-Hodgkin's lymphomas. *N. Engl. J. Med.* 1993, **329**: 987–994.

20. Gianni AM, Siena S, Bregni M, et al. High-dose sequential chemo-radiotherapy with peripheral blood progenitor cell support for relapsed or refractory Hodgkin's disease – A 6-year update. *Ann. Oncol.* 1993, **4**: 889–891.

21. Gianni AM, Bregni M, Siena S, et al. 5-year update of the Milan Cancer Institute randomized trial of high-dose sequential (HDS) vs MACOP-B therapy for diffuse large-cell lymphomas. *Proceedings of the American Society of Clinical Oncology* 1994, Vol.13, 373 (Abstract 263).

22. Reed JC, Kitada S, Takayama S, et al. Regulation of chemoresistance by the *bcl*-2 oncoprotein in non-Hodgkin's lymphoma and lymphocytic leukemia cell lines. *Ann. Oncol.* 1994, **5** (Suppl. 1): S61–S65 .

23. Miyashita T, Reed JC. *Bcl*-2 oncoprotein blocks chemotherapy-induced apoptosis in a human cell line. *Blood* 1993, **81**: 151–157.

24. Mariano MT, Moretti L, Donelli A et al. *Bcl*-2 gene expression in hematopoietic cell differentiation. *Blood* 1992, **80**: 768–775.

25. Keating MJ (guest ed.). Fludarabine phosphate: Current and future therapeutic applications. *Semin. Oncol.* 1993, **20** (Suppl. 7): 1–31.

26. Keating MJ, McLaughlin P, Plunkett W, et al. Fludarabine – present status and future developments in chronic lymphocytic leukemia and lymphoma. *Ann. Oncol.* 1994, **5** (Suppl. 2): S79–S83.

27. Redman JR, Cabanillas F, Velasquez WS, et al. Phase II trial of fludarabine phosphate in lymphoma: An effective new agent in low-grade lymphoma. *J. Clin.*

Oncol. 1992, **10**: 790–794.

28. Kay AC, Saven A, Carrera CJ, et al. 2-Chlorodeoxy-adenosine treatment of low-grade lymphomas. *J. Clin. Oncol.* 1992, **10**: 371–377 .

29. Betticher DC, Fey ME, von Rohr A, et al. High incidence of infections after 2-chlorodeoxy-adenosine (2-CDA) therapy in patients with malignant lymphomas and chronic and acute leukemias. *Ann. Oncol.* 1994, **5**: 57–64.

30. Juliusson G, Elmhorn-Rosenborg A, Liliemark J. Response to 2-chlorodeoxyadenosine in patients with B-cell chronic lymphocytic leukemia resistant to fludarabine. *N. Engl. J. Med.* 1992 327: 1056–1061.

31. O'Brien S, Kantarjian H, Estey E, et al. Lack of effect of 2-chlorodeoxyadenosine therapy in patients with chronic lymphocytic leukemia refractory to fludarabine therapy. *N. Engl. J. Med.* 1994, **330**: 319–322.

32. Tefferi A, Witzig TE, Reid JM, et al. Phase I study of combined 2-chlorodeoxyadenosine and chlorambucil in chronic lymphoid leukemia and low-grade lymphoma. *J. Clin. Oncol.* 1994, **12**: 569–574.

33. McLaughlin P, Hagemaister FB, Swan F, et al. Phase I study of the combination of fludarabine, mitoxantrone, and dexamethasone in low-grade lymphoma. *J. Clin. Oncol.* 1994, **12**: 575–579.

34. Smalley RV, Andersen JW, Hawkins MJ et al. Interferon alfa combined with cytotoxic chemotherapy for patients with non-Hodgkin's lymphoma. *N. Engl. J. Med.* 1992, **327**: 1336–1341.

35. Solal-Celigny P, Lepage E, Brousse N, et al. Recombinant interferon alfa-2b combined with a regimen containing doxorubicin in patients with advanced follicular lymphoma. *N. Engl. J. Med.* 1993, **329**: 1608–1614.

36. Horning SJ. Low-grade lymphoma 1993: State of the art. *Ann. Oncol.* 1994, **5** (Suppl. 2): S23–S27.

37. Pai LH, Pastan I. Immunotoxins and recombinant toxins for cancer treatment. In De Vita VT, Hellman S, Rosenberg SA (eds) *Important Advances in Oncology* Philadelphia: JB Lippincott Company, 1994, pp. 3–19.

38. Vallera DA. Immunotoxins: will their clinical promise be fulfilled? *Blood* 1994, **83**: 309–317.

39. Gottstein C, Winkler U, Bohlen H, et al. Immunotoxins: Is there a clinical value? *Ann. Oncol.* 1994, **5** (Suppl. 1): S97–S103.

40. Singer MF, Jones OW, Niremberg MW. The effect of secondary structure of the template activity of polyribonucleotides. *Proc. Natl Acad. Sci. USA* 1963, **49**: 392–399.

41. Pestka S, Daugherty BL, Jung U et al. Anti-mRNA: Specific inhibition of translation of single mRNA molecules. *Proc. Natl Acad. Sci. USA* 1984, **81**: 7525–7528.

42. McManaway ME, Neckers LM, Loke SL, et al. Tumor-specific inhibition of lymphoma growth by an antisense oligodeoxynucleotide. *Lancet* 1990, **335**: 808–811.

43. Magrath IT. Prospects for the therapeutic use of antisense oligonucleotides in malignant lymphomas. *Ann. Oncol.* 1994, **5** (Suppl. 1): 567–570.

CHAPTER 51

Exploitation of genetic abnormalities in the development of novel treatment strategies for hematological malignancies

KISHOR BHATIA AND IAN T. MAGRATH

Introduction

One of the ultimate benefits of basic research in oncology will be to permit the design of therapy that is targeted specifically at the tumor cell. Our abilities to conceptualize possible 'magic bullets' and to 'custom tailor' treatment strategies have changed vastly in the past 30 years *pari passu* with our ability to define individual disease entitites. Morphologically based classification systems provided few, if any, possibilities for therapeutic targeting. The use of a panoply of monoclonal antibodies permitted both improved definitions of disease and the possibility of targeted therapy, although the latter could not, with

rare exceptions, be truly disease-specific, but rather specific for the subpopulation of cells from which the tumor originated. The identification of an increasing repertoire of tumor-specific genetic lesions, along with the recognition of their direct contribution to the development and progression of the tumor, have not only further refined our ability to define diseases but have also brought into focus the distinct possibility of exploiting these very genetic abberrations, which are, by definition, unique to the neoplastic clone or its immediate precursors, to control neoplasia.

Future treatment strategies will be based on fundamental observations made in the laboratory, initially to refine current therapeutic approaches, but eventually to develop totally new therapeutic strategies directed towards the genetic lesions. Even now, knowledge of molecular aberrations that accumulate as a result of tumor progression and impart to the cell a refractory phenotype, permits screening for the presence of refractory cells in the primary tumor and the design risk-adapted therapies, in some cases choosing drugs on the basis of the molecular abnormalities. It appears, for example, that apoptosis often plays an important role in drug and radiation-induced tumor cell death [1–7]. Consequently, the functional loss of genes that are involved in triggering apoptosis, such as p53 [8], could seriously impair the cytotoxicity of such agents. In this circumstance, agents that circumvent the need of this protein to trigger apoptosis following DNA damage could be preferentially used and strategies might even be developed whereby the apoptic pathway could be restored.

Similarly the knowledge that genes like *bcl*-2 inhibit apoptosis [9,10] provides a possible explanation for the failure of current therapies to cure patients with follicular lymphomas [11], and since 20–30% of diffuse large-cell lymphomas have a 14;18 translocation [12] and thus express *bcl*-2 inappropriately, it is possible that the expression of *bcl*-2 [13] also accounts for the apparently worse prognosis that has been reported in this subgroup of large-cell lymphomas [14]. Clearly, if strategies could be developed that are directed towards abrogating the resistance to apoptosis conferred by *bcl*-2, the reason for failure could be converted to a pathway to success. Indeed, characterization of mechanisms that promote programmed cell death – a basic means of regulating lymphoid cell populations and eliminating damaged cells in a variety of settings – could eventually lead to genetic interventional strategies that shift the balance from cell accumulation to cell loss by utilising existing molecular pathways rather than blocking them.

In general, genetic targeting strategies can be divided into approaches designed to abrogate the positive influence of oncogenes involved in cellular proliferation or to restore the function of inactivated tumor suppressor genes. Of particular relevance to cancer treatment has been the recognition that the latter are intimately associated with apoptotic pathways, which can be activated at several critical points in the proliferation cycle and differentiation pathways. A normal cell is dependent upon successfully passing several such check points before it can proliferate. These controls are critical to the integrity of both the genome and the cell. In lymphoid cells and almost certainly in all cell populations, there are check points to ensure that only cells that have successfully accomplished one step in the differentiation pathway are allowed to mature further. For

example, cells that have failed to recombine their immunoglobulin genes in such a way as to produce a functional antibody molecule are selected against. Quality control is accomplished by utilizing apoptosis to delete unwanted cells. Imbalance in the expression of critical genes will also lead to cell death in a normal cell. For example, forced expression of c-*myc* in circumstances in which the cell cannot proliferate is an imbalance that leads to contradictory signals and hence triggers apoptosis. For a tumor cell, which contains a number of aberrations to survive and proliferate, mechanisms to bypass these check points must be present, i.e. surveillance or executive genes at the check points must be inactivated. Genetic repair of such check points could, thus, result in programmed cell death of the neoplastic compartment.

In this short review we will analyze the pathogenetic mechanisms that lead to the development of lymphomas and leukemias with the objective of highlighting those lesions, which, at the present state of knowledge, appear to constitute appropriate targets for tumor-specific therapy. The goal of targeted therapy is to utilize the genetic lesions that provided the tumor cell with a survival advantage, and which are, therefore, unique to the tumor cell, as an Achilles heel – rendering, in effect, the tumor cell vulnerable to treatment that should have a minimal effect on normal cells.

Pathogenetic mechanisms in hematological malignancies

A common theme in the molecular pathology of neoplasia is that tumor-associated genetic abnormalities provide the the neoplastic cell with the ability to overcome the normal controls of homeostasis. Like all other cancers, tumors of hematopoietic origin result predominantly from one of the three basic pathogenetic mechanisms – the abnormal expression of genes associated with cell proliferation, the silencing of growth inhibitory genes, or the loss of the ability of cells to self-destruct through programmed cell death (apoptosis). Frankly neoplastic cells always accumulate more than one genetic abnormality, since multiple lesions are required to provide the tumor cell with the necessary ability to avoid or pass through the check points present in normal cells, which regulate such intricately balanced events as the cell-proliferation cycle, cell differentiation, cell migration and apoptosis. Cells that are lacking in some essential attribute necessary for them to function correctly are diverted at these check points for repair or self-destruction. Examples of such check points include one in the latter part of the G_1 phase of the cell cycle, at which the integrity of DNA is examined, one in precursor B-cells at which the presence of a functional μ-chain is examined, and one in precursor T-cells at which the presence of correctly expressed major histocompatibility complex (MHC) class I or II molecules is tested.

An understanding of the advantages that hematological malignancies derive from their genetic abnormalities provides information that could be used to develop strategies for combating the tumorigenic potential of the neoplastic cells. Such a treatment strategy differs in principle from present treatment approaches that depend upon the use of cytotoxic agents to kill cells during their passage through the cell cycle. Indeed conventional treatment is dependent for its success on the presence of intact check points that lead to detection of the drug- or radiation-induced damage, and the consequent initiation of the cell death program. Most cytotoxic agents target the mitotic or the DNA synthetic machinery of the cells. None of the agents, however, do this discriminately and, as a consequence, the use of chemotherapeutic drugs is limited by their effect on normal cells – a limitation that can be expressed as a therapeutic index. As is often seen in the clinic, the requirement of presently available antitumor drugs that cells be in cycle (proliferating) means that tumors with a low growth fraction (i.e., a low proportion of cells in cycle) may not be curable. In contrast, therapy directed at the very genetic lesions that permit the neoplastic cell to bypass normal check points will be highly tumor-specific, and in some circumstances could obviate the need for the cell to be cycling. Since the primary genetic lesions differ in different malignancies, one disadvantage of targeted therapy is that it would have to be tailored to a particular molecular subtype of malignancy. It seems probable, however, that secondary genetic lesions could also be targeted for therapy, since abrogation of their potential advantage to the tumor cell could still provide a means to combat neoplasia – or render the tumor cell less resistant to conventional therapy. One advantage of this approach is that some of the secondary lesions occur frequently in diverse cancers, for example, mutations in *ras*, p53 and p16.

To devise genetic intervention strategies, however, it is first imperative to understand the pathogentic mechanisms and relate these to pathological subtypes of hematological malignancies. While present knowledge amounts only to a small beginning, numerous novel therapies have already been contemplated and several have entered clinical trials. There can be little doubt that, as knowledge of the molecular genetic lesions present in neoplastic cells increases, there will be a corresponding increase in the development of novel therapeutic approaches.

GROWTH SIGNALS INDUCED BY AN ABBERANT SIGNAL TRANSDUCTION PATHWAY

When the extracellular environment is conducive to proliferation, the cell orchestrates various sets of events that result in growth. In effect, the cell surface senses the environment through specific receptors and conveys relevant information to the nucleus via pathways specific for a given signal(s). A mutation leading to excessive production of a growth factor may lead to an 'autocrine loop' resulting in continuous cell proliferation. Although described in hyperplastic states, this situation, by itself, is unlikely to cause neoplastic transformation. On the other hand, if the molecular switches within the signal transduction pathways are locked in the 'on' position, the cell will play out all the downstream events and proliferate even in the absence of a signal. One such molecular switch that has been the subject of intense study is the G-protein, Ras. Normal Ras is a membrane-bound guanosine triphosphate (GTP) binding protein, which is activated when bound to GTP, and deactivated when GTP is converted to GDP [15]. Specific mutations in *ras*, for example, at codons 12 or 61, decrease the GTPase activity of the Ras protein and thereby result in a persistent activation of the gene [16]. Following the cloning of the viral *ras* gene, mutated *ras* was isolated from several human cancers. Accumulated evidence has highlighted the frequent involvement of *ras* in human colon and pancreatic cancers [17]. Ras pathways, however (not always directly involving the *ras* gene), also appear to be frequently involved in a variety of myeloid malignancies. Examples include *ras* mutations associated with multiple myeloma, acute myeloid leukemia (AML) and some myelodysplastic syndromes [18], perturbation of the *ras*–GTPase activating protein (GAP) resulting from neurofibromatosis-1 (NF1), mutations in juvenile chronic myeloid leukemia (CML) [19], and the *bcr–abl* translocation, which is a characteristic feature of CML and a minority of acute lymphoblastic leukemias. The chimeric proteins p210 and p190 formed as a result of a 9;22 chromosomal translocation have enhanced tyrosine kinase activity [20,21]. Normally the c-Abl tyrosine kinase is localized in the nucleus, but the fusion with Bcr allows it to migrate to the cytoplasm, where it is believed to interact with proteins which activate *ras* [22].

Several other translocations that result in the

generation of a fusion protein with consequent constitutive activation of signal-transduction mechanisms have been described [23]. One such translocation is t(2;5), observed in Ki-1 lymphomas [24], in which the cytoplasmic and part of the transmembrane domain of a novel receptor, Alk, is fused with sequences from nucleophosmin, a ubiquitously expressed gene inolved in ribosome assembly. A more recently described translocation that also involves a receptor is t(5;12) which has been described in chronic myelomonocytic leukemia [25]. This translocation creates a chimeric protein in which the platelet-derived growth factor (PDGF) receptor is fused to a transcriptional activator, Tel. This fusion may allow a constitutive activation of the PDGF receptor tyrosine kinase leading to activation of the Ras pathway and leukemogenesis.

ONCOGENESIS BY A CONSTITUTIVELY 'ON' CELL CYCLE SWITCH

Just as aberrations in the signaling pathways may transduce an inappropriate 'go' signal, the cell can develop lesions within the cell cycle commitment program, such that it is induced to proliferate even in the absence of upstream signals in the pathway that transduces information from surface receptors. A critical point in the commitment to proliferate occurs in the G_1 phase of the cell cycle [26]. Once commited to proliferate at this check point, cells continue through the cycle even in the absence of growth signals, as long as factors that support their vaibility are present. Following commitment to the cell cycle (i.e., passage from G_0 to G_1), several proteins are expressed early in the G_1 phase. These include c-Myc, c-Myb, c-Fos, c-Jun and proliferating cell nuclear antigen (PCNA) [27]. The critical role these proteins play is highlighted by the observations that when expressed inappropriately, many of them can act to promote cell transformation; deregulation of the proto-oncogene c-*myc*, for example, which occurs in both B-cell and T-cell lymphomas [28–31]. The deregulation of c-*myc* is achieved by a process that appears to occur frequently in hematological malignancies: translocation of a transcriptional activator from its normal chromosomal location to a novel location (characterized by the presence of regulatory sequences) or translocation of regulatory sequences from another locus to the c-*myc* locus [31]. Most often this translocation is associated with antigen-receptor gene loci, either because these loci are accessible in lymphoid cells or because the translocations results from a mistake in the VDJ recombinase involved with the generation of complete antigen receptor molecules [32,33]. In either case, however, the consequence of such a translocation is that the gene is juxtaposed to an immunoglobulin (Ig) or the T-cell receptor (TCR) gene and comes under the regulatory control of this locus. Ig and TCR loci are transcriptionally active in lymphoid cells, and, as a consequence, genes translocated into their vicinity are also rendered transcriptionally active.

For a cell that has suffered a translocation of a master regulatory gene such as c-*myc*, which is necessary for the G_0 to G_1 phase transition [34] and which orchestrates the expression of genes required in G_1, abnormal expression or function can have dire consequences. During normal cell proliferation, the expression of c-*myc* is tightly regulated, both at transcriptional and posttranscriptional levels [35]. Additionally, the transactivation functions of Myc (as opposed to the level of the protein itself) are also regulated by p107, a growth-suppressor protein belonging to the retinoblastoma (Rb) family of proteins, which is able to complex with and repress the activity of Myc [36].

Thus, when the cell loses its ability to regulate c-*myc*, the untimely expression of the Myc protein can initiate downstream events which result in proliferation of the cell in the absence of signals that would normally be necessary to induce the cell to cycle [37]. Interestingly, 'fine tuning' of the deregulation of c-*myc* is observed in Burkitt's lymphomas, whereby the expressed c-*myc* gene accumulates mutations [36,38–41], resulting in a protein that can now escape the control exerted by p107 over its transactivation functions. One implication of this is that the deregulated expression of c-*myc*, although necessary, may not be sufficient for lymphomagenesis [42]. Additional regulators of function may need to be disabled. It is also likely that the abrogation of additional cell cycle check points, whereby aberrant gene expression diverts the cell to the apoptosis pathway is necessary for full neoplastic transformation.

PROLIFERATION INDUCED BY ABSENCE OF A 'NEGATIVE' CONTROL

Normal cells have at least two check points in the cell cycle: one in the G_1 phase prior to S phase, and the other in the G_2 phase prior to mitosis. Both these check points serve as surveillance points to detect DNA damage in replicating somatic cells and to control untimely proliferation. These check points are coupled to cell cycle arrest genes such that cells which are in some way defective exit the cell cycle. Transformation probably requires loss of the influence of either the 'check points' or the cell cycle exit genes, either by inactivating them by mutations, by subjugating their function by complexing them with other proteins (a central strategy of some transforming DNA viruses, for example, SV40, adenoviruses and papillomaviruses), or by deleting them [43]. Mutations in, or loss of, check point genes including Rb [44], p53 [45] and p16 [46,47] are among the most frequent lesions seen in human tumors. Among these, deletion or mutation is particularly frequently observed in p53, since abrogation of p53 allows the tumor cell to bypass normal controls in cell cycle progression even if it has suffered DNA damage – thus permitting the accumulation of additional genetic lesions (i.e., 'increasing genetic instability') thereby increasing the likelihood that at least some cells will progress to a more aggressive phenotype [48].

Besides the ability to induce G_1 arrest, p53 is independently involved in triggering the apoptic pathway [8,49,50]. The involvement of p53 in inducing normal cells to undergo apoptosis under unfavorable circumstances therefore provides an incentive for the tumor cell to delete the expression of the wild-type p53 protein such that it can now survive in circumstances and environments normally not conducive to its growth.

Among the several proteins that act in concert in allowing normal progression through the cell cycle, the cyclins play a critical role. Cyclins are expressed transiently during specific phases in the cell cycle and are then degraded [51–55]. Key cyclins mediating G_1 transition (i.e., passage through G_1 to S) are cyclins D1, D2, D3 and E. Deregulation of cyclin D1 is involved in lymphomagenesis [56, 57] (i.e., in the 11;14 translocation of mantle cell lymphomas). Cyclin E, along with cyclin A, is also critical for S-phase transition. Cyclins associate with cyclin-dependent kinases (cdks) to form holoenzymes that relieve cell cycle check point blocks [58]. Cyclin D associates with cdk4 and cdk6, while cyclin E associates with cdk2 later in the G_1 phase. Once the cell has completed DNA synthesis and entered G_2, cyclins A and B are both required for progression to mitosis [58]. The molecular progression of the cycle is thus regulated by the sequential activation of the cdks by these different cyclins. Some of the substrates of the cyclin/cdk complexes are known to be involved in tumorigenesis, because they have been observed to be mutated or deleted in some tumours. A good example of this is Rb, and it is likely that related 'pocket' proteins (p107 and p130) may also be mutated in some types of neoplastic transformation. Both Rb and p107 in their hypophosphorylated state complex with and inhibit the action of at least one or more of the members of the family of transcription factors known as the E2F-like proteins [59–62]. Following activation of cyclin D/cdk complexes, Rb is phosphorylated [63–65], leading to the

relase of E2F. E2F is thus made available to transactivate genes like c-*myc*, *myb*, thymidylate kinase and thymidine synthetase, which are probably essential for the G_1–S transition. Proteins that can inhibit the activation of the cyclin/cdk complexes serve to induce cell cycle arrest [66]. p21 (also known as waf1, cip1 and Sdi1), for example, which is a universal cdk inhibitor [67], can negatively regulate D/cdk activity [68–70]. p21 expression in turn is regulated by p53. When cells sustain DNA damage, p53 can recognize the damage and prevent the cells from progressing beyond the G_1 check point. For this reason it has been referred to as the the 'guardian of the genome'.

The ability of p53 to cause G_1 arrest is mediated via its transactivating functions [71]. Following DNA damage, p53 induces the expression of p21, p21 in turn inhibits the activity of the cyclin D/cdk complex. Rb, and presumably other family members (e.g., p107), are prevented from being hyperphosphorylated by the cyclin/cdk complex and remain complexed to E2F, preventing the induction of genes necessary for the G_1–S transition and forcing the cell to remain in G_1. The G_1 arrest mediated by p53 serves to allow the cell to repair its DNA prior to entering S phase and thus to prevent the persistence of genetic defects. When the cell cannot repair all the damage prior to S-phase synthesis or in the presence of conflicting signals to proliferate in spite of the damage, p53 induces the cell to enter apoptosis. Thus the elimination of a functional p53 protein will allow abnormal cells to proliferate. The G_1 check point proteins are, clearly, crucial to tumorigenesis and progression, and also to the response to DNA damaging agents used therapeutically (many drugs and radiation). It is readily apparent why p53 functions are so commonly abrogated in neoplasms and it is likely that other mechanisms exist that tend to abrogation of this check point in tumors in which p53 is intact.

CELLULAR ACCUMULATION RESULTING FROM LOSS OR NEUTRALIZATION OF APOPTOTIC POTENTIAL

Aggressive uncontrolled proliferation of cells is one aspect of tumorigenesis, while accumulation, resulting from a loss of susceptibility to dying is another pathway to neoplasia. Normal architecture is maintained within organs from early in embryogenesis because all normal cells are subject to homeostasis [72]. An important mechanism that contributes to this regulation is an inherent ability to selectively deplete cells. This ability is derived from the capacity of cells to activate pathways that result in 'suicide'. The process of self-induced cell death is referred to as apoptosis. Morphologically, apoptosis is characterized by cell shrinkage rather than the cell swelling and osmotic rupture that is a feature of necrotic cell death. Apoptosis involves plasma-membrane blebbing, vacuolarization of the cyto-plasm and nuclear fragmentation. The genomic DNA is cleaved into small nucleosomal fragments, which give rise to the characteristic 'ladder' seen when DNA from apoptic cells is run in a gel. Apoptosis may have been critical to the evolution from unicellular to multicellular organisms and this molecular suicide program appears to be highly conserved from *C. elegans* to humans [72]. Recently, it has become apparent that the pathological loss of this program in multicellular organisms can lead to neoplasia. The first tumor in which abrogation of apoptotic pathways was shown to be relevant to pathogenesis was follicular lymphoma [73,74]. In this disease, the *bcl*-2 gene was shown to juxtaposed to an Ig locus (a commonly used mechanism of deregulation in B-cell neoplasms), resulting in the deregulated expression of Bcl-2. Later, evidence was provided that demonstrated the protective effect of Bcl-2 against apoptotic cell death resulting from certain negative stimuli, for example, starvation or DNA damage [9,10,75,76]. It now appears that resistance to death at certain stages of normal lymphoid cell differentiation relates to overexpres-sion of *bcl*-2. Recently, several other proteins with homology to Bcl-2 have been described [77,78]. Proteins in the Bcl-2 family contain at least two conserved domains, the major regions being called BH-1 and BH-2. Several members of the Bcl-2 family interact with each other in orchestrating the cell death program. The protective action of Bcl-2 in countering apoptosis, for example, is dependent upon its ability to associate with Bax. Bax can, however, also titrate out the protective function conferred by *bcl*-2, such that when overproduced (resulting in Bax:Bax dimers) it induces apoptosis [77]. It is probably the ratio of Bax and Bcl-2 that determines whether the apoptotic program is turned on or off [77]. Other members of the extended Bcl-2 family also provide both negative and positive regulation of the death cycle; thus Bcl-*x* is expressed as two separate proteins, Bcl-*x* long, which acts like Bcl-2, and Bcl-*x* short, which acts like Bax [79,80]. The loop between proliferation cycle and death cycle is further connected by common check points; p53, which exerts its effects through the G_1 check point, is a transcriptional upregulator of Bax, and can thus influence the Bcl-2/Bax ratio [81]. Another protein, Bad, can displace Bcl-2 from Bax:Bcl-2 dimers and tip the balance towards apoptosis.

In a strategy reminiscent of abrogation of the G_1

arrest functions of proteins in the cell cycle in tumorigenesis, DNA viruses also appear to target the death regulation pathway of the cell to achieve successful transformation. Thus the adenoviral protein, E1B, along with E1A, is critical to transformation. E1A, which complexes with Rb, results in uncon-trolled cellular proliferation, but the need for E1B can be substituted by Bcl-2 [82], suggesting that E1B, which complexes with p53, counteracts apop-tosis resulting from aberrant proliferation. At least one DNA virus, long associated with lymphoid neoplasia, carries an antiapoptic gene within its coding sequences. The BHRF1 gene of Epstein–Barr virus (EBV) is homologous to *bcl*-2 and can block apoptosis [83,84], although whether BHRF1 con-tributes to lymphomagenesis is, as yet, not known. At least in transformation *in vitro*, EBV may utilize the cell death neutralizing theme to contribute to immortalization of B-cells. The latent membrane protein, which is one of the few proteins expressed by EBV in latent infection, is also capable of promoting the expression of *bcl*-2 [85], although the importance of this in either the viral life cyle or oncogenesis remains unknown.

Since conventional chemotherapy is largely based upon genotoxic insults, it is also dependent upon the ability of the cell to undergo apoptosis following such insults. In those neoplasms where the transforma-tion process has abrogated the apoptotic machinery in order to ensure survival, the use of genotoxic therapy can be a losing battle unless strategies to counter the loss of resistance to apoptosis can be developed.

Therapeutic agents with a potential for genetic intervention: agents of tumor-specific destruction

The ability of the clinician to deliver tumor-specific treatment is largely dependent upon the identifica-tion of a tumor-specific target and the development of pharmacological agents that can be directed against the target. An ideal pharmacological agent must reach the relevant intracellular and very often intranuclear sites, where the targets are located, and be sustained in sufficient amounts for as long as is necessary. To meet these goals one needs to consider not only chemical substances traditionally consid-ered as drugs, but also other agents, such as nucleic acid derivatives, viruses and perhaps even geneti-cally modified cells. These may function either as the therapeutic agent itself or as a vehicle for delivery of the agent to tumor cells.

DRUGS AND PEPTIDES

A critical element in the maintenance of the neoplastic phenotype is the effective maintenance of protein interactions that drive the aberrant proliferative cycle. In some cases this interaction is between a mutated product and its substrate, for example, Ras, while in other cases the interaction is between aberrantly expressed transcriptional activators and their consensus DNA recognition sequences, for example, Myc. Since several of the known proto-oncogenes and tumor supressor genes are transcriptional activators, drugs that are capable of manipulating the interaction of these factors with their cognate DNA sequences or with other proteins could be attractive candidates for interventional therapy. The strategy of modulating transcription-based protein interactions has been successfully exploited in developing pharmacological agents, for example, compactin, which, as an inhibitor of cholesterol biosynthesis, upregulates the transcription of the low-density lipoprotein (LDL) receptor gene leading to enhanced clearance of cholesterol. The protein:protein interactions between oncogenic DNA viruses and their cellular partners also provide potential pharmacological targets, for example, the papilloma virus E6 and E7 interactions with p53 and Rb, respectively.

The development of inhibitors of protein interactions is dependent upon the careful mapping of the contact domains of the proteins. It is possible, using this information, to design peptide or drug mimics that compete with natural substrates for binding sites on the target protein. Thus, Ras peptides, derived from Ras effector region, successfully bind to GAP and block the biological function of Ras [86]. Similarly, the interaction between Rb and E7 can be reduced by using a peptide [87], and transcriptional activation of c-myc can be impaired by manipulating Myc–Max dimerization [88]. Aside from the interactions between viral proteins and host proteins, which are tumor-specific, in each of these other situations, some means of avoiding similar effects on normal cells must be found if the therapy is not to be as toxic as conventional chemotherapy.

Strategies that are dependent upon inhibitors of enzyme function may also be well suited for interventional treatment in neoplasia. Two important examples are the inhibition of *ras* farnesylation [89] and the inhibition of tyrosine kinases [90–92]. Although few advances have been made in translating peptide inhibitors of protein:protein interaction

into potent pharmacological agents, the development of inhibitors of Ras-dependant neoplasia are promising; agents capable of blocking the action of the enzyme farnesyl protein transferase have been developed [93]. The posttranslational modification of Ras brought about by this enzyme is critical for its biological function [94]. The farnesyl protein transferase itself binds farnesyl diphosphate and a protein acceptor. Four C-terminal amino acids (known as the CAAX box) of the protein acceptor are critical determinants of the catalytic activity and specificity of the complex. Using rational drug design, peptidomimic agents were developed that interfered with the interaction of the CAAX box with the enzyme farnesyl transferase. These agents have demonstrated selective antiproliferative activity in *ras*-transformed cells [89], although the basis for selectivity is unknown.

Development of ATP-competitive compounds is another avenue that appears to hold some promise. Drugs that will effectively inhibit specific tyrosine kinases may have selectivity in neoplasia based upon the importance of these tyrosine kinases in signalling pathways. These proteins, examples of which include epidermal growth factor (EGF) receptor, PDGF receptor, Alk, Abl, etc., play a role in several cancers. Selective inhibitors could, thus, allow for rational interventional approaches. One such compound is 4,5-dianilinophthalimide (DAPHI), which appears to possess selective inhibitory activity against the EGF receptor kinase [95].

Because of the nature of the targets involved in oncology, one may need to go beyond the traditional medicinal chemistry approaches in the design of interventional strategies. Screening for specific functional acitivities, or the design of molecules likely to possess such activity will be required. The use of peptide inhibitors greatly simplifies this process, but methods of favorably altering the pharmacokinetic properties of peptides will need to be found. Promising steps along this pathway have already been taken.

NUCLEIC ACID DERIVATIVES

In several genetic interventions, nucleic acids in one form or another have been used to modulate the expression of genes. When it is necessary to replace a gene function, because of loss of a gene or because of mutational inactivation of genes, strategies to transduce gene constructs using retroviral agents have been developed. Retroviral agents have also been used to deliver oligonucleotides. In such cases, because the delivery system will normally have no tumor specificity, it is necessary that the therapeutic agent has an intrinsic targeting capability. Table 51.1

Table 51.1   Targets and agents in genetic intervention of neoplasia

Tumor-specific target	Example	Agent	Mode
Abnormal DNA	Sequences across a translocation junction	Oligonucleotide	Triplex DNA
Abnormal mRNA	Leader intron sequences in t(8;14) Burkitt's lymphoma	Oligonucleotide	Antisense RNA
		Ribozyme	
Novel proteins	Oncofetal antigens Fusion proteins Mutated cellular proteins	Antibodies Peptides	Binding and inhibition of interactions Targeting
Tumor cells		cDNA	Replacement of suppressive control
			Introduction of self-destructive potential
		Lymphocytes	Immune-mediated destruction
		Heterologous cells	Tumor regression

and Figure 51.1 summarize a number of potential targets and corresponding potential agents.

Antisense molecules

Antisense molecules are probably one of the most widely explored agents used to inhibit gene expression. Several antisense constructs are at present in clinical trials. It is, however, too early to determine whether antisense molecules will prove to be effective agents, in practice, for modulating gene expression. In principle, antisense molecules can be either single-stranded DNA or RNA oligonucleotides, Most often, synthetic DNA oligomers of lengths ranging from 15 to 25 bases are used. The current interest in antisense molecules as potential antitumor agents derives mainly from their intrinsic specificity [96–100], which is based upon their length (the shorter the nucleotide sequence, the more likely it is to occur multiple times within the cell genome). Oligomers with an approximate length of 15 bases are highly specific, since 15 base sequences, unless they are repeat sequences or highly conserved within a gene family, are unlikely to occur more than once in the genome. Thus, such antisense molecules have an extremely high probability of hybridizing to a single RNA species containing the complementary sequence, and selectively affecting the expression of a single gene.

There are several mechanisms that lead to oligonucleotide inhibition of gene expression. The creation of a double-stranded RNA molecule as a result of the formation of an RNA-antisense hybrid could lead to the cleavage of the hybrid species by RNAse H. Enhanced degradation of the mRNA

species through other degradation pathways may also cause a shortening of the half-life of the transcript. In addition, it has been suggested that oligomers may interfere with the translational machinery, either by inhibiting the binding of translation complexes to the mRNA, or by interfering with the passage of ribosomes [101]. Consistent with both these possibilities, oligomer sequences directed against the translation initiation regions appear to be more effective at inhibiting gene expression than oligomers directed to other regions. Additionally, sequences in the 3'-untranslated regions of the message, presumably because of their role in maintaining the stability of the RNA, are also susceptible targets for antisense-based RNA degradation. Finally, since several oncogenes are transcriptional activators, which bind to specific consensus DNA sequences, it may be possible to deliver appropriate oligomers in sufficient quantity to the neoplastic cell for them to inhibit the binding of the oncogenic transcription factor to its targets in the genome.

Although antisense oligomers are specific, the use of these agents is associated with intrinsic problems. Oligonucleotides themselves are subject to intracellular degradation and require the accumulation of significant intracellular concentrations in order to achieve effective inhibition of gene expression. Modified oligonucleotides, which are resistant to degradation by intracellular nucleases, have been introduced to overcome this problem. However, the sustained delivery of antisense molecules poses numerous practical problems, including a financial one, and it is likely that such approaches would be more likely to be feasible if temporary inhibition of the production of a cellular protein, or of the function

USE OF OLIGONUCLEOTIDES IN GENE THERAPY

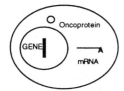

LYMPHOMA CELL THAT CONTAINS A TUMOR-SPECIFIC TRANSLOCATION RESULTING IN
A TUMOR-SPECIFIC TRANSCRIPT

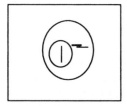

ANTISENSE APPROACH

COMPLEMENTARY OLIGONUCLEOTIDE
BINDS TO THE mRNA AND PREVENTS
THE SYNTHESIS OF THE ONCOPROTEIN

RIBOZYME APPROACH

COMPLEMENTARY OLIGONUCLEOTIDE
BINDS TO AND CATALYZES THE CLEAVAGE
OF THE TRANSCRIPT

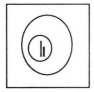

ANTIGENE APPROACH

COMPLEMENTARY OLIGONUCLEOTIDE FORMS A TRIPLEX DNA
MOLECULE AND PREVENTS EXPRESSION OF THE ONCOGENE

Figure 51.1   The figure depicts three levels of tumor-specific targets in non-Hodgkin's lymphomas, available for interventional therapy by use of oligonucleotides. Both the antisense and the ribozyme approach utilize oligonucleotides targeted at sequences in the transcript originating from a rearranged gene, such that these sequences are unique to the tumor cell. The antigene approach targets the rearrangements by the use of triplex DNA molecules at the genomic level.

of a transcription factor were to lead to an irreversible consequence, such as apoptosis.

Ribozymes

Another genetic intervention based on oligonucleotides that has significant potential for realizing gene-specific inhibition of expression is the use of ribozymes [102]. Ribozymes are short stretches of RNA oligomers that contain a catalytic domain flanked by a stretch of sequences that confer gene specificity. These molecules can bind to and cleave a complementary RNA molecule (the transcript of the targeted gene).

The construction of catalytic domains in ribozymes is based upon RNA chemistry derived either from self-splicing RNA molecules originally identified in several microorganisms, or from RNA molecules in viroids that contain the 'hammerhead' motif [103–107]. The recent identification of sim-

ilarities within the conserved domains of snRNAs involved in the splicing of precursor mRNA with the 'hammerhead' ribozyme motif has led to the utilization of these modified RNA complexes as ribozymes [108].

One potential drawback to the use of ribozymes as potential therapeutic agents is the need for a high ratio of ribozyme to substrate RNA. The ability of ribozymes to cleave mRNA molecules *in vitro* is largely dependant upon the free interactions between the ribozyme and the substrate RNA. Various strategies have been developed to increase the *in vivo* efficacy of the cleavage reaction, including the use of promoters derived from transfer RNA genes which utilize polymerase III (109), to ensure a high copy number of ribozymes. Recently ribozymes have been constructed which include 'homing' signals (retroviral packaging signals) that allow the ribozyme to be delivered to the same cellular compartment as its target molecule. Whether ribozymes (which, of course, also function as standard antisense oligomers) have any advantages with respect to the inhibition of protein synthesis remains to be seen.

Triplex molecules

The formation of hybrid molecules between antisense oligonucleotides and the mRNA transcripts of genes targeted for inhibition of expression can be extended to include the gene itself, since oligonucleotides also recognize specific sequences in the double-stranded DNA molecule. In this case, rather than forming a double helical complementary structure, as is the case with antisense oligomers, a triple helical structure occurs via Hoogsten or reversed Hoogsten hydrogen bonding between bases in the oligomer and base pairs in the duplex DNA molecule [110, 111]. The oligomer now lies in the major groove of the double helical structure, resulting in a triplex DNA molecule. The formation of a triplex molecule can occur at physiological pH and ionic strength and is very stable.

Strategies designed to inhibit gene expression by exploiting the properties of oligomers in the formation of triplex molecules take advantage of the interactions between the transcriptional machinery and regulatory regions of genes. Inhibition of transcription occurs, for example, when oligonucleotides are targeted at the transcriptional regulatory regions in transcription systems *in vitro*. An additional means whereby triplex molecules could induce downregulation of gene expression is through their ability to catalyze DNA strand breakage. Specially designed oligonucleotides complexed with various 'endonucleases' have been shown to result in the scission of DNA. Oligonucleotides capable of forming regions of triplex DNA thus have the potential of offering a permanent deletion of the oncogenic potential if localized to one or a few recognized genes. Perhaps in the future, such 'genomic surgery' will become possible [112]. Although the use of triplex molecules in genetic intervention therapy is still in its infancy, a number of advances that are likely to assist in the development of this form of targeted therapy have been made. For example, the use of circular oligonucleotides with both parallel and antiparallel complementarity to the target gene appears to increase specificity significantly compared to standard oligomers.

GENETICALLY ENGINEERED VIRUSES: DELIVERY SYSTEMS FOR INTERVENTIONAL THERAPY

Like any other pharmacological agent, the ability of the various forms of oligonucleotides discussed above to inhibit tumor growth is, of course, dependent upon these agents reaching the tumor in biologically effective concentrations. At least for *in vitro* systems, the delivery of oligonucleotides to the cell can be accomplished by either passive transfection or by active processes such as electroporation, ballistic barrage, receptor-mediated transfer, liposomal transfer or viral transduction [113,114]. In a limited number of animal experiments, systemic administration of naked DNA plasmids has also resulted in effective transfer to some tissues. It seems quite probable, however, that the insertion of novel genetic material, whether oligonucleotides or gene constructs, into cancer cells would need to be achieved through encapsulation in a vector. In circumstances where the oligonucleotides themselves do not posses intrinsic tumor specificity, this could be confered on the agent by building a targeting mechanism into the vector (see below).

Besides conventional delivery systems such as liposomes, oligonucleotides can be delivered by using viruses as vectors. Viruses, particularly the more widely used retroviruses, have a number of advantages as vehicles for agents of interventional genetic therapy [115–118]. They should be capable of serving as highly efficient delivery vehicles – the horizontal transmission of genetic information is inherent to all virus infections. Host range specificity, imparted by the viral envelope proteins, and potentially modifiable, restricts the entry of the virus to specific cell types. The viral genome can be readily modified, by genetic engineering, to express the requisite genes or oligomer sequences in the host cell. The genetic information transferred by viruses is also capable of stable integration and thus self-propagation in the host cell. Finally, the viral genome can be further modified to restrict expression of the antisense molecules, ribozymes or complete genes only to specific cell types, e.g., lymphoid cells, subsets of lymphoid cells, by making use of lymphoid-specific regulatory elements. Transduction with such viruses will thus allow an added measure of protection to normal cells.

Two major groups of viral vectors have been used in gene therapy. These include retroviral vectors and adenoviral vectors. Retroviruses are favorite vehicles for gene therapy, because their small genome renders them more easily modified than large DNA viruses. Initially adapted from the Moloney murine leukemia virus, they have been extensively used in laboratories to transduce cells and their basic biology is well characterized. The retroviral vectors can be packaged using amphotrophic particles, such that they can infect a wide variety of human cells. The viral vector consists essentially of the long terminal repeats (LTRs), which contain the viral regulatory elements and govern its insertion into the cell genome, and a packaging signal to enable the genetic material to be packaged in the viral envelope, using a packaging cell line [119]. The nucleic acid sequence of interest is engineered into the vector (with a size limitation for a foreign insert of 8 kb) and transfected into a packaging cell line. The endogenous retrovirus in the packaging cell line is devoid of the packaging signal but is equipped with the *gag*, *pol* and *env* genes. Thus, the retroviral vector, which contains packaging signals, is preferentially incorporated into virions, although the latter will be defective (i.e., cannot replicate) because they do not contain the required *gag*, *pol* and *env* genes. The virion, carrying the vector along with the sequence of interest, buds from the cell and can be now used to infect tumor cells *in vitro* or *in vivo*. Virion preparations are readily tested to ensure that the particles produced are indeed free of replication-competent viruses.

There are several disadvantages to the use of retroviruses, including the low viral titers following infection, and their requirement for the cell to be proliferating for the sequence of interest to be integrated into the cellular genome and maintained. The latter, of course, is not necessarily a limitation in the context of neoplasia, and may also confer an added element of selectively to the system. Another concern is the probability that the random integration of viral genomes into the cell genome may disrupt a tumor supressor locus or may cause activation (via the viral enhancer elements in the LTR). An additional, major disadvantage to retroviral vector systems in general, stems from the low efficiency of transfer of the genetic material into target cells *in vivo*. It is unlikely, using present systems, that one could transduce each and every tumor cell with the viral vectors. This disadvantage can be offset, to some extent, by using intervention systems in which there is a 'bystander effect'. In such systems a gene product, or drug activated by a gene product, is able to penetrate and kill adjacent cells. The potential value of the bystander effect has been demonstrated in an animal model. Direct injection of a retrovirus containing thymidine kinase, able to activate ganciclovir, although only able to infect 10% of the tumor cells, caused total regression of brain tumors in a rat model [120].

In contrast to retroviral vectors, adenoviral vectors [121], being derived from DNA viruses, can insert their sequences into nonreplicating cells (as well as replicating cells) and, although the vector does not integrate into the host cell genome in these circumstances, it is maintained as an episome in the nucleus. As a consequence of this, however, the duration of expression of the foreign sequences is limited, unless exposed to a selective pressure. For interventional therapy in cancer, this may not be a major drawback, since, if effective, the expression system should lead to the death of the neoplastic cell. The ability to infect nonproliferating cells may be valuable in neoplasms with a low growth fraction. Among other groups of viruses, the herpesviruses have also been considered as vehicles for delivery of gene therapy [122], although the large size of their genome makes them more difficult to engineer. Recently, modified versions of the EBV genome, which include only the genes required for cell transformation, have been constructed. Such constructs could be used to generate more flexible vector systems for gene therapy [123].

THERAPEUTIC STRATEGIES BASED UPON INHIBITION OF THE ONCOGENIC POTENTIAL

A familiar theme in the development of lymphomas has been the recurrent involvement of the Ig or the TCR loci in nonrandom translocations. The mechanism of translocation is not yet clear but quite frequently the consequence is deregulation of proto-oncogenes involved in either cell proliferation or cell death. Normally, the products of proto-oncogenes play an important role in the homeostatic control of growth, such that interventional strategies designed to interfere with the inappropriate expression of growth-promoting genes must be designed to have an effect *only* in the neoplastic cell if toxicity to normal dividing cells is to be avoided. An item that would top the 'wish list' for future techonology would thus be the ability to undo or circumvent the effects of the translocation. Translocations themselves, in some instances, provide a feasible target for a tumor-specific attack. An excellent example of this strategy has already been successful in the laboratory [124]. In this case advantage is taken of the position of the breakpoints in the c-*myc* gene on chromosome 8. In Burkitt's lymphomas from North America, as many as 40% of the tumors appear to carry breakpoints in the c-*myc* gene, which result in the translocation of only a part of the first intron, and the second and third exons of the c-*myc* gene, to the Ig locus. This remaining part of the translocated first intron is incapable of being spliced out of the mature message, as would normally be the case, because the splice donor and acceptor sites have been separated [125]. Thus, when c-*myc* is transcribed from this rearranged allele, the mature transcript carries with it an additional 'prefix' of nonspliced RNA from the first intron. These extra 5' RNA sequences are, of course, present only in the tumor cell. Antisense molecules directed to the intronic sequences have been shown to inhibit Myc expression in cells containing an appropriate 8;34 translocation, but not in other cells [124].

Translocations in lymphoid malignancies that that do not involve the Ig genes appear to follow an entirely separate pathogenetic mechanism. Rather than merely cause the abnormal expression of a normal protein, the chromosomal translocation in these cases results in the expression of a novel gene not found in nonmalignant cells (Figure 51.2). Translocation breakpoints are often in the introns of the two partner genes and result in the expression of a chimeric protein (Figure 51.2), which has novel properties not associated with the parent molecules. A classical example of such translocations includes the t(9;22), which results in the formation of a Bcr–Abl fusion protein [126], which has enhanced tyrosine kinase activity [20] compared to the normal Abl protein and a potential ability to inhibit apoptosis following DNA damage. Another example of this class of translocations in lymphoid malignancies is seen in a subset of pediatric ALL in which a t(1;19) results in a fusion gene product between two trans-

cription factors: the E2A gene, which is a member of the helix–loop–helix class of transcription factors, is fused to a homeobox gene, *pbx-1* [127,128]. The fusion protein in all cases examined carries the DNA binding domain of the *pbx-1* gene, but the transactivation domain of E2A. It is quite likely that the chimeric protein has acquired the ability to transactivate *pbx* target genes, although it appears that the transactivational function of E2A–Pbx is not identical to that of Pbx.

Similar fusion proteins have also been described in myeloid leukemias, notably the PML–RARα produced by a 15;17 chromosomal translocation in acute promyelocytic leukemia (APL) [129,130]. The fusion protein includes most of the normal PML protein as well as the DNA and hormone binding domains of the retinoic acid receptor, RARα. Unlike E2A–Pbx, however, the PML–RAR fusion protein appears to have a negative effect. Normally PML functions as a growth suppressor [131]. The chimeric protein, PML–RARα, however, binds to PML and appears to inhibit its suppressive properties. The PML–RARα fusion is also an excellent example of a disease in which specific correlates exist between the molecular defect and the biology and clinical behavior of the tumor. Response of APL to retinoic acid treatment is observed only in leukemias with a 15;17 translocation, i.e., in which the PML–RARα protein is expressed [132].

**TARGETS FOR GENE THERAPY IN
LYMPHOMAS ASSOCIATED WITH GENE FUSION**

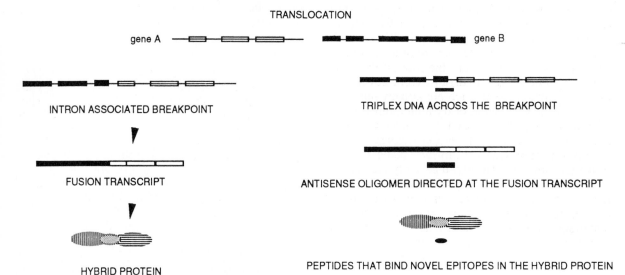

Figure 51.2 In lymphomas where chromosomal rearrangements result in a fusion of two genes, the rearranged chromosome and the transcript originating from such a rearrangement provide a unique target for gene therapy. Similarly, domains that overlap at the fusion between the two native proteins also provide a tumor-specific target that can be blocked using peptides that bind to these epitopes.

A more recent example of the involvement of a chimeric gene in lymphomas is the fusion product resulting from a t(2:5) in anaplastic large-cell lymphomas. This rearrangement, observed in approximately one-third of large-cell lymphomas, results in the fusion of a nucleolar phosphoprotein gene on chromosome 5q35 to a previously unidentified protein tyrosine kinase gene, *alk*, on chromosome 2p23 [24]. Again, it appears that the breakpoint locations on both the chromosomes may regularly involve the same introns, since identical junctions of the genes have been observed in the transcripts detected in the tumors of several patients. Similar to the *bcr–abl* fusion product, it is conceivable that this translocation also results in a constitutively activated catalytic domain of the truncated alk tyrosine kinase protein.

Since these novel chimeric proteins are found only in tumor cells and are an essential element of pathogenesis, they provide excellent tumor-specific targets. Clearly, if the expression of the fusion protein could be inhibited without disrupting the expression of either of the normal partners in nonmalignant cells, cytotoxicity would be confined to tumor cells. There are several possible means of achieving this. One approach would be to design antisense oligonucleotides or ribozymes that span the junction sequences in the mature transcript of the fusion gene (Figure 51.2); such molecules should be capable of inhibiting the expression of the chimeric protein, but because the sequences in the antisense molecule complementary to either of the parent sequences are not long enough to result in hybridization to either of the parent transcripts, there should be no effect on the normal protein levels. Using antisense molecules directed against the junction sequences it has been possible to inhibit production of the Bcr–Abl protein in myeloid leukemias. Clinical trials involving *ex vivo* therapy with antisense oligonucleotide to purge bone marrow for use in autologous transplantation are already underway [133–139]. The potential of designing oligonucleotides that will form triplex DNA molecules at the breakpoint junctions, but which are incapable of triplex formation with the reciprocal parent chromosomes raises the exciting possibility of triplex-mediated genetic intervention to deactivate the translocated chromosome. Finally, it may prove possible to synthesize drugs – perhaps based on peptides – that specifically bind to the fusion protein and inhibit its activity.

SUPPLEMENTATION OF A TUMOR SUPPRESSOR POTENTIAL

Early studies in the biology of cancer suggested that the nontumorigenic phenotype is dominant [140,141] and thus provided preliminary evidence for the existence of tumor supressor genes. Since then there has been an increased recognition of the role of tumor supressor genes in the pathogenesis of neoplasia. Tumor supressor proteins by their nature act in constraining cell growth. Thus in the process of transformation, it is their absence that is relevant to the oncogenic potential. To achieve a complete loss of growth constraint it is essential to inactivate both the alleles of a tumor suppressor gene. This usually occurs by loss of genetic information on one allele and inactivation, by mutation, of the other allele. Deprivation of the gene products of these recessive genes now make the cell unresponsive to signals that would normally cause growth arrest or activate apoptosis [142].

As opposed to gene activation, inactivation can be more readily achieved by random events, since damage to many regions of a gene can lead to loss of function. This has the corollary that a wider range of mutations may exist in tumor suppressor genes than in oncogenes, where only a limited range of lesions can lead to activation. Moreover, since the circumvention of check points is a critical element of neoplastic growth, mutations or loss of growth suppressor genes is likely to be frequently encountered. This is supported by the recent findings that the tumor suppressor gene, p53, at present appears to be the most widely mutated gene in human cancer. In the last few years the search for other tumor supressor genes has met with considerable success. The list now includes Rb, p53, APC, DCC WT1, p21, p16, p15 and NF1. The association of tumor suppressor genes appears to be more often observed with solid tumors than with leukemias and lymphomas, but this could simply reflect the state of current knowledge. Even the most frequently mutated supressor gene, p53, is rarely involved in leukemias, and among lymphomas appears to be largely restricted to the small noncleaved cell lymphomas [143]. A number of loci that demonstrate loss of heterozygosity have, however, been recognized in hematopoietic tumors, including deletions of 5q in myeloid leukemias, 12q and 6q in B- and T-cell acute lymphoblastic leukemias (B- and T-ALL), and deletions of chromosomes 2 and 6 in lymphomas (Table 51.2), indicating that supressor genes pathogenetically relevant to lymphomagenesis have yet to be identified.

Because of the influence of the functional loss of tumor supressor genes, one potential approach to

Table 51.2 Chromosomal deletions in lymphoproliferative disorders

Chromosomal loci	Lymphoproliferative disorder
2q	DLCL
3p	Plasmacytoma
5q	ANLL
6p	NHL
6q	NHL, B-ALL, T-ALL
13q	Follicular lymphoma

DLCL, Diffuse large-cell lymphoma; ANLL, anaplastic large-cell lymphoma; NHL, non-Hodgkin's lymphoma; B-ALL, B-cell acute lymphoblastic leukemia; T-ALL, T-cell acute lymphoblastic leukemia.

genetic therapy would be the replacement of mutated or deleted genes. That such a genetic manipulation is feasible has been demonstrated by recent *in vitro* experiments where the introduction of a number of recessive oncogenes has enabled the tumor cell to regain lost growth control. For example, reintroduction of Rb and p53 in several tumor cell lines has resulted in reversion of the tumorigenic phenotype [144–149].

CREATING A TUMOR-SPECIFIC SWITCH

An attractive approach to cancer therapy is to confer upon the tumor cells the ability for self-destruction. Indeed in most, perhaps all cancers, cell loss is continuously occurring, and growth results from an inbalance in proliferation and cell loss.

Several strategies can be utilized to try to elicit a suicide response from the tumor cells themselves [150–153]. Suicide gene systems, which take advantage of the herpes thymidine kinase (Tk) gene are already in clinical trials for the treatment of brain tumors [154]. Sytems that parallel the chemoselectivity available in the treatment of infectious agents may provide realistic alternatives to Tk. In such a system tumor cells are rendered susceptible to anti-infective drugs by the introduction of exogenous genes that act as bacterial/fungal specific targets, i.e., render mammalian cells as susceptible as microorganisms. Genes that may serve this role include those that code for enzymes capable of converting a relatively nontoxic prodrug in human cells to an effective cytotoxic metabolite. One such gene that has been demonstrated to be effective in preliminary animal studies is cytosine deaminase. Bacteria and fungi are capable of deaminating cytosine to uracil. This deamination is achieved by cytosine deaminase, an enzyme not present in normal mammalian cells. Cytosine deaminase is also capable of converting

5-fluorocytosine (5FC) to its toxic analog 5-fluorouracil (5FU) – hence the toxicity of 5FC to fungi with sparing of mammalian cells. Thus transfer of the cytosine deaminase gene to tumor cells will render them susceptible to the normally nontoxic drug 5-fluorocytosine [155].

Tumor selectivity for the conversion of the nontoxic 5FC to 5FU can be achieved by using a retroviral/adenoviral vector system that contains a regulatory element which ensures that the cytosine deaminase gene is expressed only under the influence of a tumor-related or tumor-specific protein. Oncofetal proteins are examples of proteins that, although not necessarily of a causal nature, are present in some tumors (hepatic, colonic) as a result of phenotypic changes related to malignancy and which, therefore, can be utilized for targeting the expression of suicide genes [156]. A genetic construct containing the regulatory sequences of α-fetoprotein as a controlling switch to express the Tk gene has been tested in suicide-based therapy for hepatoma cells. Hepatoma cells that express the kinase gene under the influence of the oncofetal regulatory regions have the capacity to convert the relatively nontoxic nucleoside analog Ara-M to the cytotoxic analog Ara-C. Treatment with Ara-M can thus be made tumor cell-specific.

USING INTRINSIC VIRUSES

In hematopoietic tumors one can take advantage of several such 'switches' to enable restricted expression and hence selectivity of the suicide gene. The association of EBV with an increasing number of subtypes of lymphomas provides another possible set of regulatory elements through which the expression of suicide genes may be targeted. Among the genes expressed by EBV in tumor cells, the nuclear protein EBV nuclear antigen-1 (EBNA1) and the small transcripts known as EBV early RNAs (EBERs) appear to be ubiquitously expressed in EBV-associated Hodgkin's and non-Hodgkin's lymphomas [157]. Although the regulatory sequences controlling EBERs may not be able to restrict the expression of the suicide genes to EBV-containing cells, the use of EBNA1 in causing selective expression of suicide genes is certainly feasible. Rather than using regulatory sequences that control EBNA1 expression, one can use EBNA1 itself as a switch, since it is a transactivating protein [158]. EBNA1 is capable of binding to the Ori-p sequence and transactivating the expression of other genes downstream [159]. Thus 'grafting' a suicide gene such as cytosine deaminase on to Ori-p sequences can lead to lymphoma-specific cell suicide in the presence of a nontoxic prodrug (Figure 51.3). A possible complication with using Ori-p sequences may result from the presence of

EBV AS A TUMOR SPECIFIC SWITCH

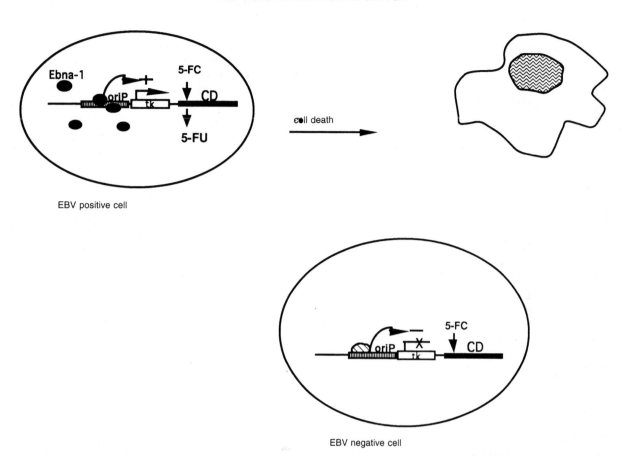

Figure 51.3   The figure is a diagrammatic representation of the use of tumor-associated proteins to express a prodrug-converting enzyme. In EBV-associated tumors, EBNA1 is always expressed. EBNA1 binds to the Ori-p sequence derived from EBV. Additionally, it also transactivates the expression of genes downstream of the Ori-p sequence. Thus, EBV-containing tumor cells can be readily engineered to express a prodrug-converting enzyme (cytosine deaminase). Exposure of these cells to the nontoxic 5-fluorocytosine (5FC) will render them susceptible to the production of 5FU. Non-EBV-containing cells will not be able to express cytosine deaminase and hence will not produce the toxic 5FU.

normal cellular proteins that can bind to Ori-p, and, theoretically, therefore, result in the transactivation of the cytosine deaminase gene even in the absence of the EBNA1. Recent experiments, however, suggest that the use of Ori-p sequences to drive suicide genes carries an additional benefit in that Ori-p acts as a supressor sequence in those cells that do not contain EBNA1 [160]. It is thus possible that cellular proteins that bind to Ori-p in the absence of EBNA1 inhibit transcription rather than activate it. This may be relevant to the host range of EBV. Because the converted prodrug may leak into the surrounding cells, the toxicity resulting from this 'bystander' effect would need to be assessed. It is not necessarily disadvantageous – tumor cells that have not been transduced with the therapeutic constructs would still be killed. This bystander effect may be very important in situations where only a small fraction of tumor cells are transduced, the situation that usually pertains with current vectors.

A further development of this strategy might parallel combination chemotherapy; both EBNA1-driven cytosine deaminase and Tk genes could be included in the construct. The lymphoma cells would then be susceptible to both Ara-M and 5FC. The advantages of using both drugs in combination would be similar to those that apply when conventional drugs are used in combination.

The use of such strategies may have an added benefit in treating the immunocompromised host. Since lymphomas are a major class of neoplasms seen in both acquired immunodeficiency syndrome (AIDS) patients and in other immunocompromised patients including allograft recipients, tumor-specific targeting of cytotoxic drugs could avoid further immune compromise.

EXPLOITATION OF A 'SELF-DESTRUCTIVE' POTENTIAL

Death by intrinsic virus activation

In EBV-associated neoplasms, EBV generally exists in a latent, i.e., nonreplicating, form [161]. Lytic infection is associated with cell death [162], although the mechanism that leads to cell death is not well understood. This provides a natural weapon that can be harnessed to cause tumor-specific lysis in EBV-containing cells. Lytic infection does occur in a small fraction of cells of EBV-associated lymphomas [163], so that it is reasonable to believe that the lytic pathway is intact in the lymphoma cells and that this process can be greatly amplified. There is a natural precedent for this in the Lucké virus-induced adeno-carcinoma in the frog. Neoplasms induced in the tadpole by the Lucké virus grow during the warm summer months, when the virus is not produced, but regress in winter, when low temperatures induce virus replication [164].

The lytic cycle in EBV appears to be controlled by the transactivating protein 'zebra' [165], which is both necessary and sufficient to induce the cascade of proteins that eventually cause virion production and cell lysis. The expression of zebra gene in EBV-containing tumor cells would therefore cause tumor cell death. In a sense, EBV proteins are used to destroy the tumor (Figure 51.4). If the expression of the zebra protein were to be linked to the expression of EBNA1, then zebra would be made only in those cells in the body that carried the EBV virus. Even if the transduction were to introduce zebra into EBV-negative and hence, normal cells, in the absence of EBNA1, these cells would be unable to synthesize significant amounts of zebra. Moreover, since the actual genes that result in cell death are encoded in the EBV genome, in the absence of EBV, there would be no effect on the cell. While nonneoplastic EBV-containing cells would also be subjected to zebra-mediated destruction, this would be unlikely to cause harm to the host. Although massive virus production would result from effective use of this system, we have shown that cell death also occurs when the virus lytic cycle is activated in the presence of acyclovir [166], a drug that inhibits viral DNA replication and hence the production of infectious virions.

Supplementation of apoptotic potential

An important feature of the mammalian lymphoid system is its ability to prevent immune reactivity against self-antigens. This is presumably achieved by check points that induce negative selection and lead to deletion of specific populations of unwanted (self-reactive) cells. There are several stages at which the activation of the programmed cell death pathway is critical for development of a functional immune system. For example, lymphoid cells that fail to rearrange their Ig or TCR genes effectively are eliminated by apoptosis [167]. Similarly, in germinal centers apoptosis is induced in cells that do not make a high-affinity antibody. In spite of these check points, however, transformation of cells that either make only low-affinity antibodies or perhaps B-cells unexposed to antigen occur and result in hemato-logical malignancies. It would seem that, analogous to the abrogation of cell cycle check points in neoplasia, circumvention of developmental check points is a mechanism used by lymphomas. For example, lymphomas of follicular center cell origin, which carry the 14;18 translocation, deregulate the *bcl*-2 gene [73,74]. Since Bcl-2 can abrogate the apoptotic pathway [75,76], it circumvents the nega-tive selection of these cells, allowing them to survive and accumulate, resulting in an indolent neoplasm. It is likely that several of the indolent lymphomas or leukemias have abrogated their differentiation apoptotic check points, in contrast to the aggressive lymphomas, which have circumvented the cell cycle check points. Reactivating these check points would be an effective means of targeting therapy in such malignancies.

The molecular pathways of the apoptosis program are just beginning to be unravelled. In addition to Bcl-2 there appears to be a family of related proteins that either interact with Bcl-2 or with each other in regulating apoptosis [77,78]. This extended family of Bcl-2-like proteins, identified by its conservation of two Bcl-2 homology domains (BH-1 and BH-2), includes Bax, Bag, Bad, Bcl-*x*-long and Bcl-*x*-short. Bax associates with itself and with Bcl-2 and the ratio of the two complexes is the switch of the apoptic program. Thus, when Bcl-2 is present, the quantity of Bax:Bax dimers decreases and Bax:Bcl-2 dimers increase, allowing the cell to survive [79]. The implication of this is that in indolent lym-phomas, the apoptotic program could presumably be switched on by manipulating Bcl-2:Bax ratios. One way to do this would be to overexpress Bax or Bad, or even Bcl-*x*-short in the lymphoma cells [168]. Bad, which is another member of the Bcl-2 family, can also allow the cell to be guided to the apoptotic pathway by neutralizing the death-sparing effects of Bcl-2. Bad associates with Bcl-2 and thus inhibits

EBV-positive tumors are latently infected with EBV and almost always make EBNA1

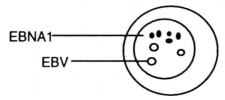

EBV also encodes a protein (zebra) that is both necessary and sufficient to induce a lytic cycle. By introducing a construct with zebra under the regulation of Ori-p, zebra production is restricted to EBV-containing cells

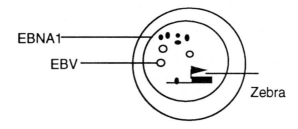

Expression of zebra in these tumor cells switches on the lytic cycle, eventually results in the lysis of the EBV-containing lymphoma

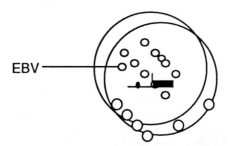

Figure 51.4 Intrinsic viruses associated with lymphomas, for example, EBV, can be used to target the tumor cells specifically. In this case, EBV, which is always associated as a latent virus in B-cell lymphomas, can be induced to undergo a lytic cycle by conditionally expressing a lysis-inducing gene (zebra) under the regulation of EBNA1.

Bcl-2:Bax complexes while promoting Bax:Bax complexes. The long and the short versions of the Bcl-*x* protein also inversely determine the cell's destiny to live or die. Thus whereas Bcl-*x*-long favors survival, Bcl-*x*-short allows cell death [80]. These various genes have more or less important roles as regulators of apoptosis in different tissues and in different circumstances.

Another set of related proteins that interact to regulate the apoptosis decision include ICH-long and ICH-short genes [169, 170]. ICH has some homology to the interleukin-1β-converting enzyme (ICE) gene. The ICE protein is a mammalian homolog of the CED-3 gene [171] of *C. elegans*. CED-3 is an effector molecule of cell death that is critical to the development of this organism [172]. Overproduction of ICE or CED 3 in mammalian cells will induce cell death, which can be prevented by Bcl-2. Both ICH long and short have a conserved sequence that includes the cysteine residue also present in ICE required for its proteolytic activity, although direct evidence that they are, like ICE, cystein proteases has not yet been observed. Deregulated expression of ICH long, like ICE, induces cell death that can be prevented either by Bcl-2 or by the short version of ICH.

The molecular lesion resulting from the *bcl*-2 deregulation in follicular lymphomas has additional prognostic significance. It has been shown that overexpression of Bcl-2 in cell lines makes them increasingly resistant to cell killing by antineoplastic agents [76]. These results have prompted speculation that the presence of deregulated *bcl*-2 in aggressive non-Hodgkin's lymphomas (NHL) may increase resistance to chemotherapy [173]. In as many as one third of aggressive lymphomas, the characteristic 14;18 translocation that results in deregulated Bcl-2 expression has been observed, while in other NHL, such as mantle cell lymphoma, Bcl-2 overexpression may occur without a characteristic translocation. Since several chemotherapeutic agents kill cells by inducing the apoptotic pathway, it is reasonable to speculate that the chemotolerance of the aggressive NHL may relate to the protective effects of Bcl-2. Strategies to overcome the Bcl-2-induced block to apoptosis may, therefore, enhance the chemosensitivity of such tumors [174].

In other hematopoietic tumors the apoptotic path-way may be blocked by either mutation or loss of genes that induce apoptosis [175]. This appears to be the case with p53 [175]. The introduction of wild-type p53 into cells that have a deleted or mutated p53 gene has been shown to result in apoptosis in these cells [176]. The presence of mutations in p53, like the overexpression of *bcl*-2, appears to correlate in a number of tumors with a poor prognosis [177–182]. In small noncleaved lymphoma, for example, there appears to be a higher frequency of p53 mutations in relapsed tumors than in primary tumor biopsies [183–185]. Preliminary results also demonstrate that both overall survival and disease-free survival is lower in patients whose tumors carry either a mutated p53 or deletion of the p53 protein [186,187].

Knowledge of the functional attributes of p53 suggests a possible mechanism to account for the association between mutated p53 and poor clinical outcome. The presence of wild-type p53 allows cells, both normal and tumor, that have incurred DNA damage to spend an extended period in G_1 and to either repair this damage or, if the damage is substantial, initiate apoptosis (Figure 51.5). The absence of a functional p53 protein prevents the cells from entering G_1 arrest and subsequent apoptosis induced by undergoing DNA damage. As a result, the cells are able to traverse the G_1 check point in spite of therapy-induced DNA damage, i.e., they are rendered more resistant to treatment.

The identification of prognostic markers of this

P53 ASSOCIATED RELAPSE IN SNCL

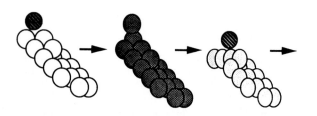

| Initial tumor contains some cells that have mutant p53 | Chemotherapy induced DNA damage incurred in all cells | Cells with wild type p53 (light hatching), undergo G1 arrest and apoptosis | Cells with mutant p53 do not undergo G1 arrest and apoptosis. They proliferate and ultimately predominate in the population |

Figure 51.5 A hypothetical schema depicting the contribution of aberrant p53 in tumor progression and resistance to therapy.

kind will ultimately help the clinician in designing risk-adapted therapies, such that patients bearing a tumor with mutated p53 may require more aggressive therapy or different therapy regardless of the extent of the disease, whereas patients with tumors that have wild-type p53 may not need as intensive a therapy as might otherwise be the case. Biological prognostic factors, however, have an advantage over purely clinical prognostic factors. If the mechanism of drug resistance is mediated by the lack of apoptosis because of loss of G_1 arrest mechanisms, drugs whose effects are not dependent upon DNA damage (spindle inhibitors, antimetabolites) or drugs that might induce a G_1 arrest following DNA damage could prove to be more effective. Such strategies could also be advantageous in the treatment of relapsed lymphomas.

References

1. Kerr JFR, Winterford CM, Harmon BV. Apoptosis, its significance in cancer and cancer treatment. *Cancer* 1994, **73**: 2013–2026.
2. Szende B, Zalatnai A, Schally AV. Programmed cell death (apoptosis) in pancreatic cancers of hamsters after treatment with analogs of both luteinizing hormone-releasing hormone and somatostatin. *Proc. Natl Acad. Sci. USA* 1989, **86**: 1643–1647.
3. Debatin KM, Goldmann CK, Banford R, et al. Monoclonal-antibody-mediated apoptosis in adult T-cell leukemia. *Lancet* 1990, **335**: 497–500.
4. Stephens LC, Schultheiss TE, Price RE, et al. Radiation apoptosis of serous acinar cells of salivary and lacrimal glands. *Cancer* 1991, **67**: 1539–1543.
5. Walker PR, Smith C, Youdale T, et al. Topoisomerase-I reactive chemotherapeutic drugs induce apoptosis in thymocytes. *Cancer Res.* 1991, **51**: 1078–1085.
6. Barry MA, Behnke CA, Eastman A. Activation of programmed cell death (apoptosis) by cisplatin, other anticancer drugs, toxins and hyperthermia. *Biochem. Pharmacol.* 1990, **40**: 2353–2362.
7. O'Conor PM, Wassermann K, Sarang M, et al. Relationship between DNA cross-links, cell cycle, and apoptosis in Burkitt's lymphoma cell lines differing in sensitivity to nitrogen mustard. *Cancer Res.* 1991, **51**: 6550–6557.
8. Yonish-Rouach E, Resnitzky D, Lotem J, et al. Wild-type p53 induces apoptosis of myeloid leukemic cells that is inhibited by interleukin-6. *Nature* 1991, **353**: 345–347.
9. Hockenbery D, Nunez G, Milliman C, et al. Bcl2 is an inner mitochondrial membrane protein that blocks programmed cell death. *Nature* 1990, **348**: 334–336.
10. Vaux DL, Cory S, Adams JM. Bcl2 gene promotes haemopoietic cell survival and cooperates with c-myc to immortalize pre-B-cells. *Nature* 1988, **335**: 440–442.
11. Dana BW, Dahlberg S, Nathwani BN, et al. Long-term follow-up of pateints with low-grade malignant lymphomas treated with doxorubicin-based chemotherapy or chemoimmunotherapy. *J. Clin. Oncol.* 1993, **11**: 644–651.
12. Offit K, Wong G, Fillpa DA, et al. Cytogenetic analysis of 434 consecutively ascertained specimens from patients with NHL. Clinical correlations. *Blood* 1991, **77**: 1508–1515.
13. Zutter M, Hockenbery D, Silverman GA, et al. Immunolocalization of the Bcl2 protein within hematopoietic neoplasms. *Blood* 1991, **78**: 1062–1068.
14. Hermine O, Haioun C, Lepage E, et al. Bcl2 protein expression in aggressive NHL. A new adverse prognostic factor? *Fourth International Conference on Malignant Lymphoma*, Lugano, Switzerland, 1994, *Annals of Oncology*, Kluwer Academic Publishers.
15. Marshall CJ. How does p21 ras transform cells? *Trends Genet.* 1991, **7**: 91–95.
16. Moodie SA, Wolfman A. The 3Rs of life Ras, Raf and growth regulation. *Trends Genet.* 1994, **10**: 44–48.
17. Kiaris HR, Spandidos D. Mutations of ras genes in human tumors (review). *Int. J. Oncol.* 1995, **7**: 413–421.
18. Janssen JW, Steenvoorden ACM, Lyons J, et al. RAS gene mutations in acute and chronic myelocytic leukemias, chronic myeloproliferative disorders, and myelodysplastic syndromes. *Proc. Natl Acad. Sci. USA* 1987, **84**: 9228–9232.
19. Shannon KM, O'Connell P, Martin GA, et al. Loss of the normal NF1 allele from the bone marrow of children with type 1 neurofibromatosis and malignant myeloid disorders. *N. Engl. J. Med.* 1994, **330**: 597–601.
20. Konopka JB, Watanabe SM, Witte ON. An alteration of the human c-Abl protein in K5G2 leukemia cells unmasks associated tyrosine kinase activity. *Cell* 1984, **37**: 1035–1042.
21. Lugo TG, Pendergast AM, Muller A, et al. Tyrosine kinase activity and transformation potency of Bcr–Abl oncogene products. *Science* 1990, **247**: 1079–1082.
22. Pendergast AM, Quilliam LA, Cripe LD, et al. BCR–ABL-induced oncogenesis is mediated by direct interaction with the SH2 domain of the GRB-2 adaptor protein. *Cell* 1993, **75**: 175–185.
23. Rabbits TH. Translocations, master genes and differences between the origins of acute and chronic leukemias. *Cell* 1991, **67**: 641–644.
24. Morris SW, Kirsten MN, Valentine MB, et al. Fusion of a kinase gene, alk, to a nucleolar protein gene, NPM in non-Hodgkin's lymphoma. *Science* 1994, **263**: 1281–1284.
25. Golub TR, Barker GF, Lovett M, et al. Fusion of PDGF receptor to a novel ets-like gene, tel, in chronic myelomonocytic leukemia with t(5;12) chromosomal translocation. *Cell* 1994, **77**: 307–316.
26. Pardee AB. G1 events and regulation of cell proliferation. *Science* 1989, **246**: 603–608.
27. Sherr CJ. Growth factor-regulated G1-cyclins. *Stem Cells* 1994, **12**: 47–55.
28. Soudon J, Bernard O, Mathieu MD, et al. C-myc gene expression in a leukemic T-cell line bearing a

t(8;14) (q24;q11) translocation. *Leukemia* 1991, **5**: 60–65.

29. Inaba T, Murakami S, Oku N, et al. Translocation between chromosomes 8q24 and 14q11 in T-cell acute lymphoblastic leukemia. *Cancer Genet. Cytogenet.* 1990, **49**: 69–74.

30. Aghib DF, Bishop JM, Ottolenghi S, et al. A 3' truncation of MYC caused by chromosomal translocation in a human T-cell leukemia increase mRNA stability. *Oncogene* 1990, **5**: 707–711.

31. Magrath I. The pathogenesis of Burkitt's lymphoma. *Adv. Cancer Res.* 1990, **55**: 133–270.

32. Aplan PD, Lombardi DP, Ginsberg AM, et al. Disruption of the human SCL locus by 'illegitimate' V–(D)–J recombinase activity. *Science* 1990, **250**: 1426–1429.

33. Lu M, Dube I, Raimondi S, et al. Molecular characterization of the t(10;14) translocation breakpoints in T-cell acute lymphoblastic leukemia: Further evidence for illegitimate physiological recombination. *Genes Chromosom. Cancer* 1990, **2**: 217–222.

34. Luscher B, Eisenman RN. New light on Myc and Myb. Part I. Myc. *Genes Dev.* 1990, **4**: 2025.

35. Marcu KB, Bossone SA, Patel AJ. Myc function and regulation. *Ann. Rev. Biochem* 1992, **61**: 809–860.

36. Gu W, Bhatia K, Magrath IT, et al. Binding and suppression of the Myc transcriptional activiation domain by p107. *Science* 1994, **264**: 251–254.

37. Keath EJ, Caimi PG, Cole MD. Fibroblast lines expressing activated c-myc oncogenes are tumorigenic in nude mice and syngeneic animals. *Cell* 1984, **39**: 339–348.

38. Bhatia K, Huppi K, Spangler G, et al. Point mutations in the c-*myc* transactivation domain are common in Burkitt's lymphoma and mouse plasmacytoma. *Nature Genet.* 1993, **5**: 56–61.

39. Albert T, Urlbauer B, Kohlhuber, et al. Ongoing mutations in the N-terminal domain of c-Myc affect transactivation in Burkitt's lymphoma cell lines. *Oncogene* 1994, **9**: 759–763.

40. Yano J, Sander CA, Clark HM, et al. Clustered mutations in the second exon of the MYC gene in sporatic Burkitt's lymphoma. *Oncogene* 1993, **8**: 2741–2748.

41. Bhatia K, Spangler G, Gaidano G, et al. Mutations in the coding region of c-*myc* occur frequently in acquired immunodeficiency syndrome-associated lymphomas. *Blood* 1994, **84**: 883–888.

42. Adams JM, Cory S. Oncogene cooperation in leukaemogenesis. *Cancer Surveys* 1992, **15**: 119–141.

43. Hartwell LH, Kastan MB. Cell cycle control and cancer. *Science* 1994, **266**: 1821–1827.

44. Weinberg RA. Tumor suppressor genes. *Science* 1991, **254**: 1138–1146.

45. Levine AJ, Momand J, Finlay CA. The p53 tumor suppressor gene. *Nature* 1991, **351**: 453–456.

46. Kamb A, Gruis NA, Weaver-Feldhaus J, et al. A cell cycle regulator potentially involved in genesis of many tumor types. *Science* 1994, **264**: 436–440.

47. Nobori T, Miura K, Wud J, et al. Deletions of the cyclin-dependent kinase-4 inhibitor gene in multiple human cancers. *Nature* 1994, **368**: 753–756.

48. Weinert T, Lydall D. Cell cycle checkpoints, genetic instability and cancer. *Cancer Biol.* 1993, **4**: 129–140.

49. Lowe SW, Schmitt EM, Smith SW, et al. P53 is required for radiation-induced apoptosis in mouse thymocytes. *Nature* 1993, **362**: 847–849.

50. Caelles C, Helmberg A, Karin M. P53-dependent apoptosis in the absence of transcriptional activation of p53-target genes. *Nature* 1994, **370**: 220–223.

51. Evans T, Rosenthal ET, Youngblom J, et al. Cyclin: A protein specified by maternal mRNA in sea urchin eggs that is destroyed at each cleavage division. *Cell* 1983, **33**: 389–396.

52. Motokura T, Bloom T, Kim HG, et al. A novel cyclin encoded by a *bcl*-1 linked candidate oncogene. *Nature* 1991, **350**: 512–515.

53. Matsushime H, Roussel MF, Ashman RA, et al. Colony-stimulating factor 1 regulates novel cyclins during the G1 phase of the cell cycle. *Cell* 1991, **65**: 701–713.

54. Xiong Y, Connolly T, Futcher B, et al. Human D-type cyclin. *Cell* 1991, **65**: 691–699.

55. Koff A, Cross F, Fisher A, et al. Human cyclin E, a new cyclin that interacts with two members of the CDC2 gene family. *Cell* 1991, **66**: 1217–1228.

56. Mokokura T, Arnold A. Cyclin D and oncogenesis. *Curr. Opin. Genet. Devel.* 1993, **3**: 5–10.

57. Rosenberg CL, Wong E, Petty EM, et al. PRAD1, a candidate BCL1 oncogene: Mapping and expression in centrocytic lymphoma. *Proc. Natl Acad. Sci. USA* 1991, **88**: 9638–9642.

58. Sherr CJ. Mammalian G1 cyclins. *Cell* 1993, **73**: 1059–1065.

59. Chellappan SP, Hiebert S, Mudryj M, et al. The E2F transcription factor is a cellular target for the RB protein. *Cell* 1991, **65**: 1053–1061.

60. Hamel PA, Gill RM, Phillips RA. Transcriptional repression of the E2-containing product promotes EIIaE, c-myc and RBI by the production of the RBI gene. *Mol. Cell Biol.* 1992, **12**: 3431–3438.

61. Helin K, Lees JA, Vidal M, et al. A CDNA encoding a PRB-binding protein with properties of the transcription factor E2F. *Cell* 1992, **70**: 337–350.

62. Shirodkar S, Ewen M, DeCaprio JA, et al. The transcription factor E2F interacts with the retinoblastoma product and a p107-cyclin A complex in a cell cycle regulated manner. *Cell* 1992, **68**: 157–166.

63. Ewen ME, Sluss HK, Sherr CJ, et al. Functional interactions of the retinoblastoma protein with mammalian D-type cyclins. *Cell* 1993, **73**: 487–497.

64. Buchkovich K, Duffy LA, Harlow E. The retinoblastoma protein is phosphorylated during specific phases of the cell cycle. *Cell* 1989, **58**: 1097–1105.

65. Lees JA, Buchkovich KJ, Marshak DR, et al. The retinoblastoma protein is phosphorylated on multiple sites by cdc2. *EMBO J.* 1991, **10**: 4279–4290.

66. Peter M, Mershowitz I. Joining the complex cyclin-dependent kinase inhibitory proteins and the cell cycle. *Cell* 1994, **79**: 181–184.

67. Xiong Y, Hannon GJ, Zhang H, et al. P21 is a universal inhibitor of cyclin kinases. *Nature* 1993, **366**: 701–704.

68. Harper JW, Adami GR, Wei N, et al. The p21Cdk-interacting protein Cipl is a potent inhibitor of G1 cyclin-dependent kinases. *Cell* 1993, **75**: 805–816.

69. Noda A, Ning Y, Venable SF, et al. Cloning of senescent cell-derived inhibitors of DNA synthesis using an expression screen. *Exp. Cell Res.* 1994, **211**: 90–98.

70. El-Deiry WS, Tokino T, Velcylescu VE, et al. Waf1 – a potential mediator of p53 suppression. *Cell* 1993, **75**: 817–825.

71. Pietenpol JA, Tokino T, Thiagalingams E. Sequence specific transcriptional activation is essential for growth suppression by p53. *Proc. Natl Acad. Sci. USA* 1994, **91**: 1998–2002.

72. Hengartner MO, Horvitz HR. *C. elegans* cell survival gene ced-9 encodes a functional homolog of the mammalian proto-oncogene bcl-2. *Cell* 1994, **76**: 665–676.

73. Cleary ML, Sklar J. Nucleotide sequence of a t(14;18) chromosomal breakpoint in follicular lymphoma and demonstration of a breakpoint-cluster region near a transcriptionally active locus on chromosome 18. *Proc. Natl Acad. Sci. USA* 1985, **82**: 7439–7443.

74. Tsujimoto Y, Cossman J, Jaffe E, et al. Involvement of the *bcl2* gene in human follicular lymphoma. *Science* 1985, **228**: 1440–1443.

75. Nunez G, London L, Hockenbery D. Deregulated Bcr-2 gene expression selectively prolongs survival of growth factor-deprived hemopoietic cell lines. *J. Immunol.* 1990, **144**: 3602–3610.

76. Miyashita T, Reed JC. Bcl-2 gene transfer increases relative resistance of S49.1 and WEH17.2 lymphoid cells to cell death and DNA fragmentation induced by glycocorticoids and multiple chemotherapeutic drugs. *Cancer Res.* 1992, **52**: 5407–5411.

77. Korsmeyer SJ, Shutter JR, Veis DJ. Bcl-2/Bax: A rheostat that regulates an anti-oxidant pathway and cell death. *Semin. Cancer Biol.* 1993, **41**: 327–332.

78. Williams GT, Smith CA. Molecular regulation of apoptosis: genetic control of cell death. *Cell* 1993, **74**: 777–779.

79. Oltvai ZN, Milliman CL, Korsmeyer SJ. Bcl-2 heterodimerizes in vivo with a conserved homolog, Bax, that accelerates programmed cell death. *Cell* 1993, **74**: 609–619.

80. Boise LH, Gonzalez-Garcia M, Postema CE, et al. Bcl-x, a Bcl-2-related gene that functions as a dominant regulator of apoptotic cell death. *Cell* 1993, **74**: 597–608.

81. Selvakumaran M, Lin HK, Miyashita T, et al. Immediate early up-regulation of Bax expression by p53 but not TGF beta 1: A paradigm for distinct apoptotic pathways. *Oncogene* 1994, **9**: 1791–1798.

82. Rao L, Debbas M, Sabbatini P. The adenovirus E1A proteins induce apoptosis which is inhibited by the E1B 19K-Da and Bcl2 proteins. *Proc. Natl. Acad Sci USA* 1992, **89**: 1742–1746.

83. Henderson S, Huen D, Rowe M, et al. Epstein–Barr virus BHRF1 protein, a viral homologue of Bcl-2 protects human B-cells from programmed cell death. *Proc. Natl Acad. Sci. USA* 1993, **90**: 8479–8488.

84. Tarodi B, Subramanian T, Chinnadura G. Epstein–Barr virus BHRF1 protein protects against cell death induced by DNA damaging agents and heterologous viral infection. *Virology* 1994, **201**: 404–407.

85. Larsen CJ, Seite P, Hillion J, et al. Some recent aspects of the molecular biology of human lymphoma. *Nouv. Rev. Fr. Hematol.* 1993, **35**: 37–40.

86. Gibbs JB. Pharmacological probes of Ras function. *Semin. Cancer Biol.* 1992, **3**: 383–390.

87. Huber HE, Koblan KS, Heimbrook DC. Protein–protein interactions as therapeutic targets for cancer. *Curr. Med. Chem.* 1994, **1**: 13–34.

88. Amati B, Brooks, MW, Levy N, et al. Oncogenic activity of the c-*myc* protein requires dimerization with max. *Cell* 1993, **72**: 233–245.

89. Gibbs JB, Oliff A, Kohl NE. Farnesyltransferase inhibitors: ras research yields a potential cancer therapeutic. *Cell* 1994, **77**: 175–178.

90. Murakami Y, Mizuno S, Hori M, et al. Reversal of transformed phenotypes by herbimycin A in sarc oncogene expressed in rat fibroblasts. *Cancer Res.* 1988, **48**: 1587–1590.

91. Dvir A, Milner Y, Chomsky O, et al. The inhibition of EGF-dependent proliferation of keratinocytes by tyrphostin tyrosine kinase blockers. *J. Cell. Biol.* 1991, **113**: 857–865.

92. Yuan CJ, Jakes S, Elliot S. A rationale for the design of an inhibitor of tyrosyl kinase. *J. Biol. Chem.* 1990, **265**: 2255.

93. Gibbs JB. Ras c-terminal processing enzymes – new drug targets. *Cell* 1991, **65**: 1–4.

94. Hancock JF, Magee Al, Childs JE, et al. All ras proteins are polyisoprenylated but only some are palmitoylated. *Cell* 1989, **57**: 1167–1177.

95. Buchdunger E, Trinics U, Meh H, et al. 4,5-Dianilinopthalimide a protein–tyrosine kinase inhibitor with selectivity for the epidermal growth factor receptor signal transduction pathway and potent *in vivo* antitumor activity. *Proc. Natl Acad. Sci. USA* 1994, **91**: 2334–2338.

96. Zon G. Innovations in the use of antisense oligonucleotides. *Ann. N. York Acad Sci.* 1190, **616**: 161–172.

97. Tidd DM. A potential role for antisense oligonucleotide analogues in the development of oncogene targeted cancer chemotherapy. *Anticancer Res.* 1990, **10**: 1169–1182.

98. Zon G. Oligonucleotide analogues as potential chemotherapeutic agents. *Pharm. Res.* 1988, **5**: 539–549.

99. Stein CA, Cohen JS. Antisense compounds: Potential role in cancer therapy. *Important Adv. Oncol.* 1989, **8**: 79–97.

100. Calabretta B. Inhibition of protooncogene expression by antisense oligodeoxynucleotides: Biological and therapeutic implications. *Cancer Res.* 1991, **51**: 4505–4510.

101. Stein CA, Cohen JS. Oligodeoxynucleotides as inhibitors of gene expression: A review. *Cancer Res.* 1988, **48**: 2659–2668.

102. Stull RA, Szoka FC. Antigene, ribozyme and aptomer nucleic acid drugs: Progress and prospects. *Pharm. Res.* 1995, **12**: 465–483.

103. Pace NR, Brown JW. Evolutionary perspective on the structure and function of ribonuclease P, a ribozyme. *J. Bacteriol.* 1995, **177**: 1919–1928.

104. Belinsky M, Dinter-Gottlieb G. Characterizing the self-cleavage of a 135 nucleotide ribozyme from genomic hepatitis delta virus. *Prog. Clin. Biol. Res.* 1991, **364**: 265–274.

105. Branch AD, Levine BJ, Boroudy BM, et al. The novel tertiary structure in delta RNA may function as a ribozyme control element. *Prog. Clin. Biol. Res.* 1991, **364**: 257–264.

106. Been MD, Cech TR. RNA as an RNA polymerase: Net elongation of an RNA primer catalyzed by the Tetrahymena ribozyme. *Science* 1988, **239**: 1412–1416.

107. Forster AC, Davies C, Hutchins CJ, et al. Characterization of self-cleavage of viroid and virusoid RNAs. *Meth. Enzymol.* 1990, **181**: 583–607.

108. Yang JH, Cedergren R, Nadal-Ginard B. Catalytic activity of an RNA domain derived from the U6-U4 RNA complex. *Science* 1994, **263**: 77–81.

109. Cotten M, Birnsteil ML. Ribozyme mediated destruction of RNA *in vivo*. *EMBO J.* 1989, **8**: 3861–3866.

110. Francois JC, Saison-Behmoaras T, Helene C. Sequence-specific recognition of the major groove of DNA by oligodeoxynucleotides via triple helix formation. Footprinting studies. *Nucl. Acids Res.* 1988, **16**: 11431–11440.

111. Chen FM. Intramolecular triplex formation of the purine.purine.pyrimidine type. *Biochemistry* 1991, **30**: 4472–4479.

112. Perrouault L, Asseline U, Rivalle C, et al. Sequence specific artificial photoinduced endonucleases based on triple helix-forming oligonucleotides. *Nature* 1990, **344**: 358–360.

113. Gray A, Morgan J. Liposomes in haematology. *Blood Rev.* 1991, **5**: 258–272.

114. Riedmann T, Xu L, Wolff J, et al. Retrovirus vector-mediated gene transfer into hepatocytes. *Mol. Biol. Med.* 1989, **6**: 117–125.

115. Uckert W, Walther H. Retrovirus-mediated gene transfer in cancer therapy. *Pharmacol. Ther.* 1994, **63**: 323–347.

116. Yung WK. New approaches in brain tumor therapy using gene transfer and antisense oligonucleotides. *Curr. Opin. Oncol.* 1994, **6**: 235–239.

117. Schreier H. The new frontier: Gene and oligonucleotide therapy. *Pharm. Acta Helv.* 1994, **68**: 145–159.

118. Miller AD, Rossman GJ. Improved retroviral vectors for gene transfer and expression. *Biotechniques* 1989, **7**: 980–982.

119. Watanabe S, Temin H. Construction of a helper-free cell line for avian reticuloendotheliosis virus cloning vectors. *Mol. Cell Biol.* 1983, **3**: 2241–2249.

120. Culver KW, Ram Z, Wallbridge S, et al. *In vivo* gene transfer with retroviral vector–producer cells for treatment of experimental brain tumors. *Science* 1992, **256**: 1550–1552.

121. Trapnell BC. Adrenoviral vectors for gene transfer. *Adv. Drug. Del. Rev.* 1993, **12**: 1815–1821.

122. Breakfield XO, DeLuca NA. Herpes simplex virus for gene delivery to neurons. *N. Biol.* 1991, **3**: 203–218.

123. Roberson E, Kieff E. Reducing complexity of the transforming EBV genome to 64 kb. *J. Virol.* 1995, **69**: 983–993.

124. McManaway ME, Neckers LM, Loke SL, et al. Tumor-specific inhibition of lymphoma growth by an antisense oligodeoxynucleotide. *Lancet* 1990, **335**: 808–811.

125. Gutierrez MI, Bhatia K, Barriga F, et al. Molecular epidemiology of Burkitt's lymphoma from South America: Differences in breakpoint location and Epstein–Barr virus association from tumors in other world regions. *Blood* 1992, **79**: 3261–3266.

126. Shtivelman E, Lifshitz B, Gale RP, et al. Fused transcripts of *abl* and *bcr* genes in chronic myeloid leukemia. *Nature* 1985, **315**: 550–554.

127. Kamps MP, Murre C, Sun X, et al. A new homeobox gene contributes the DNA binding domain of the t(1;19) translocation protein in pre-B ALL. *Cell* 1990, **60**: 547–555.

128. Nourse J, Mellentin JD, Galili N, et al. Chromosomal translocation t(1;19) results in synthesis of a homeobox fusion mRNA that codes for a potential chimeric transcription factor. *Cell* 1990, **60**: 535–545.

129. Borrow J, Goddard AD, Sheer D, et al. Molecular analysis of acute promyelocytic leukemia breakpoint cluster region on chromosome 17. *Science* 1990, **249**: 1577–1580.

130. de Thé H, Chomienne C, Lanotte M, et al. The t(15;17) translocation fuses the retinoic acid receptor α gene to a novel transcribed locus. *Nature* 1990, **347**: 558–561.

131. Liu JH, Mu ZM, Chang KS. PML suppresses oncogenic transformation of NIH/3T3 cells by activated *Neu*. *J. Exp. Med.* 1995, **181**: 1965–1973.

132. Miller WH, Jr. Differentiation therapy of acute promyelocytic leukemia: Clinical and molecular features. *Cancer Invest.* 1996, **14**: 182–183.

133. Smetsers TF, Skorski T, Van de Locht LT, et al. Antisense BCR-ABL oligonucleotides induce apoptosis in the philadelphia chromosome-positive cell line 13V173. *Leukemia* 1994, **8**: 129–140.

134. Szczylik CT, Skorski NC, Nicolaides I, et al. Selective inhibition of leukemia cell proliferation by BCR–ABL antisense oligodeoxynucleotides. *Science* 1991, **253**: 562–565.

135. Skorski T, Skorska MN, Barletta C, et al. Highly efficient elimination of Philadelphia leukemic cells by exposure to bcr/abl antisense oligodeoxynucleotides combined with mafosfamide. *J. Clin. Invest.* 1993, **92**: 194–202.

136. Gewirtz AM. Potential therapeutic applications of antisense oligodeoxynucleotides in the treatment of chronic myelogenous leukemia. *Leuk. Lymphoma* 1993, **11**: 131–137.

137. deFabritilis P, Amadori S, Calabretta B, et al. Elimination of clonogenic philadelphia-positive cells using bcr-abl antisense oligodeoxynucleotides. *Bone Marrow Transplant.* 1993, **12**: 261–265.

138. Vaerman JL, Lewalle P, Martiat P. Antisense inhibition of p210 bcr–abl in chronic myeloid leukemia. *Stem Cells* 1993, **11**: 89–95.

139. Lewalle P, Martiat P. Inhibition of p210 expression in chronic myeloid leukemia oligonucleotides and/or transduced antisense sequences. *Leuk. Lymphoma* 1993, **11**: 139–143.

140. Harris H. The analysis of malignancy by cell fusion: The position in 1988. *Cancer Res.* 1988, **48**: 3302–3306.

141. Weissman BE, Stanbridge EJ. Complementation of the tumorigenic phenotype in human cell hybrids. *J. Natl Cancer Inst.* 1983, **70**: 667–672.

142. Levine AJ. Tumor suppressor genes. *Bioessays* 1990, **12**: 60–66.

143. Prokocimer M, Rotter V. Structure and function of p53 in normal cells and their aberrations in cancer cells: Projection on the hematologic lineages. *Blood* 1994, **84**: 2391–2411.

144. Huang HJ, Yee JK, Shew JY, et al. Suppression of the neoplastic phenotype by replacement of the RB gene in human cancer cells. *Science* 1988, **242**: 1563–1566.

145. Bookstein R, Shew JY, Chen, PL, et al. Suppression of tumorigenicity of human prostrate carcinoma cells by replacing a mutated RB gene. *Science* 1990, **247**: 712–715.

146. Baker SJ, Markowitz S, Fearon ER, et al. Suppression of human colorectal carcinoma cell growth by wildtype p53. *Science* 1990, **249**: 912–915.

147. Cheng J, Yee JK, Yeargin J, et al. Suppression of acute lymphoblastic leukemia by the human wild-type p53 gene. *Cancer Res.* 1992, **52**: 222–226.

148. Cai DW, Mukhopadhyay T, Liu Y, et al. Expression of the wild type-53 gene in human lung cancer cells after retrovirus-mediated gene transfer. *Hum. Gene Ther.* 1993, **4**: 617–624.

149. Fujiwara T, Grimm EA, Mukhopadhyay T, et al. Induction of chemosensitivity in human lung cancer cell *in vivo* by adenovirus-mediated transfer of wild type p53 gene. *Cancer Res.* 1994, **54**: 2287–2291.

150. Ezzeddine ZD, Martuza RL, Platika D, et al. Selective killing of glioma cells in culture and *in vivo* by retrovirus transfer of the herpes simplex virus thymidine kinase gene. *N. Biol.* 1991, **3**: 608–614.

151. Short MP, Choi BC, Lee JK, et al. Gene delivery to glioma cells in rat brain by grafting of a retrovirus packaging cell line. *J. Neurosci. Res.* 1990, **27**: 427–439.

152. Moolten FL, Wells JM, Heyman J, et al. Lymphoma regression induced by ganciclovir in mice bearing a herpes thymidine kinase transgene. *Hum. Gene Ther.* 1990, **1**: 125–134.

153. Ram Z, Culver KW, Walbridge S, et al. *In situ* retroviral-mediated gene transfer for the treatment of brain tumors in rats. *Cancer Res.* 1993, **53**: 83–87.

154. Clinical protocol: Gene therapy for the treatment of brain tumors using intratumoral transduction with the thymidine kinase gene and intravenous ganciclovir. *Hum. Gene Ther.* 1993, **4**: 39.

155. Mullen CA, Kilstrup M, Blaese RM. Transfer of the bacterial gene for cytosine deaminase to mammalian cells confers lethal sensitivity to 5-fluorocytosine: A negative selection system. *Proc. Natl Acad. Sci.* 1992, **89**: 33–37.

156. Huber BE, Austin EA, Good SS, et al. *In vivo* antitumor activity of 5-fluorocytosine on human colorectal carcinoma cells genetically modified to express cytosine deaminase. *Cancer Res.* 1993, **53**: 4619–4626.

157. Gratma JW, Ingemar E. Molecular epidemiology of Epstein–Barr vrus infection. *Adv. Cancer Res.* **67**: 197–255.

158. Reisman D, Sugden B. Transactivation of an Epstein–Barr viral transcriptional enhancer by the Epstein–Barr viral nuclear antigen 1. *Mol. Cell. Biol.* 1986, **6**: 3828–3846.

159. Wysokenski DA, Yates JL. Multiple EBNA1-binding sites are required to form an EBNA1-dependent enhancer and to activate a minimal replicative origin within oriP of Epstein–Barr virus. *J. Virol.* 1989, **63**: 2657–2666.

160. Judde JG, Spangler G, Magrath I, et al. Use of Epstein–Barr virus nuclear antigen-1 in targeted therapy of EBV-associated neoplasia. *Human Gene Ther.* 1996, **7**: 647–653.

161. Rogers R, Strominer PJ, Speck S. Epstein–Barr virus in B lymphocytes: Viral gene expression and function in latency. *Adv. Cancer Res.* 1992, **58**: 1–26.

162. Keiff E, Leibowitz D. Epstein–Barr virus and its replication in fundamental virology. In Fieds BN, Knipe DM, et al. (eds) *Fundamental Virology.* New York: Raven Press, 1991, pp. 897–928.

163. Gutierrez MI, Bhatia K, Magrath IT. Replicative viral DNA in Epstein–Barr virus associated Burkitt's lymphoma biopsies. *Leuk. Res.* 1993, **17**: 285–289.

164. Collard W, Thornton H, Mizeel M, et al. Virus-free adenocarcinoma of the frog (summer phase tumor) transcribes Lucké tumor herpesvirus-specific RNA. *Science* 1973, **181**: 448–449.

165. Miller G. The switch between latency and replication of Epstein–Barr virus. *J. Infect. Dis.* 1990, **161**: 833–844.

166. Gutierrez M, Judde JG, Magrath I, et al. EBNA-1 dependent induction of cell lysis: A novel therapeutic approach specific for EBV-associated neoplasia. *Cancer Res.* 1996, **56**: 969–972.

167. Nossal GJV. Negative selection of lymphomas. *Cell* 1994, **76**: 229–239.

168. Yang EJ, Zha J, Jocke LH, et al. Bad, a heterodimeric partner for Bcl-Xl and Bcl-2, displaces Bax and promotes cell death. *Cell* 1995, **80**: 285–291.

169. Kumar S, Kinoshita M, Noda M. Induction of apoptosis by the mouse Nedd2 gene, which encodes a protein similar to the product of the *Caenorhabditis elegans* cell death gene ced-3 and the mammalian IL-1 beta-converting enzyme. *Genes Dev.* 1994, **8**: 1613–1626.

170. Wang L, Miura M, Bergeron L, et al. Ich-1, an Ice/ced-3-related gene, encodes both positive and negative regulators of programmed cell death. *Cell* 1994, **78**: 739–750.

171. Thornberry NA, Bull HG, Calaycay J, et al. A novel heterodimeric cysteine protease is required for interleukin-1 beta processing in monocytes. *Nature* 1992, **356**: 768–774.

172. Yuan J, Shaham S, Ledous S, et al. The *C. elegans* cell death gene ced-3 encodes a protein similar to mammalian interleukin-1 beta-converting enzyme. *Cell* 1993, **75**: 641–652.

173. Yunis JJ, Mayer MG, Arnesen MA, et al. Bcl-2 and other genomic alterations in the prognosis of large cell lymphoma. *N. Engl. J. Med.* 1989, **320**: 1047–1054.

174. Mitada S, Miyashita T, Tanaka S, et al. Investigations of antisense oligonucleotides targeted against bcl-2 RNA's. *Antisense Res. Dev.* 1993, **31**: 157–169.

175. Curtis HC, Hollstein M. Clinical implications of the p53 tumor suppressor gene. *N. Engl. J. Med.* 1993, **329**: 1318–1327.

176. Ramquist T, Magnusson KP, Wang Y, et al. Wild-type p53 induces apoptosis in a Burkitt lymphoma (BL) line that carries mutant p53. *Oncogene* 1993, **8**: 1495–1500.

177. Papadakis E, Malliri A, Linardopoulos S, et al. Ras and p53 expression in non-small cell lung cancer patients: p53 overexpression correlates with a poor prognosis. *Int. J. Oncol.* 1992, **1**: 403–413.

178. Horio Y, Takahashi T, Kuroishi T, et al. Prognostic significance of p53 mutations and 3p deletions in primary resected non-small cell lung cancer. *Cancer Res.* 1993, **53**: 1–4.

179. Thorlacius S, Borresen A-L, Eyfjord E. Somatic p53 mutations in human breast carcinomas in an Icelandic population: A prognostic factor. *Cancer Res.* 1993, **53**: 1637–1641.

180. Elledge RM, Fuqua SAW, Clark GM, et al. Prognostic significance of p53 alterations in node-negative breast cancer. *Breast Cancer Res. Treat.* 1993, **26**: 225–235.

181. Elledge RM, Fuqua SAW, Clark GM, et al. The role and prognostic significance of p53 gene alterations in breast cancer. *Breast Cancer Res. Treat.* 1993, **27**: 95–102.

182. Navone NM, Troncoso P, Pisters LL, et al. P53 protein accumulation and gene mutation in the progression of human prostate carcinoma. *J. Natl Cancer Inst.* 1993, **85**: 1657–1669.

183. Gaidano G, Ballerini P, Gong JZ, et al. P53 mutations in human lymphoid malignancies: Association with Burkitt's lymphoma and chronic lymphocytic leukemia. *Proc. Natl Acad. Sci.* 1991, **88**: 5413–5417.

184. Bhatia KG, Gutierrez MI, Huppi K, et al. The pattern of p53 mutations in Burkitt's lymphoma differs from that of solid tumors. *Cancer Res.* 1992, **52**: 4273–4276.

185. Bhatia K, Goldschmidts W, Gutierrez M, et al. Hemi- or homozygosity: A requirement of some but not other p53 mutant proteins to accumulate and exert a pathogenic event. *FASEB J.* 1993, **7**: 951–956.

186. Gutierrez M, Bhatia K, Diez B, et al. Prognostic significance of p53 mutations in small non-cleaved cell lymphomas. *Int. J. Oncol.* 1994, **4**: 567–571.

187. Venkatesh C, Adde M, Gutierrez M, et al. Prognostic value of p53 expression in Burkitt's lymphoma is significantly enhanced in tumors with high LDH. (in preparation).

Index